IMPR[illegible] MEDICINE

Providing Care in Extreme Environments

Second Edition

Kenneth V. Iserson, MD, MBA, FACEP, FAAEM
Fellow, International Federation for Emergency Medicine
Professor Emeritus, Emergency Medicine
The University of Arizona, Tucson, AZ
Founder/Director, REEME (www.reeme.arizona.edu)

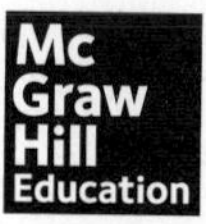

New York Chicago San Francisco Athens London Madrid Mexico City
Milan New Delhi Singapore Sydney Toronto

Improvised Medicine: Providing Care in Extreme Environments, Second Edition

1 2 3 4 5 6 7 8 9 0 DOC/DOC 20 19 18 17 16 15

ISBN 978-0-07-184762-9
MHID 0-07-184762-6

This book was set in Times LT Std by Cenveo® Publisher Services.
The editors were Brian Belval and Kim J. Davis.
The production supervisor was Richard Ruzycka.
Project management was provided by Shruti Awasthi, Cenveo Publisher Services.
The cover designer was Thomas DePierro.
Cover photo courtesy of Kenneth V. Iserson, M.D.
Caption: Dr. Iserson using improvised neonatal warmer in rural Zambia.

RR Donnelley was printer and binder.

This book is printed on acid-free paper.

NOTICE

Medicine is an ever-changing science. As new research and clinical experience broaden our knowledge, changes in treatment and drug therapy are required. The authors and the publisher of this work have checked with sources believed to be reliable in their efforts to provide information that is complete and generally in accord with the standards accepted at the time of publication. However, in view of the possibility of human error or changes in medical sciences, neither the authors nor the publisher nor any other party who has been involved in the preparation or publication of this work warrants that the information contained herein is in every respect accurate or complete, and they disclaim all responsibility for any errors or omissions or for the results obtained from use of the information contained in this work. Readers are encouraged to confirm the information contained herein with other sources. For example and in particular, readers are advised to check the product information sheet included in the package of each drug they plan to administer to be certain that the information contained in this work is accurate and that changes have not been made in the recommended dose or in the contraindications for administration. This recommendation is of particular importance in connection with new or infrequently used drugs.

Library of Congress Cataloging-in-Publication Data

Iserson, Kenneth V., author.
Improvised medicine: providing care in extreme environments/Kenneth V. Iserson.—Second edition.
p.; cm.
Includes bibliographical references and index.
ISBN 978-0-07-184762-9 (pbk.: alk. paper)
ISBN 0-07-184762-6 (pbk.: alk. paper)
I. Title.
[DNLM: 1. Emergency Medicine–methods. 2. Disaster Medicine–methods. 3. Wilderness Medicine–methods. WB 105]
RC86.7
362.18–dc23

2015026227

Contents

Preface to the Second Edition

WHY A NEW EDITION?

This second edition developed from the marked increase in published innovations applicable to medical improvisation. Clinicians throughout the world who dared to stretch their imaginations beyond the tight confines of medical conformity have produced marvelous innovations, generally stemming from the necessity to provide treatment in situations of acute or chronic shortages. Increasingly, clinicians have also recognized that the use of improvised techniques, equipment, and knowledge may be necessary not only in remote settings and in the developing world, but also in large medical centers and sophisticated emergency medical service (EMS) systems when confronted by medication and equipment shortages, localized crises, and major disasters. I am grateful for these clinicians' experiences and their support for *Improvised Medicine*, clearly an outlier from the staid teachings and guidelines of traditional practice.

HOW THE BOOK IS ORGANIZED

This book is divided into several sections, beginning with introductory chapters that describe resource-poor situations that may require medical improvisation. Subsequent sections discuss Basic Needs, Patient Assessment/Stabilization, Surgical Interventions, and Nonsurgical Interventions. The Appendices provide useful information about preparing a hospital disaster plan and assembling medical kits for different activities.

The Basic Needs section begins with communication alternatives, because difficult communication is the most frequently cited problem in resource-poor situations. Improvised methods for preventive medicine/public health come next, because supplying clean drinking water and suitable waste facilities saves more lives (in a non-dramatic way) than all the interventional medical treatments combined. After that, I discuss improvised basic equipment for health care. However, only a fraction of the book's improvised equipment is discussed in this first section: Most is described in the chapter appropriate for its use.

The final topic in Basic Needs is methods for cleaning and reusing medical equipment under resource-poor conditions. Reusing medical equipment is, rightfully, a controversial subject, because inadequate cleaning, disinfection, and sterilization lead to passing diseases from one patient to another. The best available information has been used to provide guidance about when to avoid reusing supplies and when certain cleaning methods are suboptimal.

The Patient Assessment/Stabilization section describes methods and improvised equipment to assess vital signs and to manage airways, breathing, circulation, and dehydration/rehydration (vital to saving children's lives). Also included are improvisations and alternatives for medications and medication delivery, imaging, laboratory testing, and patient movement/evacuation. Four chapters describe improvisations for analgesia, local and regional anesthesia, and general anesthesia. The Sedation and General Anesthesia chapter includes techniques for both non-anesthesiologists and anesthesiologists. The Ketamine, Ether, and Halothane chapter describes the most common anesthetics used in developing countries, including unique administration methods. Younger anesthesiologists, as well as other practitioners who may be called upon to give ketamine or ether, may be unfamiliar with these medications or alternative administration techniques.

While not everything in the Surgical Interventions section is strictly surgical (e.g., there is a chapter on Neurology/Neurosurgery), dividing the chapters in this way provides a convenient method to quickly locate information. The two Dental chapters and the Orthopedics chapter occupy significant space, because health care professionals often need to apply these skills in resource-poor environments even if they have little training in these areas. All chapters in the Surgical Interventions section describe improvised equipment and techniques that can save lives. For instance, the Otolaryngology chapter describes the old, very basic, technique of placing posterior nasal packs, whereas the Obstetrics/Gynecology chapter describes balloon tamponade for peripartum and other vaginal bleeding.

All chapters in the Nonsurgical Interventions section include improvisations that can be used in traditional medical areas (e.g., gastroenterology, infectious diseases, pediatrics/neonatal, and psychiatry), as well as other areas in which health care professionals may need to be involved when resources are limited: recognizing and treating malnutrition, assisting with rehabilitation, and doing death notification, forensic investigation, and body management.

The Appendices provide a disaster plan and suggestions for what to include in medical kits for several resource-poor situations. Although some have questioned including a disaster plan, my experience shows that it helps to have a structure to guide clinicians and others in what may be the most significant improvised situation of their career.

Hopefully, *Improvised Medicine's* contents will help you provide excellent medical care to your patients in resource-poor settings. This information has already proven valuable when I had to provide care in such settings. My experience has convinced me that medical improvisation is both possible and highly useful.

Acknowledgments

It has taken a huge international "village" to produce this strange compendium. The significant help I received is the only reason this book exists. First and foremost is the fantastic assistance and support from my wife, Mary Lou Iserson, CPA, who has also been a research medical technologist and a field member of the Southern Arizona Rescue Association. Acting as a skilled and persistent editor, she patiently explained why some sections made no sense—even before the manuscript went to the publisher.

Libby Lamb Wagner, biomedical content illustrator, created most of the new illustrations in the second edition.

Jennifer Gilbert supplied most of the great original artwork for the first edition and some additional pieces for this edition. She also was the diligent proofreader and organizer for both editions, nicely and diplomatically pointing out my errors. Any remaining errors in the drawings or a sense of incompleteness are my fault entirely, because I was the final arbiter.

As with all my books, I owe a debt of gratitude to my friends at the University of Arizona Health Sciences Library, who find sources of information in inscrutable ways. I am especially grateful to Nga T. Nguyen, BA, BS, Senior Library Specialist and to Ms. Hannah Fisher, RN, MLS, AHIP (now retired), who helped me to find obscure references that added immensely to the information I could provide.

Because many of the most valuable references are neither online nor contained in The University of Arizona's extensive collection, the Arizona Health Sciences Center's Inter-Library Loan staff provided amazing assistance in gathering hundreds of references for this book.

I also want to thank Suzanne Schoenfelt (aka, The Wordsmith) for her superb editing skills for the first edition.

Finally, I must extend my thanks to Brian Belval, Executive Editor, and Kim J. Davis, Associate Managing Editor, at McGraw-Hill Education for believing in this project and seeing it to fruition.

Chapter Reviewers

Quite a few content experts willingly gave of their time to review specific chapters and provide input. Their expertise proved invaluable in clarifying and augmenting the information provided. In alphabetical order, I sincerely thank:

Geoffrey Ahern, MD, PhD, Prof., Neurology, Psychology, Psychiatry and the Evelyn F. McKnight Brain Institute; Bruce and Lorraine Cumming Endowed Chair in Alzheimer's Research; Medical Director, Behavioral Neuroscience and Alzheimer's Clinic, The University of Arizona, Tucson, AZ

Robert (Denny) Bastron, MD, Prof., Clinical Anesthesiology, The University of Arizona, Tucson, AZ

Paul Cartter, Former Communications Chief, AZ-1 DMAT, Tucson, AZ

Julie Dixon, MD, Dermatologist, Tucson, AZ

Daniel Godoy Monzón, MD, Orthopedic Surgeon, Orthopedic and Traumatology Service; Prof., Instituto Universitario del Hospital Italiano, Buenos Aires, Argentina

Michael Grossman, DDS, General and Special-needs Dentist, Tucson, AZ

Tim B. Hunter, MD, Prof. Emeritus, Radiology, The University of Arizona, Tucson, AZ

Lawrence Hipshman, MD, MPH, Department of Psychiatry, Intercultural Psychiatric Clinic and Public Psychiatry Clinic, Oregon Health Sciences University, Portland, OR

Andrew R. Iserson, MSB, Adj. Asst. Prof., University of Maryland University College, Information Systems Management Dept (College Park); Lecturer, Georgetown School of Continuing Studies

Daniel Klemmedson, MD, DDS, DMD, Oral/Maxillofacial Surgery, Tucson, AZ
William Madden, MD, Assoc. Prof. (Retired), Clinical Pediatrics, The University of Arizona, Tucson, AZ
David Merrell, MD, Otolaryngologist, Toledo, OH; Past President, Medical Society of the US and Mexico
Joseph Miller, MD, MPH, Prof. and Department Head, Ophthalmology and Vision Science; Prof., Optical Sciences and Public Health; Murray and Clara Walker Memorial Endowed Chair in Ophthalmology, The University of Arizona, Tucson, AZ
Bernard (Barry) M. Morenz III, MD, Assoc. Prof., Clinical Psychiatry; Director, Forensic Psychiatry, The University of Arizona, Tucson, AZ
Steve Nash, JD, Executive Director, Tucson Osteopathic Medical Foundation, Tucson, AZ
Wallace Nogami, MD, Assoc. Prof., Clinical Anesthesiology and Pediatrics, The University of Arizona, Tucson, AZ
Asad (Sid) Patanwala, PharmD, Assoc. Prof., Pharmacy Practice and Science, The University of Arizona College of Pharmacy, Tucson, AZ
Alan Reeter, MSEE, Reeter Associates, Tucson, AZ
Barnett R. Rothstein, DMD, MS, Orthodontist and former Indian Health Service Dentist, Tucson, AZ
John C. Sakles, MD, Prof., Clinical Emergency Medicine, The University of Arizona, Tucson, AZ
Kenneth Sandock, MD, Consulting Radiologist, Tucson, AZ
Joe Serra, MD, Adj. Prof., Physical Therapy, University of the Pacific; Founding member of Wilderness Medical Society; National Ski Patrol (Retired)
William Sibley, MD, Prof. Emeritus, Neurology (Deceased), The University of Arizona, Tucson, AZ
Craig Steinberg, PharmD, Chairman, Pharmacy Emergency Response Team (RxERT); Pharmacy Manager, Sharp Coronado Disaster Medical Assistance Team, San Diego, CA
Matthew L. Steinway, MD, Staff Urologist, Banner Good Samaritan Medical Center, Phoenix, AZ
Bruce White, DO, JD, Director, Alden March Bioethics Institute; Prof., Center for Biomedical Ethics Education and Research, and Pediatrics, Albany Medical College, Albany, NY

Others

Many other people assisted in this book's development by providing information for techniques or equipment, reviewing specific elements, acting as test subjects for equipment, or clarifying published information. In many cases, their specific contributions have also been cited as personal communications within the text or endnotes. In alphabetical order, they are:

Alan Beamsley, DO, President, Western New Mexico Emergency Physicians; Physician, Rehoboth McKinley Christian Hospital, Gallup, NM
Manuel C. Bedoya, DMD, General Dentist, Tucson, AZ
Jamil Bitar, MD, Emergency Physician, Tucson, AZ
Jeffrey S. Blake, MD, Pediatric Emergency Medicine, Mary Bridge Children's Hospital, Tacoma, WA
Cindy Blank-Reid, RN, MSN, CEN, Trauma Clinical Nurse Specialist, Temple University Hospital, Philadelphia, PA
Leslie V. Boyer, MD, Founding Director, VIPER Institute, The University of Arizona, Tucson, AZ
Megan Brandon, PharmD, The University of Arizona, Tucson, AZ
Richard J. Bransford, MD, Assist. Prof., Orthopedics and Sports Medicine, University of Washington, Seattle, WA
Julie Brown, MD, Co-Director, Emergency Medicine Research, Seattle Children's Hospital; Assoc. Prof., Pediatrics, University of Washington School of Medicine, Seattle, WA
Singhal V. Chintamani, MS, FRCS(Edin), FRCS(Glasg), FICS, FIAMS, India

Scott Clemans, Consulting Engineer, Tucson, AZ; Member, Southern Arizona Rescue Association

Peter M.C. DeBlieux, MD, Director, Resident and Faculty Development; Prof., Clinical Medicine, LSUHSC University Hospital, New Orleans, LA

Michael Dyet, BA, RRT, Technical Specialist, Respiratory Care, Banner University Medical Center, Tucson, AZ

Gordon A. Ewy, MD, Prof. Emeritus, Internal Medicine (Cardiology); Director Emeritus, Sarver Heart Center, The University of Arizona, Tucson, AZ

Eric Fleegler, MD, MPH, FAAP, Assist. Prof., Pediatrics, Harvard Medical School; Emergency Medicine, Boston Children's Hospital, Boston, MA

Ronald Goodsite, MD, Pediatrician, Tucson, AZ

Douglas H. Freer, MD, DPM, MPH, FAAFM, FAWM, Head, Acute Care Branch Health Clinic, Marine Corps Recruit Depot, San Diego, CA

Donald "D.J." Green, MD, Assoc. Prof., Surgery, Medical Director of Trauma Services, Banner University Medical Center, Tucson, AZ

Haywood Hall, MD, FACEP, FIFEM, Founding Director, PACEMD/PACE Global Health International; Medical Director, MDLIVE, Inc., Marfil, Guanajuato, Mexico

Col. Patricia Hastings, DO, AMEDDCS; Medical Director, Joint Staff Support to Global Health, Office of the Director, Joint Staff, Joint Chiefs of Staff [JCS], US Dept. of Defense

Sri Devi Jagjit, MD, Emergency Physician, Georgetown, Guyana

Mark Hauswald, MS, MD, Prof., Emergency Medicine; Director of Global Health Programs, The University of New Mexico, Albuquerque, NM

John Jared, EMT-P, Emergency Department, Banner University Medical Center, Tucson, AZ

Harry Kraus, MD, FACS, Missionary Surgeon and Author, Tucson, AZ

Yosef Leibman MD, Physician, Soroka Hospital, Beer Sheva, Israel; Founder, *Israeli Journal of Emergency Medicine*; Editor-in-Chief, *Emergency Medicine Update*

Michael K. Levy, MD, FAAEM, Emergency Physician, Alaska Regional Hospital, Anchorage, AK

Joe Lex, MD, FACEP, FAAEM, Prof. (Retired), Emergency Medicine, Temple University, Philadelphia, PA

David Liem, PhD, Assist. Research Physiologist, David Geffen School of Medicine at UCLA, Los Angeles, CA

Mario Llurie, RN, CWCS, Wound Specialist, Banner University Medical Center, Tucson, AZ

Darrell G. Looney, MD, FACEP, FAAEM, Emergency Physician, OSF St. Joseph Medical Center, Bloomington, IL

Thomas O. McMasters, Director, US Army Medical Department Museum, Fort Sam Houston, TX

Naveen Malhotra, MD, Department of Obstetrics and Gynaecology, All-India Institute of Medical Sciences, New Delhi, India

Tawnya Meeks-Modrzejewski, Nurse Practitioner, CareMore Health Plan; Flight Nurse, Tucson, AZ

Katherine Mehaffey, BSN, RN, CWS, CWOCN, Wound, Ostomy, and Continence Nursing Service, Banner University Medical Center, Tucson, AZ

Andy Norman, MD, Assist. Prof., Obstetrics and Gynecology; Affiliated faculty member, Vanderbilt Institute for Global Health (VIGH), Vanderbilt University Medical Center, Nashville, TN

Charles O. Otieno, MD, MPH, Emergency Physician, Los Robles Emergency Physicians Medical Group, Burbank, CA

Sue Philpott, RN, Training Officer, AZ-1 Disaster Medical Assistance Team, Tucson, AZ

Farhad Pooran, PhD, PE, Vice President, Engineering, Schneider Electric, Washington, DC

Laurence H. Raney, MD, FAAEM, FACEP, Emergency Physician, Isle of Palms, SC

Mykle Raymond, Engineering Technician, Tucson, AZ; Member, Southern Arizona Rescue Association

James Riopelle, MD, Prof., Clinical Anesthesiology, LSUHSC School of Medicine, New Orleans, LA

Mohammed RM Rishard, Teaching Hospital, Kandy; GVMP Galgomuwa, Faculty of Medicine, University of Peradeniya; and K. Gunawardane, Teaching Hospital, Kandy, Sri Lanka
Karen Schneider, RSM, MD, Assist. Prof., Pediatrics, Johns Hopkins University, Baltimore, MD
Sandra M. Schneider, MD, FACEP, Prof., Emergency Medicine, University of Rochester, Rochester, NY; Physician-Editor, *AHC Media*
John J. Shaw, DMD, Emergency Preparedness Planner, JJS Consulting; Former Program Director, Capitol Region Metropolitan Medical Response System, Hartford, CT; Chair, ESF 8, Capitol Region Emergency Planning Committee
Ronald A. Sherman, MD, MSc, DTM&H, Director, BioTherapeutics, Education and Research Foundation, Orange County, CA
Farshad (Mazda) Shirazi, MD, PhD, Assoc. Prof., Clinical Toxicology; Medical Director, University of Arizona Poison and Drug Information Center; Director, Medical Toxicology Fellowship, Emergency Department, The University of Arizona, Tucson, AZ
Rhonda Shirley, EMT-P, Emergency Department, Banner University Medical Center, Tucson, AZ
John Spero, Emergency Department, Banner University Medical Center, Tucson, AZ
Daniel Tsze, MD, MPH, Assist. Prof., Pediatrics; Director, Pain Management and Sedation Program, Columbia University College of Surgeons and Physicians, New York, NY
Oren Weissman, MD, Department of Plastic and Reconstructive Surgery, Asaaf Harofeh Medical Center, Zerifin, Israel
Lara Zibners-Lohr, MD, Emergency Pediatric Physician, London, UK

Finally, I must thank everyone whose name I inadvertently omitted. While I tried to include everyone who helped me produce this enormous project, I'm sure that there were some that I omitted. Sorry. I hope you still enjoy the book.

I | THE SITUATION

1 | What Is Improvised Medicine?

As this second edition goes to press, the need for improvisation among health care workers has become more evident. Natural and human-made disasters have overwhelmed many of the world's resource-poor regions; local and international health care workers have stepped in to assist—with excellent skills, but often with less than adequate supplies and equipment. Health care workers in more developed countries also experience these shortages, even under "normal circumstances," but generally to a lesser degree. The information in this book should help to overcome some of these difficulties.

Improvised medicine encompasses a spectrum of ad hoc equipment, and special methods and knowledge for advanced health care practitioners who already work capably within their own areas of expertise. Use *Improvised Medicine* when, due to prevailing circumstances, you must reach beyond your comfort level and provide medical care usually provided by other specialists—or without the medications, equipment, and milieu to which you have become accustomed.

In the context of a disaster or a resource-poor environment, frustration may be defined as understanding what can be done, what needs to be done, and how to do it, but not having the necessary tools. Unlike paramedics, who are trained to expect the unexpected, most other health care professionals (including physicians, dentists, podiatrists, physician assistants, and nurse practitioners) who work in high-tech health care systems don't expect that the power will fail, a fire will ignite, the computer system will crash, a flood will inundate their facility, or an epidemic will erupt. Yet these events occur on a routine basis and, given the state of the world, it is likely they will occur more frequently in the future.

How do you practice medicine in a disaster, when you are confronted by increased numbers of patients, the need to extend your scope of practice beyond your comfort level, and the need to work with limited or alternative methods, equipment, and staff in unusual, often makeshift, locales? When a disaster's scope is regional or national, knowing what to do and how to improvise becomes even more crucial. For a health care provider to work, innovate, and provide leadership in resource-poor environments, especially when others are panicking, often requires superior knowledge and greater understanding. *Improvised Medicine* provides this.

Exemplifying the need to innovate and to manage limited resources is the performance of Dr. Lin and his colleagues of the Israel Defense Forces Medical Corps after the 2010 earthquake in Haiti. Just 89 hours after the massive quake struck Port-au-Prince, the IDF Medical Corps Field Hospital was fully operational. Despite having highly trained personnel and equipment adequate for prior humanitarian missions, "the vast dimensions" of the crisis forced the Corps to find creative solutions "to several problems in a variety of medical fields: blood transfusion, debridement and coverage of complex wounds, self-production of orthopedic hardware, surgical exposure, and managing maxillofacial injuries." "Under these hectic conditions," Lin wrote, "lack of specific medical equipment is expected and requires improvisation using available items."[1]

In selecting material for this book, I have tried to anticipate both short-term and long-term resource deficiencies. Therefore, some improvised techniques in the book can be used immediately in sudden critical situations; others are long-term solutions for use when equipment and facilities will be lacking for some time. The most mundane, everyday occurrences include the lack of necessary equipment and supplies (e.g., IV fluids, medications) and having difficulty with a procedure (e.g., airway, IV). If this book's improvised methods help in these situations, great. But the real emphasis is on opening your mind to ways of solving problems in a crisis and providing options for you (and your patients) when alternatives seem limited or nonexistent.

METHODS AND EQUIPMENT

Farley wrote in 1938 that "original ideas for improvising equipment have been pretty well exhausted."[2]

This book demonstrates the fallacy in Farley's thinking. *Improvised Medicine* represents both exploration and discovery. It encompasses a search through the world's medical literature, both past and current, for procedures that can be used and equipment that can be improvised in resource-poor situations. I tested many techniques to see if they actually work; some that clinicians believe should work, did not. Four major techniques that, initially, seemed like good ideas were the use of papier-mâché (paper-mâché) for casts, soda bottles as bag-valve-masks, ham or portable radios for intra-hospital communication, and the much-published auscultation for fractures. I won't bore you with the details, but trust me, these methods don't work. (Thanks to my very patient wife for acting as the subject for the casting tests, and to Scott Clemans and Mykle Raymond of the Southern Arizona Rescue Association for helping with the radio tests—multiple times.)

Creative techniques and equipment in the book include a light-bulb beaker, the "ruggedized" IV, a method to fit a child oxygen mask on infants, an improved postpartum balloon, easy DIY ultrasound gel, simplified vertical mattress sutures, makeshift medication atomizers (with and without pressurized gas), improvised stethoscope earpieces, a scalpel fashioned from a disposable razor and an improvised handle for scalpel blades, an extremely simple method of extracting additional epinephrine doses from an EpiPen, a way to improve laryngeal mask airway (LMA) placement, a nasal speculum made from a clothes hanger, and many more improvisations.

These methods and equipment were tested in clinical practice—due to necessity, both in the United States and during my stints practicing and teaching medicine on all seven continents. I learned and tested the simple and rapid method for vertically (down the stairs) evacuating patients from hospitals during a Disaster Medical Assistance Team exercise, although it does not seem to have been published before. Rapid-admixture blood warming, the amobarbital interview for conversion reactions, and hypnosis for fracture-dislocation reduction are not new (although either I originally published the rapid blood warming technique or my publications on the subject are among the most recent). A new mnemonic (PAIN for tooth pain) is included to assist in remembering these important details. This book also rescues many techniques from the obscurity of dusty books or little-known publications. While some critics might contend that they should remain there, I'm convinced that lives may be saved by resurrecting them.

Because of the medication and intravenous fluid shortages rampant in every locale, the text suggests ways to manage these crises, as well as novel medication substitutions, ways to use alternative medication administration methods, and safe ways to conserve medications and fluids.

ELEGANT IMPROVISATION

There is no one-size-fits-all in situations with limited resources. Circumstances will vary: in one, necessary equipment may be unavailable; in another, medications will be lacking; and in yet others, there will be no way to transport patients safely and quickly. Whatever the problem, the individuals making key decisions—and often the entire medical team—need to participate in fashioning the best medical treatment for their patients in that situation. As Dr. Maurice King wrote, "Failure to improvise, where this is at all possible, is never an adequate reason for not doing something."[3]

Nearly all the chapters contain material that may be familiar to specialists in that field. There is, however, a separate chapter on using ether, ketamine, and halothane, because even many anesthesiologists have had little experience with these agents, although they are commonly used in resource-poor settings. The difficult challenge has been to include enough information so that those not familiar with the field can perform adequately without a wealth of equipment or expert assistance. The goal is for any advanced clinician to be able to use the appropriate techniques in this book.

Naturally, a huge emphasis is placed on using improvised methods in less-developed countries, remote areas, and other resource-poor environments. My hope is that, while most clinicians will know many of these techniques, they will find new material that can be used to help their patients. Every effort has been made to supply enough information to perform the techniques or to make the equipment, even if the original sources lacked some necessary details.

Ultimately, this book suggests ideas that should prod you into a *How can I do this?* mind-set. Problem solving is only part of the solution. The real issues are motivation and attitude. Your motivation is to help your patient; your attitude is "The difficult we do immediately. The impossible takes a little longer."[4]

Improvised Medicine is intended to help you and your health care team to problem-solve and find a workable solution. As the old medical adage about stethoscopes says, "It's not what goes in the ears, but what's between the ears that matters." A modern update, based on military medicine, says that while "technology is important, … the best instruments on the battlefield are your hands, fingers, and brain, trained for optimal use. They seldom break, they are hard to misplace, they can be upgraded continuously, and frequently invent new solutions."[5] In austere medical situations, it is the combination of the knowledge and skills of the entire team, not just of one individual, that may save the day. One very basic (and recent) example of improvisation occurred while I was considering what to include in this introduction. I had to drain an ischemic priapism in an austere situation and discovered that no large-bore butterfly needle was available. (The butterfly tubing permits movement of the needle without dislodging it during the drainage/irrigation/medication instillation process.) Once the team decided to go ahead with the procedure and not to use a less-than-optimal piece of equipment (e.g., small-bore butterfly or fixed needle), a workable substitute was quickly devised using a large-bore hypodermic needle attached to a short piece of extension tubing.

This book can only supply ideas about how to "make-do" when dealing with shortages. Problem-solving skills will take you the rest of the way when you are faced with missing equipment, personnel, or facilities. As is typical in medicine—and in life, generally—once we recognize that something can be done, we find ways to do it better. Over time, the hot air balloon evolved into a rocket ship, a daguerreotype into a digital video movie, an abacus into a computer, and the ancients' signal fires into the Internet. Many of the techniques and much of the equipment described in this book are either retrieved from our predecessors, essentially "lost knowledge," or innovations that colleagues have developed. Nearly all can be improved upon; it only takes more people thinking about how to do it better. That is where you come in. If you develop an improvement on the techniques or equipment described in this book, please forward it to me so it can be included (with credit to you or the originator, of course) in the next edition. Mail them to me c/o Galen Press, Ltd., PO Box 64400-IM, Tucson, AZ, 85728-4400 USA; or email me: kvi@galenpress.com.

REFERENCES

1. Lin G, Lavon H, Gelfond R, Abargel A, Merin O. Hard times call for creative solutions: medical improvisations at the Israel Defense Forces Field Hospital in Haiti. *Am Disaster Med.* 2010;5(3):188-192.
2. Farley F. Improvising equipment. *Am J Nurs.* 1938;38(4, section 2):42s-43s.
3. King M, Bewes P, Cairns J, et al, eds. *Primary Surgery, Vol. 1: Non-Trauma.* Oxford, UK: Oxford Medical Publishing; 1990:9.
4. US Army Service Forces slogan. (Many others claim the slogan. This attribution is per *Bartlett's Familiar Quotations*, 14th ed.)
5. Holcomb JB. The 2004 Fitts Lecture: current perspective on combat casualty care. *J Trauma.* 2005;59(4):990-1002.

2 | What Are Resource-Poor Situations?

INTRODUCTION

In what types of situations would you need to improvise medical equipment and procedures? Experience demonstrates that physicians in the most-developed countries are most likely to need improvisation when their usual procedures fail or their equipment does not function. That is not the case outside these privileged medical practice arenas:

> The mother's blank stare and hurried manner reveals that she knows how sick the child is that she carries into the emergency department at a rural sub-Saharan district hospital. Still swaddled in a colorful cloth, the child stares unseeing from eyes with white palpebral conjunctivae; there's barely a grimace when she's stimulated. A nursing assistant quickly puts her ear to the child's chest to listen for a heartbeat and then applies a venous tourniquet in a vain attempt at finding an extremity IV site. The nurse wants to apply oxygen, but they used the last of it on the night shift; the oxygen concentrator promised for two years has never arrived. She then fashions a scalp tourniquet from a disposable glove and the physician uses an injection needle to place an IO line. The first blood sample is rushed to the lab along with the mother-donor, since the blood bank has no blood; the lab reports that the child's Hgb is <4 g/dL. More fluid is needed, so the physician starts an intraperitoneal infusion. Even with the mother as donor, the blood is not forthcoming, since the lab has run out of reagents and is having to use a coagulation test to check for compatibility.
>
> The child's respirations become labored and, using a makeshift fit with an adult mask, they assist her breathing. They improvise an endotracheal tube and prepare to intubate. They give IV quinine using aluminum foil to control the flow and IM ceftriaxone using a resterilized single-use syringe. Blood arrives; it's still warm. They begin transfusing. The child is doing a little better and the nursing aide steadfastly keeps monitoring the femoral pulse, since that's all that is available. It's going to be a long night.

Throughout the world, clinicians must practice medicine while making do with minimal resources. Material and equipment scarcity often overwhelms health care professionals, whether they are the sole medical provider at a localized event who lacks the materials to treat one or more patients, groups at a more widespread calamity that affects an entire community or region, or teams at a long-lasting degradation of care spanning entire countries. This resource scarcity may last from only minutes to many days or even weeks. Or, they may be chronic conditions. Limited-resource situations may be due to physical isolation (e.g., prisoner of war [POW] camp, airplane, ship), being in a remote area (e.g., wilderness, rural highway), being in a least-developed country with a chronic lack of health care resources, or being in a disaster/post-disaster setting.

These situations, especially when they occur in settings where resources are usually plentiful, often result in degraded levels of treatment (Fig. 2-1). But, if clinicians use their ingenuity, this need not be the case. Good medical treatment can often be provided using limited resources if clinicians willingly alter their approach and techniques to fit the circumstances.

Resource-poor situations are logically grouped into simple, extended, and complex disasters, depending on how long they are likely to last, how much help is required, and the degradation of health care and the social order (riots and unrest) that may occur.[1]

Throughout this book, methods that can and should be used in all four circumstances are discussed interchangeably. The focus in many sections is on the chronically resource-poor situations found in the least-developed countries, although these methods may be used anywhere. Each of the main limited-resource settings is briefly described later in this chapter.

Simple disasters last a short time and usually require only local resources. Examples include a multi-casualty motor vehicle crash, an apartment building collapse, a multi-casualty fire, a landslide, and a tornado going through a trailer park. The needed support systems include emergency medical services (EMS), fire services, medical services, and law enforcement. Social order generally remains intact.

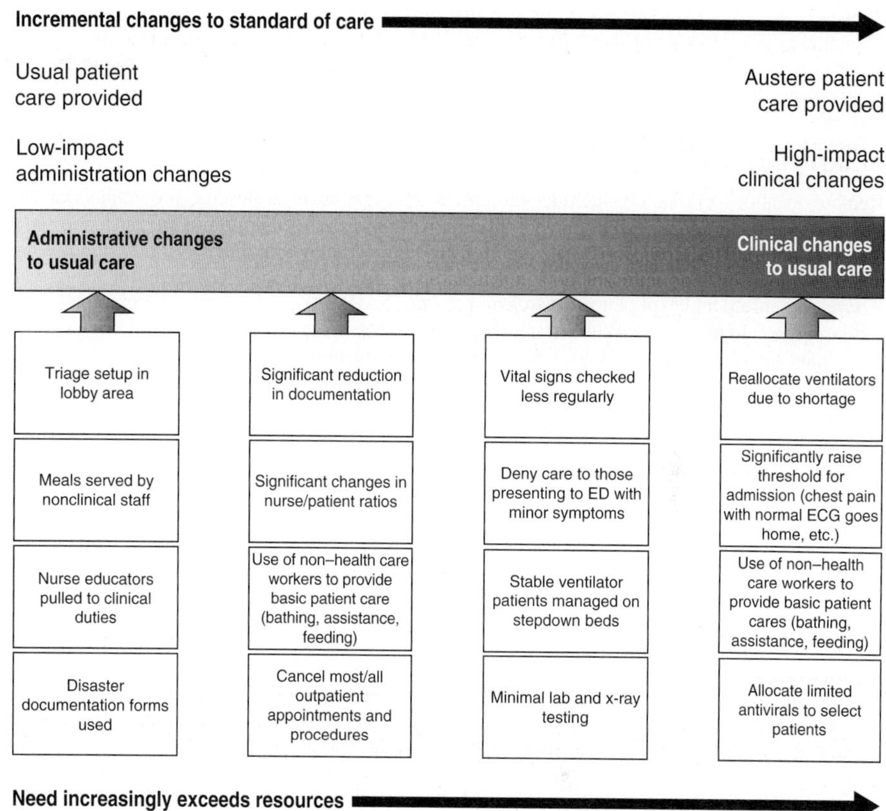

FIG. 2-1. Progression of changes in health care in resource-poor situations. *(Reproduced from Hick et al.[2])*

Extended disasters include widespread flooding, devastating hurricanes or tsunamis, massive heat waves, and major earthquakes. In these cases, the necessary support system also includes outside assistance to augment surviving local EMS, fire services, medical services, and law enforcement. The social order may be unstable.

Complex disasters are those chronic situations, usually in the least-developed countries, that often are the result of a major drought, famine, or war. A major nuclear incident would also fall into this category. Societal and social support systems are normally disrupted.

ISOLATED SETTINGS

Isolated settings are remote, without an immediate way to gather resources that are not already available. The classic isolated setting is in an internment camp, such as the World War II POW camps. However, isolated settings may also occur on a boat or an airplane or, the ultimate isolation, in space. One of the best-documented physician histories from a POW camp is that of Capt. Thomas H. Hewlett (Surgeon, US Army Medical Corps). He wrote,

> [In the camp,] our only available anesthesia consisted of several vials of dental Novocain tablets. Two of these tablets dissolved in a small amount of the patient's spinal fluid, and injected into the spine gave about forty-five minutes of anesthesia, giving us time to perform most operations that had to be done .... Dutch torpedo technicians were able to make surgical knives out of old British table silver-ware .... We treated fractures without x-rays .... We operated bare handed, [sic] the fingernails of the surgical team stayed black

as a result of our using bichloride of mercury and 7% iodine in preparing our hands before surgery … . [However,] our infection rate in surgical patients never exceeded 3% … . Sharpened bicycle spokes were used as traction wires in the treatment of hip and leg fractures. Plaster of Paris was never available.[3]

REMOTE LOCATIONS

Remote locations classically include wilderness settings, such as deserts, mountains, caves, forests, and jungles. More commonly, even in the most-developed countries, it means coming across ("on-siding") a personal injury crash or medical emergency far from a source of help. Be prepared by carrying basic materials (see Appendix 2) and being ready to improvise.

Even organized and experienced search and rescue (SAR) teams who carry equipment into the field may have to improvise. While rescuing a patient deep in a cave shaft with a back injury, our SAR team found that we could not maneuver a backboard into the narrow space where she lay. After several hours of working in the hot, humid, cramped, and relatively dark area, we improvised an immobilizer and extricated her from the cave.

LEAST-DEVELOPED COUNTRIES

Chronic shortages are the norm in the least-developed countries. Health care workers know they must make-do with whatever supplies and equipment are available and functioning. As a nurse practitioner student on a medical mission to the rural Philippines wrote, "the challenge of the lack of equipment and medications taught me that we sometimes have to deal with the resources at hand and that there are ways to improvise in order to obtain the same results."[4]

An emergency physician working at a Latin American general hospital (used by the poorest people) found that only two or three vials of medication were available for resuscitation, and only 8-mm endotracheal (ET) tubes were available. The medications would change weekly, as would the ET tube sizes. The medical team made-do with available supplies when they could; when they couldn't, patients died. Improvisation was the norm.

DISASTERS/POST-DISASTER

The key features of disasters are "threat, urgency and uncertainty, which affect not only the victims themselves, but also the organizations that have to respond."[5] Disasters can be from man-made (e.g., multivictim vehicle crashes, terrorism, radiation leaks, and war) or natural (e.g., tsunamis, earthquakes, and epidemics) forces. Both often lead to resource-poor situations. The assistance provided varies greatly, depending on a host of factors.

The vagaries of war can overwhelm what seem to be adequate medical facilities. For example, during the Spanish-American War, three-fourths of all casualties came from the assault on San Juan Hill. "A temporary hospital at Siboney, established to care for only 200 men, was overwhelmed by so many injured that soldiers slept naked on the ground until tents could be set up for them …. For five straight days, doctors treated the wounded."[6]

Terrorist attacks have become common in many areas of the world. Immediate improvisation is often required until organized EMS and medical teams take control. Dr. Wesley Shum worked in "a surreal scene" at a makeshift hospital set up close to ground zero immediately after 9/11. We lacked "basic medical supplies like bandages and painkillers … [I] was forced to use cut-up cardboard boxes and strapping tape to make makeshift casts for [my] patients."[7] All of his patients were firemen injured when the Twin Towers collapsed.

Specific problems associated with different natural disasters are listed in Table 2-1.

Presenting their own mini-disaster, health care facilities may be suddenly struck by an unexpected flood, water or power outage, computer crash, epidemic, or other occurrence that diminishes or overwhelms their capacity to treat patients. For example, when Tropical Storm Allison flooded Houston's Memorial Hermann Children's Hospital in June 1991, the facility lost all but its emergency power. As some nurses described it,

> We had no air-conditioning; garbage and medical supplies filled the hallways. Generators provided electricity as water was pumped out of the building, and the parking lot served as a cafeteria. We had only bottled water and portable toilets. The scene bordered

TABLE 2-1 Common Medical Problems in Specific Situations

Earthquakes		
Long bone fractures	Head, spine fractures	Soft tissue trauma
Dust asphyxia	Crush or compartment syndrome	Animal attacks
Infectious disease problems generally related to water and food. Usually little increase in infectious diseases.		
Tsunamis		
Drowning	Blunt injuries	High mortality-morbidity ratio
Infectious diseases may temporarily decrease, in part due to elimination of insect vectors.		
Tornadoes		
Blunt, crush, and penetrating wounds		Eye injuries
Volcanoes		
Blunt, crush, and penetrating trauma	Dust asphyxiation	Burns
Eye injuries	Little evidence of increased infectious disease	

Adapted from Rega.[1]

> on catastrophe. [The next day] the ground floor was under 4 feet of water; the basement was completely submerged .... We climbed the seven flights of stairs to the NICU in the dark and were immediately hit by hot, humid air and pitch-black darkness. The usual noises were strikingly absent: none of the cardiopulmonary monitors, ventilators, radiant warmers, or incubators worked. Every baby was covered with blankets to contain warmth.[8]

Who Should Respond to Disasters?

Many untrained and inexperienced volunteers offer their assistance after every major disaster. While well meaning, they not only are unwanted but, unlike organized teams that have their own supplies, also use resources that the affected population desperately needs.[9] Even if they connect with nongovernmental agencies providing assistance, these unsolicited, often young, and short-term volunteers are usually not covered by insurance, may not get on-site training, and commonly get post-traumatic stress disorder.[10,11]

Even senior experienced clinicians fall into the spontaneous volunteering trap. For example, after nearly 300,000 people perished in the 2004 Southeast Asia tsunami and millions were displaced from their homes, well-known author and Yale surgeon Sherwin Nuland hopped on a commercial plane with six compatriots and went to Sri Lanka to help. As he later wrote, this was a bad idea:

> I am not sure just what it was that made me drop everything on December 31 and join six colleagues on a medical relief mission to Sri Lanka. At the moment I made the decision, it simply seemed like the right thing to do, and in retrospect it still does. But it turned out that the need for our small group was very different than we had anticipated: there was far less acute disease and injury than expected, but the human misery was of a sort that will require attention for years to come. In a strictly clinical sense, we accomplished far less than we had hoped ... Disaster relief is only the most immediate kind of relief that this punished place requires ... In retrospect, we were like an amateur and astonishingly naive flying squad or rapid-response team ... I had brought with me a set of surgical instruments to be used as though in a field hospital, assuming that my principal work

> would be to treat the late consequences of major trauma. I was wrong. The tsunami had an effect similar to that of September 11, when emergency rooms all over Manhattan prepared themselves for an influx of the seriously injured, and very few came. The reason was the same: almost everyone caught up in the disaster was killed.[12]

If you are interested in disaster medicine, join a team designed to respond after global disasters. Before you do, ask enough questions to understand their mission, training, and activity level.[13]

REDUCING MEDICAL IMPROVISATION

Organized teams venturing into disaster or remote environments can try to reduce the need for and optimize any required medical treatment. The way to do this is through in-depth planning and following these 10 guidelines:

1. Optimize workers' fitness.
2. Anticipate treatable problems.
3. Stock appropriate medications.
4. Provide appropriate equipment.
5. Provide adequate logistical support.
6. Provide adequate medical communications.
7. Know the environmental limitations on patient access and evacuation.
8. Use qualified providers.
9. Arrange for knowledgeable and timely consultations.
10. Establish and distribute rational administrative rules.

Planners using these guidelines may better be able to generate a strategy that optimizes the participants' health and reduces the need to use improvisation for medical care.[14]

DISASTER MYTHS

As Jeff Arnold wrote, "At least one thing has become predictable about disasters in recent years—once a disaster begins to unfold, an outbreak of disaster mythology is likely to ensue."[15] The persistence of such myths is attested to by David Alexander,

> This reaction is particularly tragic in response to disasters, in which incorrect beliefs often are the basis for misguided actions that lead to avoidable casualties and suffering .... One of the most troublesome aspects of present-day responses to disasters is the crushing inevitability of the mistakes that are made, the myths that are propagated, and the inefficiencies that plague their management. For the people who live through them, disasters are times of accelerated learning .... Disaster myths are robust enough to survive Herculean attempts to debunk them.[16]

Many people, even experienced disaster workers, have trouble not believing all the myths in Table 2-2.

ETHICS

While it may seem obvious in retrospect, designating a significant resource-poor situation as a disaster may, at the time, be difficult, bureaucratic, financially burdensome, and ethically charged. Specific, measurable, and widely-known "triggers" must be in place so that an on-site individual can declare a disaster. This allows the mobilization of resources while they can still be most effective. See Appendix 1 for a generic all-hazards approach to identifying and responding to localized or larger disasters.

Two excellent, free, on-line disaster resources are available: The World Health Organization's Health Library for Disasters (http://helid.digicollection.org/en/) is available in English, French, and Spanish. Three short videos (in English and in Spanish) describing the method behind and the ethics of allocating scarce resources in disaster situations can be found at www.youtube.com/channel/UC-KrAtJ_TCLv05NgZUNlUuQ.

TABLE 2-2 Typical Myths and Misconceptions About Disasters

Myth: Disasters are unusual events.

Reality: Disasters occur frequently, and the same types often occur in the same locations (e.g., flooding in Bangladesh). Since 1995, on average, more than one natural disaster per day has been reported throughout the world.[a]

Myth: Disasters kill people without respect for social class or economic status.

Reality: The poor and marginalized are more at risk of death than are rich people or the middle classes.

Myth: Earthquakes commonly result in a large number of deaths.

Reality: The majority of earthquakes do not cause high death tolls. Deaths can be reduced further by constructing antiseismic buildings and teaching people how to behave during earthquakes.

Myth: People can survive for many days when trapped under the rubble of a collapsed building.

Reality: The vast majority of people extracted alive from rubble are saved within 24 hours and often within 12 hours of impact.

Myth: Panic is a common reaction to disasters.

Reality: Most people behave rationally in a disaster. While panic occasionally occurs, many disaster sociologists regard it as insignificant.

Myth: People flee in large numbers from a disaster area.

Reality: Usually, there is a "convergence reaction" and the stricken area fills with people. Few survivors leave, and even obligatory evacuations are short lived.

Myth: After a disaster, survivors tend to be dazed and apathetic.

Reality: Survivors rapidly start reconstruction. Activism is much more common than fatalism. (This is the so-called "therapeutic community.") Even in the worst scenarios, only 15%-30% of victims show passive or dazed reactions.

Myth: Disasters usually give rise to widespread, spontaneous manifestations of antisocial behavior (riots).

Reality: Generally, disasters are characterized by great social solidarity, generosity, and self-sacrifice, perhaps even heroism.

Myth: Looting is a common and serious problem after disasters.

Reality: Looting is rare and limited in scope. It mainly occurs when there are strong preconditions, as when a community is already deeply divided.

Myth: The disruption and poor health caused by major disasters nearly always cause epidemics.

Reality: Generally, the level of epidemiological surveillance and health care in the disaster area is sufficient to stop epidemics from occurring. However, the rate of disease diagnosis may increase due to a temporary increase in the availability of health care.

Myth: Disasters cause a great deal of chaos, preventing systematic management.

Reality: There are excellent theoretical models of how disasters function and how to manage them. The general elements of disaster are well known from more than 75 years of research. The same events tend to repeat themselves from one disaster to the next.

Myth: To manage a disaster well, it is necessary to accept all forms of aid that are offered.

Reality: It is better to limit acceptance of donations to goods and services that are actually needed in the disaster area.

Myth: Any kind of aid and relief is useful after disasters, provided it is supplied quickly.

Reality: Hasty and ill-considered relief initiatives create chaos. Only certain types of assistance, goods, and services are required. Not all useful resources that existed in the area before the disaster will be destroyed. Donation of unusable materials or manpower consumes resources of organization and accommodation that could more profitably be used to reduce the toll of the disaster.

(Continued)

TABLE 2-2 Typical Myths and Misconceptions About Disasters (*Continued*)

Myth: One should donate used clothes to the victims of disasters.

Reality: This often leads to accumulations of huge quantities of useless garments that victims cannot or will not wear.

Myth: Great quantities and assortments of medicines should be sent to disaster areas.

Reality: The only medicines that are needed are those that are used to treat specific pathologies, have not reached their sell-by date, can be properly conserved in the disaster area, and can be properly identified in terms of their pharmacological constituents. Any other medicines are not only useless but also potentially dangerous.

Myth: Companies, corporations, associations, and governments are always very generous when invited to send aid and relief to disaster areas.

Reality: They may be, but, in the past, disaster areas that have been used as dumping grounds for outdated medicines, obsolete equipment, and unusable goods, usually garnering tax benefits for the donors, under the cloak of apparent generosity.

Myth: Unburied dead bodies constitute a health hazard.

Reality: Not even advanced decomposition causes a significant health hazard. Hasty burial demoralizes survivors and upsets arrangements for death certification, funeral rites, and, where needed, autopsy. The living rather than the dead are contagious.

Myth: Technology will save the world from disaster.

Reality: The problem of disasters is largely a social one. Technological resources are poorly distributed and often ineffectively used. In addition, technology is a potential source of vulnerability (e.g., computer crashes, power outages).

Myth: There is usually a shortage of resources when disasters occur, and this prevents them from being managed effectively.

Reality: The shortage, if it occurs, is almost always short-lived. There is more of a problem in deploying resources well and using them efficiently than in acquiring them. Often, there is also a problem of coping with a superabundance of certain types of resources.

Myth: International rescue workers save thousands of lives during the aftermath of natural disasters.

Reality: Lives are saved only during or immediately following the event. Search and rescue effectiveness declines rapidly after 12 to 24 hours.

Myth: Foreign-run field hospitals are the primary way to provide mass casualty treatment after disasters.

Reality: Local health care providers and systems provide most casualty management. Foreign workers often supply only ancillary help.

[a]EM-DAT International Disasters Database: Natural disasters reported 1900-2006. http://www.emdat.be/disasters/img/Total%20reported%20damages%20in%202006%20billions%20from%20disasters%201900–2006.pdf. Accessed September 30, 2007.

Data from Alexander,[16] PAHO,[17] and De Ville de Goyet.[18]

REFERENCES

1. Rega P. Disaster health: health consequences and response. NDMS Response Team Training Program, September 2003.
2. Hick JL, Kelen G, O'Laughlin D, et al. Hospital/acute care. In: Phillips SJ, Knebel A, eds. *Providing Mass Medical Care With Scarce Resources: A Community Planning Guide.* Rockville, MD: Agency for Healthcare Research and Quality, 2006:66.
3. Report of Thomas H. Hewlett, MD (Col. US Army, Ret.) *"Di Ju Nana Bunshyo: Nightmare-Revisited."* Based on the original medical report from Camp 17 and presented to the Reunion of Survivors of Bataan-Corregidor, August 1978. Supplied by the US Army Medical Department Museum, Ft. Sam Houston, TX; used with their permission.

4. Christman MS. A personal account of a medical mission. *J Am Acad Nurse Pract*. 2000;12(8): 309-310.
5. Hodgkinson PE, Stewart M. *Coping With Catastrophe: A Handbook of Disaster Management*. London: Routledge; 1991.
6. National Museum of Health and Medicine. Spanish-American War (exhibit). http://www.medicalmuseum.mil/index.cfm?p=exhibits.past.spanishamericanwar.page_03. Accessed September 30, 2006.
7. Sherman T. One doctor's attempt to help. Opportunity. NYU Stern School of Business. http://pages.stern.nyu.edu/~opportun/issues/2001–2002/issue2.htm. Accessed September 14, 2006.
8. Verklan MT, Kelley K, Carter L, et al. The day the rain came down. *Am J Nurs*. 2002;102(3): 24AA-KK.
9. Iserson KV. *The Global Healthcare Volunteer's Handbook: What You Need to Know Before You Go*. Tucson, AZ: Galen Press, Ltd; 2014:27-29.
10. Sauer LM, Catlett C, Tosatto R, Kirsch TD. The utility of and risks associated with the use of spontaneous volunteers in disaster response: a survey. *Disaster Med Pub Hlth Prep*. 2014;8(01):65-69.
11. Cranmer HH, Biddinger PD. Typhoon Haiyan and the professionalization of disaster response. *New Engl J Med*. 2014;370(13):1185-1187.
12. Nuland SB. A report from a relief mission: after the deluge. *The New Republic*. April 11, 2005. www.tnr.com/article/after-the-deluge. Accessed January 21, 2015.
13. Iserson KV. *The Global Healthcare Volunteer's Handbook: What You Need to Know Before You Go*. Tucson, AZ: Galen Press, Ltd.; 2014:30-33.
14. Iserson KV. Medical planning for extended remote expeditions. *Wild Environ Med*. 2013;24(4): 366-377.
15. Arnold JL. Disaster myths and Hurricane Katrina 2005: can public officials and the media learn to provide responsible crisis communication during disasters? *Prehosp Disaster Med*. 2006;21(1):1-4.
16. Alexander DE. Misconception as a barrier to teaching about disasters. *Prehosp Disaster Med*. 2007;22(2):95-103.
17. PAHO. *Epidemiological Surveillance After Natural Disasters*. Scientific Publication #420. Washington, DC: Pan American Health Organization; 1982.
18. De Ville de Goyet C. Myths, the ultimate survivors in disasters. *Prehosp Disaster Med*. 2007;22(2):104-105.

II | BASIC NEEDS

3 | Communications

Communication means successfully exchanging information so that the message reaches the correct recipient in a timely manner and is interpreted accurately. In resource-poor situations, especially following disasters, communication difficulties are usually the major problem health care and other service/rescue providers face.

POST-DISASTER COMMUNICATION NEEDS

Relying on a predisaster or "normal" telecommunication system—such as landline telephones, cellular telephones, or pager systems—to work in austere circumstances is foolish. Communication systems fail during disasters due to network/signal problems, electrical power loss, damage to infrastructure, surviving infrastructure (telephone, cellular phones, etc.) overload, or system damage that overwhelms repair crews.

Multiple space-based satellite communication systems have been used internationally during disasters.[1] Even in the best circumstances, however, this type of communication may not be available until several hours, or even days, after major disasters, while good communication is needed immediately. Whichever makeshift methods are used will depend on what resources are still available.

Preparation for Disaster Communications

Experienced, prepared spokespeople are needed to communicate with the professional teams and the public before, during, and after disasters. They need specific skill sets that address "risk communication." (See Table 3-1 and "Hardest Decisions: Who Allocates Scare Healthcare Resources" video at https://www.youtube.com/watch?v=w2qFjRNmtX4.) Building communication capacity prior to a disaster includes prewriting public service announcements in multiple languages that address questions that frequently arise during disasters (Table 3-2) and maintaining contact lists. These lists, to be updated on a scheduled basis, should include reliable information sources in frequently affected regions, media contacts that can rapidly disseminate information, and government agencies and nongovernmental organizations that can provide assistance.

ON-SCENE COMMAND AND CONTROL

In disasters and other chaotic situations, successful control of the situation depends on obtaining adequate information and distributing messages to those with "boots on the ground." This often takes ingenuity.

For example, rather than being used for rescue or extraction, the first helicopter on the scene of a widespread disaster, such as a commercial airliner crash, may best be used as a command and control center for subsequently arriving ground rescue units. The relative positions of the victims and rescue units can be better seen from an elevated vantage point than from the ground. Experience has shown that directing rescue units from the air in these circumstances may save the lives of victims who may otherwise not have been found in a timely manner. This approach also ensures more efficient use of rescue units.

Many ambulances and rescue vehicles now have large roof markings for identification from above. If they do not have these, apply temporary markings using water-based paint or tape. Number and letter (alphanumeric) combinations should be used to minimize duplication. Symbols (star, box, tree) may also be used with or without an alphanumeric designation. Everything should be very large, so the controller can see it easily from the air.

In chaotic situations, it is often difficult to keep track of contact information for the multiple teams, agencies, and individuals. Keep and carry a personal log with this information, as well as a record of important events, directions, methods of making/procuring equipment or supplies, and so forth. During the response to Hurricane Katrina, such a log proved invaluable for tracking the constantly changing satellite and cell phone numbers for key contacts from

TABLE 3-1 Most Important Skills for Disaster Communicators

- Ability to lead a communications team composed of people from diverse cultural and professional backgrounds
- Ability to coordinate a communications strategy
- Effective writing and editing skills
- Ability to photograph, video, and edit events
- Media relations experience
- Public health competency and knowledge
- Ability to be diplomatic and respectful in complex sociocultural-political contexts
- Ability to remain calm under stress
- Ability to be flexible

Adapted from Medford-Davis and Kapur.[2]

multiple agencies. Use a small spiral notebook that can fit in your pocket, or a hardback, bound notebook, as some military personnel use.

TELEPHONES

During power outages and other crises, cell phones may often be used to bypass other failed systems. However, even with a functional system (i.e., the cell towers working), cell phones may not work inside all the areas of modern hospitals because of shielding and other dense barriers to the signals. More mundane, it may be difficult to locate cell phones or landlines designated for emergency use in the dark. Putting a piece of reflective tape on them can help, assuming that there is any light source.

Cellular Phones

Cellular phones are an excellent communication tool when they function. However, there are three problems: (a) cell towers may be down (as after Hurricane Katrina); (b) power may not be available to recharge phones; or (c) buildings in which phones must be used have too much steel, concrete, and lead for cellular service to function effectively.

Interestingly, in some affected areas after Hurricane Katrina, text messaging seemed to work when voice messaging did not. Since Katrina, some hospitals are stocking cell phones with long-distance area codes, assuming that the phones will work even if the local cell towers are down. They won't.

Drying Out a Wet Cell Phone

A cell phone that has been dropped in fresh water may be salvageable, but it takes a while. Immediately remove the battery and memory chip and put them in a bowl, completely covering

TABLE 3-2 Typical Disaster Messages to Prepare in Advance

How to sterilize water and avoid waterborne illnesses (S, F, E)
Using protection to avoid secondary injuries (S, F, E, C)
Who should and how to get vaccines/immunizations (S, F, W, E)
Low risk of disease from corpses after natural disaster (S, F, W)
How to safely stay warm/cool (S, F, W)
How to get food and water (S, F, W)
Do not come and volunteer unless asked: Directed outside affected area (S, F, W, D, C)
Do not send unrequested donations of material or medications (S, F, W)

S = Storms; F = Floods/tsunamis; W = War; E = Epidemic; C = Chemical disaster
Adapted from Medford-Davis and Kapur.[2]

them with uncooked rice. After 2 to 3 days, use a toothbrush to gently brush away any remaining rice dust so that it doesn't get trapped in the openings in the phone. Hopefully, the phone will work—if you recharge the battery.

Medical Apps

New apps to assist with diagnosis and, indirectly, with therapy (see the "Distraction Analgesia" section in Chapter 14) appear constantly. The problem is that not all functions, especially videos and illustrations, are accessible without an Internet connection. Try them out while your phone is on "airplane mode" and with "WiFi" turned off and then on to see how well they will work in those situations.

Phones in Remote Areas

While some remote areas of the world have cellular network signals, many do not. A cellular connection relies on line-of-sight radio frequency signals and may only be accessible from high points with a clear view of the surrounding area. If maps will be needed, download them prior to entering the remote or cell-service-poor area.[3]

Computer-Based Telephones

If the power is out and no batteries or generators are functioning, the computers (and thus Internet phones) will not work. If the power is on and the Internet provider is online, voice-over-Internet protocols (VoIPs) are an excellent communication method. If a strong signal is available, most provide both audio and video connections.

Field Phones

One solution to the internal hospital communication problem is to use hard-wired, directly connected phones, similar to those used in caving. If possible, install direct lines in advance between key parts of the institution, such as between the emergency department, ICU, operating room, command center, security, power station, laboratory, and medical records. In addition, use building wiring for a field phone conduit. The problem is that surplus field phones are now scarce. Wired intercoms may also be used if they can be configured to run on battery power. (Scott Clemans, Consulting Engineer, Tucson, Ariz. Personal written communication, September 11, 2008.)

After an earthquake, be sure all phone handsets on the same line are in their cradles; if one is off the hook, no calls can be made or received. If you get a fast busy signal or an "all circuits are busy" recording, hang up and try again. You may have to wait several seconds for the dial tone as the circuits are rerouted. Have at least one phone that plugs directly into the phone jack in the wall. If a phone has an AC power adapter (cordless phone), it will not work if the power is out.

Even when the local circuits are overloaded, if telephone service remains uninterrupted, it may be possible to dial a long-distance number. Call a contact outside the local area (preferably in another state) who can call back into the affected area to relay messages.

Priority Status

Another solution (in the United States) is to arrange in advance for the organization or facility to obtain priority communication status. For landline communication, qualifying agencies may obtain this through the Government Emergency Telecommunications Service (GETS) program (http://www.dhs.gov/government-emergency-telecommunications-service-gets; Tel: 866-627-2255). An equivalent service for wireless communication is the Wireless Priority Service (WPS) program (https://www.dhs.gov/wireless-priority-service-wps; Tel: 866-627-2255). These systems allow first responders, police and fire personnel, and federal, state, and local governments priority access to land and cell lines during a crisis. With GETS or WPS priority, the user dials a 710 phone number and then enters a code that grants priority to the call through the three major landline providers. If a call to the 710 number is made from a landline, the call is also granted priority on cellular providers' lines.[4]

Internet Attacks

The Internet now forms society's social, economic, management, and communication backbone. Any disruption causes havoc; widespread disruption may be a disaster. While the Internet was designed to survive a nuclear holocaust, components and institutional systems are vulnerable to power outages, programming errors, and intentional hacker attacks. So, while the Internet will not go down, it may not work as it should or you just may not be able to access it when you need it. However, if the local computers (or handheld devices), servers, and Internet providers are operating, messaging, e-mail, and VoIP (phone) are excellent communication tools.

More than 94% of health care institutions have been victims of cyberattacks, particularly data loss, monetary theft, medical device attacks, and infrastructure attacks.[5] Planning to protect these systems includes taking a comprehensive inventory of all clinical, research, and business processes and systems that depend on Internet connectivity. Work-arounds then must be developed that include not only a total loss of Internet connectivity, but also the loss of specific components or functions. Connecting to the "cloud" is now vital for many institutions, because it often hosts electronic health records. Analyzing computer threats and devising processes should systems fail is complex, expensive, and not certain to work. Yet, it is worth the effort.[6]

PATIENT–CLINICIAN COMMUNICATION

Interpreters

In resource-poor circumstances, anyone who is willing and *says* that they are able to translate is often used as an interpreter. However, in such cases, there may be problems with a translation's accuracy and completeness. In addition, the use of friends or family members as translators may interfere with patient confidentiality, cause patients to avoid sensitive issues, and disrupt established social roles.

Assessing translation skills can be difficult. Even when health care personnel are used as makeshift translators, accuracy may be an issue. About 20% of health care staff who also work as interpreters have insufficient bilingual skills to serve as interpreters in a medical encounter.[7]

Smart Phone Apps—Translators and Interpreters

The *Star Trek* point-of-care "universal translator/interpreter" is almost here. Translators convert text into another language; interpreters work with spoken language. New smart phone apps can now do both!

While most of the world's resource-poor areas still need people to do the translating and interpreting, if patients or colleagues speak or write in English, Russian, Spanish, French, Italian, German, or Portuguese, some new electronic help is available. Google, Microsoft, and others now provide services to instantly translate text using smart phone cameras. Some programs also instantly interpret and speak a translation of what you say in your language to a select other language—and then reverse the process for the other speaker. These programs are available on Android, iOS, Blackberry, Skype, and other platforms. While the programs use select major languages and the interpreter function requires Web access, the language list, as well as their functionality, platforms, and translation accuracy, will continue to improve over time.

Telephone–Human Interpreters and Pictures

Many hospitals in developed countries use telephone-based interpreter systems, although it is unclear if they will be available in disaster settings. While clinicians can find these human interpreters for any language or dialect, the service can be costly. Without specialized dual-handset phones and in austere settings, a modification of this system is calling a friend or relative who is known to speak both needed languages and putting the patient and clinicians on speakerphone. Amplify the sound using a size 5 facemask (Fig. 3-1) or nearly any solid container that is slightly larger than the phone.

Patients whose caregiver uses a different language often have limited understanding of instructions and home care plans, including correct medication dosing.[8] Without interpreters, pictorial representations may be effective for limited clinician–patient communication. It is best to prepare these pictorial representations in advance (Fig. 3-2).[9] Figure 13-2 has some useful pictorial medication instructions. You can, of course, also draw simple figures and hope that the patient understands them.

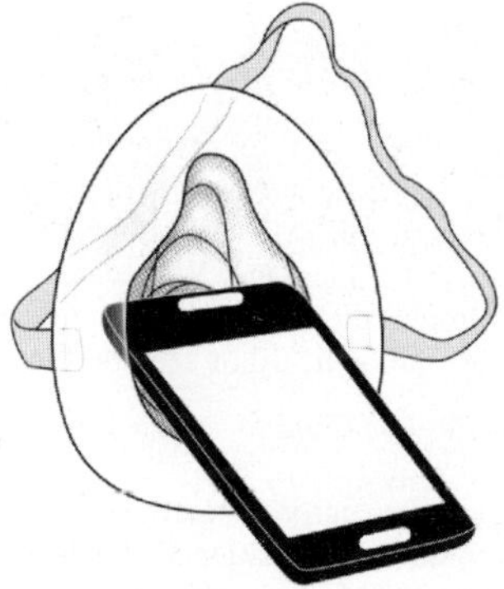

FIG. 3-1. Amplify phone sound with a size 5 facemask.

Hearing-Impaired Patients

If a sign language interpreter is not available for a profoundly hearing-impaired patient, using writing (possibly with an electronic translation program) and pictures may work. Note that sign language is specific to each language, so someone who knows it in one language cannot help in another.

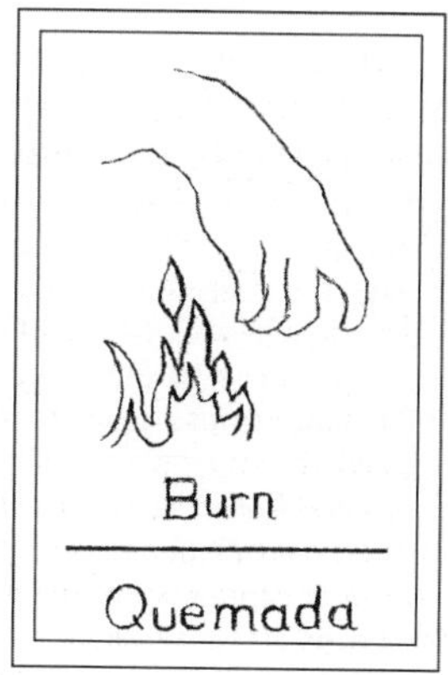

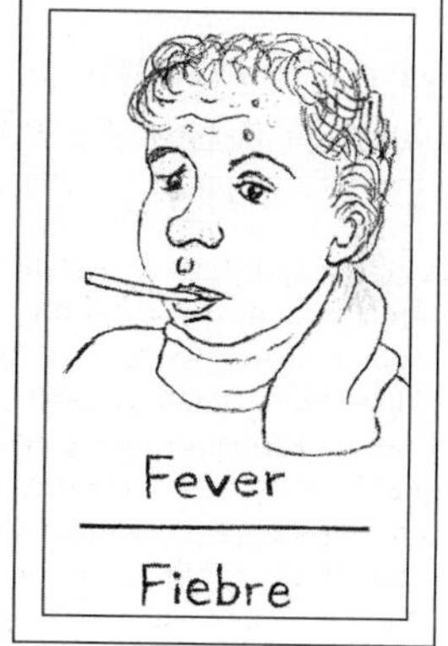

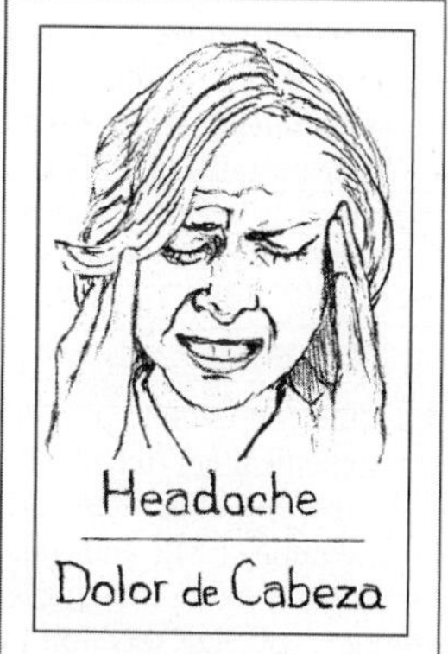

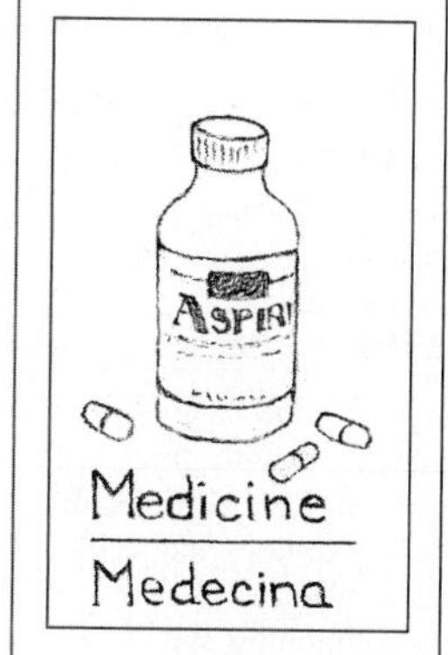

FIG. 3-2. Pictorial communication cards.

LOCAL-AREA COMMUNICATION

Makeshift Signals

In a localized area, preset signals may be used for communication. Miners and sailors have used signal bells for decades to indicate specific needs or actions (e.g., send lift down, danger, help, time, etc.). Flags, whistles, lights and mirrors, cell phone flashlights or strobe lights, or even hand signals can be used to transmit a message. With care, using a fire to produce light and smoke can also be effective. It is important that both the sender and recipients clearly understand the signals' meaning and that they can be heard or seen by the recipients.

Tracking Patients

Blackboards or white (erasable/grease marker) boards are used throughout the world to keep track of patients, personnel assignments, and patients' orders, tests, and bed assignments. These boards are used in all clinical areas, including emergency departments, operating rooms, and patient wards. It generally should have columns for the patient's room number, name, age, sex, problem/diagnostics (widest column), physician(s), nurse(s), admitting area, and consultations.

While this may seem to be the most obvious and easy solution to tracking and locating patients in the emergency, outpatient, and inpatient units, experience shows that many, if not most, providers around the world detest using it. If an unused white board has become a "white elephant," wasting space, remove the lines and turn it into a teaching board to illustrate procedures or cases ("case-of-the-day") and questions. The staff often appreciates this approach to teaching.

In recent years, boards have been replaced in many institutions with computerized tracking systems. When computers go down or the electricity fails, track down an appropriate board to use. (The best place to look is in the institution's administrative area.) Remember to grab the writing instruments and erasers needed for that type of board.

TRANSFERRING PATIENT INFORMATION

Patient medical records are the most elegant method of transferring patient information to other clinicians and helping them pursue a relatively straightforward track toward diagnosis and therapy. Records communicate to others which treatments have been performed, tests results, successes and failures with different therapies, and plans for future interventions.

When transferring a patient to the care of other clinicians, it is vital that the patient's records be transferred as well. This may mean the records are sent from a battlefield or disaster site to a medical facility, from the emergency department to the ward, from a clinic to a hospital, or to a provider or consultant hundreds or thousands of miles away.

Clothespins, safety pins, a lanyard, string, or paperclips can be used to attach information about patients to their clothing during mass casualty situations or when they are being transferred to another facility. Make a hole through the papers (or their container/envelope) and reinforce it with tape to avoid ripping. Then use a paperclip, clothespin, string, or cloth to attach the records to their clothing through a buttonhole or another part of the garment. Note that records may be lost if attached to medical equipment. Information can also be written directly on postoperative abdominal dressings (Fig. 3-3) or included on a USB (thumb) drive or sent electronically. An old, workable method of transmitting the vital information that a tourniquet has been applied to a trauma patient is to write a large "T" on the patient's forehead using lipstick, grease pencil, heavy marking pen, or the patient's blood. Similarly, after initially providing fracture care, provide the patient with a "fracture passport," the name given to writing vital information on the patient's cast (Fig. 3-4).[9]

TELECONSULTATIONS

Consultants no longer need to be on-site or even on the same continent to provide useful diagnostic information and assistance with procedures. Emergency medical service (EMS) systems, aircraft crews, ships at sea, remote expeditions, disaster relief teams, and clinicians in resource-poor areas potentially have access to knowledgeable medical consultation. EMS and others have long used telephone and radio consultations. Now, we have consultations using imaging and, in some cases, video. See the "Photographing Wounds for 'Tele-estimates' of Size" section in Chapter 25 for a description about how photos are used to assess and guide treatment in burn patients.

DAMAGE CONTROL
LIVER LACERATION
20 LAP PADS IN ABD
SKIN ONLY CLOSED

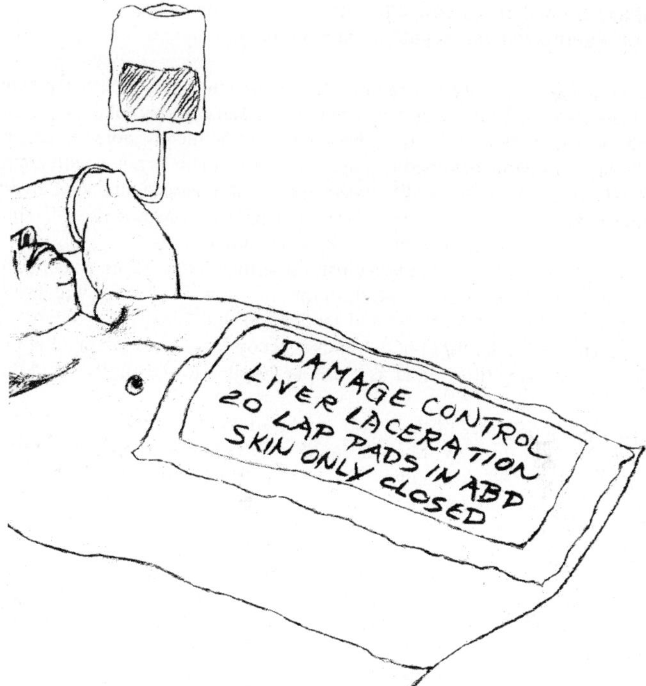

FIG. 3-3. Patient information written on postsurgical dressing.

Taking and Transmitting Digital Images

The wide availability of the Internet, digital photography, and camera phones makes transmitting images of patients and radiographs much simpler than in the past—and possible even in austere circumstances. Images can be transmitted (a) to get advice from distant consultants, (b) to avoid repeating costly and time-consuming radiography, (c) to provide sufficient information so that

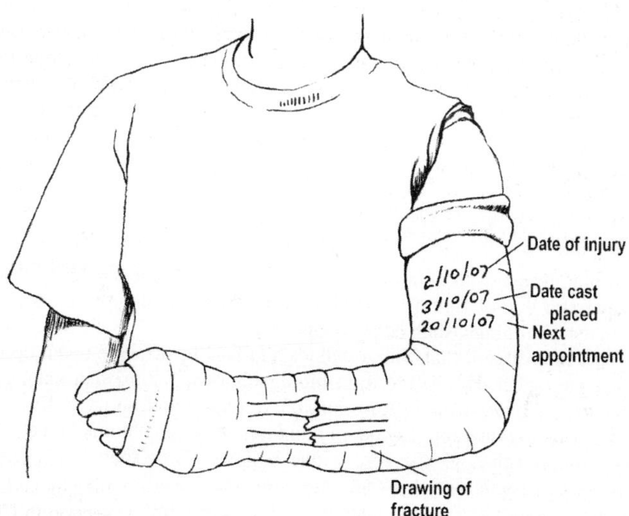

FIG. 3-4. Fracture "passport."

receiving facilities can make appropriate preparations for patients before their arrival, and (d) to post images or information on a public Internet bulletin board when bodies need to be identified.

Images and videos can be taken using the camera built into most cellular phones. They can then be downloaded to the Internet or sent through the same phone, depending on the service provider and the services available on that phone. Both ends must be able to interpret the image format, or an "image protocol conversion" may be required. (This is not usually a problem while using standard photo formats.) The quality of the image will be less than that of an original photo or the original document (e.g., electrocardiogram [ECG]). However, it still should provide enough detail so that the recipient can help make clinical decisions.

To photograph a digital radiograph, use a close-up setting and no flash; a standard radiograph, no flash; and a patient/body photograph, no flash for close-ups. For studies with multiple images, such as CT scans, it is important to select and send the most clinically significant images, rather than the whole study. To get the best photo, remain steady for at least a second after pushing the button, use the highest resolution, stand as close as possible to the subject, and do not use the digital zoom.

When working in remote areas of the world and faced with unusual cases, I have successfully used teleconsultation with images sent via email with ophthalmologists, dermatologists, and radiologists, and provided real-time audiovisual cardiac resuscitation direction. Teleconsultation has also been tested with success for evaluating and providing on-site direction to manage burns[10] and facial lacerations,[11] and with somewhat less success for evaluating child abuse.[12]

Useful Patient Information to Send

Useful patient images and information to send to other practitioners, government authorities (in the case of missing or dead patients), or to the patients themselves include identifying and relatives' contact information; graphic patient charting (e.g., vital signs, anesthesia records, or medication lists); other vital written records (e.g., the history/physical examination, discharge summary, and list of medical/surgical interventions); test and monitoring results (including ECGs, rhythm strips, electroencephalograms [EEGs], laboratory tests); images of the patient's injuries or intraoperative photos; gross pathology specimens; radiographic and ultrasound images; and information or images of unidentified bodies or noncommunicative patients.

INTRA-INSTITUTIONAL AND REGIONAL COMMUNICATION

Communicating Within Medical Facility

Paging Systems

Many modern hospitals rely heavily on their paging systems; these systems generally depend on the telephone system and the normal power supply. Without this power or when some backup generators kick in, these systems may fail. Prepare for this by keeping up-to-date contact lists, in paper and electronic forms. (Paper lists are important, because computers may not be operational.) The lists should contain telephone numbers for vital sites within the facility (especially the radio or telephone hubs), as well as contact information for physicians and other hospital staff.

Walkie-Talkies

Many hospitals plan to use walkie-talkies (low-wattage radios) for post-disaster internal communication. Except for line-of-sight (straight line without obstructions) communication, they are ineffective in modern buildings, such as hospitals.

Our tests have demonstrated that walkie-talkies and handheld radios (even up to 5 MW and with antenna repeaters placed) failed to transmit signals in any consistent manner in a modern hospital. The tests included checking transmission vertically and horizontally in the building. The only way these radios function in modern buildings is to use a "trunk" repeater (essentially, a giant antenna) running through the core of the building. Even then, experience shows that transmission is not consistent, and that there are numerous "dead" spots from which messages cannot be heard. These dead spots change daily, depending on atmospheric and other conditions.

Runners

When communication options are not available, it usually means there is (a) no electricity, (b) no Internet, and (c) no working land or cellular phones. To construct a runner system, remember that the goal is to transmit messages between specific points ("nodes" or "hubs") within an institution or a local area in a manner that maximizes efficiency, that is, that uses the fewest runners (messengers) and has the fastest transmission times. Using set nodes or hubs is the efficient model that FedEx employs. (Alan Reeter, MSEE, Tucson, Ariz. Personal verbal communication, March 26, 2008.)

The types of messages transmitted between sites typically vary in volume and urgency. System efficiency can be increased if the senders designate each message as "1" urgent/stat, "2" important, or "3" routine or delay-tolerant. Category 1 messages are urgent requests for help, equipment, or supplies; critical laboratory reports; or urgent security warnings. Most clinical messages fall into category 2, whereas category 3 messages are administrative information, general announcements, and so forth. All level 3 messages can be routed to the central node, where they may be stored until several messages are collected to send to the same location. This "store-and-forward" technique conserves resources and decreases runners' frustrations from continually delivering status 3 messages.

Assuming that the message volume between different nodes (sites) varies and no mechanism exists to signal runners at different nodes that they are needed elsewhere to carry a message, the following method is a way to determine how many runners are needed.

The general scheme is to position the "command center" so that there is minimal distance between the command center and the nodes. With the normal scarcity of runners, base most runners at busiest nodes, with a minimum of one runner at every node. Have runners go in only one direction; let another runner return to the original node. (This system generally provides a rest period for the runners.)

The number of runners based at a node also depends on the distance they need to travel (and the time it takes to do so) to reach the most distant or difficult-to-get-to site. In a hospital, this may mean running between a node in the basement and one in the 12th floor ICU. If the laboratory and pharmacy (two frequent-message sites) have satellite facilities near the busiest clinical nodes, this limits the number of messages (and runners) required.

The following formula helps to determine how many runners are needed. With a runner dedicated to each pair of nodes, the total number of runners will be N × (N – 1), where N = the number of message nodes. For example, 3 nodes require 6 runners, 4 nodes require 12 runners, and 6 nodes require 30 runners. Optimally, the number of runners at each node would be N minus 1, with each of 6 nodes having 5 runners (Fig. 3-5). Because this number is too large for most situations, either decrease the number of nodes or assign more runners to the high-priority nodes. (Be aware that doing so may decrease the system's efficiency.)

Runners need to work in shifts. Assuming that they work in 12-hour shifts, the total number of runners required will be double the number for each shift, plus extras for illnesses and time off.

Typical hospital nodes may include the command center/central administration, emergency department, ICU 1, ICU 2, ward 1, ward 2, ward 3, operating room (OR), pharmacy, laboratory,

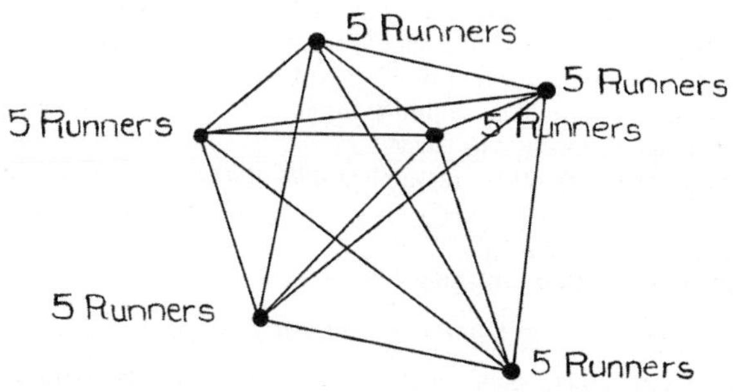

FIG. 3-5. Nodes-runner system.

personnel pool, security, food services, and ambulance bay/helipad. Adjacent areas (e.g., two wards next to each other) can share one communication node.

Regional Communication

911/Rescue Communication Techniques

Dialing "911" on a cellular or satellite telephone from a remote spot may not direct the call to the appropriate emergency call center for the caller's location. Activating a personal locator beacon (PLB), mainly used on aircraft and boats, will notify search and rescue (SAR) or public safety authorities of the location of the party, but not the nature of the emergency. Foot messengers or teams sent to get help or to find a location to improve cell or radio communication should carry a detailed written note that includes the patient's location, condition, and what type of rescue you think is indicated (ground evacuation, helicopter, etc.). For safety reasons, those leaving a party to go for help should not travel alone, unless there is no other option.[3]

Radio Communications

Mobile Radios

Although the idea of using mobile radios is appealing, several problems exist. First, they can be very expensive, although the basic models cost only about $100 each. Next, there is the question of compatibility with other radios in use, concerns about message security, and the fact that the transmitting range diminishes depending on terrain, weather, buildings, body mass, and so forth. Radio signals depend on an uninterrupted line-of-sight between transmitter and receiver, and their range is dependent on the transmitter's output power, operating frequency, and the size and location of its antenna.[3] The range can be extended with one or more repeaters that rebroadcast the signals and thus increase their range.[13]

Despite these problems, consider using low-cost Family Radio Service radios, an improved walkie-talkie radio system in the United States, to keep in touch with neighbors and family members. The range is 1 to 2 miles, and no license is required. Set up a network of these radios in your neighborhood to help each other in a disaster.[14]

Amateur Radio Operators (Hams)

Groups of amateur radio operators exist in many areas of the world to help with communications in disaster situations. In the United States, these groups are Amateur Radio Emergency Service (ARES) and Radio Amateur Civil Emergency Service (RACES). They generally have preset and tested equipment and can be activated in crises. This is an excellent method, even under austere circumstances, to communicate with others with similar amateur radio (not necessarily just ARES or RACES) capabilities.

Radio Communications Techniques

To improve radio signal strength, hold portable radios away from your body and hold both the radio and the antenna vertical and as high as possible to increase the line-of-sight range. Achieve the best transmission/reception by moving the antenna to different places, changing its angle, and, if horizontal, moving it 360 degrees to see what works best. To send a message, keep the radio about 3 inches in front of your face. Before speaking, listen for several seconds to be sure that no one else is on the channel. Then wait 1 second after pressing and holding down the push-to-talk button to prevent the first part of your message from being lost. Speak slowly and clearly in a normal voice, avoiding any jargon. Ask the message recipient to repeat key parts of the message in case it was garbled in transmission. When talking about any sensitive (including patient) information, remember that others may be monitoring your radio transmissions.[3]

Emergency Medical System Communication

Telemedical Transmission From Emergency Medical Service

EMS systems have used digital photographs with some success to transmit medical reports, medication lists, ECGs, and other "paper data" to hospitals. While this resulted in slightly longer

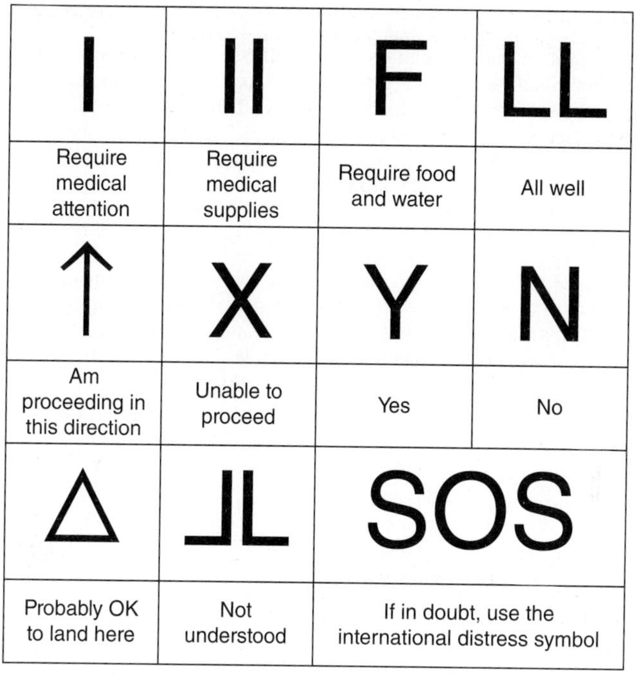

I	II	F	LL
Require medical attention	Require medical supplies	Require food and water	All well
↑	X	Y	N
Am proceeding in this direction	Unable to proceed	Yes	No
△	⅃L	SOS	
Probably OK to land here	Not understood	If in doubt, use the international distress symbol	

FIG. 3-6. Ground-to-air signals. *(Source: US Army.[18])*

on-scene and hospital arrival times, the main problem was that about 25% of the received data were of poor quality and of limited use.[15]

Amplifying Cell Phone Sounds

When using a cell phone to receive instructions during a procedure or using an audible translator app, amplify the sound by resting it in a size 5 adult facemask (Fig. 3-1). This arrangement results in a subjectively increased volume by acting as a parabolic reflector/Helmholtz resonator, changing the phone's output to approximate the center of the tonal range for the male voice and guitars.[16]

Aeromedical Communications

Miscommunication can lead to disastrous events in aeromedical transportation. Nearly all the errors, as in other critical situations, involve not making contact (equipment failure, inability, unwillingness) or misunderstanding the message ("not being on the same page").[17]

If in distress, attempt to communicate "in the blind," that is, to any station that may be able to hear the distress message. Clearly state the nature of the emergency, the location of the party, and what type of assistance is required. If help is needed immediately or the situation is dire, begin by saying "Mayday" three times, indicating a significant life-threatening illness or injury or serious or imminent danger. After stating "Mayday," give recipients the information they will need to help you.[3]

When compatible radio communication is unavailable, use the standard signals to communicate with rescue aircraft (Fig. 3-6).

LONG-DISTANCE COMMUNICATION

Depending on the extent of the disaster, telephones and radios can often be used for long-distance communication. Other options include the use of satellite phones and the Internet, assuming these are available. Any of these methods can be used in any resource-poor situation for telemedicine consultation with experts.

Satellite Phones

Depending on the system, satellite phones can be difficult to use, expensive, and subject to the vagaries of weather. Satellite communications technology offers a wide range of applications, including voice, messaging, data, and distress signaling. Direct communication is possible to and from almost any place on the planet—as long as there is a clear line-of-sight to the satellite. Always select a site that offers the least obstructed view of the sky.[3] Test the phone before you need it to be certain that it works and you know how to operate it.

REFERENCES

1. Garshnek V, Burkle FM. Applications of telemedicine and telecommunications to disaster medicine: historical and future perspectives. *J Am Med Inform Assoc*. 1999;6:26-37.
2. Medford-Davis LN, Kapur GB. Preparing for effective communications during disasters: lessons from a World Health Organization quality improvement project. *Int J Emerg Med*. 2014;7:15.
3. Worley GH. Wilderness communications. *Wild Env Med*. 2011;22(3):262-269.
4. Saucier J. Get GETS! *Arizona Response Commission Gatekeeper Newsletter*. October 1, 2007;7(10):5.
5. Perakslis ED. Cybersecurity in health care. *New Engl J Med*. 2014;371(5):395-397.
6. Nigrin DJ. When 'hacktivists' target your hospital. *New Engl J Med*. 2014;371(5):393.
7. Moreno MR, Otero-Sabogal R, Newman J. Assessing dual-role staff-interpreter linguistic competency in an integrated healthcare system. *J Gen Intern Med*. 2007;22(suppl 2):331-335.
8. Samuels-Kalow ME, Stack AM, Porter SC. Parental language and dosing errors after discharge from the pediatric emergency department. *Ped Emerg Care*. 2013;29(9):982-987.
9. King M. *Primary Surgery, Vol. 2: Trauma*. Oxford, UK: Oxford University Press; 1987:217.
10. Kiser M, Beijer G, Mjuweni S, et al. Photographic assessment of burn wounds: a simple strategy in a resource-poor setting. *Burns*. 2013;39(1):155-161.
11. Farook SA, Davis AKJ, Sadiq Z, Dua R, Newman L. A retrospective study of the influence of telemedicine in the management of pediatric facial lacerations. *Pediatr Emer Care*. 2013;29:912-915.
12. Melville JD, James L, Lukefahr JL, et al. The effect of image quality on the assessment of child abuse photographs. *Pediatr Emer Care*. 2013;29:607-611.
13. Merlin RZ, Levy MJ. Establishing the base of operations—introduction to telecommunications during disasters. NDMS Response Team Training Program, 2003.
14. Amateur Radio Emergency Service, Santa Barbara South County. Communications in a disaster: a guide for the general public. http://www.sbarc.org/publicservice/ares/pdfs/ARES_DisasterComm.pdf. Accessed November 6, 2006.
15. Bergrath S, Rossaint R, Lenssen N, Fitzner C, Skorning M. Prehospital digital photography and automated image transmission in an emergency medical service: an ancillary retrospective analysis of a prospective controlled trial. *Scand J Trauma Resusc Emerg Med*. January 16, 2013;21:3.
16. Cubitt J, Williams D. An improvised amplification device for smartphone loudspeakers. *Ann R Coll Surg Engl*. March 2014;96(2):166.
17. Dalto JD, Weir C, Thomas F. Analyzing communication errors in an air medical transport service. *Air Med J*. 2013;32(3):129-137.
18. US Army. *Field Manual No. 21-60, Visual Signals*. Washington, DC: Department of the Army; 1987:5.

4 Preventive Medicine/Public Health

Clean water and proper sanitation are two key elements to preventing diseases in health care facilities and following disasters. Immunization against preventable diseases is the third, but vaccines cannot be improvised.

WATER

Emergency Water Supply

After breathable air, water is the next vital need people have. Water is necessary for drinking and food preparation (2.5-3 L/day), personal hygiene (2-6 L/day), and cooking (3-6 L/day). Potable water is required to lessen the chance of spreading water-borne diseases and to have a functioning health care facility.[1,2]

Even if water is available, a loss of water pressure or of electricity for the pumps can mean that toilets become inoperable. Wastewater can be used to "prime" the toilets, but a plan for disposing of waste is necessary.

If large alternative water sources can be identified, a method of transporting the water must also be found. For smaller, more immediate needs in emergencies, sterile saline and sterile water may be used for hand washing, although it may be better to save the sterile water for drinking and cooking. Using waterless hand wipes or gels conserves water.

Preparing Drinking Water

Supplying sufficient amounts of clean drinking water is vital to prevent outbreaks of severe gastrointestinal disease. Nearly all springs, streams, and rivers are contaminated to varying degrees by commercial effluent, natural mineral run-off, or animal feces. Wells usually are not contaminated with microorganisms, but the water frequently has a high mineral content.

It seems logical to collect drinking water from atmospheric sources (rain, snow), but such water is often contaminated with dissolved and suspended substances. Even so, if properly collected, this water is within acceptable limits for potability. Using scrapings from the top layer of newly fallen snow is the best option. Less acceptable is collecting rainwater from a roof very shortly after a rain, using clean drainpipes. This method cannot, however, be used for snow, because it becomes contaminated prior to melting.

Improve the collected water's quality by filtering it through commercial filters or through white cotton cloth that has been boiled in soapy water and then rinsed thoroughly. Using that filter with new-fallen ground snow taken from the surface eliminates bacteria. Unfiltered ground snow has 44 bacteria/mL and cotton-cloth-filtered rainwater has 124 bacteria/mL. Unfiltered rainwater contains >1000 bacteria/mL with clumps of potentially pathogenic organisms. Filtering through filter paper, newspaper, four-layered gauze, and cotton is unsatisfactory.[3] Bangladeshi villagers use old cotton saris, folded into eight layers (mesh size ~20 μm), to filter homemade drinks. Filtering through this cloth reduces the cholera incidence by 48%.[4]

When using dirty or cloudy water, clarify it before disinfecting it. Filter the water through a cloth or sand filter, or allow it to stand so that particles and associated bacteria sink to the bottom. Another option is to fill a small-mouth water container with water and stuff one or two tampons into the neck. Then invert the container and wait for clear (not clean) water to emerge.

Disinfect the water, if necessary. Boiling or heating can be effective for small amounts (as for households). Heat water to temperatures >70°C (160°F) for 30 minutes to kill all enteric pathogens. If the water temperature is raised to 85°C (185°F), pathogens are eliminated within a few minutes. If water is brought to a boil, it is safe, even at high altitudes.[5,6] Water can be partially disinfected if left in a clear or translucent storage container for an hour or more in the very hot sun.

If using chlorine, add three drops of chlorine solution to each liter of water, mix well, and wait for half an hour before drinking it. To make the chlorine solution, mix three level of tablespoons (33 g) of bleaching powder in 1 L of water. This formula is for a bleaching powder that contains 30% concentration by weight of available chlorine. Adjust the quantity of bleaching powder to use based on the available chlorine in the powder you have.[7]

For chlorine bleach (liquid), place two drops of chlorine bleach (5.25% sodium hypochlorite) in a canteen of clear water. Let it stand for 30 minutes. If the water is cold or cloudy, wait for 60 minutes. Remember that not all bleach is of the same concentration; check the available level of sodium hypochlorite.

If using iodine tablets (tetraglycine hydroperiodide), dissolve one tablet in 1 L of water. Almost all water treated with this dose is safe for drinking. Use two tablets for heavily polluted water.[6] If 2% tincture of iodine is used, add 5 drops to 1 L of clear water; if the water is cloudy or cold, use 10 drops. Let the water stand for 30 minutes before drinking. If using 10% povidone-iodine or 1% titrated povidone-iodine, use two drops. (Betadine is usually 2% strength, so use 10 drops.) Let it stand for 30 minutes. If the water is cold and clear, wait for 60 minutes; if it is very cold or cloudy, add four drops and wait for 60 minutes.[6] Do not use iodine crystals.[8]

For formula-fed infants, use ready-to-feed formula, if available. If not, use bottled water to prepare powdered formula. Use boiled water only if bottled water is not available. A last choice is disinfected water.[9]

After purifying a canteen of water, partially unscrew the cap and turn the canteen upside down to drain unpurified water from the inside of the lid and the threads of the canteen, where your mouth touches.

While having the cleanest possible drinking water is important, "quantity is of greater importance than water quality: People are more likely to become ill as a result of having soiled hands, dirty eating utensils, or from eating food prepared with soiled hands than from drinking contaminated water. That is not to say that the quality of water is unimportant, merely that it is less important than having sufficient water. A large quantity of water that is not completely free of bacteria is better than a small amount of pure water."[10]

SANITATION

Food

Poor food handling and storage is often the cause for enteric disease outbreaks. If permeable food containers have been exposed to flood water, discard the containers and food. If a lack of power results in food being held at the wrong temperature for >2 hours, discard it. The appropriate refrigeration temperature is <40°F (4.4°C); hot food should be kept at >140°F (60°C). If there is no refrigeration, discard any perishable food items, including meat, fish, eggs, and leftovers. Also, discard any food with an unusual odor, color, or texture.[11]

Latrines

Because disease prevention can be much easier than treatment (although not as dramatic), the placement, design, and use of toilet facilities can markedly lessen the incidence of transmitted disease.

Place latrines >60 feet (20 m) from all water (wells, rivers, springs, and streams) and living quarters (Fig. 4-1). If near a water source for people, latrines must be downstream.[12]

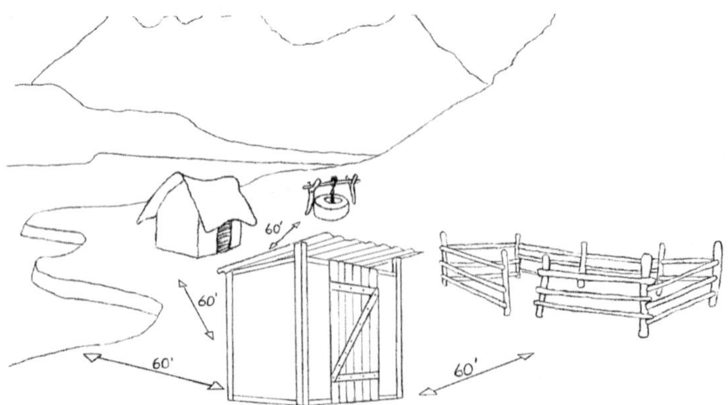

FIG. 4-1. Positioning the outhouse.

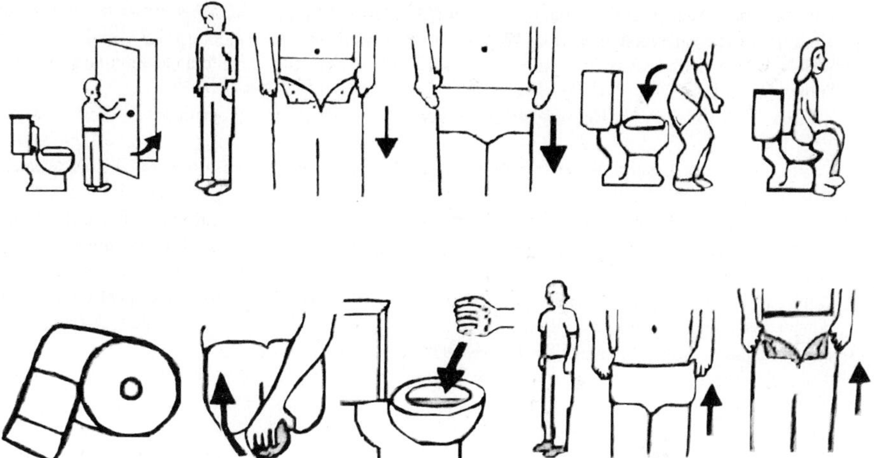

FIG. 4-2. Pictorial instructions for using flush toilets.

The simplest latrines are vertical or horizontal pits. Throwing dirt, lime, or ash into the hole after each use reduces the odor and the flies. Keep a pile of this material and a scoop or shovel next to the hole. If vertical, cover the hole with a simple outhouse that can be moved to the next hole when the current one is filled. People are more likely to use the latrine if it is at least minimally comfortable, private, easily accessible, and kept clean.

Comfort starts with a place to sit. Position a simple portable toilet seat over a deep hole (see Fig. 5-9). Place a shovel next to a dirt pile to scoop over each person's waste. In polar regions, build outdoor latrine walls with ice bricks. Place a concrete cover over the pit toilet for longer-term situations.

In general, place a minimum of 1 latrine or toilet/20 beds or 50 outpatients in short-term, disaster situations. For long-term situations, the number should increase to 1 latrine/10 beds or 20 outpatients.

Even if flush toilets are available, people in remote locations may not be familiar with them, and some instruction may be necessary. To avoid embarrassing them, it may be easiest simply to place an instruction sheet on how to use the toilet on the wall (Fig. 4-2).

Incinerators

Deeply bury or incinerate dangerous and infectious waste. Fashion an incinerator for use in a home or small clinic from an empty coffee can. Punch holes in the bottom of the can and in the cover to provide the necessary draft. Place soiled gauze dressings and other small, easily flammable items in the can and put on top of a gas stove or open fire. After the gauze starts burning, put a wire mesh screen over it. The gauze will burn easily, completely, and safely.[13] Larger amounts of medical waste require the use of a formal incinerator.

REFERENCES

1. Sphere Project. *Humanitarian Charter and Minimum Standards in Humanitarian Response.* 2011. http://www.spherehandbook.org/. Accessed August 26, 2015.
2. Gleick PH. Basic water requirements for human activities: meeting basic needs. *Water Int.* 1996;21(2):83-92.
3. Kozlicic A, Hadzic A, Bevanda H. Improvised purification methods for obtaining individual drinking water supply under war and extreme shortage conditions. *Prehosp Disaster Med.* 1994;9(1):S25-S28.
4. Colwell RR, Huq A, Islam MS, et al. Reduction of cholera in Bangladeshi villages by simple filtration. *Proc Natl Acad Sci USA*. 2003;100:1051-1055.
5. Forgey WW. *Wilderness Medical Society Practice Guidelines for Wilderness Emergency Care.* 2nd ed. Guilford, CT: Globe Pequot Press; 2001:60.

6. US Army Field Manual 3-05.70. *Survival*. Issued May 17, 2002.
7. World Health Organization. *Guidelines for the Control of Epidemics Due to Shigella dysenteriae type 1*. WHO/CDR/95.4. Geneva, Switzerland: WHO; 1995. http://www.who.int/child-adolescent-health/New_Publications/CHILD_HEALTH/WHO. CDR.95.4.pdf. Accessed December 16, 2006.
8. Zemlyn S, Wilson WW, Hellweg PA. A caution on iodine water purification. *West J Med*. 1981;135:166-167.
9. Centers for Disease Control. Water safety after a disaster. www.bt.cdc.gov/disasters/psa/video/safewater.asp. Accessed September 30, 2006.
10. Smith M, Reed R. Water and sanitation for disasters. *Trop Doct*. 1991;21(suppl 1):30-37.
11. Centers for Disease Control. Food safety after a disaster. www.bt.cdc.gov/disasters/psa/video/safefood.asp. Accessed September 30, 2006.
12. Werner D. *Where There Is No Doctor: A Village Health Care Handbook*. Palo Alto, CA: The Hesperian Foundation; 1977:138-139.
13. Farley F. Improvising equipment. *Am J Nurs*. 1938;38(4, section 2):42s-43s.

5 | Basic Equipment

AVAILABILITY AND IMPROVISATION

Be prepared to improvise even the most basic medical equipment. In developing countries and other resource-poor settings, even some of the largest medical facilities lack equipment and materials considered standard elsewhere.[1] Louis Pasteur reportedly said, "Chance favors the prepared mind." This book supplies ideas about how to make-do when faced with shortages. Problem-solving skills will take you the rest of the way.

"When improvising medical equipment, consider whether it (a) Will accomplish the purpose for which it is intended? (b) Is practical? and (c) May cause an accident or increase danger to the patient or clinician?"[2]

FACILITIES

Health care resources, whether purchased, donated, or improvised, should be matched to the skills of the practitioners and the type of facility in which they are to be used. Table 5-1 describes the spectrum of health care facilities worldwide and is the basis for the "Essentials" tables in this chapter (Table 5-2) and elsewhere in the book.

Given the rustic clinical facilities in resource-poor environments, basic ethical standards of privacy and even confidentiality may be compromised. Little or nothing provides privacy between adjacent patients in the clinic and other inpatient settings when they relate their medical histories or undergo physical examinations and procedures. However, with a little effort, sheets, blankets, and makeshift dividers can be used to provide some privacy.

Improvised (Safe) Medical Structures/Modification of Existing Structures

Any available site may be used to provide immediate health care when local facilities are overwhelmed. Generally, these will be buildings of convenience. Optimally, especially in regions prone to repeated disasters, planners will select such buildings in advance and assign them a specific use (ambulatory care, hospital or nursing home overflow, minor acute hospitalization). Control (who runs and is responsible for it) and funding (who pays) for the facility, as well as the required supplies and equipment, should be predetermined. In most cases, a contingency contract with the building's owners will be necessary.

The following elements are necessary for any health care facility to function. They may need to be improvised at alternative sites and even at regular health care facilities in disaster or austere situations.

Access

Identification as a Health Care Facility

Making the public aware of the availability of a makeshift medical facility is an often overlooked task. Workers assume that once they have set up shop, people will know where they are located. Not true! If possible, make easily visible signs with identifiable symbols (e.g., Red Cross, Red Crescent, Mogen David Adom, or Disaster Medical Assistance Team [DMAT]). Also, ask patients and others who visit the site to spread the word.

Ramps

If the facility you use has stairs at the entryway or inside the building between patient care areas, build ramps so that non-ambulatory patients and those with difficulty walking have easy access.

When elevators are not functional, use pulley systems to help get stretchers up ramps with steep inclines. Such pulley systems, similar to search and rescue haul systems, can be set up and operated by fire departments or rescue teams.

TABLE 5-1 Spectrum of Health Care Facilities

Basic	Village health posts Clinics with nurses or medical assistants Clinics with doctors
General Practitioner Hospital	General practitioner-staffed hospitals General practitioner-staffed with surgical capabilities
Specialty Hospital	Hospitals with general surgeons Hospitals with general and orthopedic surgeons Hospitals with general and orthopedic surgeons and other specialties
Tertiary Hospital	Tertiary care facilities with limited range of specialties Tertiary care facilities with full range of specialties

Adapted, with permission, from Mock et al.[3]

Light Sources

Health care facilities must have ambient lighting and specialized task lighting for workers to perform examinations and procedures. Because electrical power may be limited or nonexistent, you may need to improvise.

Sunlight

Sunlight (or even a bright moon) can provide excellent general lighting. During the US Civil War, for example, surgeons often performed operations outside. This provided them with much better light than they could get inside the hospital tent. It also was safer, because there was no need to have an open flame that could ignite the flammable anesthetic they were using.[4]

TABLE 5-2 WHO Basic Diagnostic/Monitoring Essentials

	Facility Level			
Resources/Capabilities	Basic	GP	Specialist	Tertiary
Stethoscope	E	E	E	E
Blood pressure cuff	E	E	E	E
Flashlight (torch)	E	E	E	E
Thermometer	E	E	E	E
Fetal stethoscope	D	E	E	E
Urinary catheter and collection bag	D	E	E	E
Otoscope	D	E	E	E
Ophthalmoscope	D	D	E	E
Pediatric length–based tape (Broselow)	D	D	D	D
Electronic cardiac monitoring	I	D	D	D
Central venous pressure monitoring	I	D	D	D
Right heart catheterization	I	I	D	D
Intracranial pressure monitoring	I	I	D	D

Abbreviations: D, desirable; E, essential resources; I, irrelevant.

Adapted, with permission, from Mock et al.[19]

When using sunlight for illumination, it helps to know how much time you have until sunset. Hold your palm out flat toward the Western horizon. One fingerbreadth from the horizon to the bottom of the sun = 15 minutes until the sun sets.

Headlamps/Flashlights

Powerful illumination is, of course, necessary in the operating room (OR). It is also needed for many diagnostic and therapeutic procedures, including intra-oral and gynecological procedures. Even at major medical centers during normal conditions, extra light may be needed. Carrying a powerful, small, battery-powered, and hands-free headlamp literally "saves the day" by providing sufficient light to examine patients and do procedures when the power fails or the existing light is insufficient.[5]

When choosing a headlamp, check the brightness and the focus at the distance you will need to perform procedures. Also, be sure it is comfortable to wear for several hours (or an entire shift) and that you can get extra batteries for it. (Rechargeable batteries are useless if the power is out.)

Very small flashlights, such as the penlights that health care professionals commonly carry, can be tucked into an elastic athletic headband or an elastic bandage wrapped around the head to make a headlamp. Laryngoscopes have been used for light when ORs unexpectedly lost power.

Room Lighting

Solar-powered garden lights work well as room lighting (if charged). They last for several hours and work best if put into an empty 2-L soda bottle (with a hole cut in the side). They can be carried around, and the plastic helps diffuse the light, like luminarias (paper bags half-filled with sand in which a candle sits). Just remember to put them in the sun to recharge. Another option is to put a glow stick (like divers use) into a clear plastic container with a gallon of water. The water diffuses the light, which can illuminate a small space for a short time period.

Automobile Headlamp

One group successfully used an automobile headlamp as a light for the OR. They wrote that

> The halogen headlamp is preferable to an incandescent lamp because of greater light intensity. A 12-volt automobile battery serves as the power source.... A disadvantage is the periodic need to recharge the battery. The battery may remain in a vehicle (a mobile eye unit's Land Rover, operating on a 12-volt electrical system, for example) and a constant charge maintained with the engine running. The battery leads for the operating lamp are passed into the operating theatre through a window. The halogen lamp is affixed with a small metal hinge to a 10 × 20 × 2 cm section of wood with 4 drilled holes, one in each corner. Sturdy cord passed through these holes and to an IV pole will attach and elevate the lamp above the surgical field for an excellent surgical light source. The portable operating theatre light may be used as a back-up light source for eye surgery in communities where power shortages are frequent. It is also reliable for mobile eye work and surgery in rural areas where electricity is unavailable.[6]

Flaming Light

You may need to make a fire for light. More commonly, you can use one or more candles. For a short burst of light (or as a fire starter), petrolatum (Xeroform) gauze works well, as does an alcohol swab. The swab's flame lasts only seconds, but is especially useful for warming ENT mirrors. Always be careful when using open flames because there is always danger of igniting nearby objects (such as clothing) or combustible gases.

Patient Records

To make medical records and radiographs more accessible and less likely to "walk away," tie them to the end of the patient's bed or chair. Alternatively, place radiographs and the patient's bedside chart (containing vital signs and intake/output) in a holder made from cloth or old x-ray film and taped to the head of the bed or wall.

If no other method is available, especially when there are large numbers of patients during a disaster or when transferring patients to another medical unit or facility, clip or pin patients' records and imaging studies to their clothing.

Refrigeration

The ability to keep laboratory reagents and medications cool is usually taken for granted. When there is no power, some type of system must be devised to keep them cool. It is important to remember that refrigeration is vital for vaccines, as well as for some other medications (e.g., epoetin alfa, total parenteral nutrition, some antibiotic intravenous [IV] solutions, and suppositories). Four types of refrigeration units can be improvised. Note that **storing blood requires a relatively constant temperature of 4°C: This cannot be achieved using the methods mentioned below.**

Use Refrigerators Normally Used for Other Purposes

If you have electricity, but not a standard refrigerator, try to find an alternative. The best way to store refrigerated medical supplies is in a unit with a transparent door so that the contents are visible. Other than laboratory refrigerators, only commercial-product refrigerators, such as those used to dispense soda pop and cold water, have these. Some hospitals have appropriated them for use when necessary. Of course, they put a lock on them to avoid pilferage.

Refrigeration Using Ice[7]

To make an "icebox," use a 5- or 10-gallon can or jar with a cover. Place it in the center of a wooden box or barrel. Surround the can with chopped ice mixed with sawdust, bran, flaxseed, hay, straw, or similar material. Cover the entire box with newspapers or an old raincoat, robe, or quilt. Place the material to be cooled in the can. Do not let it remain uncovered for long when you retrieve the contents.

Alternatively, you can make an "in-ground" icebox. Dig a hole in the ground big enough for a large sealed can or jar plus a 1-foot space between the can and the sides of the hole. Put the can in the center and pack cakes of ice (as big as will fit) around it. Pack crevices with sawdust, leaving a generous covering on top of the ice. Put on another covering of hay or straw, followed by a thick layer of heavy mud. Leave about 8 inches of the container above ground for easy access; cover this part to protect it from the sun. Place the articles inside the can to cool. Take special care to close the cover tightly after opening the icebox.

Refrigeration Using Cool Outside Temperature

During cold weather, a "cold box" built into a window will keep items cold. Fit a wooden or metal box to the outside of a window with a vertical sash (the pane slides up). Raise the window to access the cold box. This still allows light to enter the upper half of the window. Extend the windowsill with a shelf supported by brackets. The cold box rests on the windowsill and the extended shelf, and is fastened to the window casing by screws or nails near the top and bottom of each side of the box. The box should have a sloping top to shed rain. Cut holes for ventilation in the ends of the box and cover with screen. Shelves in the box may be made of heavy screening, poultry netting, or wood. They rest on cleats fastened to the sides of the box (Fig. 5-1). Cover anything placed in the box to protect it from dust.[7]

Refrigeration Using Evaporative Cooling

This iceless refrigerator is excellent for high-temperature, low-humidity conditions. It costs little to build and nothing to operate. Make a wooden frame 42 × 16 × 14 inches and cover it with screen wire, preferably rust-resistant. It should have a solid floor, but cover the top with wire screening. Attach the door with brass hinges and fit tightly; fasten it with a wooden latch. Wooden shelves or sheets of galvanized metal rest on side braces that can be spaced as needed. Place a 14 × 16-inch baking pan on the top and rest the frame in a 17 × 18-inch pan. Paint the wood, the shelves, and the pans with two coats of white paint and one or two coats of white enamel. Also paint the wire screen to prevent rusting.[7]

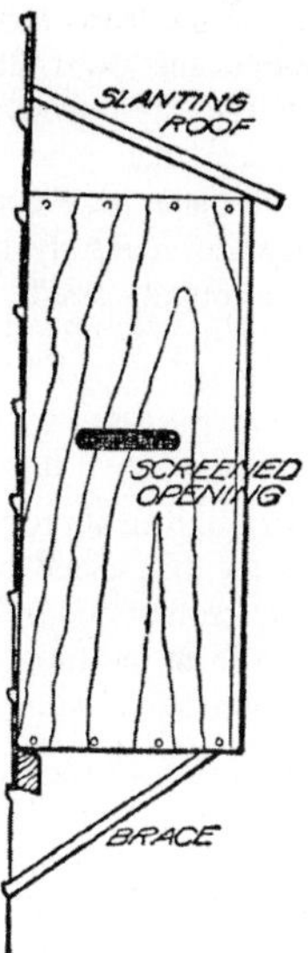

FIG. 5-1. Cold box (side view).

Make a cover of flannel, burlap, or canvas to fit the frame; this requires about 3 yards of material. If flannel is used, put its smooth side out. Secure this cover around the top of the frame and down the two sides and back using buttons, hooks and eyes, safety pins, or similar easy-to-remove methods. On the front, arrange the hooks on the top of the door, instead of on the frame, and fasten the cover along the latch side of the door, allowing a wide hem of the material to overlap where the door closes. This allows the door to be opened without unbuttoning the cover. The bottom of the cover should extend down into the lower pan. Sew four double strips, which taper to 8 or 10 inches wide, to the upper part of the cover. These strips form wicks for the water to drip down the sides from the upper pan (Fig. 5-2).

Lowering the temperature inside the refrigerator depends on the evaporation of water. Keep the upper pan filled with water. The water is drawn by capillary attraction through the wicks and

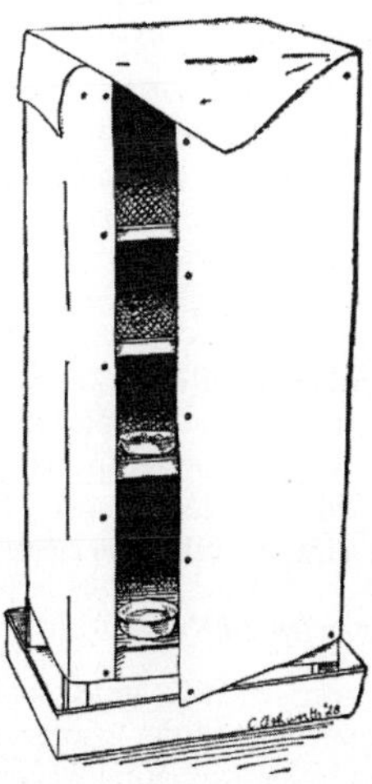

FIG. 5-2. Completed iceless refrigerator showing fitted canvas covering. *(Reproduced with permission from United States Bureau of Agriculture.[7])*

drips onto the cover, saturating it. Capillary action starts more readily if the cover is dampened with water. The greater the rate of evaporation, the lower the temperature; therefore, the refrigerator works best with rapid evaporation. Place the refrigerator in a shady spot with a strong, preferably warm and dry, breeze. Evaporation takes place continuously, and the temperature inside the refrigerator may get as low as 50°F under ideal conditions. It works less well in damp or cool conditions. Clean and dry the refrigerator regularly. If possible, make a second cover, so the first can be removed for cleaning and thoroughly dried.

Beds and Amenities

Fixing a Sagging Mattress

Sagging mattresses and poor bedsprings are a universal problem in health care facilities, as well as in other sleeping accommodations. To fix this, place two smooth boards across the bed, between the mattress and the springs. Place the first about one-third of the way down from the head and the other one-third of the way up from the foot.[8] You can also put one big piece of plywood under the entire mattress, if you have lots of wood.

Protecting Mattresses

If available, plastic trash bags of any decent thickness work well as mattress protectors—as well as shelters, rain catchers, ponchos, and boot liners. They also can double as personal protective equipment (PPE), especially gowns (see the "Gowns, Gloves, Masks, Booties, and Goggles" section below), protective covers over tables and chairs being used for medical treatment, and various first aid wraps and slings. Even if rubber, plastic, or similar impermeable materials are not available, patient mattresses can be protected from soiling. Use heavy paper such as butcher's paper or newspapers stapled together (about 10 layers thick) to protect the mattress. Smooth them out, if necessary, by sewing or stapling them to heavy cloth, which may be tucked under the mattress.[8] Pieces of old raincoats, tents, or tarps can also be used.[9]

Heating the Bed

Heating a patient's bed or sleeping bag when the external temperature is low makes them feel better and may stave off hypothermia. Just remember to wrap hot objects to avoid burning the patient. Heat bricks or smooth stones, wrap in newspapers or old cloth, and place them in the bed. Sand, salt, sawdust, bran, oats, or wheat can be heated and then placed in bags, or just placed in bags or old cotton socks and then heated. (Turn filled bags frequently so they don't burn.) You can also make "hot-water bottles" using plastic bottles or bags, canteens, or similar items filled with hot water.[10,11]

Backrest for Patient Bed

On basic beds and stretchers, the head end cannot be raised. To elevate a patient's head, use a chair placed with its legs against the headboard and the seat facing the mattress. Pad it by putting pillows under the patient's head (Fig. 5-3).

Pillows

Making a comfortable improvised pillow is difficult. Generally, after a few hours, what initially seemed like a fluffy pillow substitute is rock hard. Reportedly successful options include stuffing a clothes or laundry bag or stuff sac with clothing, especially anything made of fleece. Or, wrap clothes or a water bottle (already hard) in a fleece jacket. Carry rubber bands to try to keep it shaped. Better yet, use an inflatable airplane pillow or neck rest.

A Cradle to Support Bed Linen Over the Body or an Extremity

Make cradles to support bedsheets over sensitive areas, such as for burn patients, by tying two or more wire hangers together. Put the ends of the hangers under the mattress or other support (Fig. 5-4). (See also Fig. 25-13.) Use several supports, depending on the length needed. Another method is to string wire or twine the length of the bed above the patient and hang the sheet over the wire(s) (Fig. 5-5).[12]

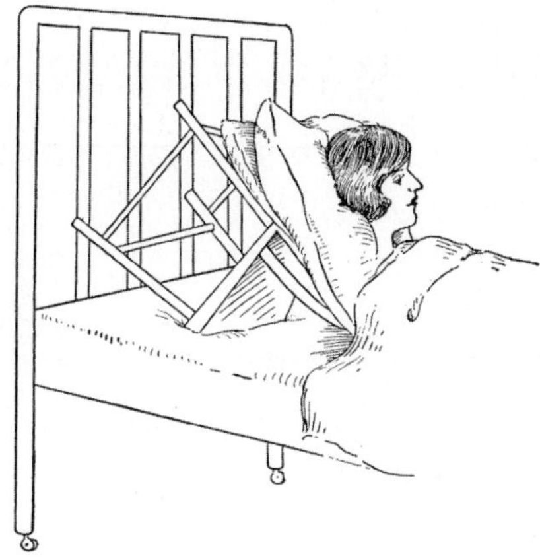

FIG. 5-3. Improvised back rest. *(Reproduced from Olson.[9])*

Bedside Table/Tray

Construct temporary tables for meals by placing a board, supported on both ends by chairs, across the patient. Alternatively, use piles of books to support the corners of a square piece of wood or metal.[9]

Bed Screen

To screen one patient from another in multi-bed rooms, including in the emergency department, tape together bed sheets or newspapers and suspend them from string or wire, or from hooks in the ceiling. For more substantial and portable screens, make two or three lightweight wood frames that are tall enough to provide privacy (at least 6 feet). Each should be about 3 feet wide. Put three hinges between the frames, one set going each way. Stretch a sheet or piece of cloth across the frames, and nail or staple it in place. When using this screen, angle the pieces slightly at the points where they are hinged, to give it stability. If desired, put small wheels on the bottom so that it can be moved.

Waste Basket

A "newspaper bag" pinned to the bedside will hold refuse and tissues. Fold a newspaper into a basket, with or without staples or adhesive, and attach it to the side of the patient's bed using safety pins or clothespins (Fig. 5-6).[13]

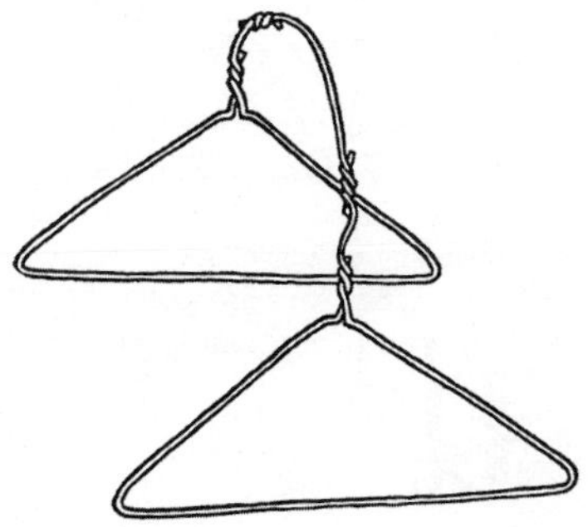

FIG. 5-4. Wire-hanger cradle for bed linen. *(Reproduced from Olson.[12])*

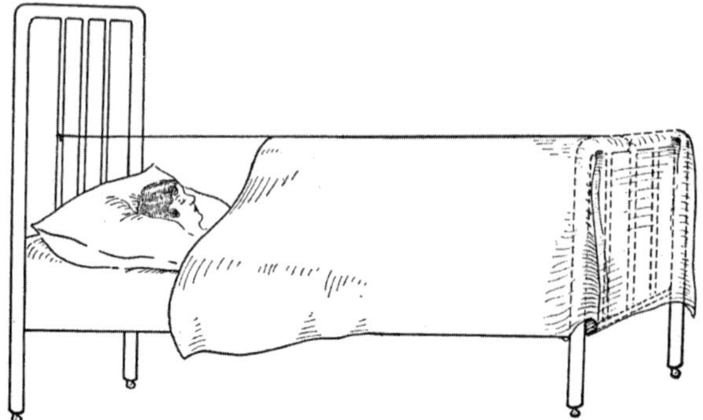

FIG. 5-5. Wire-based cradle for bed linen. *(Reproduced from Olson.[12])*

Bedpans/Urinals/Commodes

Bedpan

To improvise a bedpan, place a board (for the patient to sit on) across one end of a wide baking pan.[14] At the Nakom Paton Japanese prison camp during World War II, allied medical personnel made bedpans from giant bamboo.[15] One disaster team lined bedpans with plastic bags that, after use, were tied closed and put into a large red biohazard bag. The waste was incinerated on a daily basis.[5]

Commodes

The camp toilet for the same disaster team was a bucket lined with plastic. It had a padded toilet seat attached. Each team member was responsible for removing their bag and depositing it in the larger biohazard bag.[5]

A bedside commode or toilet also can be fashioned by cutting a hole in the seat of an old kitchen chair and then putting padding and a plastic cover on it. Place the chair over a bucket at the patient's bedside. To hide the bucket, tack a piece of heavy cloth around the chair legs (Fig. 5-7). Similarly, you can put wheels on the legs of a chair that has a hole cut into the seat, and use it over a standard toilet or a bucket. This can also double as a wheelchair to take a non-ambulatory patient to the bathroom (Fig. 5-8).[16] Attaching legs to a standard toilet seat or to a padded piece of wood with a hole cut into it works, either over a bucket or as a movable seat over a pit latrine (Fig. 5-9).

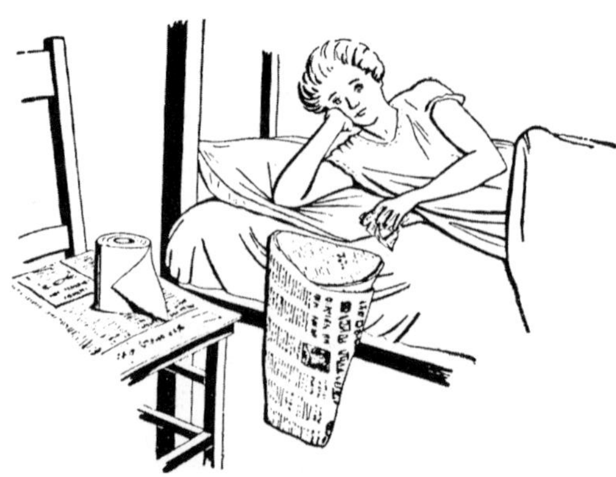

FIG. 5-6. Bedside newspaper trash can. *(Reproduced from Olson.[13])*

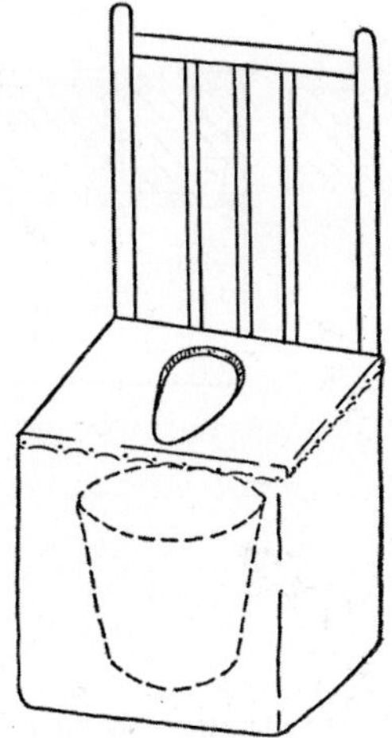

FIG. 5-7. Chair and wastebasket bedside commode. *(Reproduced from Olson.[16])*

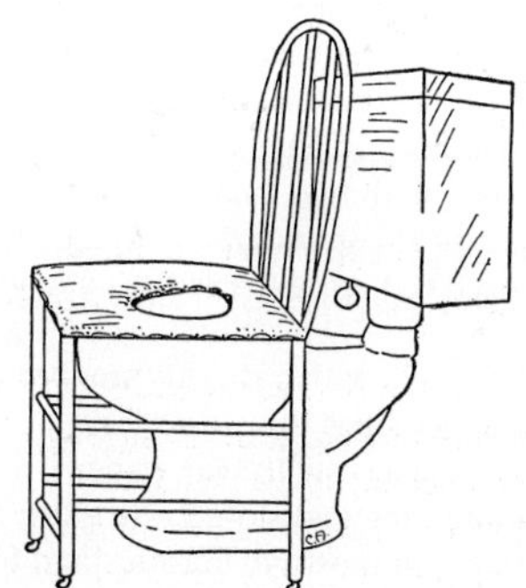

FIG. 5-8. Chair as improvised toilet seat. *(Reproduced from Olson.[16])*

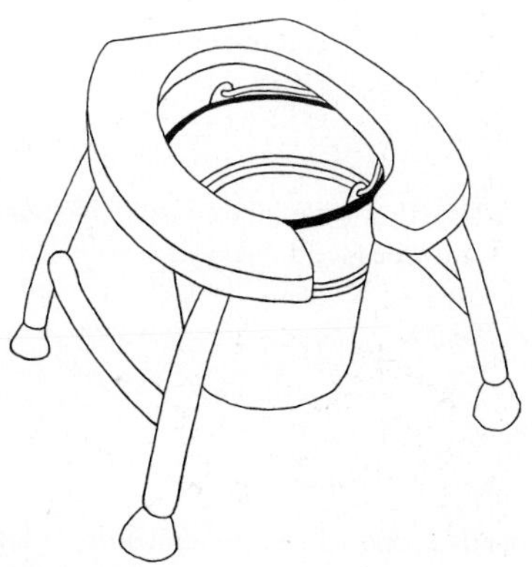

FIG. 5-9. Bedside commode from a toilet seat attached to legs.

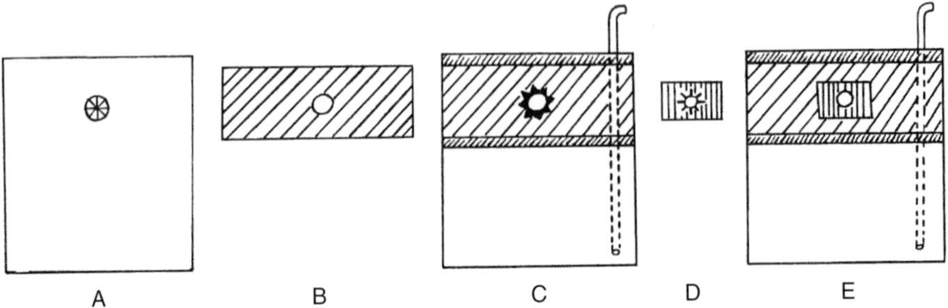

FIG. 5-10. Construction of an infant urine collection bag.

Urinals

As every trucker knows, any waterproof container can be used as a urinal. For patients, a plastic bottle or carton, cut such that the diameter of the container's mouth is at least 2 inches (5 cm), serves as an adequate urinal. One nurse described a very usable urinal made from a bleach bottle with a large oval hole cut out opposite the bottle's large handle.[17]

Construct an infant urine bag from a small plastic sandwich bag, several pieces of tape, and a small straw or piece of IV tubing. Use waxed paper to store it until needed. To make this urine bag (Fig. 5-10), follow these directions[18]:

1. Make a hole in the plastic sandwich bag using radial cuts (A). The hole should be about the size of a small child's penis for a boy or, for a girl, large enough for the urethral opening.
2. With the holes lined up, attach a piece of adhesive tape with the same-size hole (B) (adhesive side out) to the outside of the bag with two smaller pieces of tape.
3. Insert the straw or a small piece of IV tubing into the bag, and fold the top piece of tape over the top of the bag to seal it closed (C). Fold the radial cuts out and stick them to the adhesive tape.
4. Then, take a smaller piece of adhesive with a slightly smaller hole (D), line the holes up, place it adhesive-to-adhesive, and fold its sides inward to form a smooth opening (E).
5. Cover the bag's exposed adhesive piece with wax paper if it is not being used immediately. Multiple bags can be made at one time and stored. They can also be sterilized using ultraviolet irradiation, such as is available in most laboratories and ORs.

Controlling Odors

A way to disguise noxious odors is to aerosolize a beverage, such as orange juice or coffee. When the problem is chronic foot odor, put booties filled with antacid solution on the patient. If the odor cannot be disguised well enough, including when working in an area with decomposing tissues or bodies, wear a surgical mask with a dab of benzoin or two surgical face masks with a fresh tea bag sandwiched between them.

ESSENTIAL EQUIPMENT

The World Health Organization (WHO) lists what they consider the essential basic equipment for patient diagnosis and monitoring worldwide (see Table 5-2). This is in addition to the "Essentials" listed in other chapters and varies with four levels of hospital capabilities shown in Table 5-1.[19]

DIAGNOSTIC EQUIPMENT

Stethoscope

Ear to Patient

Before Laennec invented the stethoscope, direct auscultation—placing the physician's ear directly on the patient's chest—was an established practice.[20] If no other option is available, you can still put your ear directly against the chest, heart, or abdomen. The clarity of the sounds will

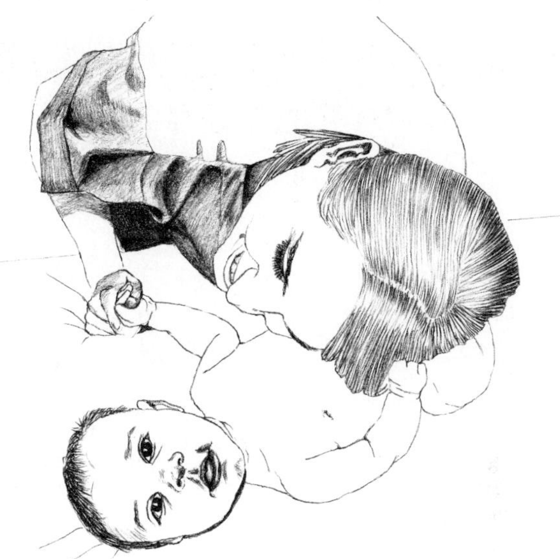

FIG. 5-11. Direct auscultation of an infant's abdomen.

not be as good as through a stethoscope (you probably cannot hear a murmur unless the murmur is also palpable), but you can get a general idea of cardiac rhythm, chest clarity, and bowel sounds (Fig. 5-11). As noted in Chapter 7, directly listening to an infant's chest is the fastest and most accurate method for assessing the presence of cardiac activity.

Improvised Standard Stethoscopes

Stethoscopes can easily be fashioned by following Laennec's original method. As first described, Laennec used his original stethoscope on a young woman "because her age and sex did not allow him to directly place his ear on her chest. "In 1816, I was consulted by a young woman presenting general symptoms of disease of the heart. Taking a sheaf of paper, I rolled it into a very tight roll, one end of which I placed over the praecordial [*sic*] region, while I put my ear to the other.'"[20]

To make a basic Laennec-type stethoscope, use a hollow wooden tube such as bamboo, or the cardboard tube from toilet paper or paper towels. Place one end on a person's chest and your ear at the other end; you can hear the heartbeat clearly, depending on ambient noise and the person's habitus. Nearly any hollow tube can be (and has been) used as a monaural stethoscope. These include short lengths of garden hose, ivory or wood tubes, and metal pipes.

Make a slightly more sophisticated stethoscope by attaching a funnel to two pieces of tubing. Use T-tubing scrounged from any source (including a juncture of IV tubing) to connect two long pieces of rubber tubing to a piece of short rubber tubing. Connect the short piece to the funnel. Put the tubing directly in your ears, or fashion earpieces as described in the section "Stethoscope Earpiece," later.

Precordial Stethoscope

One of the most useful anesthetic monitors that is also useful in prehospital care is a precordial stethoscope taped to the patient's chest. It gives the anesthetist a continuous assessment of the patient's heart rate and rhythm and breath sounds. Only one earpiece is normally used, so that the anesthetist can also monitor everything else in the OR.[21] For infants, it is best to tape the stethoscope to the left chest, so that both the heartbeat and breath sounds can be heard.[22] In adults, it can be placed over the midsternum, in the suprasternal notch, in the paralaryngeal area, or in the axilla. If in the suprasternal notch or paralaryngeal areas, it facilitates recognizing the presence of vomitus in the hypopharynx.[23]

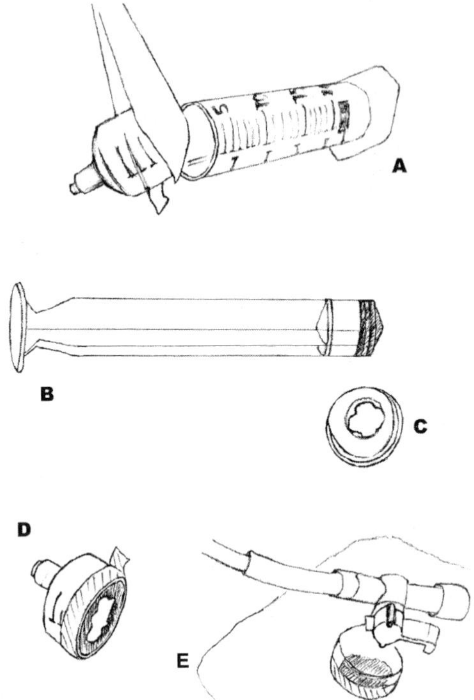

FIG. 5-12. Improvised precordial stethoscope.

Several improvised methods will produce a workable precordial stethoscope that can also be used as a regular stethoscope. The basic method is to attach a piece of rubber tubing to the top of a screw-top plastic bottle that has a narrow, tapered opening, such as a ketchup/mayonnaise dispenser. Another way is to cut off the tapered end of a rubber bulb suction syringe and connect it to a piece of rubber tubing that runs to the ear.[24] If a stethoscope head is available, make an improvised precordial stethoscope by attaching about 1 meter of IV tubing to the stethoscope head.[21]

Some California anesthesiologists produced an excellent, easily constructed precordial stethoscope when they forgot theirs at home while on a medical mission (Fig. 5-12, A-E). They cut a 20-mL syringe 1 inch (2.54 cm) from the infusion end (A). They then smoothed the edges with a file and placed adhesive tape around the syringe's cut end to further smooth it. Next, they removed the rubber sealer from the plunger (B) and cut a large hole in its center (C). They then inserted the rubber piece into the small piece they cut off the syringe barrel (D). After securing this to a three-way stopcock, they connected the stopcock to IV tubing (or other tubing) and then to an earpiece (E).[25]

Esophageal Stethoscope

Breathing and cardiac rhythm can be monitored with a tube passed into the esophagus—the esophageal stethoscope. To make an esophageal stethoscope, you need a rubber glove, a nasogastric (NG) tube, a suture, and a regular stethoscope. Cut a finger off the glove and tie the finger over the end of an NG tube (Fig. 5-13). Remove the head from the stethoscope. Pass the NG tube approximately halfway down the esophagus and connect the proximal end to the end of the stethoscope. The NG tube can also be passed through the nose (Fig. 5-14). In the OR, this stethoscope is often used with only one earpiece, so that the anesthetist can hear the rest of the surgical team.[26]

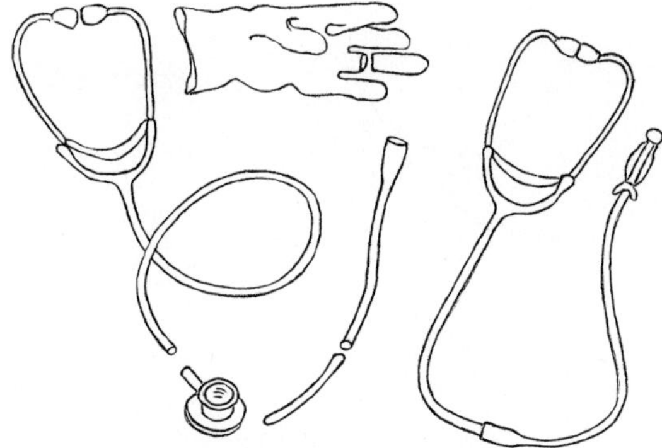

FIG. 5-13. Making an esophageal stethoscope.

Hearing Aid

A stethoscope can be a substitute for a patient's hearing aid during an examination. You simply use the stethoscope in reverse by putting the earpieces in the patient's ears and talking into the diaphragm (Fig. 5-15). Unfortunately, experience shows that it only works for patients with specific types of hearing loss. (But so do hearing aids.)

Stethoscope Earpiece

When the earpieces for a stethoscope have been lost (a very uncomfortable situation), use the nipple from a baby bottle or a "binky" (pacifier) (Fig. 5-16). Make the normal pinhole opening in the nipple slightly larger, and tie the nipple in place on the stethoscope. So you don't look ridiculous, cut the nipple so only the distal 1 to 2 cm of the rubber piece is used, rather than the entire nipple and the flange that holds it in the bottle cap. The rubber part (bulb) of a medicine- or eye-dropper can also be used in a similar fashion. Be sure to cut a hole to allow the sound to flow through it.

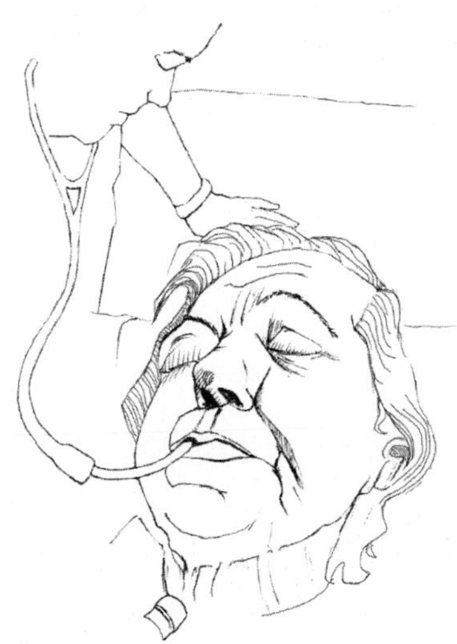

FIG. 5-14. Esophageal stethoscope in use.

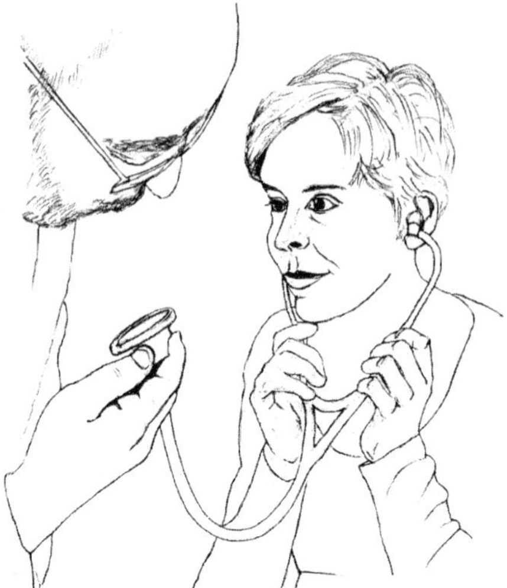

FIG. 5-15. Stethoscope used as hearing aid.

Sphygmomanometer

If you have a BP cuff, ideally it is accurate. However, aneroid devices (those without fluid) are easily damaged and can give erroneous readings without it being detected. The most common problems with these devices are that they leak, do not "zero," or go out of calibration.

To find the leak "in the system, wrap the cuff around itself and secure the end. Inflate the cuff to 250 mm Hg; watch the pointer. If it slowly drops, there is a leak—it is most likely to be in the cuff or inflation bulb. It is fairly rare for a leak to occur in the gauge itself. A small pointed brush with soapy water on it will help find the smallest leak."[27]

If the gauge does not return to zero after the cuff has been deflated, "the easiest method of adjusting it is by removing the glass from the front of the gauge and carefully taking off the pointer and replacing it in the correct position. The pointer can usually be taken off using your finger and thumbnails. If this is not successful, find two very small screwdrivers or thin flat pieces of metal and lever the pointer upward using one on each side."[27]

Aneroid systems may go out of calibration, especially if dropped. Check them on a regular basis for accuracy against a mercury sphygmomanometer. To do this, "connect the gauges

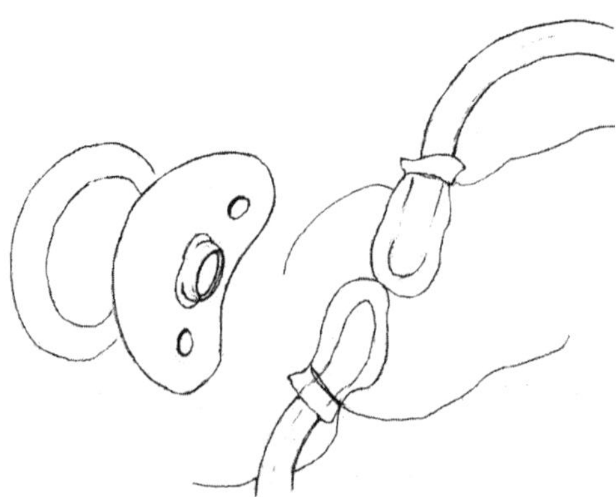

FIG. 5-16. Earpieces for a stethoscope.

together with a plastic T-piece and connect the third arm to an inflation bulb. Inflate the bulb slowly and note the readings showing on each instrument" at intervals of about 20 mm Hg. "If the readings are within a few millimeters of mercury throughout the scale this is acceptable for clinical use."[27] Someone who has experience with aneroid blood pressure machines should calibrate them.

One other common problem is that the glass breaks on the pressure gauge. Either get a watch repair person to fix it or make a cover from a thin plastic sheet.[27]

Mercury sphygmomanometers work longer and more consistently than do aneroid systems. However, if the mercury is not clean or if it continues to rise slowly after you have stopped inflating the cuff, it may need repair. Mercury is toxic. Find a reputable, qualified person to fix it.

Infant Spinal Tap Needle

If a standard infant lumbar puncture (LP) needle is not available, use a 22-gauge butterfly needle with the tubing cut short. It works as well as, or better than, the standard LP needle—as long as the child is not too chunky.

TREATMENT SUPPLIES/EQUIPMENT

Smart Phone Applications

Smart phones have become so ubiquitous that, if electricity is available to charge them, medical phone apps may be very useful. Many diagnostic devices, computational aids for fluids and medications, and problem-solving algorithms are being developed and improved for use with smart phones. Some are very expensive, whereas others may be free. The availability and quality of these apps change almost weekly as the technology and our medical knowledge improve. The primary advice is (a) if the application requires online access, this may not be available in resource-poor settings, and (b) *caveat emptor*—let the buyer beware—when purchasing or using these applications. Note that there are several useful map applications that can be used without an Internet connection.

Gowns, Gloves, Masks, Booties, and Goggles

Standard Precautions

Standard, or universal, precautions start with protecting oneself against the microbes, fluids, and detritus that haunt the health care environment. The basic equipment is PPE. In an austere environment, this paraphernalia often must be made, rather than purchased. However, experience has demonstrated that makeshift PPE is not sufficient to protect health care workers from virulent viruses, such as severe acute respiratory syndrome (SARS) and some viral hemorrhagic fevers.

Gowns

The simplest gown that is waterproof is a plastic garbage bag with head and arm holes cut out. Arm pieces can also be cut from another bag and stapled on. Note this also works well as a raincoat, although if used for that purpose, the arm connections should be folded over and secured so that they do not leak.

While not waterproof and probably better for patient use than as medical equipment, a sheet cut like a poncho will also work. Fold a flat sheet so that one-third is doubled over to form the arms. In the center of the folded edge, cut out a hole large enough for your head to pass through. The sleeve is fashioned by cutting slits on both sides of the sheet, midway down the folded section. The slits should extend to the approximate site of the axilla (Figs. 5-17 through 5-19). Once the person dons the gown, secure the arms with safety pins, staples, or tape (Fig. 5-20). Wrap the large pieces around the back under the arms, and use the flap on the back as a tie for the gown.[28] Depending on the person's girth, the tie may also need to be pinned.

Sometimes, you cope as best you can, as one disaster response team discovered: "Sterile gowns are bulky and consume precious space; therefore, the team considered other options, such as wearing one gown and changing gloves between each case, or wearing disposable aprons, sleeves, and gloves. [We] finally decided to use aprons over street clothes and boots covered with disposable covers."[5]

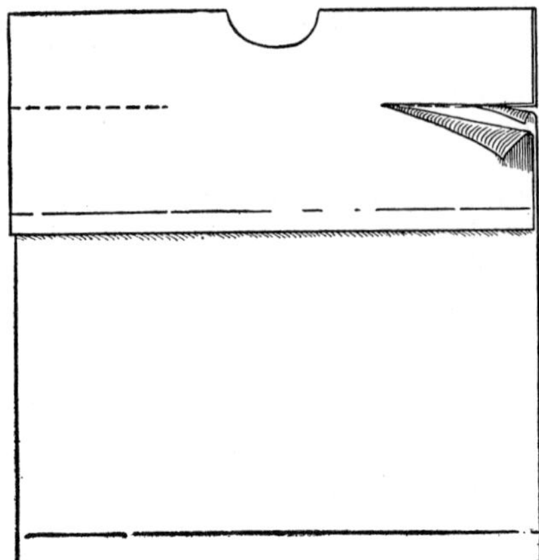

FIG 5-17. Improvised surgical/patient gown, Step 1. *(Reproduced from Olson.[28])*

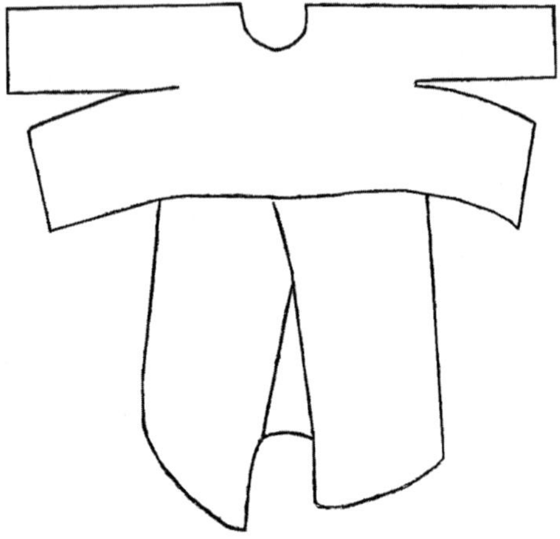

FIG. 5-18. Improvised surgical/patient gown, Step 2.

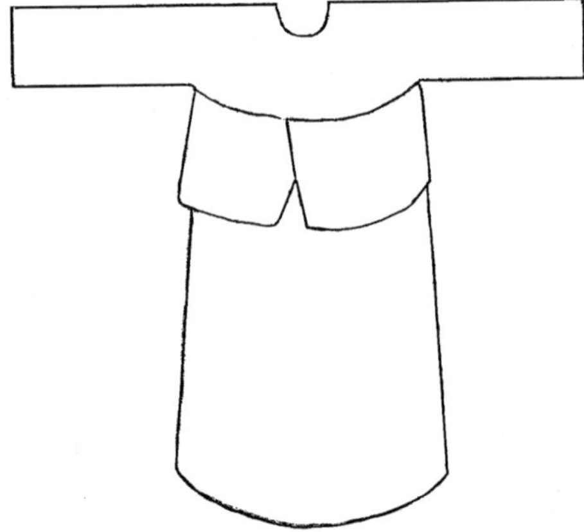

FIG. 5-19. Improvised surgical/patient gown, Step 3.

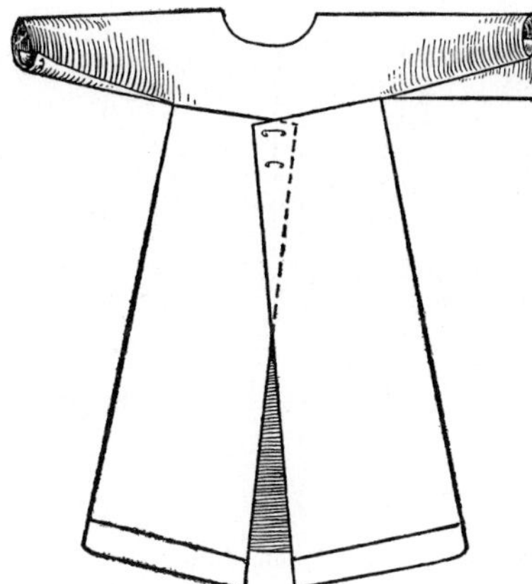

FIG. 5-20. Improvised surgical/patient gown, completed. *(Reproduced from Olson.[28])*

Caps and Masks

Masks are useful to protect both you and your patients against dust and particulate matter (i.e., inhaling ash is what often kills people after a volcanic explosion), virulent organisms that they or you carry, and nauseating smells, especially when working around decomposing bodies or opening feculent abscesses. Put some tincture of benzoin on your mask to disguise the smell. Caps protect the head and hair from any nasty stuff. They are also useful for protecting the patients' wounds from contamination by your hair. The most basic masks are towels or cloth held to the mouth and nose, either with your hand or tied in place.

HOMEMADE FACE MASKS

An improvised face mask should be viewed as the last possible alternative if a supply of commercial face masks is not available. However, in an epidemic, the supply of professional quality N95 and FFP2 masks may be limited. When common household materials were assessed to test their filtration efficiencies against organisms smaller than the influenza virus (60-100 nm; 1 nm = 1000 μm) and *Mycobacterium tuberculosis* (0.2-0.5 μm), standard surgical masks filtered 90% to 96% of the organisms; pieces of vacuum cleaner bags, 86% to 94%; tea/dish towels, 72% to 83%; cotton-blend cloth, 70% to 75%; pillowcases, 57% to 61%; and 100% cotton T-shirts, 51% to 69%. Doubling the material improved filtration only with the tea towel. Any mask will provide some benefit to the general population, but should be used with caution by health care professionals. And, no matter how efficient the mask and how good the seal, it must be used in conjunction with isolation of infected cases, immunization, good respiratory etiquette, and regular hand hygiene.[29]

To fashion an improvised surgical mask and cap, use a piece of the best available material, about 18 × 12 inches (46 × 31 cm). Cut a 4-inch (10-cm) narrow oval to fit over the eyes, about 5 inches (12.5 cm) from one end. Be certain that you can breathe as easily through the cloth as through a normal surgical mask. Attach a long piece of tape that extends over the edges of the material, at both sides of the slit. Also, attach a long piece of tape to the bottom of the short end. The wearer can adjust the slit over the eyes, flip the long piece of material over the head for a cap, and then tie both pieces of the tape behind the neck (Fig. 5-21).

Make a simple cap by covering the head with a long cloth or towel (Fig. 5-22) and pinning or taping it to the nape of the neck.

Wearing caps and masks helps protect clinicians but does not reduce the incidence of wound infection, even during surgery.[30]

Eye Protection

Wearing eyeglasses helps to protect the eyes from splattering blood and fluids. If your glasses are small or if you expect the splatter to be large, put tape around their edges. Goggles (such as

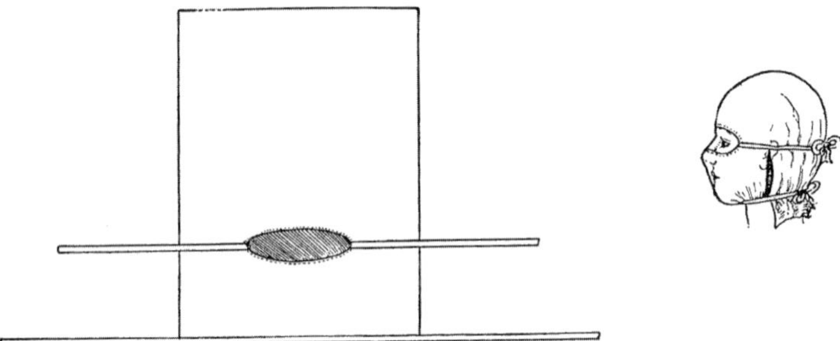

FIG. 5-21. Improvised cap-mask.

for skiing, woodworking, etc.) also work and can often be worn over eyeglasses. Another option is to purchase a cheap pair of plain glass or plastic (no refraction) glasses with big lenses.

Anti-Fog Solution for Glasses, Goggles, and Masks

Fog inside glasses, goggles, or face masks is because of higher temperature and humidity inside the goggles or shield than outside them. The following methods should solve this problem. First, clean the lenses and dry them completely, because rubbing anything over a dirty lens or face shield will invariably result in scratches.

Premixed Solution:

1. Mix 1 qt water, 4 oz rubbing alcohol, ¼ tsp liquid dish washing soap, and 1 oz sudsy ammonia in a spray bottle.
2. Spray both sides of the lenses thoroughly.
3. Use a lint-free cloth to wipe off the solution.
4. Reapply throughout the day, as necessary.

Quick alternatives that may work just as well include liquid dish soap, baby shampoo, shaving cream, and bar soap (with a few drops of water). Put a small drop on a soft cloth or a very clean finger. Apply it inside the lens, let it dry (overnight, if possible), and buff off just enough to provide clear vision.

Gloves

Sterile gloves may not always be necessary for outpatient wound repair. The infection rate in simple, uncomplicated lacerations is no different when using sterile gloves than when using

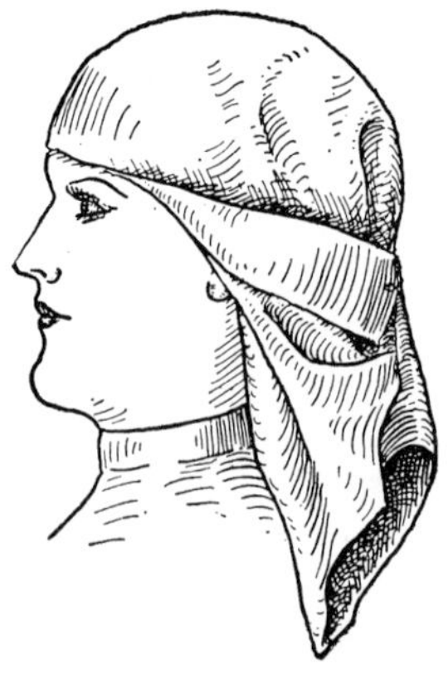

FIG. 5-22. Improvised cap. *(Reproduced from Olson.[31])*

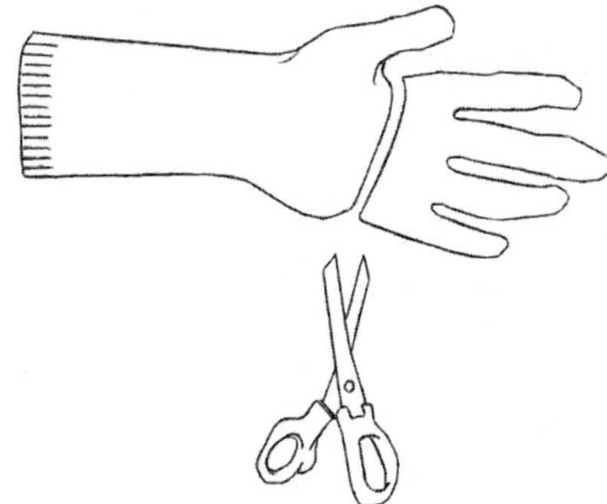

FIG. 5-23. Improvised long gloves, Step 1.

clean, nonsterile gloves in the following patients: those who are ≥1 year old with uncomplicated lacerations; those who are not immunologically compromised (diabetes mellitus, renal failure, asplenia, AIDS, immunosuppressive therapy, cirrhosis); those who do not form keloid scars; those who do not have an open fracture at the wound site; those without a tendon or nerve injury; those with no penetrating trauma; those with a late (>12 hours) presentation; or those with evidence of infection on presentation.[32,33]

If possible, clinicians should wear some type of glove to protect themselves against potential pathogens. However, to conserve examination gloves, cut the fingers off a glove and use each one as a finger cot for digital rectal examinations, allowing for five examinations with one glove.

Digital Impaction/Obstetric Gloves

Use elbow-length gloves for bimanual compression of the uterus, manual placental extraction, vaginal childbirth, disimpactions, and similar procedures where there is a great chance of contamination. When they are not available, you can make them from two pairs of standard surgical gloves. Cut the four fingers (not the thumb) off one pair of gloves just below the point where the finger portion of the glove begins (Fig. 5-23). If you are doing this sterilely, such as in the OR, or using the gloves for a disimpaction, then use the pieces as described below. Otherwise, for obstetric cases, sterilize or high-level disinfect those pieces along with a standard pair of uncut gloves. When ready to use the elbow-length gloves, first pull a fingerless piece of glove over your hand and up to the elbow. Do the same on the other arm. Then put on the surgical gloves so that the wrist portion overlaps the pieces already on the arm (Fig. 5-24). The overlapping section can be sealed with cyanoacrylate, although this is not usually necessary.[34] Rather than making long gloves, standard long kitchen or lightweight household gloves can also be used.

Booties

To fashion waterproof booties, cut a large plastic garbage bag open so that it lays flat. From that piece, cut out a portion that is as long as the distance from your foot to your knee and as wide as three lengths of your foot. Use larger dimensions if you need longer booties, such as in a bloody procedure or trauma. Secure them on your foot with duct tape. Do not make it too

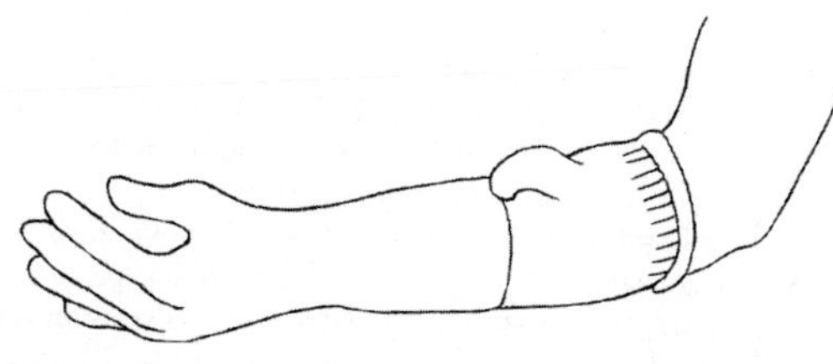

FIG. 5-24. Improvised long gloves, Step 2.

tight—you may be wearing them a while. One caveat: Take care when wearing these plastic boots; they can become very slippery on a wet or tiled surface.

Dressings and Bandages

Dressings are the materials that go on the wound. They can be adherent or nonadherent, wet or dry, and absorbent or nonabsorbent. Dressings are usually sterile and can be occlusive (airtight). Bandages cover dressings and can be adherent (such as tape) or impermeable. Bandages can also be used to place pressure on the wound. Most clean fabric can be used as a dressing or a bandage. Avoid paper products such as tissues and paper towels, because they disintegrate when wet and leave fibers in the wound.

No Dressing

To make life simpler, consider not putting a dressing on the wound! Sound like sacrilege? It's not. You do not have to put a dressing on every wound. Most clean closed wounds do not need them. Not applying a dressing allows easy inspection for infection or dehiscence. It also does not form a moist, possibly anaerobic, space in which the wound can macerate and thus increase the likelihood of infection.

Not applying a dressing also makes it much easier to keep the wound clean. Forget the voodoo about keeping it dry for 24 hours. (You think they don't sweat for that time either?) After a few hours, let patients shower or swim. Have them keep the wound clean with soap and water.

Dressing Material

Even so, some wounds do better, at least initially, if dressed. A dressing helps absorb any serosanguineous drainage, keeps the wound moist (good initially for small plastic closures), protects them from further injury, and may lessen pain by keeping the air off open wounds (e.g., paper cuts always hurt less when covered).

Use any absorbent material as a dressing. If a highly absorbent dressing is needed, such as for wounds with lots of exudate, use a menstrual pad or several tampons. Otherwise, use the more-absorbent cotton fabrics, rather than synthetics, which absorb less. In a pinch, use moss, especially sphagnum (peat) moss, that many cultures traditionally use as an absorbent dressing.

Make non-adherent dressings from sheer synthetic materials, such as parachute cloth or nylon stockings. Make occlusive dressings, such as those used over open-chest wounds from any clean piece of plastic sheeting, such as a plastic bag. If possible, first place a sterile dressing against the open wound.

One concern with dressings is their sterility. However, "provided the material used for dressings is clean, in most cases this will have very little impact on the incidence of infection."[35] If you need a sterile dressing—or need to sterilize dressings to reuse on other patients, the procedure is described in the section "Dressings and Other Textiles" in Chapter 6.

Bandages

The purpose of a bandage is to hold a dressing in place. If you need a bandage, the easiest and most available option is to use a piece of cloth that is expendable. Remember the damsel in old movies ripping up her petticoat to make bandages? She had the right idea. Another simple method is spirally cutting a shirt. If you prepackage bandages, be sure to label the package so you know what is inside.

If no cloth bandage is available, use duct tape to secure a dressing. Shave the area first, because when the tape comes off, it can hurt. Shaving can also help tape stick, which is a problem if the person's skin is wet. Poking holes in the tape (especially thick tape, like duct tape) helps by allowing fluids and sweat to escape. Clean the skin with soap and water, acetone, or alcohol to remove oils. Prepare the skin with tincture of benzoin to enhance "stickiness." To make an adhesive dressing, cover a small square of dressing with a piece of tape.

Improvise a wound-closure bandage (like a Steri-Strip), with two ends that adhere to the skin and a nonadherent bridge between them (Fig. 5-25). To make this type of bandage, take a 3½- to 4-inch-long piece of strong tape (duct, nylon cloth) and lay it on a smooth surface, such as metal, glass, or plastic. Cut two slits, about ¾ inch apart, one-third of the way across the center of the tape on both sides of the tape. Fold the pieces under to form the bridge.

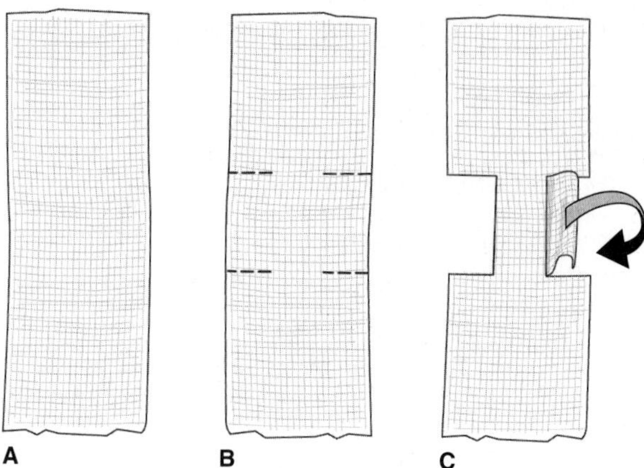

FIG. 5-25. Making a wound-closure bandage.

If necessary, use acetone to get paper tapes to adhere to the skin. First, degrease the area around the wound with acetone, then place the bandage and rub acetone onto it so that the stickiness does not extend beyond the bandage.[36] Alternatively, put cyanoacrylate over the bandage ends and adjacent skin to increase their adherence. If you need to see the wound but still want it covered, a clear bandage (like the standard Steri-Drape) can be fashioned from clear plastic wrap (e.g., Saran Wrap) or a piece of clear plastic bag. In both cases, affix the edges to the skin with tape or cyanoacrylate glue.

A pressure bandage over dressings, used when there is significant seepage or concern about hematoma development, is most easily constructed from an elastic bandage, a bungee cord (use only over fabric stiff enough to distribute the cord's force), a surgical glove,[37] or the elastic from a piece of clothing or equipment.

Syringes and Needles

Sharps Containers

Sharps containers are often in shorter supply than are the abundance of used needles, especially after disaster-mandated immunization clinics or in the homes of patients needing routine injections, such as for insulin. Sharps containers are easily improvised.

For sizeable volumes of sharps, use a large container such as a 5-gallon water bottle. Empty the container and tape a fitted piece of cardboard or thin plastic over the top. Cut an X-shaped slit in the cardboard to form a "one-way" opening. When it is full, tape the slits and dispose of it with other biohazardous waste. An alternative is to use a heavy cardboard box. Seal it completely and then cut a 3-inch "X" in one side. Push the sharps through the hole. Discard the box when it is full.

For clinic or patient (small-volume) use, get a large, empty coffee can with a plastic lid; clean and dry it. Then make two slits at 90-degree angles to each other in the center of the plastic lid. Securely tape the lid to the can. Push a syringe and needle through the opening to make sure that it easily fits through the slits, but that a small child's fingers cannot get through. When the coffee can is full, tape the slits shut and dispose of it.

Intravenous Fluids and Equipment

Venipuncture Tourniquet

Use a piece of IV tubing as a tourniquet for drawing blood or placing IVs. A rubber glove (sterile or unsterile, but "stretchy") works well as a venous tourniquet when starting intravenous lines or drawing blood. Cutting between the fourth and fifth fingers and onto the wrist part of the glove produces a nice tourniquet. Even better, cut the wrist portion off a surgical glove and slip it over

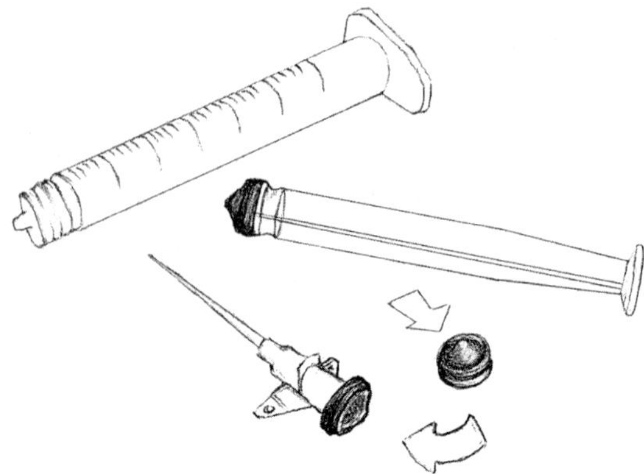

FIG. 5-26. Improvised saline lock.

the arm, as suggested by Daniel Tsze, MD, from Brown University (written communication, June 5, 2007). This is very effective as a tourniquet to locate an infant's scalp vein.

Intravenous Needles

Needles used for injection also can be used as IV needles, although they may be more difficult to thread into a vein, because the injection needle will tend to puncture the vein, rather than slide in as the plastic-coated needle on a catheter does. Also, because they have a tendency to perforate the vessel, take extra care when securing them, and always check that they cannot be jostled or moved; use an arm board or generous bandaging, if needed.

Should you reuse needles in austere situations? If so, how do you sterilize them? The answers are in Chapter 6. How to make surgical needles and suture materials is discussed in Chapter 22.

Saline Locks

Make an excellent, inexpensive saline lock by slipping the rubber end of the plunger from a 2- or 3-mL disposable syringe over the end of an IV catheter (Fig. 5-26). This also works on a straight needle, if that needs to be used as an IV catheter. Simply fill the catheter with saline (or heparin) as would normally be done. With some catheters, you first must slice off the small flanges on the hub so that the rubber fits.

Intravenous Tubing

One method for adjusting an IV flow rate is to wrap a small piece of malleable metal (e.g., heavy aluminum foil) around the tubing. The flow rate is controlled by how tightly it is wrapped on the tubing. Count the drops to get the desired rate.

Intravenous Bottles/Bags

There are multiple ways to increase the external pressure on IV or blood bags. These include inflating a blood pressure cuff around them and wrapping them with an elastic bandage, a belt ("stretchy" if possible), nylon stockings, a rope, or similar materials.

If external pressure is applied to an IV bag, it does not have to be hung. Rather, the pressurized IV bag can simply lie on, or next to, the patient. This facilitates transporting the patient. If the bag is placed under an adult patient, the pressure exerted by the body keeps the IV flowing. This is particularly useful when transporting a patient in the field.

To speed the flow of IV fluid running out of a plastic bottle, once it is hanging, insert a hypodermic needle into its uppermost part. This also helps to more accurately gauge the amount of delivered fluid, because without the needle to release the vacuum, the plastic deforms and gives a false reading on the quantity markers on the bottle's side.

With glass bottles, increase flow by inserting a needle into the stopper or end of the IV bottle to speed the flow by "venting," allowing air to enter as the fluid drips out. You can also "strip" the IV tubing by using your fingers to compress the tubing and continually running them down

TABLE 5-3 Safety Pin Size Chart

- Size 00 or 2/0 = ¾ inches
- Size 0 = 7/8 inches
- Size 1 = 1 1/16 inches
- Size 2 = 1½ inches
- Size 3 = 2 inches
- Size 4 (blanket pins) = 3 inches

Notice that the increase in length is not equivalent as the size goes up.

both sides of the IV tubing. This is marginally useful and very time consuming, but it is better than doing nothing.

If the IV pole will not accommodate the IV bag or bottle's "hanger," use a loop of IV tubing to connect the bottle's hanger to the pole or other available elevated hook.

Resuscitation/Equipment Cart

Use clear plastic bins to store clinical equipment. Israeli emergency physicians store critical equipment in clear plastic bins that contain only the most commonly used equipment and sizes at the bedside; the rest is stored across the room for use when needed. They also position most bins between adjacent beds so that they can slide them open to either side—doubling their usability and conserving space.

Safety Pins

In austere settings, safety pins have many uses, including securing an endotracheal tube (ETT) or surgical airway, closing a wound, punching holes in a can, attaching information to a patient's clothing, and improvising a tracheal hook. See appropriate chapters for more detailed instructions. However, all safety pin sizes cannot be used for all purposes (Table 5-3).

Tubing Clamp/Organizer

How many uses can you think of for the common clothespin? It works well as a tubing clamp for urethral catheters and IVs: Double the tubing over and clamp it with a clothespin. It also works great as a wire/tubing organizer (Fig. 5-27): Gather up a number of wires and tubes and

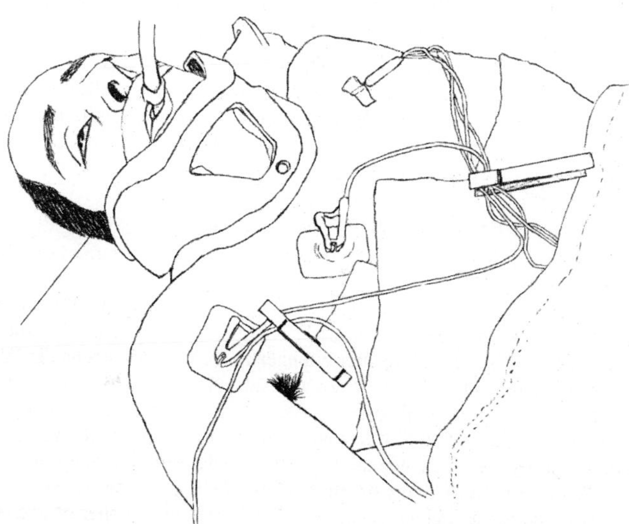

FIG. 5-27. Clothespins holding wires out of the way.

secure them with a clothespin. This is particularly helpful when transporting patients, because it keeps the extraneous equipment from becoming entangled with ambulance or helicopter equipment. Of course, these clips can also be used to attach triage tags and medical records to patients' clothing.

Lubricants (for Rectal/Pelvic Examinations and Nasal Packing)

Nearly any nontoxic lubricant works for rectal examinations if standard water-based lubricants are not available. Try vegetable oil, lard, cold cream, salad oil, sweet cream, unsalted butter, or sweet oil.[38]

For ETTs, you normally do not need lubricant unless you are doing an awake intubation or a nasotracheal intubation. In those cases, use a sterile, water-based lubricant. Similarly, it does not help much to put a little lubricant on an NG tube. It is better to apply some local anesthetic and wet the tube before insertion. Likewise, use warm water to lubricate a vaginal speculum. Sterile water is the safest, least-toxic substance.

Adhesives

Cyanoacrylate, duct or other tape, sutures, or surgical wire can be used to quickly secure, repair, and construct medical equipment. Securely fix tapes and leads on a patient using tincture of benzoin or, absent that, achieve the same effect by saturating alcohol gauze with Betadine. As the alcohol evaporates, "you're left with the same residue as tincture of benzoin. It's convenient and readily applied without using extra 4 × 4s" (Darrell G. Looney, MD. Personal written communication, June 5, 2007).

Ice/Heat Packs

There are several ways to make ice packs, but all require something cold to fill them. The easiest is to simply fill a plastic bag with a cold source, which can be ice, frozen food, cold drinks, or snow. Be certain to put a cloth between the cold source and the skin. Without a portable cold source, an option is to put an affected extremity into cold water. Alternatively, use evaporative cooling in a warm, dry climate by putting a wet cloth over the area and exposing it to a hot breeze. It will cool quickly.

When you have sufficient facilities and want to prepare ice packs in advance, fill 1-gallon plastic bags that can be securely closed with 4½ cups of water and 1½ cups of 70% isopropyl alcohol. To prevent leaks, put each bag inside another securely locking plastic bag. Place the bags in a freezer for about 4 to 6 hours.[39]

Heat packs are a bit easier to make, although, of course, you need a heat source. To make a "Wheat Pillow" hot-pack:

1. Use dry long-grain rice or wheat grain (e.g., bird food) as the filler.
2. Put it into a heavy, wool sock or, if you want to make a larger pack, a piece of strong, breathable fabric that can be put in a microwave. Tie the end closed with a string.
3. Put it in a microwave on high for 1 to 2 minutes; use a longer heating time if the microwave is less powerful. You can also put it in an oven at low heat.
4. If the smell is bothersome, add some potpourri.
5. This heating pad works for 8 to 10 minutes and can be reheated and reused.

See also "Heating the Bed" section, above, for more ideas.

Dinnerware

It may seem mundane, but being able to supply plates and cups becomes vital, especially when a horde of patients descends on a facility after a disaster. Metal cans of various sizes can be cut down, if necessary, for use as cups, plates, pots, storage containers, and a wide variety of other items. The only caveat is that whenever cans are cut down for use, their edges must be folded inward or otherwise dulled, because they are very sharp. While most cans are used to store food, it is safest to both clean and sterilize them before using them for eating. What if you need forks, knives, and spoons? In a pinch, hands work great. Emily Post is not looking, but do wash your hands before eating!

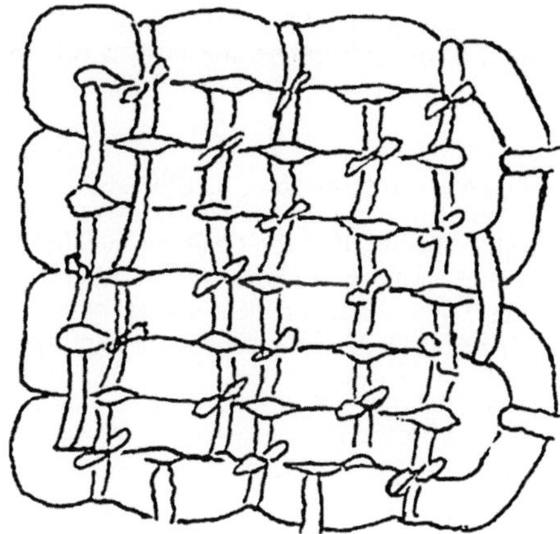

FIG. 5-28. Making a seat/stretcher cushion.

PATIENT TRANSPORT

Transportation Within Health Care Facilities

Patients must be transported within health care facilities, once they arrive. How they arrive is discussed in Chapter 21.

Cushions for Wheelchairs, Examination Tables, Stretchers, and Chairs

Any patient surface that will be used for a prolonged period should be cushioned. There are three ways to make cushions: (a) Stuff a bag with soft, quiet (feathers, cotton, etc.) materials—but use torn newspaper, if necessary—and sew up the open end. (b) Tie bicycle tire tubes or similar tubes together in an "S" pattern. Use thin pieces of the tubing to bind the tube together. If larger pieces are needed, such as to cover a gurney or a bed, use the tube strips to tie multiple "S" pieces together (Fig. 5-28). (c) Glue together multiple pieces of thick cardboard. Wet the cardboard and have someone sit on it to mold it. Then let it dry and varnish it. If rubber is available, use a 1-inch thick piece to pad it.[40]

Wheels for Gurneys, Wheelchairs, or Other Equipment

Make simple wheels from circular pieces of wood at least 2 inches thick and with a diameter to fit the equipment on which it is to be used. If this thickness of wood is not available, glue one or more pieces together. The wood grain should run across, rather than through, the wheel. Cut a hole just large enough to fit the axle. Then cover the wheel rim by either gluing or nailing on a piece of rubber from an old car tire or inner tube. Alternatively, cut a piece along the circumference of the wheel from a bicycle tire. Cutting notches in the side of the tire allows it to conform to the wooden wheel and prevents the nails from loosening.[41]

EQUIPMENT SAFETY/MAINTENANCE

Safety

Safety After Flooding

Many disasters result from flooding. Rather than simply beginning to use equipment that may have been damaged in a flood, take the following steps:

1. Check all power cords and batteries to make sure they are not wet or damaged by water. If electrical circuits and electrical equipment have gotten wet, turn off the power at the main breaker.
2. Make sure you check for water before plugging in your device. Do not plug in a power cord if the cord, the device, or the outlet is wet.

3. If there was a power outage, when the power is restored, check to make sure the settings on your medical device have not changed (often these devices reset to a default mode when power is interrupted).[42]

Generator Safety

Generators are the common source of electricity in austere circumstances. The problem is that they generate carbon monoxide. To be safe, never run a generator, pressure washer, or any gasoline-powered engine outside an open window or door where exhaust can vent into an enclosed area. Also, do not run them inside a basement, garage, or other enclosed structure, even if the doors or windows are open, unless the equipment has been professionally installed and the area properly vented.[42]

Maintenance

Heat and Humidity

Heat and humidity affect equipment anywhere, especially when electricity no longer powers air conditioning. In moist environments, frequently examine all equipment—including ophthalmoscopes, otoscopes, microscopes, tonometers, and endoscopes—for mildew. In addition, the US Food and Drug Administration offers these suggestions to protect medical devices from heat and humidity:

1. Use a dry cloth to wipe off devices regularly.
2. Keep devices out of direct sunlight.
3. Enclose medical products in plastic containers to keep them dry.
4. Do not use ice if there is a danger of water contamination; use dry ice or instant cold packs to keep your device cool.
5. Do not use disposable devices that are wet.[42]

TABLE 5-4 The French Gauge System—Comparison with the Metric and (Stub's) Gauge Systems

Gauge Number	Inch	French[a]	mm
36	0.0040	0.305	0.102
28	0.0140	1.067	0.356
23	0.0250	1.905	0.635
19	0.0420	3.200	1.067
16	0.0650	4.953	1.651
10	0.1340	10.211	3.404
8	0.1650	12.573	4.191
	0.1839	14.000	4.667
	0.2101	16.000	5.333
	0.2364	18.000	6.000
	0.2627	20.000	6.667
	0.2889	22.000	7.333
	0.3152	24.000	8.000
	0.4728	36.000	12.000

[a]Although the French gauge system is based on three times the measurement in millimeters, some of the numbers appear to be other than exactly three times the millimeter equivalent due to rounding.

Adapted with permission from Iserson.[43]

Anesthesia Hoses

Black (antistatic) anesthetic breathing hoses, used with ether anesthesia, deteriorate rapidly in high humidity. After use, they will be wet inside from the water vapor in the patient's breath. After use, hang them vertically to allow them to dry. Inspect them regularly for cracks, especially between the corrugations, where they most often develop leaks. The normal polyethylene anesthetic hoses do not deteriorate as rapidly.[44]

MEASUREMENT EQUIVALENTS

In austere situations, you use what is available. That may include catheters, tubes, and needles sized in a system with which you are unfamiliar. This conversion chart (Table 5-4) can help you decide the appropriately sized equipment for the situation. Other measurement equivalents are listed in Chapter 20. For volume and length conversions, see Chapter 7.

REFERENCES

1. Arreola-Risa C, Mock C, Vega Rivera F, et al. Evaluating trauma care capabilities in Mexico with the World Health Organization's Guidelines for Essential Trauma Care publication. *Rev Panam Salud Publica*. 2006;19(2):94-103, Table 2.
2. Farley F. Improvising equipment. *Am J Nurs*. 1938;38(4, section 2):42s-43s.
3. Mock C, Lormand JD, Goosen J, et al. *Guidelines for Essential Trauma Care*. Geneva, Switzerland: World Health Organization; 2004:15.
4. Bollet AJ. *Civil War Medicine: Challenges and Triumphs*. Tucson, AZ: Galen Press Ltd.; 2002:108.
5. Owens PJ, Forgione A, Briggs S. Challenges of international disaster relief: use of a deployable rapid assembly shelter and surgical hospital. *Disaster Manag Response*. 2005;3(1):11-16.
6. Schwab L. *Primary Eye Care in Developing Nations*. Oxford, UK: Oxford University Press; 1987:137-138.
7. US Bureau of Agriculture. *Bulletin 927*. Quoted in: Olson LM. *Improvised Equipment in the Home Care of the Sick*. Philadelphia, PA: WB Saunders; 1928:81-87.
8. Hansen HF. *Reference Handbook for Nurses: First Aid, Materia Medica, Nursing Arts, Diet Therapy, Nursing Care and Improvised Equipment*. Philadelphia, PA: W.B. Saunders; 1938:317-318.
9. Olson LM. *Improvised Equipment in the Home Care of the Sick*. Philadelphia, PA: W.B. Saunders; 1928:26-27.
10. Hansen HF. *Reference Handbook for Nurses: First Aid, Materia Medica, Nursing Arts, Diet Therapy, Nursing Care and Improvised Equipment*. Philadelphia, PA: W.B. Saunders; 1938:319-320.
11. Olson LM. *Improvised Equipment in the Home Care of the Sick*. Philadelphia, PA: W.B. Saunders; 1928:50-51.
12. Olson LM. *Improvised Equipment in the Home Care of the Sick*. Philadelphia, PA: W.B. Saunders; 1928:21-22.
13. Olson LM. *Improvised Equipment in the Home Care of the Sick*. Philadelphia, PA: W.B. Saunders; 1928:77.
14. Hansen HF. *Reference Handbook for Nurses: First Aid, Materia Medica, Nursing Arts, Diet Therapy, Nursing Care and Improvised Equipment*. Philadelphia, PA: W.B. Saunders; 1938:319.
15. Duncan I. Makeshift medicine: combating disease in Japanese prison camps (reprinted from *Med J Australia*). COFEPOW, January 1983. http://www.cofepow.org.uk/pages/medical_makeshift_medicine.htm. Accessed September 14, 2006.
16. Olson LM. *Improvised Equipment in the Home Care of the Sick*. Philadelphia, PA: W.B. Saunders; 1928:36-37.
17. Jump EP. Improvised urinal. *RN*. 1964;27(7):9.
18. Kuhan N, bin Ahmad ZA, Lip TQ. Improvised urine bag. *J Singapore Paediatr Soc*. 1977;19(3):212-213.
19. Mock C, Lormand JD, Goosen J, et al. *Guidelines for Essential Trauma Care*. Geneva, Switzerland: World Health Organization; 2004:54.
20. Carmichael AG, Ratzan RM. *Medicine: A Treasury of Art and Literature*. New York, NY: Hugh Lauter Levin Associates; 1991.
21. Dobson MB. *Anaesthesia at the District Hospital*. Geneva, Switzerland: World Health Organization; 1988:33.
22. Kamm G. Paediatric anaesthesia with the Ambu-Paedi-Valve and Bag. *Trop Doct*. 1980;10(2):66-71.
23. Greenberg RS. Facemask, nasal, and oral airway devices. *Anesth Clin N Am*. 2002;20:833-861.

24. Werner D. *Where There Is No Doctor: A Village Health Care Handbook*. Palo Alto, CA: The Hesperian Foundation; 1977:445.
25. Greenberg M, Spurlock M. Makeshift use of a syringe, scalpel blade, and a stopcock to create a precordial stethoscope bell. *J Clin Anesth*. 2006;18:79.
26. Dobson MB. *Anaesthesia at the District Hospital*. 2nd ed. Geneva, Switzerland: World Health Organization; 2000:27.
27. Yeats M. The maintenance of an aneroid sphygmomanometer. *Pract Proced*. 1993;3(8):1. http://www.nda.ox.ac.uk/wfsa/html/u03/u03_018.htm. Accessed September 13, 2006.
28. Olson LM. *Improvised Equipment in the Home Care of the Sick*. Philadelphia, PA: W.B. Saunders; 1928:98.
29. Davies A, Thompson KA, Giri K, et al. Testing the efficacy of homemade masks: would they protect in an influenza pandemic? *Disaster Med Pub Health Preparedness*. 2013;7(4):413-418.
30. Tunevall TG. Postoperative wound infections and surgical face masks: a controlled study. *World J Surg*. 1991;15(3):383-387.
31. Olson LM. *Improvised Equipment in the Home Care of the Sick*. Philadelphia, PA: W.B. Saunders; 1928:98-100.
32. Perelman VS, Francis GJ, Rutledge T, et al. Sterile versus nonsterile gloves for repair of uncomplicated lacerations in the emergency department: a randomized controlled trial. *Ann Emerg Med*. 2004;43(3):362-370.
33. Bodiwala GG, George TK. Surgical gloves during wound repair in the accident-and-emergency department. *Lancet*. 1982;2:91-92.
34. Blouse A, Gomez P, eds. *Emergency Obstetric Care: Quick Reference Guide for Frontline Providers*. Baltimore, MD: JHPIEGO Maternal & Neonatal Program; 2003:80-82.
35. The Remote, Austere, Wilderness, and Third World Medicine Discussion Board Moderators. *Survival and Austere Medicine: An Introduction*. 2nd ed. 2005:94-95. www.aussurvivalist.com/downloads/AM%20Final%202.pdf. Accessed June 8, 2007.
36. Aronberg J, Kluser F. Surgical pearl: securing surgical dressing with acetone. *J Amer Acad Derm*. 2003;48(4):611-612.
37. Mashiko T, Ohnishi F, Oka A, et al. Usefulness of surgical glove dressing: a novel technique for skin graft fixation after hand burns. *J Plast Reconst Aesthet Surg*. 2013;66(9):1304-1306.
38. Olson LM. *Improvised Equipment in the Home Care of the Sick*. Philadelphia, PA: W.B. Saunders; 1928:91.
39. RESQDOC website. http://medtech.syrene.net/forum/showthread.php?s=349d3c19041 ccaab2d90a951edc6fe34&t=963. Accessed September 14, 2006.
40. Platt A, Carter N. *Making Health-Care Equipment: Ideas for Local Design and Production*. London, UK: Intermediate Technology Pub; 1990:13.
41. Platt A, Carter N. *Making Health-Care Equipment: Ideas for Local Design and Production*. London, UK: Intermediate Technology Pub; 1990:8.
42. US Food and Drug Administration. Center for Devices and Radiological Health. FDA offers tips about medical devices and hurricane disasters. Updated August 30, 2005. www.fda.gov/cdrh/emergency/hurricane.html. Accessed September 17, 2006.
43. Iserson KV. Charriere—the man behind the 'French' gauge. *J Emerg Med*. 1987;5(6):545-548.
44. Dobson MB. Draw-over anaesthesia part 3—looking after your own apparatus. Update in anaesthesia. 1993;3:Article 5. www.nda.ox.ac.uk/wfsa/html/u03/u03_014.htm. Accessed September 14, 2006.

6 | Cleaning and Reusing Equipment

Much modern medical equipment is labeled "disposable." When resources are scarce, the luxury of not reusing serviceable medical equipment cannot be sustained. On the other hand, safety regarding equipment reuse is paramount. Patients should not be put at risk either through introducing infections from previously used equipment or by using malfunctioning equipment. This chapter discusses the guidelines and techniques for reusing, cleaning, and sterilizing medical equipment.

POLICIES ON REUSING MEDICAL EQUIPMENT

Major governments do not agree on their recommendations regarding the reuse of single-use devices (SUDs). The US policy across several agencies is that SUDs can be reused.

A US government panel of experts stated that in resource-scarce situations, equipment and supplies "will be rationed and used in ways consistent with achieving the ultimate goal of saving the most lives (e.g., disposable supplies may be reused)." However, they also said guidelines are needed on "how to use and reuse common supplies and equipment, such as gloves, gowns, and masks."[1]

The US Food and Drug Administration (FDA) found "no data to indicate that people are being injured or put at increased risk by the reuse of SUDs,"[2] while acknowledging that many SUDs are commonly reused. Among these are many types of equipment, including those used in dentistry, orthodontics, otolaryngology, and laparoscopy. Specific equipment includes needles, scalpels, forceps, trocars, saw blades, staplers, drills, scissors, masks, syringes, gowns, and biopsy devices.[3] The problems found with reusing SUDs include a "loss of elasticity in inflatable balloons, persistence of blood and biofilms, loss of original lubricants and resultant effect on catheter threading, and crystallization of liquid x-ray contrast material."[3] The FDA recently advised that "single-use sterile devices that do not have reprocessing instructions should not be reprocessed." They did not comment on resource-poor situations.[4]

The US Centers for Disease Control and Prevention (CDC) states that "in general, reusable medical devices or patient-care equipment that enters normally sterile tissue or the vascular system or through which blood flows should be sterilized before each use."[5] Except in rare and special instances, items that do not ordinarily touch the patient or that touch only intact skin are not involved in disease transmission and generally do not necessitate disinfection between uses on different patients. Special rules apply when patients are infected or colonized with drug-resistant or highly virulent microorganisms. In these cases, the CDC recommends that noncritical items be dedicated to one patient or patient cohort (someone with the same contagious illness) or that this equipment be subjected to low-level disinfection between patient uses. Reusable items that touch mucous membranes should, at a minimum, receive high-level disinfection between patients.[5]

The US Government Accounting Office (GAO) concluded that there is no evidence that reprocessed SUDs create an elevated health risk for patients. Testifying before the US Congress, Dr. Kenneth Kizer, a former undersecretary for health at the US Department of Veterans Affairs, said, "Single-use labeling is a real scam for a lot of devices, and by not using reprocessed devices where possible, it is wasteful and not environmentally responsive, since these items have to be disposed of as biomedical waste."[6]

Members of the European Community have multiple conflicting policies on reusing SUDs, with some allowing it, others regulating it, and some banning it.[7]

RISK STRATIFICATION

The infection risk that medical equipment poses to patients can be stratified according to its use into (a) high risk, (b) intermediate risk, and (c) low risk. Each group, under normal circumstances, has different decontamination requirements.

1. High-risk items (sterilization required) come into close contact with breaks in the skin or mucous membranes or are introduced into a normally sterile body area. These include

surgical instruments, needles, endoscopes used in sterile body cavities and their irrigation systems and biopsy accessories, and urinary or other catheters.[4]

2. Intermediate-risk items (disinfection required) come into close contact with mucous membranes or are items contaminated with particularly virulent or readily transmissible organisms. These include most respiratory equipment, for example, laryngoscope blades, endotracheal and tracheostomy tubes, and oropharyngeal and nasal airways.
3. Low-risk items (cleaning required) come into contact only with normal intact skin. These include stethoscopes, other physical examination equipment, stretchers and wheelchairs, and electrocardiogram (ECG) and electroencephalography (EEG) leads.[8]

DECONTAMINATION

Cleaning, disinfection, and sterilization all decontaminate medical equipment. Decontamination is the general term describing any method of reducing the risks of cross infection—passing microbes from one infected person to a previously uninfected person.[8]

Table 6-1 contains recommended processes for decontaminating and, then, cleaning different types of medical equipment that can easily be accomplished in most settings.

When using chlorine solutions, avoid prolonged exposure of the equipment, because this causes metal to rust and rubber and cloth to deteriorate. To avoid dulling the edges, do not sterilize needles or instruments with a cutting edge at temperatures >160°C (320°F).

CLEANING

Cleaning is the process of removing any visible dirt or secretions, including dust, soil, large numbers of microorganisms, and organic matter (e.g., blood, vomit) on which microorganisms grow. Cleaning must be done before equipment is disinfected or sterilized; not doing so can impede effective disinfection or sterilization.[8]

Especially in austere circumstances, "clean items are sufficient to prevent infection in the majority of cases. For the vast majority of minor cuts and lacerations, clean is fine."[9] Note that SUD needles cannot be cleaned adequately.

Method

Cleaning normally involves washing the equipment with detergent (soap) and water.[8] Mix fresh dilute soap solutions (and other disinfectant solutions) every 24 hours and store them in a cool place: Bacteria may grow in dilute solutions (but not in concentrated solutions).

Clean equipment immediately after use. First, remove blood and other visible dirt by washing equipment thoroughly with warm water without soap. Then wash thoroughly with warm water and soap, rinse with water, and dry completely. Leave scissors and forceps open while drying.[10] Clean surgical instruments with a small brush, such as a soft toothbrush.[11]

Maintenance and Packing

Once the equipment is clean, perform any necessary maintenance (e.g., tighten screws, sharpen edges) and pack them for use or prepare them for disinfection or sterilization.

DISINFECTION

Disinfection is a process used to reduce the number of microorganisms, although not usually bacterial spores. The process does not necessarily kill or remove all microorganisms, but simply reduces their number to a level that is not harmful to health.[8] The CDC recognizes three levels of disinfection: high, intermediate, and low.[5]

High-level disinfection methods kill all organisms, except when there are large numbers of bacterial spores, with a chemical germicide such as bleach or ethyl alcohol. Intermediate-level disinfection procedures kill mycobacteria, bacteria, and most viruses by using a chemical germicide registered as a "tuberculocide" by the US Environmental Protection Agency. Low-level disinfection kills some viruses and bacteria by using a chemical germicide such as soap.

TABLE 6-1 Recommended Decontamination, Cleaning, and High-Level Disinfection/Sterilization Methods

Instrument/Item	Decontamination	Cleaning	Alternatives	
			Sterilization	High-Level Disinfection
	The first step in handling used items; reduces risk of HBV and HIV/AIDS.	Removes all visible blood, body fluids, and dirt.	Destroys all microorganisms, including endospores.	Destroys all viruses, bacteria, parasites, fungi, and some endospores.
Airway (plastic)	Soak in 0.5% chlorine solution for 10 min before cleaning. Rinse and wash immediately.	Wash with soap and water. Rinse with clean water; air or towel dry.	Not necessary.	Not necessary.
Ambu bag/CPR face mask	Wipe exposed surfaces with gauze pad soaked in 60% to 90% alcohol or 0.5% chlorine solution; rinse immediately.	Wash with soap and water. Rinse with clean water; air or towel dry.	Not necessary.	Not necessary.
Bed pan, urinal, and emesis basin	Not necessary.	Use a brush to wash with disinfectant, soap, and water. Rinse with clean water.	Not necessary.	Not necessary.
Cotton cord umbilical tie	Not necessary.	Not necessary.	Not practical.	Place in small metal bowl. Place bowl in steamer, steam for 20 min. Air dry.
Exam table or other large surface areas (cart and stretcher)	Wipe off with 0.5% chlorine solution.	Wash with soap and water if organic material remains after decontamination.	Not necessary.	Not necessary.

(Continued)

TABLE 6-1 Recommended Decontamination, Cleaning, and High-Level Disinfection/Sterilization Methods (*Continued*)

Instrument/Item	Decontamination	Cleaning	Alternatives: Sterilization	Alternatives: High-Level Disinfection
Hypodermic needle and syringe (glass or plastic)	Fill assembled needle and syringe with 0.5% chlorine solution. Flush ×3 and either dispose of needle or soak for 10 min before cleaning. Rinse by flushing ×3 with clean water.	Disassemble. Then wash with soap and water. Rinse with clean water; air or towel dry syringes (only air dry needles).	Preferable. 1. Dry heat for 2 hours after reaching 160°C (320°F) (glass syringes only). —*or*— 2. Autoclave at 121°C (250°F) and 106 kPa (15 lb/in^2) for 20 min (30 min if wrapped).	Acceptable. Steam or boil for 20 min. Use of chemical disinfection is not recommended, because chemical residue may remain (even after repeated rinsing in boiled water) and interfere with the action of drugs being injected.
Instruments (e.g., scissors, forceps, vaginal speculum, needle holder, needle)	Soak in 0.5% chlorine solution for 10 min before cleaning. Rinse or wash immediately.	Using a brush, wash with soap and water. Rinse with clean water. If will be sterilized, air or towel dry.	Preferable. 1. Dry heat for 1 hours after reaching 170°C (340°F). —*or*— 2. Autoclave at 121°C (250°F) and 106 kPa (15 lb/in^2) for 20 min (30 min if wrapped). For sharp instruments, use dry heat for 2 hours after reaching 160°C (320°F).	Acceptable. 1. Steam or boil for 20 min. —*or*— 2. Use chemical to high-level disinfect by soaking for 20 min. Rinse well in boiled water and air dry before use or storage.
Manual vacuum aspirator cannula (plastic)	Soak in 0.5% chlorine solution for 10 min before cleaning. Rinse or wash immediately.	Wash with soap and water, removing all particles.	Not recommended. Heat from autoclave or dry-heat oven damages cannula.	Steam or boil for 20 min.
Plastic apron and sheet	Wipe off with 0.5% chlorine solution.	Wash with soap and hot water. Rinse with clean water; air dry.	Not necessary.	Not necessary.

Personal protective equipment (cap, mask, gown), cloth drape, cloth to dry and wrap neonates	Not necessary. (Laundry staff should wear protective gowns, gloves, and eyewear when handling soiled linen.)	Wash with soap and hot water. Rinse with clean water; air or machine dry.	Not necessary.	Not necessary.
Stethoscope	Not necessary.	Wipe with 60% to 90% alcohol.	Not necessary.	Not necessary.
Storage container for instruments, specimen cup, test tube	Soak in 0.5% chlorine solution for 10 min before cleaning. Rinse or wash immediately.	Wash with soap and water. Rinse with clean water; air or towel dry.	1. Dry heat for 1 hour after reaching 170°C (340°F). *—or—* 2. Autoclave at 121°C (250°F) and 106 kPa (15 lb/in^2) for 20 min (30 min if wrapped).	Boil container and lid for 20 min. If container is too large: Fill container with 0.5% chlorine solution and soak for 20 min. Rinse in water that has been boiled for 20 min and air dry.
Suction bulb	Soak in 0.5% chlorine solution for 10 min before cleaning. Rinse and wash immediately.	Wash with soap and water. Rinse with clean water; air or towel dry.	Not necessary.	Not necessary
Suction catheter	Soak in 0.5% chlorine solution for 10 min before cleaning. Rinse or wash immediately.	Wash with soap and water. Rinse ×3 with clean water (inside and outside).	Not recommended. Heat from autoclave or dry-heat oven will damage catheter.	Steam or boil for 20 min. Use of chemical disinfection is not recommended, as chemical residue may remain (even after repeated rinsing with boiled water) and interfere with the action of drugs being injected.
Surgical gloves	Soak in 0.5% chlorine solution for 10 min before cleaning. Rinse or wash immediately.	Wash with soap and water. Rinse with clean water and check for holes. If will be sterilized, dry inside and out (air or towel dry) and package.	If used for surgery, autoclave at 121°C (250°F) and 106 kPa (15 lb/in^2) for 20 min. Do not use for 24-48 hours.	Steam for 20 min; dry in steamer.

(*Continued*)

TABLE 6-1 Recommended Decontamination, Cleaning, and High-Level Disinfection/Sterilization Methods (*Continued*)

			Alternatives	
Instrument/Item	Decontamination	Cleaning	Sterilization	High-Level Disinfection
Thermometer, oral	Soak in 0.5% chlorine solution for 10 min before cleaning. Rinse and wash immediately.	Wash with soap and water. Rinse with clean water; air or towel dry.	Not necessary.	Not necessary.
Thermometer, rectal	Soak in 0.5% chlorine solution for 10 min before cleaning. Rinse and wash immediately.	Wash with soap and water. Rinse with clean water; air or towel dry.	Not necessary.	Not necessary.
Forceps (pick-ups)	Not necessary. Reprocess each shift or when contaminated.	Using a brush, wash with soap and water. Rinse with clean water. If will be sterilized, air or towel dry.	Preferable 1. Dry heat for 1 hour after reaching 170°C (340°F). —*or*— 2. Autoclave at 121°C (250°F) and 106 kPa (15 lb/in^2) for 20 min (30 min if wrapped).	Acceptable. 1. Steam or boil for 20 min. 2. Use chemical to high-level disinfect by soaking for 20 min. Rinse well with boiled water and air dry before use or storage.
Urinary catheter	Soak in 0.5% chlorine solution for 10 min before cleaning. Rinse or wash immediately.	Use a brush to wash with soap and water. Rinse ×3 with clean water (inside and outside).	1. Dry heat for 2 hours after reaching 160°C (320°F) (metal only). —*or*— 2. Autoclave at 121°C (250°F) and 106 kPa (15 lb/in^2) for 20 min (30 min if wrapped) (metal only).	Steam or boil for 20 min.

Abbreviations: AIDS, acquired immune deficiency syndrome; CPR, cardiopulmonary resuscitation; HBV, hepatitis B virus; HIV, human immunodeficiency virus.

Usefulness

While the effectiveness of disinfection depends on the method and the disinfectant that are used, some general principles apply[8]:

- Gram-positive bacteria are more sensitive than gram-negative bacteria.
- Mycobacteria and spores are relatively resistant.
- Non-enveloped viruses, such as *Coxsackie*, tend to be more resistant.
- Fungal spores can be killed by disinfectants. Other bacterial spores, such as *Clostridia*, are generally resistant.
- Tubercle bacteria (TB and related organisms) are more resistant to chemical disinfectants than other bacteria.
- Many common pathogenic viruses can be inactivated by exposing them for 10 minutes to 70% alcohol or for 30 minutes to 5.25% sodium hypochlorite (bleach). These include hepatitis B virus (HBV) and human immunodeficiency virus (HIV), as well as the viruses that cause rabies, Lassa fever, and other hemorrhagic fevers.

Methods

While chemical disinfectants are the norm, in austere environments, using boiling water, with or without soap, is the best disinfection method. Heat disinfection is more effective than chemicals. At 80°C (176°F), most bacteria (but not their spores) will be destroyed within a few minutes. Boiling accelerates rusting of items with a sharp edge, such as scissors and knives. Using distilled or soft water reduces this problem.

Washing instruments in soap solution and then boiling for some minutes in water is an effective method of disinfection.[12] Various concentrations of soap solution may also be used to wash hands and operating fields before surgery, to wash bedding and clothes, and for personal hygiene.

Boiling

The general rule is to boil contaminated equipment in clean water (100°C [212°F] for 10-30 minutes at sea level). This kills all organisms except for a few bacterial spores. Do not start timing it until the water has come to a full boil. At higher altitudes, the temperature at which water boils decreases, so a longer boiling time is required. In theory, the time should be increased by 5 minutes for each 300-meter (1000-foot) rise in altitude.[13] For example, at 4000 m (~12,000 foot) above sea level, water boils at 86°C (187°F), so ≥60 minutes is required for disinfection.

A way to increase the disinfectant effect of boiling is to use "double boiling." Boil the instruments for 30 to 40 minutes. Let them cool and then boil for another 30 to 40 minutes.[14]

Various techniques can be improvised to boil medical equipment, including using a sieve, a vegetable steamer, or a sling.[15] To use a sieve (or colander), place the instruments in it and put it into a pan of boiling water. When the time has elapsed, lift the sieve out and let everything air dry. With a vegetable steamer, place the instruments in it, cover it tightly, and steam the instruments. Then drain the water and the instruments can cool without being touched. Alternatively, use a sling made from gauze or other thin material. Stretch a piece of gauze, in the form of a hammock, over a pot and tie the ends to the handles. Place wrapped equipment in the hammock and put a tight-fitting lid on the pot. When finished boiling (this takes more time, up to 4 hours, because the equipment is sealed in packages), transfer the packages to a baking pan or an oven grate wrapped in heavy paper for drying. A net bag can also be used to suspend wrapped or unwrapped small equipment in a pot.

Chemicals

There are a number of chemical disinfectants available, even in austere environments. To disinfect against different organisms, the equipment must be immersed in the chemical for the appropriate amount of time.

Hypochlorite Solutions

Hypochlorite (e.g., bleach) in varying concentrations has a wide range of activity against bacteria, fungi, viruses, and bacterial spores. It is an effective disinfectant, both for equipment and for medical areas such as operating rooms.

Thoroughly clean equipment before using bleach as a disinfectant, because its activity is reduced by the presence of a biofilm or organic material. Because bleach is corrosive to metal instruments, do not leave instruments in the solution longer than 30 minutes. As soon as they are removed, rinse and dry them.

In health care facilities, bleach is used to clean environmental surfaces, disinfect laundry and equipment, decontaminate blood spills, and decontaminate medical waste prior to disposal (Table 6-2). Bleach has also been recommended as a good way for intravenous (IV) drug addicts to clean needles for reuse (see the "Needles" section later in this chapter). In the past, health care workers used bleach to clean their hands.[16]

ALCOHOLS

Alcohols (e.g., methanol, ethanol, and isopropanol) are active against bacteria and viruses. Alcohols do not inactivate bacterial spores or hydrophilic viruses (i.e., poliovirus, *Coxsackie* virus).[17] When an alcohol solution of ≥70% concentration is used, immerse the equipment in the solution for ≥10 minutes, and for ≥12 hours if possible.[18] As with bleach, use alcohol as a disinfectant only after equipment has been cleaned—or, at least after all the visible surface dirt has been removed from the area to be disinfected.[8] To prepare a 70% ethanol solution, add eight parts 90% ethanol to two parts water. To prepare a 70% isopropanol solution, add seven parts standard isopropanol to three parts water.[13]

TABLE 6-2 Uses of Hypochlorite (Bleach) in Health Care Facilities

Use on	Purpose
Potable water	Controls waterborne pathogens. Hyperchlorination controls *Legionella* spp during outbreaks
Hemodialysis water and machines	Reduce bacterial growth and prevents bacterial sepsis
Flower vase water	Reduces risk of water for fresh flowers acting as reservoir for gram-negative pathogens
Dental appliances	Disinfect contaminated dental equipment
Tonometers	Prevent cross-transmission of microorganisms, especially adenovirus and herpes viruses
Hydrotherapy tank	Reduces risk of cross-transmission from pathogens in water
Manikins	Prevent potential cross-transmission of herpes simplex virus and other pathogens when practicing mouth-to-mouth resuscitation
Syringes and needles	Reduce risk of HIV cross-transmission when the same needles and syringes are used by multiple people
Blood spills	Prevent acquisition of blood-borne pathogens, especially HIV and hepatitis B and C viruses, if there is contact with non-intact skin or there is a sharp injury
Environmental surfaces	Reduce risk of cross-transmission from health care personnel's hands during *Clostridium difficile* outbreaks
Laundry	Reduces risk of pathogen cross-transmission and laundry worker acquisition
Medical waste	Reduces microbial load associated with regulated medical waste
Antisepsis	Reduces risk of pathogen transmission from health care personnel's hands
Dental therapy	Disinfects root canal

Adapted, with permission, from Rutala and Weber.[16]

Aldehydes

Aldehydes (e.g., formaldehyde, glutaraldehyde) are potent, potentially dangerous chemicals, but they are relatively inexpensive. Formaldehyde, usually available wherever a laboratory or mortuary exists, is active against bacteria, viruses, and fungi, but has a slow action against tubercle bacilli.[8] Prepare an aldehyde disinfectant solution by adding one part 4% formaldehyde to three parts water. Soak instruments for 30 minutes or, if they were used on infected patients, for 1 hour before drying and sterilizing.[10,13]

Povidone-Iodine

Povidone-iodine (PVP; Betadine) may be used for disinfecting instruments if nothing else is available. The CDC supports its use, citing manufacturers' data demonstrating that while it is fungicidal, virucidal, and bactericidal, it may not be tuberculocidal[19] and is not sporicidal. There is more active free iodine (as iodophors, the active ingredient) in disinfectants, such as 10% scrub and solution, than in antiseptics.[20] The recommendation is to add one part 10% povidone-iodine solution to three parts water and soak instruments for 15 minutes.[13]

STERILIZATION

Sterilization removes or destroys all forms of microbial life, including bacterial spores.[8]

Methods

There are several methods for sterilization, but only the methods using heat are useful in austere environments. Clean and open instruments, then wrap them in paper (including newspaper) or tightly woven cloth. Double wrapping generally gives the equipment a shelf life of several weeks. The ideal wrap is a layer of cloth inside a paper cover.[13] If instruments or cloth packs are kept in metal boxes for autoclaving, the boxes must have multiple holes in the bottom to let the dry air "run out" of the box.[14]

Moist Heat: Pressure Cooker

Moist heat is the most effective method for sterilization in austere situations, although the necessary equipment may not be available.

If you can find one, a home pressure cooker will sterilize medical equipment very well. (Note that this is not a "double-boiler," but a sealed cooker with a pressure gauge, such as those used for home canning. The combination of steam and pressure sterilizes the equipment.) Home pressure cookers do not have a thermometer: Use time and the pressure gauge to decide when sterilization is complete. Generally, you should boil items for at least 30 minutes under 3 to 5 pounds pressure.[15] For an extra measure of safety, add another 30 minutes.

To sterilize equipment using a pressure cooker[14]:

1. Add water, preferably distilled or fresh rainwater. to lessen mineral deposits that have to be cleaned off. Add enough water so the cooker won't run dry during the process.
2. Put the equipment on the pressure cooker tray over the water and close the lid. Do not stuff the equipment in; the steam must circulate to be effective. Put any metal container containing equipment on its side with the top removed, so the steam will circulate.
3. Open the valve and apply heat. Bring the cooker to a full boil. It will begin whistling like a tea kettle when ready. When it stops expelling air and water from the valve, close it.
4. Only at that point should you begin timing. (The sterilization process will be ineffective if you begin timing before it is boiling.)
5. Once the process is done, take the cooker off the heat and, when it has cooled and the steam is out, open the valve. Unlock the cooker and let the equipment dry by evaporation as it cools. Equipment packs may need to be placed on a drying rack. The time required to cool off depends on the material, but usually is at least 30 minutes. Glass and culture media can take several hours to cool. To cool the equipment quickly, run cool (sterile) water over it. Caution: this may cause any glass to shatter.
6. Clean the pressure cooker with distilled water or fresh rainwater after each use; do not use detergents. Check the gasket, pressure vent, gauge, and other parts; you don't want it to

explode on you. If the cooker has a manual, read it to determine any special maintenance requirements, time variations for sterilization, how much water to add, and how to tell when it is safe to open it.[13]

Dry Heat

OVEN

An oven is normally used for hot air sterilization, but this takes a long time. Equipment must be able to withstand temperatures of at least 160°C (320°F) for 120 minutes or 170°C (340°F) for 60 minutes.[21] Do not start timing until the desired temperature has been reached. Be careful not to exceed 170°C (340°F) or metal instruments may be damaged.

To eliminate most moisture and decrease the chance of metal equipment rusting, leave the door open for a few minutes while heating the oven. Use this method for surgical instruments and high-temperature glass or plastics, but not for textiles. (See the "Dressings and Other Textiles" section in this chapter.) Heat the oven to 160°C (320°F) to disinfect oils, ointments, waxes, and powders. Bake them for 2 hours.

FIRE

Equipment "soused" and "flambéed" are two common methods to quickly disinfect small metallic medical equipment in austere settings. The recipients of this affection are usually pins (e.g., to trephine nails or open blisters), knives (e.g., to incise and drain abscesses or remove foreign bodies), and needles (e.g., to suture or remove foreign bodies). Dip the instrument in alcohol, preferably the highest concentration available, and set fire to it. This is not a completely reliable sterilization method and will damage the instruments. If alcohol is not available, heat the "business end" of the instrument with an open flame until it glows red. This is an effective sterilization method, but it will also damage any instrument on which it is used.[13]

REUSING SPECIFIC EQUIPMENT—METHODS AND SAFETY

Syringes

There are two types of syringes: disposable and reusable. The main differences relate to the material used to make the barrel and plunger of the syringe.

Reusable Syringes

A reusable syringe's body and plunger are made of either glass or a plastic that can be autoclaved. Even though these instruments may sometimes be called "permanent," autoclaving eventually breaks down the rubber on a "reusable" plastic plunger and the glazing on the glass plunger wears out.[9]

STERILIZATION

The best method to sterilize syringes is to use a rack to suspend the barrel and plunger. The World Health Organization (WHO) reports a 40% failure rate with other methods—probably because the syringe surfaces in contact with the tray are not accessible to the steam; thus, some organisms survive.

Make a holder by bending metal in an "S" configuration so that the syringe bodies, plungers, and needles can be suspended with minimal contact with the rack itself; they should hang freely. Be sure to take the plungers out of the syringes or they may break.

An alternate sterilization method is to wrap the plungers and cylinders in an operating room (OR) towel and push the needles through the cloth. No item should be in contact with another. Fold to make a pack and autoclave, or use a pressure cooker as described previously.[9]

Single-Use Syringes

The danger of reusing syringes, even though this practice is common throughout the world, appears to negate any good produced by medical treatment. Every year the reuse of dirty syringes infects millions of people with acquired immune deficiency syndrome (AIDS) and hepatitis and "causes 1.3 million early deaths, a loss of 26 million years of life, and an annual burden of US $535 million in direct medical costs."[22] Young adults are most affected.

If you still plan on trying to sterilize disposable syringes, understand that they will generally melt when heated to sterilizing temperatures, but they can be autoclaved several times before deforming beyond usefulness.[9]

Needles

Reusable Needles

Reusable needles generally have a Luer lock attachment to fasten to the syringe (as do many disposable ones) and are made of a harder metal than the disposable needles so that they can be sharpened. They also come with a needle plunger so anything trapped in the needle cylinder can be removed.[9]

Sharpening Permanent Needles

According to the editors of *Survival and Austere Medicine*, this is how to sharpen a permanent needle[9]: Place a drop of light oil (sewing machine, light machine, or gun oil) on a fine sharpening stone. Draw the bevel of the needle (flat part of tip) back and forth at a uniform angle with no rocking. The goal is to keep the bevel the same length as on a new needle. Any rocking side to side will cause the bevel to become rounded, which needs to be corrected. Changing the angle of attack against the stone will cause, at best, a dull needle and, at worst, a hook on the point. After sharpening for a bit, a burr will form on the sides of the bevel—this is a thin edge of metal. Remove it by gently drawing the needle on the side to the top, forming two facets along the top of the point.

Always finish by giving one rub along the bevel and one to each facet. When finished, check it with a magnifying glass. Needles should be soaked overnight in trichloroethylene to remove any oil. Then, polish with a soft cloth and push water through the needle to make sure the cylinder is clear. If you do not have access to oil and a solvent to remove it, then sharpen and clean the needle using hot soapy water (including inside the barrel using fine wire). This procedure should be done only when the needle seems to be getting dull, not after every use.[9] Maurice King's *A Medical Laboratory for Developing Countries* (Oxford University Press, 1973) contains more complete instructions and good illustrations.

Single-Use Needle on Same Patient

Patients with diabetes routinely reuse the same syringe for up to 1 week, which is fine if it is kept in a clean container. During this time, they do not decontaminate the syringe. Likewise, in situations of scarcity, a needle should be able to be used on the same patient over a short time period (e.g., 1 week). This assumes that care will be taken to keep the needle clean and that it won't be used on anyone else.[9]

Reuse of Single-Use Device Needles

Unsterilized SUD needles are responsible for 1.3 million deaths per year, mostly in developing countries.[23] In addition, it is estimated that 160,000 new HIV infections and millions of new cases of hepatitis B and C are caused each year from the use of dirty needles.[24]

Disinfection Method for Needles and Syringes

It is not possible to clean the interior of disposable syringes and needles well enough to use them safely on multiple patients. Although syringe reuse is a common practice throughout the world, it is so dangerous that it negates any good produced by medical treatment. Only when no other option exists should cleaning and reusing syringes be considered. If that is the case, the best option is one that the US governmental agencies recommend for needles and syringes potentially contaminated with HIV. That is, they should be thoroughly cleaned and then immersed in full-strength bleach (5.25% sodium hypochlorite) for 10 minutes.[16,25-27] Presumably, they would be allowed to dry, although injecting small amounts of bleach is harmless.[28]

Respiratory, Anesthesia, and Resuscitation Equipment

In general, it is unnecessary to sterilize respiratory and anesthetic equipment, because spore-bearing organisms are not a cause of respiratory infections.[8] High-level disinfection, or even a lower level of decontamination, often suffices.

Anesthesia Equipment

The internal circuit in mechanical ventilators can often be autoclaved. The external (or patient) circuit should be changed every 48 hours or between patients. Both the external circuit and the humidifiers require high-level disinfecting. Heated-water humidifiers, however, need only be cleaned, dried, and refilled with sterile water every 48 to 72 hours.[8]

Nebulizers should be cleaned and rinsed in alcohol every 48 hours.

Resuscitation/Respiratory Equipment

Bag-valve-masks (BVMs) should be washed and cleaned as soon as possible after each use. Laryngoscope blades should be washed after each use, ideally using hot, soapy water to remove secretions. A surgical brush helps to clean the blade. High-level disinfection should follow.[29]

SUD endotracheal tubes can be reused if they are cleaned and given high-level disinfection. Note that using heat will probably damage them, so immerse them in a 70% alcohol solution for 10 minutes. Allow the tubes to dry before reuse.[8]

Suction catheters can be difficult to clean. The best method is to suction clean water through them. Then use a high-level disinfectant and allow them to air dry before reuse.

Surgical Instruments

Sharp/Delicate Instruments

Sharp or delicate instruments should be chemically sterilized using alcohol. Acetone can also be used if the equipment does not contain plastic or polymers. Rinse them in hot, sterile water and let them dry before reuse.[11]

Lightweight Surgical Instruments

Lightweight surgical instruments, such as ophthalmic or plastic instruments, can be sterilized in a pressure cooker or autoclave. Heavier surgical instruments (without a fine tolerance or sharp edges), such as mosquito clamps, towel clips, and large needle holders, may be disinfected in boiling water.[11]

Endoscopic Equipment

Laparoscopic or arthroscopic telescopes (optic portions of the endoscopic set) should be sterilized before each use. Do not use iodophors, chlorine solutions, alcohols, quaternary ammonium compounds, or phenolics, because they lack proven efficacy against all microorganisms found on these instruments or have materials incompatibility.[19] If this is not feasible, use high-level disinfection. Sterilize heat-stable endoscopic accessories, such as trocars, using an autoclave/pressure cooker or dry-heat oven.[5]

Dressings and Other Textiles

Disinfection can be accomplished with the following methods[9,13]:

Ironing: Cover a table with a cloth that has previously been ironed. Then, dampen that cloth and the one to be disinfected with boiling water and press with a very hot iron for several passes. Steam as you iron.
Solar: Hang the textile in full sunlight for 6 hours per side.
Washing: When dressings are in short supply, they can be disinfected by (a) washing and then boiling them for 5 minutes or (b) washing, rinsing, and then soaking them for 30 minutes in a 0.1% chlorine solution or a 5% Lysol solution.

"Sterile" Dressings

Clean and disinfect cloth for a dressing by boiling it in water for 15 minutes or by saturating it with alcohol. Let it dry before use. Using any of the sterilization methods described previously will also sterilize it. Normally, clean and disinfected is sufficient. If using dry-heat (oven) sterilization, remember that the exact time and temperature required will vary according to the volume of material treated, volume of the autoclave, contamination level, and moisture content of the cloth: the minimum is 160°C to 170°C (320°F–340°F) for 2 to 4 hours.[30]

When reusing dressings (common in austere battlefield conditions), wash the gauze dressings (or immerse in saline) to remove stains, dry them, and then sterilize using dry heat.[31]

To make sterilization easier, wrap dressings in aluminum foil and place the package on a flat pan in the oven. Bake at 350°F (177°C) for 3 hours. When they have cooled, label each dressing with its size.[32]

Gloves, Tubing, and Plastic Items

Gloves

While disposable gloves are preferred, they may not be available—or may be too expensive to use only once. Single-use surgical gloves may be reused up to three times if they are not obviously torn. After that, additional autoclaving breaks down the rubber and the gloves develop microscopic tears that put the patient and clinician at risk.

To prepare disposable gloves for reuse, first blow into them to ensure they do not leak. If there are holes, patch them from the inside. Next, decontaminate the gloves by soaking them in a 0.5% chlorine solution for 10 minutes, or simply wash and rinse them. Cover the inside with talcum powder and let them dry thoroughly; otherwise, they will stick together and be unusable. Sterilize by autoclaving or perform high-level disinfection using steam or boiling.[33]

Rubber and Plastic

Rubber and plastic deteriorate with repeated sterilization. Wash all tubes, catheters, gloves, and other rubber or plastic equipment for reuse in cold water immediately after use, next, wash in warm water with soap, and, finally, rinse in water. Dry rubber equipment thoroughly. It sticks to itself and becomes damaged if stored moist.[34]

Plastic Items (Airways, Syringes, and the Like)

How to sterilize plastic equipment depends on the type of plastic.[9] Unfortunately, that may be difficult to discern. General guidelines are as follows:

- *High-density polyethylene (HDPE):* Translucent. Autoclave at 121°C (250°F) for no more than 15 minutes.
- *Polypropylene (PP):* Translucent. Autoclave at 121°C (250°F).
- *Polymethylpentene (PMP):* Clear, brittle at room temperature, can crack or break if dropped. Autoclave at 121°C (250°F).
- *Polycarbonate (PC):* Clear. Autoclave at 121°C (250°F).
- *Polytetrafluoroethylene (PTFE):* Not translucent. Autoclave at 121°C (250°F) or put in oven at 160°C (320°F) for 2 hours or 170°C (340°F) for 1 hour.

Glassware

In general, clean and then sterilize glassware used for laboratory or patient care. Use a pressure cooker or autoclave. However, note that glassware can crack or shatter if the autoclave or pressure cooker is opened too soon or if cool water is poured over hot glass (known as speed cooling). In addition, some glassware, especially pipettes, may not fit in a pressure cooker.

REFERENCES

1. *Altered Standards of Care in Mass Casualty Events*. Prepared by Health Systems Research Inc., under Contract No. 290-04-0010. AHRQ Publication No. 05-0043. Rockville, MD: Agency for Healthcare Research and Quality; April 2005:10-13.
2. Feigal DW, Director, Center for Devices and Radiological Health, Food and Drug Administration. Testimony on Reuse of Medical Devices before the Senate Health, Education, Labor and Pensions Committee, June 27, 2000.
3. Lewis C. Reusing medical devices: ensuring safety the second time around. *FDA Consumer Mag*. September-October 2000. www.fda.gov/fdac/features/2000/500_reuse.html. Accessed September 17, 2006.

4. Center for Biologics Evaluation and Research, Center for Devices and Radiological Health Office of Device Evaluation, Food and Drug Administration, U.S. Department of Health and Human Services. *Reprocessing Medical Devices in Health Care Settings: Validation Methods and Labeling Guidance for Industry and Food and Drug Administration Staff.* Document issued March 7, 2015. www.fda.gov/downloads/MedicalDevices/DeviceRegulationandGuidance/GuidanceDocuments/UCM253010.pdf. Accessed August 25, 2015.
5. CDC. Sterilization or disinfection of medical devices. August 20, 2002. www.cdc.gov/ncidod/dhqp/bp_sterilization_medDevices.html#. Accessed September 18, 2006.
6. Landro L. Hospitals reuse medical devices to lower costs. *Wall Street J.* March 19, 2008:D1.
7. Schröer P. Reuse of single-use medical devices. *Regulatory Affairs Focus Mag.* July 2000. www.raps.org/s_raps/rafocus_article.asp?TRACKID=&CID=61&DID=6222. Accessed September 17, 2006.
8. Skilton R. Decontamination procedures for medical equipment. *Update in Anesthesia.* 1997;7(5):1. http://tabula.ws/archive/a_day_after/medical/nuclear_biologic_chemical/deconmedequip.pdf. Accessed September 13, 2006.
9. The Remote, Austere, Wilderness and Third World Medicine Discussion Board Moderators. *Survival and Austere Medicine: An Introduction.* 2nd ed. 2005:44-48. www.aussurvivalist.com/downloads/AM%20Final%202.pdf. Accessed June 8, 2007.
10. Husum H, Ang SC, Fosse E. *War Surgery: Field Manual.* Penang, Malaysia: Third World Network; 1995:69.
11. Schwab L. *Primary Eye Care in Developing Nations.* Oxford, UK: Oxford University Press, 1987:143-144.
12. Husum H, Ang SC, Fosse E. *War Surgery: Field Manual.* Penang, Malaysia: Third World Network; 1995:656-657.
13. The Remote, Austere, Wilderness and Third World Medicine Discussion Board Moderators. *Survival and Austere Medicine: An Introduction.* 2nd ed. 2005:50. www.aussurvivalist.com/downloads/AM%20Final%202.pdf. Accessed June 8, 2007.
14. Husum H, Ang SC, Fosse E. *War Surgery: Field Manual.* Penang, Malaysia: Third World Network; 1995:658-659.
15. Olson LM. *Improvised Equipment in the Home Care of the Sick.* Philadelphia, PA: W.B. Saunders; 1928:17, 96-97.
16. Rutala WA, Weber DJ. Uses of inorganic hypochlorite (bleach) in health-care facilities. *Clin Microbiol Rev.* 1997;10(4):597-610.
17. Klein M, DeForest A. The inactivation of viruses by germicides. *Chem Specialists Manuf Assoc Proc.* 1963;49:116-118.
18. The Remote, Austere, Wilderness and Third World Medicine Discussion Board Moderators. *Survival and Austere Medicine: An Introduction.* 2nd ed. 2005:50-54. www.aussurvivalist.com/downloads/AM%20Final%202.pdf. Accessed June 8, 2007.
19. Rutala WA, Weber DJ, CDC Healthcare Infection Control Practices Advisory Committee. Guideline for disinfection and sterilization in healthcare facilities, 2008. www.cdc.gov/hicpac/pdf/guidelines/Disinfection_Nov_2008.pdf. Accessed February 28, 2015.
20. Favero MS, Bond WW. Chemical disinfection of medical and surgical materials. In: Block SS, ed. *Disinfection, Sterilization, and Preservation.* Philadelphia, PA: Lea & Febiger; 1991:617-641.
21. World Health Organization. Waste minimization, recycling, and reuse. In: Prüss A, Giroult E, Rushbrook P, eds. *Safe Management of Wastes From Health-Care Activities.* Geneva, Switzerland: WHO; 1999:58-60. www.who.int/water_sanitation_health/medicalwaste/058to060.pdf. Accessed September 18, 2006.
22. World Health Organization. Fact sheet #321: Injection safety. www.who.int/injection_safety/toolbox/en/InjectionFactSheet2002.pdf. Accessed February 18, 2009.
23. Manalo K. WHO says 1.3 million die annually due to unsterilized syringes. *AHN News.* October 23, 2007. http://www.allheadlinenews.com/articles/7008919926. Accessed June 5, 2008.
24. Carlsen W. Lethal injection: when medical devices kill. *Amnesty Int Mag.* Winter 2002. www.amnestyusa.org/magazine/winter_2002/lethal_injection/html. Accessed September 17, 2006.
25. Klein M, Deforest A. Antiviral action of germicides. *Soap Chem Specialist.* 1963;39:70-72, 95-97.
26. Klein M, Deforest A. Principles of viral inactivation. In: Block SS, ed. *Disinfection, Sterilization, and Preservation.* Philadelphia, PA: Lea & Febiger; 1965:422-434.
27. Klein M, Deforest A. The chemical inactivation of viruses. *Federation Proceedings.* 1965;24:319.
28. Froner GA, Rutherford GW, Rokeach M. Injection of sodium hypochlorite by intravenous drug users [letter]. *JAMA.* 1987;258(3):325.

29. Yeats M. Maintaining your laryngoscope. *Pract Proced.* 1004;4(9):1. www.nda.ox.ac.uk/wfsa/html/u04/u04_018.htm. Accessed September 13, 2006.
30. Biosafety Program. Sterilization. Environment, Health, & Safety Division, Lawrence Livermore Laboratories. www.lbl.gov/ehs/biosafety/Biosafety_Manual/html/sterilization.shtml. Accessed December 8, 2006.
31. King M, Bewes P, Cairns J, et al, eds. *Primary Surgery, Vol. 1: Non-Trauma.* Oxford, UK: Oxford Medical Publishing; 1990:10.
32. The Remote, Austere, Wilderness and Third World Medicine Discussion Board Moderators. *Survival and Austere Medicine: An Introduction.* 2nd ed. 2005:96. www.aussurvivalist.com/downloads/AM%20Final%202.pdf. Accessed June 8, 2007.
33. Blouse A, Gomez P, eds. *Emergency Obstetric Care.* Baltimore, MD: JHPIEGO; 2003:79.
34. Husum H, Ang SC, Fosse E. *War Surgery: Field Manual.* Penang, Malaysia: Third World Network; 1995:70.

III PATIENT ASSESSMENT/ STABILIZATION

7 | Vital Signs, Measurements, and Triage

PEDIATRICS

Age

Knowing a child's age is important to determine normal vital signs, disease prevalence, and the appropriate medications. It is also an indicator of social milestones. The easiest way to determine a child's age is to ask the parent or check available records. However, in cultures where birth records are unavailable, as well as during acute out-of-hospital or emergency department (ED) events, this information may not be easy to get.

Without records, one way to estimate a child's approximate age is to count the number of teeth present and then add six to derive the age in months.[1] Another way is to have the child sit upright (with the head in a neutral position), then raise one arm over his head and try to touch the opposite ear (Fig. 7-1). This "overhead test" has a sensitivity of 90% and a specificity of 78% (positive predictive value 93%, negative predictive value 68%). If the child successfully performs this test, he is most likely ≥6 years old, which is the age to begin school and to receive other benefits in many cultures. If a child fails this test, there is a good chance that he is <6 years old, but it is less clear, because other factors, such as malnutrition, may influence the results. The test works because a 6-year-old child's humerus is long enough to raise the elbow so that the forearm extends across the head and allows the fingers to reach the opposite ear.[2]

Height

Any firm surface can be marked in 1-cm (or 0.5-inch) increments to measure a patient's height. For ambulatory patients, use a vertical surface, such as a wall or the side of a doorway. For infants, children, and bedridden patients, mark the side rails of stretchers and beds with indelible ink. Once a child's height is known, the weight can be estimated.

Weight

Correct weight estimates are crucial in determining pediatric medication and fluid doses. When asked, the parents of children aged from 1 to 11 years old can estimate their child's weight within 10% of the measured weight only 78% of the time. All other forms of guessing a child's weight, including the Argyll, the Advanced Pediatric Life Support (APLS), and the Best Guess methods, perform poorly.[3] If the parents aren't available, use the following formula for children 1 to 13 years old:

$$(3 \times \text{age in years}) + 7 = \text{weight in kilograms (kg)}$$

This formula underestimates weight by about 7%, as opposed to > 33% for the APLS formula.[4]

Although many clinicians still use the Broselow tape, it is inaccurate in most children >10 years old, falls within 10% of the measured weight only 61% of the time, and is less accurate with older children.[5-9] A much better method is to use the Mercy TAPE (Fig. 7-2), which integrates mid-arm circumference (MAC) and humeral length (HL), a surrogate of height, to dramatically improve its predictive performance.[10] The Mercy TAPE works well with children not only in developed countries, but also has been shown to be accurate in India and Mali.[11]

In children, measure the MAC at the midpoint of the humerus with the arm hanging down at the child's side. Measure the HL from the upper edge of the posterior border of the acromion process to the tip of the olecranon process. Record the measurements to the nearest millimeter.[12]

Beam Scale for Infants

When standard scales to weigh infants are not available, make a beam scale (Fig. 7-3). If finely calibrated, the beam scale may also be used to weigh smaller items, such as medications.

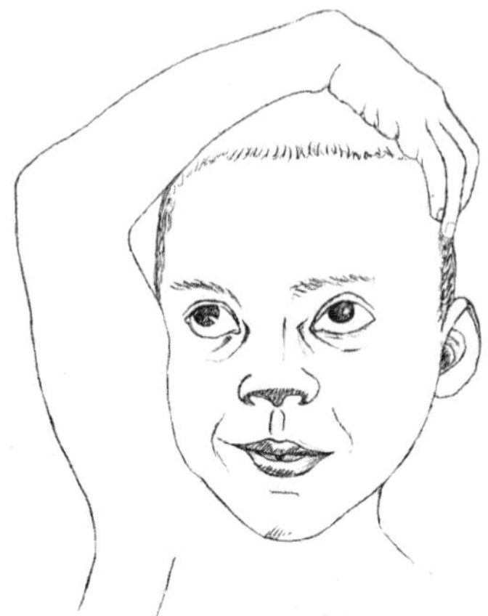

FIG. 7-1. A child <6 years old cannot reach his opposite ear.

Humeral Length (cm)	Partial Weight A (kg)	Mid-Upper Arm Circumference (cm)	Partial Weight B (kg)
9	0.5	10	2.8
10	0.7	11	3.8
11	0.9	12	4.6
12	1.5	13	4.9
13	2.0	14	5.3
14	2.8	15	5.9
15	3.4	16	6.5
16	4.2	17	7.4
17	5.0	18	8.0
18	6.1	19	9.4
19	7.2	20	10.9
20	8.1	21	12.4
21	9.1	22	14.3
22	10.4	23	16.5
23	11.4	24	18.0
24	12.6	25	20.5
25	13.7	26	23.4
26	14.7	27	25.5
27	16.6	28	27.8
28	18.3	29	30.5
29	19.6	30	33.3
30	21.4	31	36.3
31	23.7	32	39.6
32	25.5	33	44.8
33	27.3	34	46.5
34	29.2	35	50.2
35	31.0	36	53.2
36	33.5	37	55.7
37	34.5	38	60.3
38	36.5	39	61.1
39	38.2	40	67.0

FIG. 7-2. Mercy TAPE. Add "partial weight A" and "partial weight B" to get the child's weight. *(Reproduced with permission from Abdel-Rahman and Ridge.[13])*

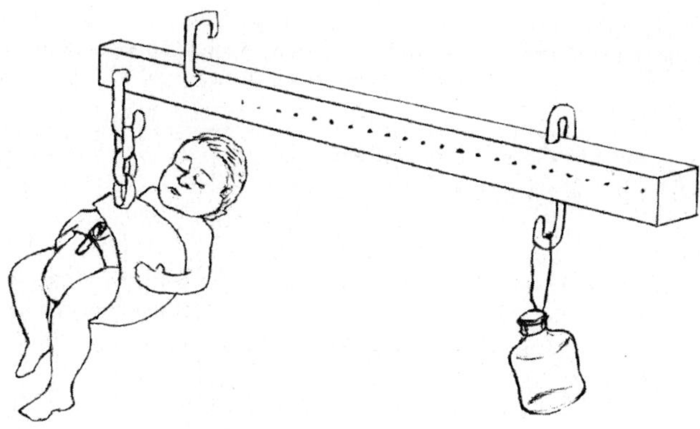

FIG. 7-3. Improvised beam scale to weigh infants.

To make a beam scale, use a straight, rigid pole of bamboo, metal, or dry wood, ~1 m long. Mount a hook close to one end from which the beam will be suspended. Put another hook about 5 cm away, between the first hook and the nearest end of the beam. This is where the infant or substance to be weighed is suspended. A fixed weight is also suspended from the beam, but on a moveable slide (e.g., metal wire). The weight can be a bag, bottle, or other container filled with sand. Mark gradations on the beam for each weight increment. Use standard weights to calibrate the scale initially, so the gradations are accurate. Hang the known weight at the end of the scale (i.e., where the infant would be) and mark the point on the beam where the sliding weight is when the scale balances evenly.[14] Large increments (1 L of water weighs 2.2 kg, 0.5 L weighs 1.1 kg, etc.) and smaller increments (use the weight of a common coin and its multiples) can be easily determined. If a local merchant (jeweler, grain dealer, etc.) has standard weights, try to borrow them for more accurate calibration of the scale.

ADULTS

Height

If an adult's height can be measured only in a sitting position, such as with a wheelchair-dependent patient, measure each arm span in centimeters, from midsternum to the end of the extended middle finger (half-arm span). Use the longer of these measurements in the following formula: Height ≅ (0.73 × [2 × half-arm span]) + 43 cm.[15] A simpler method is to double the longest measurement from midsternum to the tip of the patient's long finger.[16]

Patient-reported height is the best bedside method to estimate true height and can be used to calculate ideal body weight (IBW). Physician and nurse estimates of true height are substantially less accurate, as is true height obtained from a regression formula that uses measured tibial length.[17]

Actual Weight

A patient's own weight estimate is the most accurate method to approximate true actual body weight. Clinicians' bedside estimate of a patient's weight is unacceptably low, and the conventional 70-kg/60-kg male/female IBW standard misclassifies most patients by 5 kg, and many by 10 kg. The following method is a good way to estimate adults' actual body weights. These formulas can be preprogrammed in a computer for easier use.[18]

$$\text{Male's weight (kg)} = [\text{knee height (cm)} \times 1.10] + [\{\text{MAC (cm)} \times 3.07\} - 75.81]$$

$$\text{Female's weight (kg)} = [\text{knee height (cm)} \times 1.101] + [\{\text{MAC (cm)} \times 2.81\} - 66.04]$$

Knee height: The distance between the thigh prominence with the knee bent at 90 degrees proximally and the plantar aspect of the foot at the heel with the ankle bent at 90 degrees distally.

MAC: In adults, palpate the humeral head proximally and the lateral humeral condyle distally. Wrap a tape measure around the arm midway between these landmarks so that it contacts the skin at all points but does not compress the soft tissue.

Use the actual weight to determine the patient's body mass index (BMI), which correlates with nutritional status. The formula to calculate BMI is body weight (kg) divided by [height (m) squared], or [kg ÷ m^2].[15] In adults, a BMI ≥18.5 is normal; BMI <16 is severe malnutrition.[19]

Ideal Body Weight

Knowledge of a patient's ideal body weight (IBW) can be important for drug dosing and for calculating ventilator volume settings. It can be calculated from the patient's height using the Devine formula, which is most applicable for people ≥60 inches (152 cm) tall[17]:

- IBW for men (kg) = 50 + [2.3 × (height in inches – 60)]
- IBW for women (kg) = 45.5 + [2.3 × (height in inches – 60)]

MEASURING TEMPERATURE WITHOUT A THERMOMETER

In austere circumstances, a thermometer normally is not available. Generally, caregivers notice a tactile fever in only about half of all children with a measurable fever. Elevated tactile temperatures, as measured at home by mothers touching their child's forehead, have moderate (46%–73%) correlation with fevers recorded in the ED or hospital.[20,21] However, for children >2 years old with a temperature ≥38.9°C (102°F), tactile assessment can determine that a child has a fever 98% of the time.[20]

If you do have a thermometer and you need to convert the numbers from Celsius (Centigrade; C) to Fahrenheit (F) or vice versa, use these formulas:

$$°F = (°C \times 1.8) + 32°$$

$$°C = (°F - 32°) \div 1.8$$

An Osborn or J wave on an electrocardiogram (ECG) can suggest hypothermia, especially in elderly patients in whom the diagnosis is not suspected. This elevation at the QRS-ST junction (Fig. 7-4) occurs in about 80% of hypothermic patients (a core body temperature ≤95°F [35°C]) and in nearly all patients whose temperature is <90°F (32.2°C). The waves' sizes appear to be inversely related to temperature, but otherwise they do not appear to have any prognostic value.[22]

PULSE AND RESPIRATIONS

Measuring Time

To time pulse or respiration measurements without a watch, clock, or other timepiece, you must either count the pulse beats or respirations yourself or make a timer.

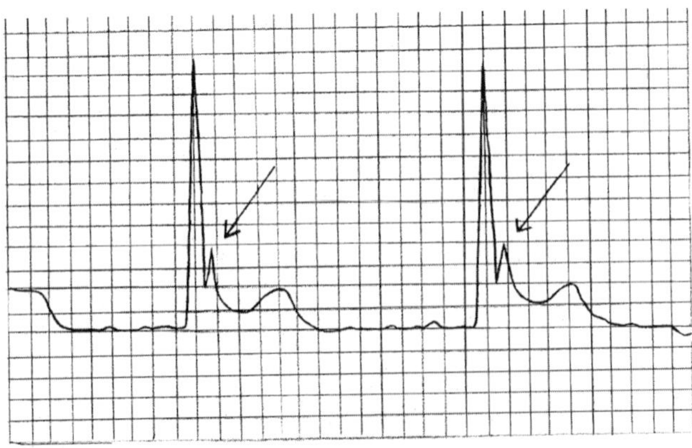

FIG. 7-4. Osborn or J wave.

Counting is not as accurate as using a watch, but time may be measured by counting in any situation: Simply count "one-thousand-one, one-thousand-two," and so on, while someone else counts the pulse. To calculate pulse rate per minute, count to "one-thousand-six" (about 6 seconds), then multiply the counted pulsations by 10. Simply estimating time without counting always results in underestimation.

To make a simple, portable sand timer, use a blood collection tube or other piece of glass that can be molded when heated. Heat the middle of the tube and stretch to narrow the diameter. Then, if both ends of the tube are open, seal one end by heating it over a flame. Next, sift some sand through a fine strainer. Dry the sifted sand completely by using sunlight or an oven. Stand the tube upright and put enough sand in the top part so that the sand takes 1 minute to run from the top, through the narrow middle, to the bottom section (Fig. 7-5). During construction, you will need a watch, a clock, or a previously calibrated timer to check the initial timing. After the correct amount of sand is in the tube, seal the open end either by heating or with a stopper. Because these tubes break easily, store the timer in a padded box.

Water timers also work well. Heat the end of a long, narrow glass tube. Stretch that end and break it, leaving a very tiny opening. A micropipette with a very tiny opening may also suffice without the need to work with heated glass. In either case, make a narrow mark near the top (near the wide opening) of the tube with nail polish, tape, or another marker, or by etching the glass. Cover the narrow end of the tube and fill the tube with water exactly to the level of the mark. Let the water drip out of the tube for 1 minute. Mark the tube again at the exact water level after 1 minute (Fig. 7-6). Voilà, you have a timer!

Finally, if you have no clock or wristwatch for measuring pulse and respirations, use the clock or timer function on the now ubiquitous (even in the least-developed regions of the world) cell phones—if it has a second hand—or download a free stopwatch app.

Alternate Sites to Palpate the Pulse

When you cannot palpate a pulse at the typical wrist or femoral areas, try one of these sites:

Carotid artery: Slide your fingers from the midline to the opposite side of the neck from where you are standing and stop at the anterior border of the sternocleidomastoid muscle. The carotid should be palpable. Do not press too hard and cause a vagal response.

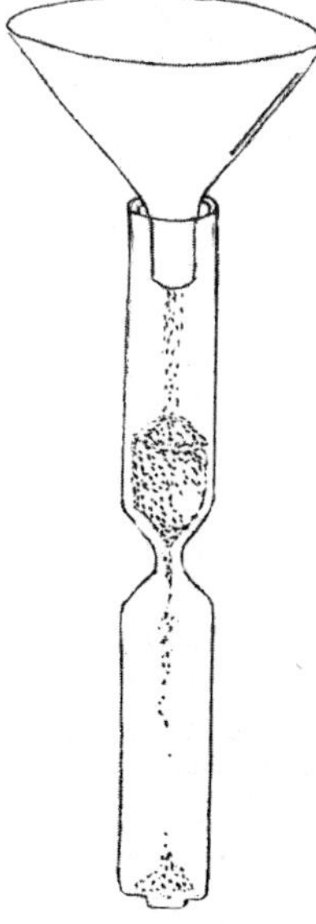

FIG. 7-5. Making a sand timer.

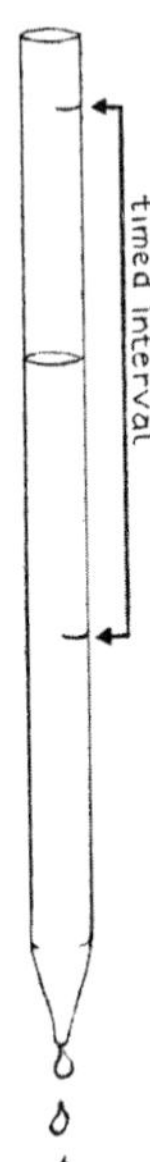

FIG. 7-6. Homemade water timer.

Superficial temporal artery: This is accessible in nearly all patients. Put two fingers just anterior to the ear at the superior part of the tragus. The finger most proximal to the ear will normally feel the pulsation without difficulty.

Dorsalis pedis and posterior tibial (foot/ankle) arteries: These are often used to check for peripheral vascular integrity, and also to monitor the pulse, especially when the other sites are inaccessible. These arteries can also be used when drawing arterial blood gasses; it is much easier and safer to draw from these arteries than, for example, from the femoral arteries.

Palpating an Infant's Pulse

Palpating an infant's pulse, especially when they are critically ill and a decision must be made immediately about whether to begin resuscitation, can be very difficult. The easiest, fastest, and most successful method of determining infant cardiac activity can be applied in any situation, because it requires no equipment. It does not even require finding and palpating a pulse: Simply place your ear against the infant's chest wall and listen for heart sounds—direct auscultation (Fig. 7-7).

A study with experienced pediatric nurses trying to find a pulse in infants showed that the mean time to correctly identify the pulse rate using direct auscultation was 2.4 ± 1.2 seconds, with a 100% success rate. Palpation methods took longer and were less successful. The frequently used femoral pulse rate took 9.1 ± 5.9 seconds to find, with only a 43% success rate.[23]

Radial Pulse and Trauma Prognosis

A weak radial pulse in most trauma patients (at least those 18-50 years old without a head injury) indicates a markedly increased mortality (29%) compared to only 3% of those with a normal pulse (odds ratio: 15.2). There is also a strong likelihood that these patients will require intubation (odds ratio: 7.5) and admission to the intensive care unit (ICU) (odds ratio: 5.3). Patients with an absent radial pulse are usually dead or soon will be dead.[24] In addition, tachycardia is a much more reliable sign of hypovolemia than is blood pressure (BP).

BLOOD PRESSURE

"The ability to obtain a blood pressure measurement in an austere environment is often limited by time constraints, equipment availability, and noisy conditions."[24]

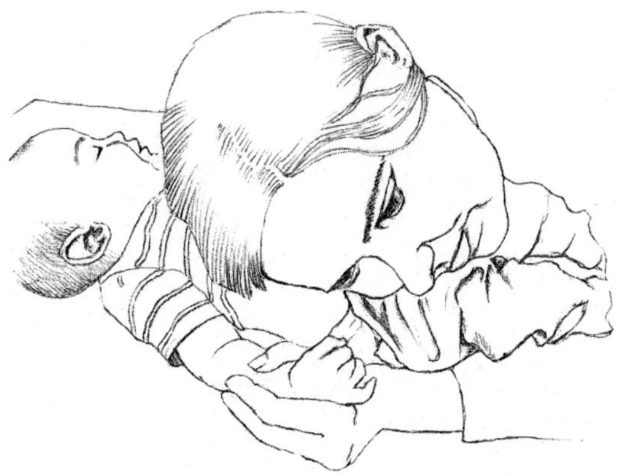

FIG. 7-7. Direct precordial auscultation.

Measuring Blood Pressure Without a Cuff

Estimating BP from a palpable pulse, for example, radial (>80 mm Hg), femoral (70-80 mm Hg), or carotid (60-70 mm Hg), overestimates the patient's actual BP.[25]

A useful finding is that patients with palpably cool extremities as compared with those of other patients have hypoperfusion. Especially when found in an arm and a leg, such patients have low cardiac indices, low pH, low bicarbonate levels, low mixed venous oxygen saturation (SvO_2), and elevated lactate levels.[26]

Measuring Blood Pressure Without a Stethoscope

When transporting patients by air or in a noisy ambulance, Korotkoff sounds (BP) may not be audible through a stethoscope. When a stethoscope is not readily available or cannot be used, palpate the systolic pressure. If done carefully, this method is as accurate as using a stethoscope.

If a pulse oximeter is available, it also can be used to measure the systolic BP when there is too much noise or vibration either to use a stethoscope or to palpate a pulse. Place the sensor on a finger, get a good waveform, inflate the sphygmomanometer until the waveform disappears, and then slowly deflate the cuff until the waveform reappears. This measurement is an accurate measure of the systolic pressure.[27]

Makeshift/Alternative Blood Pressure Cuff

Neonatal arm BP cuffs can be used successfully on adult forefingers, producing a "finger cuff." Only the mean BP equates to that taken on the arm.[28] If a manometer is available, some disposable (or non-disposable) pressure pumps for intravenous (IV) fluids and blood can be used as (a) a BP cuff if attached to a manometer or (b) an extremity tourniquet (clamp the tube when inflated). In large adults, these devices may only fit on their calf or forearm.

Wrist and Calf Blood Pressures

Blood pressure cuffs placed on the forearm (Fig. 7-8) and above the ankle (Fig. 7-9) deliver the same or nearly the same BP as when placed at the brachial artery (arm). Forearm or ankle measurement comes in handy with obese patients on whom the standard adult cuff is too small, for adults when only a child-sized cuff is available, or to avoid compressing an area with trauma. In addition, use a forearm or ankle BP to avoid periodically occluding an arteriovenous fistula (in dialysis patients) or an IV line. The mean and diastolic pressure readings are essentially equal in the arm and the ankle, but the systolic pressures are not. So, use the mean BP with a calf BP cuff. (Calculate this by multiplying the diastolic pressure by two and adding the systolic pressure. Then divide the result by three. Alternatively, take one-third of the difference between the systolic and diastolic pressures and add it to the diastolic pressure.)

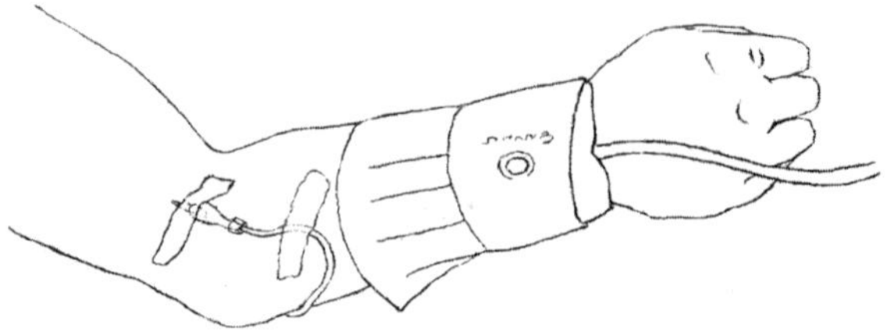

FIG. 7-8. BP cuff on forearm.

This difference between the calf and the arm BP readings is reflected in the normal ankle–brachial index (ABI), used to test for vascular compromise in the leg. The calf's systolic pressure is normally higher than that in the arm. To calculate ABI, divide the systolic pressure in the leg by that in the arm. Use a Doppler for accuracy. In the supine patient, the normal result is generally 0.9 to 1.2.

Preventing an Intravenous Tube From Backing Up

To prevent an IV from backing up and possibly contaminating the IV solution when the BP cuff inflates on the same extremity, run the IV tubing under the cuff, so that when it inflates, the IV stops. When the cuff deflates, the IV starts flowing again.[29]

Falsely High Blood Pressure Readings

Falsely high BP measurements result in patients taking unnecessary and potentially harmful medication. The following factors can result in inaccurate BP readings[30]:

If the:	BP can be falsely elevated by:
1. Patient has a full bladder.	10-15 mm Hg
2. Patient's back is unsupported.	5-10 mm Hg
3. Patient's feet are unsupported.	5-10 mm Hg
4. Patient's legs are crossed.	3-8 mm Hg
5. Sphygmomanometer cuff is over clothing.	10-40 mm Hg
6. Patient's arm is unsupported.	10 mm Hg
7. Patient is talking or has not had at least 3 minutes of quiet time prior to the measurement.	10-15 mm Hg

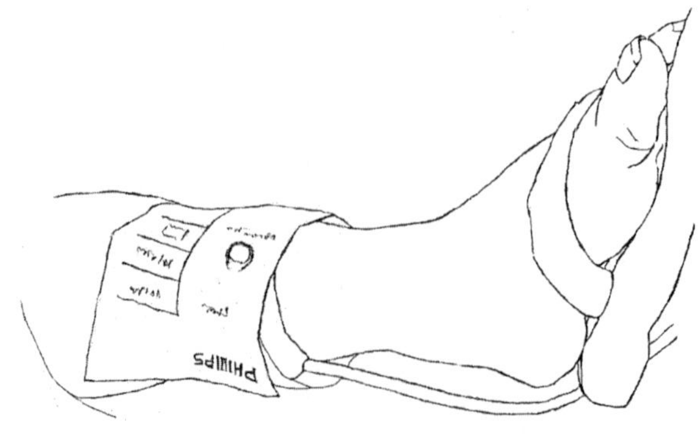

FIG. 7-9. BP cuff on the calf above the ankle.

GERIATRIC VITAL SIGNS

Elderly patients (≥75 years old) are frequently under-triaged, and sometimes over-triaged, on the basis of their vital signs. In this population, vital signs may not accurately reflect the severity of dehydration, pneumonia, acute blood loss, or other injuries. Vital sign abnormalities that are associated with increased morbidity and mortality are respiratory rate <8 breaths/min, oxygen saturation <90%, systolic BP <100 mm Hg, and heart rate >100 beats/min. Low temperatures are not strongly predictive of serious injury or illness. Preexisting diseases, vital sign-altering medications, and cognitive impairment often complicate assessing these patients.[31]

PEDIATRIC VITAL SIGNS

Children are not small adults; they have the disturbing habit of continually changing their height, weight, and normal vital signs as they grow. Therefore, it helps to have some idea of what these are supposed to be (Tables 7-1A and 7-1B), especially when calculating fluid and medication requirements. This section includes both some simple formulas and more specific tables for various pediatric parameters.

Formulas for Quick Estimates (Normals)

Systolic BP in Children Aged >1 Year (Approximation)[32]

Median systolic BP = 90 mm Hg + (2 × age in years)

Minimum systolic BP = 70 mm Hg + (2 × age in years)

The Foot as a Vital Sign

In neonates, the sole of the foot may provide a general idea about the child's status. Cold or dusky soles can indicate one or all of the following: (a) hypothermia, (b) hypoxemia, or (c) hypotension, especially in a child with delays in capillary refill and without respiratory distress who does not respond to rewarming.[33]

TABLE 7-1A Normal Pediatric Vital Signs

	Pulse (beats/min)	Systolic BP (mm Hg)	Diastolic BP (mm Hg)
Newborn	95-145	60-90	30-45
Infant	125-170	75-100	30-70
Toddler	100-160	80-110	40-90
Preschool	70-110	80-110	45-85
School age	70-110	85-120	45-88
Adolescent	55-100	95-120	60-90

TABLE 7-1B Normal Pediatric Vital Signs

	Respiration (breaths/min)	Weight (kg)	Blood Volume (mL/kg)
Newborn	30-60	3.5	90
Infant	30-60	4-10	90
Toddler	24-40	12-14	90
Preschool	22-34	16-18	80
School age	18-30	20-26	80
Adolescent	12-16	>50	70

Pediatric Milestones in Development

All parents question whether their children are normal. The answer to this question is that no child is "normal," but the child may be developing normally. When assessing the child's development, an easy way of remembering some basic developmental milestones is that a 1-year-old does one action, a 2-year-old does two actions, etc. An alternative method is as follows:

1-year-old	Can say single words
2-year-old	Uses two-word sentences
	Understands two-step commands
3-year-old	Uses three words together
	Repeats three digits
	Rides tricycle (three-wheel bike)
4-year-old	Draws square (four sides)
	Counts four objects

MEASURING LENGTH, AREA, AND VOLUME

The practitioner needs to be able to judge the size of wounds and incisions, as well as skin and internal lesions. Yet, clinicians usually make inaccurate size estimates, with male clinicians more likely to overestimate the size and women more likely to underestimate it.[34]

This can be improved with measurements, rather than estimates. Mark standard measurements, in centimeters or in inches, on personal medical equipment that you normally carry, such as the metal eartubes (binaurals) on a stethoscope (Fig. 7-10), the reflex hammer's handle, penlights, and scissors.

Since antiquity, practitioners have used their own body parts to make these measurements. Table 7-2 gives some approximate lengths and areas for the sites described on one's own body. These correspond most closely to adult Caucasian males. In practice, reasonable approximations such as these usually suffice. However, because body sizes vary greatly, especially between men and women, practitioners should measure these sites on their own body to use for approximations. (Figures 7-11 through 7-15 demonstrate how to take these measurements.) The area measurements are particularly useful for estimating the size of skin lesions.

Volume Measurement

Measuring volume is useful, not only to determine the output of urine and other secretions or bodily losses (such as blood), but also to measure fluids and medications to give patients.

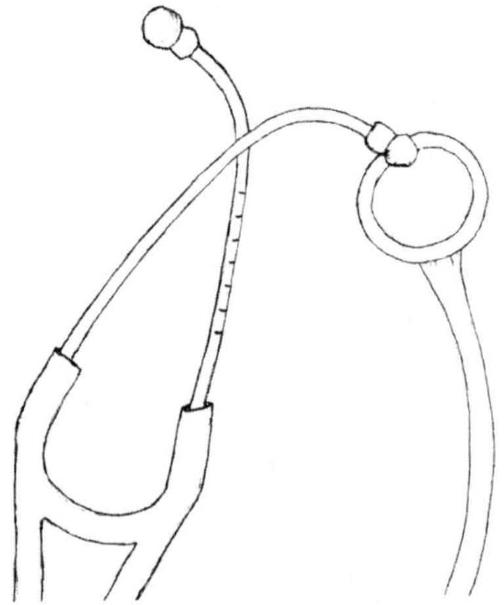

FIG. 7-10. Stethoscope marked to measure lengths.

TABLE 7-2 Clinical Measurements Using Body Parts

Approximate Length (inch, cm)	Measurement Site(s)
0.5, 1.26	Finger width: greatest width of the distal phalanx of the small finger
0.75, 1.90	Finger width: width of the small finger at the MP crease
1, 2.54	Phalanx: length of the middle phalanx of the small finger (Fig. 7-11) Phalanx: from the palmar MP crease to the proximal IP joint of the long (middle) finger Thumb: width of thumb at the IP joint
6, 15.24	Span: when opening the hand and spreading the fingers widely, from the tip of the thumb to the tip of the index finger (Fig. 7-12)
12, 30.48	Forearm: from the point of the elbow to the distal palmar crease
18, 45.72	Cubit: from the point of the elbow to the tip of the extended long (middle) finger (Fig. 7-13)
36, 91.44	Yard/ ~ meter: from the tip of the nose to the end of the extended long (middle) finger
Diameter (inch, cm)	
1.5, 3.81	Grasp: the greatest diameter of the circle formed with the thumb and index finger (Fig. 7-14)
4, 10.16	Contracted-finger circle: the greatest diameter when forming a circle with both hands, the thumbs touching, and with the first metacarpals of the index finger overlapping (Fig. 7-15)

Abbreviations: IP, interphalangeal; MP, metacarpal-phalangeal.

Data from White.[35]

Most food containers (cans, cartons, bottles) have their volume on the label. When empty and cleaned, use them to accurately measure volumes. They need not be sterilized to measure bodily fluids, unless the specimen also has to go to the laboratory. Sterility, of course, is vital for anything used to measure material for injection. For items that will be taken orally, containers should be "potable clean," meaning that you could safely drink from them. The volume measures on some containers may not easily equate to those that you know (or need); Table 7-3 provides common conversions.

Kitchen measuring devices can also be used to measure volume. Those with a capacity of ≥32 ounces (oz) or 1L are especially good for measuring urine output. A transparent container

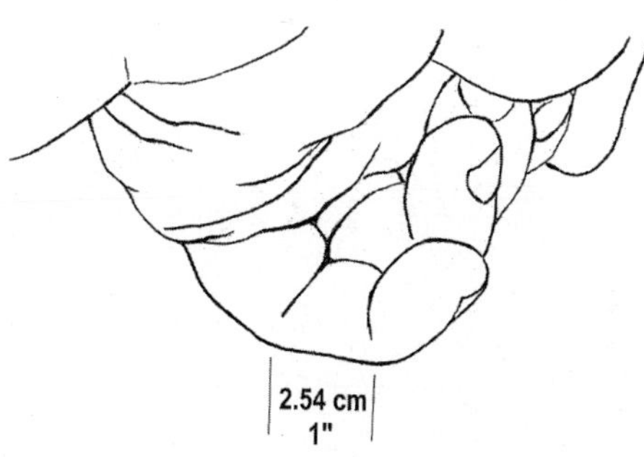

FIG. 7-11. Phalanx (1 inch, 2.54 cm).

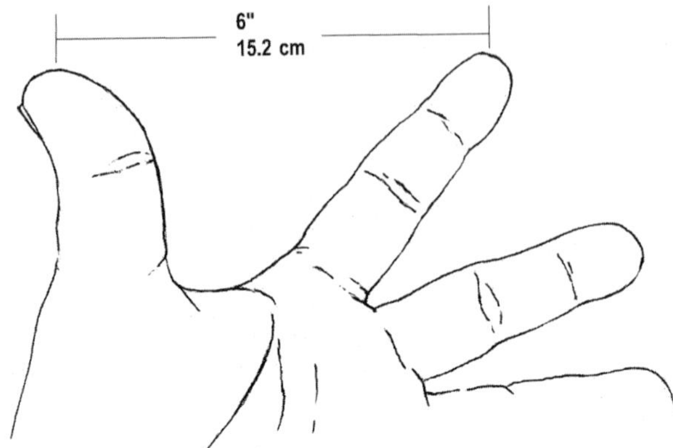

FIG. 7-12. Span (6 inches, 15.24 cm).

with measurement markings makes the task much easier. The container may be used a lot, so use something durable.[36]

Most glass or plastic containers are not marked with volume increments. Mark them either by fastening a piece of tape from the bottom of the container along its side, or by etching or marking them with an indelible marker. Add 1 mL (or 1 oz) at a time from a syringe or other source of known quantity. Mark the tape or the container at the level reached after adding each quantity. Repeat the process until the container is full.

COLOR

A patient's overall color can provide valuable information, especially in critical situations or in surgery. Abnormal skin coloring, including jaundice (yellow), plethora (red), and paleness (blanched), can signify a wide variety of diseases. One of the most important clues is the

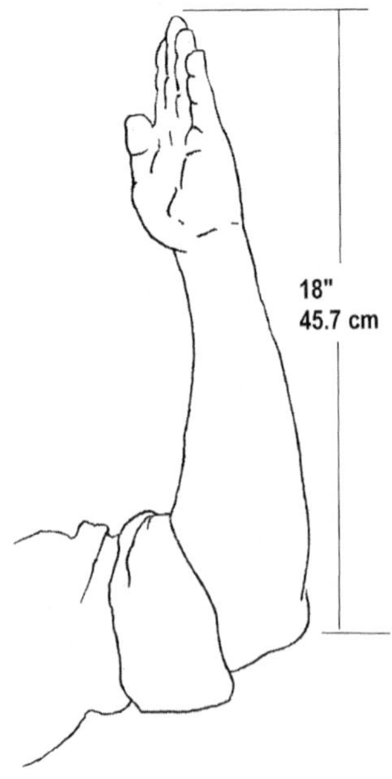

FIG. 7-13. Cubit (18 inches, 45.72 cm).

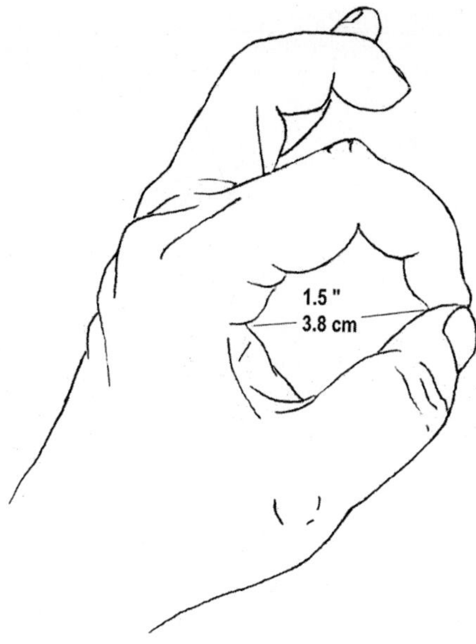

FIG. 7-14. Grasp (1.5 inches, 3.81 cm).

presence of cyanosis (blue), often indicating decreased oxygenation. Recognition of central cyanosis (due to deoxygenated hemoglobin) is best done by viewing the tongue. It is more sensitive for this finding than are the earlobes, conjunctivae, or nail beds.[37,38] Cyanosis of the tongue also can be recognized in dark-skinned patients, in whom skin color is not useful when making the diagnosis.[39]

In the operating room, "a patient breathing or being ventilated with air will not look as pink as the "supersaturated" patient familiar to the modern anesthetist using high concentrations of oxygen, but his arterial oxygenation is nonetheless likely to be adequate. Lighting conditions, green drapes, the reflecting quality and color of the walls, vasospasm, and venous congestion

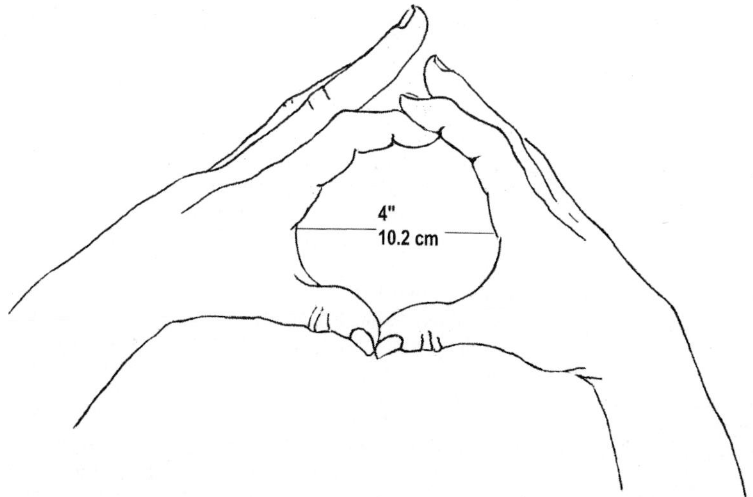

FIG. 7-15. Contracted-finger circle (4 inch, 10.16 cm).

TABLE 7-3 Conversion of US Volume Measures to Metric

US/English Volume	Metric Volume	Other
Gallon US	3.785 liters	4 quarts 16 cups 0.8333 imperial gallon
Quart	0.9463 liters	4 cups 32 fluid ounces US
Pint	473.2 milliliters	2 cups 16 fluid ounces US
Fluid ounce	29.57 milliliters	6 teaspoons 2 tablespoons
1 liter	1000 milliliters	2.1 liquid pints US 1.057 liquid quarts US 0.26 gallon US 33.8 fluid ounces US
1 milliliter	1 cubic centimeter (cm^3)	0.34 fluid ounces US 0.002 liquid pint US
1 tablespoon	14.8 milliliter	3 teaspoons 0.5 fluid ounces US
1 teaspoon	4.93 milliliter	80 drops 0.1667 fluid ounces US

due to position can all cause an appearance of cyanosis. When there is any doubt, the color of the open wound is the most reliable clinical indication of oxygenation of the patient."[40]

BLOOD LOSS

The amount of blood a patient has lost determines whether he will receive blood (and how much) for resuscitation. Initially, clinicians may need to estimate this, especially in the ED or in other uncontrolled situations. In the operating room, it should be possible to measure at least some of the blood loss.

Estimates

After blood loss, an inability to stand secondary to postural dizziness or a large postural pulse change (≥30 beats/min) strongly suggests that a patient is significantly hypovolemic. After moderate blood loss—or loss over a long period of time (e.g., slow gastrointestinal [GI] bleed)—a patient may not have this symptom. Postural hypotension is much less useful for hypovolemia due to dehydration.[41]

Excluding closed fractures and stab wounds, the patient's fist and open hand can be used to help estimate blood loss from soft tissue wounds.[42,43] The volume of an adult male's fist is about 500 mL (one unit of whole blood; two units of packed erythrocytes); an adult female's fist is between 250 and 350 mL. Use this measurement when the blood loss can be seen or place a fist over areas of the body where there is soft tissue swelling to approximate occult blood loss.[44]

Likewise, tissue damage equal to one of the patient's fists or skin loss equal to the area of one of the patient's open hands equates to a blood volume loss of ~10% (i.e., 500 mL in an adult, where normal blood volume = 80 mL/kg). This figure includes both the initial loss at the time of injury and the continuing loss through exudation and into tissue (swelling) in the first 48 hours.[44]

TABLE 7-4 Body Area Injured and Estimated Blood Loss

Body Part Injured	Estimated Blood Loss
Hand injury (crush)	1.6 L
Ulnar artery at wrist	0.5-2 L
Upper extremity fracture	500 mL
Pelvic fracture	1-3 L
Femoral shaft fracture	0.4-1.7 L
Tibial/fibula fractures	0.5-2 L, depending on swelling
Rib fracture (each)	100 mL
Crushed chest	1.5-2 L
Any open fracture	+ Additional 250-500 mL
Abdominal or thoracic injury (adult)	>3 L

While this is a rough estimate, wounds with more than five "hands" of tissue damage lost ≥50% of the total blood volume.[42] Table 7-4 gives the approximate blood loss from injuries to various areas of the body.[44,45]

Measurements

To maintain adequate blood volume during surgery, it is essential to continually assess blood loss throughout the procedure, especially in neonates and children, where even a small amount lost can represent a significant proportion of blood volume. Weigh blood-soaked swabs and suction bottles, and estimate the blood lost into surgical drapes and onto the floor; then subtract the volume of irrigation fluids. An alternative is to use the estimate that 10 well-soaked large abdominal swabs represent a blood loss of from 1.0 to 1.5 L.[45]

MONITORING PATIENTS

Repeat Physical Examinations

In resource-limited situations, the repeat physical examination remains one of the best tools in the clinician's armamentarium. When the same clinician examines the patient over time, diagnoses for abdominal and, often, chest and neurological conditions become clearer.

DISASTER TRIAGE

Prehospital

A disaster involves multiple casualties that require more resources than are currently available. Triage is the system for quickly allocating the few medical resources.

Patient Classification

Patients are generally classified into one of four groups, depending on the gravity of their medical problem: Immediate/Emergent (Red), Delayed/Urgent (Yellow), Minor/Non-urgent (Green), and Dead/Unsalvageable/Expectant (Black).

Triage Tags

Use easily recognized triage tags to avoid confusion, to accurately transmit information to other providers, and to avoid duplicated triage efforts. At least initially, premade (formal) triage tags may not be available. Informal tags include using lipstick or grease pencils to mark patients (usually on the forehead) with the generally accepted triage term, such as "Immediate" or "Delayed." Another option is to tie ribbons that are the triage color onto their extremities.

Secure paper tags to the patient's clothing with a clothespin or safety pin, and to an extremity with twine or a rubber band.

An alternative is to use the system the Japanese developed after the sarin subway attack. They use large colored clothespins not only to indicate the standard triage categories, but also to separate patients into those who need "wet" or "dry" decontamination after a chemical exposure. The simple triage and rapid decontamination of mass casualties with colored clothes pegs (STAR-DOM-CCP) system uses inexpensive (~5 cents each, US) plastic clothespins in the typical triage colors: red, yellow, green, and black, and adds white for patients needing dry decontamination and blue for wet decontamination. Each patient gets a standard (welfare) and decontamination clothespin.

The clothespins are large enough to be easily handled and recognized by responders in protective gear. Clothespins also survive wet decontamination, although the patients must often hold the pins after their clothes are removed. They recommend having a large sign on-site describing the triage process and the colors.[46] This type of triage tag can be quickly fashioned from standard clothespins and colored markers or paint.

Simple Triage and Rapid Treatment (START)

This system (Table 7-5), designed for adult patients in the prehospital setting, ideally allows providers to triage each patient in <30 seconds, with the goal of finding the sickest or "immediate" patients.[47] In real disasters, this system (and those who use it) overestimates ("over-triage") the severity of the patients evaluated.[48] The Australians use an almost-identical system that they call Triage Sieve/Triage Sort.[49]

JumpSTART

For children, use JumpSTART (rather than START) for triage (Table 7-6), because children may normally have a respiratory rate >30/minute, may not follow commands (age and behavioral), and may have a "salvageable period" where they are apneic with a pulse.

TABLE 7-5 START Triage Method (Adults)

1. Ask everyone who can walk to move to another safe location. They can be reassessed there as conditions and resources allow. Walking makes them a "Green," unless a secondary triage finds otherwise.
2. Begin triaging (use the RPM method) where you stand. Spend 30-60 seconds with each patient.
3. If possible, begin transporting "Immediate" patients first. Track where they are going.

RPM (Respiration, Perfusion, Mental Status) Method

Respiration

- Not breathing? Clear mouth and open airway
- If they breathe or need airway assistance = Immediate. If still not breathing = Dead
- >30/min = Immediate; <30/min → Assess Perfusion

Perfusion

- Radial pulse absent or irregular = Immediate
- Radial pulse present and regular → Assess Mental Status
- Note: Capillary refill >2 seconds is sometimes used as the discriminatory criteria, but that can be difficult to assess in many low-light situations.

Mental status

- Follows simple verbal commands (i.e., "squeeze my hand," "open your eyes") = Delayed
- Unresponsive or cannot follow commands = Immediate

Abbreviations: RPM, respiration, perfusion, mental status; START, simple triage and rapid treatment.

TABLE 7-6 JumpSTART Triage Method (Children)

1. Ask everyone who can walk to move to another safe location. They can be reassessed there as conditions and resources allow. Walking makes them a "Green," unless a secondary triage finds otherwise. Infants being carried should initially be assessed in the Green area.
2. Begin triaging (using the RPM method) where you stand. Spend no more than 1 minute with each patient.
3. If possible, begin transporting "Immediate" patients first. Track where they are going.

RPM Method (Children)
Respiration
Respiratory rate <15/min or >40/min = Immediate
Respiratory rate 15/min to 40/min → Assess Perfusion
If apneic, open airway
If begins breathing = Immediate
If no breathing and no pulse = Dead
If no breathing, but pulse present, ventilate × 15 seconds
If begins spontaneous breathing = Immediate
If still not breathing = Dead
Perfusion
A peripheral pulse absent = Immediate
A peripheral pulse present → Assess Mental Status
Note: Capillary refill >2 seconds is sometimes used as the discriminatory criteria, but may be difficult to assess in many low-light situations.
Mental status (AVPU method)
Alert? Responds to Voice? Responds to Pain? Unresponsive?
Unresponsive or inappropriate response to pain = Immediate
Alert, responds to voice or localizes pain = Delayed/Urgent

Abbreviations: AVPU, alert, voice, pain, unresponsive; RPM, respiration, perfusion, mental status; START, simple triage and rapid treatment.

Secondary Assessment of Victim Endpoint (SAVE)

SAVE triage is designed for catastrophic disasters where there are limited transportation and medical resources.[50] Transport may be delayed for days and prolonged when it occurs, and the patient's condition may deteriorate during the interim. This is a secondary (and tertiary) triage system and assumes that START triage has already been done. The system's priorities are based on the following equation:

$$\text{Value} = (\text{Benefit expected} \div \text{Resources required}) \times \text{Probability of survival}$$

PATIENT CLASSIFICATION (IN ORDER OF PRIORITY)

1. Those who will benefit from limited, immediate field intervention. Provide treatment based on two questions:
   a. What is the patient's prognosis with minimal treatment?
   b. What is the patient's prognosis with treatment using available resources?
2. Those who will survive whether or not they receive treatment. Provide basic care, as available. Periodically reassess patient status.
3. Those who will die regardless of treatment. Periodically reassess for improvement.

Patients who fail to respond to treatment should be reclassified. Identify and mark those who would benefit most from transportation to a medical facility (should transportation become available).

Hospital/Health Care Facility

The following criteria, drawn from the 2011 emergency medical services (EMS) triage guidelines from the Centers for Disease Control and Prevention (CDC), suggest which trauma patients may require the most available resources.[51]

Physiologic Criteria

- Glasgow Coma Scale <13; or
- Systolic BP of <90 mm Hg; or
- Respiratory rate of <10 or >29 breaths/min (<20/min in infants aged <1 year) or need for ventilatory support

Anatomic Criteria

- All penetrating injuries to head, neck, torso, and extremities proximal to the elbow or knee
- Chest wall instability or deformity (e.g., flail chest)
- Two or more proximal long-bone fractures
- Crushed, degloved, mangled, or pulseless extremity
- Amputation proximal to the wrist or ankle
- Pelvic fractures
- Open or depressed skull fractures
- Paralysis

Mechanism of Injury

- Falls
  - Adults: >20 feet (one story = 10 feet)
  - Children: >10 feet or two to three times the height of the child
- High-risk auto crash
  - Intrusion, including roof: >12 inches occupant site; >18 inches at any site
  - Ejection (partial or complete) from automobile
  - Death in the same passenger compartment
- Telemetry data consistent with a high risk for injury
- Automobile versus pedestrian/bicyclist thrown, run over, or with significant (>20 mph) impact
- Motorcycle crash >20 mph

Special Considerations

- Older adults
  - Risk for injury/death increases after age 55
  - Systolic BP <110 might represent shock after age 65
  - Low-impact mechanisms (e.g., ground-level falls) might result in severe injury
- Children
  - Should be triaged preferentially to pediatric-capable trauma centers
- Anticoagulants and bleeding disorders
  - Patients with head injury are at high risk for rapid deterioration
- Burns
  - Without other trauma mechanism: triage to burn facility
  - With trauma mechanism: triage to trauma center
- Pregnancy >20 weeks
- EMS provider judgment

The Israelis use a "continuous" triage method to avoid under-identifying seriously injured patients. They have found that, although experienced triage officers may not be able to initially identify as many as 50% of the victims who suffered life-threatening injuries, the continuous triage system reduced that number to <4%.

The Israeli method incorporates both the decisions made by the triage officers and the primary evaluations performed in the ED. The Israelis divide their EDs into three sections according to the severity of injury: (a) mild, (b) moderate, and (c) severe. The decisions made by the triage officer help distribute the victims between the various sections. Once the casualty arrives at the appropriate site, medical personnel quickly perform primary and secondary surveys to identify the severely injured victims. The medical team refrains from using diagnostic resources on those whose examination suggests that they are not seriously injured. If they identify a patient as suffering a life-threatening injury, the trauma surgical team assumes care and transfers the patient to a secondary treatment site. This method has worked well in >20 multi-casualty incidents involving >600 patients, missing only 3.8% of those suffering from life-threatening injuries. Those patients all had distracting injuries.[52]

ICU Admission Triage in Disasters

The most useful criteria for deciding which patients should not receive limited intensive care resources come from those developed for use in pandemics (Table 7-7). These patients should then receive standard medical and, when appropriate, palliative care.[53-55]

TABLE 7-7 Patients *NOT TO RECEIVE* ICU Treatment

A. SOFA score >11
B. Severe trauma
C. Severe burns of patient with any two of the following: Age >60 years >40% of total body surface area affected Inhalation injury
D. Cardiac arrest with any of the following: Unwitnessed cardiac arrest Witnessed cardiac arrest, not responsive to electrical therapy (defibrillation or pacing) Recurrent cardiac arrest
E. Severe baseline cognitive impairment
F. Advanced untreatable neuromuscular disease
G. Metastatic malignant disease
H. Advanced and irreversible immunocompromise
I. Severe and irreversible neurologic event or condition
J. End-stage organ failure meeting the following criteria: *Heart*: NYHA class III (marked limitation of activity; they are comfortable only at rest) or class IV (should be at complete rest, confined to bed or chair; any physical activity brings on discomfort and symptoms occur at rest) heart failure. *Lungs*: (1) COPD with FEV_1 <25% predicted, baseline PaO_2 <55 mm Hg, or secondary pulmonary hypertension; (2) cystic fibrosis with post-bronchodilator FEV_1 <30% or baseline PaO_2 <55 mm Hg; (3) pulmonary fibrosis with VC or TLC <60% predicted, baseline PaO_2 <55 mm Hg, or secondary pulmonary hypertension; (4) primary pulmonary hypertension with NYHA class III or IV heart failure, right atrial pressure >10 mm Hg, or mean pulmonary arterial pressure >50 mm Hg. *Liver*: Child-Pugh score ≥7 (equating to moderate, or Class B, dysfunction).
K. Age >85 years
L. Elective palliative surgery

Abbreviations: COPD, chronic obstructive pulmonary disease; FEV_1, forced expiratory volume in 1 second; ICU, intensive care unit; NYHA, New York Heart Association; PaO_2, partial pressure of arterial oxygen; SOFA, Sequential Organ Failure Assessment; TLC, total lung capacity; VC, vital capacity.

Data from Christian et al,[53] Vincent et al,[54] and Ferreira et al.[55]

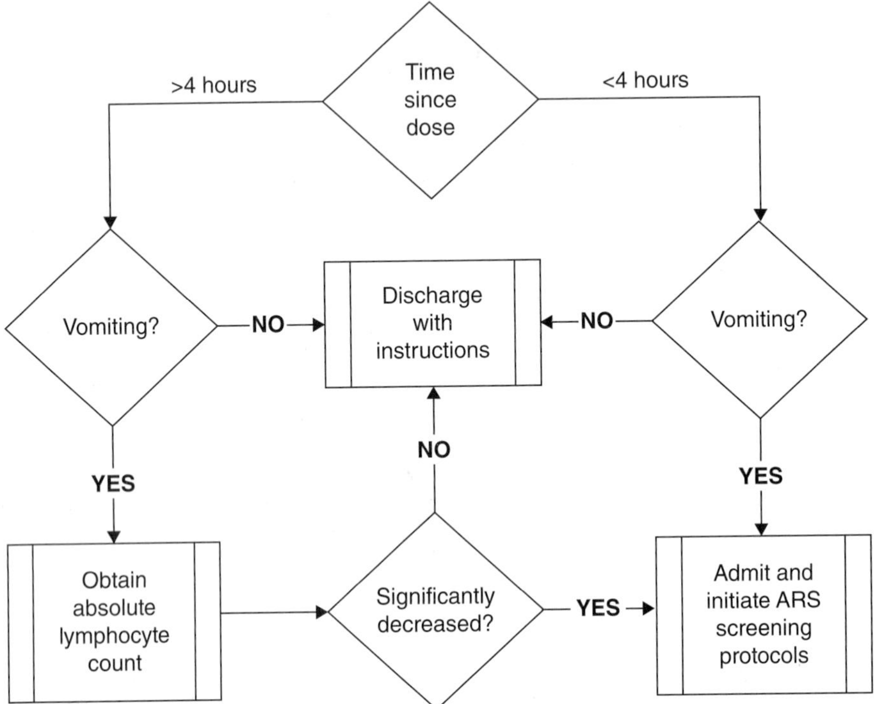

FIG. 7-16. Screening method to identify high-risk patients after RDD detonation. *(Modified from Reynolds et al.[56])*

Triage After a Radiological Dispersal Device

If a radiological dispersal device (RDD, or "dirty bomb") detonates, a large influx of potential patients will present, including many who will not have not suffered any radiation exposure. Figure 7-16 provides a way to quickly identify patients who may need further intervention—assuming that an absolute lymphocyte count can be performed.

DIAGNOSING DEATH

When to Abandon Resuscitation

If an attempt has been made to resuscitate a patient, it is pointless to continue when it becomes obvious that there is no hope of recovery. The following signs, if present after 30 minutes of intensive resuscitation, indicate a poor prognosis: fixed and dilated pupils, impalpable femoral and carotid pulses, and no respirations.[57]

Death Diagnosis With Limited Resources

With limited resources, especially with no access to an ECG, cardiac monitor, or ultrasound, clinicians must rely on their clinical examinations to determine whether death has occurred, or will quickly and inevitably occur (the "Expectant" [or black] triage category). Without an ECG, mistakes have and will be made. The ECG was the first advance for diagnosing death since biblical times, and it remains the most useful method to accurately determine death—although the absence of cardiac activity using an ultrasound is replacing the ECG in many hospitals.[58]

Other ways physicians can diagnose death at the bedside are to listen with a stethoscope, feel a carotid or femoral pulse, and use an ophthalmoscope to see whether blood in the vessels in the eye has broken into the stationary segments ("boxcars") that signal the absence of cardiac activity.[59,60]

Even better are the basic signs used by ambulance crews to determine which patients cannot be resuscitated: rigor mortis, livor mortis (purplish color changes in dependent areas), algor mortis (cooling to room temperature), or an injury incompatible with survival. Note that, when a patient has been exposed to very cold temperatures, severe hypothermia may simulate death. In that situation, warm the patient, if possible, to check for signs of life. Within reason, patients should not be considered dead until they are warm and dead.

REFERENCES

1. Baily KV. Dental development in New Guinean infants. *J Pediatr.* 1964;64:97-100.
2. Tindall AJ, Lavy CBD, Msamarti B, Igbigbi P. Overhead cubital angle as a measure of age. *Trop Doct.* 2005;35(2):89-90.
3. Krieser D, Nguyen K, Kerr D, et al. Parental weight estimation of their child's weight is more accurate than other weight estimation methods for determining children's weight in an emergency department? *Emerg Med J.* 2007;24(11):756-759.
4. Luscombe MD, Owens BD, Burke D. Weight estimation in paediatrics: a comparison of the APLS formula and the formula 'Weight=3(age)+7'. *Emerg Med J.* 2011;28(7):590-593.
5. Lubitz D, Seidel J, Chameides L, et al. A rapid method for estimating weight and resuscitation drug dosages from length in the pediatric age group. *Ann Emerg Med.* 1988;17:576-581.
6. Hofer C, Ganter M, Tucci M, et al. How reliable is length based determination of body weight and tracheal tube size in the paediatric age group? The Broselow tape reconsidered. *Br J Anaesth.* 2002;88: 283-285.
7. Black K, Barnett P, Wolfe R, et al. Are methods used to estimate weight in children accurate? *Emerg Med.* 2002;14:160-165.
8. Argall J, Wright N, Macway-Jones K, et al. A comparison of two commonly used methods of weight estimation. *Arch Dis Child.* 2003;88:789-790.
9. Cattermole, GN, Leung PYM, Graham CA, Rainer TH. Too tall for the tape: the weight of schoolchildren who do not fit the Broselow tape. *Emerg Med J.* 2014;31:541-544.
10. Abdel-Rahman SM, Ridge A, Kearns GL. Estimation of body weight in children in the absence of scales: a necessary measurement to insure accurate drug dosing. *Arch Dis Child.* 2014;99(6):570-574.
11. Dicko A, Alhousseini ML, Sidibé B, Traoré M, Abdel-Rahman SM. Evaluation of the Mercy weight estimation method in Ouelessebougou, Mali. *BMC Public Health.* 2014;14(1):270.
12. Abdel-Rahman S, Ahlers N, Holmes A, et al. Validation of an improved pediatric weight estimation strategy. *J Ped Pharm Therap.* 2013;18(2):112-121.
13. Abdel-Rahman SM, Ridge AL. An improved pediatric weight estimation strategy. *Open Med Dev J.* 2012;4:87-97.
14. Werner D. *Where There Is No Doctor: A Village Health Care Handbook.* Palo Alto, CA: The Hesperian Foundation; 1977:445.
15. World Health Organization. *Management of Severe Malnutrition: A Manual for Physicians and Other Senior Health Workers.* Geneva, Switzerland: WHO; 1999:37.
16. Lamparelli J. Outstretched arms equal height. *Postgrad Med.* http://www.postgradmed.com/pearls.htm. Accessed September 23, 2007.
17. Stehman CR, Buckley RG, Dos Santos FL, et al. Bedside estimation of patient height for calculating ideal body weight in the emergency department. *J Emerg Med.* 2011;41(1):97-101.
18. Lin BW, Yoshida D, Quinn J, et al. A better way to estimate adult patients' weights. *Am J Emerg Med.* 2009;27:1060-1064.
19. World Health Organization. *Management of Severe Malnutrition: A Manual for Physicians and Other Senior Health Workers.* Geneva, Switzerland: WHO; 1999:38, adapted from Table 13.
20. Banco L, Veltri D. Ability of mothers to subjectively assess the presence of fever in their children. *Am J Dis Child.* 1984;138:976-978.
21. Bergeson PS, Steinfeld HJ. How dependable is palpation as a screening method for fever? *Clin Pediatr.* 1974;13:350-351.
22. Mattu A, Brady WJ, Perron AD. Electrocardiographic manifestations of hypothermia. *Am J Emerg Med.* 2002;20(4):314-326.
23. Inagawa G, Morimura N, Mlwa T, et al. A comparison of five techniques for detecting cardiac activity in infants. *Paediatr Anaesth.* 2003;13:141-146.

24. McManus J, Yershov AL, Ludwig D, et al. Radial pulse character relationship to systolic blood pressure and trauma outcomes. *Prehosp Emerg Care*. 2005;9:423-428.

25. Deakin CD, Low JL. Accuracy of the advanced trauma life support guidelines for predicting systolic blood pressure using carotid, femoral, and radial pulses: observational study. *Br Med J*. 2000;321: 673-674.

26. Kaplan LJ, McPartland K, Santora TA, et al. Start with a subjective assessment of skin temperature to identify hypoperfusion in intensive care unit patients. *J Trauma*. 2001;50:620-628.

27. McCluskey B, Addis M, Tortella BJ, et al. Out-of-hospital use of a pulse oximeter to determine systolic blood pressures. *Prehosp Disaster Med*. 1996;11(2):105-107.

28. Khan SQ, Wardlaw JM, Davenport R, et al. Use of a neonatal blood pressure cuff to monitor blood pressure in the adult finger: comparison with a standard adult arm cuff. *J Clin Monit Comput*. 1998;14(4): 233-238.

29. Deva C, Bansal S. Kinking to cut the backflow. *Postgrad Med*. http://www.postgradmed.com/pearls.htm. Accessed September 23, 2007.

30. Pickering TG, Hall JE, Appel LJ, et al. Recommendations for blood pressure measurement in humans and experimental animals part 1: blood pressure measurement in humans: a statement for professionals from the Subcommittee of Professional and Public Education of the American Heart Association Council on High Blood Pressure Research. *Hypertension*. 2005;45(1):142-161.

31. LaMantia MA, Stewart PW, Platts-Mills TF. Predictive value of initial triage vital signs for critically ill older adults. *West J Emerg Med*. 2013;14(5):453.

32. Moses S. *Pediatric vital signs*. http://www.fpnotebook.com/cv/exam/pdtrcvtlsgns.htm. Accessed September 2, 2015.

33. Daga SR. Simplified monitoring of sick newborns. *Trop Doct*. October 1998;28(4):232-234.

34. Peterson N, Stevenson H, Sahni V. Size matters: how accurate is clinical estimation of traumatic wound size? *Injury*. 2014;45(1):232-236.

35. White J, ed. *Handbook of Indians of Canada*. Published as an Appendix to the Tenth Report of the Geographic Board of Canada, Ottawa; 1913:280-281. http://faculty.marianopolis.edu/c.belanger/quebechistory/encyclopedia/MeansofMeasurementbyIndians.htm. Accessed November 11, 2007.

36. The Remote, Austere, Wilderness, and Third World Medicine Discussion Board Moderators. *Survival and Austere Medicine: An Introduction*. 2nd ed. 2005:148. www.aussurvivalist.com/downloads/AM%20Final%202.pdf. Accessed June 8, 2007.

37. Marx JA, Hockenberger RS, Walls RM, et al, eds. *Rosen's Emergency Medicine: Concepts and Clinical Practice*. 6th ed. Philadelphia, PA: Mosby Elsevier; 2006:268-274.

38. Keady MT. Respiratory distress. In: Cline DM, Ma OJ, Tintinalli JE, et al, eds. *Just The Facts in Emergency Medicine*. New York, NY: McGraw-Hill; 2001:113-117.

39. King MH, ed. *Primary Anaesthesia*. Oxford, UK: Oxford University Press; 1986:18.

40. Boulton TB, Cole PV. Anesthesia in difficult situations. 2. General anesthesia—general considerations. *Anesthesia*. 1966;21(3):379-399.

41. McGee S, William B, Abernethy III WB, et al. Is this patient hypovolemic? *JAMA*. 1999;281:1022-1029.

42. Grant RT, Reeve EB. Observations on the general effects of injury in man. *Med Res Council Special Report No. 277*. London, UK. 1951:228. As cited in: Boulton TB, Cole PV. Anesthesia in difficult situations. 8. Special preparation–blood, fluids, electrolytes and drugs. *Anesthesia*. 1968;23(3):385-411.

43. Davies JWL. Methods of assessment of blood loss in the shocked and injured patient. *Br J Anaesth*. 1966;38:250-254.

44. King M. *Primary Surgery, Vol. 2: Trauma*. Oxford, UK: Oxford University Press; 1987:17.

45. Boulton TB, Cole PV. Anesthesia in difficult situations. 8. Special preparation—blood, fluids, electrolytes and drugs. *Anesthesia*. 1968;23(3):385-411.

46. Okumura T, Kondo H, Nagayama H, et al. Simple triage and rapid decontamination of mass casualties with colored clothes pegs (STARDOM-CCP) system against chemical releases. *Prehosp Disaster Med*. 2007;22(3):233-236.

47. Super G. *START: A Triage Training Module*. Newport Beach, CA: Hoag Memorial Presbyterian Hospital; 1984.

48. Kahn CA, Schultz CH, Miller KT, Anderson CL. Does START triage work? an outcomes assessment after a disaster. *Ann Emerg Med*. 2009;54:424-430.

49. NSW Ministry of Health. Policy Directive: Mass casualty triage pack - SMART triage pack. NSW Government: North Sydney, Australia, 2011:4. http://www0.health.nsw.gov.au/policies/pd/2011/pdf/PD2011_044.pdf. Accessed September 5, 2015.

50. Benson M, Koenig KL, Schultz CH. Disaster triage: START, then SAVE—a new method of dynamic triage for victims of a catastrophic earthquake. *Prehosp Disaster Med*. 1996;11(2):117-124.

51. Sasser SM, Hunt RC, Faul M, et al. Guidelines for field triage of injured patients: recommendations of the National Expert Panel on Field Triage, 2011. *MMWR Recomm Rep*. 2012;61(RR-1):1-20.
52. Ashkenazi I, Kessel B, Khashan T, et al. Precision of in-hospital triage in mass-casualty incidents after terror attacks. *Prehosp Disaster Med*. 2006;21(1):20-23.
53. Christian MD, Hawryluck L, Wax RS, et al. Development of a triage protocol for critical care during an influenza pandemic. *CMAJ*. 2006;175(11):1377-1381.
54. Vincent JL, Moreno R, Takala J, et al. The SOFA (Sepsis-Related Organ Failure Assessment) score to describe organ dysfunction/failure. On behalf of the Working Group on Sepsis-Related Problems of the European Society of Intensive Care Medicine. *Intensive Care Med*. 1996;22:707-710.
55. Ferreira FL, Bota DP, Bross A, et al. Serial evaluation of the SOFA score to predict outcome in critically ill patients. *JAMA*. 2001;286:1754-1758.
56. Reynolds SL, Crulcich MM, Sullivan G, Stewart MT. Developing a practical algorithm for a pediatric emergency department's response to radiological dispersal device events. *Ped Emerg Care*. 2013;29(7): 814-821.
57. Dobson MB. *Anaesthesia at the District Hospital*. 2nd ed. Geneva, Switzerland: World Health Organization; 2000:21.
58. Arnold JD, Zimmerman TF, Martin DC. Public attitudes and the diagnosis of death. *JAMA*. 1968;206: 1949-1954.
59. Iserson KV. *Death to Dust: What Happens to Dead Bodies?* 2nd ed. Tucson, AZ: Galen Press Ltd.; 2001: 13-60.
60. Ludwig J. *Current Methods of Autopsy Practice*. Philadelphia, PA: W.B. Saunders; 1972:12.

8 | Airway

BASIC AIRWAY MANAGEMENT

Establishing or maintaining a patent airway is one of the most fundamental lifesaving skills. Clinicians must be able to secure an airway regardless of the circumstances, that is, with limited or unusual equipment. Depending on a single technique or device is potentially dangerous for the patient.[1]

Positioning for Safe Airway

It is much better to prevent aspiration than to treat it. When there is concern about a patient maintaining his airway, especially if there are copious secretions or vomitus, place the patient in the "rescue" or "recovery" position—on his side with his face aimed toward the bed to prevent aspiration. If possible, also raise the foot of the bed so that the patient is in the head-down position.

Even patients with extensive and penetrating facial injuries may not need endotracheal intubation if they are put into the recovery position.[2]

If the individual has a suspected cervical spine injury, use the High Arm IN Endangered Spine (HAINES) position (Fig. 8-1). This differs from the recovery position in that the dependant upper limb is fully abducted and lies under the head, where it reduces lateral neck flexion, and both lower limbs are flexed at the hip and the knee, resulting in one lying on top of the other, possibly reducing torque on the thoracolumbar spine. A single rescuer can easily put a patient in the HAINES position.[3]

Opening the Airway

Chin Lift/Jaw Thrust

Perhaps the easiest method to maintain an open airway is to simply push the chin up. For somnolent and sedated patients, this is often all that is needed to keep the airway patent. If a cervical spine injury is suspected, push the jaw forward from the mandibular angles.

Head Turn

Head turn is a simple, but rarely used, procedure to open an airway. In patients with significant amounts of redundant tissue in the pharynx and hypopharynx (and no history of possible acute cervical spine injury), simply turn the head to one side to improve airflow.[1]

Positioning the Tongue

If the patient's tongue still blocks the airway after positioning the head, or if the head cannot be repositioned because of a suspected cervical spine injury, grasp the tongue with gauze and pull it forward. This is a temporizing measure only. For better control over longer periods, put a heavy (~2-0) suture or a wire or suture substitute (such as fishing line) vertically through the tip of the tongue in the midline (Fig. 8-2). Placing it anterior and midline avoids significant bleeding. An assistant can hold the suture or it can be passed through the skin of the lower lip and then tied.[4] A towel clip (Fig. 8-3) or a safety pin (Fig. 8-4) can also be placed vertically in the midline to hold the tongue. Do not use a clamp or forceps that "may in the excitement of the moment be

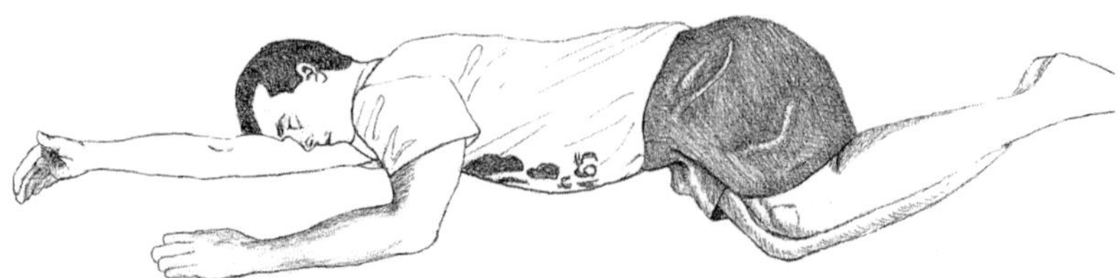

FIG. 8-1. HAINES position.

so firmly applied as to nip a piece out of the tongue."[5] Physicians, surgeons, and anesthetists have used these methods since at least the 19th century without complication.[6]

Opening a Clenched Mouth

If the mouth is clenched and the patient needs to be ventilated, first ventilate through the nose. Try to open the mouth by putting pressure on the temporomandibular joints. If neuromuscular blockers are available and you are comfortable with your advanced airway skills, use them to relax the jaw.

If the patient is apneic with a clenched jaw, press your fingers between his teeth and gums, behind the last molars. This will usually open the jaw wide enough to pass a laryngoscope or to place an airway.

Nasal Airways

A nasal airway, or "trumpet," is one of the most useful pieces of airway equipment. However, for some reason, clinicians rarely use it, even though it is easy to improvise.

To make a nasal airway, use any soft piece of rubber tubing that is the appropriate size for the patient's nose and put a safety pin through the end so that it cannot disappear down their nose (Fig. 8-5). Most adults do well if the length of the tube beyond the safety pin equals the length from their nares to the meatus of their ear (4.5 to 5 inches; 11.5 to 13 cm). This device has been termed a "Goldman's nasopharyngeal airway."[7] The Goldman's airway can be made to fit any nose. Some clinicians cut an uncuffed endotracheal tube (ETT) to size. It can be sutured to the nasal septum (midline between the cartilage and skin) to keep it in place.[1]

If one nasal airway works, two may sometimes work better. Consider using a "binasal airway"—you need only an extra piece of tubing and a second safety pin or suture. When placing a nasal airway, lubricate it well and pass it along the floor of the nose (straight back, not cephalad).

EVALUATE FOR DIFFICULT INTUBATIONS

Total Laryngectomy Patients

Total laryngectomy patients cannot be ventilated through their mouths; they are obligate neck breathers and usually have no tube in their stoma. Airway assessment and control and supplementary oxygenation must be done through the stoma. If it is unclear whether the patient is an obligate neck breather, place supplemental oxygen over both the face and the neck. Use a tracheostomy mask or a pediatric face mask placed over the stoma. Assess stomal and tracheal patency by passing a suction catheter into the trachea and, if patent, use it to suction the patient. If the suction catheter cannot be passed, deflate any tube cuffs and remove a laryngectomy tube, if present. Oxygenate through the stoma and ventilate using a pediatric face mask or with mouth-to-stoma ventilation. To intubate, use a 6-mm ETT through the stoma. If necessary, pass it over a bougie or fiberoptic scope. (Algorithms for treatment can be found at http://www.tracheostomy.org.uk/.) Use a tracheostomy mask or a pediatric face mask placed over the stoma to deliver nebulized drugs to patients with a total laryngectomy. After giving the medications, wash and dry the skin surrounding the stoma to prevent skin reactions.[8]

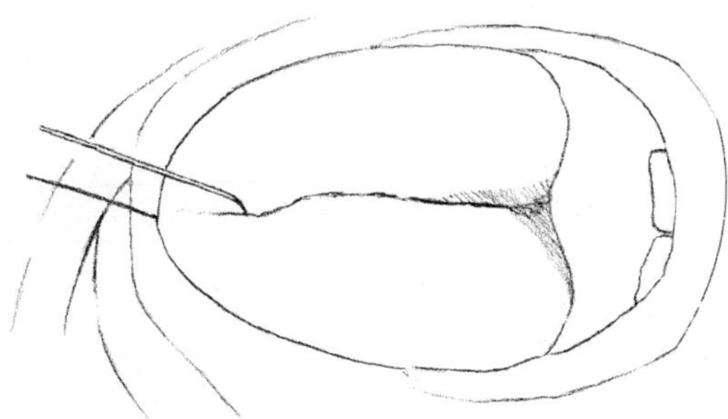

FIG. 8-2. Suture used to hold tongue out.

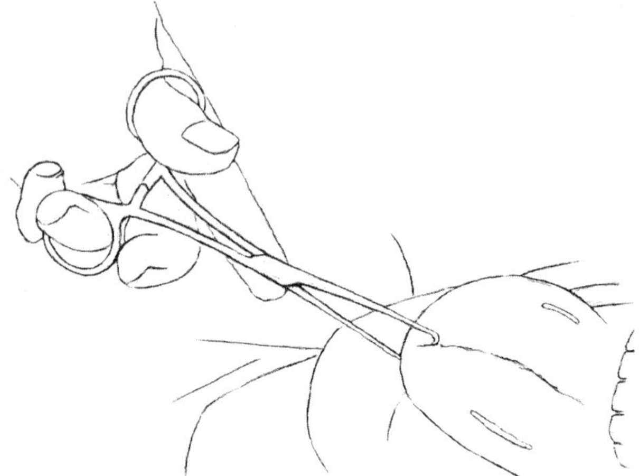

FIG. 8-3. Towel clip holding tongue out.

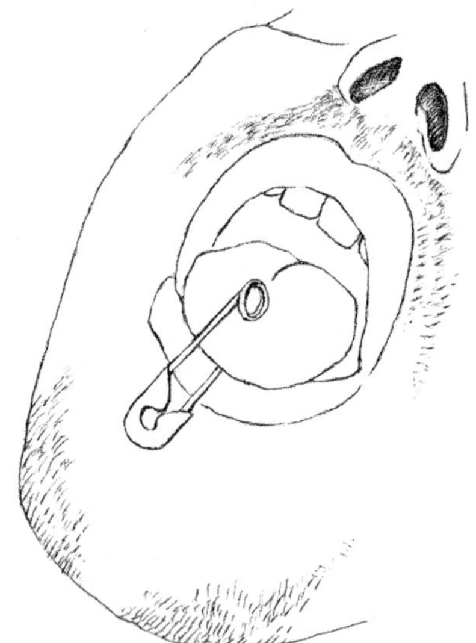

FIG. 8-4. Safety pin holding tongue out.

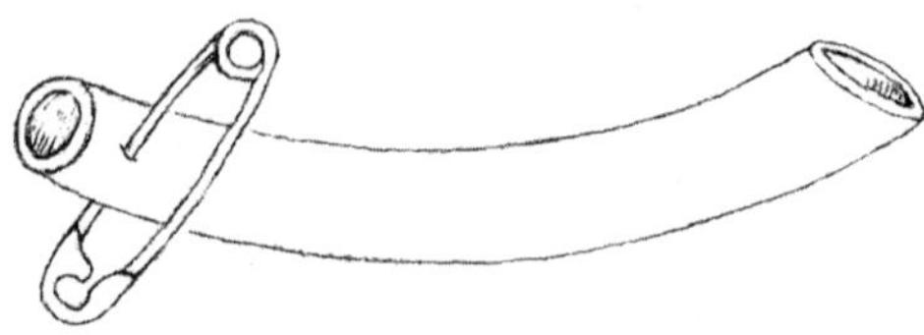

FIG. 8-5. Goldman's nasopharyngeal airway.

TABLE 8-1 Pediatric Endotracheal Tube Sizes and Weights

Age (years)	Weight Using "Simple" Method (kg)	Tube Internal Diameter (mm)				
		Uncuffed Tubes			Cuffed Tubes	
		Standard	Formula #1	Formula #2	Standard	Formula #3
Newborn		3.0	4.5	—	3.0	3.0
1	10	3.5-4.0	4.5	—	3.5	3.0
2		4.5	5.0	4.5	4.0	3.5
5	20		5.5	5.0	5.0	4.0
10	30	6.0	7.0	6.5	6.0	5.5
10-15		6.0-7.5	5.5-8.0	6.5-7.5	6.5-7.0	5.5-7.0

Formula #1: ETT size (mm internal diameter [ID]) = (age in years/4) + 4.5
Formula #2 (for children from 2 to 10 years old): ID (mm) = (age + 16)/4
Formula #3: ID (mm) = (age in years/4) + 3

Pediatric

When intubating children, the two key elements are (a) using the laryngoscope correctly and (b) correctly estimating the ETT size.

No matter what type of laryngoscope is used, the most common reason practitioners cannot intubate a child is that they advance the laryngoscope too far. If the laryngoscope does not immediately produce a view of the cords, keep looking into the larynx and slowly back the laryngoscope out. The epiglottis usually pops into view.

For pediatric intubations, you need to have the correct ETT size. Because cuffed tubes are now being used for most children and for infants other than neonates (and even for some neonates), many of the older formulas for uncuffed tubes do not work. See Table 8-1 for the standard and formula-calculated sizes for cuffed and uncuffed pediatric ETTs. The size of a cuffed tube will be smaller than an uncuffed tube, because only the balloon, not the tube itself, needs to occlude the airway. Keep cuff inflation pressure <20 cm H_2O to avoid tracheal necrosis.

The ETT should be inserted to a distance (in centimeters) equal to (10 + age in years) or (3 × ETT size) at the lips. Table 8-2 gives the placement for newborns.

Adult

Adults have anatomical, physiological, and situational issues that may complicate intubation (Table 8-3). However, improvised solutions are available, as described later.

Special Situations

Most intubations won't be dramatic. However, patients may be in a variety of unusual positions, especially in out-of-hospital situations. Knowing some alternative positions to use for intubation can lessen the stress.[9]

TABLE 8-2 Position of ETT at Lips for Newborn

Weight (kg)	Distance to Insert Tube (cm)
1	7
2	8
3	9
4	10

TABLE 8-3 Predictors of Difficult Direct Laryngoscopy

- Limited mouth opening
- Limited mandibular protrusion
- Narrow dental arch
- Decreased thyromental distance
- Modified Mallampati class 3 or 4
- Decreased submandibular compliance
- Decreased sternomental distance
- Limited head and upper neck extension
- Increased neck circumference

Adapted from Law et al.[10]

Obesity and Airway

Obesity alone predicts that ventilating with a laryngeal mask airway (LMA) may fail. In addition, its use in obese patients is relatively contraindicated, because it doesn't protect the airway from aspiration, causing increased morbidity and mortality.

Obesity *does not necessarily* predict impossible mask ventilation or difficult laryngoscopy/intubation. However, the combination of obesity and abnormal upper teeth or a large neck circumference measured at the level of the superior border of the cricothyroid cartilage may predict difficult laryngoscopy.

Direct laryngoscopy can be optimized in obese patients by aligning their external auditory meatus with their sternal notch. Achieve this by placing obese patients in the "ramped" position, either with multiple pillows or folded blankets or towels under their upper body, shoulders, and head (Fig. 8-6), or by elevating the head of the stretcher to 30 degrees.[11] An added benefit in obese patients is that the head-up (or even simple reverse-Trendelenburg) position slows desaturation during apnea when compared to the supine position, thus increasing the time available to obtain a definitive airway.

Seated Vehicular Entrapment

When patients are trapped in a sitting position, face the victim when managing the airway. Even in this position, if bag-valve-mask (BVM) or mouth-to-mask ventilation is necessary, an adequate mask seal may be difficult to achieve. If a controlled airway is necessary and the patient is still breathing, use blind nasotracheal or digital intubation (see the "Non-Laryngoscopic Intubation" section later), a Combitube, an LMA, retrograde intubation (often unsuccessful), or a cricothyrotomy. If the patient has lost muscular tone and can no longer bite down, use digital intubation. If a patient is not breathing, perform an "inverted" intubation by holding the laryngoscope handle toward the patient's lap with the blade facing upward like an ice-pick and visualizing the glottis from the front. Gently pull on the laryngoscope handle to visualize the vocal cords. It may be easier to perform this maneuver by using the laryngoscope in the nondominant hand and guiding the tube with the dominant hand.

For a patient strapped into stretcher with rigid sides (e.g., a Stokes basket), straddle the patient and face him or her, then do the intubation as with a seated vehicular entrapment.

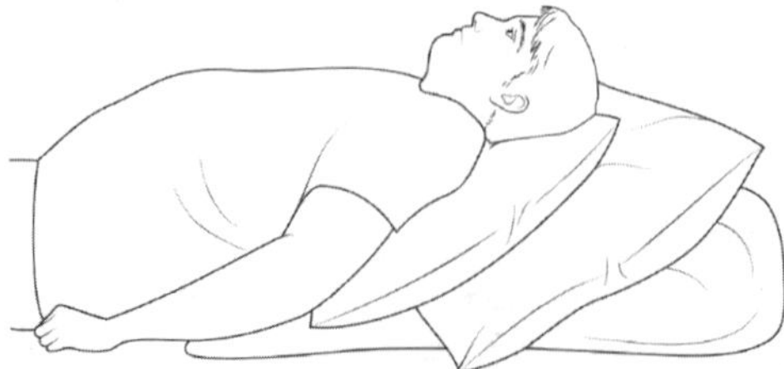

FIG. 8-6. Obese patient "ramped" using towels and pillows.

Difficult Airway—What Next?

If the patient is difficult to intubate, stop trying and return to using bag-and-mask ventilation. The maximum time allotted to intubate should be no longer than the time you can hold your breath; the patient who needs intubation can't hold his or her breath that long. This time can be slightly longer if the patient is preoxygenated with 100% oxygen for 3 minutes of tidal volume breathing or with eight vital capacity breaths over 60 seconds, or until FEO_2 (Fraction of Expired Oxygen) exceeds 90%. Preoxygenation is most effective if done with the patient in the semi-seated (Fowler's) or reverse Trendelenburg position. Also, consider using a nasopharyngeal catheter or nasal cannula to provide apneic oxygenation.[10]

If you can use a BVM to ventilate the patient, use that to buy yourself time to consider any adjuncts or procedures that may help you to intubate.

If you are unable to ventilate the patient despite using the adjuncts mentioned, consider trying one of the airway methods described in the following paragraphs and call for help. If none of these is an option, wake the patient if appropriate (such as in the operating room [OR; theatre]) or prepare for an emergency cricothyroidotomy.

IMPROVISED NON-INTUBATION AIRWAYS

Poor-Man's Laryngeal Mask Airway

The Poor-man's LMA consists of blindly passing an appropriately sized cuffed ETT into the oropharynx so that the cuffed portion of the tube lies between the tongue and the posterior pharyngeal wall (Fig. 8-7). Insert the ETT with the balloon fully inflated. Then pinch the patient's nose closed and seal the lips around the tube, while an assistant bags the patient through the tube in the normal fashion.[12] This does not work as well as a normal LMA, so replace this with another airway method as soon as possible.

Transtracheal Ventilation in Children

Transtracheal (percutaneous jet) ventilation (TV) generally does not work well in adults.[13] Use this method only in children, as a temporizing measure to provide oxygenation until a definitive airway can be obtained; do a surgical cricothyrotomy on everyone else who needs this type of intervention.

The problems with doing a TV are (a) placing the needle/catheter correctly, (b) preventing the catheter from kinking, and (c) obtaining adequate flow through the catheter. So, the guiding principle is that if the cricothyroid membrane will be violated in austere circumstances, use a knife, not a needle, whenever possible.

If opting for TV, insert the needle/catheter into either the cricothyroid space or the trachea, directing it inferiorly while aspirating for air. Determining where to place the needle can be

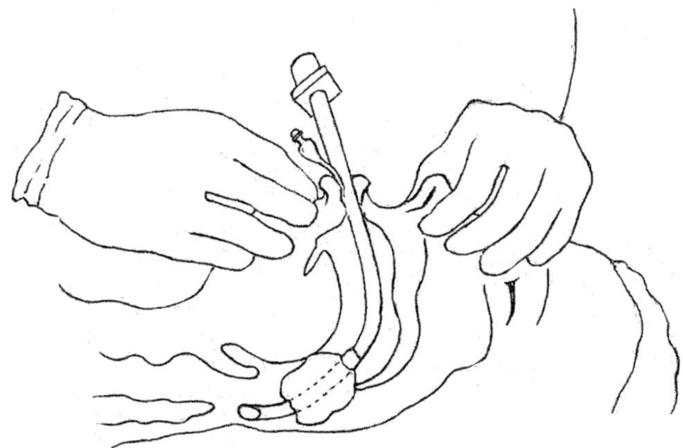

FIG. 8-7. Poor-man's laryngeal mask airway.

daunting for those not familiar with the process. The key is to find the midline. (See the "Cricothyrotomy" section for more details.)

Catheters

The catheters used for jet ventilation range from 14 to 18 gauge, but most clinicians use 14-gauge intravenous (IV) catheters for the procedure. These standard over-the-needle IV catheters may kink at their hub due to the acute angle as they pass into the trachea.[14] This may be ameliorated somewhat by holding the catheter at its hub.[15]

An alternative is to use a larger (13-Fr/ > 4-mm outside diameter [OD]; 9-Fr/3-mm internal diameter [ID], ~6-inch) catheter, which is about the same size as an ETT for a newborn (12-Fr/4-mm OD; 2.5-mm ID). These catheters generally are used as central lines or as "introducers" for large lines. While they may not provide much better oxygenation or ventilation than a 14-gauge catheter, the polyvinyl chloride structure and the length provide enough strength to prevent collapse and decannulation. It also avoids the catheter slipping into the subcutaneous space where, if the oxygen is being delivered under pressure, it can result in a massive buildup of subcutaneous air, leading to collapse of the tracheal lumen and death.[16] A real benefit is that these catheters also can be easily turned cephalad and used to do a retrograde intubation.[17]

Flow

Once the catheter is placed and functions, the real problem begins: how to oxygenate/ventilate the patient without a standard transtracheal jet ventilator. High pressures are required, so clinicians must hold the catheter tightly to prevent it from kinking or dislodging. This method doesn't work well in adults because a 70-kg patient requires a flow rate of >1100 mL/second to be adequately ventilated. The only makeshift method that supplies this flow through a 14-gauge catheter is unregulated wall oxygen that delivers about 1400 mL/second at about 65 psi. (This is not oxygen from a "wide-open" regulator that delivers only about 350 mL/second.[17]) Flow through a simple catheter can be controlled using a simple "Y" device in the tubing, which connects the oxygen source and the patient (Fig. 8-8). When using this device, occlude the opening for 1 second to allow inspiration and release it for 3 seconds during expiration.[18]

In addition, in the OR, the catheter can be connected to the "oxygen flush valve" on the anesthesia machine; this is essentially a jet ventilator.[19] To do this, connect stiff tubing to the common gas outlet with a standard 15-mm ETT connector. Most modern machines, however, are fitted with a safety valve to prevent overpressure and therefore may not be suitable for this purpose.[20]

Another option is to use a needle connected to a standard T-piece that allows flow control by occluding one end with the thumb (Fig. 8-9).

The danger when using an unregulated oxygen source is that it can cause barotrauma to the lungs. However, adequate jet ventilation is just that—ventilation. The high flow rate not only supplies oxygen, but also forces CO_2 out of the lungs.[21] It also appears to protect against aspiration at least as well as a cuffed ETT does.[22]

How about connecting a 15-mm ETT adapter and using a BVM? This has been suggested repeatedly in the literature and in medical protocols. Any IV catheter can be attached to a 3.5-mm ETT adapter, although removing the adapter from the tube may require cutting it off, because it is very firmly attached. An easier method is to insert a 6.5- to 8.5-mm cuffed ETT into a 5-, 10-, or 20-mL syringe barrel, inflate the balloon, and connect the syringe to the IV catheter. The ETT provides the 15-mm BVM adapter.[23]

The problem, then, is that ventilating with a BVM is not only physically challenging, but also quickly results in hypercarbia, even when a 4-mm ID catheter is used (about three times the ID of a 14-gauge catheter). However, if doing TV with a jet ventilator, patients may have the same respiratory and hemodynamic variables after 20 minutes as those with surgical cricothyroidotomies,

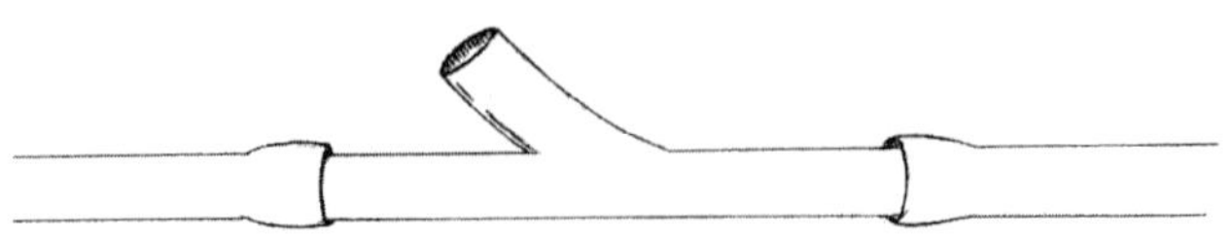

FIG. 8-8. Flow control for direct oxygen connection to cricothyrotomy.

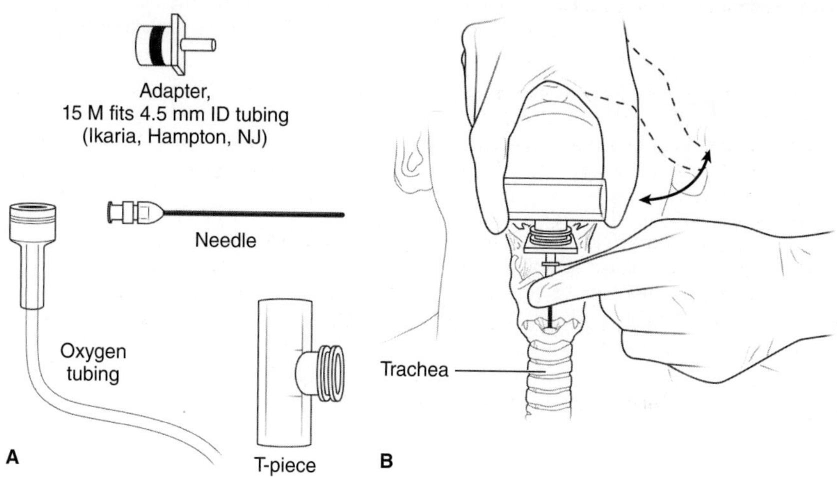

FIG. 8-9. (A) Equipment needed to use T-piece for transtracheal ventilation; (B) T-piece "closed" to provide flow through needle and "open" (dotted figure) to allow exhalation.

if they are allowed adequate time for exhalation.[24] Therefore, unless a jet ventilator, unregulated wall oxygen, or an anesthesia machine's oxygen flush valve is used, consider TV a temporizing method, to be used for no more than a few minutes. In most adult patients, this makes it not worth the trouble. Use another method!

Easier Laryngeal-Mask-Airway Insertion

LMA insertion may be made easier if you make a 90-degree angle close to the laryngeal portion of the LMA by using the malleable metal ETT stylet (sometimes doubled over to be stiffer). For safety, do not extend the stylet into the mask. The bend is about 3 cm proximal to the mask, and the result looks similar to a commercial intubating LMA (Fig. 8-10). To insert the modified LMA, partially inflate the mask, lubricate it normally, and slide the tip along the hard palate.

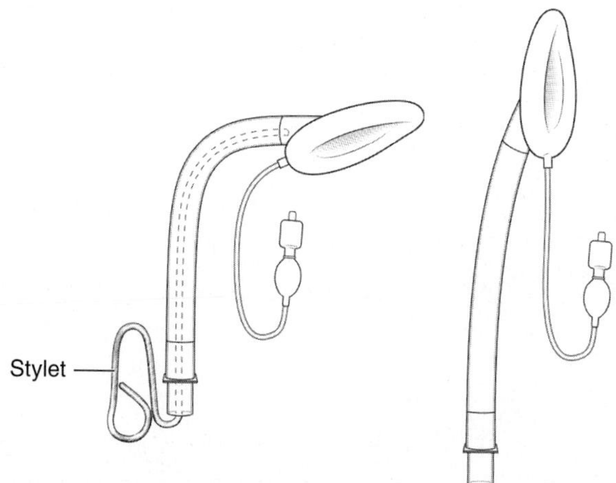

FIG. 8-10. Comparison of LMA with (left) and without (right) a stylet and 90-degree angle curve.

Then use the same motion as when inserting a laryngoscope and rotate the LMA so that the mask follows the airway's curvature into its final position in the pharynx. Once the mask is inserted, remove the stylet so the tube can bend to match the patient's anatomy. Lubricating the stylet makes it easier to remove once the LMA is inserted.[25,26]

INDICATIONS TO INTUBATE

Intubation is probably used far too often in Western tertiary care centers and not often enough elsewhere. However, ask yourself why you are *not* intubating a patient who

- Tolerates an oral airway
- Is too agitated to fully evaluate and cannot be easily or safely sedated
- Is not oriented to time, place, person, or events after head trauma
- Is not maintaining, or may not be able to maintain, a patent airway
- Cannot or may not be able to handle his or her secretions without aspirating
- Has had an acute mental status change

While many of these patients may not need intubation immediately, make a conscious decision to either intubate them or carefully observe them.

IMPROVISED INTUBATION EQUIPMENT

Suction Device

It is possible, and often necessary, to remove airway debris manually with your fingers or by sucking it out with a bulb syringe or large-mouth (Toomey) syringe. However, the best option for long-term use is to build a simple foot-operated suction device (Fig. 8-11). One way to do this is to modify an automobile or truck tire pump so that its valves suck instead of pump. Attach this to two wide-mouth, unbreakable 1-L bottles and then to the sucker.[27]

Improvised Endotracheal Tubes

Many tubes can be used as uncuffed endotracheal, cricothyrotomy, and tracheostomy tubes in emergency situations. The wide variety of medical tubing available in hospitals and clinics offers the benefits of cleanliness and various degrees of flexibility. For example, connector tubing for suction devices and chest tubes are useful for this purpose. Even though very large urethral

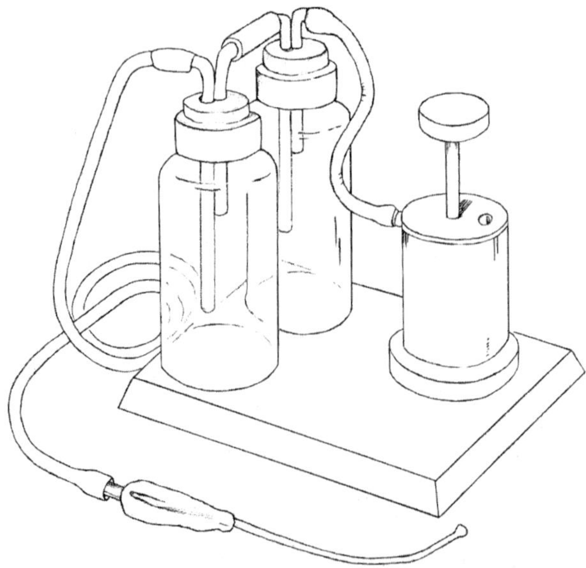

FIG. 8-11. Improvised foot-operated suction device. (*Redrawn from King.*[27])

catheters could be used for infant ETTs if their tips are cut off, their soft rubber walls may collapse. Some polyvinyl tubes and heavier rubber tubes offer less flexibility than others (e.g., chest tube). Typical chest tube sizes (OD = ETT size) that work appropriately as ETTs are 10 Fr (3.3 mm), 12 Fr (4.0 mm), 16 Fr (5.3 mm), 20 Fr (6.7 mm), and 24 Fr (8.0 mm). Cut any tube to the appropriate length before use.

Any hollow tubing that can go through the airway also can be used as an ETT, at least temporarily. If the tube is straight and rigid (like a rigid bronchoscope), such as a small pipe or a piece of bamboo, the patient must be kept fully sedated and, if possible, paralyzed, to avoid breaking the teeth or causing other trauma. The patient must also be in a condition to have his head extended (i.e., no neck injury).

The biggest problem with makeshift ETTs is how to connect them to a BVM or a ventilator. Whatever tubing is used, and no matter what size is needed—from neonatal to large adult—the tube can quickly and easily be adapted to fit a standard ventilator or bag-valve connector using the technique described in the following section.

Endotracheal Tube Adapter

If an alternative tube is used as an ETT, if the standard ETT you have does not fit the ventilation device being used, or if the standard adapter that fits the ventilation device is lost or broken, a simple fix is at hand. Made from the nipple of a standard infant feeding bottle, this adapter is similar to a Foregger-Racine adapter and other, more complex equipment described for the same purpose.[28] Enlarge the nipple hole so that the ventilator end of the ETT can just fit through with a tight seal. Push the tube through the hole so that the BVM/ventilator end is inside the nipple. The other (bottle) end of the nipple connects to the ventilation device (Fig. 8-12). Experience shows that any size pediatric or adult ETT, or any equivalent that is being used as a makeshift endotracheal, cricothyrotomy, or tracheostomy tube, will fit.[29]

Improvising an Endotracheal Tube "Cuff"

ETTs work best if they are cuffed. If an ETT (regular or improvised) is not cuffed or if its balloon breaks, there may be a significant air leak, which may increase the chance of aspiration. In those

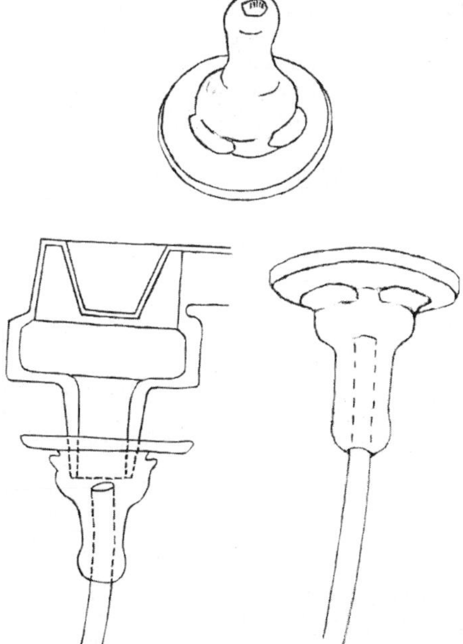

FIG. 8-12. Improvised endotracheal tube and 15-mm adapter. Use any hollow tube, but preferably flexible polyvinyl.

cases, pack the pharynx under direct vision with moist 2-inch roller gauze or cloth soaked in saline, using Magill or similar forceps. Moisten the pack in water and squeeze the water out. Don't use petroleum jelly (e.g., Vaseline) or other petroleum-containing products to soak the gauze, because that might cause pneumonitis.[30] As when packing the nose or an abscess, use only one length of packing material so that, when it is removed, there is no chance of leaving an unobserved second piece behind. Tie one end of the packing to the ETT to ensure its removal when the tube is removed.[7] It is safest to write "PACK" on a piece of tape and place it on the patient's forehead to let other clinicians know that a pack is in place. This method can also be used if an ETT cuff develops a leak after a successful intubation and changing the tube is too dangerous.[31]

Fixing an Endotracheal Tube

If a polyvinyl ETT is torn, the best solution is not to use it. If it is already in place, replace it. However, if this is not possible or is too dangerous for the patient, two temporizing methods exist: (a) To quickly seal a small hole, put a moist sponge over it; (b) For a more permanent seal, use a small amount of cyanoacrylate (i.e., superglue, Dermabond) to immediately and completely seal the hole. Before using the glue, thoroughly dry the torn portion of the tube so that it will seal properly.[32]

Stylet

Stylets are invaluable for keeping an ETT in the shape desired by the intubating clinician. But, when stylets are used repeatedly, especially those used for neonatal intubations, they can break at their tip from constant bending.[33] To make an improvised stylet, take a piece of any malleable wire and put it into a nasogastric (NG) tube or a small urethral catheter. Voilà! A stylet.

A coat hanger slips into a 12-Fr NG tube, thus producing stylets for ETTs size 5 and greater. Fashion stylets for smaller tubes using smaller NG tubes. These can be easily resterilized for repeated use.[34] Alternatively, batches of stylets can be made from copper wire that is the appropriate diameter for the ETT in which they will be used.

To keep a tube rigid without using a stylet, and if there is time to wait, put the ETT in ice water or freeze it. This tends to work better for smaller caliber ETTs. (Daniel Tzse, MD, Brown University. Personal written communication, June 5, 2007.)

Bougies

Bougies, also known as introducer guides, intubation guides and Eschmann-type guides, have been available to facilitate orotracheal and nasotracheal intubations since Macintosh described them in 1949. They are semirigid thin rods that can be inserted with blind technique into the airway of patients with poor glottic visualization. Table 8-4 describes the technique.

To use a bougie for endotracheal intubation without assistance, use the "pistol grip" technique. Preload the ETT onto the bougie, leaving about one-quarter of the introducer exposed at the ETT's proximal (ventilation) end. Have the bent (Coudé) tip facing anteriorly. Bend the proximal bougie so that the clinician can hold both that end of the introducer and the ETT simultaneously in one hand. Once the tip of the introducer passes the cords, release the proximal part and pass it, and then the ETT, into the trachea, making the counterclockwise (left-hand) turn so that it does not hang up on an aretynoid cartilage.

Sterilized bougies can also be used to assist with chest tube insertions, cricothyrotomies, and peritoneal lavages. Although they are listed as single-use items, commercial guides that have sealed ends are often cleaned with a disinfectant, such as glutaraldehyde, and reused. Autoclaving melts them. If there are no bougies available, they may need to be improvised, as the following section details.

Improvising Bougies

According to Dr. James Riopelle of Louisiana State University Dept. of Anesthesiology, one can make an intubation guide using any type of plastic rod, although it should be about 15-Fr diameter (4.7 mm; 3/16 inches) for a child, and slightly larger for an adult. The tighter the fit the introducer has in the ETT, the less chance it has of catching on the ariepiglottic fold. The length can be 60 cm (less chance for over-insertion) or the more common 70 cm. The plastic must be malleable when heated so that the tip can be bent into a Coudé tip. Some people have used

TABLE 8-4 Protocol for Intubation With Introducer Guide

1. Using laryngoscopy, insert the introducer guide through the cords; feel for palpable vibrations (or clicks).
2. If the vocal cords are *not* visible, insert the introducer guide in the most anterior position possible, until palpable clicks are felt.
3. Advance the endotracheal tube over the introducer (without removing the laryngoscope), until it "locks" or to a maximum distance of 45 cm.
4. If no vibrations (or clicks) are perceived or there is no feeling of resistance after passing the tube 20-40 cm (the "lock"), assume that the introducer is in the esophagus. At that point, either leave the tube in the esophagus (blocking the unwanted passage) or remove it. Repeat laryngoscopy.
5. When the vibrations (or clicks) are felt, rotate the endotracheal tube 90 degrees (either direction) to prevent it from catching on the arytenoids and pass it through the vocal cords.
6. Remove the guide, while holding the endotracheal tube in place.
7. Confirm proper endotracheal tube position.

Adapted from Dexheimer Neto et al.[35]

esophageal temperature probes, guide wires for passing electrical wire through conduits (i.e., thread guides) or NG tubes. Two commonly available materials are Teflon fluorinated ethylene propylene (FEP) and polyethylene rods. The latter are stiffer than Teflon, and so may be more dangerous in the hands of novices. In either case, sandpaper the ends to make a bullet-shaped tip. Then add the kink about 2.5 cm from the end by dipping one end of the guide into boiling water for about a minute, withdrawing it, and holding the tip under cold running water to "fix" the kink in place. Use a permanent marker (or tape in the case of Teflon) to make a prominent mark 23 to 25 cm from the tip to warn against passing the introducer further than this distance past the lips (and less in a very small patient). (Personal communication, July 28, 2014.)

Improvising Bougie/Jet Stylets

A 14- or 18-Fr or a Salem Sump NG tube can also be used to improvise a bougie, or used as a "jet stylet," to insufflate oxygen or simply to provide nasopharyngeal oxygen to a breathing patient. To fashion this device, insert an unbent paper clip through the NG tube's most distal hole (eyelet). Then use a forceps to push the paperclip into the most distal end of the NG tube (Fig. 8-13). Bend this end into a 40-degree "hockey stick" angle. Cut the proximal end of the NG tube so that it is 60- to 70-cm long. Place the NG tube with the desired curvature into a basin of ice. Within 30 seconds, the tube will be sufficiently rigid so that it can be used as a bougie. An 18-Fr NG tube is suitable for 8.0 mm and larger ETTs, whereas the 14-Fr tube can be used for a 6.0- to 7.0-mm ETT.[36] Dr. Riopelle has used this device a few times in infants, using a very thin paperclip.

To convert the NG bougie into a jet stylet, insert a 14-gauge IV catheter into the proximal end and attach it to a transtracheal jet ventilator. When using an 18-Fr NG tube, fully insert the catheter to ensure an adequate seal. To provide oxygen to a spontaneously breathing patient, insert a standard 3-mm ETT adapter into the end of the 18-Fr tube or a 2.5-mm adapter into a 14-Fr tube. Provide oxygen by attaching the adapter to a conventional anesthetic circuit, BVM (compressing the bag), or similar device.[36]

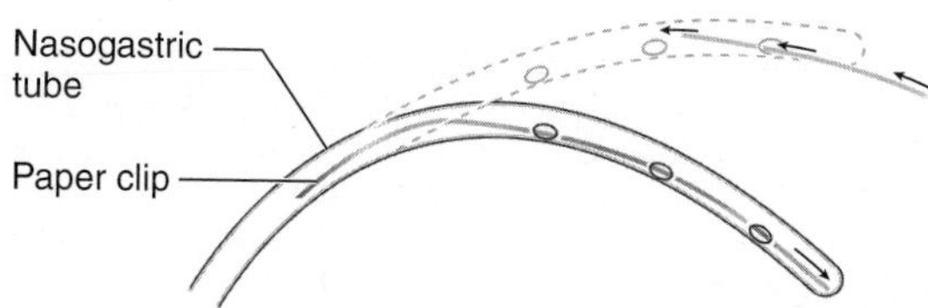

FIG. 8-13. Unbend a paperclip and insert it into the distal hole in a NG tube; then move it into the tube's distal end.

Makeshift Laryngoscope

Transillumination With Makeshift Laryngoscopes

A common problem when you need to intubate a patient urgently is that either there is no laryngoscope or the laryngoscope light doesn't work. In these cases, use either the dead laryngoscope or an alternative made from a tongue depressor, shoehorn, spatula, or spoon. If using a nonmalleable improvisation, use it to extend the tongue out of the mouth as far as possible, or grasp and pull the tongue to achieve the same result. The larynx should be visible if illuminated. A spoon handle can be bent to act as a laryngoscope blade to facilitate this view (Fig. 8-14). Illuminate the larynx either directly through the mouth using, for example, a penlight or an OR light, or by transillumination through the cricothyroid membrane using a portable light, such as a flashlight or headlamp.[37-39] Boulton wrote that "the larynx is seen as a brightly illuminated area in a black field."[7] John C. Sakles, MD, a colleague at the University of Arizona who has used the transillumination method, commented, "It is extremely dark in there. Not much light gets through. Red light works best." (Written communication, September 5, 2008.)

Homemade Laryngoscope

Gillett and Patkin developed an inexpensive laryngoscope constructed of simple materials for situations where standard laryngoscopes are too expensive or unavailable (Fig. 8-15).

> The handle is made of oak or beech, and two penlight batteries are attached to it by Sellotape [heavy clear tape] or by two light aluminum bands. At one end they are held by the blade, and at the other by a small piece of Perspex [acrylic glass; Plexiglas] which bears a simple pivot switch. The blade is of twin-track aluminum from which one of the three flanges have been removed entirely, while the other two have been partly cut away towards the tip. It is shaped by bending in a heavy vice. In the track that is left there is an inexpensive prefocused torch bulb with a lead soldered to its base. The rest of this track has in it some hard rubber tubing about this lead, and this stops the metal of the blade knocking on to the upper teeth or the gum when the instrument is in use. The bulb lies in a shallow hammered recess. The blade is held on to the wooden handle with two strong chrome screws.[40]

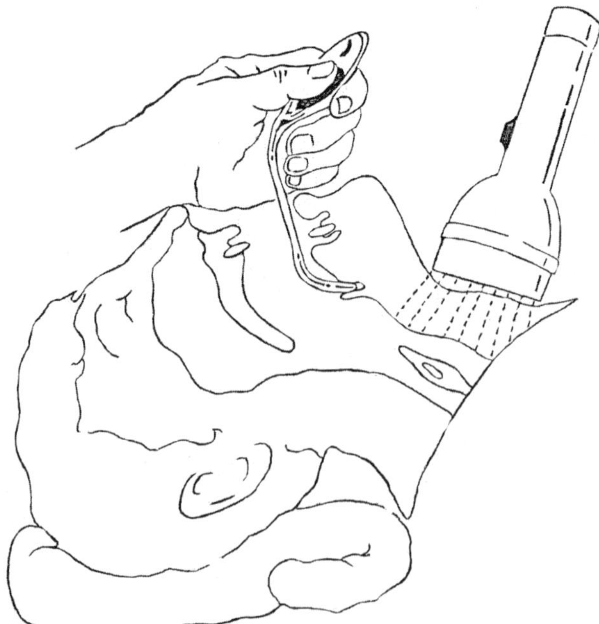

FIG. 8-14. Cricothyroid membrane transillumination and spoon laryngoscope.

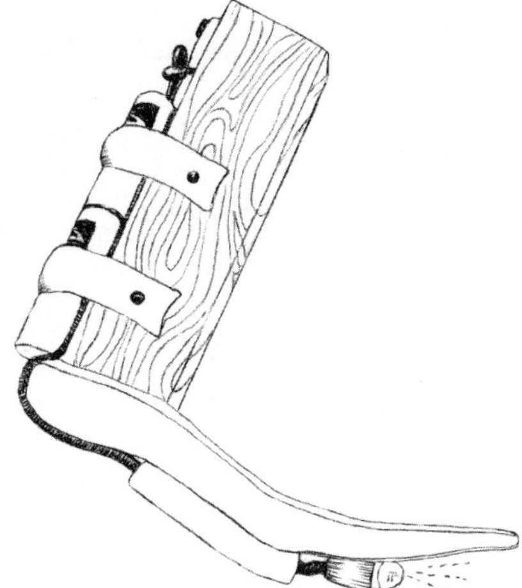

FIG. 8-15. Makeshift laryngoscope.

This device costs almost nothing to make, and "in a well-equipped workshop an inexperienced person can make a batch of these instruments at the rate of two an hour." This laryngoscope was successfully used on 88 patients in its initial trial.[40] Similar inexpensive laryngoscopes have been made at other small hospitals.[41]

Laryngoscope Problems

If the laryngoscope light fails to work, it may be due to a loose or faulty bulb, dead batteries, or an electrical problem. First, tighten the bulb; this is the most common problem. Second, clean the little pins (contacts) on both the blade and the handle. (These meet to complete the electrical circuit for the light.) A pencil eraser should work, but the contacts may need to be scraped with a sharp-edged implement. Third, insert fresh batteries. Fourth, replace the bulb, remembering that light bulbs for laryngoscopes come in large and small sizes that are not interchangeable. Having a spare light means having one that not only works, but also fits the laryngoscope blade you are using. Finally, if the laryngoscope is still not working, check the electrical pathway with an electrical meter.

Corrosion of disposable batteries may cause electrical problems. To prevent this, remove them if the laryngoscope will not be used for a few days. (Do not remove rechargeable, nickel–cadmium batteries.) If corroded batteries are stuck in the handle, boil the handle in a pan of water to try to loosen them. If unsuccessful, use a large drill to remove them, being careful not to drill deep enough to damage the contact at the top of the handle. Then clean the inside of the handle as thoroughly as possible.[42]

To quickly provide a light source for the laryngoscope, place a cystoscope, arthroscope, or any other small fiberoptic scope into the groove of a Miller blade or through the introducing hole in a Macintosh blade (Fig. 8-16). Then use the blade in the normal fashion.[43]

Chrome that is peeling off the laryngoscope may seem to be a mundane problem—until the sharp edge cuts a patient. Carefully remove loose chrome with a scalpel blade and then use fine sandpaper (an emery board or a nail file will also work) and some water to smooth the remaining chrome. Check for smoothness by running cotton over the laryngoscope; any rough edges will catch the cotton.[42]

NON-LARYNGOSCOPIC INTUBATION

Blind Nasotracheal Intubation

The only tools necessary to do a blind nasotracheal intubation are an ETT (called a nasotracheal tube [NTT] for this procedure), skill, and a breathing patient, either awake or not awake. Attempt

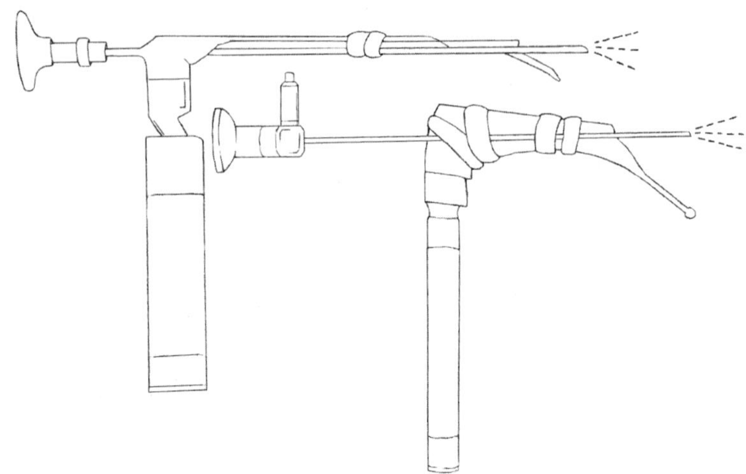

FIG. 8-16. Cystoscope/arthroscope used to supply light to Miller and Macintosh laryngoscope blades.

the procedure only in patients who are spontaneously breathing; the patient's exhalations are the guide to placing the tube. Clinicians experienced in this technique have a success rate of about 90%. Neophytes often use the "push-and-hope" method (not using exhalations as a guide), which works about 40% of the time.[44,45]

Procedure

Before beginning the procedure, wipe the connector and the tube with alcohol and firmly push the 15-mm connector at the end of the tube into the long part of the tube; it is surprising how many times the connector and tube come apart and the tube has to be "fished out" using the pilot balloon.

To do this procedure, anesthetize both nostrils thoroughly using a local anesthetic. In an emergency, simply lubricate the tube. If there is time (at least 8 minutes) and it is available, 4% cocaine is the optimal drug, because it is an excellent anesthetic/vasoconstrictor. Position the patient's head in a neutral position—with the patient supine (usual) or sitting (in severe congestive heart failure). With firm, steady pressure, introduce the tube—about 0.5 to 1 mm smaller than would be used endotracheally—through the nose and into the nasopharynx. Similar to placing an NG tube, the NTT goes straight back into the nasopharynx. At that point, resistance lessens and the breath sounds through the tube become a little harsher.[44]

Once the tube is in the nasopharynx, patience and skill are necessary to place it properly. While watching the patient's chest for exhalation and putting an ear next to the tube to hear exhalation, push the tube 0.5 to 1 inch each time exhaled breath is heard and felt through the tube. If this exhaled air is not heard or felt each time after the tube is advanced, back up the tube the same amount it was just advanced, reposition the tube (by twisting) or the patient's head (generally, more flexed), and advance it a small distance again. If the patient coughs, the tube has hit the vocal cords and should be quickly pushed into the trachea. Often, this does not occur, and the tube is fully advanced to its hub (a normal position for a nasotracheal intubation), with breath sounds still audible. That means the tube has been successfully placed. Another indication of success is that the patient cannot speak. Patients with severe congestive heart failure often seem to suck the tube into their trachea. They are the easiest patients on whom to perform this procedure. Asthmatics, with their poor breath sounds, are the most difficult.[44]

Teaching/Learning the Technique

A model[46] has been devised to teach this technique that uses an intubating head model with one of the "lungs" removed and replaced with a BVM to simulate breathing (Fig. 8-17).

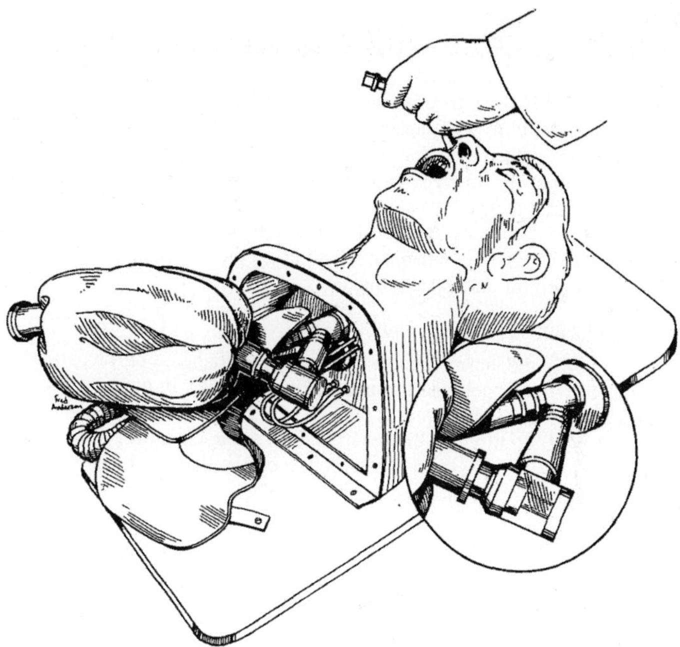

FIG. 8-17. Model to teach blind nasotracheal intubation. (*Reproduced with permission from Iserson.*[46])

Improving Nasotracheal Intubation Success Rate

Boggy Balloon

Once the tube (the same tube is used for endotracheal and nasotracheal intubation) enters the oropharynx, inflate the cuff with 15 to 20 mL of air (Fig. 8-18). Then, when a slight resistance is felt as the cuff contacts the vocal cords, deflate the cuff and advance the tube into the trachea. This technique has up to a 95% success rate, but often only after three attempts (which is not unusual in blind nasotracheal intubations).[47-49]

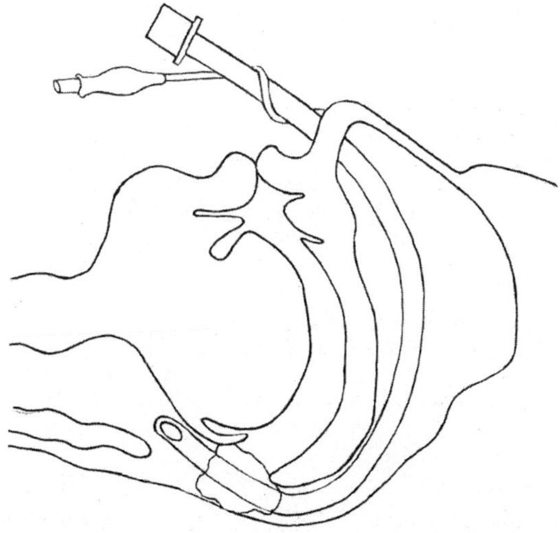

FIG. 8-18. Balloon partially inflated during blind nasotracheal intubation.

Lighted Tube

This method, a forerunner of the lighted stylet, can easily be improvised. Using an insulated wire, attach a small bulb from a pediatric laryngoscope to a laryngoscope handle or other low-voltage electrical source. Put the wire through the NTT until it just barely protrudes from the end; mark that spot on the wire with tape. Next, insert the tube into the pharynx and insert the light through the tube up to the taped line. This positions the bulb just past the tip of the tube. In a darkened room, the tip of the tube can be visualized, and you will see if it goes off midline. If the light vanishes, it is in the esophagus. To prevent aspiration, the bulb must be tightly secured to the wire. This method could also be used for oral intubations if the stylet is run through the ETT next to the wire. In that case, either tie the stylet to the wire or remove the stylet first, so that the light does not pop off and get aspirated.

Nasogastric Tube or Bougie Used as a Guide

If the NTT seems to be at the larynx (coarse breath sounds are heard or the patient coughs when the tube is advanced) but will not pass through it, hold the NTT in position and pass an NG or suction tube or a bougie through the cords (Fig. 8-19). This should easily go into the trachea. Then, withdraw the NTT slightly and either pass it into the trachea over this "guide" or remove it and pass a smaller tube over the guide.[50-52] Another option that can be used simultaneously is to rotate the tube to move the tip off the arytenoid cartilage.

Is the Tube Going Into the Right Place?

To detect breathing through the tube during blind nasotracheal intubation, cut a finger from a rubber glove and attach it to the end of the tube. Cut a small hole in the other end. It will give you "the finger" as it fills with each exhalation (Fig. 8-20). Once the tube is in the trachea, remove the glove finger quickly, or the patient will become hypoxic and hypercarbic.

Digital/Tactile Intubation

This technique, used since the 18th century, has the clinician palpate the larynx while guiding the tube into it.[53]

Adult Digital Intubation

As with blind nasotracheal intubation, digital intubation requires only the ETT and experience with the technique. As opposed to blind nasotracheal intubation, these patients are (preferably) not breathing and have no gag reflex (and no ability to bite the clinician's hand). Clinicians

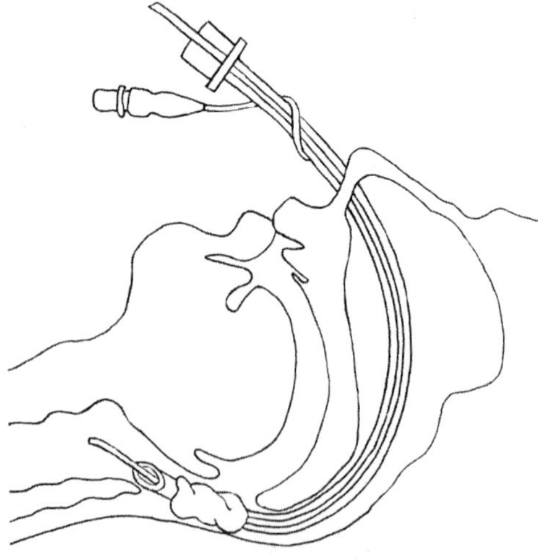

FIG. 8-19. Nasogastric tube passed through ETT as a guide.

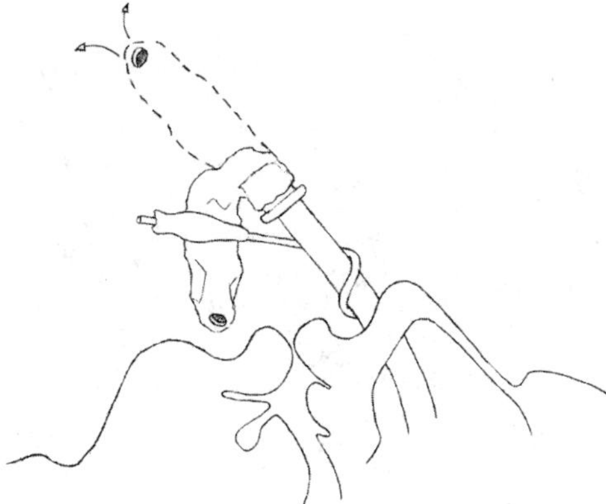

FIG. 8-20. Breathing detection device for blind nasotracheal intubation.

commonly complain that their fingers are too short, their hands are too large, or the patient's mouth is too small to do digital intubation successfully. This is not true. Experience has shown that most in-hospital and prehospital clinicians can use this method to digitally intubate a majority of adult, pediatric, and neonatal patients. With minimal instruction, physicians and emergency medical service (EMS) personnel have been able to successfully intubate ~90% of patients using this method.[54,55] One benefit of the procedure is that it can be performed with only an ETT and, preferably, a stylet and gloves. Other benefits are that c-spine immobilization can be maintained and that the clinician is not at the head of the bed, where other activities may be occurring.

Reasons to use this method include being unable to visualize vocal cords with a laryngoscope due to copious secretions, structural abnormality, or technical reasons; no or a nonfunctioning laryngoscope; cramped quarters; apnea during blind nasotracheal intubation; both intubation and cervical immobilization are required; or it is a clinician's preferred intubation method.[54,56,57]

To perform digital intubation in an adult or an older child, position yourself on the patient's RIGHT side, and slide the volar surface of your LEFT index and middle fingers over the base of the tongue into the hypopharynx. Drag down the corner of the mouth until the epiglottis can be palpated with both fingers and, if necessary, flipped up. Before advancing the tube with your right hand, push the intraoral fingers farther into the hypopharynx, posterior to the larynx (Fig. 8-21). Your fingers then act as a "backstop" for the tube—forcing it anteriorly through the glottis as it advances. Flexing the index finger may help guide the tube through the glottis. If a stylet is used, acutely flexing the tip of the tube anteriorly improves the success rate. If the patient is able to bite your fingers during the procedure, use a bite block between the molar teeth.[54,56,57]

Pediatric/Neonatal Digital Intubation

Digital intubation has been successfully used in neonates for more than 75 years. Because neonates are edentulous and have a shorter distance to their airway than adults, the procedure is both less risky and potentially easier.

To do the procedure, stand on either side (or at the head or the feet) of the child, holding an ETT with or without a stylet. (Most clinicians initially prefer using a stylet.) Put a slight bend in the end of the tube. Moisten the index finger of your left hand and put it into the pharynx beyond the epiglottis, so that the fingertip lies behind and superior to the larynx and the nail touches the posterior pharyngeal wall. In a limp newborn infant, the epiglottis feels like a band running across the base of the tongue. Moisten the ETT tip with saline and, holding it like a pencil with the right hand, pass it over your finger until the tip lies in the midline of the distal phalanx. Use the index finger to shift the catheter until the tip is just above and in line with the glottic opening. At that point, with the index finger still in place, put your left thumb on the infant's neck just below the cricoid cartilage, in order to grasp the body of the larynx between your thumb and finger (Fig. 8-22). While the thumb and finger gently steady the larynx to prevent side-to-side motion, the right hand advances the tube through the glottis for a distance of about 1 cm. You will feel a slight give or tightening as the catheter passes the glottis, but no force is needed for

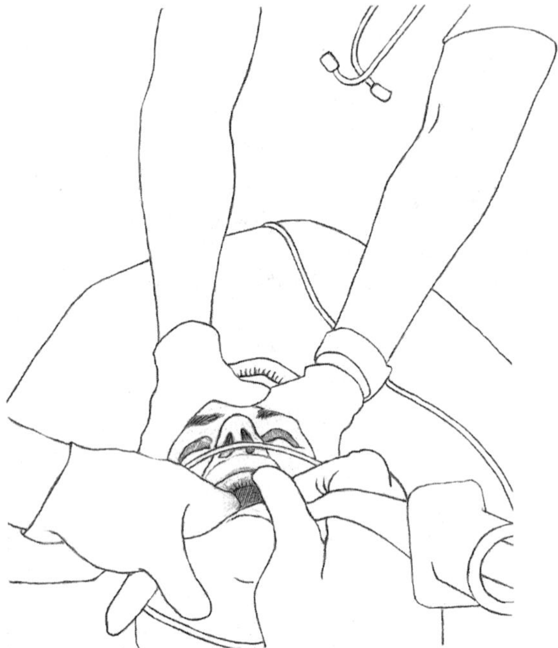

FIG. 8-21. Digital intubation, adult. Note that the intubating clinician is on the patient's right side and dragging down the right side of the mouth with the left hand.

insertion. If the tube slips into the esophagus, it can also be felt between the finger and the larynx. Leave your finger in the infant's mouth to maintain tube position during resuscitation.

Most infants weighing >2 kg, and many as little as 1.5 kg, can also be intubated using this method, although the clinician may need to use his small, rather than index, finger. This method can also be used for tracheal suctioning, changing ETTs, and quickly reintubating an accidentally extubated baby. It can be done anywhere, even in cramped quarters, so that neither the child nor other equipment needs to be moved, and the clinician does not have to stoop or bend to do the procedure.[58,59] Experienced practitioners can do this in a few seconds.

Retrograde Endotracheal Intubation

Retrograde intubation can be used to obtain a controlled airway when other methods have failed or to convert a needle cricothyrotomy into an orotracheal intubation. The technique is very useful

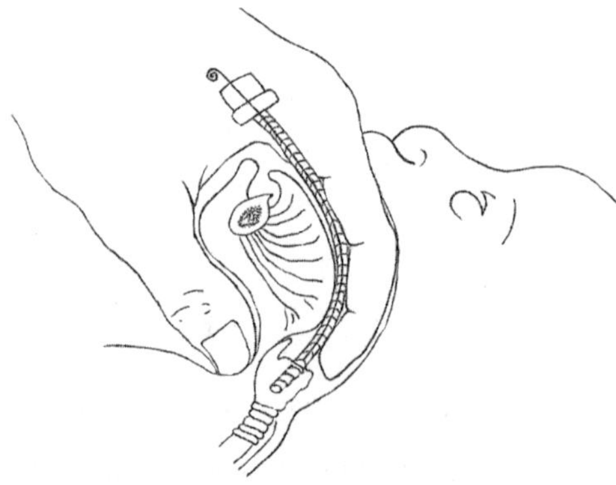

FIG. 8-22. Digital intubation in neonate.

when all else has failed, but it can also be used as a planned procedure (Fig. 8-23). It can be done with only basic equipment. Contraindications are few, but include infection, the presence of a large hematoma or tumor in the area, and clotting disorders. Unlike fiberoptic bronchoscopy, the presence of blood in the airway does not hinder the procedure.[20]

As with a number of other airway procedures, a question naturally occurs: If the cricothyroid membrane has been identified and will be violated, why not simply open it and introduce the ETT, which is a much simpler procedure?

Procedure

Do a cricothyroid puncture using a 12- to 16-gauge needle, with the bevel facing cephalad to help direct the wire toward the oropharynx. Attach a syringe to aspirate air and confirm positioning in the trachea. It is important to make sure that the needle used is large enough to allow the guidewire to pass through it easily; using a central intravenous line kit works well. An IV over-the-needle catheter may kink and thus not allow the guidewire to pass, even if it is an appropriate diameter. Once the needle is positioned, the syringe is removed and the guidewire is passed through it toward the oropharynx.

Whatever retrograde guide is used, it must be at least twice the length of the ETT, and preferably longer. It may be an epidural catheter or a vascular guidewire, such as those used for the insertion of a central venous catheter. These are stiffer wires and have a "J" tip that is less traumatic to the airway.

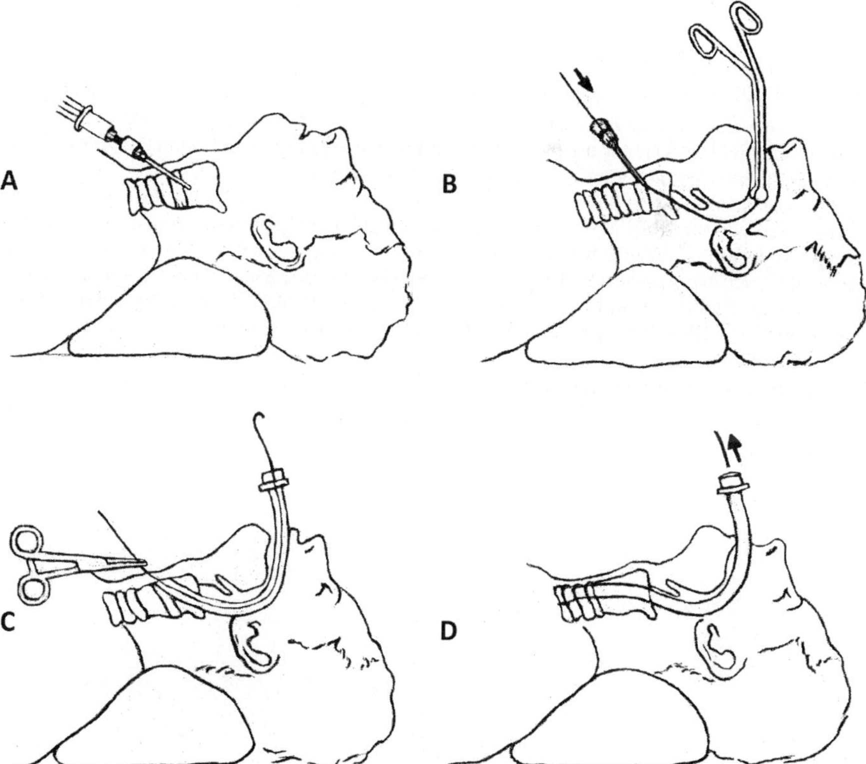

FIG. 8-23. Retrograde intubation procedure: (A) introducing the needle through the cricothyroid membrane; (B) passing the wire through the needle and out the mouth, using a Magill forceps or similar device to grab it; (C) passing an endotracheal tube over the wire while holding the neck end of the wire with a forceps; and (D) withdrawing the wire with the endotracheal tube in place.

Many other types of makeshift guides have been suggested for this procedure, including central venous through-the-needle catheters or guidewires, and guidewires for several other types of medical procedures. Many of these are too supple to pass easily, frequently become stuck in the soft tissues, make their own false passages, or reverse direction when they strike an obstruction.

When the wire is visualized in the oropharynx, it is pulled out through the mouth with a forceps or, if necessary, with one's fingers. The needle should be removed from the neck and the wire clamped at the insertion point, so an assistant can hold it in place. Some clinicians insert their needle just below the cricoid cartilage, rather than through the cricothyroid membrane. They have found that this location is preferable, partly due to less vascularity, but mostly because it allows a longer depth of insertion for the ETT, which prevents it from dislodging when inserted over the retrograde guidewire.

At this point, one option that may increase the likelihood of a successful intubation is to pass an NG tube over the wire, after first cutting it to about two-thirds the length of the guidewire and removing any side ports. The NG tube is a stiffer and more reliable guide for the ETT. The guidewire still must remain in place.

If only a guidewire is used, the wire is passed through the distal-side port (Murphy eye) of the tube; if the guidewire–NG tube is used, it passes up through the end of the tube. As the ETT is passed over the guidewire or guidewire–NG tube, it will meet resistance, either at the point where the guidewire curves up toward the skin puncture site or at more proximal structures. If the tube is at the point where the guidewire curves toward the skin, trying to advance it further pulls on the guidewire at the larynx. If unsure that the tube has passed the vocal cords, withdraw it slightly, turn it 90 degrees and advance it again.[60]

The procedure can be performed on an awake patient after appropriate local anesthesia is applied to the airway. Sedation makes the procedure more comfortable for the patient.

Intubation Through a Non-Intubating Laryngeal Mask Airway

The use of an LMA has become a routine practice in the ED, the prehospital setting, and the OR. Often, especially in critically ill patients, the LMA is changed to an ETT for long-term ventilation. This is usually done through an intubating LMA that is specifically designed for this purpose. It uses an accompanying special, and very expensive, ETT.

If this special ETT or the intubating LMA is not available, intubation can be successfully accomplished with a 6-mm-ID ETT passed through a size 3 or 4 LMA.[61] Two difficulties are encountered. The first is that the normal ETTs are not long enough to pass through the LMA and completely through the vocal cords. Standard ETTs are about 28.5 cm long and need to be about 32 cm to accomplish the task. The solution is to cut a 3.5-cm long piece of ETT and, using cyanoacrylate, bond the two together (Fig. 8-24). This adhesive should take only a few minutes to dry; test the adhesive and bonding time in advance. The second difficulty is that, unlike an intubating LMA, the distal end of the standard LMA has plastic "bars" that impede the passage of the ETT. The solution, opening the web at the patient end of the LMA, requires only a few snips of a scissors.

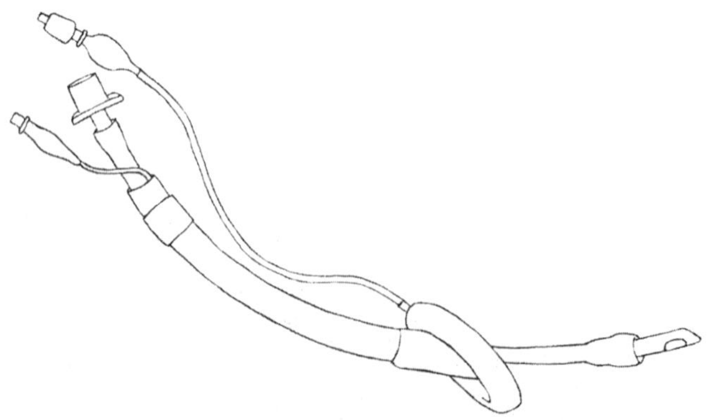

FIG. 8-24. Long endotracheal tube made from standard endotracheal tubes.

Once the patient is intubated, the LMA can be left in place with a small risk of soft tissue injury, or it can be removed using a variety of methods. Improvised methods to remove the LMA include using another ETT of the same or slightly smaller size as a buttress to hold the ETT steady as the LMA is withdrawn over it. Once the LMA is partially withdrawn, it is often possible to grasp the ETT in the posterior pharynx to stabilize it.[62] A tube changer can also be used to remove the LMA, although, if the ETT slips out, it may need to be passed over the tube changer ("railroaded") and back into the trachea.[63]

LARYNGOSCOPIC INTUBATION

Exposed Trachea

In cases where an injury to the neck or face exposes the larynx or trachea to direct visualization, an ETT can simply be placed into the airway without any manipulation except for holding the soft tissues away from the hole.

Intraosseous Rapid Sequence Intubation

Even if you have no IV access, you can give rapid sequence intubation (RSI) drugs through the intraosseous (IO) route. After IO administration of drugs for RSI, the view with direct laryngoscopy and the number of attempts at intubation are comparable to those after IV drug delivery. In a study with young trauma patients, there were no adverse events, and failure of IO infusion was only seen in the presence of traumatic wounds in the vicinity of the IO insertion site.[64]

Unanesthetized Intubation

When safety takes precedence over patient comfort, the simplest and safest way to intubate a patient in an emergency, including for emergency surgery, "is with the patient awake, and this is almost always possible with neonates and infants <2 months, in whom it is the technique of choice. Many adults, especially if they are sick, will also tolerate intubation while awake if you explain what you intend to do and why. Use a well-lubricated laryngoscope blade, and insert it gently and slowly. When you can see the larynx (it may take a minute or two), pass the tracheal tube through it, trying not to touch the sides of the pharynx on the way down, because this may make the patient gag and you will have to start again. On intubation the patient will probably cough, and your assistant may need to restrain the patient's hands. Immediately after intubation, you can safely [sedate the patient or] induce anesthesia."[65]

Experience has demonstrated that it is almost always possible to at least use local anesthetic on awake patients before intubating them orotracheally using the methods described next.

Oropharyngeal Anesthetic

One of the safest ways to intubate orally is by using local oropharyngeal anesthetics. Apply them via gargle, spray, or inhalation.

Cooperative patients can gargle 30 mL of 2% to 4% lidocaine as either a topical liquid or a mixture of the liquid and viscous forms. Gargling is best done in three or four stages, using a portion of the 30 mL for each gargle, and the patient spitting out the residual anesthetic after each gargle to avoid excessive drug exposure. Allow at least 1 minute between gargles for the anesthetic to take effect. Local spray anesthetic can be used before and after the gargles.[66]

Oral intubation can be done (carefully) after locally anesthetizing the posterior tongue, palate, uvula, tonsillar pillars, and the posterior pharynx. Options include a commercial lidocaine aerosol spray (10 mg per spray), up to 3 to 4 mL of 2% lidocaine, or a similar anesthetic, administered using an improvised atomizer (see Figs. 14-5 and 14-6) or syringe and blunt needle or plastic IV catheter. (Be careful not to overdose the patient.) The key is that local anesthesia takes a few minutes to act; don't hurry. Lidocaine, for example, takes about 1 minute to take effect when applied to the mucosal surface, has a peak effect in 2 to 5 minutes, and lasts between 30 and 45 minutes.[66]

Initially direct the spray onto the mouth and throat. After careful laryngoscopy, spray additional anesthetic onto the laryngopharynx, larynx, and trachea. Anesthetize the area below the cords, if necessary, by spraying the area using a curved hollow stylet under direct vision.[66-69] Inhaling lidocaine can quickly produce anesthesia in the nasopharyngeal cavity, pharynx, larynx, trachea, and nose. (See Chapter 28 for more details.) Experience shows that this is also a safe and effective technique to use with direct laryngoscopy, either for examination or for foreign body removal.

Transcricoid Anesthesia

Transcricothyroid or transtracheal injection is an excellent method of anesthetizing the whole tracheobronchial tree for intubation or endoscopy—especially in emergency situations. Patients are told to hold their breath while a 21- or 22-gauge needle is inserted either through the cricothyroid space or immediately above the cricoid cartilage. Aspirate air to ensure proper position, immediately inject 2 mL of 4% lidocaine, and remove the needle. For the patient to tolerate this, it must be done rapidly. The patient will immediately cough due to the presence of the lidocaine, spreading the analgesic up and down the trachea. Anesthesia reaches the superior aspect of the cords in 95% of cases.[70] Intubation is often possible after this procedure alone. If necessary or if bronchoscopy is to be done, also spray the laryngeal structures as described in the preceding text. Contraindications include neck infections.[71-74] Complications are very rare.[66,75,76]

Improving Glottic Visualization

The Colleague Assisted Laryngoscopic Maneuver (CALM) improves the first-pass success with direct laryngoscopy. While the laryngoscope is held in place with the left hand, first lift the occiput to the optimal sniffing position and put sheets under the patient's head. Then, place the right hand over an assistant's hand that is on the thyroid cartilage and move it to achieve the best glottis view. Tell the assistant when the position is optimal and hold his or her hand in that position. If necessary, use the free right hand to help pull the laryngoscope in line with the axis. Once visualized, the assistant's other hand can replace the clinician's right hand, which will be used to pass the tube.[77]

TESTS FOR ENDOTRACHEAL TUBE IN TRACHEA

Detecting Esophageal and Endobronchial Intubations

Unrecognized esophageal and endobronchial intubation causes significant morbidity and mortality. While sophisticated (and expensive) devices have proven reliable at recognizing this, clinicians may often be in situations in which they must use alternative methods (Table 8-5).

Listening over both the upper abdomen and the lungs during ventilation provides a reliable method for determining whether the ETT is in the lungs. Listening over only the lungs results in mistakes 15% of the time.[79] Alternatively, the ETT can be advanced into the right mainstem bronchus while listening for unilateral breath sounds. Providing accurate identification 91% of the time, it can be a useful adjunct to other methods.[80] If the ETT is not placed into the trachea correctly, withdraw it to its proper position above the carina after the test.

For those comfortable with using a gum-elastic bougie for intubation, the clinician can confirm tracheal placement by passing the bougie through the ETT and at ~30 cm, feeling its "hockey stick" end pass over the tracheal rings, which is sometimes described as "a hold up" of the bougie.[81]

An in-line stethoscope inserted between the ETT and the BVM has also been used successfully to determine esophageal versus tracheal intubation (Fig. 8-25). To make this device, remove the bell and diaphragm (head) from an ordinary stethoscope. Cover the end of the stethoscope tubing with a finger cot or a finger cut from a surgical glove; tape it on tightly so that it forms a new diaphragm for the stethoscope. Insert the covered tubing end into an airway connector normally used for fiberoptic bronchoscopy. The stethoscope fits where the bronchoscope normally enters. Connect the ETT to the connector at the distal end; the other end goes to the BVM.

When placed in-line during ventilation, the stethoscope allows the clinician to assess the type and quality of sounds in the system. When using the device, give six breaths to the patient. An ETT in the trachea produces loud breath sounds with a rapid decrease in volume during the expiratory phase. Esophageal intubation is indicated by an absence of sound or by the presence of squeaks, flatus-like noises, or any sound heard in expiration that does not rapidly decrease in volume. This device is accurate 95% to 99% of the time. It can also be used to monitor patients during helicopter transport and, because it is less invasive than the esophageal stethoscope, to monitor patients during surgery.[82]

TABLE 8-5 Tests for Tracheal Intubation

Test	Result	Significance	Reliability
Look			
At patient	Pink after intubation	Tracheal placement	Good (for those with good color vision)
At patient	Cyanotic after intubation	Esophageal placement	Excellent (reposition in trachea)
With laryngoscope	Tube between vocal cords	Tracheal placement	Excellent
At tube for condensation	Condensation seen if in trachea	Tracheal placement	Unreliable
Ultrasound			
Examine pleura	Pleural sliding	Tracheal placement	False positives and false negatives
Listen/Feel			
At proximal end of tube	Breathing through tube	Tracheal placement	Good
Listen			
Over lung apices, axillae, bases	Good air entry	Tracheal placement	Unreliable; ~15% error
Over lung apices, axillae, bases	Air entry only or better on one side (usually right)	Tube in mainstem bronchus	Unreliable; ~10% error (withdraw tube to get equal breath sounds)
Over stomach	Air entry, "gurgling" sound	Esophageal placement	Good (reposition in trachea)
Over lungs and stomach	Air entry into chest; no sound in stomach	Tracheal placement	Good
	-or- "gurgling" sound in stomach	Esophageal placement	Good (reposition in trachea)
Inflate With BVM			
And observe chest	Chest rises and falls	Tracheal placement	Good
And listen over stomach	"Gurgling" sound	Esophageal placement	Good (reposition in trachea)
Esophageal Detection Device			
	Air returned or reinflates	Tracheal placement	Good (patients ≥2 years old)
	No air returned, does not reinflate, or unusual noise heard	Esophageal placement	Good (reposition in trachea)

Abbreviation: BVM, bag-valve-mask, also known as a self-inflating bag.

Data from Dobson.[78]

Ultrasound Confirmation

Bilateral pleural sliding on an ultrasound lung examination suggests correct ETT placement, although subcutaneous emphysema or bilateral pneumothorax can cause false-negative examinations. Esophageal intubation may cause false positives due to increased thoracic pressure from increased air in the stomach.[83]

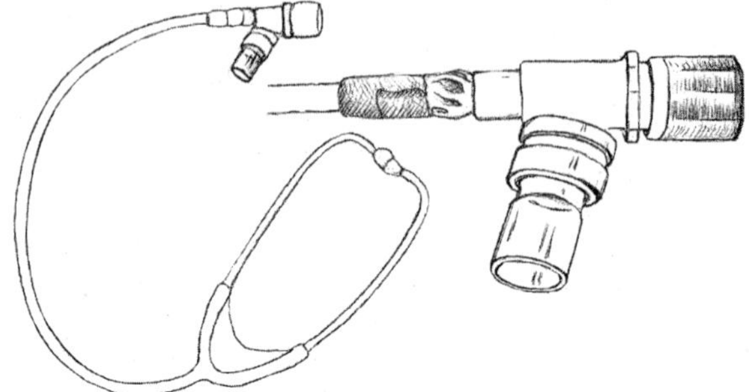

FIG. 8-25. In-line stethoscope (overview and close-up).

A more direct method to confirm correct ETT placement is to use ultrasound to visualize it during or after intubation. Initially, saline-filled cuffs were used to easily visualize ETTs within the trachea after intubation. This method may still be useful for those with limited ultrasound skills or equipment.[84] The modern technique uses a standard ETT and a high-frequency probe placed transversely just above the suprasternal notch. Correct ETT position is identified by a hyperechoic air-mucosa interface with posterior reverberation artifact, which looks like several parallel arcs. If two of these structures exist (double tract sign), the ETT is within the esophagus.[85]

Esophageal Detector Devices

The simple and reliable esophageal detector devices (EDDs) can generally differentiate esophageal from tracheal intubations. EDDs aspirate air through the ETT, using the differences in tracheal and esophageal anatomy to indicate tube placement.[86,87] If air can be aspirated easily through the tube, it is in the non-collapsible trachea; failure to aspirate air means that the tube is in the collapsible esophagus.

The two major nonelectronic EDDs are a syringe type (Fig. 8-26) and a bulb type (Fig. 8-27). The syringe-type EDD is made by using a short length of rubber tubing attached to a 60-mL catheter-tip (Toomey) syringe using a right-angled ETT connector, such as is found at the end of a BVM. The Mapleson C (anesthesia) disposable breathing system also contains soft plastic adapters for wall-mounted oxygen delivery that can form the connection.[81]

A baby bottle nipple also works well as a connector from the ETT to the syringe. Enlarge the hole slightly in the nipple and insert the syringe toward the nipple's wide bottle-end opening. Slip the bottle-end opening over the ETT; it fits perfectly.

A mechanical EDD must be airtight to work correctly. Test it by occluding the open end with a finger and pulling back on the syringe plunger. If you feel resistance or a negative pressure, it is ready for use. Once the device is joined to an ETT, use the syringe to aspirate. An esophageal

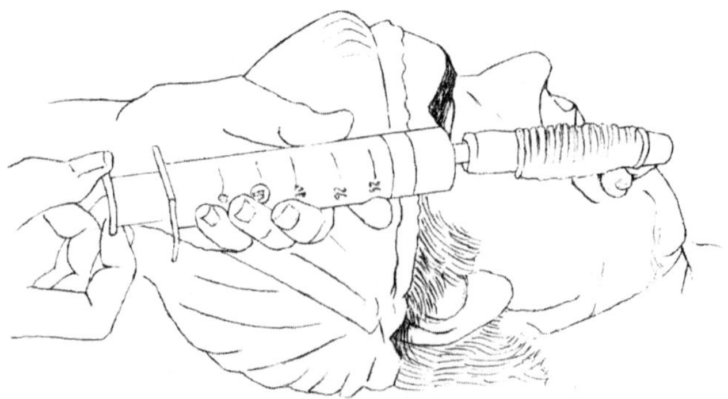

FIG. 8-26. Syringe endotracheal detection device.

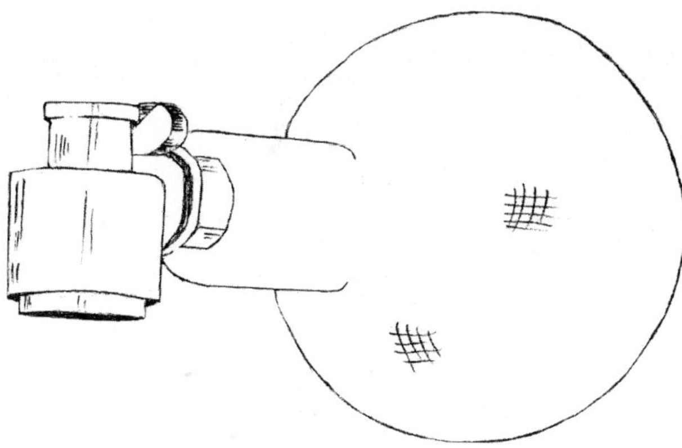

FIG. 8-27. Bulb endotracheal detection device.

intubation usually causes resistance when the syringe is aspirated and the esophagus collapses with the negative pressure; the plunger usually rebounds to its original position when released. Aspirating 30 mL of air without the plunger rebounding when released generally indicates a tracheal intubation.[86,87]

A simpler way to construct an EDD is to attach a self-inflating rubber bulb (such as may be used for newborn suctioning) directly to a right-angled ETT connector (see Fig. 8-27). Cut the suction end to accommodate the attachment. Squeeze the bulb and attach it to the ETT. Rapid passive reinflation indicates a tracheal intubation. When placed on a tube that is in the esophagus, it fails to reinflate due to esophageal collapse with the negative pressure, often producing a "flatus-like noise."[88]

The advantages of EDDs are that they (a) can be easily and inexpensively constructed with commonly available equipment; (b) are both portable and reusable; (c) do not require electricity; (d) are easy to use in hospital or prehospital settings with minimal instruction; and (e) produce highly reliable results rapidly, even during resuscitation efforts after a cardiac arrest.[89]

The disadvantages of EDDs include both false-positive and false-negative results, although the incidence of either is extremely low.[90] False-positive results (showing that the ETT is in the trachea when it is actually in the esophagus) are due to the regurgitation of gas from the stomach, esophageal distension with gas, or an EDD with a leak. False-negative results (showing that the ETT is in the esophagus when it is actually in the trachea) can occur when thick secretions block the ETT, when the end of the ETT is occluded by the tracheal wall, in obese patients, or with bronchial intubation, bronchospasm, tracheal compression, and chronic obstructive pulmonary disease.[89]

The devices are unreliable in infants <1 year old, although they work well in children ≥2 years old, even when using uncuffed tubes.[91,92] In children, use the device before any breaths are given through the tube, because extra air in the esophagus or stomach can give a false result. Only 10 cc should be aspirated if using a syringe device. Begin with the syringe plunger at the 10-mL mark, rather than at "0," to avoid an initial suction effect from the syringe.[91]

POST-INTUBATION MANAGEMENT

Securing the Endotracheal Tube

When securing an ETT, carefully note the depth, so that if the tube slips, it can be repositioned correctly.

Use interdental wiring (small-gauge wires or wire sutures) or heavy silk sutures to secure ETTs in place. This becomes particularly useful in patients with severe burns or injuries to the face. Loop a wire around an anterior tooth, usually an incisor, and twist it until it is tight. A needle holder or pliers helps to hold the wire ends when tightening them (Fig. 8-28). Then loop the free ends of the wire around the ETT and twist it until an indentation is noted in the tube.[93] When using a heavy ("0") silk suture, remove the needle and tie the suture very tightly around

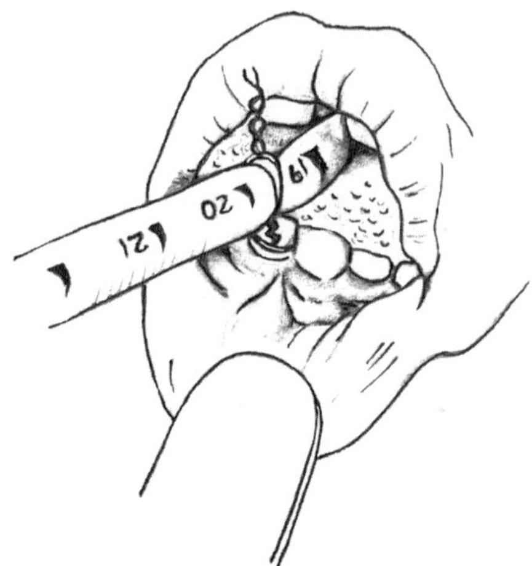

FIG. 8-28. Interdental wire securing endotracheal tube.

the base of the tooth. Tie in the ETT as with the wire suture, but add an additional tie on the ETT. A problem with using a silk suture is that it may break with intraoral manipulation, or it may slide down the silastic ETT, predisposing to unplanned extubation.[94]

Suctioning an Endotracheal Tube

If an ETT suction catheter is not available, use a number 10 rectal tube. This size works well for adult ETTs.[7]

Bite Block

To rapidly fashion a bite block, use a syringe barrel. When using it to protect the ETT, the safest method is to cut the end of the syringe barrel and slip it over the ET tube. Place it between the teeth, either before intubation or afterward, by temporarily removing the 15-mm adaptor and slipping the pilot balloon through, followed by the tube. Then, reinsert the 15-mm connector. When no longer needed, slide the barrel up on the tube and tape it in place so that it stays out of the mouth. From that position, it can be reinserted if necessary. To ensure that neither the bite block nor the ETT is displaced without recognizing it, tape them together.

Tube Changer

ETTs may need to be changed due to leaking cuffs, overly small tubes, or inspissated secretions that cause partial obstructions. Simply repeating the intubation may be a daunting task, especially if the airway has become edematous, the original intubation was difficult, or the clinician is inexperienced.

To lessen the chance that a problem will occur during the change—such as not being able to reintroduce the tube into the trachea—use a tube changer. A tube changer is a long guidewire, coated with a lubricant, which passes through the ETT currently in place and into the trachea. After preoxygenating the patient, pass the guidewire through the ETT and into the trachea. Carefully remove the ETT tube without displacing the guide. Then, gently elevate the jaw and slide the replacement tube over the guidewire into the trachea. If the tube gets hung up, withdraw it slightly, rotate it 90 degrees, and advance again.

Tube changers are normally gum-elastic bougies. Multiple pieces of equipment have been used as tube-changing guides. These include NG tubes with the flared ends and side ports cut off, feeding tubes, angiography catheters, or any piece of wire at least 2.5 times as long as the ETT. If using a wire such as an unwound coat hanger, cover it with an NG tube or double over the ends of the wire to avoid cutting the tissues. Cut off the "twisty" end of a coat hanger (the part that cannot be straightened easily). Then bend the wire to conform to the ETT that is in the patient. Success with improvised tube changers varies with their diameter relative to the ETT and their stiffness.[95]

SURGICAL AIRWAYS

Surgical airways, once common, are rarely used in emergency situations in developed countries. With their wide variety of intubating medications and sophisticated airway devices, clinicians usually have no need to apply a knife to the neck to get an emergent airway. Yet, when a patient needs an immediate airway and no other method is practicable, a surgical airway may be the best option. Some type of knife and a tube—even if they are not the optimal choices—are nearly always available. Having to perform a surgical airway is much more likely in austere medical situations than in normal circumstances.

Prediction of a Difficult Surgical Airway

A quick assessment can determine whether obtaining a surgical airway may be problematic. These are not contraindications, but simply observations that suggest that a surgical airway may be difficult, using the mnemonic "SHORT": Does the patient have (a) evidence of previous neck **S**urgery? (b) a **H**ematoma or abscess in the anterior neck? (c) **O**besity or other neck enlargement, such as from subcutaneous emphysema or edema? (d) prior **R**adiation to the neck area? or (e) a **T**umor in the neck area?[96]

In reality, in an emergency, the answers to those questions may not matter: You have to get an airway no matter what the situation. Knowing that these potential problems exist, however, may sway you toward another airway option, if it is available.

Cricothyrotomy

Cricothyrotomy is lifesaving: "This is an emergency procedure to be done at the site of injury, without anesthesia, with any sharp knife at hand."[97] A systematic review showed that no commercial cricothyrotomy kit demonstrated better results than any other or than traditional surgical and needle techniques.[98] The Israeli Defense Force provides a rule for when to do a cricothyrotomy (cric) in the prehospital setting: "After the first orotracheal intubation attempt, success with subsequent attempts tended to fall, with minimal improvement in overall intubation success seen after the third attempt. Because cric exhibited excellent success as a backup airway modality, we advocate controlling the airway with cric if intubation efforts have failed after two or three attempts. We recommend that providers reevaluate whether definitive airway control is truly necessary before each attempt to control the airway."[99]

Position

Physicians may have significant difficulty identifying the cricothyroid membrane correctly, especially in obese patients.[100] Consider locating the correct site for a cricothyrotomy using the "4-finger rule." When you lay the tip of the small finger in the sternal notch, the tip of the index finger lies over the cricothyroid membrane. This works for most adults. For a child, lift his or her hand to their neck to use their fingers. An alternative method in adults is to place one's index and long fingers on either side of the trachea (touching the anterior sternomastoid muscles) halfway down the anterior neck. Pushing posteriorly, the cricothyroid notch appears at the midline.

Procedure

Emergency cricothyroidotomies have been performed with scissors, pocket or hunting knives, razor blades, broken glass, and the jagged edges of the lid from a tin can. If using a scalpel, simply turning the scalpel blade's handle in the cricothyroid incision is as effective as using an intraoperative Trousseau dilator (the formal piece of equipment used in the OR to dilate the hole for a tracheostomy) to widen the hole to insert the tube. Using a skin hook allows a slightly larger-size ETT to be placed.[101] (For a skin hook fashioned from a bent needle, see Fig. 22-5.)

Another method of putting the tube in the trachea is to use the Seldinger technique. As soon as entry is made into the trachea, pass a guide, such as a wire or bougie, through it. Then, using the eyehole at the end of the ETT, pass the tube into the trachea.

Hold the Hole Open

Once the cricothyroid membrane is opened, if the patient is breathing spontaneously, such as when an upper airway obstruction has been relieved, the hole only needs to be held open manually. In these cases, the incision through the cricothyroid membrane needs to be slightly larger than normal. Airways also have been held open in these circumstances with paper clips and nail clippers.

Cricothyrotomy Tubes

Endotrachael and Tracheostomy Tubes

Placing an ETT through an emergency cricothyrotomy is optimal. It is easily handled, is readily available in most health care settings, is long enough not to slip out, and has a small enough balloon so that it does not tear as it passes into the trachea. A tracheostomy tube, if available, is a good alternative, although it is shorter and has a bulky balloon, potentially increasing complications in stressful situations.

Other Tubes

A wide variety of tubes has been suggested; some have even been tested. Some will be available only in health care facilities. Others are designed for use in out-of-hospital austere circumstances. The problem is that some do not work, but in these circumstances, you have to use what is available. Research shows that in critical situations when a cricothyrotomy tube is needed, it is best to use the largest hollow tube available that will fit through the hole. Be creative.

Syringe Barrel

An excellent cricothyrotomy tube can be fashioned from the flanged portion of a 2- or 3-mL syringe barrel cut to 45 degrees (Fig. 8-29). Remove the syringe plunger and cut the barrel at an approximate 45-degree angle, at a point one-third of the way toward the tip (needle end). Insert the cut end of the syringe through the surgical opening at a right angle to the trachea, with the long end entering through the upper part of the incision (Fig. 8-30). The flanges on the barrel act as a stopper and provide a site for securing the tube. The problem that arises with this device, as with many other improvised cricothyrotomy tubes, is how to attach a BVM, if one is available. Mouth-to-tube ventilation may be the only option for an apneic patient.[102]

Sports Bottle Straws

Not only have the relatively rigid and large-bore sports bottle straws been successfully used for emergency cricothyrotomies, but also both the ribbed and flat types had about the same airway resistance as do 7.0-mm ETTs and 8.0-mm tracheostomy tubes when tested. Moreover, a standard adapter from a 7.0-mm ETT can be inserted into the straw, if subsequently available, so that a bag-valve device can be used without reintubating the patient. Of course, as with all improvised devices, the straw lacks a cuff, so the patient's mouth must be sealed during mouth-to-straw ventilations. It is, however, long and flexible enough to fit into the trachea with enough extra length for the operator to perform ventilations.[103]

Tubes and Small Hollow Objects

Consider any available hollow tubing as a possible cricothyrotomy tube when doing an emergency procedure. Many small hollow objects have been suggested, including small flashlight or penlight casings, very small pill bottles, plastic throat swabs containers with the bottom cut out, and pen barrels, although they are not often used.

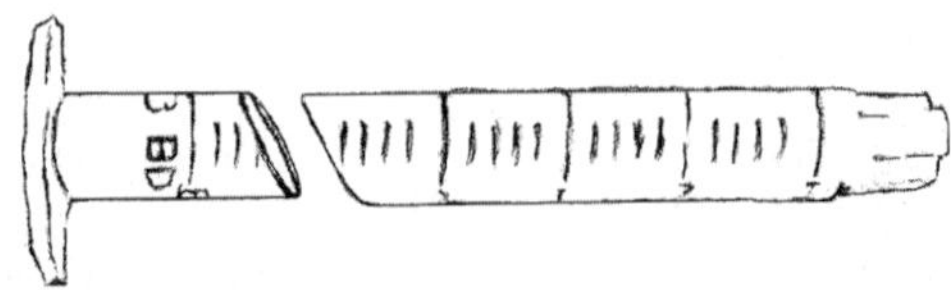

FIG. 8-29. Cricothyrotomy tube cut from 3-cc syringe.

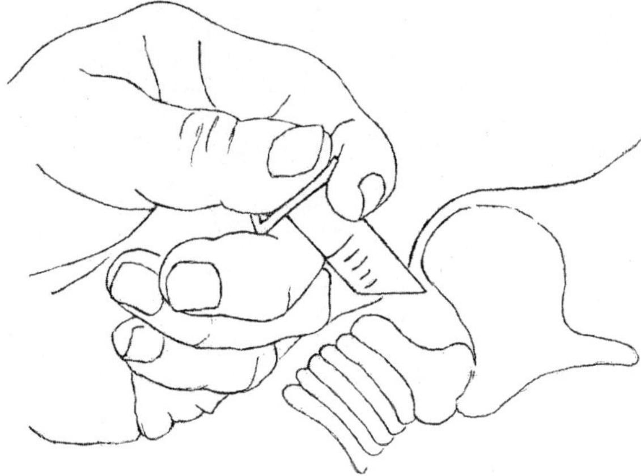

FIG. 8-30. Improvised cricothyrotomy tube inserted (lateral view).

Pen barrels have actually been tested. Although they are discussed in medical texts as being useful, at least the standard-issue US military ballpoint pen (Skilcraft, Alexandria, VA) produces so much airway resistance, even with the tapered tip cut off, that it is essentially useless as an airway—except, perhaps, as a route for transtracheal jet ventilation or for temporary apneic oxygenation.[103]

Intravenous Drip Chamber

The drip chamber from either regular intravenous tubing or one part of the "Y" from blood tubing has been suggested as a cricothyrotomy cannula.[104,105] The drip chamber is cut ~3 cm distal to the spike that goes into the IV bag/bottle. After cutting through the skin over the cricothyroid membrane (a vertical incision is best if uncertain of the landmarks), insert the spike through the membrane.[106]

Although the drip chamber supposedly fits well onto a standard BVM, tests show that it only works with some IV tubing. Even with tubing that is too small to fit well, "V-shaped" cuts can be made on both sides of the drip chamber and the BVM can be forced into or around it. Test this before inserting it into the neck, so that modifications can be made before it is in place. Also, consider attaching the BVM before inserting the tube, because attaching it may require more leverage than is possible once the tube is in place.

Post-Procedure Bleeding

Protect yourself, if possible, from the spray of blood that invariably accompanies opening the trachea. If you are midline, you can control any bleeding after the tube is in place by packing the area around it with petroleum jelly impregnated or other gauze. Sutures or cautery are rarely needed to control this bleeding. If you have strayed off midline, however, you may be into the major vessels of the neck—and will not find the trachea. Use a vertical incision and, once through the skin, feel for the cricothyroid membrane, or use the needle-guided method (as with an emergency tracheostomy, described next) if you are concerned about staying in the midline.

Emergency Tracheostomy

Because of its difficulty and potential complications, a true emergency "crash" tracheostomy should be the last option if no other method of establishing an adequate airway is available. An emergency tracheostomy is also useful in children needing an immediate surgical airway, because their cricothyroid area is generally too small for a cricothyrotomy. It can also be used (and the author has used it successfully) for patients in whom massive neck swelling from bleeding or from subcutaneous emphysema obscures the cricothyroid landmarks. The basic principle is to stay in the midline. The following technique provides a solution and has proved easy to learn and to use.

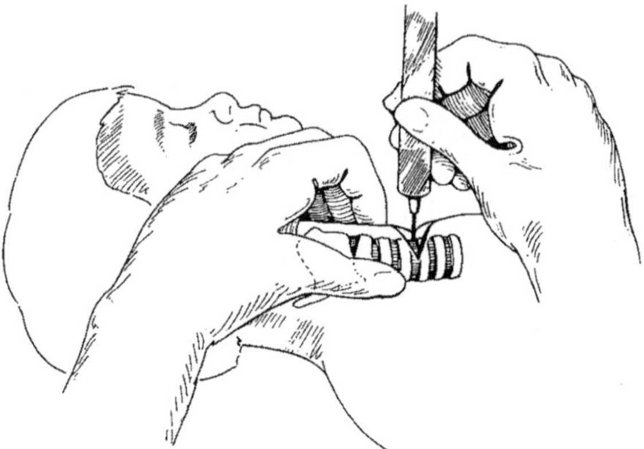

FIG. 8-31. Insert fluid-filled syringe with needle into midline until there is no resistance when pushing the plunger. (*Reproduced with permission from McLaughlin and Iserson.*[107])

This emergency tracheostomy technique requires only a fluid-filled syringe, a needle, a knife, and a tube. To perform the tracheostomy using this technique[107]: Locate the midline of the neck and secure the trachea between the thumb and index finger of the nondominant hand. Incise the overlying skin transversely. Use a finder needle, attached to a saline (or any nontoxic fluid)-filled syringe, to locate and stabilize the tracheal lumen prior to incision and cannulation. Insert the needle into the midline between the prominent thyroid cartilage and the sternal notch, aiming for the anterior trachea (Fig. 8-31). Inject the fluid gently; when it flows without resistance, the needle has entered the trachea. Aspiration of air confirms correct positioning within the lumen. While holding the needle steady, make a vertical stabbing incision lateral to and against the needle (Fig. 8-32). Using the knife handle to open the stoma, remove the needle and insert a standard ETT (Fig. 8-33). Secure the tube with tape and, if necessary, pack the wound to control bleeding.

Another slower tracheostomy method, only appropriate in nonurgent situations, requires some equipment that may not be readily available. Based on the method described previously, it uses the Seldinger (wire-through-needle) technique. With the larynx firmly stabilized with the nondominant hand, make a 1.5- to 2.0-cm transverse or vertical incision just below the cricoid cartilage. Then pass a large-gauge needle through the incision and into the trachea. Optimally, the

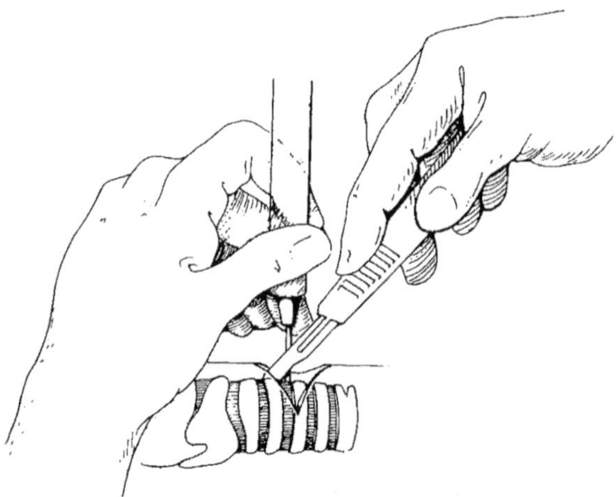

FIG. 8-32. Vertical incision in trachea. This is done with the needle still in place, "cutting down on" the needle. (*Reproduced with permission from McLaughlin and Iserson.*[107])

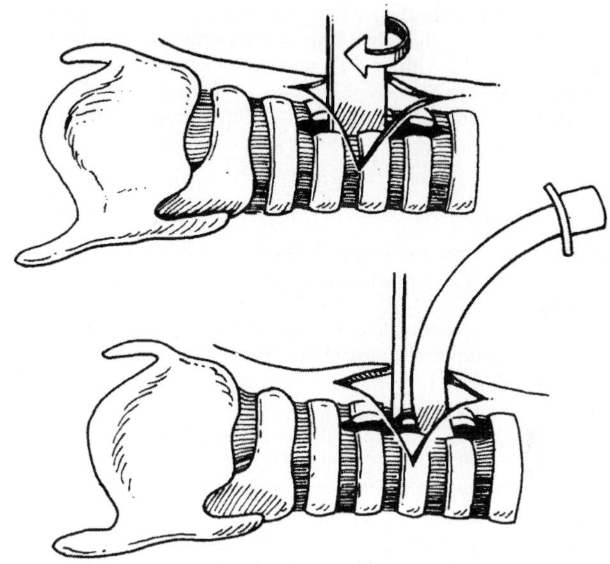

FIG. 8-33. Opening stoma with knife handle and introducing endotracheal or tracheostomy tube. (*Reproduced with permission from McLaughlin and Iserson.*[107])

needle is specifically designed to accommodate the wire, such as with an arterial line or a central line kit. Using a fluid-filled syringe attached to the needle simplifies locating the trachea with the needle, as described previously. Once the trachea is entered, carefully remove the syringe and pass the wire through the needle into the trachea. Pass small (artery-dilating Howard-Kelly) forceps along the wire through the soft tissues of the neck until you feel resistance at the outside of the trachea. Open the forceps to dilate the opening down to the trachea. Then close the forceps and pass them over the wire through the tracheal wall. Advance the forceps until the tip is in the long axis of the trachea; spread the forceps and pass the tracheostomy tube or, if the wire is long enough, pass an ETT over the guide wire.[108,109]

Dislodged Tracheostomy Tube

The only sign that the tracheostomy tube is dislodged may be the inability to pass a suction catheter through it, although this can also occur when concretions block the tube.

A mature (>30 days) tracheostomy tube can usually be replaced without too much difficulty if no granulation tissue or foreign body blocks the passage. Simply replace the obturator and pass it into the mature stoma. With tracheostomies <1 month old, it may be difficult to put a dislodged tube back into the trachea due to stoma closure; trying to do so may cause a false passage. In these cases, place an ETT, rather than the shorter tracheostomy tube; a tracheostomy tube can be placed once the airway is again secure.

As a guide, use a urethral catheter with the tip cut off, a suction catheter, or similar tubing connected to an oxygen source. Pass it through the ETT and then gently into the trachea. If the trachea cannot be visualized, pass a pediatric laryngoscope into the trachea, followed by the tube/guide. Once the tube is in the trachea, remove the guide.[110]

Post-Tracheostomy Bleeding

Post-tracheostomy bleeding can be deadly. While mild incision bleeding is typical 1 to 3 weeks post tracheostomy, 85% of tracheo-innominate artery fistula bleeds also occur in the first month. They have a mortality rate of 80% even with treatment. Post-tracheostomy bleeding often occurs due to granulation tissue in the stoma or trachea or erosion of the thyroid vessels or gland, or the tracheal wall due to overzealous suctioning.[111]

Methods to help control the bleeding while getting the patient to the OR or interventional radiology include hyperinflating the tube's cuff, putting mild anterior traction on the tube, or replacing the tracheostomy tube with an ETT and hyperinflating the balloon, which should be placed, if possible, just distal to the site of bleeding to tamponade it. The best technique is to stick one's finger into the stoma and apply local digital pressure to compress the innominate artery. If this does not work on one side, go to the other side.[112]

REFERENCES

1. Greenberg RS. Facemask, nasal, and oral airway devices. *Anesthesiol Clin N Am.* 2002;20(4):833-861.
2. Holcomb JB. The 2004 Fitts Lecture: current perspective on combat casualty care. *J Trauma.* 2005;59(4):990-1002.
3. Blake WE, Stillman BC, Eizenberg N, et al. The position of the spine in the recovery position–an experimental comparison between the lateral recovery position and the modified HAINES position. *Resuscitation.* 2002;53:289-297.
4. Husum H, Ang SC, Fosse E. *War Surgery: Field Manual.* Penang, Malaysia: Third World Network; 1995:136.
5. Foote EM. *A Text-book of Minor Surgery.* New York, NY: Appleton; 1912:723-724.
6. Aronson E. Notes on anaesthesia. *Med Record: A Weekly J Med Surg.* 1899;55(Feb 18):236-238.
7. Boulton TB, Cole PV. Anesthesia in difficult situations. 2. General anesthesia-general considerations. *Anesthesia.* 1966;21(3):379-399.
8. Townsley RB, Baring DE, Clark LJ. Emergency department care of a patient after a total laryngectomy. *European J Emerg Med.* 2014;21:(3):164-169.
9. Miller K. Trauma and injuries: airway management. NDMS Response Team Training Program, 2003.
10. Law JA, Broemling, N, Cooper RM, et al. The difficult airway with recommendations for management–Part 2–the anticipated difficult airway. *Can J Anesth.* 2013;60(11):1119-1138.
11. Murphy C, Wong DT. Airway management and oxygenation in obese patients. *Can J Anesth.* 2013;60(9):929-945.
12. Boyce JR. Poor man's LMA: achieving adequate ventilation with a poor mask seal. *Can J Anaesth.* 2001;48(5):483-485.
13. Hooker EA, Danzl DF, O'Brien D, et al. Percutaneous transtracheal ventilation: resuscitation bags do not provide adequate ventilation. *Prehosp Disaster Med.* 2006;21(6):431-435.
14. Metz S, Parmet JL, Levitt JD. Failed emergency transtracheal ventilation through a 14-gauge intravenous catheter. *J Clin Anesth.* 1996;8(1):58-62.
15. Smith RB, Albin MS, Williams RL. Percutaneous transtracheal jet ventilation. *J Clin Anesth.* 1996;8(8):689-690.
16. Boyce JR, Peters GE, Carroll WR, et al. Preemptive vessel dilator cricothyrotomy aids in the management of upper airway obstruction. *Can J Anaesth.* 2005;52(7):765-769.
17. Patil VU, Atlas GM, Woo P. Use of a large bore cricothyroidotomy catheter for emergency airway management (abstract). *J Trauma.* 1993;35(2):323.
18. Wrathall G. The management of major trauma. *Update Anaesth.* 1996;6:1-19.
19. Scuderi PE, McLeskey CH, Comer PB. Emergency percutaneous transtracheal ventilation during anesthesia using readily available equipment. *Anesth Analg.* 1982;61(10):867-870.
20. Dhara SS. Aids to tracheal intubation. *Pract Proced.* 2003;17(3):1. http://e-safe-anaesthesia.org/e_library/05/Tracheal_intubation_aids_Update_2003.pdf. Accessed September 4, 2015.
21. Smith RB, Schaer WB, Pfaeffle H. Percutaneous transtracheal ventilation for anaesthesia and resuscitation: a review and report of complications. *Can Anaesth Soc J.* 1975;22(5):607-612.
22. Yealy DM, Plewa MC, Reed JJ, et al. Manual translaryngeal jet ventilation and the risk of aspiration in a canine model. *Ann Emerg Med.* 1990;19(11):1238-1241.
23. Reich DL, Schwartz N. An easily assembled device for transtracheal oxygenation. *Anesthesiology.* 1987;66(3):437-438.
24. Manoach SC, Corinaldi C, Paladino L, et al. Percutaneous transcricoid jet ventilation compared with surgical cricothyroidotomy in sheep airway salvage model. *Resuscitation.* 2004;62:79-87.
25. Yodfat UA. Modified technique for laryngeal mask airway insertion. *Anesth Analg.* 1999;89:1327.
26. Jaffe RA, Brock-Utne JG. A modification of the Yodfat laryngeal mask airway insertion technique. *J Clin Anesth.* 2002;14(6):462-463.
27. King MH, ed. *Primary Anaesthesia.* Oxford, UK: Oxford University Press; 1986:16-17.

28. Grosshandler S, Vlazny F. Universal adapter for endotracheal tubes. *Anesthesiology*. 1964;25:727.
29. Albert SN. A "homemade" endotracheal-tube adaptor. *Anesth Analg*. 1973;52(1):79-80.
30. King MH, ed. *Primary Anesthesia*. Oxford, UK: Oxford University Press; 1986:102.
31. Brock-Utne JG. A leaking endotracheal tube in a prone patient. *Clinical Anesthesia: Near Misses and Lessons Learned*. New York, NY: Springer; 2008:127-128.
32. Briskin A, Drenger B, Regev E, et al. Original method for in situ repair of damage to endotracheal tube. *Anesthesiology*. 2000;93(3):891-892.
33. Choi PT-L, Rhyddercb G. An unusual cause of elevated airway pressures. *Can J Anaesth*. 1998;45:381.
34. Bern MJ, Wilson IH. Coathanger wire, as an aid to endotracheal intubation. *Trop Doct*. 1991;21(3):122-123.
35. Dexheimer Neto FL, de Andrade JMS, Raupp ACT, et al. Use of a homemade introducer guide (bougie) for intubation in emergency situation in patients who present with difficult airway: a case series. *Brazilian J Anesth (English Ed.)*. March 2014, online.
36. Manos SJ, Brock-Utne JG, Jaffe RA. An alternative to the gum elastic bougie and/or the jet stylet. *Anesth Analg*. 1994;79:1017.
37. Tate N. Transillumination of the larynx. *Lancet*. 1955;ii:980.
38. Essien CK. What do you do when the laryngoscope bulb fails during intubation? *Pract Proced*. 1995;5(9):1. http://www.nda.ox.ac.uk/wfsa/html/u05/u0509_015.htm. Accessed September 13, 2006.
39. Ayim E, Bewes PC, Cory C, et al. *Primary Anaesthesia*. Oxford, UK: Oxford University Press; 1986:102.
40. Gillett GB, Patkin M. A laryngoscope for emergency use. *Anaesthesia*. 1964;19:595-597.
41. Staff of CMC Hospital Vellore. The Vellore laryngoscope. *J Christ Med Assoc India*. 1965;40:459.
42. Yeats M. Maintaining your laryngoscope. *Pract Proced*. 2004;4:(9)1. www.nda.ox.ac.uk/wfsa/html/u04/u04_018.htm. Accessed September 13, 2006.
43. Roark GL. Use of a fiberoptic cystoscope to facilitate intubation in a difficult airway. *Trop Doct*. 2006;36:104-105.
44. Iserson KV. Blind nasotracheal intubation. *Ann Emerg Med*. 1981;10(9):468-471.
45. Tintinalli FE, Claffey J. Complications of nasotracheal intubation. *Ann Emerg Med*. 1981;10(3):142-144.
46. Iserson KV. Blind nasotracheal intubation—a model for instruction. *Ann Emerg Med*. 1984;13(8):601-2. Reprinted in: *Can J Prehosp Med*. 1986;1(3):30-31.
47. Van Elstraete AC, Pennant JH, Gajraj NM, et al. Tracheal tube cuff inflation as an aid to blind nasotracheal intubation. *Br J Anaesth*. 1993;70:691-693.
48. Van Elstraete AC, Mamie JC, Mehdaoui H. Nasotracheal intubation in patients with immobilized cervical spine: a comparison of tracheal tube cuff inflation and fiberoptic bronchoscopy. *Anesth Analg*. 1998;87:400-402.
49. Casals-Caus P, Mayoral-Rojals V, Canales MA, et al. El inflado del neumotaponamiento como ayuda para la intubación nasotraqueal a ciegas en pacientes con predicción de laringoscopia difícil. [Inflation of the cuff as an aid to blind nasotracheal intubation in patients with predicted difficult laryngoscopy.] *Rev Esp Anestesiol Reanim*. 1997;44:302-304.
50. Dryden GE. Use of a suction catheter to assist blind nasal intubation (letter). *Anesthesiology*. 1974;45:260.
51. Sloan EP, VanRooyen MJ. Suction catheter-assisted nasotracheal intubation. *Acad Emerg Med*. 1994;1:388.
52. Findlay CW, Gissen AJ. A guided nasotracheal method for insertion of an endotracheal tube. *Anesth Analg*. 1961;40(6):460-462.
53. Kite C. *An Essay on the Recovery of the Apparently Dead*. London, UK: C. Dilly in the Poultry; 1788.
54. Hardwick WC, Bluhm D. Digital intubation. *J Emerg Med*. 1984;1(4):317-320.
55. Young SE, Miller MA, Crystal CS, et al. Is digital intubation an option for emergency physicians in definitive airway management? *Am J Emerg Med*. 2006;24(6):729-732.
56. Stewart RD. Tactile orotracheal intubation. *Ann Emerg Med*. 1984;13:175-178.
57. Cook RT. A modification to the standard digital intubation technique. *Am J Emerg Med*. 1992;10:396.
58. Woody NC, Woody HB. Direct digital intratracheal intubation for neonatal resuscitation. *J Pediatr*. 1968;73(6):903-905.
59. Hancock P, Peterson G. Finger intubation of the trachea in newborns. *Pediatrics*. 1992;89:325-327.
60. Benumof JL. Management of the difficult airway. *Anesthesiology*. 1991;75:1087-1110.

61. Breen PH. Simple technique to remove laryngeal mask airway "guide" after endotracheal intubation (letter). *Anesth Analg*. 1996;82:1302.
62. Breen PH. An alternative way to remove the laryngeal mask airway "guide" after intubation (letter). *Anesth Analg*. 1997;85:948-949.
63. Kyama S. An alternative way to remove the laryngeal mask airway "guide" after intubation (letter). *Anesth Analg*. 1997;85:948-949.
64. Barnard EBG, Moy RJ, Kehoe AD, Bebarta VS, Smith JE. Rapid sequence induction of anaesthesia via the intraosseous route: a prospective observational study. *Emerg Med J*. June 24, 2014 (online).
65. Dobson MB. *Anaesthesia at the District Hospital*. 2nd ed. Geneva, Switzerland: WHO; 2000:76-77.
66. Morris IA. Pharmacologic aids to intubation and the rapid sequence induction. *Emerg Med Clin North Am*. 1988;6(4):753-768.
67. Kenny JF, Molloy K, Pollack M, et al. Nebulized lidocaine as an adjunct to endotracheal intubation in the prehospital setting. *Prehosp Disaster Med*. 1996;11(4):312-313.
68. King M. *Primary Surgery, Vol. 2: Trauma*. Oxford, UK: Oxford University Press; 1987:11.
69. Pearson JW, Safar P. General anesthesia with minimal equipment. *Anesth Analg*. 1961;40(6):664-671.
70. Walts LF, Kassity KJ. Spread of local anesthesia after upper airway block. *Arch Otolaryngol*. 1965;81: 77-79.
71. Boulton TB. Anesthesia in difficult situations. The use of local analgesia. *Anaesthesia*. 1967;22(1): 101-133.
72. Duncan JAT. Intubation of the trachea in the conscious patient. *Br J Anaesth*. 1977;49:619-623.
73. Dobson MB. *Anaesthesia at the District Hospital*. 2nd ed. Geneva, Switzerland: World Health Organization; 2000:89.
74. Prior FN. Anaesthetic household hints. *J Christian Med Assoc India*. 1964;39:282-287.
75. Danzl DF, Thomas DM. Nasotracheal intubation in the emergency department. *Crit Care Med*. 1980;8: 677-682.
76. Gold MI, Buechel DR. Translaryngeal anesthesia: a review. *Anesthesiology*. 1959;20:181-185.
77. Botha MJ, Wells M. Ujuzi (Practical Pearl/*Perle Pratique*). *African J Emerg Med*. 2014 (in press).
78. Dobson MB. *Anaesthesia at the District Hospital*. 2nd ed. Geneva, Switzerland: World Health Organization; 2000:14, Table 1.
79. Andersen KH, Hald A. Assessing the position of the tracheal tube: the reliability of different methods. *Anaesthesia*. 1989;44:984-985.
80. Baigel G, Safranske J. Clinical test to confirm tracheal intubation: a new method to confirm endotracheal intubation in the absence of capnography. *Eur J Anaesth*. 2003;20:475-477.
81. Sellers SF, Holesworth SP. Updating Wee's oesophageal detector. *Anaesthesia*. 2003;8(6):615-616.
82. Nicoll SJB, King CJ. Airway auscultation: a new method of confirming tracheal intubation. *Anaesthesia*. 1998;53:41-45.
83. Kaldirim U, Tuncer S, Eyi YE. Does ultrasonographic lung sliding sign always verify the success in endotracheal tube intubation? *Am J Emerg Med*. 2014;32:472.
84. Raphael DT, Conard FU. Ultrasound confirmation of endotracheal tube placement. *J Clin Ultrasound*. 1987;15:459-62.
85. Sun JT, Sim SS, Chou HC, et al. Ultrasonography for proper endotracheal tube placement confirmation in out-of-hospital cardiac arrest patients: two-center experience. *Crit Ultrasound J*. 2014;6(suppl 1); A29.
86. Wee MYK. The esophageal detector device: assessment of a new method to distinguish esophageal from tracheal intubation. *Anaesthesia*. 1988;43:27-29.
87. O'Leary JJ, Pollard BJ, Ryan MJ. A method of detecting esophageal intubation or confirming tracheal intubation. *Anaesth Intensive Care*. 1988;16:299-301.
88. Nunn JF. The esophageal detector device (letter). *Anaesthesia*. 1988;43:804.
89. Haridas RP. Oesophageal detector devices. *Update Anaesth*. 1997;7(6). www.nda.ox.ac.uk/wfsa/html/u07/u07_016.htm. Accessed September 14, 2007.
90. Zaleski L, Abello D, Gold MI. The esophageal detector device. *Anesthesiology*. 1993;79:244-247.
91. Wee MYK, Walker AKY. The oesophageal detector device: an assessment with uncuffed tubes in children. *Anaesthesia*. 1991;46:869-871.
92. Haynes SR, Morton NS. Use of the oesophageal detector device in children under one year of age. *Anaesthesia*. December 1990;45(12):1067-1069.
93. Jensen Neils F. Securing an endotracheal tube in the presence of facial burns or instability (letter). *Anesth Analg*. 1992;75:633-646.

94. Botts J, Srivastava KA, Matsuda T, et al. Interdental wire fixation of endotracheal tube for surgery of severe facial burns. *Ann Burns Fire Disasters*. 1998;11(3):168-170.

95. Kumar R, Mittal S, Kumar S, et al. An easily available device as a makeshift tube changer. *J Anaesth Clin Pharmacol*. 2004;20(4):417-418.

96. Murphy MF, Walls RM. Identification of the difficult and failed airway. In: Walls RM, Murphy MF, eds. *Manual of Emergency Airway Management*. 3rd ed. Philadelphia, PA: Lippincott Williams & Wilkins; 2008:81-92.

97. Husum H, Ang SC, Fosse E. *War Surgery: Field Manual*. Penang, Malaysia: Third World Network; 1995:139.

98. Langvad S, Hyldmo PK, Anders Rostrup Nakstad AR, et al. Emergency cricothyrotomy—a systematic review. *Scand J Trauma Resusc Emerg Med*. 2013;21:43.

99. Katzenell U, Lipsky AM, Abramovich A, et al. Prehospital intubation success rates among Israel Defense Forces providers: epidemiologic analysis and effect on doctrine. *J Trauma Acute Care Surg*. 2013;75(2):S178-S183.

100. Murphy C, Wong DT. Airway management and oxygenation in obese patients. *Can J Anesth*. 2013;60(9): 929-945.

101. Bramwell KJ, Davis DP, Cardall TV, et al. Use of the Trousseau dilator in cricothyrotomy. *J Emerg Med*. 1999;17(3):433-436.

102. Jackson AS. Emergency care of the trauma patient in remote regions of Papua New Guinea. *Papua New Guinea Med J*. 2002;45(3-4):222-232.

103. Adams BD, Whitlock WL. Bystander cricothyroidotomy performed with an improvised airway. *Mil Med*. January 2002;167:76-78.

104. Fisher JA. A "last ditch" airway. *Can Anaesth Soc J*. 1979;26:225-230.

105. Blanas N, Fisher JA. A "last ditch" airway revisited. *Can J Anaesth*. 1999;46(8):809-810.

106. Platt-Mills TF, Lewin MR, Wells J, et al. Improvised cricothyrotomy provides reliable airway access in an unembalmed human cadaver model. *Wild Environ Med*. 2006;17:81-86.

107. McLaughlin JH, Iserson KV. Emergency pediatric tracheotomies—a usable technique and model for instruction. *Ann Emerg Med*. 1986;15(4):463-465.

108. Griggs WM, Gilliagan JE, Myburg JA. A simple percutaneous tracheostomy technique. *Surg Gynecol Obstet*. 1990;170:543-545.

109. Soni N. Percutaneous tracheostomy: how to do it. *Br J Hosp Med*. 1992;57(7):339-345.

110. Bailitz JM. *Tracheostomy tubes in the emergency department: tricks & troubleshooting. ACEP Scientific Assembly*, Seattle, WA, October 11, 2007.

111. Berrouschot J, Oeken J, Steiniger L, et al. Perioperative complications of percutaneous dilational tracheostomy. *Laryngoscope*. Nov 1997;107(11 Pt1):1538-1544.

112. Allan JS, Wright CD. Tracheoinnominate fistula: diagnosis and management. *Chest Surg Clin North Am*. May 2003;13(2):331-341.

9 | Breathing/Pulmonary

LUNG SOUNDS

Clinicians are exhorted to always place their stethoscopes directly on a patient's skin. Yet, when patients are examined in hallways and prehospital settings or in locations where cultural norms prevent patients from disrobing, this rule is often violated. That is not a problem: By applying pressure on the stethoscope head, clinicians can hear all the sounds normally heard on bare skin, through up to two layers of indoor clothing—including double-layered flannel shirts. Of course, inspection and percussion cannot be done through clothing, and clothing-induced acoustic artifacts may create problems.[1]

QUANTIFYING PLEURAL FLUID USING ULTRASOUND

Estimate the amount of pleural fluid using an ultrasound examination on supine patients. Elevate the chest to 15 degrees and move the probe perpendicular to the body axis along the posterior axillary line. Measure the maximal pleural separation, which is usually visible at the lung base. The simplified formula is: Volume of pleural fluid (mL) = 20 × Maximal distance between parietal and visceral pleura in end expiration (mm).[2]

PULMONARY TREATMENT

Aerosols and Spacers

The use of aerosol spacers more than doubles the amount of medication delivered to the lungs from metered-dose inhalers (MDIs); for steroid inhalers, an aerosol spacer diminishes the incidence of oral candidiasis by decreasing deposition in the oropharynx. The tube from a roll of toilet paper works well as an aerosol spacer, as does a piece of ventilator tubing.

Dr. Lara Zibners-Lohr wrote that in remote areas of the world, she uses large Styrofoam cups. The cup lip (open end) goes over the nose and mouth. The MDI goes through a hole in the bottom end of the cup. She uses just the blue tubing from a nebulizer for older children: they close their mouth around one end and put the MDI in the other. (Personal written communication, June 5, 2007.)

Dr. Karen Schneider uses a dry water bottle with a hole in the bottom for the MDI. The hole is sealed with tape, leaving a small opening to allow air movement from the outside when the child inhales. The inside of the bottle must be dry; otherwise, the aerosolized particles will stick to the water. When the MDI is activated, the child places his or her mouth over the drinking end and inhales a few times until the mist is cleared (Fig. 9-1). It is important that the child not exhale into the bottle because this will blow the mist out the small hole. (Written communication, June 5, 2007.)

Improvised spacers have been shown to be just as effective as the expensive commercial spacers.[3]

Treating Persistent Cough

An unremitting cough may be due to airway hyperirritability caused by an upper respiratory infection, toxic inhalation, asthma (sometimes unrecognized), allergens, or the use of angiotensin-converting enzyme (ACE) inhibitors. The cough is uncomfortable for the patient and may worsen bronchospasm. For adults and children, add 0.5 mg/kg of lidocaine to 0.3 mL of albuterol solution in 3 mL of normal saline; administer the combination by aerosol nebulization. Lidocaine suppresses the cough reflex while the sympathomimetic agent relieves the bronchospasm.[4]

Positioning to Improve Lung Function and Maximize Oxygenation

In patients with unilateral lung disease, positioning the healthy lung down—in the most dependent position possible—may improve the ventilation–perfusion mismatch and raise oxygen saturation levels. This may buy valuable time, turning an emergent situation into an urgent one.[5]

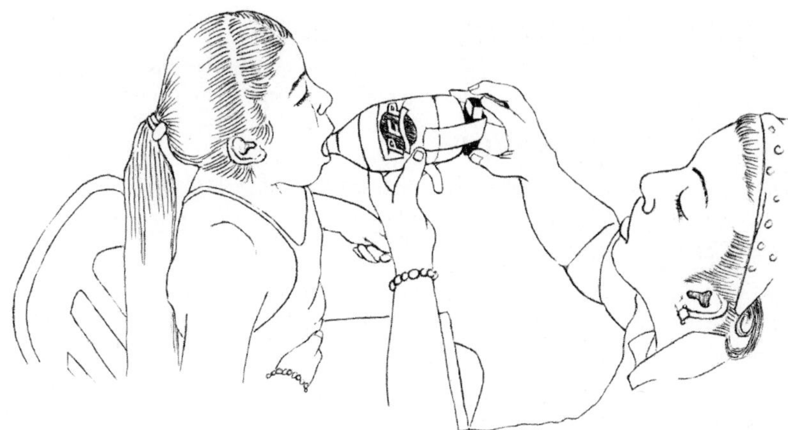

FIG. 9-1. Water bottle used as spacer by Dr. Schneider in Peru. (*Drawn from a photo contributed by Dr. Karen Schneider.*)

The FiO_2 can be doubled by combining nasal oxygen (15 liters/minute) and non-rebreather face mask oxygen (15 L/min) (Fig. 9-2). The technique delivers close to 100% FiO_2 (rather than the typical 60%) by eliminating the accumulation and rebreathing of CO_2 in the mask, hypopharynx, and nasopharynx. This method is useful to buy time to set up formal noninvasive ventilation (NIV) equipment or to more quickly preoxygenate before intubation. If using a bag-valve-mask (BVM), attach a positive end-expiratory pressure (PEEP) valve (set the dial at 5 mm Hg) to produce a slightly positive end-expiratory pressure through the ventilation cycle.[6]

Under anesthesia, and probably in other critical care situations, morbidly obese patients have a wide alveolar–arterial oxygen gradient [$P(A\text{-}a)O_2$]. However, when they are placed in the reverse Trendelenburg position (RTP), with their head higher than their feet, their A-a gradient shows a significant improvement and a return toward baseline. In addition, total respiratory system compliance is significantly higher in RTP, suggesting that RTP is an appropriate position

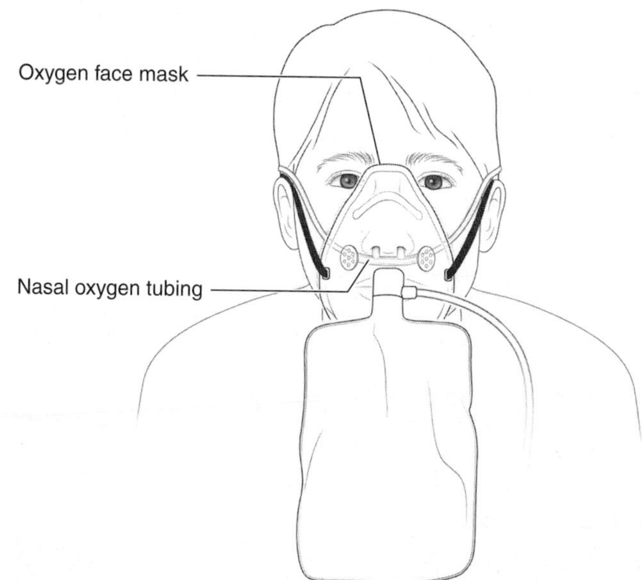

FIG. 9-2. Nasal prongs combined with non-rebreather face mask.

for obese subjects who can tolerate it, because it causes minimal arterial blood pressure changes and improves oxygenation.[7]

Sitting a ventilated patient up also helps avoid gastric aspiration. Use this simple maneuver in any patient whose blood pressure can tolerate a semi-recumbent or upright position.[8]

Makeshift Noninvasive Ventilation (NIV)

Clinicians now commonly use noninvasive ventilation to avoid or delay intubating patients.

Guidelines for Appropriate Use Outside Critical Care Areas (from University Medical Center, Tucson, Ariz., 2014)

1. Stable patients who require NIV for obesity hypoventilation syndrome, obstructive sleep apnea, or other chronic, stable conditions. The patient can go to an unmonitored inpatient bed.
2. Palliative care use of NIV to alleviate suffering at the end of life. The patient can go to an unmonitored inpatient bed.
3. Acute or acute-on-chronic respiratory distress, including patients listed under #1, above, with progressive or new problems. The patient must go to a monitored inpatient bed.

Noninvasive Ventilation in Chest Trauma

A meta-analysis suggests that early use of NIV in chest trauma patients may reduce mortality and the intubation rate without increasing complications. However, the patient selection criteria and timing for NIV remain unclear.[9]

Bi-level Positive Airway Pressure

Bi-level positive airway pressure (BiPAP) is becoming an increasingly useful modality to avoid intubations. In settings with ventilators but no BiPAP equipment, BiPAP can be improvised. For example, after Hurricane Katrina, Peter DeBlieux, MD, FACEP, reported that physicians at Charity Hospital improvised BiPAP machines from mechanical ventilators: "We used a pressure-cycled ventilator with pressure support of 10 cm H_2O and PEEP [positive end-expiratory pressure] of 5 cm H_2O and attached it to the circuit. [However,] ventilators do not tolerate the leak associated with noninvasive ventilation (NIV or NIPPV) and the alarms sound frequently with mouth opening and poor mask fit. A full-face mask is necessary when using this system, rather than a smaller nasal mask. Using BiPAP as invasive ventilators is not the standard, but could be used in a pinch for pressure supported ventilation." (Written communication, February 2008.)

Continuous Positive Airway Pressure Using a Nasopharyngeal Airway

Use a nasopharyngeal airway (NPA) to generate positive-pressure oxygenation when other methods will not work. This method can provide NIV in patients with a poor mask seal and apneic oxygenation during procedures, including intubation. It also allows positive-pressure oxygenation without obstructing airway visualization. To use this method, insert an NPA into the nostril and connect it, using standard wall suction tubing, to an oxygen regulator opened to >25 L/min, if the regulator goes that high (Fig. 9-3). Excessive pressure exits through the open nare and mouth. Aspiration and gastric insufflations are the primary risks, as with other NIV methods.[10]

Alternative Neonatal Continuous Positive Airway Pressure

In neonates and infants, an infant feeding tube (IFT) can deliver continuous positive airway pressure (CPAP) simply, economically, and with fewer adverse effects than with traditional methods. Insert an IFT into the nasopharynx, approximately the distance between the tip of the nose and the tragus. Connect the tube to an oxygen flow meter (usually 2-6 L/min) with a humidifier. This method is used in many developing countries with few complications (e.g., nasal mucosal injury, stomach distension, aspiration, hyperinflation, and pulmonary air leaks) that can be avoided with humidification and gastric decompression.[11]

MAKESHIFT SPIROMETERS

To encourage patients to breathe deeply after surgery, trauma, or illness, use an incentive spirometer, such as a balloon or a surgical glove. Have the patient blow one up several times an hour while awake. It works, however, only if the patient has received adequate analgesia.[12]

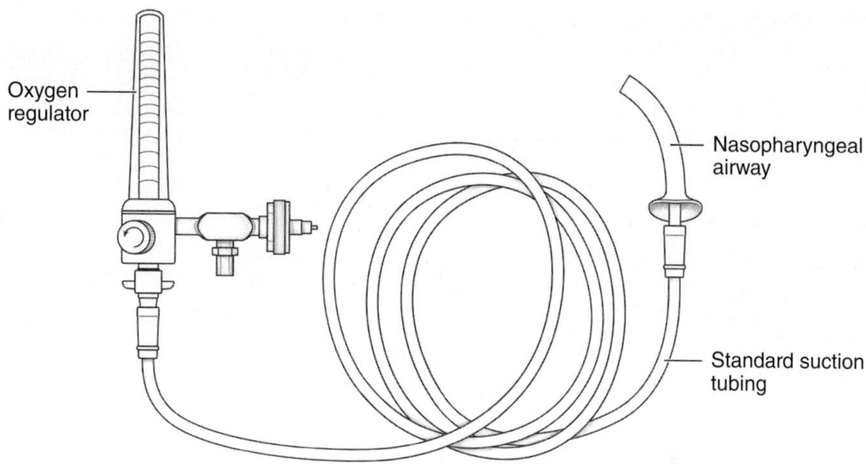

FIG. 9-3. NIV setup after inserting the tubing into an NPA.

Incentive spirometers can also be made from plastic bottles, such as those for milk or soda. Fill the bottle about halfway with water. Insert a tube with an internal diameter (ID) of at least 0.5 cm so that the resistance is not too great (Fig. 9-4). Insert the tube into the bottle's open mouth; this can be messy if the bottle tips over. Instead, you can insert the tube through a hole drilled in the resealed cap, although, in that case, either the cap must be left loose or a small additional hole must be made so that air can escape. Adjust the water height (resistance) for the patient; less water may be necessary for children and for the elderly and infirm. Have the patient blow bubbles. Coloring the water with food coloring makes it more fun for children. Spirometers improvised to measure lung function produce unreliable measurements.

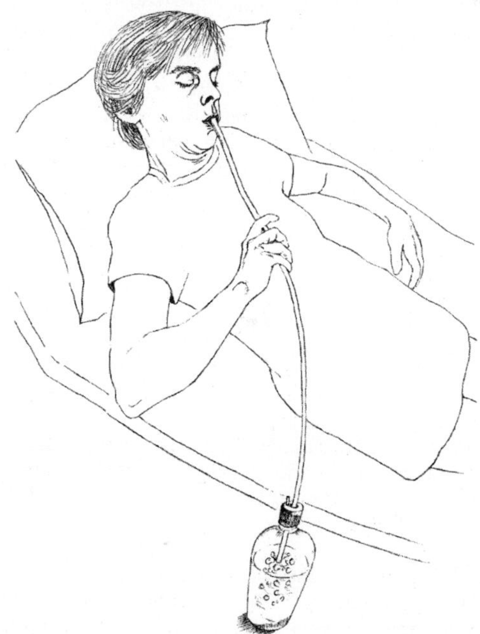

FIG. 9-4. Incentive spirometer made from cola bottle.

OXYGEN

Oxygen is one of the most basic drugs we have. In many acute illnesses, such as acute respiratory infections, asthma, fetal asphyxia, and shock, the availability of an oxygen supply can save a patient's life. It becomes especially important during resuscitations, in the operating room, or when treating cardiopulmonary illnesses and any illness (including acute mountain sickness) at altitude.

Industrial Oxygen

In austere medical situations, industrial (or research or aviation) oxygen can be used instead of medical oxygen. Oxygen gas is produced from the boiling-off of liquid oxygen, so it would appear that industrial oxygen is the same as medical oxygen. However, there is an ongoing controversy about whether there is any difference between four kinds of oxygen that are sold: aviation, medical, welding, and research. They are all at least 99.5% pure (usually 99.9% pure) and all are produced from an identical—often the same—system. Any humidity present in medical oxygen is added at the bedside. Purity is not an issue, because the purity required for welding is more critical than that for breathing. The major differences between medical oxygen and industrial oxygen are how it is filtered and the amount of liability insurance paid by the manufacturer. Microscopic filtration is used to remove air particles from both, but medical oxygen is run through filters that can also remove bacteria, and so is considered sterile.[13-15]

Oxygen Cylinders

Oxygen often comes in bulky, expensive cylinders. It may be difficult to identify which cylinders contain oxygen. The international standard requires oxygen cylinders to be painted white. In the United States, however, they are green, and in British Commonwealth countries, they are usually black with white shoulders. Industrial oxygen cylinders may be painted almost any color, so don't rely on the cylinder's color to identify its contents.[16] Note that you may see one of two terms used in descriptions of flow rates, either the term psi (pounds-force per square inch) or psig (pounds-force per square inch gauge; i.e., pressure related to the surrounding atmosphere). For medical purposes, they are generally equivalent. In this book, I will use the term "psi."

Oxygen cylinders vary in size, from the small portable D or E cylinders, which supply 1 to 10 hours of oxygen, to the larger stationary M, H, or K cylinders, which, at very low flow rates, supply oxygen for up to 56 hours. The duration depends on the oxygen flow rate. For example:

D cylinder: 350 L @ 2200 psi (23 min @ 15 L/min)
E cylinder: 625 L @ 2200 psi (42 min @ 15 L/min)
M cylinder: 3000 L @ 2200 psi (200 min @ 15 L/min)
H and K cylinders: 6900 L @ 2200 psi (690 min @ 10 L/min; ~33 hours @ 3 L/min)

Therefore, it is helpful to know how much oxygen each type of cylinder commonly contains and how long it will last.

Oxygen Concentrators

Oxygen concentrators extract the nitrogen from room air to produce 95% oxygen. They do this by using zeolite granules to adsorb the nitrogen from compressed air.[17] Zeolite crystals can be expected to last at least 20,000 hours—about 10 years' use.[15] Oxygen concentrators have been effectively used for surgery and related medical uses at extremely high altitudes (3650 m = 11,000 feet).[18]

Concentrators are available in sizes ranging from domestic models with flows of up to 4 L/min to very large installations that supply an entire hospital. They typically deliver 2 to 5 L/min of oxygen.[19] Oxygen concentrators require 350 to 400 W of electric power and can run off a small gasoline generator, a solar- or wind-powered system with battery storage, or a domestic or commercial power source.[20] However, the machine's power requirements must match the available power supply.

The price to purchase an oxygen concentrator is about half that of purchasing a 1-year supply of oxygen in cylinders.[15] The cost (electricity) to run it, regardless of the oxygen flow, is about 2.5 p/hr (UK) or 5 ¢/hr (US). This is much cheaper than using cylinder oxygen, which costs from 10 p/hr (UK) or 20 ¢/hr (US) at a flow rate of 0.5 L/min, up to £1.00/hr (UK) to $2/hr (US) at 5 L/min.[15]

Anesthesia

Oxygen concentrators can be used to supplement oxygen to anesthetized patients, but the outlet pressure is insufficient to power an anesthesia machine.[15] A flow splitter allows oxygen from a concentrator to be supplied to up to four separate sites simultaneously if required, depending on the concentrator's capacity and the patients' needs.[17]

The oxygen must be introduced upstream from the vaporizer in a drawover system or it will dilute the inspired vapor concentration.[17] If added using a reservoir attachment above the vaporizer inlet, the 95% oxygen at a flow rate of 1 L/min produces a FiO_2 from 35% to 40%; a rate of 5 L/min produces an FiO_2 of up to 80%.[21]

To increase the FiO_2 even more and provide an improved margin of safety, prefill a large plastic sack (e.g., trash bag) with concentrator oxygen and then attach this reservoir to the inlet side of the drawover system during preoxygenation. Remove the empty sack as soon as preoxygenation and intubation are completed.[22,23]

Oxygen Delivery

Improvised Oxygen Tent

Oxygen tents are not the best way to administer oxygen. But, when nothing else is available, the top of a plastic cake server with a hole cut out of the side for the neck works well as an oxygen tent for infants (Fig. 9-5).

Splitter

High-pressure oxygen sources (25 or 50 psi) can be split for use by up to seven patients with commercially available devices. These can also be "jury-rigged" by knowledgeable respiratory therapists. Low-pressure oxygen sources (cylinders/concentrators) can also be split, depending on the patients' needs.

Mouth-to-Mouth/Mouth-to-Tube Resuscitation

For mouth-to-mouth resuscitation, make a shield by cutting out about half the length of the third (long) finger from a medical glove. Extend the part of the finger still on the glove into the

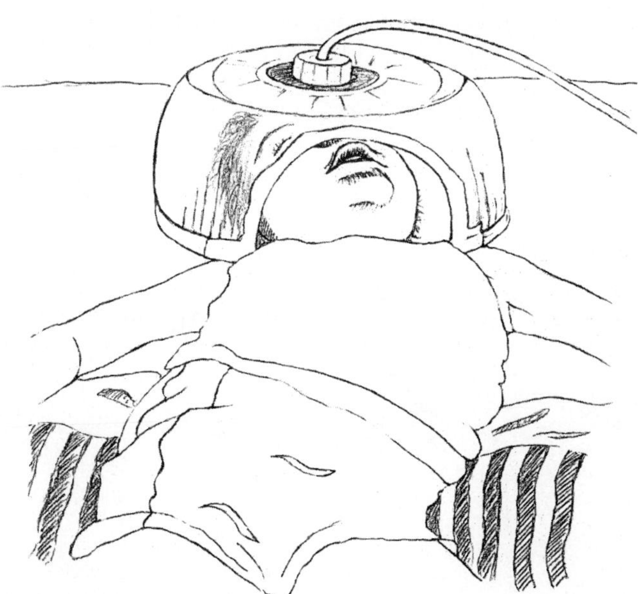

FIG. 9-5. Improvised pediatric oxygen tent.

patient's mouth, and stretch the remainder of the glove over the mouth and nose as a protective shield.[24] This works, but a handkerchief draped over the mouth and nose might work as well or better to protect the rescuer from at least the "big stuff." With the new, "continuous" cardiopulmonary resuscitation (CPR), rescue breathing is taking a back seat to chest compressions, at least for cardiac events.

Often forgotten is that, if no other means is available, patients can be given mouth-to-tube ventilation through an endotracheal tube (ETT), a laryngeal mask airway (LMA), a tracheostomy tube, an esophageal obturator airway (EOA), a Combitube, a makeshift cricothyrotomy tube, or a similar device. The problem is, other than covering the tube's end with a thin cloth (e.g., a handkerchief) to avoid contact with large amounts of blood or other secretions, none of these devices provides infectious protection to the rescuer.

VENTILATION

Cannot Ventilate: Semisolid Obstruction

If the airway is open but the patient cannot be ventilated due to inhalation of a semisolid material, such as muddy water, rapidly irrigate the ETT with 100 mL 0.9% saline (adult). Immediately suction the fluid with an NG tube and ventilate.[25]

Masks

Even the most experienced clinicians under optimal conditions have difficulty using a mask to ventilate in 2% to 5% of patients because of poorly fitting masks.[26]

Incorrect Mask Size: Adults

When a mask is too small for the patient, place the mask over only the nose. Seal the mouth by placing your long finger under the chin, or even with a piece of transparent dressing. With very large patients (BMI >26), hold the mask with both hands over the mouth and nose, or just the nose, while someone else ventilates the patient.[27]

Incorrect Mask Size: Infants and Children

When trying to use a small child's oxygen mask on a neonate, simply turn it upside down and it fits well (Fig. 9-6).

If the ventilation mask is too large for a child's face, bring the bottom of the mask below the chin (i.e., between the underside of the chin and the hyoid). This forms an adequate seal until the

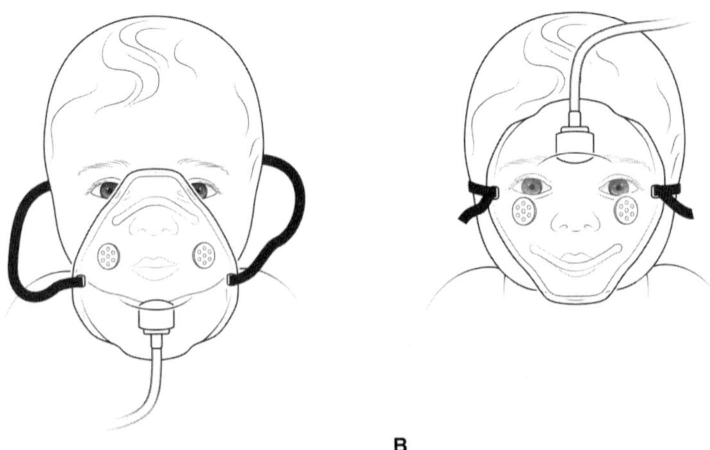

FIG. 9-6. (A) Child size does not fit neonate. (B) Turned 180 degrees, the mask fits well.

properly sized mask can be found. Occasionally, turning the mask upside-down so that the nasal angle is caudad (toward the feet) and the more rounded edge of the seal is across the nasal bridge may help achieve a seal.[27]

Lack of Teeth

It may be difficult to establish an effective seal in patients with no, or few, teeth. If the patient has dentures, leave them in place (as long as they are firmly attached) until the patient is ready for laryngoscopy, at which time the upper teeth should be removed. Not only is this safe, but it also decreases the incidence of difficulty with mask ventilation from 16% to 4% in this group.[27,28]

If the patient lacks teeth and dentures, place a large oral airway down the midline of the tongue. Then use a large mask to cover the lateral aspects and angle of the mouth. Put your third finger across the bottom of the jaw to keep the mouth closed and ventilate mainly through the nose.[27]

Beard

In wartime, during disasters, and in many remote areas, many male patients have a beard. If a beard is causing problems with getting a good mask seal, "simply shaving the beard may solve the problem."[27]

Another option is to apply petroleum, KY jelly, or other soluble grease around the edge of the mask. The beard has to be "filled" with the lubricant, which makes the mask slippery. It does not work as well as shaving the beard, but the following method works almost as well. Apply a large defibrillator pad or transparent sticky plastic dressing (i.e., Tegaderm or another clear plastic adhesive sheet) with a hole cut in it to expose the nose and mouth. The sheet keeps the beard in check as the mask is applied.[29,30] This also works well for CPAP/BiPAP masks.

A simpler solution may be to insert cotton between the mask and the skin. After administering anesthesia for operations near the front lines during World War I, Flagg wrote: "The great majority of the patients one sees are unshaven. In this connection it might be well to emphasize the great advantage of placing a layer of cotton between the skin and the face piece [mask]."[31]

Restoring the Seal of an Anatomical Face Mask

With repeated use, the seal of the anatomical facemask commonly used for anesthesia becomes flattened due to the cushion losing air, resulting in a poor fit on the patient's face. The loss of air is due to damage to the filling tube or to the plug. To at least temporarily re-inflate the mask, inject air through the filling tube by either using a 50-mL syringe or blowing into it. If the plug is nonfunctional, insert a needle cap to plug the filling tube.[32]

Flavoring the Mask for Pediatric Patients

Whether a mask is used for oxygenation, to deliver medications, or for anesthesia, children seem to tolerate both it and procedures better if it smells good. Liberally coat the inside of the mask with a flavored lip balm, which is inexpensive and readily available. The child can pick the flavor. It is also useful to have the child breathe through a flavored mask before and after the instillation of intranasal medication, or when emerging from procedural sedation.[33]

Bag-Mask-Valves

Caring for a Bag-Valve-Mask (Ambu) Valve

Regularly inspect your reusable bag-mask-valves (BVMs) to be certain that the valves function properly. If the BVM valve is stuck or needs cleaning, unscrew the two ends that do not go to the patient. Then remove the lugs on the leaflets. Don't pull on the flaps—they are fragile and you may tear them. Wash the inside and outside of the valve with warm, soapy water and allow the parts to dry thoroughly. Most of these BVMs can be disinfected with antiseptics or autoclaved, but this is only necessary if the bag has been used on an infected patient. Carefully reassemble the valve, making sure that the flaps are not wrinkled. Also, check the bag for cracks and for deterioration of the rubber. This is almost impossible to repair, although you should be able to make a temporary patch with cyanoacrylate.[34]

The disposable BVMs have sealed valve chambers that cannot be opened without breaking the equipment. These are designed for one-time use, but in settings with limited resources they may be used many times. Use either a moist cloth or steam to try to clean disposable BVMs between uses; however, this may be less than adequate for infection control.

Improvising a Bag-Valve-Mask

Nothing seems to work well as a substitute to a BVM other than mouth-to-mouth ventilation. A number of alternatives, including using a plastic soda bottle, have been suggested; they do not work. Do not waste precious time trying them.

However, if a rebreathing bag fails in a neonatal anesthesia circuit, a size 7.5 latex surgical glove can be used temporarily to provide a tidal capacity of 500 to 600 mL. Make a 2-cm diameter hole in the tip of the middle finger as a release valve.[35]

Improvised One-Way Valves

One-way valves in ventilation devices allow the exhalation to the atmosphere of "used" air to prevent a buildup of CO_2. While various types of one-way valves are commercially available, they also can be improvised, although the system requires both hands, and is somewhat cumbersome.

Pearson and Safar wrote about one such system: "A large hole, in the wall of the tracheal tube adapter, to permit exhalation through the hole and inflation while the hole is occluded with the finger … systems are relatively clumsy, as they occupy both hands of the anesthesiologist."[36] Although described for use with an endotracheal tube, this could also be used for a patient who is undergoing anesthesia with only a mask.

Mechanical Ventilation: Lung-Protective Strategies

Use the following methods when starting mechanical ventilation for patients who do not have acute respiratory distress syndrome: (a) Prevent volume trauma (keep tidal volume 4-8 mL/kg predicted body weight with plateau pressure <30 cm H_2O); (b) Prevent atelectasis (keep positive end-expiratory pressure ≥5 cm H_2O); (c) Maintain adequate ventilation (respiratory rate at 20-35 breaths/min); and (d) Prevent hyperoxia (titrate inspired oxygen concentration to peripheral oxygen saturation (SpO_2) levels of 88%-95%). Most patients tolerate these measures without excessive sedation.[37]

Mechanical Ventilator Use With Multiple Patients

Short-term mechanical ventilation can be lifesaving. The lack of ventilators represents a major limitation on medical treatment capabilities, both acutely during pandemics and chronically in many areas of the world. It is unlikely that medical facilities or governments will be able to stockpile sufficient mechanical ventilators (and, in the case of governments, distribute them in a timely manner) to meet the need during pandemics or other widespread disasters involving agents that affect the respiratory system.

While not the optimal solution, one ventilator can, theoretically, be used to ventilate four patients simultaneously in both pressure- and volume-controlled modes. This may be a temporizing measure when alternatives are not available—or when the only alternative is to not ventilate a patient and let him die. This design is for "last-ditch ventilation," and only a simulation model has been published. I describe the method used in detail, to provide the maximum information in case it needs to be used clinically.[38]

Four sets of standard ventilator tubing (Hudson) are connected to a single ventilator (Puritan-Bennett, 840 series) via two flow splitters, one on the patient inflow limb of the circuit, the other on the patient exhaust limb. Each flow splitter is constructed from three Briggs T-tubes with included connection adapters (Hudson) (Fig. 9-7), but with the valves removed. The Briggs T-tube is used clinically (and is generally available) to provide flow-by oxygen to a patient with an endotracheal or a tracheostomy tube and for in-line aerosol treatments of ventilated patients. The T-tubes are arranged so that the two side ports of a central T-tube are attached to the bottom ports of the two side T-tubes via adapters that come with the T-tube. Standard ventilation tubing connects this device to the ventilator. This configuration (Fig. 9-8) allows air flowing from the

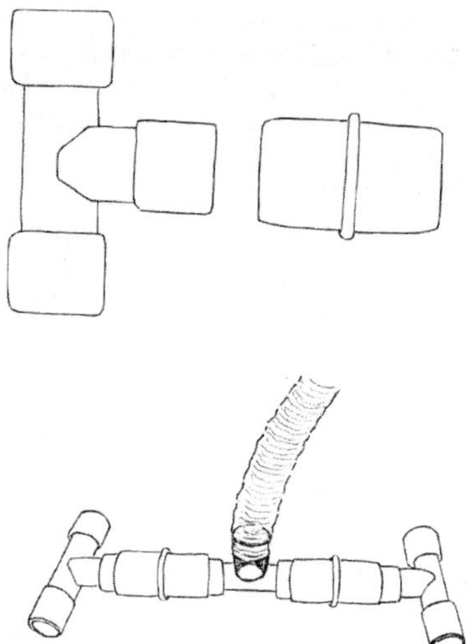

FIG. 9-7. Detail of circuit for multiple-patient ventilation.

ventilator to be split evenly to four patients and the air returning from the four patients to flow back into the single exhaust port on the ventilator.[38]

For pressure control, the ventilator settings were dialed to a peak pressure of 25 cm H_2O, 0 cm of PEEP, and a respiratory rate of 16 breaths/min. The ventilator software chose an inspiratory/expiratory ratio of 1:2 automatically. For volume control, settings of 2000-mL tidal volume (500 mL per test lung) and a respiratory rate of 16 breaths/min were chosen to approximate physiologic parameters. The ventilator software chose an inspiratory/expiratory ratio of 1:1

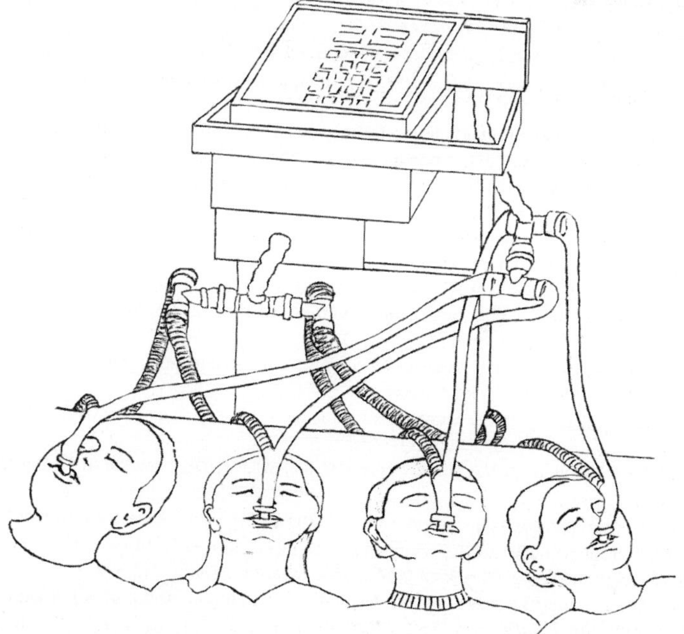

FIG. 9-8. Multiple patients ventilated by one machine.

automatically. In the model, the four simulated lungs' pressures did not exceed 35 cm H_2O and tidal volumes approximated 7 mL/kg for a 70-kg patient.[38]

Potential problems with this system include the differences in the four patients' lung compliance, the risk of passing infection from one patient to another, the different tidal volumes required by patients of differing sizes, and the need for constant supervision by a knowledgeable health care provider. Patients will probably need to be completely sedated and chemically paralyzed, require frequent suctioning (airway toilet), and be able to be temporarily removed from the system to use bag-valve ventilation, if necessary.[38]

REFERENCES

1. Kraman SS. Transmission of lung sounds through light clothing. *Respiration*. 2008;75(1):85-88.
2. Balik M, Plasil P, Waldauf P, et al. Ultrasound estimation of volume of pleural fluid in mechanically ventilated patients. *Intensive Care Med*. 2006;32(2):318-321.
3. Panicher J, Sethi GR, Sehgal V. Comparative efficiency of commercial and improvised spacer device in acute bronchial asthma. *Indian Pediatr*. 2001;38(4):340-348.
4. Roberge RJ, Martin TP. Relief of cough. *Postgrad Med*. www.postgradmed.com/pearls.htm. Accessed September 23, 2007.
5. Dacey MJ. Keep the healthy lung down. *Postgrad Med*. http://www.postgradmed.com/pearls.htm. Accessed September 23, 2007.
6. Levitan R. Strategies for maximizing O_2 delivery. *Emerg Phys Monthly*. February 2014:10-11.
7. Perilli V, Sollazzi L, Bozza P, et al. The effects of the reverse Trendelenburg position on respiratory mechanics and blood gases in morbidly obese patients during bariatric surgery. *Anesth Analg*. 2000;91: 1520-1525.
8. Torres A, Serra-Batlles J, Ros E, et al. Pulmonary aspiration of gastric contents in patients receiving mechanical ventilation: the effect of body position. *Ann Intern Med*. 1992;116(7):540-543.
9. Hua A, Shah KH. Does noninvasive ventilation have a role in chest trauma patients? *Ann Emerg Med*. 2014;64(1):82-83.
10. Engström J, Hedenstierna G, Larsson A. Pharyngeal oxygen administration increases the time to serious desaturation at intubation in acute lung injury: an experimental study. *Crit Care*. 2010;14(3):R93.
11. Babu TA. A simple and cheap alternative approach to administering continuous positive airway pressure in resource limited settings. *Trop Doct*. October 2012;42:240.
12. Husum H, Ang SC, Fosse E. *War Surgery: Field Manual*. Penang, Malaysia: Third World Network; 1995:630.
13. C-F-C StarTec. http://www.c-f-c.com/specgas_products/oxygen.htm. Accessed December 12, 2006.
14. Aerox Aviation Oxygen Systems. https://aerox.com/frequently-asked-questions/. Accessed September 3, 2015.
15. Dobson MB. Oxygen concentrators for district hospitals. *Pract Proced*. 1999;10(11):1. http://www.nda.ox.ac.uk/wfsa/html/u10/u1011_01.htm. Accessed September 13, 2006.
16. Dobson MB. *Anaesthesia at the District Hospital*. 2nd ed. Geneva, Switzerland: World Health Organization; 2000:67.
17. Eltringham R. The oxygen concentrator. *Pract Proced*. 1992;1(6):1. http://www.nda.ox.ac.uk/wfsa/html/u01/u01_009.htm. Accessed September 14, 2006.
18. Masroor R, Iqbal A, Buland K, Kazi WA. Use of a portable oxygen concentrator and its effect on the overall functionality of a remote field medical unit at 3650 meters elevation. *Anaesth Pain Intensive Care*. 2013;17(1):45-50.
19. McCormick BA, Eltringham RJ. Anaesthesia equipment for resource-poor environments. *Anaesthesia*. 2007;62(suppl 1):54-60.
20. Litch JA, Bishop RA. Oxygen concentrators for the delivery of supplemental oxygen in remote high-altitude areas. *Wild Environ Med*. 2000;11:189-191.
21. Dobson MB. *Anaesthesia at the District Hospital*. Geneva, Switzerland: World Health Organization; 1988:67.
22. Johnson TW. Preoxygenation attachment for the Triservice apparatus. *Anaesthesia*. 1988;43:713.
23. Wilson IH, Van Heerden PV, Leigh J. Domiciliary oxygen concentrators in anaesthesia: preoxygenation techniques and inspired oxygen concentrations. *Br J Anaesth*. 1990;65:342-345.
24. Weiss EA. *Backcountry 911: 1001 uses for duct tape and safety pins. Talk at ACEP Scientific Assembly*. Seattle, WA: October 11, 2007.

25. Schober P, Christiaans HM, Loer SA, Schwarte LA. Airway obstruction due to aspiration of muddy water. *Emerg Med J*. 2013;30(10):854-855.
26. Kheterpal S, Tremper KK, Mashour GA. Bag and mask ventilation (letter). *N Engl J Med*. 2007;357(2): 2091.
27. Greenberg RS. Facemask, nasal and oral airway devices. *Anesthesiol Clin N Am*. 2002;20:833-861.
28. Conlon NP, Sullivan RP, Herbison PG, et al. The effect of leaving dentures in place on bag-mask ventilation at induction of general anesthesia. *Anesth Analg*. 2007;105:370-373.
29. Simpson S. Drawover anaesthesia review. *Pract Proced*. 2002;15(6):1-10. http://www.nda.ox.ac.uk/wfsa/htmL/u15/u1506_01.htm. Accessed September 14, 2006.
30. Peter DeBlieux, MD, FACEP. Personal written communication with author, received February 2008.
31. Flagg PJ. Anaesthesia in Europe on the Western battlefront. *Int Clin*. 1918;3:210-228.
32. Singhal S, Lal J. Restoring the seal of an anatomical face mask. *Trop Doct*. 2011;41:190-191.
33. Mell H. Why choose when you can have both? *ACEP NOW*. April 2014;26.
34. Dobson MB. Draw-over anaesthesia part 3—looking after your own apparatus. *Update Anaesthesia*. 1993;3(5). www.nda.ox.ac.uk/wfsa/html/u03/u03_014.htm. Accessed September 14, 2006.
35. Oyinpreye JA, Ofejiro OB, Osemwegie OA. An urgent necessity under general anaesthesia surgical gloves made into re-breathing bag. *Trop Doct*. 2011;41:121-122.
36. Pearson JW, Safar P. General anesthesia with minimal equipment. *Anesth Analg*. 1961;40(6):664-671.
37. Kilickaya O, Gajic O. Initial ventilator settings for critically ill patients. *Crit Care*. 2013;17:123.
38. Neyman G, Irvin CB. A single ventilator for multiple simulated patients to meet disaster surge. *Acad Emerg Med*. 2006;13(12):1246-1249.

10 | Circulation/Cardiovascular

Few improvised methods are available for diagnosing and treating cardiovascular abnormalities. The most basic treatment, cardiopulmonary resuscitation (CPR), can be performed without extra equipment. However, not even MacGyver would really be willing to try cardioversion without a defibrillator, and the most basic treatments used for cardiovascular care require at least certain medications and equipment.

DIAGNOSIS: ELECTROCARDIOGRAM

No Calipers

To measure electrocardiogram (ECG) intervals without calipers, mark a card or piece of paper with vertical lines: | | | | | | | | |. The marks can be spaced to match the top of the R or the P waves, depending on what you are looking for. Move the marks to another part of the ECG to determine if the rates are constant or to find a P wave hidden in a QRS complex.

Alternate Electrocardiogram Positions and Leads

If there is no room to lay a patient down, do the ECG with the patient in a standing position (Fig. 10-1). The resulting ECG is just as interpretable as one done in a supine position.

Attaching Electrocardiogram Leads

If an ECG or a cardiac monitor is available, but the way of attaching the leads to the patient is missing, several methods work well. The key is to pull off any device hiding the bare metal leads (that usually are covered by devices that attach to tape leads on Western ECG machines). After removal, place the leads directly on small alcohol or saline pads or a lubricant (oil, K-Y jelly)

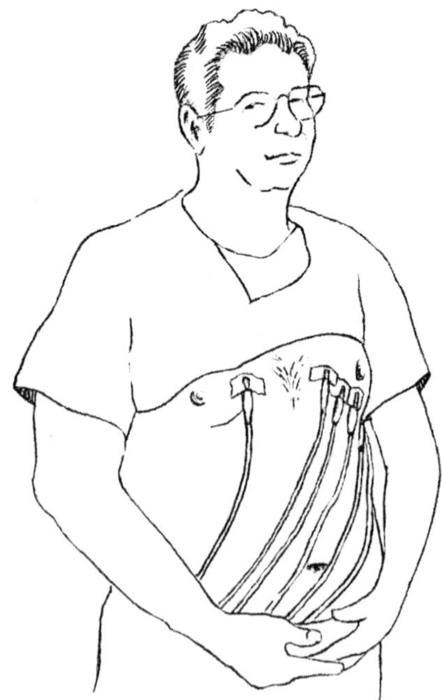

FIG. 10-1. Standing ECG with improvised leads.

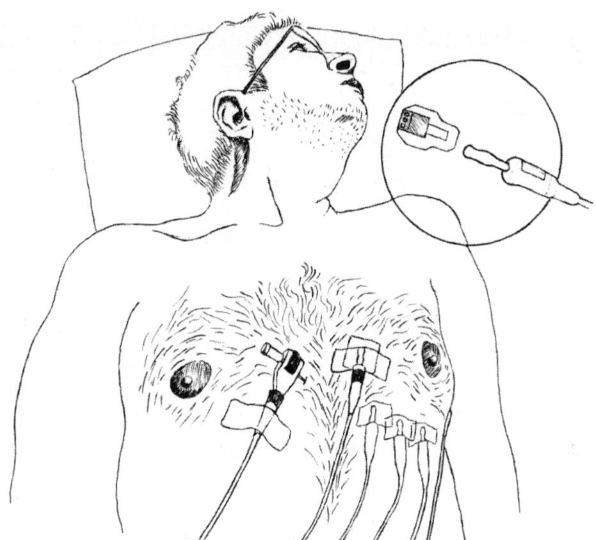

FIG. 10-2. Electrocardiogram leads attached using a variety of improvised methods.

between the skin and the lead, but that is not essential to obtain a good ECG reading. Affix them in the normal locations using phlebotomy tourniquets. If chest leads are needed, place these on the skin in the same manner, using tape to temporarily secure them. If they must be kept on for some time or if the patient has injuries (e.g., burns) precluding the use of tape, insert small-gauge needles just beneath the epidermis and use alligator clips to make a connection (Fig. 10-2).

"12-Lead" Electrocardiogram Using 3 Leads

Normal 12-lead ECG machines may not be available when additional ECG information is needed for a diagnosis. In this situation, clinicians can use a 3-lead machine to obtain an ECG tracing that produces most of the information provided by a 12-lead ECG. To do this, do a tracing with the ECG pads placed in the normal 3-lead positions:

White = right chest just below the clavicle
Black = left chest just below the clavicle
Red = left lower abdomen just above the umbilicus

Then, do four more tracings, each time moving the red (left leg) lead to the V1, V2, V3, or V6 positions (Fig. 10-3).[1] Many monitors can also show leads II, III, aVL, aVR, and aVF by moving a dial on the machine with the leads kept in their normal position.

Improve ECG Diagnostic Accuracy

Standard ECG machines run at 25 mm/second. Doubling the paper output speed to 50 mm/second makes subtle ECG findings more evident and improves diagnostic accuracy of narrow complex tachycardias. A way to visualize this is to think about stretching the ECG tracing like a rubber band. One group of physicians improved their diagnostic accuracy from 63% at the standard rate to 71% with the faster tracings. Also, inappropriate use of adenosine decreased from 18% to 13%. Everything, including the QRS complex and intervals, gets wider.[2]

Measure Central Venous Pressure

Both the catheters and the manometers used for central venous pressure (CVP) monitoring are disposable, but, if necessary, they can be boiled (disinfected) and reused. The danger in reusing catheters is that particulate matter may remain within them, so the disinfection may not be effective.[3]

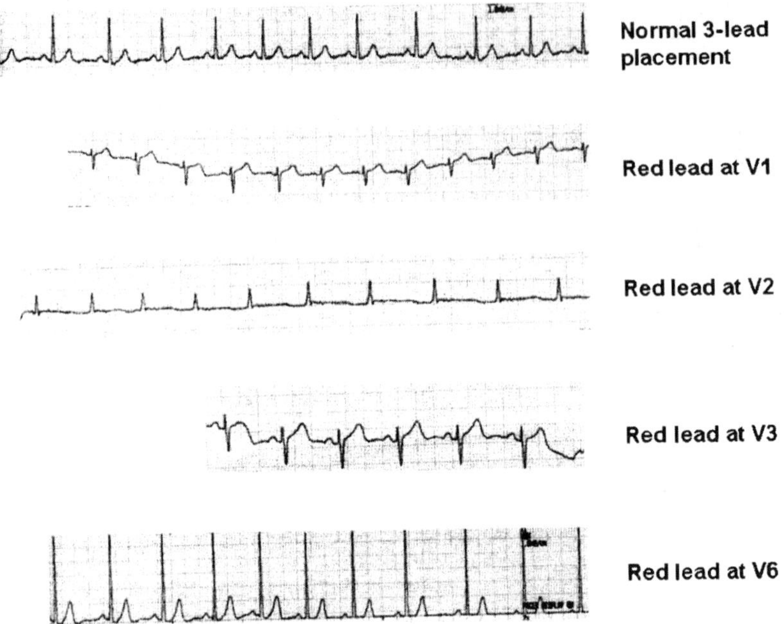

FIG. 10-3. A normal ECG (I, V1, V2, V3, V6) done using only the three leads from a monitor. The additional limb lead tracings taken by changing settings on the monitor are not shown. The "normal" tracing is lead I, although on most machines it also can do tracings of the other limb leads.

For measuring CVP, attach a manometer to either a three-way stopcock or a sterile "Y" tube. Construct a manometer from another intravenous set taped over or beside an upright ruler or cardboard marked in centimeter increments. Fill the manometer from the intravenous bottle and then connect it via a central line to the patient. Any drip going through the line is stopped. The zero point is the mid-axillary line, with the patient in a supine position.[4] (The normal reading is 5-10 cm H_2O.)

To be accurate, the zero ("0") mark on the CVP manometer must be level with the supine patient's mid-axillary line. Use a long piece of wood with a level taped on top, so you can check that it is parallel with the floor. Place one end of the wood at the patient's mid-axillary line and, while watching the level, attach the CVP manometer to an intravenous (IV) pole so that the zero ("0") is even with the wood's other end. An alternative is to use a piece of IV tubing that has been half-filled with colored water and then formed into a loop by connecting the two ends. The two menisci (where the water meets the air) in the tube will always be at the same level if the loop is held vertically. Figure 10-4 illustrates how to use such a tube to adjust the manometer height.[3]

Pulmonary Embolism Diagnosis

Even if you cannot calculate the probability of a patient having a pulmonary embolus (PE) using one of the standard clinical decision rules (Wells and revised Geneva scores), your gestalt assessment will be sufficient. In fact, physicians' gestalt assessment is better at selecting patients with a low or high probability of PE than are the scoring systems.[5]

TREATMENT

Paroxysmal Supraventricular Tachycardia

The simplest and most available method to convert paroxysmal supraventricular tachycardia (PSVT) is to use vagal maneuvers. However, if the patient is unstable, cardiovert immediately if

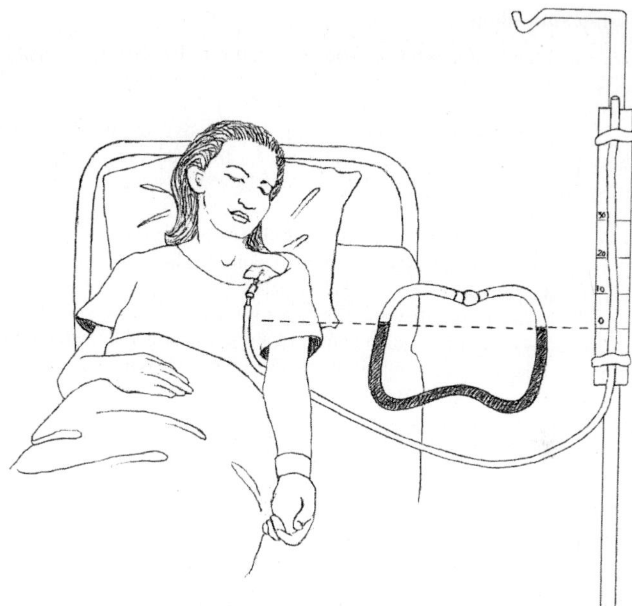

FIG. 10-4. Makeshift CVP monitor with leveling loop.

that option is available. If using paddles, make contact with the patient using either saline pads or the same gels that are used for ultrasound examinations.

Valsalva Maneuvers

The Valsalva maneuver (VM), bearing down against a closed glottis, is the most consistently effective vagotonic technique. Optimize the VM by placing the patient in a supine position, which generates greater vagal tone than Trendelenburg posturing. This position produces the largest transient heart rate decrease. Its efficacy can be increased further by pressing firmly over the right hypochondrium (over the liver) while the patient exhales and bears down. This increases venous return to the right side of the heart and augments the effect on cardiac stretch receptors, thereby increasing the chance of successfully terminating the arrhythmia.[6]

Older Vagal Stimulation Methods

Other useful vagal maneuvers include blowing into a tube connected to a sphygmomanometer for 15 seconds to achieve a pressure of 40 mm Hg and stimulating the human dive reflex by applying a cold pack to a patient's face for 30 seconds.[7]

Stimulating the diving reflex works best on children. Ask children who are old enough to cooperate to hold their breath and dunk their face into a pan of ice water resting on their lap. Do not force their head into the water or hold it under! For younger children, have a parent hold a towel that has been dipped in ice water over the child's face. Be sure to keep the airway clear.

Pressor drugs can occasionally terminate atrioventricular (AV) nodal reentry by inducing reflex vagal stimulation mediated by baroreceptors in the carotid sinus and aorta. This requires the systolic blood pressure (BP) to be elevated to about 180 mm Hg, and so should be used carefully or not at all in the elderly and in patients who have structural heart disease, significant hypertension, hyperthyroidism, or an acute myocardial infarction. Given over 1 to 3 minutes, the adult doses for these agents are phenylephrine 1%, 1 (0.1 mL) to 10 mg (1 mL); methoxamine, 3 to 5 mg; or metaraminol, 0.5 to 2.0 mg. If edrophonium is used, administer it over 15 to 30 seconds—it is very short acting.

Adenosine Dosing Simplified

The advanced cardiovascular life support (ACLS)-recommended dosing strategy of 6, 12, and 12 mg for adenosine may not be appropriate in every situation. Caffeine is an adenosine blocker and can interfere with the successful reversion of PSVT. In fact, ingestion of caffeine <4 hours before a 6-mg adenosine bolus significantly reduced its effectiveness in the treatment of PSVT. An increased initial adenosine dose may be indicated for these patients. In those cases, consider using 12 mg (instead of 6 mg) for the first dose, and 18 mg (instead of 12 mg) for the second and third doses.[8]

Use a lower dose of adenosine if administering it through a central line or if the patient has a transplanted heart or takes carbamazepine or dipyridamole. In those cases, administer 3 mg (instead of 6 mg) for the first dose and 6 mg (instead of 12 mg) for subsequent doses.[9]

Rather than push adenosine and then the flush, combine them in one syringe. Using a 20 mL or a 30 mL syringe, draw up both the adenosine and the saline bolus. Push them rapidly through a proximal peripheral line. The adenosine is stable in saline and even a 12-mg adenosine dose is only 4 mL.[10]

Ineffective Congestive Heart Failure Treatments

The hallmark of improvised treatment methods to treat pulmonary edema accompanying heart failure is preload reduction, that is, reducing the volume of blood entering the heart. However, none of the old treatment methods are effective in austere situations.

"Congesting cuffs" or "rotating tourniquets" were often applied to the extremities to treat patients with acute pulmonary edema secondary to left heart failure. The theory was that rotating tourniquets would provide some benefit until medications could be administered. They don't work.[11-13]

Practiced since biblical times, the removal of volumes of blood to treat heart failure (therapeutic phlebotomy) continued into the late 20th century. Unfortunately, the technique is ineffective, except in patients with hemochromatosis or polycythemia.

Thrombolytics Through an Intraosseous Line

Patients who need immediate thrombolytics for a massive pulmonary embolus, but who do not have standard venous access, can have the medication administered through an intraosseous (IO) line. This has been done for both patients in cardiac arrest and those with cardiac activity.[14]

Peripheral Edema/Lymphedema

Developed by Dr. Robert Jones to help treat fractures, the Jones compression dressing also effectively eliminates edema caused by systemic problems, such as chronic venous insufficiency, lymphedema, and other illnesses causing lower extremity swelling.[15] However, because the dressing does not treat the underlying problems, when possible, these should also be treated.

To make your own compression dressing, apply three to five rolls of 4-inch cast padding, or equivalent material, with minimal compression: Going distal to proximal creates a pressure gradient that permits the swelling to increase. Over these layers, wrap a 6-inch elastic bandage, again in a distal to proximal manner so that it also creates a compression gradient. With severe edema, place cotton between the toes.

Repeat the padding layer with three to five more padding rolls, followed by another 6-inch elastic bandage. Apply each layer with increasing tightness to maintain the compression gradient effect. The result is that each layer is applied with greater pressure distally and less pressure proximally. A layer of plaster can be added if additional support is needed. If plaster is added as a splint, it is generally not used posteriorly.

Change the dressing every 5 to 7 days. When used for a fracture, this dressing virtually eliminates the need to remove a cast that becomes "too tight." However, burning or numbness with application may indicate tissue ischemia. If that occurs, remove the dressing and reapply it.

CARDIOPULMONARY RESUSCITATION

Cardiopulmonary resuscitation (CPR) can be improved using telephonic instruction and easily available devices to time CPR.

Cardiopulmonary Resuscitation Telephonic Instructions

CPR now can be quickly understood as "Push Hard, Push Fast." This may not suffice for patients located where there is a prolonged EMS response time or no EMS services. In those situations, either no benefit or harm may result if bystanders use only chest-compression resuscitation.[16]

Telephonic instructions to laypeople performing CPR may increase the likelihood that they place their hands in the correct chest position. Instructions that seem to optimize CPR are: "Lay the patient's arm which is closest to you, straight out from the body. Kneel down by the patient and place one knee on each side of the arm. Find the midpoint between the nipples and place your hands on top of each other."[17]

When trying to instruct a layperson on CPR technique via phone, using a landline may result in instructions and CPR occurring sequentially. Using a speaker function (cell phone or landline) allows the rescuer to receive instructions and encouragement from the dispatcher simultaneously while performing CPR. However, in one study, two-thirds of elderly people could not quickly activate their cell phone speaker function.[18]

Metronome-Guided Cardiopulmonary Resuscitation

A systematic review showed that the use of metronomes to guide the rate at which external chest compressions are delivered is associated with improved rates closer to those recommended in the current resuscitation guidelines.[19] Metronome sound guidance during dispatcher-assisted compression-only CPR (DA-COCPR) improved untrained bystanders' chest compression rates, but was associated more with shallow compressions than the conventional DA-COCPR in a manikin model.[20]

Strobe Light-Guided Cardiopulmonary Resuscitation

Strobe light-guided CPR is particularly advantageous for maintaining a desired minimum compression rate during hands-only CPR in noisy environments, where metronome pacing might not be clearly heard. The strobe light guidance device should be set to emit light pulses at the rate of 100 flashes/min. Many free smart phone strobe light apps are available.[21]

Ultrasonography to Determine Cardiac Death

The current evidence does not support using ultrasonography alone to predict outcomes in cardiac arrest patients. A systematic review yielded a survival-to-admission rate of 2.4% in patients with cardiac standstill. Although these results seem to indicate that resuscitation in such patients is not futile, longer-term outcomes should be considered. In previous resuscitation research, survival-to-hospital admission has proven to be a poor surrogate for survival-to-hospital discharge or neurologic outcomes.[22]

Optimal Cardiopulmonary Resuscitation Performance

Rescuers' positions determine how well they can generate standard CPR. Lightweight people may have difficulty achieving the full compression depth of 5 to 6 cm in adults that standard guidelines prescribe. Improvement results from maximally using their body mass by positioning their shoulders directly over the sternum. Both kneeling on the bed beside the patient and standing on a 20-cm-high footstool equally increased the chance that compression depths would be ≥5 cm over a 2-minute period. These positions do not change the compression rate or the percentage of correctly released compressions.[23,24]

Team leaders should not rely on rescuers to self-report fatigue. Because rescuer fatigue affects chest compression delivery within the second minute of CPR, those doing compressions should switch with another team member after delivering CPR for 2 minutes.[25]

Pediatric Cardiac Arrest Post-Trauma Outcome

Children with post-traumatic out-of-hospital cardiac arrest do poorly. Those most likely to survive and who should receive maximal resources, arrive with high or normal BP, normal heart rate, sinus rhythm, urine output of >1 mL/kg/hr, and non-cyanotic skin color. Among survivors, those most likely to have a good neurologic outcome had initial Glasgow Coma Score (GCS) scores >7.[26]

Hypothermia after Return of Spontaneous Circulation

Therapeutic hypothermia after return of spontaneous circulation (ROSC) improves survival and neurologic outcomes, especially in patients presenting with shockable rhythms (ventricular fibrillation/pulseless ventricular tachycardia). Both infusing cold intravenous fluids and surface cooling have been used successfully, although, with the latter, there is more temperature variation during the maintenance phase. The optimal desired temperature is still unclear, but it seems to be less important than preventing the patient from becoming hyperthermic. Most clinicians attempt to get their patients to a core temperature of 32°C to 36°C (89.6°F to 96.8°F). The prehospital sector has also had success with induced hypothermia, both during resuscitation and after ROSC. Methods to induce hypothermia in both settings include infusing ice-cold IV fluids (500 mL to 30 mL/kg of 0.9% saline or Ringer's lactate) and applying surface cold packs or cooling blankets. Whenever possible during the cooling process, monitor core temperature using an esophageal thermometer or a bladder catheter temperature probe. Axillary and oral temperatures are inadequate. Continue induced hypothermia for 12 to 24 hours, or until the patient awakens.[27]

Disinfecting Cardiopulmonary Resuscitation Manikins

Manikins are used throughout the world to teach CPR. To prevent a possible transmission of herpes simplex virus and other pathogens among those who share manikins for mouth-to-mouth resuscitation training, disinfect the manikin's contact surfaces at the end of each class. To do this, wet all surfaces with a 500 ppm sodium hypochlorite (bleach) solution, leave it on for 10 minutes, rinse with fresh water, and immediately dry. Between students or after the instructor demonstrates a procedure, wipe the face and interior of the manikin's mouth with 500 ppm hypochlorite solution or 70% alcohol.[28]

REFERENCES

1. Personal communication and testing with Capt Shelley Metcalf, RN, USAF, McMurdo Station, Antarctica, September 2009.
2. Accardi AJ, Miller R, Holmes JF. Enhanced diagnosis of narrow complex tachycardias with increased electrocardiograph speed. *J Emerg Med.* February 2002;22(2):123-126.
3. King MH, ed. *Primary Anesthesia.* Oxford, UK: Oxford University Press; 1986:142.
4. Eggleston FC. Simplified management of fluid and electrolyte problems. *Trop Doct.* 1985;15:111-117.
5. Penaloza A, Verschuren F, Meyer G, et al. Comparison of the unstructured clinician gestalt, the Wells Score, and the Revised Geneva Score to estimate pretest probability for suspected pulmonary embolism. *Ann Emerg Med.* 2013;62:117-124.
6. Mitchell ARJ. Augmented Valsalva's maneuver terminates tachycardia. *Postgrad Med.* www.postgradmed.com/pearls.htm. Accessed September 23, 2007.
7. Smith G, Broek A, Taylor DM, Morgans A, Cameron P. Identification of the optimum vagal manoeuvre technique for maximising vagal tone. *Emerg Med J.* 2015;32:51-54 (online June 5, 2014).
8. Cabalag MS, Taylor DM, Knott, JC, et al. Recent caffeine ingestion reduces adenosine efficacy in the treatment of paroxysmal supraventricular tachycardia. *Acad Emerg Med.* 2010;17(1):44-49.
9. Neumar RW, Otto CW, Link MS, et al. Part 8: adult advanced cardiovascular life support: 2010 American Heart Association Guidelines for Cardiopulmonary Resuscitation and Emergency Cardiovascular Care. *Circulation.* 2010;122(18 suppl 3):S729-S767.
10. Choi SC, Yoon SK, Kim GW, et al. A convenient method of adenosine administration for paroxysmal supraventricular tachycardia. *J Korean Soc Emerg Med.* 2003;14(3):224-227.
11. Habak PA, Mark AL, Kioschos JM, et al. Effectiveness of congesting cuffs ("rotating tourniquets") in patients with left heart failure. *Circulation.* 1974;50;366-371.
12. Bertel O, Steiner A. Rotating tourniquets do not work in acute congestive heart failure and pulmonary edema. *Lancet.* 1980;8:171:762.
13. Roth A, Hochenberg M, Keren G, et al. Are rotating tourniquets useful for left ventricular preload reduction in patients with acute myocardial infarction and heart failure? *Ann Emerg Med.* 1987;16:764-767.

14. Taylor R, Spencer TR. Intraosseous administration of thrombolytics for pulmonary embolism. *J Emerg Med*. 2013;45(6):e197-e200.
15. Yu GV, Schubert EK, Khoury WE. The Jones compression bandage. Review and clinical applications. *J Am Podiatr Med Assoc*. 2002;92(4):221-231.
16. Orkin AM. Push hard, push fast, if you're downtown: a citation review of urban-centrism in American and European basic life support guidelines. *Scand J Trauma Resusc Emerg Med*. 2013;21:32.
17. Birkenes TS, Myklebust H, Kramer-Johansen J. New pre-arrival instructions can avoid abdominal hand placement for chest compressions. *Scand J Trauma Resusc Emerg Med*. 2013;21:47.
18. Birkenes TS, Myklebust H, Kramer-Johansen J. Time delays and capability of elderly to activate speaker function for continuous telephone CPR. *Scand J Trauma Resusc Emerg Med*. 2013;21:40.
19. Tar C. Can metronomes improve CPR quality? *Emerg Med J*. 2014;31(3):251-254.
20. Park SO, Hong CK, Shin DH, Lee JH, Hwang SY. Efficacy of metronome sound guidance via a phone speaker during dispatcher-assisted compression-only cardiopulmonary resuscitation by an untrained layperson: a randomised controlled simulation study using a manikin. *Emerg Med J*. 2013;30:657-661.
21. You JS, Chung SP, Chang CH, et al. Effects of flashlight guidance on chest compression performance in cardiopulmonary resuscitation in a noisy environment. *Emerg Med J*. 2013;30:628-632.
22. Cohn B. Does the absence of cardiac activity on ultrasonography predict failed resuscitation in cardiac arrest? *Ann Emerg Med*. 2013;62(2):180-181.
23. Krikscionaitiene A, Stasaitis K, Dambrauskiene M, et al. Can lightweight rescuers adequately perform CPR according to 2010 resuscitation guideline requirements? *Emerg Med J*. 2013;30:159-160.
24. Hong CK, Park SO, Jeong HH, et al. The most effective rescuer's position for cardiopulmonary resuscitation provided to patients on beds: a randomized, controlled, crossover mannequin study. *J Emerg Med*. 2014;46(5):643-649.
25. McDonald CH, Heggie J, Jones CM, Thorne CJ, Hulme J. Rescuer fatigue under the 2010 ERC guidelines, and its effect on cardiopulmonary resuscitation (CPR) performance. *Emerg Med J*. 2013;30:623-627.
26. Lin YR, Wu HP, Chen WL, et al. Predictors of survival and neurologic outcomes in children with traumatic out-of-hospital cardiac arrest during the early postresuscitative period. *J Trauma Acute Care Surg*. 2013;75:439-447.
27. Peberdy MA, Callaway CW, Neumar RW, et al. Part 9: post-cardiac arrest care: 2010 American Heart Association Guidelines for Cardiopulmonary Resuscitation and Emergency Cardiovascular Care. *Circulation*. 2010 Nov;122(18 suppl 3):S768-S786.
28. Rutala WA, Weber DJ. Uses of inorganic hypochlorite (bleach) in health-care facilities. *Clin Microbiol Rev*. 1997;10(4):597-610.

11 | Dehydration/Rehydration

Sir William MacGregor, MD, at the end of his term as Papua New Guinea's colonial governor, wrote: "Dysentery causes more deaths than any other disease in tropical countries. No other malady is so universally distributed and of such constant occurrence … [Dysentery has become] the chief agent in the rapid depopulation of the Pacific."[1]

Rehydration does not have the drama of other medical interventions—but it saves more lives than all other disease treatments combined.

ASSESSMENT

Diarrhea

Diarrhea causes most cases of lethal dehydration, especially among infants and children. Acute diarrhea is three or more loose or watery stools per day or a definite decrease in stool consistency and an increase in stool frequency for the individual. The volume of fluid lost through stools can vary from 5 mL/kg body weight/day (approximately normal) to ≥200 mL/kg body weight/day.[2] Because of the use of oral rehydration therapy (ORT), the annual worldwide deaths from diarrhea have decreased from >5 million in 1978 to 2.6 million in 2009 (1.1 million people >5 years old and 1.5 million children <5 years old).[3]

Pediatric Dehydration

Assessing a child's level of dehydration is a clinical diagnosis. This assessment should be no harder in austere situations than in standard practice—except that the confounder of malnutrition may play a big role in a child's appearance. Laboratory studies, including serum electrolytes, are usually unnecessary.[4] Stool cultures are indicated in dysentery, but are not usually indicated in acute, watery diarrhea for an immunocompetent patient.

Although studies in Africa and the United States have shown dehydration assessment scales to be relatively unreliable, they give clinicians a starting point to evaluate these children. Tables 11-1 and 11-2 are two scales that are easy to use in austere settings and have good inter-rater reliability.[5,6]

Dehydration Versus Septic Shock in Malnourished Children

In children with severe malnutrition, dehydration and septic shock are difficult to differentiate. Both present with signs of hypovolemia and worsen without treatment. Rather than using the

TABLE 11-1 Clinical Pediatric Dehydration Scoring System

	Points for Physical Findings		
Finding	**1**	**2**	**3**
Alertness	Normal	Restless, irritable, abnormally quiet, drowsy, or floppy	Delirious, comatose, or shocky: "very ill"
Pulse	Strong, <120/min	120-140/min	>140/min
Respirations	<30/min	30-40/min	>40/min
Skin elasticity	Normal	Moderately reduced	Extremely reduced
Eyes: sunken eyeballs	Normal	Moderate	Extreme, hypotonic

<6 points = normal to mild dehydration
6-10 points = moderate dehydration
11-14 points = severe dehydration
15 points = critical/impending death

TABLE 11-2 WHO Scale for Dehydration in Children 1 Month to 5 Years Old

	A	B	C
General Condition[a]	Well, alert	Restless, irritable	Lethargic or unconscious
Eyes[b]	Normal	Sunken	Sunken
Thirst	Drinks normally, not thirsty	Thirsty, drinks eagerly	Drinks poorly or not able to drink
Skin Pinch[c]	Springs back quickly	Goes back slowly	Goes back very slowly

[a]A lethargic child is not simply asleep. The child's mental state is dull, the child cannot be fully awakened, and s/he may appear to be drifting into unconsciousness.

[b]Ask the mother if the child's eyes are normal or more sunken than usual.

[c]The skin turgor, as estimated by pinch, is less useful in infants or in children with marasmus or kwashiorkor.

SCORING: < 2 signs from columns B and C = <5% dehydration

≥ 2 signs in column B = 5%-10% dehydration

≥ 2 signs in column C = ≥10% (severe/critical) dehydration

Data from World Health Organization.[7]

normal signs to assess dehydration, use the signs and symptoms presented in Table 11-3. Otherwise, dehydration will be overdiagnosed and its severity overestimated, and it will be difficult to recognize and treat children with both dehydration and septic shock.[8]

Ultrasound Assessment of Dehydration in Children—Not Useful

Bedside ultrasound measurements of the inferior vena cava (IVC) diameter do not correlate with central venous pressure (CVP) measurements, so they cannot be used to assess the intravascular volume status in severely ill pediatric patients.[9]

TABLE 11-3 Differentiation of Dehydration and Shock in the Malnourished Child

Clinical Sign	Some Dehydration	Severe Dehydration	Incipient Septic Shock	Developed Septic Shock
Watery diarrhea	+	+	+/–	+/–
Thirst	Drinks eagerly	Drinks poorly	No	No
Hypothermia	–	–	+/–	+/–
Sunken eyes	+	+	–	–
Weak or absent radial pulse	–	+	+	+
Cold hands and feet	–	+	+	+
Urine flow	+	–	+	+
Mental status	Restless/irritable	Lethargic/comatose	Apathetic	Lethargic
Hypoglycemia	+/–	+/–	+/–	+/–

Data from World Health Organization.[8]

REHYDRATION PLAN

Use available resources to provide the maximal benefit for dehydrated, usually pediatric, patients. That generally means reserving non-oral hydration for the sickest patients and for those who fail a good trial of oral therapy. Then, escalate treatment methods, depending on the patient's condition, the clinician's skills, and the available resources.

Treatment includes two phases: rehydration and maintenance. In the rehydration phase, replace the fluid deficit quickly, that is, within 2 to 4 hours. In the maintenance phase, administer the normally required amounts of calories and fluids, accompanied by rapid realimentation.[10]

Mild Dehydration

Unless they also have another significant disease, patients with mild dehydration rarely present to health care facilities in austere settings. For mild dehydration, oral rehydration solution (ORS) (up to 50 mL/kg over 12-24 hours) is generally the first and only treatment needed.[11] One method is to give 20 mL/kg over the first hour and 10 mL/kg over the next 6 to 8 hours.[12] Give the remaining balance over the following 16 to 18 hours. Some children will not respond to the oral method. In these cases, use one of the alternative parenteral methods discussed below in this chapter. However, keep trying to hydrate patients orally and switch them back to ORT alone as soon as possible.

Moderate Dehydration

Start patients with moderate dehydration on ORS (25-50 mL/kg over 6-12 hours) with or without simultaneous intravenous (IV) or other parenteral intervention.[11] A common method is to give 20 mL/kg and the balance over the next 5 to 11 hours.[12] If patients don't respond quickly, start fluids via a parenteral method. Keep trying to hydrate patients orally; switch them back to ORT alone as soon as possible.

If IV therapy is needed, give from 20 to 40 mL/kg normal (0.9%) saline (NS) or lactated Ringer's solution over 1 to 2 hours. Administer additional boluses of 10 to 20 mL/kg/hr NS or Ringer's to normalize heart rate and blood pressure, as needed. Once patients stabilize, calculate maintenance fluids using the "4-2-1 rule": 4 mL/kg/hr for the first 10 kg, plus 2 mL/kg/hr for every kilogram between 10 and 20 kg, plus 1 mL/kg/hr for each kilogram >20 kg. (This may be easier to remember than the equivalent 24-hour rule: 100 mL/kg for the first 10 kg of body weight, 50 mL/kg for every kilogram between 10 and 20 kg, and 10 mL/kg for each additional 10 kg of body weight.)

Severe Dehydration

Table 11-4 describes the general plan for rehydrating severely dehydrated patients. Some patients may need more parenteral fluid than noted in the chart. Also, while intraperitoneal rehydration

TABLE 11-4 Progressive Treatment for Severe Dehydration

Fluid Type	mL/kg	Time Until Fluid Administration Completed
Infant		
1. Normal saline or Ringer's lactate IV/IO	30	<1 hour
2. Normal saline or Ringer's lactate IV	40	Next 2 hours
3. ORS (po)	40	Next 3 hours
Older Child/Adult		
1. Normal saline or Ringer's lactate IV/IO	110	<4 hours; initially as fast as possible until palpable radial pulse
2. ORS (po)	15-30	Next 3-4 hours, depending on ongoing fluid loss

Abbreviations: IO, intraosseous; IV, intravenous; ORS, oral rehydration solution; po, by mouth.

Data from Ree and Clezy.[13]

works well for mild-to-moderate dehydration, the fluid is not absorbed quickly enough to be the sole method of treating severe dehydration.

In cases of severe dehydration, especially if hypotension is present, parenteral rehydration is optimal. Successful treatment depends on replacing fluids and electrolytes at least as fast as they are being lost. In general, use parenteral rehydration for patients:

- Who present with severe dehydration
- With continued, frequent vomiting despite small, frequent feedings
- With worsening diarrhea and an inability to keep up with fluid losses
- In stupor, in coma, or who are unable to swallow without aspirating
- With intestinal ileus (no bowel sounds heard)

See Table 12-2 for the composition of standard IV fluids.

Note that in one large study in southern Africa, children with severe febrile illness and impaired perfusion but with no hypotension, malnutrition, or gastroenteritis (generally suffering from malaria) who received fluid boluses of 20 to 40 mL/kg of 5% albumin solution or 0.9% saline upon admission had increased mortality compared to those that did not receive a fluid bolus.[14]

Even in patients with severe dehydration, supplement parenteral therapy with oral rehydration if they are conscious and able to drink. Oral rehydration has been effective in many cases of severe dehydration when parenteral methods were not available.

RAPID REALIMENTATION

Use rapid realimentation after rapid rehydration to return the patient to an age-appropriate, unrestricted diet, including solids. Gut rest is not indicated. Breast-feeding should be continued at all times, even during the initial rehydration phases. Increase the patient's diet as soon as tolerated, to compensate for lost caloric intake during the acute illness. Lactose restriction is usually not necessary, although it might be helpful in cases of diarrhea among malnourished children or among children with a severe enteropathy. Changes in formula usually are unnecessary. Full-strength formula usually is tolerated and allows for a more rapid return to full energy intake.[10]

Other Additives

Adding zinc to the diet of a patient with diarrhea can have significant benefits, including a reduction in the duration of the acute phase, reduced stool output and frequency, and decreased recurrence. Naturally available sources of zinc include beans, lentils, yeast, nuts, seeds, and whole grain cereals. Pumpkin seeds are one of the most concentrated sources of zinc.

Diarrhea reduces the absorption of, and thus increases the need for, vitamin A. Zinc deficiency exacerbates vitamin A deficiency, which can lead to blindness and death. Supplementing vitamin A decreases the severity of, and the number of, deaths from diarrhea (and measles). Dairy products, raw carrots, sweet potatoes, cantaloupe, and spinach are good dietary sources of vitamin A.

If an antiemetic is available inexpensively and there are no contraindications to its use, it may improve the success of ORT in children with acute gastroenteritis and dehydration by reducing emesis.[15] However, 3 to 5 children must be treated for one not to need IV hydration. Between 6 and 100 children must be treated to prevent one hospitalization.[16]

Breast-feeding

Nipple Shield

If a mother is breast-feeding and has a nipple too sore for the child to use, use a breast pump or manually drain the breast into a bottle, or use a nipple shield until the nipple heals. The shield must fit tightly and form a seal around the breast. It can be fashioned from the rubber nipple from a baby's bottle. Use vegetable oil to help form the seal, although the mother may still have to hold it in place. The shield must be boiled between uses.[17]

Supplementing Breast-feeding Neonates

Families with exclusively breast-fed newborns, especially during those first few days of life when mother's milk production has not yet been well established, often present with concerns about poor feeding, adequate urine output, and insufficient milk supply. The solution is to make a supplemental nursing device to allow the infant to continue to breast-feed. It provides the needed stimulation to increase milk production and ensures that the infant will get at least 1 to 2 oz of volume per feeding, preventing some infants from needing an IV or switching to bottle feeding, which can foil attempts to breast-feed.

Method

Jeffrey S. Blake, MD, a physician at Mary Bridge Children's Hospital in Tacoma, Wash, suggests this method for supplemental nursing. Attach a 5-Fr feeding tube or an equivalent size urethral catheter to a 30- or 60-mL syringe filled with pumped breast milk or formula. Do one of the following: (a) tape the tip of the feeding tube along the breast with the tip positioned alongside the nipple so that the infant will latch onto both the nipple and the tube tip or (b) have the parent insert the tip of the tube ~1 to 2 cm into the corner of the infant's mouth after the child has already latched onto the breast. Because the tube is so small, neither method interferes with the infant's latch to the breast. Then, hold the syringe elevated above the infant's head or hang it around the mother's neck with string, like a necklace. Allow gravity to help slowly trickle the formula/breast milk in as the infant sucks at the breast. With the infant's sucking, along with help from gravity, pushing the syringe plunger is usually not necessary. Adjust the syringe height so that only the sucking is needed to regulate the flow. (Personal written communication, June 5, 2007.)

Disinfecting Baby Bottles/Nipples

Because small children often use baby bottles to take ORS, it is important to clean the bottles, especially in an austere environment where no replacements may be available. Both of the methods described in the following paragraphs disinfect, rather than sterilize, the nipples and bottles; that is sufficient.

Boiling

After washing the bottles and nipples with a brush, put several bottles and nipples in a pan filled with clean water. Cover and bring it to a boil. At sea level, leave the bottles in the water for an additional 30 minutes. (For more information, see the section "Boiling" in Chapter 6.) Then drain the water and leave the bottles and nipples in the pan until needed.

Sodium Hypochlorite/Bleach

After washing the bottles and nipples with a brush, put several bottles and nipples in a plastic bowl covered with clean water. Be sure that the air is out of the bottles. For every liter (quart) of water, add two teaspoons (10 mL) of household bleach (sodium hypochlorite). Leave the bottles and nipples in the solution for at least 1 hour or until the next feeding. Remove the bottle and nipple using clean hands, and empty the sodium hypochlorite out of the bottle. The bottle need not be rinsed. Make new solution each day.[18]

ORAL REHYDRATION

More lives are saved throughout the world by rehydrating children with acute diarrhea than by any other medical intervention except for immunization. Worldwide, there are approximately 1.7 billion cases of diarrhea annually that kill about 760,000 children, nearly all of whom are <5 years old and living in developing countries.[19] Up to 70% of these deaths are due to dehydration.

More than 90% of patients with acute infectious diarrhea can be successfully resuscitated using ORS correctly.[20] Yet <25% of those who could benefit from appropriate ORT receive it.[21] Oral rehydration therapy generally results in rehydration and the resumption of solid food intake in 4 to 8 hours.[22]

Administering Oral Rehydration Solutions

For infants, use a clean eyedropper or a syringe without the needle. Drop small amounts into the mouth every 1 to 2 minutes. Also, continue breast-feeding. An alternative is to make a tiny puncture at the tip of a rubber glove finger, fill the finger or glove with ORS (while holding the hole closed), and use that as a nipple. The plastic sheath in which some 3-mL disposable syringes are still packed also works well as a mini-bottle for small-volume liquids or medications.[23] Slip a standard baby bottle nipple over the open end; it holds 9 cc.

For children or adults, give the ORS using a clean spoon or cup. Do not use feeding bottles unless they can be properly cleaned. Offer children <2 years old a teaspoonful every 1 to 2 minutes. Alternate other fluids, such as breast milk and juices, with the ORS. Older children and adults should sip from the cup every 1 to 2 minutes. Adults and large children should drink at least 3 L (3 quarts) per day until the diarrhea stops. Chilling the ORS before giving it to the patient may make it more palatable.

Continue to try to feed the drink to the patient slowly, small sips at a time. The body will retain some of the fluids and salts needed, even though there is vomiting. If the patient vomits, wait for 10 minutes and then begin again. Have the patient slowly sip ORS after every loose bowel movement.

In severely dehydrated, but conscious, patients, have them sip ORS every 5 minutes until urination returns to normal (four to five times per day and yellow color) and they no longer feel thirsty.

Oral Rehydration Solutions/Oral Rehydration Therapy

Standard and Reduced-Osmolarity Oral Rehydration Solutions

Oral rehydration solutions come as premade commercial packets, hospital-made solutions, or homemade solutions. In 2002, the World Health Organization (WHO) began recommending a new, low-osmolarity ORS containing less sodium and glucose (Table 11-5). This change has led to some cases of severe hyponatremia, while not significantly changing patients' disease course.[24] The solution does, however, replace bicarbonate with citrate, improving its stability in tropical climates. When stored in temperatures up to 60°C (140°F), no discoloration occurs and the solution has a shelf life of about 3 years.

Preparing Oral Rehydration Solutions

Commercial Oral Rehydration Solution Packets

To reconstitute a commercial ORS packet, add one packet to 1 L (1 quart; 5 cupfuls) of clean water. (Filter the water using cloth or gauze and boil it, if necessary; let it cool.) Stir the mixture until all the contents dissolve. Even if the powder clumps or hardens, there should be no difficulty in producing a satisfactory solution.[26]

Homemade Oral Rehydration Solutions

Three methods for making homemade ORS are described in the following paragraphs. Once prepared, store the ORS in a cool place. If you have a refrigerator, store it there. If the patient

TABLE 11-5 Composition of the WHO Oral Rehydration Solutions (ORS)

	Standard ORS (1975)	Reduced-Osmolarity ORS (2002)
Na^+, mEq/L	90	75
K^+, mEq/L	20	20
Cl^-, mEq/L	80	65
Citrate^{-3}, mmol/L	10	10
Glucose, mmol/L[a]	111	75
Osmolarity, mOsm/L	311	245

[a] In some areas, locally produced ORS uses rice instead of glucose. When patients eat a rice-based diet soon after correction of dehydration, the glucose-based ORS leads to less need for additional ORS than with rice-based ORS, and also shortens the duration of diarrhea and decreases stool volumes.

Data from Fayad et al.[25]

still needs ORS after 24 hours, make a fresh solution. Do not use too much salt or the patient may refuse to drink it. A rough guide to the amount of salt is that the solution should taste no saltier than tears. Too little salt is less effective in restoring the needed chemicals to the body—and may lead to hyponatremic seizures. If only a 0.5-L (1-pint) container is available, use only half the listed amounts of ingredients to prepare ORS.

Method #1

To prepare 1 L (1 quart) of homemade ORS, start with 1 L (1 quart; 5 cupfuls) clean water. (Filter the water using cloth or gauze and boil it, if necessary; let it cool.) Add one level teaspoon of salt and eight level teaspoons of sugar. Mix the solution. Add 0.5 cup orange juice or half a mashed banana to provide potassium and improve the taste.[26]

Method #2

To prepare 1 L (1 quart) of homemade ORS, start with 1 L (1 quart; 5 cupfuls) clean water. (Filter the water using cloth or gauze and boil it, if necessary; let it cool.) Add one-fourth teaspoon baking soda (bicarbonate of soda) and one-fourth teaspoon salt. Double the amount of salt (to one-half teaspoon) if baking soda is not available. Mix the solution. Add two tablespoons sugar or honey and mix until everything dissolves. Add 0.5 cup orange juice or half a mashed banana to provide potassium and improve the taste.[26]

Method #3

Plantain-based ORS. Plantain flour-based ORS uses green Hartón plantain (*Musa paradisiaca*), which is common in Columbia and elsewhere. (There are many plantain/banana varieties; several can be used for ORS.) Remove the plantain's peel and cut it into very thin slices. Dry these slices in the sun and grind them into powder. Add 50 g plantain flour to 1100 mL water and 3.5 g sodium chloride. Mix these and boil the mixture for 12 minutes. This results in an ORS with a mean osmolarity of 134 mOsm/L.

This ORS formulation was shown to decrease diarrhea frequency by one-third and the volume by one-half over that in children taking the WHO formula. However, some children taking this formula had nonclinically significant hyponatremia and hypokalemia.[27]

Alternatives to Oral Rehydration Solution

If ORS is not available or cannot be made, reasonable alternatives are breast milk, vegetable or chicken soup with salt, other salted drinks (e.g., salted rice water, salted yogurt drink), or other normally unsalted drinks to which 3 g/L salt has been added.

Two pinches of salt using three fingers (thumb, index, and long fingers coming together) are often said to equal about 3.5 g, and this measure is used as an improvised salt measure for homemade ORT solutions.[12] However, this commonly used measure is highly inaccurate and can vary by a factor of 30 between individuals, meaning that it can deliver a negligible amount of salt or nearly 4 g with each pinch.[28] A more accurate measure is to use one-fourth teaspoon iodized salt, which equals 1.5 g and which, in 1 L of water, produces a concentration of 90 mmol/L; using slightly less will yield the currently recommended ORS concentration of 75 mmol/L.

As can be seen in Table 11-6, some alternative rehydration solutions commonly used at home (e.g., apple juice, Coca Cola Classic) are not suitable due to their osmolarity, electrolyte composition, or both.

Self-Administered Oral Rehydration

ORS can be self-administered with a straw. For adults and cooperative older children, a simple and inexpensive method exists for them to administer their own ORS—if they can resist the temptation to drink too much or too often. Self-administration markedly reduces staff time associated with managing nasogastric (NG) feedings or parenteral infusions, especially for children without an adult family member who can administer ORS. Simply fill a disinfected or sterile IV container, another bottle, or a commercial ORS bottle with the desired liquid and hang it (inverted) from an IV pole or hook.

Hang a loop of the tubing higher than the fluid level in the bottle and give the other end to the patient. Depending on the size of the bottle and the tubing, adjust the bottle's height until there

TABLE 11-6 Composition of Commonly Used Rehydration Solutions

Solution	Carbohydrate[a] (g/L)	Sodium (mmol/L)	Potassium (mmol/L)	Chloride[b] (mmol/L)	Base[c] (mmol/L)	Osmolarity (mOsm/L)
WHO ORS (2002)	13.5	75	20	65	30	245
WHO ORS (1975)	20	90	20	80	30	311
Commercial Sugar-Electrolyte Solutions						
Pedialyte	25	45	20	35	30	250
Pedialyte Freezer Pop	25	45	20	35	30	250
Enfalyte	30	50	25	45	34	200
Rehydralyte	25	75	20	65	30	305
Cerealyte	40	50-90	20	—	30	220
Gatorade (premixed)	46	20	3	3	20	330
The following solutions are generally *not* appropriate for rehydration due to their osmolarity, electrolyte content, or both.						
Commercial Clear Liquids						
Jell-O	20	22-27	1.3-2.0	26	—	570-640
Coca Cola (Classic)	112	1.6	—	—	13.4	650
Ginger ale	53	2.7	0.1-1.5	0.2	4	520-540
7-Up	74	5.0-5.5	1-2	6.5	—	520-560
Kool-Aid (sugarless)	—	0.5-1.2	0.1-1.3	—	—	250-590
Popsicles	180	4.7-5.6	0.5-2.0	6	—	670-720
Fruit Juices						
Apple (liquid)	120	0.4	44	45	—	730
Grape (concentrate)	151	0.8-2.8	31-44	4	32	1170-1190
Orange (concentrate)	86	0.1-2.5	46-65	20	50	540-710
Other Liquids						
Beef bouillon (cubes)	—	110-170	5.5-11	130	—	300-390
Chicken broth (canned)	—	170-250	2.2-8.2	210	—	380-500
Tea (unsweetened)	—	0	5	5	—	~0
Milk	4.9	22	36	58	30	260

Abbreviation: ORS, oral rehydration solution.

[a]Glucose, fructose, or corn syrup.
[b]Chloride, in most cases the Cl^- content is calculated from other ingredients.
[c]Actual or potential bicarbonate, such as citrate, lactate, or acetate.
Data from Centers for Disease Control and Prevention[10] and Synder.[29]

is no spontaneous flow. (No flow controller is needed.) When the patient sucks on the tube, a mouthful of fluid comes out; when suction stops, the fluid flow stops. Do not use this for patients who cannot suck the fluid or who have difficulty swallowing.[30]

Use a piece of orthopedic stockinet, stretch bandage, or even the sleeve from a shirt to hang bottles or bags without hooks or handles. Insert the bottle into the material, and tie the end at the bottom of the container (the end away from the IV tubing) to a pole or hook. Cut a slit in the other end so it can be tied—and retied—tightly around the end with the IV tubing. Many Pedialyte bottles now come so a straw can be inserted. An IV tubing connection fits this hole perfectly.

Wounded Patients

Under normal circumstances, adult surgical patients are kept NPO (nothing by mouth) and are not allowed to ingest oral food or liquid for hours prior to surgery. But, in rudimentary environments, some latitude is needed so as not to exacerbate the situation.

Boulton and Cole, writing about care in austere circumstances, noted that stomach "emptying time for fluids is often overestimated—2 hours for water or clear fluids is normally adequate. Nonmedical auxiliaries and first aid workers should be encouraged to give moderate amounts of water to injured patients who are conscious and not vomiting; this is especially necessary in isolated circumstances where evacuation is likely to be prolonged and medical aid delayed."[31]

NASOGASTRIC REHYDRATION

Uses

Nasogastric rehydration with commercially prepared or homemade ORS can be used for patients who are moderately to severely dehydrated and who are vomiting or refuse to drink.[32] It can be used in cases of both primary dehydration (e.g., gastroenteritis) and secondary dehydration (e.g., malnutrition, measles, pneumonia).

Many malnourished or dehydrated children will not take sufficient oral intake, due to poor appetite, weakness, and painful stomatitis. Feed these children with an NG tube after they have taken as much as they can by mouth. Stop the NG feeds when the child is taking three-fourths of the daily requirements orally or takes two consecutive full feedings orally. If sufficient fluids and calories are not taken orally in the following 24 hours, reinsert the tube.[33]

If postoperative patients need an NG tube but there is a limited ability to provide IV hydration (i.e., a shortage of fluids or equipment), insert a short (gastric) and longer (distal duodenal or jejunal) tube. These can be fashioned from IV tubing, if necessary. To reduce the need for hydration while preventing aspiration in these patients, suction through an NG tube while reinfusing the aspirate and additional fluids into the distal tube.[34]

Patients with extensive burns can also be fluid resuscitated using NG (or even oral) salt solutions. This method can be used when IV therapy is unavailable or delayed, such as in mass disasters and combat casualties. Enteral resuscitation of burn shock is effective for patients with from 10% to 40% body surface area (BSA) burned and for some patients with more severe injuries. Even when not used exclusively, hypovolemic burn and trauma patients can benefit from enteral resuscitation as an initial alternative and as a supplement to IV therapy. Use this method if there is no bowel injury or no plan for immediate anesthesia. Vomiting is a complication of enteral resuscitation; it occurs less often in children than in adults, and much less often when therapy is initiated within the first postburn hour.[35]

Method

If other methods are not suitable, use a slow NG drip to rehydrate a child or adult. A modification of oral rehydration, this economical method can be easily accomplished with few adverse consequences, even with few resources and basic staff. Available NG equipment is employed, including used but cleaned/sterilized IV tubing (the NG tube) and fluid bags/bottles.

Fill the bags with standard ORS and continuously drip in, with the total amount based on the patient's weight, level of dehydration, and symptoms. The following drip rates are a good approximation[36]:

<6 kg = 25 drops/min (~1.25 mL/min; 75 mL/hr)
6 to 12 kg = 35 drops/min (~1.75 mL/min; ~100 mL/hr)
>12 kg = 50 drops/min (~2.5 mL/min; 150 mL/hr)

For adult patients, add any estimated fluid losses or deficits to their hourly maintenance. This may be most easily calculated as: Weight in kg + 40. For example, for a 70-kg man, 70 kg + 40 = 110 mL/hr maintenance fluids.

Commercial and homemade ORS (see recipes given earlier) are much cheaper to use than IV fluids. The ORS can be put into an old IV bottle (clean, not necessarily sterile) and connected to IV tubing, which is used both as the NG tubing and to drip in the solution. If the tube is curled or kinked, straighten it by holding a small flame (such as a match) under it for a moment. The IV drip chamber and rate control device on the IV tubing are used to adjust the drip rate. Once it is certain that the NG tube is in the stomach, securely attach it to the patient's face to prevent irritation from movement and accidental removal. A piece of tape across the bottom of the nose that covers the tubing and extends to the hairline near one ear is usually effective.[36] Dripping fluid through an NG tube to feed premature infants (gavage feeding) can also be done in this manner.

Encourage mothers to continue breast-feeding or else provide ORS by mouth during NG rehydration. Discontinue NG feeding when the child is able to drink and no longer appears seriously dehydrated. Nasogastric tubes can be left in the stomach for up to 3 days without adverse effects.

INTRAVENOUS FLUIDS

Shortages

Discussing how to stretch supplies, Colin Carthen of Satellite Healthcare said, "Pie is a good analogy. Now I'm going to use 16 slices of pie instead of eight slices of pie, and I'll be able to feed 16 people instead of eight."[37] With recurrent or, in some areas of the world, chronic medication and IV fluid shortages, we should recognize that "clinicians must regularly negotiate unfamiliar drug alternatives, concentrations, or dosing strategies.... In many ways, [normal saline] is more the lifeblood of hospital care than blood itself."[38] Yet, there are reasonable methods to conserve IV solutions (Table 11-7).

Saline Lock: A Simple Conservation Method

A simple way to conserve IV fluids is to use a saline lock. Use this to give intermittent fluid boluses or to decrease the amount of unnecessary equipment during patient transport. (See the "Intravenous Fluids and Equipment" section in Chapter 5 for an easy way to improvise a saline/heparin lock.) This avoids the need for nursing personnel to constantly monitor infusions in small children and allows the child, if not too ill, to return home between bolus infusions. Do not use this for an intraperitoneal line because the risk of infection is great and, if one results, it can be devastating.

Administering Intravenous Fluids Safely

When infusion pumps or burettes are unavailable, use a dark indelible-ink pen to mark the IV bag with the amount of fluid to be infused and the time when that amount of infusion should be done. If that is not possible (or bottles are being used for the fluid), put the marks along the length of the bottle using a piece of tape. Write the date an IV was placed on a piece of white tape over the catheter.

Coconut Water as Intravenous Solution

Green coconut water (GCW) has been used successfully as an IV fluid by the British in Ceylon, and by the Japanese in Sumatra during World War II. While not an optimal fluid for long-term use, it has primarily been used as a temporizing alternative in urgent situations, such as cholera epidemics, and for other ill and dehydrated adults and children in wartime. In 1942 in Havana, Cuba, Pradera administered 1000 to 1870 mL GCW IV over 24 hours to each of 12 pediatric patients without adverse reactions, and parenterally administered up to 500 mL GCW in 13 others with only a local inflammatory reaction. Subsequently, filtered GCW was successfully administered in Thailand, St. Louis (MO), Ceylon, and (unfiltered) Malaysia—all without significant reactions other than local discomfort at high infusion rates.

The procedure uses fresh, intact coconuts. Husk them, leaving the one large and two smaller "eyes" intact until ready to use. Insert a 20-gauge needle through one of the smaller eyes to equalize pressure within the coconut. If the coconut meat blocks the needle lumen, pass a second needle through the same port. Insert single chambered blood transfusion tubing through the large

TABLE 11-7 Intravenous Solution Conservation Strategies

What Can Clinicians Do to Conserve?

- Use oral hydration whenever possible.
- Substitute comparable IV solutions based on availability (Table 11-8).
- Frequently, or at minimum once each shift, evaluate the clinical need to continue intravenous fluid therapy. Consider identifying specific clinical personnel to actively monitor usage for each patient.
- Discontinue infusions as soon as appropriate. Consider stop orders for infusions, e.g., 24-48 hr automatic stops, if not reordered.
- Frequently, or at minimum once each shift, assess need to continue "keep vein open" (KVO) orders.
- Consider using a saline or heparin lock rather than infusing fluids at a KVO rate.
- Consider flushing central venous access devices 1-3 times per week rather than daily.
- Evaluate total fluid requirements for surgeries. The *American College of Surgeons: Principles and Practice 2014* notes that total volume replacement needs for elective surgeries are much less (500-3000 mL total) than previously thought (4500-6000 mL total).

Product Conservation

- Use small-volume bags for slow infusion rates (Table 11-9).
- Consider deferring elective procedures and surgeries requiring solutions in short supply.
- Consider hang times longer than 24 hr for solutions, weighing the risk of infection against the need to conserve IV solutions.
- Evaluate the clinical practice of using flush bags for intermittent medications when no primary solution is being administered. 0.9% sodium chloride flush syringes are an alternative.
- Use commercially available dialysis solutions whenever possible, instead of compounding them with 0.9% sodium chloride.

Inventory Control Strategies

- Minimize stocks of large-volume IV fluid bags except where they are an essential emergency supply.
- Ensure smaller-volume bags are stocked in other supply areas, especially pediatric areas.
- Limit quantities of bags placed in warmers.

Caveat/Safety Information

- Compounding sodium chloride solutions from sterile water for injection and concentrated sodium chloride injection is error prone, labor intensive, and may worsen the existing shortage of concentrated sodium chloride injection.
- Avoid using sodium chloride irrigation solution for IVs. Sterility requirements and limits on particulate matter differ between these two products.

Modified from American Society of Health-System Pharmacists and University of Utah Drug Information Service. See disclaimer in reference.[39]

eye and suspend the coconut in netting. Secure it to the netting with tape (Fig. 11-1).[40] Because the drip rate may be slow, use IV boluses by aspirating fluid from the tubing distal to the blood filter.

Green coconut water is hypotonic, with a specific gravity similar to plasma (SG 1.020), but it is more acidic than plasma. Even after infusions of 3 L of GCW, patients have shown no pH change within 24 hours of the infusion. Resembling intracellular fluid more closely than extracellular plasma, it is higher in potassium, calcium, and magnesium than it is in sodium, chloride, and phosphate. The high osmolarity is due to GCW's glucose and fructose (immature) and sucrose (mature). While rich in many essential amino acids, including lysine, leucine, cystine, phenylalanine, histidine, and tryptophan, it is a poor source of vitamins and protein.[41] Nevertheless, GCW

TABLE 11-8 Comparison of Selected Intravenous Fluids

	mOsm/L	Na (mEq/L)	Cl (mEq/L)	Dextrose (g/L)	K (mEq/L)	Ca (mEq/L)	Lactate (mEq/L)
0.9% Sodium chloride	308	154	154	—	—	—	—
0.45% Sodium chloride	154	77	77	—	—	—	—
5% Dextrose - 0.225% sodium chloride	329	38.5	38.5	50	—	—	—
5% Dextrose - 0.45% sodium chloride	406	77	77	50	—	—	—
5% Dextrose - 0.9% sodium chloride	560	154	154	50	—	—	—
5% Dextrose	252	—	—	50	—	—	—
Lactated Ringer	273	130	109	4	2.7	28	—
Lactated Ringer - 5% dextrose	525	130	109	50	4	2.7	28

Modified from American Society of Health-System Pharmacists and University of Utah Drug Information Service. See disclaimer in reference.[39]

TABLE 11-9 Recommended Container Volumes Based on Infusion Rates

Infusion Rate	Bag Size
<20 mL/h	250 mL
21-40 mL/h	500 mL
≥41 mL/h	1000 mL

Modified from American Society of Health-System Pharmacists and University of Utah Drug Information Service. See disclaimer in reference.[39]

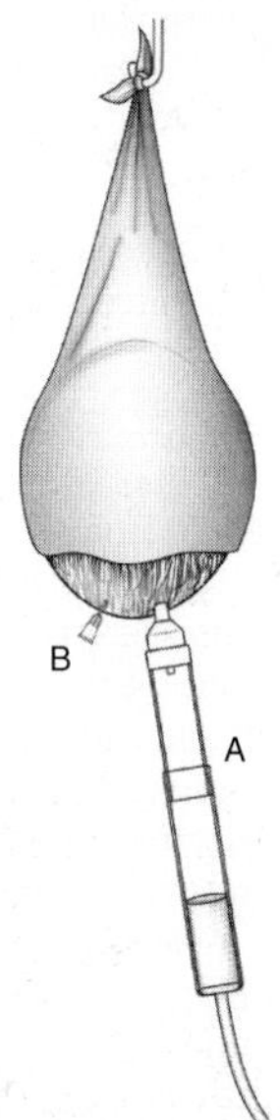

FIG. 11-1. Intravenous coconut set-up. The coconut has (A) single-chambered blood transfusion tubing attached and (B) a second needle to equalize intraluminal pressure, and is then placed in orthopedic netting.

TABLE 11-10 Macro- and Micro-Infusion Drip Rates

Macro-Infusion Set—10 drops/mL	
Solution per Hour (mL)	Drop Rate Interval (sec)
50	7.2
100	3.6
150	2.4
200	1.8
250	1.4
300	1.2
360	1
Micro-Infusion Set—60 drops/mL	
Solution per Hour (mL)	Drop Rate Interval (sec)
10	6
20	3
30	2
40	1.5
50	1.2
60	1

Adapted from Canadian Air Division.[45]

could be used for total parenteral nutrition (TPN) in resource-poor situations. As measured by thrombelastography (TEG), GCW's effect on hemostasis does not differ from that of the same volume of physiological saline.[42]

Intravenous Drip Rates

If you must calculate IV drip rates, macro-infusion (adult) drip sets are generally set for 10 drops/mL; micro-infusion (pediatric) rates are 60 drops/mL (Table 11-10).

Increasing Infusion Rate

Intravenous infusion rates depend on the internal diameter (ID) of the equipment. The size of the smallest element of the system (IV catheter, connector, IV tubing) is the rate-limiting factor.[43,44] The other factors are the viscosity of the fluid (blood generally flows slower than crystalloid) and the external pressure on the system. The pressure is often the easiest component to adjust when a high-flow infusion is needed, such as during resuscitation.

Pressurize IV solution bags by wrapping them with elastic bandages, standing on them, or inflating blood pressure cuffs around them. During patient transport, laying the (adult) patient on the IV bag generally supplies sufficient pressure to keep the fluid flowing.

One method of increasing the speed of infusion using IV bottles (rather than bags) is to use a three-way stopcock attached to the IV near the catheter. A syringe is alternately filled from the drip set while closing the line to the patient and then closing the line to the bottle and injecting the fluid into the patient. Increasing the air pressure by injecting air into the bottle and closing the air inlet also works. Finally, either with bottles or bags, the drip chamber in the IV line can be pumped; the ball valve closes the inlet when external pressure is applied.

Warming Intravenous Fluids

Three methods of warming IV bags have been advocated in cold, austere circumstances: using body heat, soaking in hot water, and applying external heat packs. Carrying IV bags next to one's body to warm the solution in a cold environment, even when the person carrying them is doing vigorous exercise, warms the bags only about 10°C (50°F), if the bags are initially cold (~5°C [23°F]). If the bags are prewarmed, they still lose their warmth steadily.[46,47]

When IV bags were warmed to 58°C (136°F), their temperatures dropped to 35°C (95°F) in 2 hours, even though they were kept in a pouch against a thin undergarment while rescuers were hiking. If this method is used, you will need to apply external chemical heat packs to the bags to augment the saline's temperature before administering it.

Researchers in two studies warmed 500-mL bags of normal saline in a pot over a wood stove to an external bag temperature of 75°C (167°F). Bags in one study reached an initial 58°C (136°F) fluid temperature, while the other researcher obtained temperatures of 39°C (102°F) to 40°C (104°F). This suggests that great care must be taken when employing this method so as not to overheat the fluids.[46,47]

A technique that does produce body-temperature fluid is to tape two meals-ready-to-eat (MRE) heating bags to the outside of a 5°C (41°F) 500-mL saline bag for 10 minutes. Then remove the MRE bags and wait 10 more minutes for some cooling to occur before infusion. It helps to cover the bag and the proximal IV line with insulation such as a coat or sleeping bag.[47]

REFERENCES

1. MacGregor W. Some problems of tropical medicine. *Lancet*. October 1900;13:1055-1061.
2. World Health Organization. *The Treatment of Diarrhoea: A Manual for Physicians and Other Senior Health Workers*. Geneva, Switzerland: WHO; 1995.
3. UNICEF/WHO. *Diarrhoea: Why Children Are Still Dying and What Can Be Done*. Geneva, Switzerland: UNICEF; 2009.
4. Nager AL, Wang VJ. Comparison of nasogastric and intravenous methods of rehydration in pediatric patients with acute dehydration. *Pediatrics*. 2002;109:566-572.
5. King M, King F, Martodipoero S. *Primary Child Care*. Oxford, UK: Oxford University Press; 1978. Cited in: Green SDR. Treatment of moderate and severe dehydration by nasogastric drip. *Trop Doct*. 1987;17(2):86-88.
6. Pringle K, Shah SP, Umulisa I, et al. Comparing the accuracy of the three popular clinical dehydration scales in children with diarrhea. *Int J Emerg Med*. 2011;4:58.
7. World Health Organization: *Treatment of Diarrhea: A Manual for Physicians and Other Senior Health Workers*. Geneva, Switzerland: WHO; 2005.
8. World Health Organization. *Management of Severe Malnutrition: A Manual for Physicians and Other Senior Health Workers*. Geneva, Switzerland: WHO; 1999:8-10.
9. Ng L, Khine H, Taragin BH, et al. Does bedside sonographic measurement of the inferior vena cava diameter correlate with central venous pressure in the assessment of intravascular volume in children? *Pediatr Emerg Care*. 2013;29(3):337-341.
10. Centers for Disease Control and Prevention. Managing acute gastroenteritis among children: oral rehydration, maintenance, and nutritional therapy. *MMWR Recomm Rep*. November 21, 2003;52(RR16): 1-16.
11. Holliday MA, Friedman AL, Wassner SJ. Extracellular fluid restoration in dehydration: a critique of rapid versus slow. *Pediatr Nephrol*. 1999;13:292-297.
12. Rehydration Project. Oral rehydration solutions. http://rehydrate.org/ors/ort.htm. Accessed October 22, 2015.
13. Ree GH, Clezy JK. Simple guide to fluid balance. *Trop Doct*. 1982;12(4 Pt 1):155-159.
14. Maitland K, Kiguli S, Opoka RO, et al. Mortality after fluid bolus in African children with severe infection. *N Engl J Med*. 2011;364(26):2483-2495.
15. Freedman SB, Adler M, Seshadri R, et al. Oral ondansetron for gastroenteritis in a pediatric emergency department. *N Engl J Med*. 2006;354(16):1698-1705.
16. Weinstein E. What is the role of antiemetics in the treatment of children with acute gastroenteritis? *Ann Emerg Med*. 2011;58(4):371-372.

17. King M, King F, Martodipoero S. *Primary Child Care: A Manual for Health Workers*. Oxford, UK: Oxford University Press; 1978:262.
18. King M, King F, Martodipoero S. *Primary Child Care: A Manual for Health Workers*. Oxford, UK: Oxford University Press; 1978:264.
19. World Health Organization. Diarrhoeal disease. Fact sheet No. 330, April 2013. http://www.who.int/mediacentre/factsheets/fs330/en/. Accessed September 4, 2015.
20. Centers for Disease Control and Prevention. The management of acute diarrhea in children: oral rehydration, maintenance, and nutritional therapy. *MMWR Recomm Rep*. 1992;41:9.
21. Myers A. Outpatient oral rehydration. *Ann Emerg Med*. 1997;29:551-553.
22. International Study Group on Reduced-Osmolarity ORS Solutions. Multicentre evaluation of reduced-osmolarity oral rehydration salts solution. *Lancet*. 1995;345:282-285.
23. Glassman SK, Measel CP. A makeshift mini-bottle: accurate small volume fluid or oral medication administration to infants. *Neonatal Netw*. 1989;7(4):29-31.
24. CHOICE Study Group. Multicenter, randomized, double-blind clinical trial to evaluate the efficacy and safety of a reduced-osmolarity oral rehydration salts solution in children with acute watery diarrhea. *Pediatrics*. 2001;107(4):613-618.
25. Fayad IM, Hashem M, Duggan C, et al. Comparative efficacy of rice-based and glucose-based oral rehydration salts plus early reintroduction of food. *Lancet*. 1993;342:772-775.
26. World Health Organization. *Oral Rehydration Salts: Production of the New ORS*. Geneva, Switzerland: WHO; 2006:46-47.
27. Arias MM, Alcaráz GM, Bernal C, et al. Oral rehydration with a plantain flour-based solution in children dehydrated by acute diarrhea: a clinical trial. *Acta Paediatr*. 1997;86(10):1047-1051.
28. Wilcox WD, Miller JJ. Inaccuracy of three-finger pinch method of determining salt content in homemade sugar salt solutions. *Wild Environ Med*. 1996;2:122-126.
29. Snyder JD. From Pedialyte to Popsicles: a look at oral rehydration therapy used in the United States and Canada. *Am J Clin Nutr*. 1982;35:157-161.
30. Bamford JDR, Gibbs K. Oral regulated feeding and hydration. *Trop Doct*. 1988;18:45.
31. Boulton TB, Cole P. Anesthesia in difficult situations. 7. Routine preparations and pre-operative medication. *Anaesthesia*. 1968;23(2):220-234.
32. World Health Organization. *A Manual for the Treatment of Acute Diarrhoea* (unpublished). WHO/CDD/SER/80.2. Geneva, Switzerland: WHO; 1980.
33. World Health Organization. *Management of Severe Malnutrition: A Manual for Physicians and Other Senior Health Workers*. Geneva, Switzerland: WHO; 1999:14.
34. King M, Bewes P, Cairns J, et al, eds. *Primary Surgery, Vol. 1: Non-Trauma*. Oxford, UK: Oxford Medical Publishing; 1990:11.
35. Kramer GC, Michell MW, Oliveira H, et al. Oral and enteral resuscitation of burn shock: the historical record and implications for mass casualty care. *J Burns Wound Care*. 2003;2(1):19. http://www.journalofburns.com. Accessed June 25, 2008.
36. King M, King F, Martodipoero S. *Primary Child Care: A Manual for Health Workers*. Oxford, UK: Oxford University Press; 1978:120-122.
37. Dembosky A. Shortage of saline solution has hospitals on edge. Medscape. www.medscape.com/viewarticle/827468_print. Accessed June 26, 2014.
38. Hick JL, Hanfling D, Courtney B, Lurie N. Rationing salt water—disaster planning and daily care delivery. *New Engl J Med*. 2014;370(17):1573-1576.
39. Modified from American Society of Health-System Pharmacists and University of Utah Drug Information Service. *Intravenous Solution Conservation Strategies*. March 20, 2014. www.ena.org/about/media/Documents/ConservationStrategiesForIVFluids.pdf. Accessed March 30, 2014. This information was developed by the Drug Information Center of University of Utah in collaboration with the American Society of Health-System Pharmacists. ASHP and the University of Utah neither endorse nor recommend the strategies for the use of any drug or product, nor assume any liability for persons providing medications or other medical care in reliance upon this information. Users of this information must exercise their independent professional judgment when using this information to make decisions regarding the use of drugs and drug therapies.
40. Campbell-Falck D, Thomas T, Falck TM, Tutuo N, Clem K. The intravenous use of coconut water. *Am J Emerg Med*. 2000;18(1):108-111.
41. Petroianu GA, Kosanovic M, Shehatta IS, et al. Green coconut water for intravenous use: trace and minor element content. *J Trace Element Exp Med*. 2004;17:273-282.

42. Pummer S, Hell P, Maleck W, Petroianu G. Influence of coconut water on hemostasis. *Am J Emerg Med.* 2001;19:287-289.

43. Iserson KV, Reeter AJ, Criss E. Comparison of flow rates for standard and large bore blood tubing. *West J Med.* 1985;143(2):183-185.

44. Iserson KV, Criss E. The combined effect of catheter and tubing size on fluid flow. *Am J Emerg Med.* 1986;4(3):238-240.

45. Canadian Air Division. *Search and Rescue Technician: Pre-hospital Protocols and Procedures*. Ottawa, Canada: 1st Canadian Air Division, A1 Division Surgeon; June 2003:8.8.

46. Mortimer RB, Hurtt H. Intravenous fluid warming with body contact in a wilderness setting. *Wild Environ Med.* 2008;19(2):144-145.

47. Platts-Mills TF, Stendell E, Lewin MR, et al. An experimental study of warming intravenous fluid in a cold environment. *Wild Environ Med.* 2007;18(3):177-185.

12 Vascular Access—Intravenous, Intraosseous, Clysis, and Peritoneal

In some cases, patients cannot tolerate oral therapy or they need immediate medications, rehydration, or fluid/blood-product resuscitation. Clinicians must then be prepared to use intravenous and other parenteral infusion methods. Some of the following methods are not well known, but all can be used safely when needed.

INTRAVENOUS HYDRATION

Why Use Intravenous Hydration?

Intravenous hydration is a rapid method that ensures that the fluid enters the vascular space. In addition, it is appropriate for administering at least one form of nearly all parenteral medications and fluids. In severely dehydrated patients, rapid volume replacement, also called rapid rehydration therapy, saves lives.[1-4] Patients who present with severe dehydration (indicated by a weight loss of ≥10%), with impaired circulation (as measured by rapid pulse and a reduced capillary fill time), and evidence of interstitial fluid loss (including loss of skin turgor and sunken eyes) should be rehydrated intravenously over 1 to 2 hours with isotonic saline. To rapidly restore extracellular fluid (ECF), administer intravenous (IV) lactated Ringer's solution and/or normal saline (NS) at 40 mL/kg over 1 to 2 hours. If skin turgor, alertness, or the pulse does not return to normal by the end of the infusion, infuse another 20 to 40 mL/kg over 1 to 2 hours. Repeat that infusion as needed. Initiate oral rehydration therapy (ORT) as soon as tolerated.[5]

In situations of scarcity, multiple problems exist with using IV hydration, including lack of equipment, skilled personnel, and ability to monitor patients adequately. The most obvious problem is scarcity of equipment and personnel trained to place IV catheters and administer IV solutions. The lack of adequate patient monitoring can lead to critically over-hydrating patients, especially infants and the elderly.

Need for Rapid Venous Access in Sick Children

Rapidly establishing peripheral IV access in the sickest children is vital, because delaying "fluid resuscitation is associated with increased mortality. In septic shock, every hour that passes without restoration of normal blood pressure has been associated with at least a 2-fold increase in mortality."[6]

Reusing Intravenous Tubing

Reusing either IV tubing or needles poses a serious risk of passing on blood-borne diseases, a result that may not be immediately obvious. Reusing IV tubing may be the safer of the two, because, if tubing has not been contaminated with patient secretions or blood, it may be relatively safe to use if disinfected. To disinfect IV tubing, first try to boil it for 5 minutes. If that destroys the tubing, disinfect subsequent tubing by soaking it in sodium hypochlorite (bleach) or another antiseptic for several hours. Be sure to also soak the inside of the tubing, which can be done by sucking the solution into the tube with a syringe. Before using the tubing on a patient, wash it thoroughly with boiled water, inside and out, to remove the disinfectant.

Reusing needles is more problematic. Classed as high-risk devices, needles must be sterilized, not just disinfected, before reuse.[7] That can be a challenge, because the interior is difficult to clean of residual materials, a prerequisite to adequate sterilization. See Chapter 6 for further details on cleaning, disinfecting, and sterilizing equipment.

Making Intravenous Equipment

Necessity is the mother of invention, and making IV equipment is a good example. Physician–prisoners working in prisoner of war (POW) camps along the Thai/Burma Railway during World

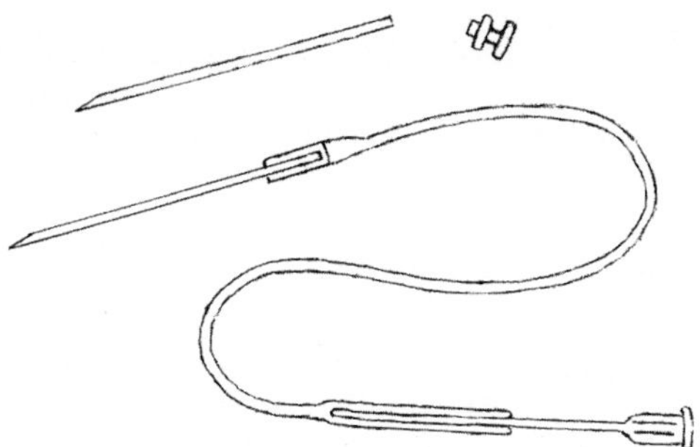

FIG. 12-1. Making a scalp vein IV.

War II, for example, made IV sets "from stethoscope tubing and sharpened bamboo sticks."[8] Injection needles can be used as IV needles after slightly bending the needle so that the hub will not exert as much tension on the skin.[9]

To make a scalp vein IV unit, break off the adapter of a short needle of the appropriate gauge (Fig. 12-1). Insert the needle's broken end into the end of a short piece of thin plastic tubing. (This type of tubing is often used in laboratory equipment.) If the tube fits loosely over the needle, soften the plastic by heating it over a small flame (e.g., match). When soft, squeeze it tightly around the needle. Put an ordinary injection needle into the other end of the tubing; that end may also need to be crimped. Nearly all IV tubing adapters fit the ends of these needles. When constructing this equipment, use forceps to hold the pieces. Disinfect this unit before use. Generally, it is best to have the scalp vein filled with fluid when entering a vein so that the blood does not clot.[10]

METHODS OF LOCATING AND DILATING PERIPHERAL VEINS

Neonates and Infants

Multiple methods have been suggested to increase the chance of finding a child's vein to access; most do not work well. The most useful in austere settings is to warm a hand or extremity to produce vasodilation. Also, alcohol swabs reflect the light off the skin, making vessels easier to see, especially in darker skinned patients. While transilluminators, including penlights, may help in visualizing vessels, their clinical benefit is marginal. Applying nitroglycerin ointments to locate and dilate IVs actually may decrease the chance of success and is associated with adverse effects, including increased infiltration, bleeding, and hypotension.[11]

Children and Adults

Seeing or feeling the vein obviously helps when inserting the IV catheter. If applying a standard venous tourniquet does not produce a vein, inflate a blood pressure cuff above diastolic pressure with the arm supported at the level of the heart. This produces the largest increase in basilic vein size. Esmarch (hard rubber) bandages also work well, as do standard IV tourniquets, although their effect lessens if the arm is below heart level.[12] If that does not work, drop the extremity below the level of the heart and apply a blood pressure cuff. Inflate it first to about 35 mm Hg. If that doesn't produce a vein, inflate the cuff to halfway between the systolic and diastolic pressures. If the cuff's tubes leak, clamp them to keep the cuff at that pressure.

Applying heat to the limb also helps. Use a hot, wet towel, but squeeze out the water before applying it to the limb so you do not burn the patient. The distal extremity can also be immersed in warm water for 10 minutes, as they once did for donors in person-to-person transfusions.[13]

In patients with peripherally constricted veins, apply a tourniquet above the elbow and establish IV access in the dorsum of the hand with a small (e.g., 22 gauge) catheter. Leave the tourniquet in place and immediately infuse NS (100 mL in adults) under pressure. The bigger proximal veins of the cubital fossa engorge so that a larger catheter can be placed.[14]

SECURING INTRAVENOUS CATHETERS

Scalp Veins

Put a paper cup over a scalp vein to protect it, cutting a notch so that the cup's lip does not crimp the tubing.

Ruggedized Intravenous

"Ruggedized" IV systems prevent catheters from being accidentally pulled out, a common occurrence.[15] Developed by military medics, they are excellent for seriously ill and injured patients in all settings in which the loss of an IV may pose serious harm. To place a ruggedized IV, insert either the largest possible needle or IV catheter (recommended) into a vein. Convert it into a saline lock and cover it completely with a clear dressing (e.g., Tegaderm). Insert a slightly smaller IV catheter into the first catheter (saline lock) and begin infusing. If the tubing gets snagged and the infusing catheter is pulled out, the saline lock remains so that a new catheter can immediately be inserted. The downside to this system is that the flow will be limited by the size of the smaller catheter. If trying to infuse fluids rapidly, pressurize the IV bag.[16]

Many austere settings may not have clear surgical dressings or standard catheters for saline locks. In that case, use a large amount of tape and gauze to secure the initial catheter, keeping only the hub exposed. To make a saline lock from an IV catheter and the rubber from the end of a 2- or 3-mL syringe plunger (see Fig. 5-26), shave off the flanges around the hub of some IV catheters. The system then works so well that nearly all critical patients and those with altered mental status can have their IVs started in this fashion.

INTRAOSSEOUS INFUSION

Intraosseous (IO) infusion is one of the quickest ways, both in children and in adults, to establish access for the rapid infusion of fluids, drugs, and blood products in emergency situations.[17-19] However, in some cultures, almost any other method, including intraperitoneal infusion, is preferable to IO infusion.[20]

Use

Placing an IO needle and beginning the infusion generally takes <1 minute; this is much faster than placing an IV in critical situations, especially in infants/small children or in any patient in shock or in cardiac arrest.[18,21] Standard practice is to use an IO needle in resuscitation situations when venous access cannot be obtained after either three attempts or within 90 seconds of starting the procedure, or when the clinicians do not believe they can quickly get venous access.

Because the marrow cavity is contiguous with the venous circulation, the IO route can be used to infuse fluids and medications, and to take blood samples for crossmatch. Any fluid, blood product, or medication (except for cytotoxic agents, such as chemotherapeutic drugs) can be given through the IO route. The onset of action and drug levels during cardiopulmonary resuscitation (CPR) using the IO route are similar to those given intravenously.[19]

Contraindications

Intraosseous infusion is contraindicated when (a) there is a proximal fracture on the ipsilateral side of the extremity that will be the site of needle placement, (b) the bone where the needle will be placed is fractured, or (c) osteomyelitis exists in the bone to be used.[19]

Intraosseous infusion is also contraindicated in patients with osteogenesis imperfecta or osteopetrosis, with an infection or burn overlying the infusion site, with a bleeding diathesis, and who have already had multiple IO needles or attempts at the same site.

Needles

Ideally, IO infusions are done through a special IO needle or a bone marrow aspiration needle with an obturator. Alternatively, use any needle with a stylet. A large-gauge spinal needle and stylet can be cut down to a 3-cm length, beveled, sharpened, resterilized, and packaged in advance for IO use.[22,23]

In emergencies or situations of scarcity, use a standard 14- to 20-gauge butterfly/injection/IV needle (without a stylet); all connect to syringes and standard IV tubing. Using smaller-gauge or longer needles, however, risks their being too fragile or flexible to penetrate the bony cortex. Occasionally, when using such a needle, the lumen becomes plugged with bone. If aspiration or running fluid under pressure does not clear the obstruction, another needle can immediately be placed in the same hole—although this may be more difficult than it sounds.

However, experience shows that needles from some large-bore catheter-over-needle cannulas may not work because the needle retracts if pressure is applied distally. Rather than entering the bone, the needle simply moves back into the hub. Test them in advance. Also, pediatric bone marrow needles may not be long or strong enough to penetrate adult bone, even at the supramaleolar site.

Sites

Common sites for IO placement are the proximal anteromedial tibia (1-3 cm below the tibial tuberosity on the anteromedial surface) or distal anterior femur in children, the proximal humerous (the greater tubercle of the anterior humeral head 1 cm proximal to the surgical neck of the humerus), the anterior-superior iliac spine or above the medial malleolus (adult or child), and the sternum (in adults with special equipment).

Without special equipment, the thickness of the bone precludes the use of the tibia or distal femur in children, and almost always in adults. Using the sternum has the potential for lethal injuries, so avoid this site unless using a sternum-specific needle or an IO drill. However, using most injection needles, the area just above the medial malleolus has proven to be easy to use in both pediatric and adult patients (Fig. 12-2). Enter the bone at a 90-degree angle (perpendicular) to the skin.[18]

Method

Use aseptic technique and a sterile needle. Placing a bone marrow needle without using aseptic technique increases the chance of osteomyelitis and cellulitis. Clean the skin. In awake patients, inject a small amount of local anesthetic in the skin and continue to infiltrate down to the periosteum. Hold the insertion site firmly to stabilize it. Do not put your hand behind the insertion site; it could get stabbed with the needle.

Insert the needle with a pressing and twisting (or "drilling") motion until you feel a "give" as the needle passes through the cortex.

Remove the obturator (if there is one) and attach a 5-mL syringe to aspirate a blood sample—both to confirm placement and to draw a sample for analysis. (A larger syringe may not be able to generate sufficient negative pressure.)

Another method to confirm needle placement is that the needle remains upright without support, although this may not be as obvious in infants because they have softer bones than older children or adults. Also, with correct placement, fluid flows freely through the needle without swelling of the subcutaneous tissue.[19]

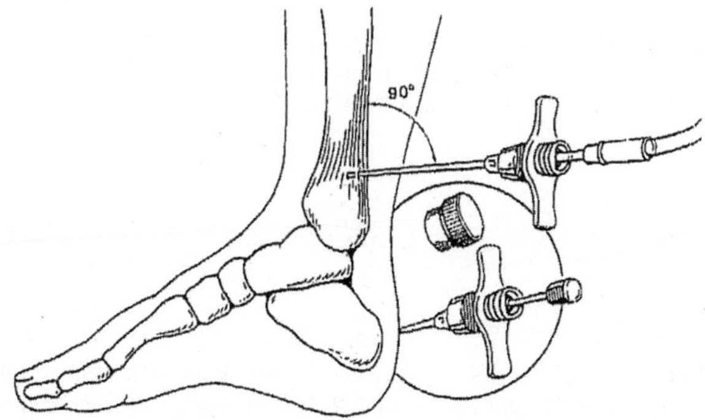

FIG. 12-2. Intraosseous needle insertion at ankle: pediatrics or adult. *(Reproduced with permission from Iserson.[18])*

Even if blood cannot be aspirated, which occurs about one-third of the time, attach IV tubing or a syringe and infuse solution, generally 0.9% saline or the equivalent, under pressure. If it flows easily, the needle is in the correct location. Pressure can be applied to the system by putting a three-way stopcock on the IO needle and using a syringe to push the fluid. This is especially useful if the IV solution is in a bottle that cannot be pressurized.

If no blood can be aspirated, the needle may be blocked with marrow. To unblock the needle, slowly inject 10 mL of NS. Check that the limb does not swell and that there is no increased resistance. If the tests are unsuccessful, remove the needle and try another site, use another needle at that site, or use a more proximal site.

Secure the needle if necessary with adhesive tape or, if the needle is longer than the short IO needle, clamp the needle where it enters the skin and tape it to the patient.

Complications

Complications are rare, the most common being local skin or bone infections, fluid extravasation, tibial fracture (especially in neonates), and compartment syndrome. The most common complication is putting an IO needle distal to a fracture or a prior IO infusion site: The infused fluid leaks out.[19]

Lidocaine Reduces Pain in Intraosseous Lines

Injecting lidocaine both before and after flushing an intraosseous (IO) needle is an effective method of reducing the pain of fluid infusion via this route.[24]

Barriers to Using Intraosseous Lines

Many physicians are reluctant to use IO lines due to misinformation, the perception that nurses are not familiar with or supportive of IO access, and a lack of confidence regarding the appropriate indications. They continue to use the relatively dangerous and lengthy technique of central venous access as a second-line technique. Yet now, the American College of Surgeons (in Advanced Trauma Life Support [ATLS]), the American Heart Association (in Advanced Cardiac Life Support [ACLS]), and the International Liaison Committee on Resuscitation recommend IO access as the first alternative to failed or delayed IV access.[25]

ALTERNATIVE PARENTERAL HYDRATION

Hypodermoclysis (Subcutaneous Hydration)

Hypodermoclysis is a well-tested, safe, inexpensive, and easy method for hydrating adult and pediatric patients; it was used from the late 19th century until IV hydration became common in the mid-20th century.[26,27] Hypodermoclysis is used acutely if starting an IV is difficult and for chronic hydration in patients who cannot take sufficient oral fluids due to nausea and vomiting, intestinal obstruction, neurological disease, or a diminished level of consciousness. In at least one case, it was used in a wilderness setting to resuscitate an adult in shock from gastrointestinal bleeding.[28]

The advantages of this method are that it has a relatively low cost, is easy to administer without skilled personnel, and is generally more comfortable for the patient than having an IV. In addition, it does not cause thrombophlebitis, generally does not cause local or system infection, and can be stopped and restarted at any time without fear of the needle clotting or the system failing (Table 12-1).[29]

Limitations

The primary limitation to hypodermoclysis is that it is generally slower (~1 mL/min) than IV hydration.

Medications via Hypodermoclysis

Any medications that can be given subcutaneously can also be given via this route. These include potassium chloride (up to 40 mmol or mEq/L), opiates (hydromorphone requires only a very small volume, although morphine also works), antiemetics (such as metoclopramide, lorazepam, diphenhydramine, dexamethasone, or promethazine), and sedative/anxiolytics (such as lorazepam

TABLE 12-1 Hypodermoclysis—Advantages and Disadvantages Compared to IVs

Advantages
Technically easier to insert and manage at any location
Less expensive
Better tolerated
Useful in agitated patients
Useful long-term management with low infection risk
Can administer most intramuscular (IM)/subcutaneous medications through this route
Disadvantages
Not useful for acute rehydration
Not useful for administration of resuscitation medications
Ineffective for administering blood and colloids
Unfamiliar technique for most modern healthcare workers

and midazolam). Other medications that have been reported to be successfully given via hypodermoclysis—but using an infusion pump—include atropine, haloperidol, hydroxyzine, methadone, methotrimeprazine, metoclopramide, octreotide, phenobarbital, and scopolamine.[30,31] In some countries, it is not unusual to give other medication classes through this route: antipsychotics (levomepromazine; UK), antibiotics (ceftriaxone, amikacin; France), and other analgesics (tramadol, demerol/pethidine, buprenorphine; Switzerland, Germany, UK, France).[32]

Method

Clean the skin with antiseptic and insert a 23- to 25-gauge butterfly needle or other small-gauge needle for injection into a subcutaneous site at a 45- to 60-degree angle, with the bevel up. These needles fit onto the end of standard IV tubing. If the needle is too deep (e.g., in the muscle), the infusion causes pain. If blood appears, a vessel has been entered; apply pressure and select another infusion site.[30]

Generally, infusion sites are the medial or lateral abdominal wall, along the iliac crest, in the anterior chest wall below or lateral to the breast, around the scapula, or in the anteromedial or anterolateral thigh. The abdominal wall and iliac crest areas are said to cause the least discomfort.[33] In extremely agitated patients, the inter- or sub-scapular area can be used to prevent them from pulling at the needle.[30] The pectoral region may be used in males, but not in women, who find this area is very painful. Typical sites for needle placement in infants and children are shown in Fig. 12-3.

Attach intravenous tubing to the needle and secure it with an occlusive clear plastic dressing, if available. Normal (0.9%) saline is most commonly used, although 0.45% saline and 5% dextrose in 0.45% saline ($D_5$1/2NS) have also been used, often at two infusion sites. The infusion rate is typically 1 mL/min/site (1.5 L/day/site), 1 to 2 L overnight, or 500 mL over 1 to 2 hours three times a day (tid). The recommended maximum infusion rate is 125 mL/hr and the minimum is 20 mL/hr to keep the needle open. The maximum daily amount should not exceed 3 L per patient and 2 L per site, to avoid local edema.[34] Hypotonic (e.g., D_5W) and hypertonic (e.g., D_5NS) solutions should not be given subcutaneously, because the body must convert the administered fluid pool into its normal fluid and electrolyte composition before it can be absorbed.[35,36] Hypotonic solutions, including 5% dextrose in water (D_5W), have caused hyponatremia. Blood and colloids are ineffective via this route.[37]

In infants and children, infuse no more than 200 mL/injection site. In premature infants during the neonatal period, fluid should not exceed 25 mL/kg body weight at no more than 2 mL/min.[38]

Ideally, you should change the needles and tubing every 1 to 4 days. Change the site after each liter of fluid and sooner if there are signs of local reaction.[33] Families and nonclinical caregivers can be instructed how to provide this therapy at home.

Although it does not seem to be very effective, some clinicians use hyaluronidase to reduce local edema and pain and to increase the fluid absorption rate. If used in adults, add 150 to 300 units to each liter of infusate or inject 75 to 150 units combined with 1 mL of anesthetic at

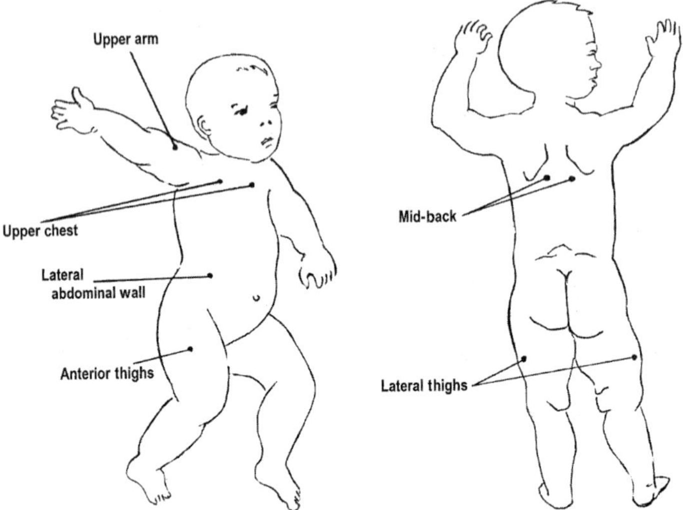

FIG. 12-3. Sites for hypodermoclysis needle placement in infants and children.

the infusion site.[33,39] For infants and children, add up to 30 units of hyaluronidase to each 200 mL of infusate.[38] Periodically massaging the infusion site increases absorption and minimizes discomfort.

Complications

Check the infusion site for evidence of edema or infection. Edema can often be relieved by massaging the area. Infection at the infusion site is rare, although at remote locations without professional medical supervision, a significant number of abscesses, presumably resulting from poor cleansing of the injection sites, have been noted.[29] Observe all patients for signs of fluid overload.

Rectal Rehydration/Proctoclysis

Rectal hydration (proctoclysis) can be used to instill fluids into children or adults who do not have profuse diarrhea. Use rectal hydration in patients who cannot tolerate hypodermoclysis because of generalized edema, pain on injection, or bleeding disorders.[40]

This method of fluid administration was popular into the 1930s, but its use declined with the development of IV technology.[33] Recently, rectal hydration has been used in the terminally ill, but it may also be of value in survival situations, for postoperative patients, and in those with mild dehydration where other routes of hydration are not available. It is safe, inexpensive, and so easy to use that it is generally administered by relatives to homebound patients.[33,40]

Method

Place the patient on his side with the buttocks raised on two pillows or folded blankets. Gently insert a well-lubricated 22-Fr NG tube or a large Foley catheter 10 to 40 cm into the rectum. Do not force the tube, because the primary danger is perforating the bowel. After taping the tube to the buttocks, attach a longer length of tubing (e.g., IV tubing) and an IV bag, enema bag, or a funnel. Elevate the bag, clamp the tube, and add warm fluid to the bag. Use this to infuse NS, standard oral rehydration fluid, or tap water, taking care to limit the amount, especially in children. Sodium and potassium may be added to the fluid.[41] Note that infusing cool fluid often causes the patient to immediately expel it.

Start the infusion at 100 mL/hr and increase it to a maximum of 400 mL/hr, or until fluid leak from the rectum appears. Another method is to start by infusing 200 mL of fluid over 15 to 20 minutes. (If >400-500 mL is administered faster than over 20 minutes, reflex abdominal cramping will expel it.) Then clamp the catheter and leave it in place. Instill another 200 mL every 4 hours, delivering up to 1200 mL/24 hr in an adult. After the infusion of a desired total daily volume of fluid, the catheter is removed; it can be reinserted daily for weeks or more at a time.[33,40,42]

In children, insert the smallest available catheter to minimize local irritation. Place it 8 to 12 cm beyond the anal sphincter. Begin instilling fluid at 1 drop/second.[43]

Complications include discomfort, leakage, tenesmus, and stool production (enema effect). If there is stool production after an infusion, decrease the infusion rate.

Emergency Use

One successful method for using proctoclysis for resuscitation employed a surgical glove with one fingertip cut off, which was secured to the end of a 14-Fr urethral catheter with waterproof tape. The glove supposedly acted as a "reservoir," although it also probably caused some added discomfort. Unlike other methods, these clinicians inflated the catheter bulb and then pulled down to seat it against the rectum. They administered 1 L of double-strength ORT and then 2 L of standard ORT over a 3-hour period. Oral rehydration followed.[28]

Fluid Maintenance

Rectal drips can be valuable in cases when maintenance or perioperative fluids are needed. Postoperatively, this can often be done for 2 or 3 days. One suggestion is to instill up to 2.5 L tap water into the (adult) anesthetized patient over 2 to 3 minutes at the end of the operation. Two hours later, begin a slow rectal drip of tap water or other appropriate solution at the rate of 2.5 L/24 hr.[44]

Using tap water conserves sterile fluids if they are scarce. Better than plain tap water is to add 0.5 teaspoon of sodium chloride/L and 0.25 teaspoon of potassium citrate/L for maintenance fluids. Replace gastric losses with an equal quantity of saline (1 level teaspoonful of salt/L tap water) that contains 20 mmol of potassium per liter.[45]

Intraperitoneal Infusion

Use

Intraperitoneal instillation of saline is a simple, safe, and effective technique to rehydrate adult and pediatric patients with ongoing fluid losses when the patient cannot tolerate oral or NG fluid administration or when clinicians cannot easily establish an IV.[20,46,47] It is most commonly used in children up to 3 years old (and older, if they are small for their age).

The procedure can be repeated and also may be used for continuous rehydration in postoperative patients.[48] Benefits of using this technique when resources are limited are that (a) it can be done in 5 to 10 minutes once a day using only one health care worker, and (b) it lessens the discomfort and the danger of over-hydration from IV infusions.

Intraperitoneal rehydration is useful for the mild to moderately dehydrated child. The procedure itself is fast (<10 minutes) and usually permits the child to return home for the next 24 hours. The patient normally returns the next day to assess whether the procedure must be repeated. However, the method does not allow fluid to be absorbed fast enough (it takes about 4 hours to be absorbed) to be the only method used for resuscitating those who are severely dehydrated. The other drawbacks are that it uses expensive IV fluids and it must be done aseptically, using sterile equipment.[49]

Method

The child can be restrained or mildly sedated, if necessary.[47] Lay the patient supine and palpate (or ultrasound) the abdomen to be certain that the liver, spleen, and bladder are not distended; if these organs are enlarged, they can be perforated during needle entry.

Use a 16-gauge needle to transfuse blood or an 18-gauge needle to administer fluids. Optimally, use a catheter-over-needle (typical IV catheter), although a hypodermic needle also works. Try to use a catheter that is at least 18 gauge; smaller ones have a tendency to kink, so may need to be held in place or readjusted several times during the infusion. Leaving the needle in the catheter (pulled back so that the needle tip is within the plastic) may not be an option, because the IV tubing may not connect to it.

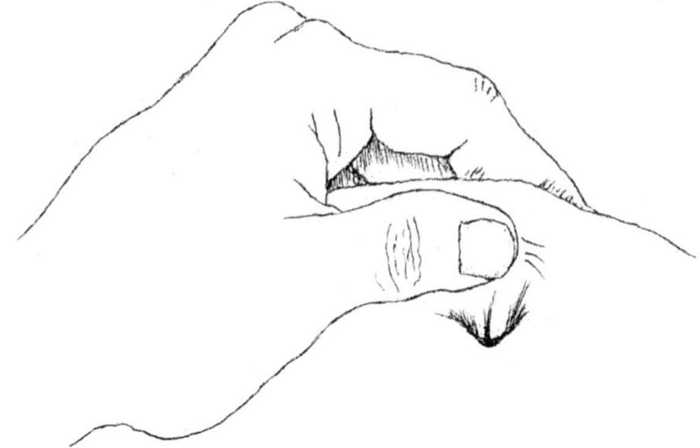

FIG. 12-4. Pinch abdominal wall and lift.

After thoroughly cleansing the overlying skin, pinch a fold of skin in the midline. After injecting local anesthetic, insert the needle either 2 cm below or 2 cm above the umbilicus in the midline. Alternatively, because the abdominal wall is generally lax in dehydrated (and especially emaciated) children, insert a thumb into the umbilicus pointing cephalad, pinching and lifting the abdominal wall between the thumb and index finger (Fig. 12-4). Apply traction and push the needle obliquely and cephalad through the abdominal wall (Fig. 12-5). Some clinicians hold the needle vertically; others insert it at an angle. In part, this depends on the thickness of the abdominal wall. Note that introducing the needle midway between the umbilicus and the symphysis pubis, which was once advocated, has resulted in severe hemorrhage from puncture of the iliac arteries.[50]

If an ultrasound machine is available, use it to guide needle entry. For additional safety, as soon as the needle enters the subcutaneous tissue, the fluid line is opened so that entering into the peritoneal cavity is marked by free flow of fluid—effectively pushing away any bowel. Run

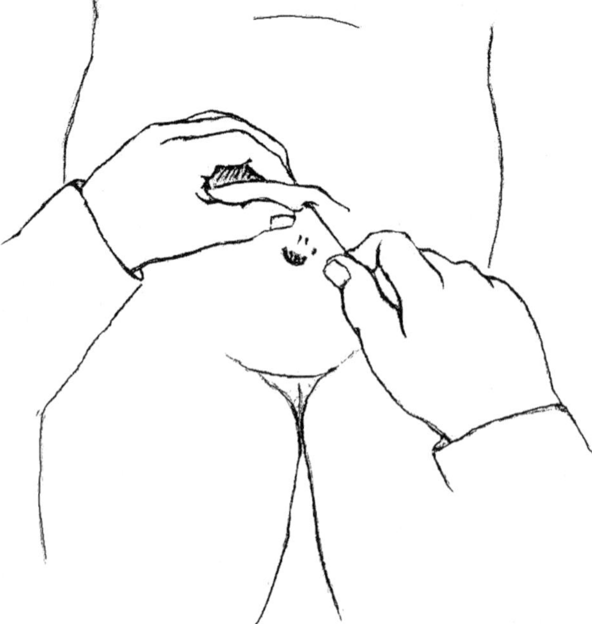

FIG. 12-5. Push needle through abdominal wall.

fluid "wide open," using gravity. Once the needle is in the abdominal cavity, the fluid will flow very fast; the fluid pushes any bowel loops out of the way of the needle. If the catheter kinks because of its small caliber (larger sizes may not be available), lift the umbilicus so that the catheter is clear of any bowel obstructing its flow. Use the initial "pinch" to both grab and lift the umbilicus. The technique is so safe that technicians and nurses have repeatedly performed this procedure independently.[47]

Fix the needle with adhesive tape. Cover it with gauze, if available.

Infuse crystalloids after the bottle or bag has been carefully warmed in an oven or hot water bath. Blood can be warmed using the rapid admixture method described in Chapter 18. Because many infants and children with emaciation and dehydration are also relatively hypothermic, the warm fluid also helps that condition.[20]

For blood, give 20 to 25 mL/kg as fast as possible, usually over 5 to 15 minutes. For fluids, give 40 to 70 mL/kg as fast as possible.[51] If the child is still in the medical facility and remains dehydrated, administer another intraperitoneal bolus 4 hours later.[49]

Infants weighing 12 lb (5.45 kg) usually tolerate about 235 mL (0.5 pint; 43 mL/kg) of fluid. Children weighing 20 lb (9.1 kg) usually tolerate about 473 mL (1 pint; 52 mL/kg). Any discomfort they experience stems from abdominal distention. Adding hyaluronidase does not seem to be of any benefit. The rate of fluid absorption varies, although fluid overload does not seem to occur.[20]

After infusing the fluid, remove the needle. Keep a child in a half-sitting position, preferably on mother's lap, for about 2 hours after infusion. Note that even if the needle pierces the intestine (which is rare), it will not cause any harm but may cause some rectal blood to appear.[51]

Fluids

In children <15 years old, infuse hypotonic crystalloids; in adults, administer isotonic solutions (e.g., 0.9% saline).[20] Other solutions that have been used include half-strength Darrow's solution with glucose (sodium, 61 mmol; potassium, 17 mmol; chloride, 52 mmol; lactate, 27 mmol; glucose, 50 g; and calories, 200/L), lactated Ringer's solution (Na^+, 130 mEq/L; K^+, 4 mEq/L; Ca^{++}, 3 mEq/L; Cl^-, 109 mEq/L; lactate, 28 mEq/L), normal (0.9%) saline (Na^+,154 mEq/L; Cl^-, 154 mEq/L), and 0.45% saline (28 mEq KCl/L).[35,52] Table 12-2 shows the composition of standard IV fluids.

Note that hypotonic solutions should not be used to treat shock.[52] Blood transfusion through this route is beneficial for the treatment of chronic anemia, rather than for resuscitation due to acute blood loss (i.e., shock).[54,55]

Contraindications

Do not perform this technique on children with ascites, distended and tympanitic abdomens, cellulitis over the abdomen, or who may have adhesions from infection (e.g., tuberculosis) or prior surgery.[50,53] If there is concern about adhesions from prior abdominal surgery or injury,

TABLE 12-2 Composition of Standard Intravenous Fluids

	Electrolyte Concentration (mEq/L)						
	Na^+	K^+	Ca^{++}	$HCO3^-$	Cl^-	Glucose (g/L)	Osmolarity
Normal (0.9%) saline	154				154		308
Dextrose 5%; 0.45% normal saline	77				77	50	406
Dextrose 5%						50	252
Ringer's lactate (Hartmann's solution)	131	5	4	28	112		275
Half-strength Darrow's solution	60	18		26	52		273

Data from Ree and Clezy.[53]

insert the needle under ultrasound guidance or using a semi-open technique as is done for peritoneal lavage. Also consider other hydration methods, including IO infusion.

REFERENCES

1. Carcello JA, Davis AL, Zaritsky A. Role of early fluid resuscitation in pediatric septic shock. *JAMA*. 1991;266:1242-1245.
2. Blickell WH, Wall MJ Jr, Pepe PE, et al. Immediate versus delayed fluid resuscitation for hypotensive patients with penetrating torso injuries. *N Engl J Med*. 1994;331:1105-1109.
3. Hirschhorn N, McCarthy BJ, Ranney B, et al. Ad libitum oral glucose electrolyte therapy for acute diarrhea in Apache children. *J Pediatr*. 1973;83(4):562-571.
4. AAP Provisional Committee on Quality Improvement, Subcommittee on Acute Gastroenteritis. Practice parameter: the management of acute gastroenteritis in children. *Pediatrics*. 1996;97:424-430.
5. Holliday MA, Friedman AL, Wassner SJ. Extracellular fluid restoration in dehydration: a critique of rapid versus slow. *Pediatr Nephrol*. 1999;13:292-297.
6. Sturgeon J, Lifford R, Cantle F. Intravenous access in children in the emergency department. *Ped Emerg Care*. 2014;30(3):226.
7. Skilton R. Decontamination procedures for medical equipment. *Pract Proced*. 1997;7(5):1. http://tabula.ws/archive/a_day_after/medical/nuclear_biologic_chemical/deconmedequip.pdf. Accessed September 3, 2015.
8. Gill G. Coping with crisis: an investigation into disease and death on the Thai/Burma Railway. *COFEPOW*. 1942:45. www.cofepow.org.uk/pages/medical.html. Accessed September 14, 2006.
9. Boulton TB. Anaesthesia in difficult situations. 3. General anaesthesia-technique. *Anaesthesia*. 1966; 21(4):513-545.
10. King M, King F, Martodipoero S. *Primary Child Care: A Manual for Health Workers*. Oxford, UK: Oxford University Press; 1978:124-125.
11. Heinrichs J, Fritze Z, Klassen T, Curtis S. A systematic review and meta-analysis of new interventions for peripheral intravenous cannulation of children. *Ped Emerg Care*. 2013;29(7):858-866.
12. Mahler SA, Massey G, Meskill L, Wang H, Arnold TC. Can we make the basilic vein larger? maneuvers to facilitate ultrasound guided peripheral intravenous access: a prospective cross-sectional study. *Int J Emerg Med*. 2011;4:53.
13. Kule A, Hang B, Bahl A. Preventing the collapse of a peripheral vein during cannulation: an evaluation of various tourniquet techniques on vein compressibility. *J Emerg Med*. 2014;46(5):659-666.
14. Quinn LM, Sheikh A. Establishing intravenous access in an emergency situation. *Emerg Med J*. 2014;31: 593
15. Reades R, Studnek JR, Vandeventer S, Garrett J. Intraosseous versus intravenous vascular access during out-of-hospital cardiac arrest: a randomized controlled trial. *Ann Emerg Med*. 2011;58:509-516.
16. Morgan TR. Evaluation of fluid bolus administration rates using ruggedized field intravenous systems. *Wild Environ Med*. 2014;25:204-209.
17. Spivey WH. Intraosseous infusions in adults. *J Pediatr*. 1987;111(5):639-643.
18. Iserson KV. Intraosseous infusions in adults. *J Emerg Med*. 1989;7(6):587-592.
19. Vreede E, Bulatovic A, Rosseel E, et al. Intraosseous infusion. *Pract Proced*. 2000;12(10):1. www.nda.ox.ac.uk/wfsa/html/u12/u1210_01.htm#equi. Accessed September 13, 2006.
20. VanRooyen MJ, VanRooyen JB, Sloan EP. The use of intraperitoneal infusion for the outpatient treatment of hypovolemia in Somalia. *Prehosp Disaster Med*. 1995;10(1):57-59.
21. Iserson KV, Criss E. Intraosseous infusions: a usable technique. *Am J Emerg Med*. 1986;4(6):540-542.
22. Kruger C. Intraosseous access in paediatric patients in a developing country setting. *Trop Doct*. 2001; 31:118.
23. Awojobi OA. Epidural needle and intraosseous access. *Trop Doct*. 2003;33:59.
24. Philbeck TE, Miller L, Montez D. Pain management during intraosseous infusion through the proximal humerus. *Ann Emerg Med*. 2009;54:S128.
25. Cheung, WJ, Rosenberg H, Vaillancourt C. Barriers and facilitators to intraosseous access in adult resuscitations when peripheral intravenous access is not achievable. *Acad Emerg Med*. 2014;21(3):250-256.
26. Anon. Treatment of scarlatinal nephritis. *JAMA*. 1900;34:1408-1409. Reprinted in: JAMA 100 years ago. *JAMA*. 2000;283(21):2765.
27. Kleinman RE, Barness LA, Finberg L. History of pediatric nutrition and fluid therapy. *Pediatr Research*. 2003;54(5):762-772.

28. Grocott MPW, McCorkell S, Cox ML. Resuscitation from hemorrhagic shock using rectally administered fluids in a wilderness environment. *Wild Environ Med.* 2005;16:209-211.
29. Green SDR. Treatment of moderate and severe dehydration by nasogastric drip. *Trop Doct.* 1987;17(2):86-88.
30. Sasson M, Shvartzman P. Hypodermoclysis: an alternative infusion technique. *Am Fam Phys.* 2001;64:1575-1578.
31. Woodall HE. Alternatives to rehydration during hypodermoclysis (letter). *Am Fam Phys.* 2002;66(1):28.
32. Vukasovic C, Fonzo-Christe C, Wasilewski-Rasca AF, et al. Subcutaneous administration of drugs in the elderly: survey of practice and systemic literature review. *Palliative Med.* 2005;19(3):208-219.
33. Nanson J. Methods of fluid administration for resuscitation and hydration under difficult circumstances: part 2, alternative routes. *Trop Doct.* 2000;30(3):172-175.
34. Lopez JH, Reyes-Ortiz CA. Subcutaneous hydration by hypodermoclysis. *Rev in Clin Gerontology.* 2010;20(2):105-113.
35. Sweeney MJ. Tonicity and its clinical application to parenteral fluid therapy. *J Pediatr.* 1955;47:237-248.
36. Abbott WE, Levey S, Foreman RC, et al. The danger of administering parenteral fluids by hypodermoclysis. *Surgery.* 1952;32(2):305-315.
37. Steffey JM. The complications of hypodermoclysis in infants and children. *J Iowa Med Soc.* 1963;53(7):393-396.
38. Daily Med. *Vitase (hyaluronidase) injection.* http://dailymed.nlm.nih.gov/dailymed/drugInfo.cfm?id=1403. Accessed December 7, 2006.
39. Bruera E, Neumann CM, Pituskin E, et al. A randomized controlled trial of local injections of hyaluronidase versus placebo in cancer patients receiving subcutaneous hydration. *Ann Oncol.* 1999;10(10):1255-1258.
40. Bruera E, Schoeller T, Pruvost M. Proctoclysis for hydration of terminal cancer patients. *Lancet.* 1994;344:1699.
41. Blouse A, Gomez P, eds. *Emergency Obstetric Care: A Quick Reference Guide for Frontline Providers.* Baltimore, MD: JHPIEGO; 2003:10.
42. The Remote, Austere, Wilderness, and Third World Medicine Discussion Board Moderators. *Survival and Austere Medicine: An Introduction.* 2nd ed. 2005:172. www.aussurvivalist.com/downloads/AM%20Final%202.pdf. Accessed June 8, 2007.
43. Campbell WF, Kerr LG. *The Surgical Diseases of Children.* New York, NY: D. Appleton; 1912:96-97.
44. Tovey F. Fluid and electrolyte balance for adults (without a biochemical laboratory). *Trop Doct.* 1999;29:49-53.
45. King MH, ed. *Primary Anesthesia.* Oxford, UK: Oxford University Press; 1986:121.
46. Ransome-Kuti O, Elebute O, Agusto-Odutola T, et al. Intraperitoneal fluid infusion in children with gastroenteritis. *Br Med J.* 1969;3:500-503.
47. Carter FS. Intraperitoneal transfusions. *East Afr Med J.* 1953;12(30):499-505.
48. Kraft AR, Tompkins RK, Jesseph JE. Peritoneal electrolyte absorption: analysis of portal, systemic venous, and lymphatic transport. *Surgery.* 1968;64:148-153.
49. King M, King F, Martodipoero S. *Primary Child Care: A Manual for Health Workers.* Oxford, UK: Oxford University Press; 1978:123.
50. Ravenel SF. The hazards of intraperitoneal injections. *JAMA.* 1933;100(7):473-475.
51. van Bemmel JAG, de Vries HR. Intraperitoneal blood transfusions. *Trop Doct.* 1988;18(2):89-91.
52. Molyneux EM, Maitland K. Intravenous fluids: getting the balance right. *N Engl J Med.* 2005;353(9):941-944.
53. Ree GH, Clezy JK. Simple guide to fluid balance. *Trop Doct.* 1982;12(4 Pt 1):155-159.
54. Florey H, Witts LJ. Absorption of blood from the peritoneal cavity. *Lancet.* 1928;211(5470):1323-1325.
55. Cole WCC, Montgomery JC. Intraperitoneal blood transfusion: report of 237 transfusions on 117 patients in private practice. *Am J Dis Child.* 1929;37(3):497-510.

13 | Medications/Pharmacy/Envenomations

SIX PROBLEMS INVOLVING MEDICATION

Six primary problems regarding medications arise in austere medical situations. In some cases, more than one of these exist simultaneously. You can have (a) no medications; (b) medication, but have no clue what it is for or how to use it; (c) some medication, but not the primary choice for the condition you need to treat; (d) medication, but in the wrong form; (e) only outdated medication; or (f) medication that might have been contaminated or that has degraded. Each of these is discussed separately.

Have No Medication

If you have no medication, you will have to use local herbal remedies, physical treatments (osteopathic manipulation, thermal treatment, surgery), street drugs, or donated medications.

Managing Drug Shortages

When clinicians face medication and intravenous (IV) fluid shortages, pharmacy supervisors should not only communicate understandable information about the shortages to clinicians, but also build safeguards into their system. Use standard triage terms such as red, yellow, and green to categorize the severity of the shortage and its probable effect on clinical practice. Pharmacists should also help clinicians safely use unfamiliar substitute medications, including compounding medications and drips in the pharmacy.[1]

Donated Medications

After disasters and in developing countries, the management of drug donations becomes extremely important. The key issue is to specify what you want and need, how much, and when it should arrive. Managing large quantities of unwanted and unneeded pharmaceuticals consumes valuable personnel time and space. After Hurricane Katrina, for example, the area was awash not only in water but also (figuratively) in cartons of ridiculously inappropriate donated medications. Safely disposing of this mountain of useless pharmaceuticals became an unwanted headache.

Similar problems occur across the globe. A Harvard School of Public Health study found that about 30% of donated medications had an expiration date <1 year from the time they were shipped; 6% had <100 days left before they (officially) expired. Up to 42% of the drugs were not on either the country's list or the World Health Organization's (WHO) list of essential drugs, nor were they therapeutic alternatives for the essential drugs.[2]

To help lessen problems with international drug donations, WHO has developed the following *Guidelines for Drug Donations*[3]:

1. All drug donations should be based on an expressed need and be relevant to the disease pattern in the recipient country. Drugs should not be sent without prior consent of the recipient.
2. All donated drugs or their generic equivalents should be approved for use in the recipient country and appear on the national list of essential drugs, or, if a national list is not available, on the *WHO Model List of Essential Drugs* (www.who.int/medicines/publications/essentialmedicines/en/), unless specifically requested otherwise by the recipient.
3. The presentation, strength, and formulation of donated drugs, as much as possible, should be similar to those of drugs commonly used in the recipient country.
4. All donated drugs should be obtained from a reliable source and comply with quality standards in both donor and recipient country. The WHO *Certification Scheme on the Quality of Pharmaceutical Products Moving in International Commerce* (www.who.int/medicines/areas/quality_safety/regulation_legislation/certification/en/index.html) should be used.

5. No drugs should be donated that have been issued to patients and then returned to a pharmacy or elsewhere or that were given to health professionals as free samples.
6. After arrival in the recipient country, all donated drugs should have a remaining shelf life of at least 1 year. An exception may be made for direct donations to specific health facilities, provided that: The responsible professional at the receiving end acknowledges that (s)he is aware of the shelf life and that the quantity and remaining shelf life allow for proper administration prior to expiration. In all cases, it is important that the date of arrival and the expiration dates of the drugs be communicated to the recipient well in advance.
7. All drugs should be labeled in a language that is easily understood by health professionals in the recipient country; the label on each individual container should at least contain the International Nonproprietary Name (INN) or generic name, batch number, dosage form, strength, name of manufacturer, quantity in the container, storage conditions, and expiration date.
8. As much as possible, donated drugs should be presented in larger quantity units and hospital packs.
9. All drug donations should be packed in accordance with international shipping regulations and be accompanied by a detailed packing list, which specifies the contents of each numbered carton by INN, dosage form, quantity, batch number, expiration date, volume, weight, and any special storage conditions. The weight per carton should not exceed 50 kg. Avoid mixing drugs with other supplies in the same carton.
10. Recipients should be informed of all drug donations that are being considered, being prepared, or are actually underway.
11. The declared value of a drug donation should be based on the wholesale price of its generic equivalent in the recipient country or, if such information is not available, on the wholesale world-market price for its generic equivalent.
12. Costs of international and local transport, warehousing, port clearance, and appropriate storage and handling should be paid by the donor agency, unless specifically agreed otherwise with the recipient in advance.

What Is This Medication?

Medications are worthless if clinicians do not know what they are or how to use them. Describing this situation at a World War II prisoner of war (POW) camp where Allied prisoners were in desperate condition, Dr. Ian Duncan wrote: "It was ironic that immediately after cessation of hostilities, a large carton of penicillin was dropped almost on top of the hospital in Camp 17, Omuta, Japan. Unfortunately, we had never heard of it and, as no instructions were enclosed, it was never used though we had many men suffering from pneumonia, osteomyelitis, infected wounds and boils."[4]

Even when clinicians are familiar with a medication, if they can't decipher the label due to an unfamiliar language or an unknown brand name, they will not be able to use it. Many common medications have different names in different countries. For example, US physicians would not recognize pethidine unless you told them that it was meperidine or know how to use paracetamol/panadol unless they knew that it was acetaminophen. Common drugs with alternative names exist throughout the world. If you face this problem, local practitioners, pharmacists, or Internet sources may provide a solution.

Some medications may no longer be used for their original indication in the most-developed countries, but are still in common use around the world. Four, as examples, are aspirin, scopolamine, chloramphenicol, and chlorpromazine.

Now relegated to the role of antiplatelet drug in developed countries, aspirin can still be used as a potent analgesic and anti-inflammatory agent when other nonsteroidal anti-inflammatory drugs (NSAIDs) are unavailable. The standard dose is 325 to 650 mg (po or rectally) q4-6hr prn; or 650 to 1300 mg (enteric coated) po q8hr (adult); 40 to 60 mg/kg/day divided q6hr po or rectally (pediatric). For juvenile rheumatoid arthritis, the dose can be up to 60 to 110 mg/kg/day divided q6-8h.

Scopolamine (Buscopan), common in "seasickness patches," is a potent anticholinergic often used for stomach cramps, renal calculi, and bladder spasms. As hyoscine butylbromide, the dose is 10 to 20 mg intramuscularly (IM). Chlorpromazine (Thorazine, Largactil), a potent antipsychotic, antiemetic, and antihiccup medication, may be the only antipsychotic available. The adult dose is 50 to 100 mg parenterally. While it is generally administered intramuscularly (IM), it can also be given slowly intravenously (IV). Chloramphenicol (parenteral only) is an excellent antibiotic. It is recommended by WHO for severe infections and commonly used in the world's least-developed regions.

Other medications are not used in some countries (such as the United States) or may be older versions of those currently used. These include flucloxacillin (antibiotic), quinine, a wide variety of artemisinin-based medications to treat malaria, and equine snake antivenin.

Medication Is Not the Primary Choice for Condition

Alternative Drugs

MULTI-USE MEDICATIONS

If you don't have what you need, use what you have. A number of standard medications can be used for a variety of purposes. Use your normal pharmacology references, poison/drug information center, and pharmacist to determine all the possible uses for available medications.

Some commonly available medications with a wide variety of uses (not all listed) include the following:

- Diphenhydramine: Sedative, antiemetic, antihistamine, local anesthetic
- Chlorpromazine: Antipsychotic, hiccup therapy, local anesthetic, migraine treatment
    - Epinephrine/adrenaline: Asthma treatment, cardiac stimulant, vasoconstrictor, allergy/anaphylaxis treatment
    - Dexamethasone: Reduces tumor edema, bronchiolitis/croup treatment, allergy/anaphylaxis treatment, antiemetic, inflammatory/vasculitis treatment, chronic obstructive pulmonary disease (COPD) treatment
    - Lidocaine: Antiarrhythmic, local/regional anesthetic
    - Dextrose solution: Medication admixture, hypoglycemia treatment, osmotic diuretic, sedative ($D_{25}W$) on a child's pacifier (i.e., binky)
    - Oxygen: Hypoxia treatment, carbon monoxide poisoning treatment, cluster headache treatment, antiemetic[5]

USING STREET DRUGS AS MEDICATIONS

With the caveat that the purity and even the identity of medications purchased from nontraditional sources may be in doubt, they may be beneficial when nothing else is available. Some uses for commonly available street drugs (most of which may be available as commercial medications or commodities) include:

- Marijuana: Antiemetic, sedative
- Heroin, fentanyl (and other narcotics): Analgesic, local anesthetic, cough suppressant
- Ketamine: Analgesic, anesthetic, antidepressant
- Cocaine: Local anesthetic, vasoconstrictor
- Benzodiazepines (various): Antiepileptic, sedatives, antianxiety, muscle relaxant
- Barbiturates (various): Sedative/hypnotic, antiepileptic
- Ethanol: Sedative, disinfectant, antidote for methanol poisoning, anesthetic
- Lysergic acid diethylamide (LSD) or psilocybin: Cluster headaches[6]

Zinc for Colds

Healthy people who begin taking oral zinc within 24 hours of onset of common cold symptoms have a shorter duration of illness. However, zinc lozenges commonly produce adverse side effects, while not diminishing symptom severity. Used prophylactically, oral zinc is associated with a reduced cold incidence in children, but it has not been studied in adults.[7]

Medication Substitutions

While many medications have therapeutic substitutes, medications in the following drug classes may be more amenable to substitution than others[8]:

Calcium channel blockers	Angiotensin-converting enzyme (ACE) inhibitors	Tricyclic antidepressants
Nonsteroidal anti-inflammatory drugs (NSAIDS)	Diuretics	H_2 antagonists
Sympathomimetic bronchodilators	Benzodiazepines	Topical agents
Cough and cold medications	Phenothiazines	Antibiotics (most)

When substituting another medication, put a note on the medication label or give it to the patient, saying: "As a result of the recent emergency, your medication is very similar, but not the identical medication to the one you normally take. When possible, please go to your usual pharmacy to continue with your previously prescribed medication."

Veterinary Drugs for Human Use

Veterinary medications that are the same generics as those prescribed for people and that are labeled "USP" (pharmaceutical grade) are equivalent to those that human pharmacies distribute, although the dose may vary. In general, veterinary medications (excluding dietary supplements) are subject to the same good manufacturing practice regulations imposed by the Food and Drug Administration (FDA) as human medications. Examples that are commonly found include penicillin, amoxicillin, ciprofloxacin, doxycycline, and cephalexin.

A large percentage of the US rural population has used veterinary medication for their own medical needs, usually due to a self-sufficient attitude, availability, lower cost, and a belief that veterinary medications are stronger than comparable human medications. Most often, these are people involved with rodeo, horse racing, and health care; rural area residents; and those lacking health insurance. They most commonly use analgesics, anti-inflammatory medications, anti-arthritis medication, systemic and topical antibiotics, and topical corticosteroids.

Some deaths and serious reactions have been reported from humans using veterinary drugs. The most common complications have been from taking phenylbutazone (Butazolidin, "Bute"), a veterinary analgesic used for racing animals, which at one time was available to treat humans in the United States. Severe adverse effects have included aplastic anemia, gastrointestinal hemorrhage or ulcers, renal insufficiency, seizures, hepatitis, and respiratory failure.[9] Those veterinary medications that have caused minor side effects when taken by humans include (o = oral, t = topical, p = parenteral): albendazole (o,t), amoxicillin (o,t), butorphanol (o,p), clindamycin (o,t,p), cyclosporine (o,t), dexamethasone (o), diclofenac (t), ketamine (t), mebendazole (o), and progesterone (t). Other common antibiotics and anti-inflammatory agents have not been reported as causing problems in humans. However, fenbendazole (o), isoflurane (inhalation), pentobarbital (p), roxarsone, tiletamine (unknown), monensin (o), and tilmicosin (o, unknown) have all caused deaths, although some were suicides.[10]

Have Medication, But in Wrong Form

Often, medications will be available, but in the wrong form or dose for the patient and circumstances. Encourage the pharmacy staff to improvise (and search their literature) for ways to solve these problems. Powders may be used to produce injectables under emergency circumstances. Parenteral drugs can usually be administered rectally at the IV/IM dose. Consider using oral, rectal, and transmucosal medications when patients need analgesics, antimicrobials, and sedative-hypnotics. If IV etomidate, propofol, or succinylcholine is unavailable, consider using IV ketamine, methohexital, rocuronium, or vecuronium.[11] Alternatives for local anesthetics are discussed in Chapter 15.

Nitroglycerine Drip

When a university pharmacy announced that they would be unable to procure IV nitroglycerine (NTG) for several months, some older physicians asked why they couldn't simply compound it, as they had done when it was first being used. They came up with the following method (Megan Brandon, PharmD, University Medical Center, Tucson, Ariz. Personal communication, March 22, 2008.):

Prepare an NTG drip from tablets as follows:

1. Dissolve 125 tablets of 0.4 mg NTG sublingual (SL) in 50 to 60 mL of 5% dextrose. The pharmacy typically does this in a 60-mL syringe. The solution will be cloudy due to excipients (undissolved materials in the tablets).
2. Using a 0.22-micron filter needle, add the solution to a glass container of D_5W and dilute to a final total volume of 250 mL.
3. This solution will be at its final concentration of 50 mg/250 mL.

If administering a continuous IV NTG drip, protect it from light by winding black tape around the IV tubing. (Sri Devi Jagjit, MD, Emergency Medicine, Georgetown, Guyana. Personal Communication, September 2014.)

NITROGLYCERINE—ALTERNATIVE ORAL TITRATIONS

Continuous SL administration: When a patient presented to the emergency department (Casualty; ED; A&E) in resource-poor rural Ghana with severe congestive heart failure and chest pain, it appeared as if he would soon die. Almost no options were available to us and we lacked sufficient NTG tablets—and a filter and a glass D_5W container—to make a drip. Instead, we had his wife administer a tablet of 0.4 mg NTG SL about every 5 minutes for the next 6 hours. By morning, he was over the acute episode and was moved to the ward.

Nitroglycerine slurry: The following is the method used at Georgetown, Guyana's Public Hospital (GPHC) to provide continuous NTG administration when IV NTG is unavailable.

- Crush five tablets of 0.4 mg NTG.
- Mix the powder in 5 cc normal saline.
- Place the slurry in a 5-mL syringe and administer 1 mL sublingually every 3 minutes.
- Monitor the blood pressure to maintain the Systolic BP ≥110 mm Hg.

Penicillin Solution to Instill in Newborn's Eyes

A penicillin solution is used particularly to treat gonococcal conjunctivitis in newborns. To make a penicillin solution of 10,000 units/mL, use one of these two methods:

(a) Boil a clean cup and let it cool. Then add 100 mL sterile water and one level teaspoon of salt or add 100 mL sterile saline. Dissolve 600 mg benzylpenicillin in the saline.
(b) Dissolve 600 mg benzylpenicillin in 10 mL water for injection. Then mix 1 mL of this solution with another 10 mL of water for injection.[12]

Converting Tablets/Capsules Into Palatable Form

Some patients (especially children, the elderly, and the less-than-conscious patient) cannot swallow tablets. Some medications don't come as a liquid; in austere situations, you may not have the liquid form even if a medication is manufactured as a liquid.

There are several ways to convert tablets to a more palatable form. For non-extended-release drugs, break or crush tablets into sections—or open up the capsule and pour out the contents. Crush tablets using a hammer, after first putting the tablet in a plastic bag or wrapping it in a paper towel so the pieces do not escape. You can also use a mortar and pestle, a similar implement used to grind grains, or a coffee grinder.

If necessary, administer the medications through a nasogastric tube. Patients can dissolve the powder in liquid to drink, or sprinkle the powder onto food and eat it. Another alternative is simply to mix larger pieces into mashed potatoes, applesauce, or foods of similar consistency.

Tablet Splitting

Splitting drug tablets not only is common among the general population, but also may be necessary when there is a limited supply of medications. It may also be needed to increase dosing flexibility, facilitate swallowing medication for patients, and reduce health care costs. The danger in doing this is that the doses in the two parts may not be equivalent, because the active drug may not be evenly distributed through many tablets, and tablets may break unevenly. How well a tablet splits depends on whether it has score marks and its size, shape, and fragility, as well as the splitter's visual acuity, strength, dexterity, and cognitive ability.[13] The accuracy of cutting a tablet in half varies. Many people cannot break scored tablets manually, so they use tablet splitters, razor blades, or kitchen knives. However, tablets could not consistently be accurately and precisely split into equal parts, even in studies with a tablet optimally designed for splitting (large, elongated tablets with deep score marks on both sides), an experienced splitter, and optimal equipment.[14]

Once-A-Day HIV Therapy During Religious Fasts

When patients with human immunodeficiency virus (HIV) infection want to celebrate a cultural or religious fast over several days or weeks (e.g., Lent, Ramadan), clinicians can suggest that treatment-experienced stable patients take once-daily rather than twice-daily dosed ritonavir-boosted lopinavir, along with a once-daily fixed-dose tenofovir–emtricitabine. With this regimen, no changes have been found in adherence, diarrhea, CD4 cell counts, viral load, hematocrit, kidney, liver, and lipid tests. However, clinicians must carefully select patients for whom this regimen is appropriate.[15]

Medication Is Outdated

Don't believe the expiration date you see on the pharmaceutical packaging. It has little relationship to the quality, potency, or safety of most medications. "Medical authorities uniformly say it is safe to take drugs past their expiration date—no matter how 'expired' the drugs purportedly are. Except for possibly the rarest of exceptions, you won't get hurt and you certainly won't get killed."[16]

Two types of expiration dates may be on medications. The first is a manufacturer's or pharmacist's date, which generally has no major significance. The second type is placed on a partially used, often liquid, medication; pay close attention to this date.

"Manufacturers put expiration dates on for marketing, rather than scientific, reasons. It's not profitable for them to have products on a shelf for 10 years. They want turnover," said one FDA pharmacist.[16] "Two to three years is a very comfortable point of commercial convenience," stated Mark van Arandonk, senior director for pharmaceutical development at Pharmacia & Upjohn Inc. "It gives us enough time to put the inventory in warehouses, ship it and ensure it will stay on shelves long enough to get used."[17] In addition, many US states require that pharmacists assign a "beyond-use" date to medications dispensed in a container; this is routinely set at 1 year shorter than the manufacturer's date.[18]

A long-term FDA program studying the shelf life of medications for the US military and the Strategic National Stockpile (of medications) has shown that nearly all medications last far beyond their official expiration dates. Some, despite being kept in markedly suboptimal conditions, retained their original quality for decades. Many of the so-called degraded medications undergo only a change in their appearance, rather than in their potency. Even when a medication loses potency over time, it often can still be used. In austere situations, use the medication despite the stamped expiration date. Generally, if you need more medication due to lack of adequate effect, it will become evident. However, there are some exceptions.

The practice, for example, has been to avoid using expired tetracycline. Nitroglycerine tablets lose potency over time, as does insulin, some liquid antibiotics, water-purification tablets, and mefloquine hydrochloride (for malaria).[17] Ointments and creams may lose potency quickly and topical ophthalmic medications are dangerous to use after their expiration dates, because any bacteria growing in them may have devastating consequences.

In an obvious effort to avoid having pharmaceutical manufacturers "dump" nearly outdated and unsellable medications by donating them, WHO's guidelines (as previously discussed) disallow the donation of drugs within a year of expiration; many companies, of course, routinely ignore that rule. However, these medications are, for the most part, still effective. It's sort of a Catch-22 situation.

In sum, as Army Col. George Crawford, a pharmacist who oversaw the government's program to test drug stability, said, "Nobody tells you in pharmacy school that shelf-life is about marketing, turnover, and profits."[17]

Pay close attention, however, to "beyond-use" dates that clinicians write on partially used medications. Some medications for injection and irrigation come in multiple-dose vials or large irrigation bottles containing enough medication to be administered several times. Both drug stability and sterility affect how long these medications can be used after being opened. The stability of many medications decreases once the package has been opened—or once medications have been reconstituted from a powdered form. Such medications must be used within a specific time; that time should be marked on the vial or bottle. After that, they must be discarded.

As for sterility, when a sterile medication is opened and exposed to air, the potential exists for bacteria to grow in the vial or bottle. Some medications have a preservative in them; others do not. For example, large irrigation bottles typically do not have a preservative. If the contents are used for sterile irrigation, the bottle should be discarded within 24 hours of being opened.[19]

Medication Is Possibly Contaminated or Spoiled

Contamination

Medications may become contaminated if they have been exposed to floodwater, seawater, or unsafe municipal water. If they are not lifesaving medications, or if replacements are readily available, they should be discarded. If, however, they are lifesaving medications that cannot easily be replaced and, although the container is contaminated, the medication seems to be unaffected (such as tablets being dry, intact, and the normal color), then use them until they can be replaced. If the medication itself appears contaminated, discard it.[20]

Temperature Control

When possible, keep pharmaceutical products at the temperature specified by the manufacturer. For general purposes, the *US Pharmacopeia* definitions suffice[8]:

Controlled room temperature: 59°F to 86°F (15°C to 30°C)
Refrigeration: 39°F to 46°F (3.9°C to 8°C)
Freezing: –4°F to 14°F (–20°C to –10°C)

Medications That Do Not Need Cooling

Some medications, such as insulin, may not need refrigeration to maintain clinical efficacy. Regular insulin has been tested after being stored at 25°C (77°F) for 12 months; it lost only about 2% bioactivity.[21] Intermediate-acting insulin was tested after being stored at 25°C (77°F) and at 34°C (93°F) for 60 days; it lost no biological activity.[22] Lente insulin (insulin zinc suspension) has been found to take 5 weeks to lose 2% of its bioactivity and 14 weeks to lose 5%. Even at 40°C (104°F), soluble porcine insulin takes 14 weeks and lente takes 4 weeks to lose 5% of bioactivity; most patients use a vial of insulin within this time.[21]

Medications That Require Refrigeration

Some medications, such as succinylcholine (suxamethonium chloride), require refrigeration, and deteriorate if left unrefrigerated. Disasters can occur if the deterioration goes unrecognized, as it did in the following remote setting. "During a surgery on what turned out to be a huge hernia, the anesthetist tried to use the 'Sux' that was on the shelf as he hastily converted an operation under local anesthesia to one under general. The 'Sux' had deteriorated to the extent that he had to use 20 vials to get an effect."[23]

Refrigeration is usually available, even in remote areas. For example, in Africa's poorest regions, more than one-third of diabetics have access to refrigeration for their medications (which may not need cooling), although the refrigerator often may belong to friends, relatives, or even the local butcher shop or beer parlor.[24]

Medications That Require Freezing

Many medications and vaccines require a "cold chain" to exist between the manufacturer and the end user. In the case of live virus vaccines, for example, this means that there must be a way of keeping them frozen throughout their journey to the patient. Two vaccines that are particularly vulnerable are the measles-mumps-rubella (MMR) vaccine and the varicella virus vaccine live. MMR may retain potency at room temperature. The varicella vaccine, however, must remain continually frozen (–15°C [5°F] or colder). The Centers for Disease Control (CDC) recommends that if any refrigerated or frozen vaccines are warmed, the manufacturer or CDC should be contacted for advice before the vaccines are used.[25] Other medications, especially other types of vaccines, must be kept at cool temperatures throughout their travels.

Keeping Liquid Medications/Vaccines Cold

In many areas of the world, electricity for refrigeration may be unreliable or nonexistent; this may even occur in the most-developed countries or regions after a disaster. But, refrigerators can be improvised. (See the "Refrigeration" section in Chapter 5.)

The use of traditional cooling methods may not be an effective method to refrigerate medications. For example, porous, unglazed clay pots have often been used as cooling mechanisms in parts of Africa. They are partially filled with soil and water, then buried in a shady place. Tests show that even under optimal circumstances, these lower the inside temperature only by 1°C or 2°C.[26]

Most vaccines require refrigeration or freezing, and so do not do well in power outages. While most refrigerated vaccines are relatively stable at room temperature for a limited period of time, it is best not to open the refrigeration units until power has been restored or the vaccines are to be transferred to a functioning cooling unit. The best method to preserve refrigeration- or freezer-dependent medications is to have alternative refrigeration/freezing sites available. When planning to store medications in disaster situations, alternative locations may include any site that has a dependable generator as well as the required cooling devices. To be useful, medical personnel must not only be aware of the availability of such facilities, but they must also have access to them during a disaster. "Access" means they should know the floor plan (to be able to find the cooling units), have portable lights (in case no light is available), have any keys or access codes to unlock doors and equipment, and be aware of any alarm systems that might be activated—and how to deactivate them.

For example, in St. Bernard Parish, Louisiana (adjacent to New Orleans' Ninth Ward), after Hurricane Katrina destroyed nearly everything in the vicinity (including the hospital), quick-thinking physicians took their supply of vaccines to the refrigerators in the telephone switching station, which they knew had a reliable generator. The vaccines survived, and they were used to inoculate thousands of people.

Alternatively, refrigerated trucks or train cars can provide temporary storage, as can an available supply of dry ice.

Keeping Pharmaceuticals Warm

A major problem in cold climates is preventing medications and IV solutions from getting too cold or even freezing. Prehospital personnel often use their own body heat for this. Refrigerators or freezers (when turned off), with their excellent insulation, can also function to prevent liquids from freezing.

Storing Parenteral Medication for Reuse

In resource-poor situations, the temptation is to "cap" open vials containing partially used medication. In some parts of the world, medical staff routinely seal partially used medication vials with sterile gauze and tape. Even when the resource is scarce, this is a bad idea, because it promotes bacterial growth and can seriously harm subsequent patients. Rather, store the extra medication in a labeled syringe with a capped needle. Ideally, this can be placed in a cool area for short-term storage.[27,28]

THE PHARMACY

Pharmacy Layout

While the concept of setting up a field/improvised pharmacy may seem to be a "no-brainer," it may be a challenge to meet the requirements for storage and safe dispensing. Limited workspace may be available, and pharmaceuticals may be mixed together, sometimes in a multitude of unlabeled boxes and bags. Among these may be many donated pharmaceuticals that are unrecognizable or useless.

Basic principles to follow when planning a field pharmacy include the following:

- The pharmacy should be situated so that access is limited and be arranged so that the personnel and pharmaceuticals within it are secure. If possible, have a locked box or area for controlled substances such as narcotics.
- For confidentiality, place the dispensing area away from, or at the end of, the flow pattern for patients and personnel.

- Store medication so that pharmaceuticals can quickly be identified and dispensed. Additional materials for dispensing, recordkeeping, and reference should also be easily accessible.
- When possible, separate the larger storage area from the dispensing area.
- Store everything off the ground to prevent water damage. Placing boxes on pallets or empty litters usually suffices.
- Whenever possible, ensure a secure source of electricity for lighting, refrigeration, computers, and other equipment.

Medication Organization

In patient care areas, it may be difficult to keep medications organized. One method is to use a cardboard egg carton to sort medications (Fig. 13-1). Another alternative is to cut down the height of a typical cardboard box in which small bottles are shipped. Both make excellent medication organizers for wards and clinics. In Guyana, ED nurses store medications in clean labeled urine containers.

Calculating Drug Doses

Basic medication math that many people forget is how to calculate correct doses. While others may do that for you in routine circumstances, the following may help if you are dispensing or administering medications without much help.

1. To calculate the correct dose of drugs expressed as mg/kg or mcg/kg or as $mg.kg^{-1}$ or $mcg.kg^{-1}$, multiply the drug dose by the patient's weight.
   Example: The dose of atropine is 20 mcg/kg.
   For a 25-kg patient, give: 20 mcg/kg × 25 kg = 500 mcg = 0.5 mg.
2. When using drugs prepared in solution, calculate the number of milligrams of the drug per 1 mL. Do this by multiplying the number in the percentage of the solution by 10.
   Examples:
   For a 2% lidocaine solution, use: 2 × 10 = 20 mg/mL
   0.5% bupivacaine = 0.5 × 10 = 5 mg/mL
   2.5% thiopental = 2.5 × 10 = 25 mg/mL

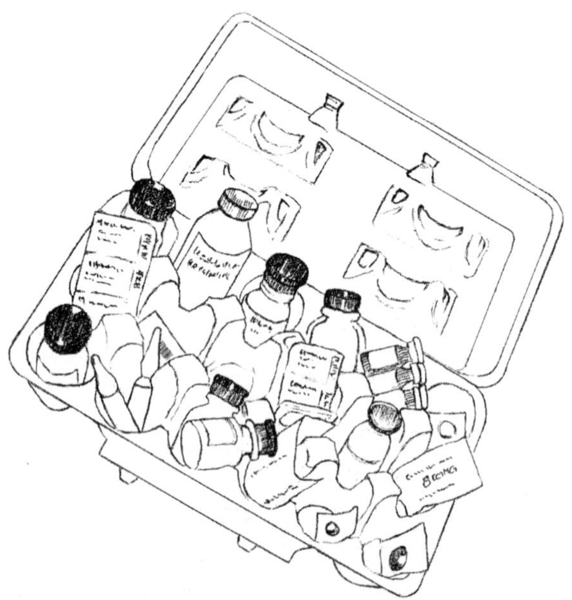

FIG. 13-1. Egg carton medication organizer.

3. Some solutions, such as adrenaline (epinephrine), may be expressed as 1:1000, or 1:10,000 or 1:100,000. This means that in a 1:1000 adrenaline ampule, there is 1 part adrenaline to 1000 parts solution. To work out how many milligrams of adrenaline are present, use the following equation:

   1:1000 solution adrenaline = 1 g adrenaline in 1000 mL solution = 1000 mg adrenaline in 1000 mL solution = 1 mg/mL

   1:10,000 solution adrenaline = 1 g adrenaline in 10,000 mL solution = 1000 mg adrenaline in 10,000 mL solution = 1 mg/10 mL, which can also be expressed as 100 mcg/mL

Weighing Medications

To make a balance scale for weighing medications, use tin cans or the bottoms from two plastic bottles attached to each end of a wood or metal rod by string or wires. Suspend the rod at its center from a fixed point. Have a nail or other indicator sticking up from the center of the rod. When the balance is empty, mark the indicator's "balance point" position. Ideally, it will point up along the suspension wire. Put an unknown quantity in one side of the scale. Then put objects of known weight (such as small coins) on the other, adding weight until the marker returns to the original "balance point" position. Coins and similar items can be "weighed" by putting them in water and measuring the amount of water they displace. Water has a known weight per volume of 1 kg/L. It may be easier to weigh an object using a known volume/weight of water as a counterweight.

Prescription Amounts for Topical Preparations

If prescribing topical preparations, use the following approximations to determine how much to prescribe:

- 1 g covers 100 cm^2 (10 cm × 10 cm).
- 22 g will cover an average-sized body.
- 1 fingertip unit (FTU) dispenses 0.5 g, which covers the area of two adult palms.
- 42 g covers one arm if applied twice daily (bid) for 1 week.
- 400 to 800 g covers the entire adult body if applied bid for 1 week.

Containers for Dispensing Medication

Medications dispensed to patients do not always have to be in the standard packaging. Rather, the container, the label with instructions, and the manner in which they are packaged may all vary with the situation.

The first concern is the container. Some acceptable containers for various forms of medications include:

- Pills/capsules: Small plastic bag, envelope, old pill bottle (relabled)
- Powders: Envelope, sealable plastic bag, bottle
- Liquids: Clean empty bottle (glass or plastic) with tight cap

Encourage patients to bring these types of containers with them. When refilling medications, ask patients to bring the container from the last time they got the pills.

Label medication containers in the patient's native language, as well as in the country's national language (e.g., English, Chinese, Russian, French, Spanish, Arabic). Include both the generic and the brand names; this allows other practitioners to identify the medication. The label should also contain the total medication dispensed, the patient's and prescriber's names, and the date. The dose and how to take it may need to be illustrated. The medication's expiration and storage information (e.g., refrigerate) may also be useful.

Language difficulties between the practitioner and patient often complicate prescribing medications—either due to differences in language or because the patient cannot read. Use illustrations to specify how much of each medication should be taken at specific times. Figure 13-2 shows a system where each label has symbols illustrating four times of day (sun rising = morning; sun high = noon; sun setting = evening; moon up = night). Beneath each symbol is another box that can be filled in with a picture of one or more tablets, portion of a tablet, capsule(s), or spoon(s) to show how much of the medication should be taken at that time.[29]

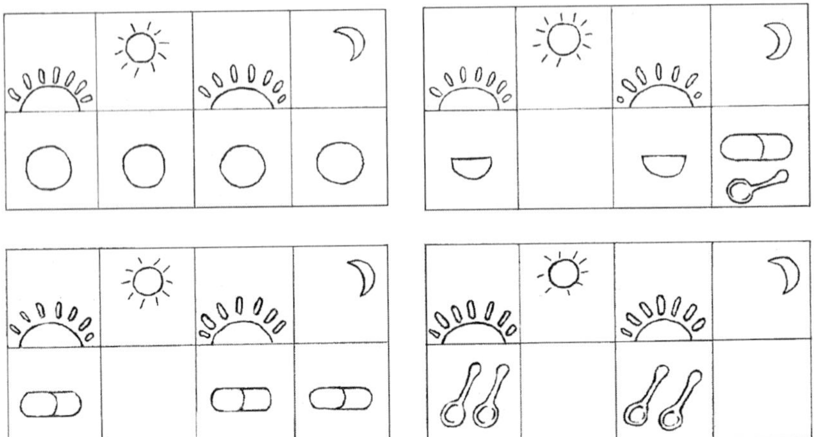

FIG. 13-2. Pictorial patient instructions for medication use. *(Redrawn from Werner.[29])*

To specify which medication goes with which instructions, use different colors of paper or use a crayon or marker to put a stripe on the instructions that is the same color as the stripe on the corresponding medication. Alternatively, use treatment-related pictures on medication labels and instructions that are culturally relevant and that can be drawn or duplicated—for example, a picture of a heart (cardiac medicine), a drop of water (diuretic), a lightning bolt (analgesic), or a thermometer (antipyretic).

Prepackaged Medications

Prepackaged "pill packs" provide a rapid method of dispensing commonly used medications to many patients or to groups of patients that may encounter similar problems (e.g., soldiers in battle). They are especially helpful when clinics are inundated with patients during a disease outbreak (e.g., flu season) and when a large number of patients need appropriate antibiotic packs, potassium iodide, or self-injector antidotes as treatment for exposure to a specific toxin (e.g., anthrax, radiation, or nerve agent). On the battlefield, the US military now supplies Special Operations troops with a package of antibiotics and analgesics for them to take if wounded.[30]

Estimating Counts: Tablets and Capsules

When preparing to dispense huge numbers of the same medications to a population, such as during an epidemic, approximating the number of tablets and capsules may be much more expeditious than counting them out. One method, successfully used by the pharmacy staff aboard the USNS Comfort hospital ship, is to use scoops cut from paper cups or plastic medication bottles. Cut the first one so that it can hold the proper number of tablets/capsules (or perhaps 10% more, to allow for error). Then cut more of the same size for each person to use when filling baggies, envelopes, etc., with the medications.

Making a Tablet/Capsule Counter

An improvised device to count tablets and capsules for dispensing to patients can be built easily and inexpensively (for a few dollars) from wood. It consists of a two-floor, varnished wooden box, with two exits and a sliding wall.[31] The box's interior dimensions are 20 cm long by 10 cm wide, the height to the groove for the slide is 4.5 cm, the height of the upper floor is 2.5 cm, and the dispensing holes have a diameter of 2 cm. The sliding separator is 2 cm vertical by 5 cm horizontal. Sand the slide so that it is smooth and moves easily; the wood varnish facilitates cleaning the box (Fig. 13-3).

Operate the counter by first sliding the separator to the middle of the box. This allows sufficient space to place medications from a larger container while blocking them from passing to the lower space where they go when counted (Fig. 13-3A). Then slide the separator to the extreme

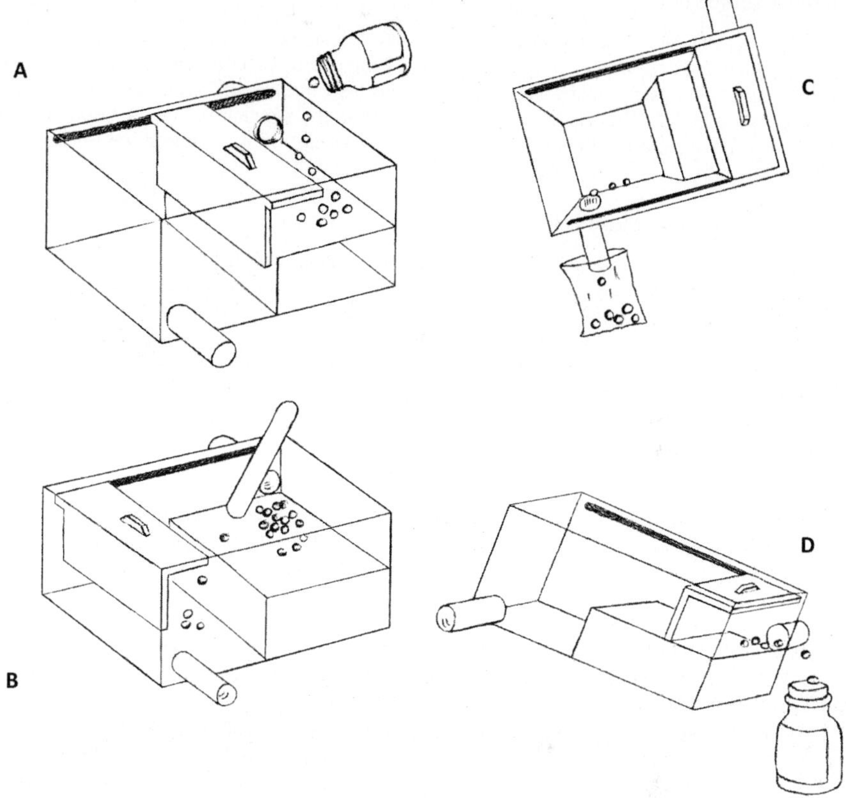

FIG. 13-3. Operation of improvised medication counter.

left to allow the medication to fall into the lower space when counted (Fig. 13-3B). When the correct number of tablets has been pushed to the lower space, move the slider to cover any medication remaining from the original stock. Put a dispensing container under the tube next to the patient's medication and pour the tablets into the container (Fig. 13-3C). Then put the medication stock bottle under the tube at the upper ledge and tilt the box, returning the medication to stock (Fig. 13-3D).

Sterile Water for Injection

To prepare sterile water for injection, fill a bottle with distilled water, close and sterilize it in an autoclave. Use it to dissolve powdered drugs for injection.[32]

Intravenous Admixtures

Experience shows that in situations where inventory or electrical resources are limited, most IV solutions should be prepared immediately prior to use rather than in large batches on a daily basis.[8]

TOXICOLOGY TREATMENT

Oral Mannitol for Overdoses

Oral mannitol is a good substitute for sorbitol if needed for overdoses (ODs), such as when treating a body packer.

Nebulized Naloxone

Nebulized naloxone is a safe and effective alternative to parenteral naloxone in spontaneously breathing patients with a suspected opioid OD. Mix 2 mg of naloxone in 3 mL normal saline for a total of 5 mL. Administer it using a nebulizer (see the "Mouth/Pharynx" section in Chapter 28). Repeat or continue the nebulizations as needed, based on the amount and type of opioid used (some have a longer half-life than others). The results may not be as complete or as prompt as with IV naloxone.[33,34]

Ethanol for Alcohol Withdrawal

A common myth says to administer ethanol for alcohol withdrawal. Do not do it, but do give it for methanol and ethylene glycol toxicity if there is no other treatment available. Studies show that ethanol for alcohol withdrawal does not help withdrawal syndrome or prevent delirium tremens, and often produces serious complications.[35] A 1953 review demonstrated that not only should it not be used, but also that physicians had discouraged this practice since the early 20th century.[36] However, as recently as 2006, a major trauma center still recommended its use.[37]

Ethanol for Methanol and Ethylene Glycol Poisoning

Ethanol has approximately 10 times greater affinity for alcohol dehydrogenase than do methanol and ethylene glycol. Therefore, ethanol competitively inhibits their metabolism into toxic substances by occupying the receptor sites for alcohol dehydrogenase. Fomepizole (usually not available in resource-poor settings) or ethanol should be administered as soon as possible after methanol or ethylene glycol ingestion. Fomepizole is given as a loading dose of 15 mg/kg IV infusion over 30 minutes; then 10 mg/kg IV q12hr for four doses; then increase to 15 mg/kg q12hr.

Ethanol is absorbed rapidly from the gastrointestinal tract, primarily from the duodenum, with food variably delaying absorption. Typical ethanol elimination rates average about 15 to 20 mg/dL/hr (150-200 mg/L/hr) but are usually higher in ethanol abusers. The serum ethanol concentration needed to treat these poisonings is ~100 to 150 mg/dL. For severe adult poisonings, immediately give about four 1-oz oral doses of 80-proof whiskey. Use the following equation to calculate oral and IV dosing, but calculate the IV dose as 100% ethyl alcohol (ETOH), the usual medical formulation:

> Goal: Serum ethanol concentrations of 100 mg/dL (1000 mg/L)
> **Loading dose (grams ethanol)** for patient weighing Y kg = 1 g/L × 0.6 L/kg × Y kg = Z g
> **Amount of ETOH required** = Z g/amount ethanol in solution being given per mL
> Note that % ETOH = proof/2; 80 proof ETOH (whiskey) = 40% ETOH = 31.6 g/100 mL; 10% ETOH (wine) ≈ 8 g/100 mL

Ethanol therapy should continue until the serum methanol concentration is 20 mg/dL (200 mg/L) and the patient is asymptomatic with a normal arterial pH. The maintenance dose varies between about 10% of the loading dose per hour (nondrinkers) and 20% per hour for chronic drinkers (averaging 110 mg ethanol/kg/hr [1.4 mL 10% ethanol/kg/hr]).

Whiskey (~86 proof) is often used for this therapy, because 2 mL ≈ 1 mL of 100% ETOH. The volume when using wine or other spirits is much greater.

Hypoglycemia in children and malnutrition in adults is the main complication of this treatment. Also, IV 10% ethanol can cause local phlebitis.[38,39]

Obtaining Additional Epinephrine (Adrenaline) Doses From an Autoinjector

Multiple doses of epinephrine may be needed to treat anaphylaxis.[40] With either the new or old (pre-2010) type of epinephrine autoinjector (e.g., EpiPen), obtain three or four additional doses by removing the end of the tube opposite the needle. Cut the plastic tube circumferentially about 1 inch from the non-needle end of the tube, pointing the end being cut off in a safe direction. When the non-needle end comes off, a tightly coiled spring shoots out very forcefully. Then slip the syringe with the additional epinephrine out of the case. After the first dose, the needle retracts into the tube and is mostly covered by a removable rubber sleeve, so it will neither be contaminated nor injure anyone during this procedure. Pull off the needle sleeve (identical to those on many preloaded injectable medication syringes) and point the needle upward. Withdraw the syringe plunger to its original position, aspirating air into the syringe. Administer another dose of epinephrine, if needed, and then repeat the process. The syringe has no markings, so giving about one-third of the volume should be adequate for an adult. Inject smaller doses if using an adult epinephrine autoinjector for a child.[41]

VENOMOUS BITES AND STINGS

Marine Envenomations

Jellyfish

All members of this large group envenomate through thousands of tiny stinging nematocysts whenever an object (such as a person's skin) comes into contact with their tentacles. Most cause immediate, severe pain and some cause a rash. Treatment for the common box jellyfish sting is the immediate, liberal use of vinegar (4%-6% acetic acid) over any area where stingers adhere to the skin. This inactivates the nematocysts' discharge. Avoid using vinegar on Portuguese man-of-war stings.[42] If vinegar is not available, a baking soda slurry may suffice. Then, remove any tentacles with a forceps or gloved hands, because even dry nematocysts can be reactivated if later exposed to water.[43] Then, if possible, treat the pain by taking a hot shower or immersing the part in water as hot as tolerable, or 45°C (113°F), for 20 minutes or as long as the pain persists. Hot packs or dry cold packs may work if hot water is not available. Traditional topical agents are relatively ineffective, including aluminum sulfate, papain, commercially available aerosol products, and a fresh water wash.[44]

Venomous Fish Stings

Pain from stings often can be relieved by putting the affected area in water that is as hot as can be tolerated (generally 40°C to 43°C [104°F to 110°F]), but take care not to burn the patient. Also, remove any foreign bodies.[43]

Stingray Wounds

Dozens of types of stingrays live in the world's coastal waters; they are venomous. Many have more than one stinger on their tail. Stingrays whip their tails backward in a defensive reflex action that, depending on the animal's size, may be powerful enough to penetrate leather boots, a diver's wetsuit, rubber, or even the side of a wooden boat. Most of those injured have either been wading in the surf or they are fishermen who have inadvertently landed a stingray. The wound may be a puncture or a laceration with or without an observable foreign body. Victims describe the pain as like "being prodded by a soldering iron"; the pain is generally out of proportion to what appears to be a trivial wound. Treat by immersing the affected part in hot (up to 113°F [45°C]) water. Remove any obvious foreign bodies as soon as possible; be aware, as with all penetrating injuries, that some may require intraoperative removal if they are near vital structures. Debride and irrigate the wound, give potent analgesics and antibiotics, and advise the patient that healing may take many months.[45]

Land-Based Envenomations

While topical therapies are often useful for marine envenomations, little evidence supports using either hot or cold therapy for most land-based envenomations. (Potential exceptions include ice for *Hymenoptera* [bee] and heat for *Chilopoda* [centipede] envenomations.) Applying other topical therapies for envenomations (e.g., *Hymenoptera, Solenopsis invicta* [fire ants]) has shown no benefit, including the application of aspirin, aluminum sulfate, papain, or bicarbonate.[46]

Arthropods

Arthropods include bees, wasps, centipedes, fire ants, and spiders. Treat anaphylactic reactions with available or improvised resources, including extra doses from EpiPens, as described above.

Scorpion stings can be extremely painful, with the pain requiring opioids over an extended period (sometimes months). In little children, and sometimes in the elderly, scorpion venom can produce acute delirium. Treat this with sedation, if possible; otherwise carefully observe patients and protect them from self-harm, as they may throw themselves around the bed. Delirium usually passes in 24 hours.

Reptiles

VIPERIDAE: TRUE VIPERS AND PIT VIPERS (SUBFAMILY CROTALINAE)

With the notable exception of bites to inebriated men who try to play with (and, yes, even kiss) pit vipers (e.g., rattlesnakes, moccasins, puff adders), most of these injuries occur in austere wilderness circumstances. About half of these snakes' bites do not inject venom. Of the others, most patients will live, albeit with some deformity of the bitten extremity, even if they do not get antivenin. Victims of most concern are little children and the elderly.

The real key is to know what *not* to do. Do *not* put a tourniquet, ice, or anything else on the wound. Do *not* cut the wound to try to suck out the venom; this is not only ineffective, but also injects flora from your very dirty mouth into the wound.[47]

Ideally, the victim should keep their limb at heart level and remain calm until help arrives. When no help is available, assist the patient to slowly walk to get help.

If antivenin is available but there is no a laboratory to do clotting tests, perform a whole-blood clotting assay. Use a glass-walled test tube and let a sample of the patient's blood sit at room temperature for 20 minutes. If no clot forms, it indicates that there is a coagulopathy and antivenin should be administered.[48] The coagulopathy should begin to resolve 4 to 6 hours after antivenin administration. (Leslie Boyer-Hassen, MD, Director, Arizona Poison and Drug Information Center, Tucson, Ariz. Personal written communication, March 6, 2009.)

ELAPIDAE

These include the mamba, cobra, coral, and sea snakes. This family produces neurotoxic venom. Unfortunately, other than supportive care, there is nothing much you can do without antivenin. These are nasty envenomations.

Suturing Dog Bites

Dog bite wounds should be treated with debridement, sufficient irrigation, povidone-iodine cleansing, and antibiotic administration. They should be primarily sutured when seen soon after the bite (<8 hours); this leads to improved cosmetic appearance (over the non-suturing approach) and there is no significant increased infection rate.[49]

Surgical Tick Removal

There is no absolutely effective and safe tick removal technique, although using continuous and steady traction while holding the tick with a blunt, medium-tipped angled forceps or fine point tweezers for extraction commonly works. In more complicated cases, such as a smashed or small tick or for bites >24 hours old, use excision to remove the tick without damaging it, as this could release disease-causing organisms into the skin. After locally anesthetizing the area, excise the epidermis and dermis 2 to 3 mm (diameter and depth) around the tick and remove it and the skin en bloc. Close the wound with a single suture or wound tape.[50]

REFERENCES

1. Hick JL, Hanfling D, Courtney B, Lurie N. Rationing salt water—disaster planning and daily care delivery. *New Engl J Med*. 2014;370(17):1573-1576.
2. Reich MR, ed. *An Assessment of US Pharmaceutical Donations: Players, Processes, and Products*. Boston, MA: Harvard School of Public Health; 1999.
3. World Health Organization. *Guidelines for Drug Donations*. 2nd ed. Geneva, Switzerland: WHO; 1999.
4. Duncan IL. Makeshift medicine: Combating disease in Japanese prison camps (reprinted from *Med J Australia*). *COFEPOW*. January 1983;1:29-32. http://www.cofepow.org.uk/pages/medical_makeshift_medicine.htm. Accessed September 14, 2006.
5. Smith E. Oxygen for reducing nausea and vomiting during emergency ambulance transportation: a systematic review of randomised controlled trials. *J Emerg Primary Health Care*. 2003;1(1-2). http://ajp.paramedics.org/index.php/ajp/article/viewFile/77/76. Accessed September 9, 2015.

6. Sewell RA, Halpern JH, Pope HG Jr. Response of cluster headache to psilocybin and LSD. *Neurology*. 2006;66:1920-1922.
7. Das RR, Singh M. Oral zinc for the common cold. *JAMA*. 2014;311(14):1440-1441.
8. Gonitzke M. *Field Pharmacies*. NDMS Response Team Training Program, September 2003. US Dept of Homeland Security.
9. Erramouspe J, Adamcik BA, Carlson RK. Veterinarian perception of the intentional misuse of veterinary medications in humans: a preliminary survey of Idaho-licensed practitioners. *J Rural Health*. 2002;18(2):311-318.
10. Woodward K. Adverse reactions in humans following exposure to veterinary drugs. *Veterinary Pharmacovigilance: Adverse Reactions to Veterinary Medicinal Products*. Hoboken, NJ: John Wiley & Sons; 2009:475-515.
11. Mazer-Amirshahi M, Pourmand A, Singer S, Pines JM, Anker J. Critical drug shortages: implications for emergency medicine. *Acad Emerg Med*. 2014;21(6):704-711.
12. King MH, Savage-King F, Martodipoero S. *Primary Child Care: A Manual for Health Workers*. Oxford, UK: Oxford University Press; 1978:277.
13. Editors. Tablet splitting. *Med Letter*. 2012;54(1396):63.
14. van Riet-Nales DA, Doeve ME, Nicia AE, et al. The accuracy, precision and sustainability of different techniques for tablet subdivision: breaking by hand and the use of tablet splitters or a kitchen knife. *Int J Pharmaceutics*. 2014;66(1):44-51.
15. Yakasai AM, Muhammad H, Babashani M, et al. Once-daily antiretroviral therapy among treatment-experienced Muslim patients fasting for the month of Ramadan. *Trop Doct*. 2011;41(4):233-235.
16. Altschuler R. *Do medications really expire?* (repost from a September 2, 2002, post on www.redflagsweekly.com/altschuler/200). Medscape General Medicine, posted August 21, 2003. http://www.medscape.com/viewarticle/460159. Accessed September 17, 2006.
17. Cohen LP. Many medicines are potent years past expiration dates. *Wall Street J*. Posted April 2, 2000. www.endtimesreport.com/Prescription_longevity.html. Accessed September 17, 2006.
18. American Medical Association. *Report 1 of the Council on Scientific Affairs: Pharmaceutical Expiration Dates*. Chicago, IL: AMA; June 2001.
19. Englebert D. Expiration dating. *Pharmacy NewsCapsule*. Wisconsin Dept Health and Family Services, July/August 2003 http://dhfs.wisconsin.gov/rl_DSL/Publications/pharmJulAug03.pdf. Accessed September 17, 2006.
20. US Dept Health and Human Services. Medication Safety. *HHS Broadcast News Service*. Posted September 25, 2005. www.hhs.gov/emergency/MedicationSafety.html. Accessed September 30, 2006.
21. Pingel M, Volund A. Stability of insulin preparations. *Diabetes*. 1972;20:805-813.
22. Fisch A, Leblanc H, Cisse H, et al. Etude de l'aterabilité d'insulines ordinaires dans les conditions climatiques africaines. [Study of changes in ordinary insulins in African climatic conditions.] *Med Afr Noir*. 1987;34:1043-1048.
23. King MH, ed. *Primary Anaesthesia*. Oxford, UK: Oxford University Press; 1986:24.
24. Famuyiwa OO. Insulin storage by diabetic patients (letter). *Int Diabetes Digest*. 1996;7:28.
25. Centers for Disease Control and Prevention. *National immunization program: emergency procedures for protecting vaccine inventories*. http://www.cdc.gov/nip/news/vacc_weather_emerg.htm. Accessed November 9, 2006.
26. Gill G, Price C, English P, et al. Traditional clay pots as storage containers for insulin in hot climates. *Trop Doct*. 2002;32(4):237-238.
27. Driver Jr RP, Snyder IS, North FP, et al. Sterility of anesthetic and resuscitative drug syringes used in the obstetric operating room. *Anesth Analg*. 1998;86(5):994-997.
28. Gonzalez S, Miller D, Murphy SP. Maintenance of sterility in 1-mL polypropylene syringes. *Am J Health Syst Pharm*. September 2007;64(18):1962-1964.
29. Werner D. *Where There Is No Doctor: A Village Health Care Handbook*. Palo Alto, CA: The Hesperian Foundation; 1992:63-64.
30. Holcomb JB. The 2004 Fitts lecture: current perspective on combat casualty care. *J Trauma*. 2005;59(4): 990-1002.
31. Bosch-Capblanch X, Loscertales MP, Memndigide A, et al. The 'handy tablets delivery device.' *Trop Doct*. 1999;29(1):31-32.
32. Monson MH, Mertens PE. A system for making hospital solutions in the Third World. *Trop Doct*. 1988;18(2):54-59.
33. Baumann BM, Patterson RA, Parone DA, et al. Use and efficacy of nebulized naloxone in patients with suspected opioid intoxication. *Am J Emerg Med*. 2013;31(3):585-588.

34. Weber JM, Tataris KL, Hoffman JD, Aks SE, Mycyk MB. Can nebulized naloxone be used safely and effectively by emergency medical services for suspected opioid overdose? *Prehosp Emerg Care*. 2012;16(2):289-92.
35. Golbert TM, Sanz CJ, Rose HD, Leitschuh TH. Comparative evaluation of treatments of alcohol withdrawal syndromes. *JAMA*. 1967;201(2):99-102.
36. Smith JA. Methods of treatment of delirium tremens. *JAMA*. 1953;152(5):384-387.
37. Dissanaike S, Halldorsson A, Frezza EE, Griswold J. An ethanol protocol to prevent alcohol withdrawal syndrome. *J Amer Coll Surg*. 2006;203(2):186-191.
38. Barceloux DG, Bond GR, Krenzelok EP, Cooper H, Vale JA; American Academy of Clinical Toxicology Ad Hoc Committee on the Treatment Guidelines for Methanol Poisoning. American Academy of Clinical Toxicology practice guidelines on the treatment of methanol poisoning. *Clin Tox*. 2002;40(4): 415-446.
39. Brent J. Current management of ethylene glycol poisoning. *Drugs*. 2001;61(7):979-988.
40. Järvinen KM, Sicherer SH, Sampson HA, Nowak-Wegrzyn A. Use of multiple doses of epinephrine in food-induced anaphylaxis in children. *J Allergy Clin Immun*. 2008;122(1):133-138.
41. Hawkins SC, Weil C, Baty F, Fitzpatrick D, Rowell B. Retrieval of additional epinephrine from auto-injectors. *Wild Environ Med*. 2013;24(4):434-444.
42. Fernandez I, Valladolid G, Varon J, Sternbach G. Encounters with venomous sea-life. *J Emerg Med*. 2011;40(1):103-112.
43. Forgey WW. *Wilderness Medical Society Practice Guidelines for Wilderness Emergency Care*. 2nd ed. Guilford, CT: Globe Pequot Press; 2001:60-65, 81.
44. Markenson D, Ferguson JD, Chameides L, et al. Part 17: First aid. 2010 American Heart Association and American Red Cross Guidelines for First Aid. *Circulation*. 2010;122:S582-S605.
45. Auerbach P, from a talk. Cited in: Boschert S. Stingray wounds excruciatingly painful, slow to heal. *ACEP News*. November 2007:11.
46. Lovecchio F, Thomas SH. Bites and stings – terrestrial. In: Thomas SH, ed. *Emergency Department Analgesia: An Evidence-Based Guide*. New York, NY: Cambridge University Press; 2008:124-132.
47. Markenson D, Ferguson JD, Chameides L, et al. Part 13: First aid: 2010 American Heart Association and American Red Cross International Consensus on First Aid Science With Treatment Recommendations. *Circulation*. 2010;122(suppl 3):S768-S786.
48. Punguyire D, Iserson KV, Stolz U, Apanga S. Bedside whole-blood clotting times: validity after snakebites. *J Emerg Med*. 2013;44(3):663-667.
49. Paschos NK, Makris EA, Gantsos A, Georgoulis AD. Primary closure versus non-closure of dog bite wounds. a randomised controlled trial. *Injury*. 2014;45(1):237-240.
50. Roupakias S, Mitsakou P, Nimer AA. Surgical tick removal. *Wild Environ Med*. 2012;23(1):97-99.

14 | Analgesics

Pain is one of the most common reasons for a patient to visit a clinician, and pain relief is one of the most consistently useful interventions clinicians make. With limited resources, the goal is to provide the best analgesia using the fewest and cheapest resources.

ASSESSING PAIN

To treat patients' pain, it is vital to assess it. There are several common methods to do this, including the following:

1. The five-point pain scale using words, in which patients point to the word that best expresses their pain level (Fig. 14-1). However, to use this, the patient must understand each of the terms for gradations of pain. (The words in the figure are provided in several languages.)
2. Faces pain scales (Figs. 14-2 and 14-3), which can be used by nonverbal patients or when language difficulties exist.[1]
3. Pain Assessment for Children (Table 14-1) can be used for children <4 years old and for children who are nonverbal or noncommunicative. It provides a rough guide to their discomfort level.

Intravenous Drug Challenges

The potential effect of analgesic treatment on pain can be assessed rapidly using intravenous (IV) drug challenges in conjunction with repeated use of the pain scales. Such evaluations can be done with minimal equipment and with commonly available medications. In addition, they can often be combined with sequential sensory neurological examinations. The two most

It sometimes helps, especially to communicate the pain level to other providers, if numbers are also assigned to the words, as in the English example, below.

	No Pain 1	Mild 2	Moderate 3	Severe 4	Excruciating 5
Spanish	No hay dolor	Leve	Moderada	Severa	Insoportable
French	Pas de douleur	Légère	Modérée	Sévère	Atroce
German	Ohne Schweiss	Mild	Moderat	Schwere	Quälenden
Russian	Не болей	Мягкий	Умеренная	Тяжелая	Мучительной
Chinese	沒有疼痛	輕度	溫和	嚴重	痛苦
Arabic	لا ا الألم	معتدل	معتدل	حاد	طاحنه
Japanese	痛み	軽い	穏健派	重度	耐え難い
Portuguese	Não Dor	Leve	Moderado	Grave	Dor tão mau

FIG. 14-1. Five-point pain scale using words.

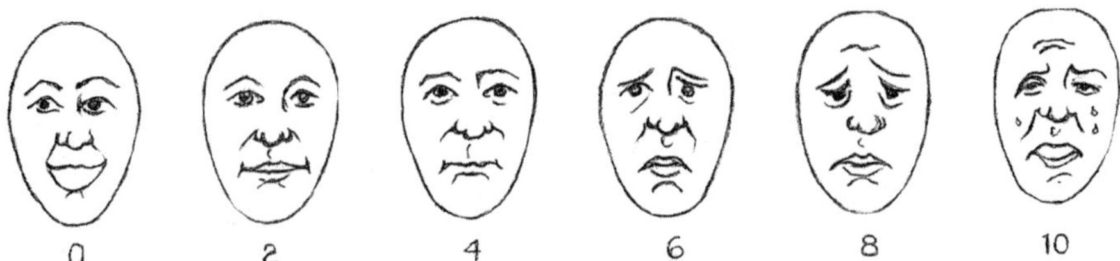

FIG. 14-2. *Faces pain scale: adult.* This scale can be used (a) with patients without language ability, (b) where a language barrier exists between the patient and health care provider, (c) with preverbal children, or (d) with those who are deaf. The numbers 1 to 10 on this scale correlate to those used on the other linear scales.

common drugs used for this test are lidocaine and ketamine. If they significantly reduce a patient's pain, this can indicate additional treatment options.

Lidocaine Infusions

These are often successful, especially in treating peripheral nerve pain. The safest, especially in patients with a history of arrhythmias or seizures, is a 4-hour infusion of 2 mg/kg IV. Dilute the lidocaine in 240 mL of normal (0.9%) saline (NS) and run it at 1 mL/min. Monitor pain scores every 15 minutes. If available, use cardiac monitoring and oximetry. If the patient has a positive response (less pain) with the lidocaine infusion, additional periodic lidocaine infusions will probably be an effective analgesic. Positive response to lidocaine indicates that mexiletine (an oral medication in the same class) may be effective.[2]

Ketamine Infusions

Ketamine has successfully treated a wide variety of pain syndromes, including those that have become resistant to opioids. The method is to administer 0.15 mg/kg over 20 minutes. Diluting the ketamine in 20 mL of NS or glucose (D_5W) allows administration of 1 mL/min. Monitoring and pain testing should be as with the lidocaine infusion. Terminate the infusion (positive test) if the pain scale is ≤2 out of 10. With a positive response, consider using oral ketamine. Calculate a starting dose as 10% to 20% of the amount needed to lessen the patient's pain significantly, with a maximum adult starting dose being 100 mg/day.[2] (See the "Ketamine" section in this chapter and in Chapter 17 for more information.)

TREATING PAIN

Treat pain whenever possible. An unreasonable fear of analgesia's side effects or of addiction, coupled with minimal staff and training, may propagate "a culture of nonintervention," in which nontreatment of pain becomes the norm. In addition, although narcotics are the gold standard for

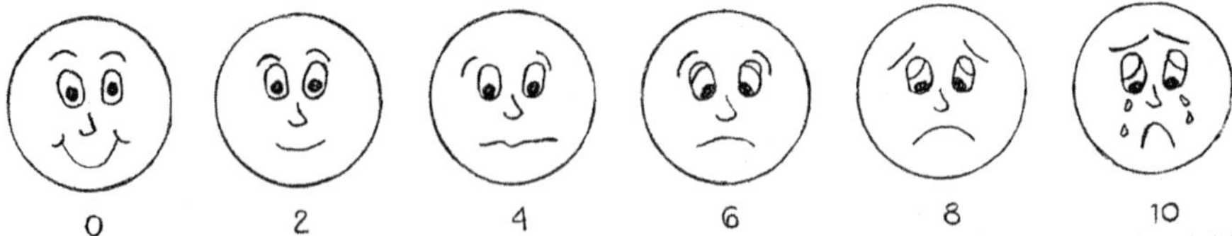

FIG. 14-3. *Faces pain scale: children.* This figure may work well with children.[1] Explain to the child that each face is for a person who feels happy because he has no pain (hurt) or who feels sad because he has some or a lot of pain. Ask the child to point to the face that best describes how he is feeling. The numbers correlate to those used on the other linear scales.

Face 0 is very happy because he doesn't hurt at all.
Face 2 hurts just a little bit.
Face 4 hurts a little more.
Face 5 hurts even more.
Face 8 hurts a whole lot more.
Face 10 hurts as much as you can imagine, although you do not have to be crying to feel this bad.

TABLE 14-1 Pain Assessment for Children <4 Years Old

If the child is asleep, no further assessment is needed. If the child is awake, check the following:

		Score
1. Cry?	Not crying	0
	Crying	1
2. Body position?	Relaxed	0
	Tense	1
3. Facial expression?	Relaxed or happy	0
	Distressed	1
4. Response?	Responds when spoken to	0
	No response	1

Total score: 1 = slight pain; 2 = moderate pain; 3 = severe pain; 4 = the worst pain possible.
Adapted with permission from Charlton.[3]

treating moderate to severe pain, many countries either ban their use outright or have so many restrictions or regulations governing their importation and use that clinicians rarely employ them.

Pain Treatment Ladders

A treatment pain ladder describes an optimal treatment strategy that starts with the weakest medications and progressively increases the strength of the medication. The Wilderness Medical Society recommends using acetaminophen with a nonsteroidal anti-inflammatory drug (NSAID) as the first-line medication for acute pain in remote settings.[4] If the patient has no relief, they are moved from an NSAID or another non-opioid drug to a weak opioid with or without another agent, and, finally, to strong opioids. Codeine and propoxyphene are weak opioids.[5]

A system that has been advocated for use with this pain ladder is "by the mouth" (use oral medications, if possible), "by the clock" (don't wait until the pain develops and is hard to control: use the medications on a fixed schedule to avoid getting the pain), and "by the ladder" (use the progressive system).[6]

The World Federation of Societies of Anaesthesiologists (WFSA) Analgesic Ladder uses regional anesthesia and a limited number of analgesics in a three-step approach.[3] A combination of these two methods (Fig. 14-4) represents the way clinicians should actually deliver analgesia to achieve optimal results. The type of analgesic intervention begins along the continuum, depending on the acuity, severity, and nature of the pain.

Pain in Children

Rather than parenteral administration, whenever possible, give analgesics by mouth (po) or via the rectum in children. Avoid aspirin, because of its association with Reye's syndrome.

Analgesic Effectiveness

If supplies are or will be limited, it helps to know which analgesics provide the most "bang for the buck." Although clinicians most often use analgesics based on tradition, the Oxford League's Table of Analgesic Efficacy provides some rational guidelines.

The Oxford League Table of Analgesic Efficacy

Based on published reviews, the Oxford League Table of Analgesic Efficacy (Table 14-2) lists commonly used analgesic medications (not IV) and the percentage of patients achieving at least 50% pain relief over 4 to 6 hours as compared with a placebo in randomized, double-blind, single-dose studies in patients with moderate to severe pain. Drugs were oral, unless specified. Note that commonly used medications such as tramadol, codeine (alone or in combination with paracetamol/acetaminophen, aspirin, or dextropropoxyphene), dextropropoxyphene alone, and

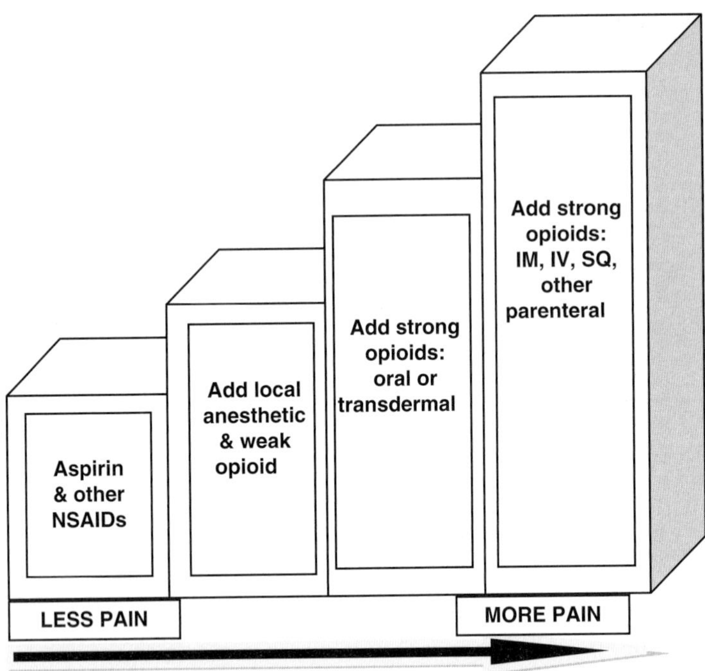

FIG. 14-4. Combined pain ladder.

lower doses of the listed medications were less effective in relieving pain than were many others that are commonly available.[7]

Although clinicians regularly administer opioid analgesics, those may not always be available or parenteral narcotics may need to be used orally. Table 14-3 lists the equianalgesic doses when using parenteral opioids by mouth.

UNCOMMON ANALGESICS AND ADJUVANTS

Sucrose for Pain in Children

Sucrose or other sweet solutions (e.g., glucose) offer a safe and effective nonpharmacologic way to decrease pain in infants during procedures. Children achieve the greatest analgesic effect when they receive 2 mL of at least 24% sucrose ~2 minutes before the painful stimulus. The analgesic effect lasts ~4 minutes.[9] These solutions are easy to administer, inexpensive (approximately US $1 per dose), have few to no adverse effects, and have been shown to decrease pain scores and crying time during painful procedures such as heel lances and immunizations.[10] At least in premature infants (32-37 weeks), the combination of sucrose with nonnutritive sucking provides better pain relief than both methods separately.[9]

Diamorphine (Heroin)

If available (~60% of UK emergency departments use it), intranasal diamorphine is a safe option that works at least as well as IV or intramuscular (IM) morphine in children with severe pain. For maximal absorption, administer it in small volumes (0.1 mL) of saline.[11]

Ketamine

Ketamine is available throughout the world as an anesthetic (see Chapter 17 for that use). Its availability combined with its effectiveness as an analgesic makes it an excellent choice for treating severe pain. Ketamine provides good analgesia when administered intramuscularly (IM), intravenously (IV), and, in much lower doses, via the oral, intranasal, transdermal, rectal, and

TABLE 14-2 The Oxford League Table of Analgesic Efficacy

Analgesic (mg)	Percentage With ≥50% Pain Relief (%)
Ibuprofen 800	100
Piroxicam 40	80
Ibuprofen 600	79
Valdecoxib 40	73
Oxycodone IR 15	73
Valdecoxib 20	68
Diclofenac 100	67
Oxycodone IR 10 + acetaminophen 1000	67
Oxycodone IR 10 + acetaminophen 650	66
Acetaminophen (paracetamol) 1500	65
Rofecoxib 50	63
Diclofenac 50	63
Piroxicam 20	63
Bromfenac 100	62
Aspirin 1200	61
Acetaminophen 500	61
Oxycodone IR 5 + paracetamol 500	60
Naproxen 220/250	58
Ketorolac 20	57
Acetaminophen 1000 + codeine 60	57
Ketorolac 60 (IM)	56
Lumiracoxib 400	56
Ibuprofen 400	56
Oxycodone IR 5 + paracetamol 1000	55
Diclofenac 25	54
Meperidine (Pethidine) 100 (IM)	54
Bromfenac 50 mg	53
Ketorolac 30 (IM)	53
Bromfenac 25	51
Naproxen 440	50
Ketorolac 10	50
Morphine 10 (IM)	50

Abbreviations: IM, intramuscular; IR, intrarectal.

Data from the Oxford League Table of Analgesics in Acute Pain.[7]

TABLE 14-3 Equianalgesic Oral-Parenteral Opioid Dosing Chart

	Equianalgesic Dose (mg)	
Opioid	Oral	Parenteral
Morphine	30	10
Fentanyl	N/A	0.1
Hydromorphone	7.5	1.5
Methadone	20 (acute) 2-4 (chronic)	10 (acute) 2-4 (chronic)
Oxycodone	20	N/A
Codeine	200	120
Meperidine	300 (not recommended)	75
Propoxyphene	N/A	130-200

Adapted with permission from Amabile and Bowman.[8]

subcutaneous routes. It has proven effective for refractory neuropathic pain, such as postherpetic neuralgia, postamputation pain, spinal ischemia, brachial plexopathy, and HIV and cancer neuropathies. It is also effective in nociceptive pain, including myofascial and ischemic pain.[12-15]

Subanesthetic concentrations of ketamine also provide effective analgesia for short, painful procedures, such as burn-dressing changes, radiotherapeutic procedures, bone marrow aspiration, and minor orthopedic procedures.[16]

Note that ketamine analgesia (1 mg/kg IV) has a pressor effect in circulatory shock and is the analgesic of choice for trauma patients in shock, especially if it is being used within 6 to 12 hours after injury. More care is needed if the patient is farther out from the injury, when it may cause hypotension. In patients with eye injuries, it may cause increased intraocular pressure at low doses.[17]

Oral and Parenteral Administration

Oral ketamine in a dose of 0.5 mg/kg has an analgesic effect at about 30 minutes postingestion. Because it tastes terrible, dilute the parenteral preparation in orange juice or cola to make it more palatable.[15]

Use subcutaneous ketamine to control both acute and chronic pain. Ketamine 0.1 mg/kg subcutaneously controls acute trauma pain better than IV morphine. In addition, it produces less drowsiness, causes no nausea or vomiting, and requires no breakthrough medications.[18] In adult cancer patients with intractable pain, either give an initial subcutaneous injection of 10 mg ketamine followed by a continuous subcutaneous infusion of 10 mg/hr, or 0.05 to 0.5 mg/kg/hr (IV or subcutaneous). An additional 2.5 mg/day can be added, up to a rate of 15 mg/hr. Alternatively, use 0.2 to 0.5 mg/kg/dose oral ketamine two to three times daily with a maximum of 50 mg/dose three times daily.[19] Most patients obtain pain relief; the side effects are site inflammation, salivation, and insomnia. Over 5 to 7 months, some patients develop a tolerance to ketamine's analgesic effect.[14]

Ketamine is frequently given IV or IM at a dose of 0.1 to 0.5 mg/kg, which produces rapid and profound analgesia.[20] Follow this with half the initial dose (0.05-0.25 mg/kg), as necessary.[16] In most patients, the higher dose produces more reliable analgesia.

Intranasal Administration

In children (usually, ages 3 to 13 years old) intranasal ketamine provides rapid, excellent analgesia. In addition, it eliminates the time, pain, cost, and equipment needed for IV or IM administration. The dose is from 0.5 to 0.8 mg/kg via an atomizer. Pain reduction occurs within 15 minutes and lasts about 3 hours. If the child needs additional pain relief at that point, administer another 0.5 mg/kg. Side effects do not differ from other administration routes and are transient.[21,22]

In Combination With Other Medications

Ketamine safely reduces the amount of morphine needed to treat acute severe pain in trauma patients.[23] In patients whose pain is poorly controlled with IV morphine, administer 0.25 mg/kg IV ketamine. This improves analgesia and reduces their nausea and vomiting.[20,23]

About one-third of patients with constant neuropathic trigeminal pain who have not responded to other modalities get long-term relief from 0.4 mg/kg IM ketamine (with 0.05 mg/kg midazolam).[24]

Postoperative Analgesia

Postoperative patients, especially those who have a tolerance to opiates, get good analgesia from low-dose ketamine.[25-27] While both IV infusions and oral ketamine have been effective, patients appear to experience fewer side effects with oral ketamine.[28]

For adult patients in severe pain, give a loading dose of 0.5 to 1 mg/kg IM ketamine. Follow this with an infusion of 60 to 180 mcg/kg/hr (4 to 12 mg/hr for a 70-kg adult). A practical regimen is to add 50 mg of ketamine to a 500-mL bag of NS or dextrose (0.1 mg/mL of ketamine) and run this at 40 to 120 mL/hr (i.e., over 4-12 hours for a 70-kg adult). This regimen is safe, because even the total volume will not deeply anesthetize the patient.[28]

Local Anesthetics: Intravenous and Blocks

Local anesthetics are underused. While frequently used for surgery, they are often not used either postoperatively or in other situations needing analgesia. Lidocaine (1.5 mg/kg IV), for example, appears to be at least and possibly more effective than morphine (0.1 mg/kg IV) in treating pain from renal calculi.[29] When an appropriate anatomical region is involved and the clinician has the skills, consider giving local or regional anesthetics, especially blocks with the long-acting anesthetics. Some useful blocks are described in Chapters 15 and 26. While these might not result in perfect analgesia, they usually lessen the pain enough for other analgesics to be effective.

Neuropathic Pain

Neuropathic pain is much more common that clinicians recognize. It stems from damage to or dysfunction of the peripheral or central nervous system (CNS) and results in pain far greater than that which would be expected from the injury. It is usually characterized by dysesthesias (burning pain, often with a "stabbing" component) and, sometimes, a deep ache. There may also be hyperesthesia (increased sensitivity to sensory stimuli), hyperalgesia (abnormally increased sensitivity to pain), allodynia (pain due to a benign stimulus), and hyperpathia (a particularly unpleasant, exaggerated pain response). Symptoms typically persist after resolution of the primary cause due to CNS remodeling. Although neuropathic pain may respond to opioids, the most effective treatment is often to give antidepressants, ketamine, anticonvulsants, baclofen, and topical medications.

Tricyclic antidepressants effectively treat most types of neuropathic pain and will often be available and inexpensive. Their analgesic effect may begin immediately (unlike their delayed action when used for depression). This group of medications includes amitriptyline, imipramine, desipramine, and nortriptyline. Their use is contraindicated in patients with liver, renal, or cardiac disease and in those with orthostatic hypotension. To reduce side effects, start amitriptyline at 25 to 50 mg hs (before bed) and increase it, as necessary, to 100 mg hs after a week. As with other analgesics, these medications are not effective for all patients. For every two patients treated, only one may get >50% pain relief. Other effective agents that may not be available, and that are more expensive, include antiepileptics (e.g., gabapentin at 300 mg twice a day [bid] to a maximum of 1200 mg tid).[30,31]

Ketamine successfully treats chronic pain states, such as complex regional pain syndromes,[32] phantom-limb pain,[33] and central and peripheral neuropathic pain.[34] Use 50 mg po tid in adults three times a day (tid). Increase this to 100 mg tid as needed. Problems with hallucinations and excessive salivation are rare. Gradually decrease the dose after about 3 weeks of good pain relief to see if it is still needed. It can be reinstituted, if necessary.[28]

Hypnosis

Hypnosis provides significant pain relief for most patients, sometimes even better relief than from traditional medications. This relief is different from the relief obtained from acupuncture and that from placebos. Hypnosis offers a moderate to large analgesic effect for many types of pain.[35-37] See the "Hypnosis" section in Chapter 15 for instructions on doing clinical hypnosis.

Distraction Analgesia

Reduce children's pain during injections, phlebotomy, or lumbar punctures by using a variety of distraction techniques. These require little, if any, equipment. Theoretically, distraction uses up cognitive capacity, leaving fewer resources to devote to pain. The techniques should be age-appropriate. For infants up to 1 year old, use music, cuddling, rocking, and a soothing, quiet tone of voice. For preschoolers aged 1 to 5 years old, use singing, picture books, puppets, and stories. For school-aged children 6 to 12 years old, use creative imagery, such as blowing an imaginary feather off the doctor's nose, playing with a kaleidoscope or 3D viewer, or blowing bubbles. Adolescents often respond to music.[38] Other methods of cutaneous stimulation or counter irritation include applying hot or cold packs (although these do not work[39]), superficial massage, acupuncture, and transcutaneous electrical nerve stimulation (TENS).

Cell Phone Movies

Movies, available for a minimal cost for smart phones, usually are the most effective distraction technique for children >1 year.[40]

Mechanoanesthesia (Vibration)

Vibrating devices placed on the site or manually pinching or shaking sites of painful procedures can markedly decrease the patient's pain perception.[41] Multiple vibration "apps" are available for smart phones—often labeled as "women's vibrators." Hold the vibrating device slightly inferior, but contiguous to, the desired injection site. Use the manual method by rapidly pinching the skin where an injection will occur between the thumb and forefinger just before inserting the needle.[42] The exact mechanism of action is unknown, but it appears that the nervous system is unable to fully receive or perceive two different types of sensory input (e.g., pain and vibration) simultaneously.[43]

Music

Music, whether sung or heard through a player, has been shown to reduce both pain and anxiety during medical procedures. This includes both short and long procedures such as suturing and burn debridement.[44-46]

Face on Glove

Another common passive distraction is drawing a face on an inflated hospital glove. It seems to be most effective if the face is drawn on the palm, rather than on the side, of the glove.[47]

"Street" Drugs

When official drug supplies are extremely limited, alternatives may be available from unusual local sources. Whenever medications are obtained from nontraditional sources, be extremely careful, because confirming the drug's identity, dose, and purity may be difficult. Find additional information about using street drugs in Chapter 13.

Methadone

Methadone is both a prescription medication and a drug used and sold by opiate addicts. When purchased in tablet form, it can usually be identified as coming from a legitimate pharmaceutical company. Methadone has the same actions as morphine and meperidine. Its unique quality is that it is well absorbed orally. It has a prolonged duration of action, making it more suitable for use in chronic, rather than acute, pain, although it has been used successfully for acute pain. Orally, the dose ranges from 2.5 to 25 mg given every 6 to 12 hours. The parenteral formulation can be administered IM at from 7.5 to 10 mg every 4 to 6 hours.[3]

ALTERNATIVE ADMINISTRATION METHODS

In areas of the world where strong opioids are available (they are not permitted for medical use in some countries and are unbelievably expensive in others[48]), IM administration may be the best method for clinical use. Generally, administer them on a scheduled, rather than an as-needed, basis. With outpatients, oral administration may be the easiest and the best tolerated.

However, normal methods of drug delivery or the forms generally used for that type of delivery (e.g., tablets, capsules, liquid) may not be available. In those cases, if the patient needs the medication or analgesic effect, consider alternative administration routes.

Oral Administration

Some opioids, although generally not given orally, can be very effective through that route (see Table 14-3). Oral fentanyl, for example, can be self-administered over 15 minutes. Between 25% and 50% of the fentanyl dose is absorbed through the oral mucosa. It has a rapid onset (5-10 minutes) and reaches its maximum serum level in 10 to 20 minutes.[49]

As mentioned previously, ketamine works very well as an oral analgesic.

Rectal Administration

Rectal administration of drugs results in direct systemic absorption, usually producing greater drug availability than through the oral route, although this varies with the medication, the presence of feces, and other factors. If it is in suppository form, place the drug in the middle or inferior rectum to avoid absorption through the superior rectal vein (directly to the portal system).

Morphine in solution given rectally is absorbed more slowly than oral morphine or a morphine hydrogel suppository. If the suppository is inserted into a colostomy, there is wide variability in absorption. NSAIDs as rectal suppositories are associated with ~20% fewer adverse gastrointestinal (GI) effects.[50] Codeine also has good rectal absorption, although it is slower than with IM administration and results in lower blood concentrations. Consider increasing rectal doses of acetaminophen and NSAIDs in children because the doses normally given often do not produce an effective blood level, depending on their formulation.[51]

To administer parenteral analgesics rectally, use a 2 mL syringe (without needle). Administer the IV formulation, generally at the same dose as would be given IV, and leave the syringe in for 2 minutes to prevent the medication from leaking out. The effect is generally rapid.[52]

Nasal Administration

Improvised Atomizers

Nasal absorption of medications is highly dependent on obtaining a small-particle mist, rather than the droplets normally produced by squirting a medication through an IV cannula into the nose. Construct improvised atomizers using commonly available medical equipment: either with or without a source of pressurized air or oxygen.[53]

If an air/oxygen supply is available, quickly assemble an atomizer (Fig. 14-5) from a piece of oxygen tubing, IV extension tubing, and a 22-gauge plastic IV catheter (with the needle removed). Place one end of the oxygen tubing on either the air or the oxygen port and set the flow to 3 L/min. Attach the female end of the IV extension tubing to the oxygen tubing by pressing them together firmly. Attach the 22-gauge catheter to the male end of the IV extension tubing. Attach the syringe with the medication to be administered to one of the access ports on the IV extension tubing. Slowly introduce the medication; it will atomize at the catheter into a fine mist. At higher air/oxygen flow rates, it becomes more difficult to push the medication out of the syringe.

If an air/oxygen supply is not available, make an atomizer by attaching a 22-gauge catheter (with the needle removed) to the male end of an IV extension set (Fig. 14-6). A 1 cc syringe containing the medication is attached to the farthest port (not the female end) of the extension tubing. On the female end of the tubing, attach a 60 cc syringe filled with air, and inject approximately 1 to 3 cc of air for every 0.1 to 0.2 cc of medication from the 1 cc syringe pushed into the tubing. This creates several very small air bubbles in the line. The medication is now in the tubing distal to the 60 cc syringe. Next, disconnect the 60 cc syringe and fill it with air again. Push this volume of air through the extension tube, thus delivering nebulized medication to the patient. While this does work, it does not atomize quite as well as when it is connected to oxygen.

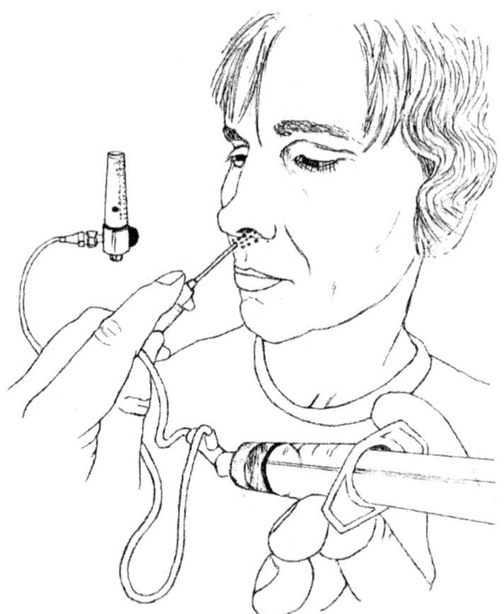

FIG. 14-5. Improvised atomizer with pressurized air/oxygen supply.

Nasal Opioid Administration

Nasally administering fentanyl, alfentanil, sufentanil, butorphanol, oxycodone, buprenorphine, meperidine, and diamorphine for analgesia in acute pain situations is highly effective, if done correctly (Table 14-4).

Nasal analgesic administration avoids the need to establish parenteral vascular access and is much kinder to patients, especially children and chronically ill patients. Nasal analgesic can be as effective as IV analgesia, and it provides a method for patient-controlled analgesia without the fancy equipment. The medications have rapid onset, bypass GI and hepatic presystemic elimination, and are useful in nauseated and vomiting patients. The same side effects exist as with the parenteral administration of these drugs. Nasal effects may include a bad taste for some drugs (not fentanyl) and, after a few days of use, nasal congestion, irritation, and epistaxis.

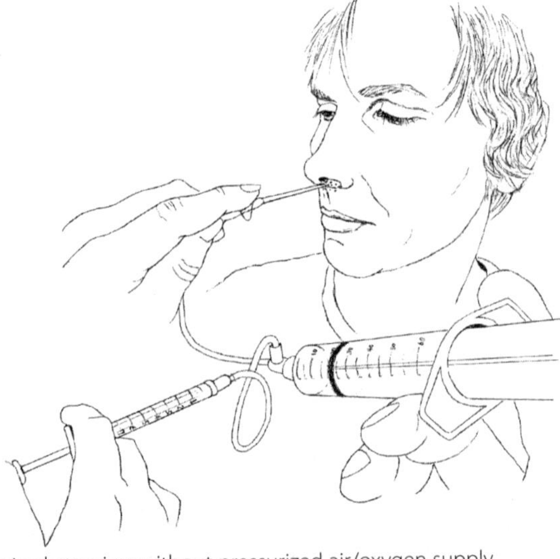

FIG. 14-6. Improvised atomizer without pressurized air/oxygen supply.

TABLE 14-4 Nasally Administered Opioids

Drug	Nasal Dose (mg)	Frequency of "As Needed" Administration	Mean Time to Pain Control (minutes)
Alfentanil	0.54		
Fentanyl	2 mcg/kg (adult) 0.5-1.5 mcg/kg (child)	q5min	30
Sufentanil	0.015		
Oxycodone	0.1		
Buprenorphine	0.3		
Butorphanol	1-2	q1-4hr	45
Meperidine/pethidine	27	q5min	30
Diamorphine/heroin	0.1 mg/kg	q20min	5

Data from Russell et al,[4] Kendall et al,[54] and Dale et al.[56]

The basic principles are: (a) a potent medication must be delivered in small quantities; (b) a higher dose should be used, because the nasal mucosa does not absorb all the medication; (c) the drug must be delivered so the nasal mucosa can optimally absorb it (i.e., as a spray rather than as drops); and (d) the maximum surface area should be used, which means using both nostrils in some patients.[55]

The ideal volume for each nostril is from 0.2 to 0.4 mL. Giving >1 mL causes the medication to run into the throat or out of the nose, making the actual dosage administered uncertain. Because intranasal drug availability is about 71%, use 1.4 times the usual IV fentanyl dose. It can be pulsed in divided doses if the total volume is too large. One alternative is to use a powdered opiate, such as diamorphine, diluting the proper dose in 0.2 mL NS. Another option is to use the more potent sufentanil, which is inexpensive and eight times as potent as fentanyl.[56] (Nasal ketamine administration was described previously.)

Nasal Administration of Other Medications

Other medications (Table 14-5) can be delivered intranasally using cotton swabs, a syringe with an IV catheter (often acts more like a dropper than an atomizer), or an atomizer. Use an improvised atomizer (see "Improvised Atomizers" earlier in this chapter) or one that is normally used

TABLE 14-5 Nasal Medication for Nonanalgesic Use

Indication	Drug	Nasal Dose/Volume	Additional Information
Sedation	Midazolam	0.4-0.5 mg/kg	Titrate for effect
	Sufentanil	0.2-1.0 mcg/kg	
	Fentanyl	1.5-3.0 mcg/kg	
	Ketamine	3-8 mg/kg	
Seizures	Midazolam	0.2-0.3 mg/kg (10 mg in teenagers and adults)	Use 5 mg/mL form Effect in ~6 min
	Lorazepam	2 mg (adults)	~10 min
Opiate reversal	Naloxone	2 mg	Use 1 mg/mL form
Nasal procedures and epistaxis	4% Lidocaine plus oxymetazoline (Afrin)	1.5 mL 0.5 mL	
	4% Cocaine	Up to 4 mL in adults	

Data from Wolfe and Bernstone,[58] Wermeling et al,[59] Lahat et al,[60] and Abrams et al.[61]

for other purposes (e.g., perfume) that has been thoroughly cleaned. The intranasal route, particularly traversing the olfactory epithelium, allows many drugs to bypass the blood-brain barrier.[57]

Inhalation

Inhaled morphine provides analgesia within 5 minutes, but requires 6 to 20 times as much for an equianalgesic effect to IM morphine. Part of this is due to the amount that does not reach the lungs with a typical inhaler.[50]

Sublingual, Buccal, and Transmucosal

Sublingual, buccal, and transmucosal routes of administering medications provide direct drug entry to the systemic circulation without first being metabolized or going through gastric emptying. Buprenorphine (Stadol) and fentanyl are quickly (~2.5 minutes) absorbed in the mouth. In contrast, it takes 6 hours for morphine to be absorbed through the oral mucosa. Buprenorphine administered transnasally results in >50% bioavailability, with onset of analgesia within 15 minutes and peak concentrations reached in 30 to 60 minutes.[50]

Transdermal

Transdermal absorption works for highly lipid-soluble drugs, such as fentanyl, sufentanil, salicylates, and certain other NSAIDs.[50]

Lidocaine patches (homemade, if needed) effectively treat acute herpes zoster pain and postherpetic neuralgia. See the "Topical Anesthetics" section in Chapter 15 for more information.

Continuous Subcutaneous

Continuous subcutaneous opioid infusions are effective, even if their absorption is unpredictable. Change the infusion site about every 4 days. These infusions are interchangeable with IM injections.[50] Note that they can be used in conjunction with hypodermoclysis (see Chapter 12).

REFERENCES

1. Wong DL, Hockenberry-Eaton M, Wilson D, et al. *Wong's Essentials of Pediatric Nursing*. 6th ed. St. Louis, MO: Mosby; 2001:1301.
2. Baranowski AP. Pharmacological diagnostic tests. In: Breivaik H, Campbell W, Eccleston C, eds. *Clinical Pain Management: Practical Applications & Procedures*. London, UK: Arnold; 2003:40-47.
3. Charlton E. The management of postoperative pain. *Update Anaesth*. 1997;7:2-17. http://www.nda.ox.ac.uk/wfsa/html/acrobat/update07.pdf. Accessed May 9, 2008.
4. Russell KW, Scaife, CL, Weber DC, et al. Wilderness Medical Society Practice guidelines for the treatment of acute pain in remote environments. *Wild Environ Med*. 2014;25(1):41-49.
5. Tran MI, Warfield C. Opioid analgesics. In: Breivaik H, Campbell W, Eccleston C, eds. *Clinical Pain Management: Practical Applications & Procedures*. London, UK: Arnold; 2003:59-76.
6. The WHO Pain Relief Ladder. www.who.int/cancer/palliative/painladder/en. Accessed May 1, 2008.
7. *Oxford League Table of Analgesics in Acute Pain*. http://www.medicine.ox.ac.uk/bandolier/booth/painpag/Acutrev/Analgesics/Leagtab.html. Accessed May 1, 2009.
8. Amabile CM, Bowman BJ. Overview of oral modified-release opioid products for management of chronic pain. *Ann Pharmacother*. 2006;40(7/8):1327-1335.
9. Simonse E, Mulder PG, van Beek RH. Analgesic effect of breast milk versus sucrose for analgesia during heel lance in late preterm infants. *Pediatrics*. 2012;129(4):657-663.
10. Michiels EA, Hoyle JD Jr. Sweet solutions and needle-related pain in infants. *Ann Emerg Med*. 2014;63(3):300-301.
11. Regan L, Chapman AR, Celnik A, et al. Nose and vein, speed and pain: comparing the use of intranasal diamorphine and intravenous morphine in a Scottish paediatric emergency department. *Emerg Med J*. 2013;30(1):49-52.
12. Akporehwe NA, Wilkinson PR, Quibell R, et al. Ketamine: a misunderstood analgesic? *BMJ*. 2006;332:1466.

13. Prommer E. *Ketamine Use in Palliative Care*. www.eperc.mcw.edu. Accessed November 1, 2006.
14. Oshima E, Tei K, Kayazawa H, et al. Continuous subcutaneous injection of ketamine for cancer pain. *Can J Anesth*. 1990;37(3):385-386.
15. Grant IS, Nimmo WS, Clements JA. Pharmacokinetics and analgesic effects of I.M. and oral ketamine. *Br J Anaesth*. 1981;53:805-809.
16. World Health Organization. *Model Prescribing Information: Drugs Used in Anesthesia*. Geneva, Switzerland: WHO; 1989:18-20. www.who.int/medicinedocs/en/d/Jh2929e.4.5.
17. Husum H, Ang SC, Fosse E. *War Surgery: Field Manual*. Penang, Malaysia: Third World Network; 1995:149, 334.
18. Gurnani A, Sharma PK, Rautela RS, et al. Analgesia for acute musculoskeletal trauma: low-dose subcutaneous infusion of ketamine. *Anaesth Intensive Care*. 1996;24(1):32-36.
19. Bredlau AL, Thakur R, Korones DN, Dworkin RH. Ketamine for pain in adults and children with cancer: a systematic review and synthesis of the literature. *Pain Med*. 2013;14(10):1505-1517.
20. Stevenson C. Ketamine: a review. *Update Anaesth*. 2005;20:25-29.
21. Andolfatto G, Willman E, Joo D, et al. Intranasal ketamine for analgesia in the emergency department: a prospective observational series. *Acad Emerg Med*. 2013;20(10):1050-1054.
22. Yeaman, F, Oakley E, Meek R, Graudins A. Sub-dissociative dose intranasal ketamine for limb injury pain in children in the emergency department: a pilot study. *Emerg Med Australasia*. 2013;25(2): 161-167.
23. Galinski M, Dolveck F, Combes X, et al. Management of severe acute pain in emergency settings: ketamine reduces morphine consumption. *Am J Emerg Med*. 2007;25(4):385-390.
24. Rabben T, Skjelbred P, Øye I. Prolonged analgesic effect of ketamine, an *N*-methyl-D-aspartate receptor inhibitor, in patients with chronic pain. *J Pharmacol Exp Ther*. 1999;289(2):1060-1066.
25. Subramaniam K, Subramaniam B, Steinbrook RA. Ketamine as adjuvant analgesic to opioids: a quantitative and qualitative systematic review. *Anesth Analg*. 2004;99(2):482-495.
26. Schmid RL, Sandler AN, Katz J. Use and efficacy of low dose ketamine in the management of acute postoperative pain: a review of current techniques and outcomes. *Pain*. 1999;82:111-125.
27. Bell RF. Low dose subcutaneous ketamine infusion and morphine tolerance. *Pain*. 1999;83:101-103.
28. Craven R. Ketamine. *Anaesthesia*. 2007;62(suppl 1):48-53.
29. Soleimanpour H, Hassanzadeh K, Vaezi H, et al. Effectiveness of intravenous lidocaine versus intravenous morphine for patients with renal colic in the emergency department. *BMC Urol*. 2012;12(1):13.
30. Sindrup SH, Bach FW. Antidepressants, antiepileptics, and antiarrhythmic drugs. In: Breivaik H, Campbell W, Eccleston C, eds. *Clinical Pain Management: Practical Applications & Procedures*. London, UK: Arnold; 2003:101-109.
31. Roche SI, Goucke CR. Management of acutely painful medical conditions. In: Rowbotham DJ, Macintyre PE, eds. *Clinical Pain Management: Acute Pain*. London, UK: Arnold; 2003:369-391.
32. Correll GE, Maleki J, Gracely EJ, et al. Subanaesthetic ketamine infusion therapy: a retrospective analysis of a novel therapeutic approach to complex regional pain syndrome. *Pain Med*. 2004;5:263-275.
33. Nikolajsen L, Hansen CL, Keiler J, et al. The effect of ketamine on phantom pain: a central neuropathic disorder maintained by peripheral input. *Pain*. 1996;67:69-77.
34. Backonja M, Arndt G, Gombar KA, et al. Response of chronic neuropathic pain syndromes to ketamine. *Pain*. 1994;56:51-57.
35. Montgomery GH, DuHamel KN, Redd WH. A meta-analysis of hypnotically induced analgesia: how effective is hypnosis? *Int J Clin Exp Hypnosis*. 2000;48:138-153.
36. Stewart JH. Hypnosis in contemporary medicine. *Mayo Clin Proc*. 2005;80(4):511-524.
37. Iserson KV. An hypnotic suggestion: review of hypnosis for clinical emergency care. *J Emerg Med*. 2014;46(4):588-596.
38. O'Donnell J, Maurice S, Beattie T. Emergency analgesia in the paediatric population. Part III non-pharmacological measures of pain relief and anxiolysis. *Emerg Med J*. 2002;19(3):195.
39. Hogan ME, Smart S, Shah V, Taddio A. A systematic review of vapocoolants for reducing pain from venipuncture and venous cannulation in children and adults. *J Emerg Med*. 2014;47(6):736-749.
40. MacLaren JE, Cohen LL. A comparison of distraction strategies for venipuncture distress in children. *J Ped Psychol*. 2005;30(5):387-396.
41. Reed ML. Mechanoanesthesia for intralesional injections. *J Am Acad Dermatol*. 1984;11:303.
42. Fosco SW, Gibney MD, Harrison B. Repetitive pinching of the skin during lidocaine infiltration reduced patient discomfort. *J Am Acad Dermatol*. 1998;39:74-78.

43. Reed ML. Surgical pearl: mechanoanesthesia to reduce the pain of local injections. *J Am Acad Derm.* 2001;4(4):671-672.
44. Klassen JA, Liang Y, Tjosvold L, Klassen TP, Hartling L. Music for pain and anxiety in children undergoing medical procedures: a systematic review of randomized controlled trials. *Ambul Pediatr.* 2008;8(2):117-128.
45. Fratianne RB, Prenser JD, Huston MJ, et al. The effect of music-based imagery and musical alternate engagement on the burn debridement process. *J Burn Care Rehabil.* 2001;22:47-53.
46. Miller AC, Hickman LC, Lemasters GL. A distraction technique for control of burn pain. *J Burn Care Rehabil.* 1992;13:576-580.
47. Fogarty E, Dunning E, Koe S, Bolger T, Martin C. The 'Jedward' versus the 'Mohawk': a prospective study on a paediatric distraction technique. *Emerg Med J.* 2014;31(4):327-328.
48. Taylor AL, Gostin LO, Pagonis KA. Ensuring effective pain treatment: a national and global perspective. *JAMA.* 2008;299(1):89-92.
49. Blankenship R. *Innovation in Combat Casualty Care: Civilian Application.* Talk at ACEP Scientific Assembly, Seattle, WA, October 8, 2007.
50. Cashman J. Routes of administration. In: Rowbotham DJ, Macintyre PE, eds. *Clinical Pain Management: Acute Pain.* London, UK: Arnold; 2003:205-218.
51. Anderson BJ, Wooolard GA, Holford NH. Pharmacokinetics of rectal paracetamol after major surgery in children. *Paediatr Anaesth.* 1995;5:237-242.
52. Husum H, Ang SC, Fosse E. *War Surgery: Field Manual.* Penang, Malaysia: Third World Network; 1995:150.
53. Kenneth V. Iserson, John Spero, and Rhonda Shirley. Dr. Iserson developed both devices with the help of these two paramedics (night shift), University Medical Center Emergency Department, Tucson, Arizona, 2008.
54. Kendall JM, Reeves BC, Latter VS. Multicentre randomized controlled trial of nasal diamorphine for analgesia in children and teenagers with clinical fractures. *BMJ.* 2001;322:261-265.
55. Wolfe T. Intranasal fentanyl for acute pain: techniques to enhance efficacy (letter). *Ann Emerg Med.* 2007;49(5):721-722.
56. Dale O, Hjortkjaer R, Kharasch ED. Nasal administration of opioids for pain management in adults. *Acta Anaesthesiol Scand.* 2002;46:759-770.
57. Illum L. Transport of drugs from the nasal cavity to the central nervous system. *Eur J Pharm Sci.* 2000;11:1-18.
58. Wolfe TR, Bernstone T. Intranasal drug delivery: an alternative to intravenous administration in selected emergency cases. *J Emerg Nurs.* 2004;30(2):141-147.
59. Wermeling DPH, Miller JL, Archer SM, et al. Bioavailability and pharmacokinetics of lorazepam after intranasal, intravenous and intramuscular administration. *J Clin Pharmacol.* 2001;41:1225-1231.
60. Lahat E, Goldman M, Barr J, et al. Comparison of intranasal midazolam with intravenous diazepam for treating febrile seizures in children: prospective randomized study. *BMJ.* 2000;321:83-86.
61. Abrams R, Morrison JE, Villasenor A, et al. Safety and effectiveness of intranasal administration of sedative medications (ketamine, midazolam, or sufentanil) for urgent brief pediatric dental procedures. *Anesth Prog.* 1993;40:63-66.

15 | Anesthesia—Local and Regional

Use local and regional anesthetic techniques when the equipment, supplies, and experienced personnel to give deep sedation or general anesthesia are unavailable. This is frequently the case during initial disaster responses and in limited-resource settings. As one experienced anesthesiologist wrote, "We must assume that supplies of compressed gases will soon run out and replacements will be unobtainable. This leaves us with local techniques, spinal and epidural analgesia, all of which can be given by the surgeon in the absence of a trained anesthetist."[1]

TOPICAL ANESTHETICS

Pharmacology

Topical anesthetics are slowly absorbed through normal skin. However, they are rapidly absorbed through the mucosa, as well as through abraded, burned, and denuded skin. When using topical anesthetics in these areas—especially if used in the tracheobronchial tree—the maximum dose should be considerably less than that used for infiltration.[2,3] Tetracaine, for example, produces higher blood levels at 5 minutes with mucosal application than with subcutaneous infiltration.[4] When used in dentistry, topical anesthetics generally anesthetize only the outer 1 to 3 mm of mucosa.[5] That, however, makes them effective to dull the pain of intraoral injections.

Common Anesthetics

Good topical anesthetics include lidocaine (lignocaine), cocaine, and tetracaine. Some anesthetics, such as procaine and mepivacaine, are not effective topically due to poor mucous membrane penetration.[3]

Lidocaine (amide) (2% to 10% [20 to 100 mg/mL]) has a peak anesthetic effect in from 2 to 5 minutes. Its maximum safe total dose (without epinephrine) in a healthy 70-kg adult is ~250 mg and it is 3 mg/kg in children. Anesthetic effect lasts 30 to 45 minutes.[2,3] Lidocaine gel 4% can be made by adding 2 mL of 2% lidocaine without epinephrine to 1 mL of a water-soluble jelly (e.g., K-Y). This gel works well, if placed under an occlusive dressing, to ease the pain of herpes zoster and other skin lesions.

Bupivacaine (amide) (0.25% to 0.5% [2.5 to 5 mg/mL]) has a peak anesthetic effect in 2 to 5 minutes. Its maximum safe total dose in a healthy 70-kg adult is 400 mg/24 hours; it is 2 mg/kg in children, although it is not officially recommended for use in children <12 years old. Similarly, it is not recommended as a spinal anesthetic in those <12 years old. Anesthetic effect lasts 4 to 8 hours.

Cocaine (ester) (4% [40 mg/mL] is the usual concentration) has a unique vasoconstricting effect. It reaches peak anesthetic effect in 2 to 5 minutes. However, it is addictive. The maximum safe total dose in a healthy 70-kg adult is 200 mg (2 to 3 mg/kg) and it is 2 mg/kg in children. The anesthetic effect lasts from 30 to 45 minutes.[2,3] Staying within the maximum adult dose is easy if the standard package of 4 mL of the 4% solution is used. While making your own topical solution with cocaine obtained from noncommercial vendors may seem logical in an emergency, the problem is that neither the strength nor the purity of the ingredient is known.

Tetracaine (ester) (0.5% [5 mg/mL] is the usual concentration) has a peak anesthetic effect in 3 to 8 minutes. The maximum safe total dose in a healthy 70-kg adult is 50 mg and it is 0.75 mg/kg in children. Its anesthetic effect lasts 30 to 60 minutes.[2,3]

Toxicity

Local anesthetics can produce allergic reactions, tissue damage, and systemic toxicity. Allergic reactions are most common with the ester preparations (e.g., procaine, tetracaine). There is no cross-reactivity between the esters and amides (e.g., lidocaine, bupivacaine, mepivacaine).

Allergic reactions to local anesthetics are rare, with most reported allergies not representing actual allergic reactions. Local tissue neurotoxicity can also occur, but it is rare.

Usually associated with inadvertent intravenous (IV) or intra-arterial injections, systemic toxicity is the most common and significant problem associated with local anesthetic use. Mental status changes may be the only resulting sign or symptom that occurs before seizures begin. Classically, the progression of systemic toxicity is tongue numbness, light-headedness, visual disturbances, muscular twitching, unconsciousness, and seizures. Patients who receive local anesthetics while sedated may have muscular twitching as the only sign before seizures. The treatment is to stop local anesthetic use, manage the airway, control the seizures, and support the patient until the central nervous system (CNS) effects of the drug wear off. The local anesthetics themselves do not cause CNS damage. Rather, the damage stems from hypoxia during the seizure and the associated coma.[6]

Viscous Lidocaine and "Magic Mouthwash"

Many topical oral anesthetic formulations ease the pain from mucosal lesions. Young children's inability to spit after gargling is a primary reason that plain oral lidocaine (usually 2%, or 20 mg/mL) is rarely used in this age group, although it is generally safe and appropriate in older children. In very young children, even a single dose of swallowed viscous lidocaine may cause toxicity and death (toxic dose is 6 mg/kg).[7] While it may reduce the pain, viscous lidocaine does not improve oral intake in children with painful infectious mouth ulcers.[8]

A topical agent that seems to work well, and that uses commonly available ingredients, is a mixture of equal parts of 2% viscous lidocaine, diphenhydramine elixir, and Maalox or Kaopectate (as a binder).[2] Swish for 1 to 2 minutes and spit. This is especially useful in older children with oral lesions that prevent the child from drinking or eating.

Sprays

Lidocaine for injection can be nebulized as an effective topical mucosal anesthetic. Some patients experience a strong bitter taste when lidocaine is administered this way; however, the taste is usually transient and this should not prevent the patient from receiving the medication. (Angela M. Plewa, PharmD. Personal communication, April 8, 2008.) To use it, the best course is to dilute it to a 0.5% solution so that the maximum safe dose is not exceeded.

Creams

Anesthetic creams are useful to reduce pain before suturing, phlebotomy, or IV insertions. They are primarily used in children.

LET (lidocaine 4%, epinephrine 0.1%, and tetracaine 0.5%), which can be compounded locally, can be used to anesthetize small lacerations on the face and scalp before repair. This works particularly well in children and has less toxicity than TAC (tetracaine 0.25% to 0.5%, adrenaline 0.025% to 0.05%, and cocaine 4% to 11.8%), which was previously widely used. In an emergency, either works well. They both work in about 75% to 90% of patients. An older formulation mixing epinephrine in cocaine, termed "cocaine mud," had a very high complication rate; don't use it.

For LET solution, mix 100 mL 20% lidocaine HCl, 50 mL 2.25% racemic epinephrine (HCl salt), 125 mL 2% tetracaine HCl, 315 mg sodium metabisulfite, and 225 mL water. Make the gel by mixing the solution with methylcellulose.

The LET formula is effective both in a solution and as a gel. For the solution, paint it onto the wound edges with a cotton-tipped applicator. Then apply a cotton ball saturated with the solution to the wound. In about 20 minutes, the wound appears blanched and is ready to suture. Apply the gel to both the wound edges and the wound with a cotton-tipped applicator. As with the solution, the wound edges look blanched and the wound is ready to suture in about 20 minutes. Remove the gel before suturing.[9]

Patches

Anesthetic patches effectively anesthetize the skin and underlying area of painful lesions. They can be used for herpetic, post-herpetic, and rib fracture pain. They only have a placebo effect when applied for joint pain.

To improvise a topical anesthetic patch for abrasions and wounds, soak gauze with a mixture of injectable lidocaine, tetracaine, and epinephrine, and place it directly onto the wound for approximately 5 minutes.[10] For rib fractures, use 700 mg lidocaine under a 10 × 14 cm occlusive dressing.

LOCAL ANESTHETIC INFILTRATION

Local anesthetic infiltration generally works well, even when administered by novices and those who do not use it regularly. This is because it diffuses through the tissues without the clinician needing to know the specific neuroanatomy.

The key to giving successful local infiltration (also for regional blocks) is to wait long enough for the anesthetic to take effect. There is a delay, a latent period, of up to 15 minutes between when the anesthetic is administered and when the area is anesthetized. (A good practice is to do the block, leave and do any paperwork associated with the case, and then return to do the procedure.) If pain—not pressure or touch sensation—still exists after 15 minutes, administer additional anesthetic. You can also give the patient mild sedation, such as an anxiolytic (a paramedication). The most common reason that local anesthesia and anesthetic blocks do not work is that the clinician does not wait long enough.

Infiltration anesthesia uses larger volumes of weaker anesthetics (e.g., 100 mL of 0.5% lidocaine). Regional blocks of larger nerves use smaller volumes of more concentrated anesthetics (e.g., 10 mL of 2% lidocaine). Table 15-1 shows how to mix 1% and 2% lidocaine with normal saline (NS) and epinephrine to produce various quantities of 0.5% lidocaine with 1:200,000 epinephrine.

To maximize efficiency when large numbers of patients require procedures done under local anesthesia, group them together. Do not interpose cases under general anesthesia, because this will only slow patient flow. Block the next patient while the surgeon is scrubbing for the first patient.[12] When you must do a series of very short procedures under local or regional anesthesia, you can often block several patients at once using a longer-acting anesthetic (often containing epinephrine 1:200,000).

Local Anesthetic Medications

If a patient tells you that he or she is allergic to a local anesthetic, avoid that class of medications (usually an ester). Anesthetics in the ester class do not have an "I" before "caine" in their name (e.g., procaine, cocaine). The names of anesthetics in the amino amide class have an "I" before "caine" (e.g., lidocaine/lignocaine, mepivacaine). If you can't use an anesthetic from the class that the patient is not allergic to (or if the patient does not know the drug he or she is allergic to), use one of the alternative medications described in the next section.

Anesthetics come as percent concentrations, with 1% equaling 10 mg/mL or 1 g of anesthetic per 100 mL. To dilute a local anesthetic, add sterile injectable saline. For example, adding 1 mL of anesthetic to 1 mL of saline changes a 1% solution into a 0.5% solution. If 3 mL of saline were added, it would become a 0.25% solution. An easy way to calculate the dose in milligrams is to use the formula: Volume (mL) × Concentration (%) × 10 = Dose (mg).[13]

When medication is scarce, reduce the needed dose of anesthetic either by diluting the solution or, except for cocaine, by adding epinephrine (adrenaline). Vasoconstriction increases an anesthetic's length of action. Except for cocaine, local anesthetics without epinephrine added are vasodilators. Do not add epinephrine to cocaine; it is unnecessary and dangerous.

TABLE 15-1 Preparing 0.5% Lidocaine Solutions Containing 1:200,000 Epinephrine

Desired Amount of Local Anesthetic	Normal Saline/ Lidocaine 2%	Normal Saline/ Lidocaine 1%	Add Epinephrine 1:1000
20 mL	15 mL/5 mL	10 mL/10 mL	0.1 mL
40 mL	30 mL/10 mL	20 mL/20 mL	0.2 mL
100 mL	75 mL/25 mL	50 mL/50 mL	0.5 mL
200 mL	150 mL/50 mL	100 mL/100 mL	1.0 mL

Adapted from the World Health Organization.[11]

Premixed lidocaine with epinephrine (adrenaline) may not be available. The epinephrine concentration in lidocaine may be expressed as 1:1000, 1:10,000, 1:100,000, or 1:200,000. This means that a

- 1:1000 solution epinephrine = 1 part epinephrine to 1000 parts solution = 1 g epinephrine in 1000 mL solution = 1000 mg epinephrine in 1000 mL solution = 1 mg/mL
- 1:10,000 solution epinephrine = 1 g epinephrine in 10,000 mL solution = 1000 mg epinephrine in 10,000 mL solution = 1 mg/10 mL, which can also be expressed as 100 mcg/mL.
- 1:100,000 concentration means 1 mg of epinephrine for every 100 mL anesthetic.
- 1:200,000 concentration means 1 mg of epinephrine for every 200 mL anesthetic.

If lidocaine premixed with epinephrine is not available, use the following method to determine the amount of epinephrine to add to the local anesthetic:

To make a 1:200,000 epinephrine-lidocaine solution, add 0.1 mL (0.1 mg) epinephrine 1:1000 to 20 mL of lidocaine. To do this, take 1 mL of epinephrine 1:1000 and dilute it to 10 mL with saline. Then take 1 mL of this mix, which is now 1 mL of 1:10,000 epinephrine, and add 19 mL lidocaine. The total solution is now 20 mL, and the original epinephrine has been diluted 200 times = 1:200,000 solution.[14]

The maximum safe dose of epinephrine = 4 mcg/kg. Therefore, the dose for an 80-kg man = 320 mcg = 64 mL of a 1:200,000 solution.

To reduce burning from most local anesthetics, add 1 mL sodium bicarbonate (1 mEq/mL) to every 10 mL of 1% lidocaine.[15] While the traditional teaching is that local anesthetics are unreliable when used in the acidic environment of an abscess, reports suggest that a "double-buffered" solution of 2 mL of bicarbonate with 8 mL of lidocaine works well.[16] Heating the anesthetic to body temperature also helps reduce pain.[17]

Alternatives to Local Anesthetics

If standard local anesthetics are not available or if the patient claims to be allergic to local anesthetics, use one of the available alternatives. These include medications with antihistamine activity, bacteriostatic normal saline (NS) with benzyl alcohol, sterile water, local cold, and pressure.

Antihistamines

Most injectable medications with antihistamine activity can be used as local anesthetics if diluted to a 0.05% solution with NS. None are as effective as standard local anesthetics, but they will certainly do if nothing else is available.[18]

Diphenhydramine hydrochloride (Benadryl) works for dermal, urological, and dental anesthesia. Because it is very soluble in water, prepare a 1% solution by diluting 1 mL of a standard 5% diphenhydramine solution for injection with 4 mL single-use NS solution for injection (without preservatives).[15] It should not be used in concentrations >1%, because that may cause ulcerations or tissue necrosis. Its duration of action is less than that of lidocaine with epinephrine and, even if buffered, it is more painful than lidocaine. A 0.5% solution can also be used, but it is considerably less effective than 1% lidocaine. Complications include sedation (occasional), local erythema (common), persistent soreness lasting up to 3 days (common), and skin sloughing (rare).[15,19] Dimenhydrinate (Dramamine) also has local anesthetic activity.[18]

Tripelennamine (aka Pyribenzamine [PBZ]), a highly water-soluble antihistamine, is effective for a wide variety of regional nerve blocks in a 1% solution. As clinically effective as diphenhydramine, tripelennamine has fewer and less severe side effects. It can be used for urethral anesthesia[20] and, in a 4% solution, as a mucosal anesthetic on the gums. In powdered form, it immediately relieves toothaches in a decayed tooth. As a 1% solution, it has been used for topical anesthesia in the mouth and esophagus and, usually with epinephrine, for skin and dental block infiltration.[21] The addition of epinephrine reduces local reactions and lengthens the anesthetic's effect up to four times. For pain relief, use between 5 mL (lingual nerve block) and 20 mL (dorsal sympathetic nerve block). For surgery done with a tripelennamine nerve block, use between 10 mL (finger block) and 35 mL (tendon graft). The anesthetic effect is prolonged by adding 1:100,000 epinephrine.[22]

Phenothiazines (e.g., promethazine [Phenergan], chlorpromazine [Thorazine]) are 23 times more potent than procaine as a local anesthetic.[23] Chlorpromazine is effective as a local anesthetic at concentrations of between 0.1% and 0.2%. It has a wide safety margin, but should not be used with epinephrine. Even without a vasoconstrictor, it has a longer duration of action than most local anesthetics. One complication, orthostatic hypotension, usually occurs when chlorpromazine is used IV or in large doses.[24] Although it has significant local anesthetic properties, chlorpromazine has never been generally used as a local anesthetic in humans.[23-25]

Water

Sterile water is a suitable anesthetic. Known to our predecessors as "aquapuncture," this method uses unpreserved sterile water produced by simply boiling distilled water. As with other local anesthetic infiltration, injecting water works better on loose tissues and is less painful when the water is at body temperature and injected slowly. The analgesia lasts 10 to 15 minutes.[26]

Allen described the procedure he used: "To obtain the full analgesic effect, it is necessary to infiltrate the tissues to the point of producing a glassy edema, the skin or mucous membrane must be infiltrated intradermally and the infiltration carried down the full depth of the proposed incision; when this is done, analgesia is usually as profound as after infiltration with the weaker anesthetic solution, but tactility is little or not at all affected; the after-pain or discomfort is about the same as that following the use of other anesthetic solutions."[26]

Bacteriostatic Normal Saline

Benzyl alcohol, the preservative in bacteriostatic NS, is an ideal alternative local anesthetic. Inexpensive and readily available, bacteriostatic NS is frequently used to flush IV catheters and to dilute or reconstitute medications for parenteral use. Another formulation is to mix benzyl alcohol (0.9%) with 1:100,000 epinephrine by adding 0.2 mL epinephrine 1:1000 to a 20-mL vial of multidose NS solution containing benzyl alcohol 0.9%.[15] This formulation is less painful, but slightly less effective, than 0.9% buffered lidocaine. In children, the pain on injection is about the same as that with lidocaine.[27] Without epinephrine, the anesthetic effect of benzyl alcohol lasts only a few minutes; with epinephrine, anesthesia lasts about 20 minutes.[28]

Antidepressants

Some antidepressants, such as amitriptyline, have shown good activity as both topical and injectable anesthetics. When the need is desperate, these can be used, although questions about their safety preclude their use under normal circumstances.[29]

Narcotics

Neither morphine nor meperidine (Demerol, Pethidine) works well as a local anesthetic. They have a potency about half that of chlorpromazine and slightly less than that of promethazine.[25,30]

Cold/Freezing (Local Anesthesia)

Apply cold to tissues to produce either local or regional anesthesia. (See also "Refrigeration Anesthesia: Amputations" below in this chapter.)

Locally applied cold provides extremely short-acting superficial anesthesia for "stab" abscess drainages, venipunctures, injections, and similar procedures. If ice is used, it must be in direct contact with the skin for at least 10 seconds immediately before the procedure. The effect lasts only a few seconds.[31]

Cold sprays for local anesthesia were developed in the mid-19th century. Various substances with low boiling points can be used, including ether, and alcohol cooled to –23°C (–10°F).[32]

Ethyl chloride (chloroethane) spray effectively anesthetizes a very small area of intact skin for a few seconds—approximately enough time to do a stab incision for an abscess. It works by "freezing" the skin. Because of its potent and potentially dangerous general anesthetic effect with abuse potential, never use it on the mucosa. It is available commercially as a cleaner (e.g., for computer keyboards) and as a medical spray. This chemical is flammable and fires have occurred while using it with diathermy.[33] Tetrafluoroethane spray, used to remove dust from personal computers, can serve as a handy substitute.[34] (Don't inhale it; you'll pass out.)

Use an atomizer to spray ethyl chloride. Directions for two homemade atomizers are in Chapter 14. Hold the atomizer just far enough from the body part being anesthetized to maximize the amount of spray reaching the skin before dissipating. If held too far away, the spray evaporates without anesthetizing. Protect sensitive parts, such as the eyes and anus, before spraying the anesthetic on surrounding areas.

Pressure

Direct pressure over an area produces transient anesthesia. As Allen wrote in 1918, "The benumbing effect of long-continued pressure upon any part of the body is well known; although some pain may be produced in the surrounding parts, it is possible to carry it to a point of depressing both tactile and painful impressions to a considerable degree; this is brought about in two ways, first the compression directly paralyzes the nerve-endings of the part, and, secondly, the anemia [actually, tissue hypoxia] intensifies this effect."[35]

Local Infiltration Techniques

Injection

Inject the anesthetic slowly. This markedly diminishes the patient's discomfort. Using buffered lidocaine also decreases pain, as described previously.

Field Block

Use a simple field block for circumscribed lesions, such as cysts or small abscesses, and for larger structures, such as ears. Visualize a diamond surrounding the area to be anesthetized, and then inject two small wheals at the apex of the diamond (Fig. 15-1). Next, block the four sides of the diamond through those wheals.

Local wound infiltration is effective for inguinal and umbilical hernia surgery, dental procedures, strabismus (eyes) surgery, and burr holes/craniotomies.[36] For craniotomies, anesthetize the scalp surrounding the entire surgical area, as well as the underlying muscles and the periosteum (Fig. 15-2).[37] Use the greatest possible anesthetic dose, because the scalp is so vascular. Always use anesthetic with epinephrine.

Infiltrate-and-Cut Anesthesia

In situations where there is no alternative, almost any surgical procedure can be done by cutting through a site that has been locally infiltrated with anesthetic, with continued anesthetic injections given as the operation proceeds.

The Vishnevsky technique, an "inject-and-cut" procedure once employed extensively in Russia, is possibly the simplest use of local anesthetics, because no knowledge of anatomy is required. The technique works very well for surgery outside the abdomen and chest. Abdominal surgery is not quite as easy; it is simple enough to open the abdomen with this technique, but handling the viscera is a different matter. The technique is to inject unlimited volumes of weak procaine solutions (0.25% to 0.5%) without epinephrine. Procaine is the only completely safe anesthetic to use for this procedure, because it is metabolized very rapidly. Other local

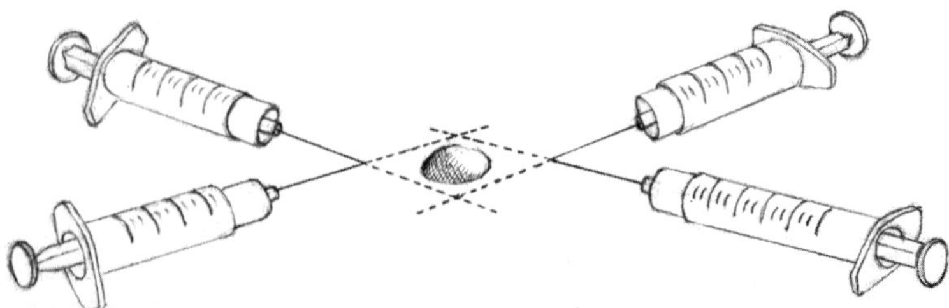

FIG. 15-1. "Diamond" block around lesion.

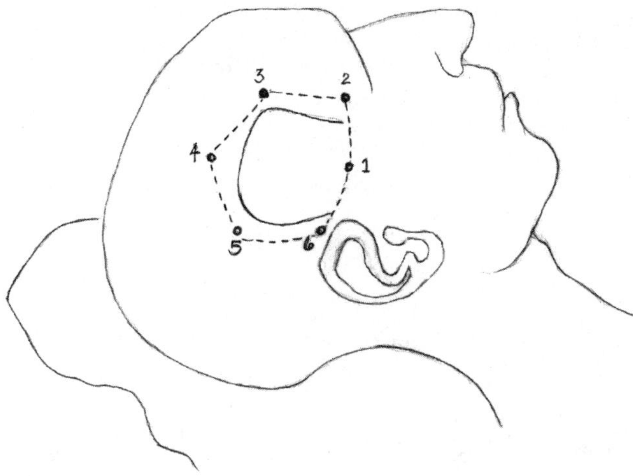

FIG. 15-2. Local anesthesia for craniotomy. *(Adapted from Allen.[37])*

anesthetics are metabolized more slowly, and the patient can become toxic.[38] If lidocaine is used, the limit is 200 mL of 0.25% lidocaine with adrenaline 1:500,000.

The primary danger of the Vishnevsky technique is inadvertent intravascular injection, which can be avoided by aspirating before injecting and keeping the needle moving.[39]

Premedication/Paramedication

Premedicating patients may be useful when giving either regional or general anesthesia. It reduces patient anxiety and often lessens the amount of anesthetic that is needed. The drugs used for premedication, such as benzodiazepines, phenothiazines (especially the commonly used promethazine), and barbiturates, are commonly available. Administer them orally, parenterally, or rectally.[40] Benzodiazepines and barbiturates have the added benefit of raising the seizure threshold.

Hypnosis, even if patients use a hypnosis recording, is effective as a premedication. The significant benefits of hypnosis include decreased anxiety, decreased blood pressure (BP), reduced blood loss, enhanced postoperative well-being, improved intestinal motility, shorter hospital stays, reduced postoperative nausea and vomiting, and a reduced need for analgesics.[41] Hypnotic techniques are described below in this chapter.

If patients become anxious or experience pain during a regional block or the subsequent procedure, give them an analgesic or an anxiolytic as paramedication. Commonly available paramedications include mild sedatives, opioids, and ketamine.

REGIONAL BLOCKS

Regional blocks are more problematic for inexperienced practitioners than infiltration anesthesia. Nevertheless, simple nerve blocks are effective for a wide variety of procedures and operations. The blocks described here will usually provide good analgesia, even when the practitioner does them for the first time. Note that this book is not designed to describe the wide variety of regional blocks, even though they are remarkable tools when resources are scarce. Find descriptions of many of the blocks you may need at the New York School of Regional Anesthesia's free website (www.nysora.com).

Scalp Block

All the nerves to the forehead and scalp run upward from about the line of the eyebrow anteriorly and from the base of the skull posteriorly. Therefore, to block a region above this line you need only to inject a horizontal line of anesthesia through this area.[42] The key is to make the anesthesia

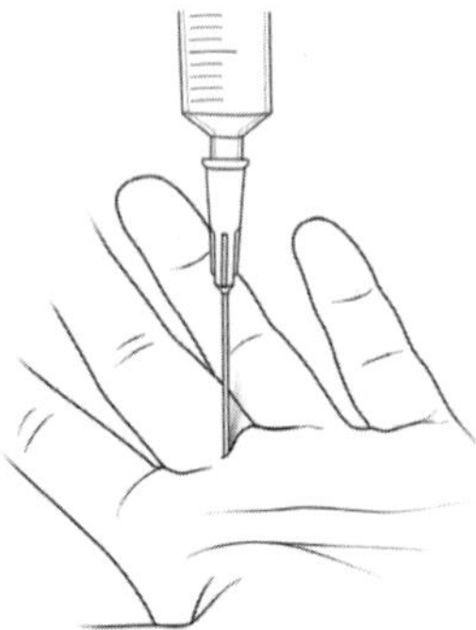

FIG. 15-3. Site of the SIMPLE block.

line long enough to block the cross innervation from nerves that are lateral to the site of injury. A good rule is to block both sides of the face or scalp for any lesion near the midline.

Single Subcutaneous Finger Block

The traditional finger and toe blocks (ring or intermetacarpal) involve at least two injections. The SIMPLE (single subcutaneous injection in the midline of the proximal phalanx with lidocaine and epinephrine) block is easier, faster, and simultaneously conserves anesthetic and reduces patient discomfort.[43] To do this block, inject about 2 to 3 mL lidocaine 1% with epinephrine 1:100,000 just above the tendon sheath at the midpoint of the crease where the finger joins the palm, on the volar (palmar) side (Fig. 15-3).[44] The block works on fingers and toes at least as well as traditional blocks. It may not, however, work as well on the thumb.[45]

Hematoma Block

A hematoma block can provide sufficient analgesia in the distal forearm and some areas of the face, such as the nose, to reduce fractures. Useful in both adults and children, it is easier to perform but is less effective for forearm fractures than is an IV regional block (e.g., intravenous regional anesthesia [IVRA], Bier block).[46] Nevertheless, if the necessary equipment or skilled personnel are unavailable to do IVRA, then a hematoma block offers a quick and easy method to obtain at least some, if not very good, anesthesia.

This block may be particularly useful in mass casualty situations, but it is not effective to treat fractures >24 hours old, because by then the hematoma has begun to organize.[38]

Technique

Palpate the fracture site and, under aseptic conditions, place the needle into the fracture hematoma. Aspirate to ensure that blood returns. Unlike other regional blocks, you want to aspirate blood before injecting to ensure that the needle is in, and that the anesthetic can diffuse through, the fracture hematoma. Then, very slowly inject 5 to 10 mL of 2% lidocaine without epinephrine. Buffered lidocaine may cause less pain than unbuffered solution.

The block should take effect in approximately 5 minutes. This technique, useful both in adults and children, is most successful when applied as soon as possible after injury, because clotted blood will limit the spread of the analgesic. Infection is not a hazard if sterile solutions and apparatus are used and adequate skin preparation employed.[39] The US military has found it occasionally useful to use ultrasound to locate the hematoma and guide needle placement.

Intra-Articular Anesthesia

If anesthesia (other than hypnosis) is needed to reduce a shoulder dislocation, an easy technique is to inject 20 mL of 1% plain lidocaine into the joint.[47,48] This must be done under aseptic conditions. The technique is remarkably simple, because the joint space is easily identified (it's where the shoulder used to be) and accessible. However, multiple studies have demonstrated that this technique usually has a lower success rate than IV sedation.[49]

Intravenous Regional Anesthesia

Intravenous regional anesthesia (IVRA) involves administering a local anesthetic into an upper or lower extremity while blocking arterial flow and venous return with an inflated cuff.[50] Used for more than 100 years, the technique is successful in >95% of cases. The advantages of this block, especially in austere situations, are that it is easy to perform; is not dependent on anatomical knowledge; requires minimal personnel; avoids the potential side effects of general anesthesia and systemic sedation; provides rapid and complete anesthesia, muscle relaxation, and a bloodless field; and is very safe.[51,52] Disadvantages include the limited duration of anesthesia (60 minutes), the relatively large dose of local anesthetic required, and the fact that it provides no postoperative analgesia.

Method

Place an IV line in the hand or the foot, depending on which extremity requires anesthesia. Place one or, preferably, two inflatable cuffs over padding on the proximal extremity, and secure them by wrapping them with strong adhesive tape so they do not accidentally come off when inflated. Then exsanguinate the extremity by lifting it straight up and wrapping it tightly, starting distally and moving proximally, with an Esmarch or other elastic bandage. If placement of an elastic bandage on the extremity is too painful due to trauma, compress the axillary or femoral artery for 5 minutes with the extremity elevated.

While the extremity is still elevated and wrapped, inflate the most proximal cuff to well above arterial pressure (palpated at the distal extremity) or, if there is an attached manometer, to 100 mm Hg above systolic BP and to at least 250 mm Hg. Use a hemostat to clamp the inflation tube on the cuff, because the valves tend to leak (Fig. 15-4).

Remove the constricting bandage on the extremity and slowly inject (60 to 90 seconds) 0.5 mL/kg 0.5% lidocaine, without preservative or epinephrine for upper extremity procedures; use 1 mL/kg for the lower extremity.[39,53] (Do not use >4 mg/kg lidocaine: For a 70-kg patient, the maximum dose is 280 mg or 56 mL of 0.5% lidocaine.) The limb becomes blanched. At that point, inflate the more distal cuff, which is now over an anesthetized area, to the same pressure as the first cuff and deflate the first cuff. This usually reduces the patient's discomfort from the tourniquet.

Tourniquet pain usually begins about 20 minutes after single tourniquet inflation, although this can be delayed by using adjuvant medications (described in the subsequent text). Using the second, more distal tourniquet, significant pain typically occurs about 40 minutes after

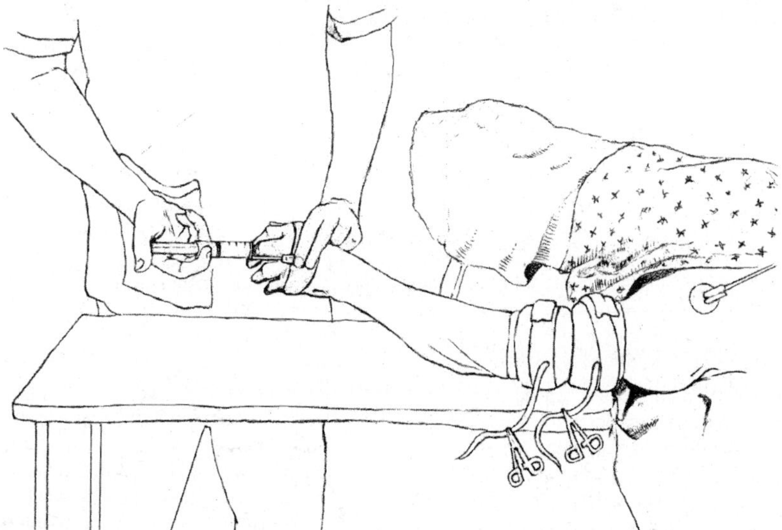

FIG. 15-4. Intravenous regional anesthesia using two blood pressure cuffs with tape wrapped around them for safety.

tourniquet inflation.[54] Tourniquet pain is usually the limiting factor for how long the block can be used.[50] There is also a minimum time for the tourniquet to remain in place. To prevent toxic effects from the anesthetic, do not release the tourniquet for at least 20 minutes after the injection, even if the procedure has been completed in less time. After 20 minutes, release the tourniquet for 5 seconds and reinflate it for 30 seconds three or four times. This permits a gradual release of the anesthetic into the circulation.

Because of the rapid reperfusion of the limb after tourniquet deflation, IVRA has typically provided minimal analgesia after surgery. Postoperative analgesia has traditionally been a major advantage of brachial plexus analgesia compared to IVRA.

This technique is contraindicated in patients with peripheral artery or sickle cell disease, with hypersensitivity to the anesthetic (although an alternative can be used), and with cellulitis at the injection site.[55]

Alternate/Improvised Methods

Improvised IVRA equipment can be fashioned from two normal BP cuffs, enough adhesive tape to wrap completely around the cuffs several times so they don't "pop" off during the procedures, clamps for the BP cuff tubing so it doesn't leak during the procedure, an elastic bandage or similar elastic cloth (such as nylon stockings) to help exsanguinate the arm, an IV, a syringe, and the medications.

If BP cuffs are not available, you can use other cuffs, such as those often used to pressurize IV fluids. If there is no inflatable cuff, wrap a wide tourniquet around the extremity and use a dowel as a windlass to tighten it (similar to the tourniquets described in Chapter 24). The absence of a distal pulse that was previously palpable determines when arterial pressure has been exceeded. Carefully secure the windlass so it does not accidentally unwind during the procedure.

Forearm tourniquets may be an option for some distal upper extremity procedures. Several advantages are evident. Forearm tourniquet pain occurs later and is less severe than with an upper arm tourniquet. In addition, approximately 50% less local anesthetic solution can be used with a forearm tourniquet, lowering the risk of toxicity. Finally, only half the amount of any adjuvant medication needs to be used to prolong the anesthetic effect or to decrease tourniquet pain.[39,54] Calf tourniquets work well for foot and ankle anesthesia. Use them in a similar manner to a forearm tourniquet. Concerns regarding increased risk of nerve injury or poor tourniquet function with a forearm tourniquet have never been substantiated.[54]

For very short foot or hand/wrist cases, a "super-low" IVRA method is applicable. Prepare the patient as usual and inflate the cuff on the upper arm or upper leg. Just before injecting the anesthetic, place a 2-cm wide rubber tourniquet, like the ones used to draw blood, above the wrist or ankle. Use about half the amount of anesthetic that would normally be injected for a standard IVRA. Both the upper leg and the upper arm tourniquet can be removed within 10 minutes. The benefit is that less anesthetic is used.[56] The drawback may be pain from the tourniquet.

Alternative Anesthetics

A number of other anesthetics can be used if lidocaine is not available. Prilocaine seems to be the safest, although it is no longer widely unavailable. When bupivacaine, rather than lidocaine, is used for Bier blocks, the block's onset is slower, but analgesia is continued for 3 to 4 hours into the postoperative period.[54,57] Alternative anesthetics used for IVRA are listed in Table 15-2.

Adjuvant Medications

A number of medications can be added to the injected solution to reduce the tourniquet and postprocedure pain associated with IVRA. They also decrease the amount of anesthetic needed.

Ketamine 0.1 mg/kg added to the anesthetic solution dramatically reduces tourniquet pain and decreases the need for paramedication during IVRA. Ketorolac (0.1 to 0.02 mg/kg, up to 20 mg) added during a standard IVRA reduces tourniquet pain and also provides 12 to 16 hours of postoperative analgesia; there is no further benefit with larger doses. Using a forearm tourniquet, 10 mg ketorolac IVRA provides even better postoperative analgesia than 20 mg of ketorolac does with an upper arm tourniquet.[54]

TABLE 15-2 Local Anesthetics for Intravenous Regional Anesthesia

Anesthetic	Concentration (%)	Volume (mL)	Dose (mg/kg)	Severe Adverse Effects
Prilocaine	0.5-1	40-50	3-4	Methemoglobinemia
Lidocaine	0.25-0.5	40-50	3	Seizures
Bupivacaine	0.25-0.5	40-50	1.5-3	Cardiac arrest
Chloroprocaine	0.25-2	40-50	8	Thrombophlebitis
Ropivacaine	0.2-0.375	40-50	1.2-1.8	Seizures

Adapted with permission from Barry et al.[55]

Adding clonidine (1 to 2 mcg/kg) to IVRA significantly reduces tourniquet and postoperative pain. While better than local anesthetic alone, it is a less effective adjunct than ketamine.[54,55,58] Narcotics should not be added. It is not clear that they are beneficial and all produce nausea, vomiting, and dizziness when the cuff is deflated.[54]

Abdominal Operations

Several options are available to provide anesthesia for abdominal surgery other than using general anesthetics. These include abdominal field blocks, spinal or caudal blocks, local infiltration, and "tie and cry." The benefit is that these methods may avoid the need to use muscle relaxants and controlled respiration, which may not be possible with the available resources. These techniques are particularly valuable for operations in the lower abdomen.

Intra-abdominal

Local Abdominal Anesthesia

When patients are very ill and equipment, skills, or both are in short supply, consider using local anesthesia plus appropriate preanesthetic medication to do abdominal procedures. (Also see the Vishnevsky technique, discussed above.) Allen wrote, "All simple operations, such as gastrostomy, gastrotomy, colostomy, appendectomy, and gallbladder drainage, are quite satisfactorily performed on suitable subjects (when not too nervous or apprehensive) when the parts are fairly easily accessible, and not matted down by inflammation or adhesions to the parietal peritoneum or surrounding organs."[59]

Thin patients with relaxed abdominal walls are ideal for this type of anesthesia. However, "as a general rule all very stout individuals and those with tense rigid abdominal walls are difficult to handle in any serious intra-abdominal operation, for as soon as the abdomen is opened the contents bulge out."[59] During laparotomies using only a local anesthetic block, patients sense a vague intra-abdominal weight or fullness that becomes crampy if the surgeon puts traction or pressure on the internal organs. If you encounter an inflamed appendix or diseased gall bladder while using local anesthetic for a midline incision, make a separate incision to take them out rather than displacing them toward the midline.[59]

Field Block

Use a rectus muscle block to provide anesthesia for a laparotomy incision. This can be combined with sedation or light general anesthesia. To do the block, place anesthetic beneath the rectus muscle in each of its 10 compartments (5 on each side). Using a 20-gauge, 5-cm needle, enter the abdominal wall through anesthetic skin wheals (marked * in Fig. 15-5) raised at the center of each compartment. After aspirating, inject 10 mL of 0.5% lidocaine with 1:500,000 epinephrine at each site. Insert the needle vertically into each compartment, feeling the resistance from the anterior sheath as it is penetrated. After traversing the muscle, resistance from the posterior sheath is felt. At that point, after aspirating, inject the anesthetic. Infiltrate a midline or paramedian surgical incision line with 0.25% lidocaine with 1:500,000 epinephrine. This only blocks the abdominal wall for the incision. Blocking visceral reflexes requires the surgeon to block the vagus and the splanchnic plexus once the abdomen is open and the viscera mobilized.[39]

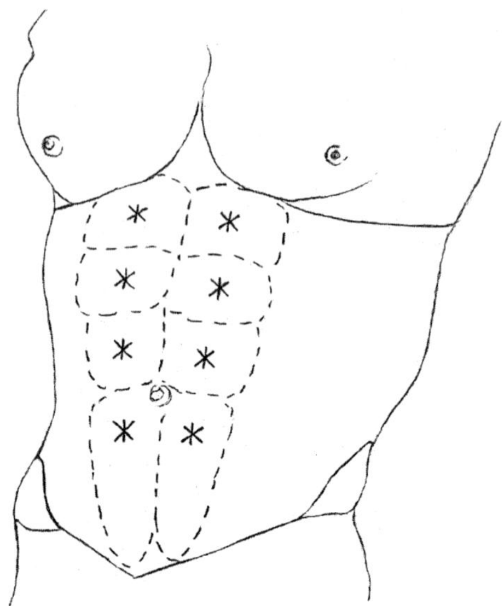

FIG. 15-5. Anesthetic for abdominal incision.

BRAUN'S METHOD

Another method to anesthetize the abdominal wall for an abdominal midline incision is to inject around the field in a more-or-less rhomboid shape (Fig. 15-6, method illustrated on upper abdomen). Inject anesthetic two or three fingerbreadths on each side of the midline. Starting on this line,

> At two or more points, depending upon the extent of the proposed incision, a long needle is directed obliquely outward, injecting as it is advanced, piercing the rectus sheath, which is recognized by its slight resistance to the needle, and advancing some little distance within this muscle until it is quite freely injected; the needle is then partially withdrawn,

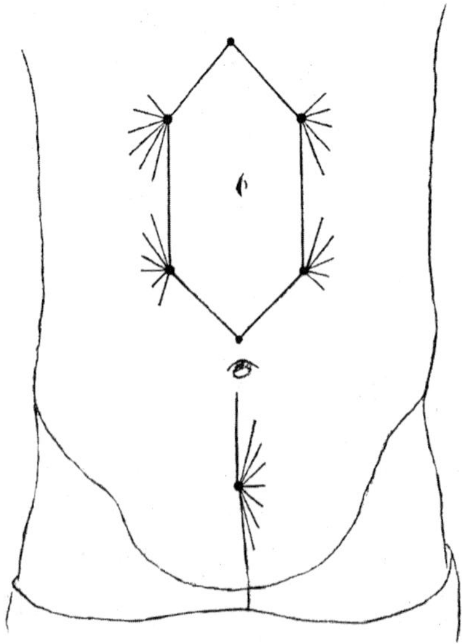

FIG. 15-6. Abdominal infiltration for laparotomy. (Braun's method is illustrated superiorly; Allan's method, inferiorly).

when it is advanced again in two or more directions above and below, slightly increasing the angle each time, thus making the injection in something of a fan-like shape; this is done along the line of cutaneous anesthesia at two or more points, having the fan-like areas of infiltration come in contact with the one above or below. The same procedure is repeated on the opposite side. These two lateral lines of infiltration are joined above and below by subcutaneous infiltration.[59]

Allen's Method

While Braun's method works well in thin subjects, a better technique in obese patients is to establish a wall of anesthesia along the proposed incision line from the skin to the peritoneum. Raise an intradermal wheal midway along the proposed incision line. Insert a long needle through the wheal and liberally inject anesthetic superiorly and inferiorly, and then into the rectus sheath on either side (Fig. 15-6, method illustrated on lower abdomen). As with the other methods, make deeper injections once the abdomen is open.[59]

Inguinal Hernia Repair

Inguinal hernia repair is very common in non-Western countries. As one group of surgeons wrote, "Local anesthesia has been identified as the most favorable anesthesia for elective inguinal hernia repair with respect to complication rate, cost-effectiveness, and overall patient satisfaction.... All surgeons in resource-poor countries should be encouraged to use local anesthesia more frequently for elective inguinal hernia repair. Valuable resources in sub-Saharan African hospital could be saved, especially if used in combination with outpatient surgery."[60]

The simplest anesthetic technique for inguinal and femoral hernia repair is for the surgeon to continuously infiltrate the area of incision, then directly infiltrate the neck of the sac.[39] This infiltrate-and-cut, or Vishnevsky, technique was described above in this chapter.

Amid and colleagues describe a more precise method of using local anesthesia for elective hernia repair: (a) subdermal infiltration along the line of incision (~5 mL), (b) intradermal injection along the line of incision (~3 mL), (c) deep subcutaneous injection (~10 mL), (d) subfascial infiltration immediately underneath the aponeurosis of the external oblique to anesthetize all three major subfascial nerves (~8 to 10 mL), (e) pubic tubercle and hernia sac injection—as much as required for complete anesthesia, and (f) splashing local anesthetic into the canal and in the subcutaneous space before closing to reduce postoperative pain (optional).[61]

Tie-and-Cry/Burrito and "Superhero Cape" Methods

Tie-and-cry anesthesia may be the safest way of anaesthetizing a child if there is no access to either special pediatric anesthesia equipment or ketamine. The general principle is that if your skills are limited, do only what is safe for the child. In many places in the world, physical restraint is still the most common technique during painful emergency procedures.[62]

Two methods seem to work to restrain a child. The first, "tie-and-cry," entails wrapping the child in a sheet like a burrito (Fig. 15-7) or tying the arms and legs to splints or to a papoose board. Secure the child's limbs, but provide access to the airway, chest, and abdomen. The descriptive name for this procedure comes from the child remaining at least partly conscious and crying.

The second method, referred to as the "superhero cape," is often easier to accomplish and more successful at immobilizing the child's arms. First, remove the child's clothes, shoes, and socks. Then, help the child put his arms into a pillowcase behind his back, with the open end at the top (Fig. 15-8A). While the child may cooperate with this because the action is similar to putting his arms into the sleeves of a jacket, also suggest that he is putting his arms in a cape so that he can "fly like a superhero." Then, help the child lay down on the stretcher over a folded sheet that has been placed horizontally (Fig. 15-8B). Roll the child to one side and tuck the sheet on that side behind their back. (Fig. 15-8C). Finally, roll the child to the other side, tucking the sheet under the opposite side.[63]

Abdominal Procedures—Sedation and Local Anesthesia in Children

While seemingly barbaric, when no anesthetists exist, the safest anesthesia for an abdominal operation in a child weighing >15 kg is to use an intramuscular (IM) injection of midazolam

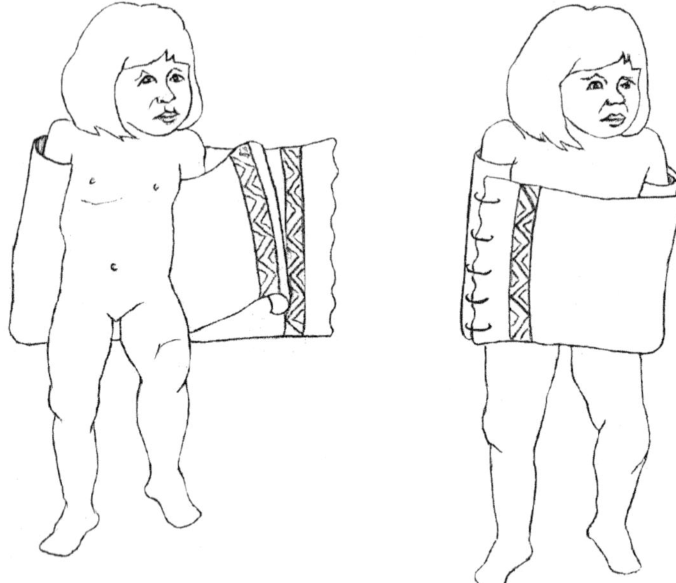

FIG. 15-7. Tie-and-cry restraint with sheet.

0.15 mg/kg or lorazepam 0.05 mg/kg. (Intramuscular diazepam has erratic absorption.) Combine this mild sedation with local lidocaine infiltration, being careful not to exceed the maximum safe dose.

As previously noted, the problem with this technique is that returning the intestines to the peritoneal cavity may be difficult because the abdominal muscles are not relaxed. As King wrote, "Such anesthesia is far from ideal, but when anesthetic skills really are minimal, it probably gives the child the best chance of living. It really is a procedure for desperate emergencies only."[64]

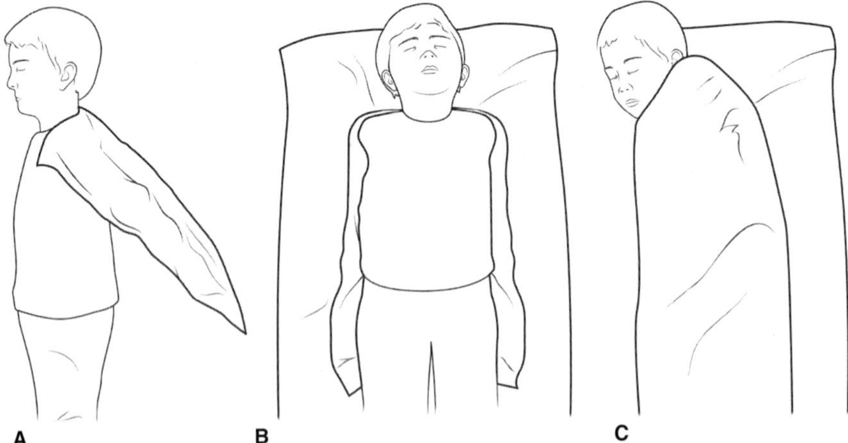

FIG. 15-8. (A) Insert the child's arms into the pillowcase behind their back. (B) Lay the child over a sheet placed horizontally on the bed. (C) Roll the child to one side and tuck the sheet on that side behind their back.

Fascia-Iliaca (Ilio-fascial) Block

The fascia-iliaca compartment block (FICB) is an excellent method to relieve pain from a fractured hip and, in many cases, knee pain. Unlike the 3-in-1 block, the FICB is simpler to perform, safer (being distant from any major structures), faster acting, and more effective (at least in adults) for simultaneously blocking the lateral femoral cutaneous nerve of the thigh and the femoral nerves.[65] It is ideal for austere situations, because it can easily be done by novices, and remedies the difficult problem of analgesia without monitoring for fractured hips and femurs. Studies have demonstrated its safety and effectiveness in the prehospital setting[66] and its superiority over standard systemic pain control in the pediatric emergency setting.[67]

To do the block, place the patient in the supine position and identify the inguinal ligament. Prepare the skin and drape the site. Identify the (imaginary) line that joins the middle of the pubic tubercle to the anterior superior iliac spine. Find the point 1 cm below the juncture of the lateral and medial two-thirds of that line. Insert a 21-gauge, 2-inch injection needle perpendicular to the skin at that point (Fig. 15-9). Insert the needle until you feel a loss of resistance as the needle passes through the fascia lata. Keep advancing the needle until a second loss of resistance occurs as the fascia iliaca is pierced (often described as two "pops"). With an attached syringe, first aspirate to exclude intravascular injection, and then inject approximately 0.3 mL/kg of 0.25 bupivacaine or 1% lidocaine.[65]

Foot/Ankle Blocks

Because, in my experience, most clinicians cannot remember the intricacies of foot and ankle blocks, I teach the following simple method. Blocking completely around the ankle at the level of the top of the malleoli (along with one deep injection to block the hallux [big toe] if necessary) completely blocks the entire foot.

A 4-cm long, 23-gauge needle works for all injections. Low concentrations of local anesthetic (e.g., 0.25% bupivacaine) will suffice in most cases, because it is necessary to block only the smaller sensory nerves.[17]

All five nerves can be blocked with the patient supine, although it is often easier to block the posterior tibial and sural nerves with the patient prone and the foot hanging off the end of the stretcher. To block the posterior tibial nerve in a supine position, flex the knee and place the ankle on top of the contralateral shin. This allows access to the medial and lateral malleolus.

Plantar (Sole) Surface

All ankle blocks are at the level of superior portion ("top") of the malleoli. Enter at the border of the Achilles tendon and aim the needle toward the tibia (medially) and fibula (laterally). If the

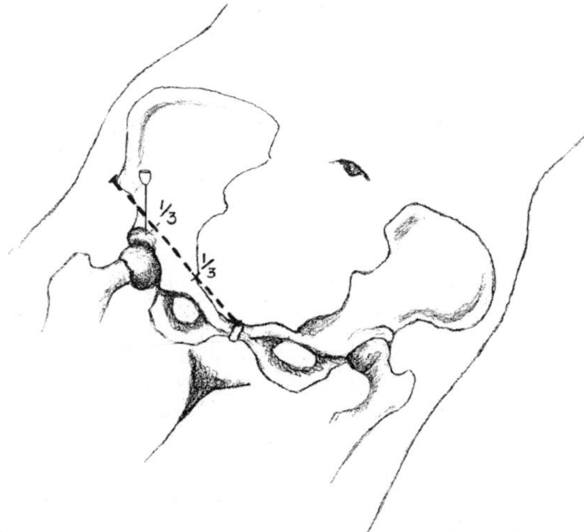

FIG. 15-9. Insertion point for the fascia-iliaca compartment block.

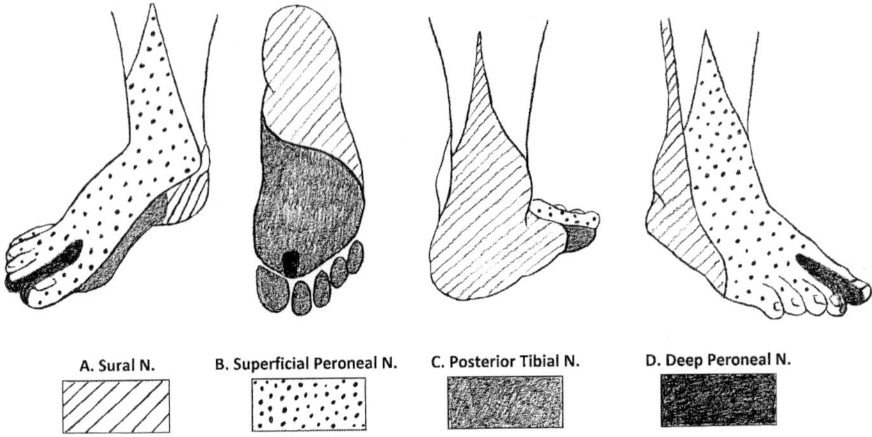

FIG. 15-10. Ankle and foot block anesthetic areas (A-D).

patient gets paresthesia with either insertion, withdraw the needle slightly and inject 3 to 5 mL of a local anesthetic, such as 0.25% bupivacaine. If not, for posterior tibial infiltrations (Fig. 15-10, shading C), advance the needle until it contacts the tibia, withdraw 0.5 cm, and inject 5 to 7 mL of anesthetic. For the sural nerve (Fig. 15-10, shading A), if the patient does not experience paresthesia, advance to the fibula and inject 5 to 7 mL as you withdraw the needle to the skin.

Dorsum of the Foot

The three other blocks, all done from one injection site, anesthetize the dorsum of the foot. For all three blocks, insert the needle 1 cm lateral to the extensor hallucis longus tendon or just lateral to the anterior tibial artery, if it can be palpated.

To block the deep peroneal nerve (blocking the area between the hallux and second toe; see Fig. 15-10, shading D), insert the needle at 90 degrees to the skin and inject 3 to 5 mL of 0.25% bupivacaine deep to the fascia on either side of the tibial artery. This is an important block for any surgery on the hallux, such as removing an ingrown toenail.

For the superficial peroneal nerve (most of the dorsal surface of the foot; see Fig. 15-10, shading B), withdraw the needle to just below the skin surface and aim it toward the lateral malleolus. Inject 5 mL subcutaneously between the lateral malleolus and the anterior border of the tibia.

To block the saphenous nerve (the medial malleolus area), inject 5 mL as the needle progresses toward the medial malleolus, trying not to enter the saphenous vein.[17]

Acupuncture

Acupuncture works well in the hands of clinicians with superb training in the technique. However, that is not true for treatment from those who dabble in it. Although the only necessary equipment is needles, the real requirement is skill and practice. Unfortunately, acupuncture is not a technique that a novice can improvise.

REFRIGERATION ANESTHESIA: AMPUTATIONS

Background

Direct application of cold to a body part can produce temporary anesthesia. For example, Baron Larrey, Napoleon's chief surgeon, reported that soldiers' wounds barely hurt and that amputations were "practically painless" if the limbs were exposed to the cold air. (The ambient temperature at the Battle of Eylau, February 1807, was –28°C [–18.4°F].) Arnott first used ice bags with salt to anesthetize limbs during surgery. In most settings, ice bags are preferable to, and more readily available than, cold exposure, although both work. Cooling also intensifies the action of all local anesthetics.[32]

In the early 1940s, surgeons at major US hospitals and in the US Navy found that they could perform lower extremity amputations on elderly and unstable patients using ice for intraoperative anesthesia and postoperative analgesia.[68]

Use

The following method provides complete surgical anesthesia for about 1 hour. The anesthesia is sufficient to perform extremity amputations without pain.[69,70]

This method is not truly a "freezing" technique, because the temperature of ice is 0°C (32°F), and a body's tissues have a freezing point below 0°C. In addition, a film of water at 0°C, rather than the ice, is in contact with the skin. After the ice has been applied for four hours, the skin temperature measures 20°C.[69]

Most often used on patients with infected or gangrenous limbs, refrigeration anesthesia has proved to be a safe option in aged and high-risk patients. Patients with ischemic limbs do the best with the technique, because the cooling does not drop their core temperature. (Little of the extremity's cold blood ever circulates. That is why the limb is being amputated.) Using this procedure, the general diabetic status of the patients did not deteriorate, even when the amputations were done through infected areas. The patients did well postoperatively, and they were usually hungry and ate soon after the operation. They generally had no appreciable change in their vital signs during refrigeration, the operative procedure, or postoperatively. Overall, the mortality and morbidity in these patients were reduced at the major hospitals using this method.[69]

Adjunctive Meds

Little adjunctive analgesia is necessary for this procedure. Some protocols routinely administer a narcotic before doing anything. In some cases, narcotics were administered as the leg was being manipulated or immediately after preoperative tourniquet placement, but that was rarely necessary.[68,69,71]

Nearly all patients experienced pain during only the first 15 to 20 minutes after immersion in the ice pack, before the extremity got numb. After this period, the patient often read, rested, or slept.[71]

Preparing for Refrigeration

Because the basic idea is to immerse the extremity in ice, a suitable container is needed. For feet and ankles, use a bucket. For more proximal surgery, a metal tank with a removable lid to add ice and a padded hole through which to place the leg is required. (A wooden box or a rubber bag—such as a body bag—can also be used, but these will deteriorate with repeated use.) The metal troughs (Fig. 15-11) have a round padded (with sponges or rubber) opening at their upper end, with a sliding top through which the extremity is inserted. At the lower end of the tank, there is a hole for drainage with a spigot, which can be closed when en route to the operating room.[68,71]

To prepare the supine patient, first protect his or her bed with a full-length rubber sheet and place a thin blanket under him or her for warmth.[71] Then elevate the limb and apply three bags of cracked ice to an area just above where the amputation is to occur. Secure them with a dressing; leave them in place for 15 minutes. This is where a tourniquet will be applied. Just before the 15 minutes are up, apply an Esmarch (or other elastic) bandage from above the area of inflammation to the tourniquet site.[68,69] Then immediately remove the ice bags, put cotton batting or a bandage over area to protect the skin, and apply the tourniquet.

Tourniquet

Wrap rubber tourniquets around the limb twice and secure with a surgical clamp. Some physicians apply two tourniquets, in case one loosens. Once the tourniquet is in place, remove the Esmarch bandage.[68] The tightness of constriction necessary to stop circulation differs with the patient, the location on the limb, and other variables. Difficulties seem to be less in the thigh, in spite of its thickness, than in the upper part of the calf, where the main artery is protected between bones.[70] It is unclear whether the tourniquet should be placed close to the amputation site so as to leave the narrowest possible zone of chilled and bloodless tissue, or whether it can be placed higher, for example, above the knee for amputation through the calf.

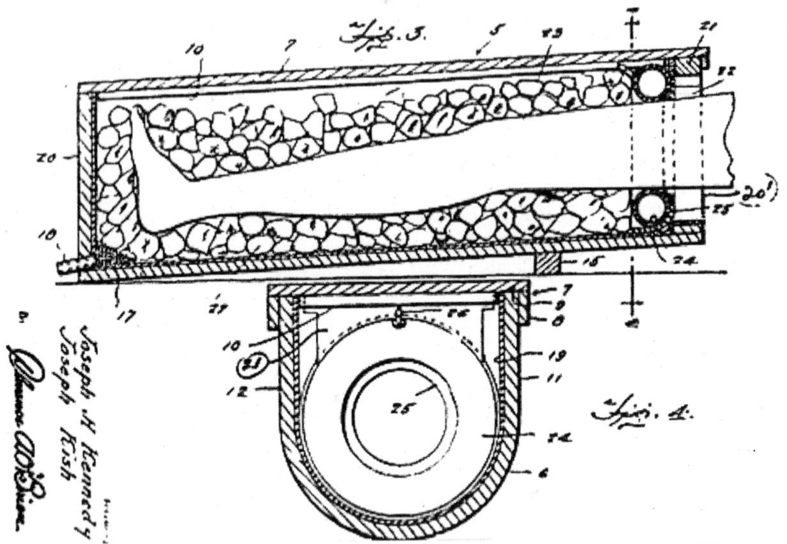

FIG. 15-11. Sagittal and transverse sections of ice trough. *(Reproduced from Kennedy.[68])*

Ice

Immediately after the application of the tourniquet, immerse the extremity in ice. If patients can sit up, those needing amputations of the foot and lower leg can immerse the area in a bucket of ice water and cracked ice. For amputations of the thigh, pack the extremity in finely cracked ice with the patient lying in bed and, usually, in one of the troughs described previously.

Using the trough, place a thin layer of chipped ice (approximately 1 to 2 inches deep) in the bottom. Gently place the leg on the ice, taking care that no sharp pieces pierce the skin. Place the tank as high into the groin as possible, using the padding for protection. Protect the genitals with a bath blanket or Turkish towel. Cover the entire limb with crushed ice (about 150 lbs is sufficient). The ice must extend to 2 inches above the tourniquet. Because of the size and awkward shape of the trough, it is difficult to anesthetize the upper thigh. However, you can form a pouch by pulling a rubber draw sheet through the hole in the upper end and then fill it with ice.[68,69,71]

Raise the head of the bed by placing small blocks under the bed frame at that end; this tilts the bed and facilitates drainage from the foot of the bed (Fig. 15-12). The bevel in the ice container at the proximal end may be used as a urinal or bedpan.[68] Place hot water bottles (49°C [120°F]) around the genitals and along the unaffected leg to protect them from the cold. Use care to prevent burning the patient. Remake the top of the bed with a bath blanket next to the patient.[71]

Because the metal tank "sweats," wrap it in a large rubber sheet with a hole connected to a tube going to the bucket at the foot of the bed.[71] Completely cover the tank by drawing the large rubber sheet around it.

It is prudent to inspect the limb one or more times 20 or 30 minutes after beginning refrigeration. Blanching of the foot is the rule, especially if the leg was elevated before applying the tourniquet. If any sizable arteries remain open, the foot will be darkly cyanosed, and the tourniquet should be readjusted. Any influx of blood makes for incompleteness or delay of anesthesia.[70]

The optimum length of preoperative refrigeration varied with the amputation level. In the typically thin, weak patients with arteriosclerosis, the optimum length of preoperative limb refrigeration for amputations at the thigh was 2 to 2.5 hours;[68-70] for disarticulation at the knee or through the middle of the leg, 2 hours; for the lower half of the leg or the foot, 1.5 hours;[69,70] and for the metatarsus or the toes, 1 hour.[70] The limbs were examined at intervals, and ice was added as necessary.

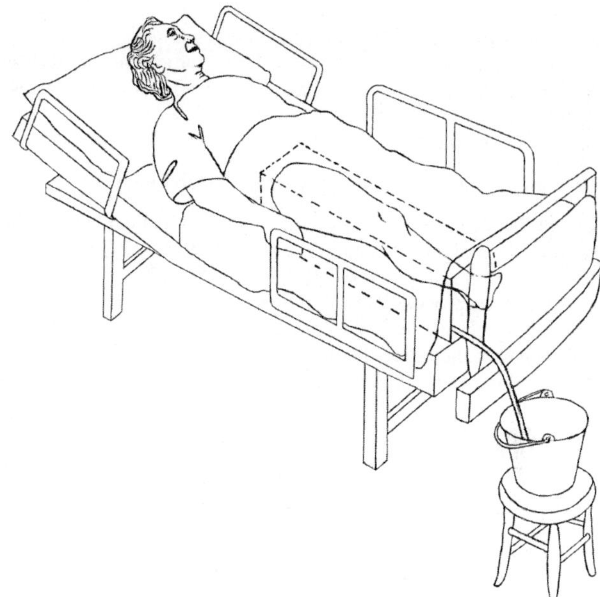

FIG. 15-12. Ice-box drainage system. *(Redrawn from Van Blarcom.[71])*

Operating Room

Bring the patient to the operating room with the extremity in ice.[69,71]

When the surgical team is ready, place the patient on the table and unpack his or her extremity from the ice. Remove the limb from the ice, dry it off, and it is ready for amputation. Do not remove the tourniquet, but prepare the extremity as usual and amputate. If the tourniquet is properly applied and securely fastened and the chilling is continuous to all parts at the correct temperature, there is complete local anesthesia so that the patient is not aware when the nerve is cut or the bone is sawed.[70]

After removing the limb, ligate the large vessels, remove the tourniquet, and then ligate other small bleeders. It is imperative to use cold instruments and cold NS solution in the procedure. About half of the cases are closed without drains. In the face of definite infection, the stump can either be drained or be left open.[69]

Postoperative Care

The usual dressing consists of one layer of petroleum jelly gauze across the wound, then a few layers of dry gauze, surrounded by bare ice bags. For example, place one bag beneath the stump and two sloping tent-like bags at the sides to avoid pressure on the limb.[70] Pain can usually be controlled with the ice bags and a small bandage over the incision.[69]

The nurses should prepare the routine postoperative bed for the patient, who is often placed in a semi-Fowler's position immediately. Because no nausea or shock is present, the patient can immediately begin progressing to a normal diet.[71]

Gradually warm the wound over several postoperative days. One method to raise the temperature is to make the dressings a little thicker each day.[70] Another is to apply three ice bags to the stump for the first 24 hours, then two ice bags for the second 24 hours, and one ice bag for the third postoperative day.[68]

Both the degree and the duration of cooling are entirely empiric, guided by the wound's appearance.[70] The warming time for the extremity depends on the blood supply and the degree of infection present. In the presence of good blood supply, remove the ice bags in 24 hours. Infection lengthens the time of postoperative thawing.[69] Sutures are normally left in for an unusually long time, because healing is slowed proportionally with the low temperature.[70]

Crossman and colleagues found that no harm was caused by either the duration or the extent of refrigeration. Tourniquet marks were visible for a day or two without significance; neither contractures nor paralysis was seen. Likewise, there was no sign of thrombosis or other damage to blood vessels, and no special tendency to necrosis or infection indicating lowered tissues resistance.[70]

TESTING AN ANESTHETIC BLOCK

Testing an anesthetic block is a two-edged sword. Boulton advised that

> Elaborate testing of the block with needles is undesirable. A patient will tolerate a surgical incision felt by him as light touch on a numb area and will be surprised and pleased when he is told that the operation is in progress but, if he is repeatedly asked, 'do you feel that', before or at the start of the procedure, he will give a positive answer even if he feels only the slightest sensation because he loses confidence thinking that the doctor himself is unsure of the efficiency of the block. Testing should be surreptitious; if a needle is boldly inserted through the skin of the surgical area, and the patient does not react, all is well![39]

In practice, minimal testing, such as touching the skin with the back of the scalpel at the incision point, allows the patient an opportunity to receive additional anesthetic, if needed.

SPINAL ANESTHESIA

Spinal anesthesia is an excellent, safe technique that has a wide range of uses, especially in austere situations. One caution in hypovolemic or seriously ill patients is that spinal blocks cause vasodilation. A rule of thumb is first to give patients 500 to 1000 mL NS (0.9%). At that point, if a patient's pulse rate is higher than their systolic BP, do not use this technique.[72]

Spinal anesthesia is one procedure you might not be willing to do without prior experience. Non-anesthesiologists who have experience performing lumbar punctures (spinal taps) may be able to provide anesthesia with these blocks with little difficulty. Administering epidural blocks requires some prior hands-on experience under supervision.

Medications for Spinal Anesthesia

Local anesthetic agents are either heavier (hyperbaric) or have the same specific gravity (isobaric) as the cerebral spinal fluid (CSF). Hyperbaric solutions tend to spread down (due to gravity) from the level of the injection, while isobaric solutions do not. It is easier to predict the spread of spinal anesthesia when using a hyperbaric agent. Add dextrose to make isobaric preparations hyperbaric.

Any medication injected into the thecal space must be taken from a previously unopened vial. Do not use anesthetics from multidose vials, because they contain potentially harmful preservatives, and solutions may be infected from prior use.

Lidocaine and bupivacaine are commonly used for spinal anesthesia, although tetracaine and procaine are used occasionally if the procedures are very short (procaine) or very long (tetracaine). They usually come as regular (isobaric) or "heavy" (hyperbaric) solutions (Table 15-3). Administering increasing amounts of the same anesthetic preparation results in higher levels being blocked.[73] The amount of anesthetic needed varies with the medication used, the level to be blocked, and whether the medication is isobaric or hyperbaric. Even with the same amount and type of medication, however, the level blocked varies with the patient's position and characteristics (age, height, weight, pregnancy, sex), site and speed of injection, and direction of the needle's bevel.[74] Table 15-4 lists typical types of solutions and patient positions to block the appropriate levels for several typical surgical procedures.

If available, isobaric bupivacaine 0.5% is best for lower limb surgery. It provides longer anesthesia than lidocaine. Hyperbaric 0.5% lidocaine or bupivacaine is useful for lower abdominal and pelvic/urogenital surgery. Add 5% glucose (D_5W) to the anesthetic to make the heavy solution, if it is not premixed. As they are dependent on gravity, hyperbaric medications localize based on the patient's position.

A number of alternative local anesthetics can be used for spinal anesthesia. If standard solutions are not available, modifying some of these medications with epinephrine, dextrose, or NS may be necessary.

TABLE 15-3 Medications for Spinal Anesthesia

Hyperbaric (Heavy)	Isobaric (Regular)	Dose (mg)[a]	Usual Volume (mL)[a]	Time Until Block Effects Diminish (min)	Time Until Block Effects Are Gone (min)
Tetracaine 0.5% in 5% dextrose	Tetracaine 0.5% in NS	5-20	1-4	90-140	240-380
Bupivacaine 0.75% in 8.25% dextrose	Bupivacaine 0.75% in NS	5-20	1-3	90-140	240-380
Lidocaine 5% in 7.5% dextrose	Lidocaine 5% in NS	25-100	1-2	40-100	140-240
Procaine 10% in water	Procaine 10% in NS	50-200	1-2	30-50	90-120

Abbreviation: NS, normal saline.
[a]Lowest doses are for saddle blocks.
Data from Covino et al[75] and Barash et al.[76]

Bupivacaine 0.5% hyperbaric (heavy bupivacaine) is the best agent to use if it is available. Plain (isobaric) 0.5% bupivacaine can also be used. Bupivacaine usually lasts from 2 to 3 hours. Cinchocaine 0.5% hyperbaric (heavy) solution is similar to bupivacaine.

Lidocaine/lignocaine achieves its best results when using a 5% hyperbaric (heavy) lidocaine solution. This lasts 45 to 90 minutes. Isobaric lidocaine 2% can also be used, but it has a shorter duration of action. Add 0.2 mL epinephrine 1:1000 to lidocaine to prolong its duration of action. Mepivacaine, if used as a 4% hyperbaric (heavy) solution, is similar to lidocaine.

Tetracaine 1% solution can be prepared with dextrose, NS, or water for injection. It has a long duration of action.

If typical spinal anesthetics are unavailable, use meperidine/pethidine 5% solution (50 mg/mL), which has local anesthetic properties and is a versatile agent. The standard IV preparation is preservative-free and isobaric. A dose of 0.5 to 1 mg/kg is usually adequate for spinal anesthesia. It has a rapid onset but can also wear off quickly.[77] Using meperidine is less expensive than using bupivacaine for spinal anesthesia.[78]

Technique

Premedicate the patient, if possible. Some patients may be very anxious about being awake during surgery, especially for amputations or other mutilating procedures. Do a lumbar puncture with the needle's bevel facing toward the patient's head. (While the official doctrine is to have

TABLE 15-4 Spinal Levels and Technique for Various Procedures

Spinal Level	Procedure	Solution and Patient Position
L1-L2	Perianal, perirectal	Hyperbaric solution, sitting position Isobaric solution, lying horizontally
T10	Lower extremity and hip Genitourinary (e.g., TURP) Vaginal/cervical	Isobaric solution
T6-T8	Herniorrhaphy Pelvic procedures Appendectomy	Hyperbaric solution, lying horizontally
T4-T6	Abdominal, C-section	Hyperbaric solution, lying horizontally

Abbreviation: TURP, transurethral resection of the prostate.

Data from Barash et al.[76]

the bevel aimed laterally, experienced anesthesiologists have found that this forces the needle to move laterally as it passes through the tissues. (Denny Bastrom, MD, oral communication, September 1, 2008.) If a caudal (saddle) block is desired, place the patient in the sitting position.

To reduce the incidence of a post-spinal tap headache, use a large IM injection needle as an introducer through the skin and muscle if a Sise introducer is unavailable. Insert the needle through the interspinal ligament (not through the dura) and then pass a small-gauge spinal needle through this larger needle. However, before doing this, be certain that the first needle is large enough to allow the spinal needle to pass through it. Insert the needle through the dura into the subarachnoid space, keeping the bevel lateral.[79]

When CSF appears, immobilize the needle by resting the back of the nondominant hand firmly against the patient while using the thumb and index finger to hold the needle's hub. Tightly attach the syringe with the anesthetic to the needle. Hyperbaric solutions are viscous and, with a high resistance to injection, may spill if the syringe is not firmly connected. Gently aspirate to check if CSF can still be withdrawn; then slowly inject the local anesthetic. Once injected, withdraw the needle.[77]

Hyperbaric solutions tend to settle in the dependent portions of the sac, whereas isobaric solutions usually will stay where they were injected, diffusing slowly in all directions. When hyperbaric agents have been used, putting a patient "head-down" can cause the block to extend cephalad for about 20 to 30 minutes after it was performed.[77] Using this principle, a saddle (perineal) block using a hyperbaric anesthetic is best done in the sitting position, with the patient remaining in that position until the anesthetic level has become "fixed."[73]

Testing the Spinal Block

To test the block's effectiveness, ask the patient to lift his or her legs. If he or she can't, the block is at least at the level of the mid-lumbar region. To test sensation, first test for a loss of temperature sensation using an ether or alcohol-soaked swab. Touch the patient's chest or arm where they can feel the cold swab. Then test the legs, moving up to the lower abdomen until the patient again feels the swab's coldness. If this is ambiguous, gently pinch blocked and unblocked areas until the level can be ascertained. Do not touch the patient and ask, "Do you feel this?" Touch sensation may persist even if there is no pain.[77]

Several problems can occur with spinal blocks: having no apparent effect, being too low, affecting only one side, or being too high. Note that moving a patient in any way in the first 10 to 20 minutes following injection increases the height of the block.

No Block

If the patient still has full power in his or her legs and normal sensation after 10 minutes, repeat the block.

Not High Enough

If using a hyperbaric solution, tilt the supine patient's head down so the solution runs up the lumbar curvature. Also, raise the patient's knees to flatten the lumbar curvature. If using a plain solution, turn the patient 360 degrees, from supine to prone and back to supine.

One-Sided or Too Low on One Side

If using a hyperbaric solution, place the patient on the inadequately blocked side for a few minutes and tilt the table into a slightly "head-down" position. If using an isobaric solution, place the patient on the side that is blocked.

Too High

While rare, this can occur quickly. These patients often complain of difficulty breathing or of tingling in their arms or hands. Do *not* tilt the table "head-up." *Get help; this is life threatening.* Treat this by monitoring, assisted ventilation, treating hypotension (raising legs and using a vasopressor, such as ephedrine or phenylephrine), and treating bradycardia (atropine first, then ephedrine or epinephrine).

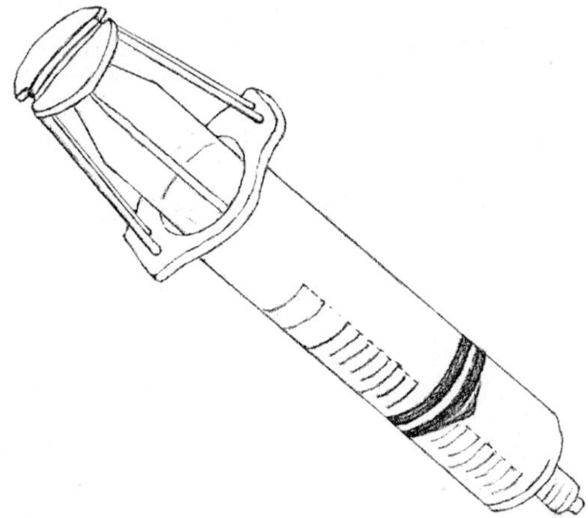

FIG. 15-13. Improvised epidural syringe.

EPIDURAL BLOCKS

For those experienced in doing epidural blocks, some improvisation may be necessary. For example, because the block should be done using a fairly thick needle with a rounded, not-too-sharp point, if the standard Touhy needle with a Huber point is not available, make one by bending the end of an ordinary spinal needle at a 45-degree angle. Grind off the tip so that only a small part of the bent end remains and then smooth it with a grindstone or file. Be certain that the lumen remains open so that the plastic catheter can pass through.[79]

A simple and cheap alternative to the standard spring-loaded syringe used to identify the epidural space can be easily improvised (Fig. 15-13). Make two wedge-shaped slots on opposite sides of a standard disposable syringe plunger. Then carefully make two holes on each side of the syringe barrel's flange. The holes on each side and the slot in the plunger should line up. Cut a rubber band, pass it through one set of holes, and insert the ends through the holes on the other side of the syringe. Tie the rubber band's ends. Then slip the rubber band over the top of the plunger, lodging it in the plunger's slots so that it does not slip off.[80]

If a standard epidural medication is not available, use ketamine, either alone or as an adjunct to local anesthetics. Using ketamine greatly prolongs the analgesia provided by single-shot epidural techniques, although preservative-free ketamine preparation must be used to avoid neurotoxicity.[81]

HYPNOSIS

Hypnosis is perfectly suited to be an anesthetic technique in austere circumstances, fulfilling nearly all requisites of the ideal minimal-resource intervention. Easy to learn, the technique requires no equipment, has a rapid onset, can be used for anesthesia and analgesia, and has no complications. In addition, it is safe, rapidly done, readily available, cost-effective, and has no risks. It can be used in any age group, including the elderly, with children aged 7 to 14 years old being particularly susceptible. Men and women are equally hypnotizable.[82] In addition, patients can later use it themselves for post-procedure pain relief.

Hypnosis, a state of wakeful suggestibility, has been used for millennia in medical and religious practices under various names. In the 19th century, the English surgeon John Elliotson and the Scottish surgeon James Esdaile performed hundreds of surgical procedures with hypnosis as the sole anesthetic, with decreased mortality compared with other methods.[83] On the battlefield, Podiapolsky found that nearly all wounded soldiers, no matter what their nationalities, responded "with exceptional facility" to hypnosis, although he did not use it for major operations.[84]

Hypnosis is being used successfully to anesthetize patients for a wide variety of operations and procedures requiring conscious sedation.[85,86] Much of the benefit is due to the patient's relaxed state and to distraction, rather than to specific suggestions to not feel discomfort.[41]

Potential symptom-oriented uses of hypnosis include: (a) to treat possible conversion reactions; (b) to treat pain associated with dislocation and fracture reductions; (c) to treat acute stress reactions, posttraumatic stress disorders, and factitious seizure; (d) to relieve the anxiety of needle phobias; (e) to treat the pain of burns; (f) to treat headaches; (g) to prepare patients for surgery, pelvic or post-rape examinations, or labor; and (h) to relieve pain and anxiety prior to emergency department (ED) procedures, such as suturing or incisions and drainage. If no other option exists, it can also be tried as anesthesia, although it works best as an adjunct to low-dose anesthesia.[47,48]

Technique

In general, a hypnosis session consists of the following:

- Explaining the process and obtaining consent
- Inducing the trance-like state
- Deepening the hypnotic state
- Delivering acceptable suggestions
- Emerging from the hypnotic state[82]

Although practitioners use many methods for inducing hypnosis, physicians and emergency medical services personnel have found the following method extremely easy to learn and use. The process is described to the patients as a way to relax, so any misconceptions they have about hypnosis will not interfere with their cooperation.[47,48] As Boulton described it, "In the particular context of 'difficult circumstances' hypnosis is often best practiced without the patient being aware that it is being employed; all that is necessary is that the patient should not be actively hostile to the technique. A tranquil and secure atmosphere and warm, comfortable conditions are important in promoting the successful practice of hypnosis."[39]

The clinician first explains the concept of patient and clinician cooperation, frequently described as permissive hypnosis. This helps allay the common adult fear of domination, control, or coercion by the clinician; children rarely experience this.[47,48]

During the "preinduction" phase, establish rapport with the patient. (In adults having prior experience with or exposure to hypnosis, discuss their experiences and the relationship between this technique and their experiences.) A key element in all cases, but especially in a noisy prehospital or ED environment, is to reinforce that the patient should listen only to the clinician and that the process will proceed at the patient's pace without pressure. The clinician should speak in a firm, quiet manner, in no way reacting to any of the noisy or distracting activities in the immediate vicinity.[47,48]

Induction

Begin by instructing the patient to close his or her eyes and to relax. Unlike adults, children in stressful conditions are already considered in Stage 1 hypnosis, and so are generally more susceptible to hypnotic suggestions. Then ask the patient to concentrate on his or her toes, imagining/producing sensations of heaviness and pleasant warmth in the limbs as "all of the muscles in your toes relax." For most people, feelings of heaviness are easier to imagine than warmth, but this is not consistent. The clinician should continue to suggest both sensations. Spend a significant amount of time (30 to 45 seconds) helping the patient to concentrate on and relax the toes. If this can be accomplished, the remainder of the procedure is much easier.[47,48]

The clinician then suggests that the patient feel the warmth or heaviness flow up into the feet, then the legs, thighs, and so forth. A significant indication that the technique has been successful is the regularization of the patient's breathing. At this point, tell the patient to slow his or her rate of breathing and further allow the entire body to relax. Suggest that with each exhalation, he or she will become more and more relaxed. Then tell the patient that he or she will feel relaxed and sleepy, and will "travel in your mind to a very pleasant place, perhaps a beach or mountain." A suggestion can be made that the patient will not remember the process of and the pain during the upcoming procedure.[47,48] Then do the procedure.

Testing the depth of hypnosis is pointless in a clinical setting; results are what matter. The key is whether the patient cooperates with the procedure, relaxes enough (e.g., joint reductions), or has diminished pain.

Emergence

The techniques related to getting patients to emerge from a hypnotic state may not be needed. If hypnosis is being used alone for the manipulation associated with reducing forearm fractures (or joint dislocations), the patient normally arouses immediately following the procedure. However, if a posthypnotic suggestion for pain relief or selective amnesia has been given, this still may be in effect. It can be reversed before the end of hypnosis, if desired.[47,48]

For those patients in very deep hypnosis (~15% of patients), it may be necessary to deliberately awaken them at the end of the procedure. The simplest method is to say: "I am going to count to ten and your eyes will open and you will feel perfectly normal. 1, 2, beginning to wake, 3, 4, lighter and lighter, 5, 6, eyes beginning to open, 7, 8, nearly awake, 9, 10, quite awake."[39]

REFERENCES

1. Moore PH. Comments in: Soper RL. Anaesthesia for major disasters. *Proc R Soc Med.* 1958;52: 239-246.
2. McGee D. Local and topical anesthesia. In: Roberts JR, Hedges JR, eds. *Clinical Procedures in Emergency Medicine*. 4th ed. Philadelphia, PA: W.B. Saunders; 2004:543-551.
3. Catterall WA, Mackie K. Local anesthetics. In: Brunton LL, Lazo JS, Parker KL, eds. *The Pharmacological Basis of Therapeutics*. 11th ed. New York, NY: McGraw-Hill; 2006:369.
4. Adriani J, Campbell D. Fatalities following topical application of local anesthetics to mucous membranes. *JAMA*. 1956;162:1528.
5. Blanton PL, Jeske AH. Dental local anesthetics: alternative delivery methods. *J Am Dent Assoc.* 2003;134:228-234.
6. Mulroy MF. *Regional Anesthesia*. Boston, MA: Little Brown; 1989:31-42.
7. Hoffman RJ. Viscous lidocaine treatment for painful oral infections in children: disappointingly dismissive of pediatric pain. *Ann Emerg Med.* 2014;64(1):96-97.
8. Hopper SM, McCarthy M, Tancharoen C, et al. Topical lidocaine to improve oral intake in children with painful infectious mouth ulcers: a blinded, randomized, placebo-controlled trial. *Ann Emerg Med.* 2014;63:292-299.
9. Kennedy RM, Luhmann JF. The 'ouchless emergency department' getting closer: advances in decreasing distressful procedures in the emergency department. *Pediatr Clin North Am.* 1999;46:1215-1247.
10. Buttaravoli P, Stair T. Traumatic tattoos and abrasions. *Common Simple Emergencies*. Washington, DC: Longwood Information. http://www.ncemi.org/cse/cse1018.htm. Accessed September 9, 2015.
11. World Health Organization. *Managing Complications in Pregnancy and Childbirth: A Guide for Midwives and Doctors*. Geneva, Switzerland: WHO; 2000:C-40.
12. King MH, ed. *Primary Anaesthesia*. Oxford, UK: Oxford University Press; 1986:23.
13. Revis DR, Seagel MB. Local anesthetics. Emedicine. http://www.emedicine.com/ent/topic20.htm. Accessed September 18, 2007.
14. Barker L. An introduction to pharmacology and drug doses. *Update in Anaesthesia.* http://e-safe-anaesthesia.org/e_library/03/Pharmacology_and_drug_doses_an_introduction_Update_2008.pdf. Accessed September 9, 2015.
15. Bartfield JM, Jandreau SW, Raccio-Robak N. Randomized trial of diphenhyrdramine versus benzyl alcohol with epinephrine as an alternative to lidocaine local anesthesia. *Ann Emerg Med.* 1998;32(6): 650-654.
16. Hansen E. Local anesthetics for abscess? *Postgrad Med.* http://www.postgradmed.com/pearls.htm. Accessed September 23, 2007.
17. McCormick BA. Ankle blocks. *Update Anesth.* 1999;10(13):66-69. http://www.nda.ox.ac.uk/wfsa/html/u10/u1013_01.htm. Accessed April 27, 2008.
18. Landau SW, Nelson WA, Gay LN. Antihistaminic properties of local anesthetics and anesthetic properties of antihistaminic compounds. *J Allergy Clin Immunol.* 1951;22:19-30.
19. Singer AJ, Hollander JE. Infiltration pain and local anesthetic effects of buffered vs plain 1% diphenhydramine. *Acad Emerg Med.* 1995;2:884-888.
20. Fitzpatrick RJ, Orr LM, Stubbart FJ. Antihistamines as local anesthetic agents for urethral manipulation. *JAMA*. 1952;150:1092.
21. Meyer RA, Jakubowski W. The anesthetic properties of antihistamines. *Am J Hosp Pharm.* 1963;20: 136-139.
22. Betcher AM, Tang ZT. Pyribenzamine: evaluation of effectiveness as an analgesic agent in regional anesthesia. *Anesthesiology*. 1955;16(2):214-223.

23. Naranjo P, Naranjo EB. Los antihistaminicaos como anesthesicos locales. [Antihistamines as local anesthetics]. *Boletín de Informaciones Científicas*. 1957;9:33-41.
24. Bowles WH. Chlorpromazine as a possible local anesthetic in dentistry. *J Dent Res*. 1971;50(4): 906-910.
25. Kopera J, Armitage AK. Comparison of some pharmacological properties of chlorpromazine, promethazine, and pethidine. *Br J Pharmacol*. 1954;9:392-401.
26. Allen CW. *Local and Regional Anesthesia*. 2nd ed. Philadelphia, PA: W.B. Saunders; 1918:63-66.
27. Windle PE, Kwan ML, Warwick H, et al. Comparison of bacteriostatic normal saline and lidocaine used as intradermal anesthesia for placement of intravenous lines. *J Perianesth Nurs*. 2006;21(4):251-258.
28. Wrightman MA, Vaughan RW. Comparison of compounds used for intradermal anesthesia. *Anesthesiology*. 1976;45(6):687-689.
29. Stumper D, Durieux MD. Antidepressants as long-acting local anesthetics. *Reg Anesth Pain Med*. 2004;29(3):277-285.
30. Gilly H, Kramer R, Zahorovsky I. Local anesthetic effects of morphine and naloxone. *Anesthesist*. 1985;34:619-626.
31. Smith DW, Peterson MR, DeBerard SC. Local anesthesia. *Postgrad Med*. 1999;106(2). http://www.postgradmed.com/issues/1999/08_99/smith.htm. Accessed September 12, 2006.
32. Allen CW. *Local and Regional Anesthesia*. 2nd ed. Philadelphia, PA: W.B. Saunders; 1918:60-63.
33. Lawson JIM. Ethyl chloride. *Br J Anaesth*. 1965;37:667-670.
34. Baum N. Ethyl chloride substitute found in office product. *Postgrad Med*. http://www.postgradmed.com/pearls.htm. Accessed September 23, 2007.
35. Allen CW. *Local and Regional Anesthesia*. 2nd ed. Philadelphia, PA: W.B. Saunders; 1918:59.
36. Howard RF. Acute pain management in children. In: Rowbotham DJ, Macintyre PE, eds. *Clinical Pain Management: Acute Pain*. London, UK: Arnold; 2003:437-462.
37. Allen CW. *Local and Regional Anesthesia*. 2nd ed. Philadelphia, PA: W.B. Saunders; 1918:524.
38. King MH, ed. *Primary Anaesthesia*. Oxford, UK: Oxford University Press; 1986:26.
39. Boulton TB. Anesthesia in difficult situations. 4. The use of local analgesia. *Anesthesia*. 1967;22(1): 101-133.
40. Boulton TB, Cole P. Anesthesia in difficult situations. 7. Routine preparations and pre-operative medication. *Anaesthesia*. 1968;23(2):220-234.
41. Stewart JH. Hypnosis in contemporary medicine. *Mayo Clin Proc*. 2005;80(4):511-524.
42. Allen CW. *Local and Regional Anesthesia*. 2nd ed. Philadelphia, PA: W.B. Saunders; 1918:519.
43. Williams JG, Lalonde DH. Randomized comparison of the single-injection volar subcutaneous block and the two-injection dorsal block for digital anesthesia. *Plast Reconstr Surg*. 2006;118(5):1195-1200.
44. Hamelin ND, St-Amand H, Lalonde DH, Harris PG, Brutus JP. Decreasing the pain of finger block injection: level II evidence. *Hand*. 2013;8(1):67-70.
45. Cannon B, Chan L, Rowlinson JS, Baker M, Clancy M. Digital anaesthesia: one injection or two? *Emerg Med J*. 2010;27(7):533-536.
46. Handoll HHG, Madhok R, Dodds C. Anaesthesia for treating distal radial fracture in adults. *Cochrane Database Syst Rev*. 2002;(3):CD003320.
47. Iserson KV. Reducing dislocations in a wilderness setting: use of hypnosis and intraarticular anesthesia. *J Wild Med*. 1991;2(1):22-26.
48. Iserson KV. Hypnosis for pediatric fracture reduction. *J Emerg Med*. 1999;17:53-56.
49. Aronson PL, Mistry RD. Intra-articular lidocaine for reduction of shoulder dislocation. *Ped Emerg Care*. 2014;30(5):358-362.
50. Mohr B. Safety and effectiveness of intravenous regional anesthesia (Bier block) for outpatient management of forearm trauma. *Can J Emerg Med*. 2006;8:247-250.
51. Koenig KL. Bier block for upper-extremity anesthesia. *Journal Watch*. (Distributed September 27, 2006, by Epocrates.)
52. Jakeman N, Kaye P, Hayward J, Watson DP, Turner S. Is lidocaine Bier's block safe? *Emerg Med J*. 2013;30:214-217.
53. Blasier RD, White R. Intravenous regional anesthesia for management of children's extremity fractures in the emergency department. *Pediatr Emerg Care*. 1996;12:404-406.
54. Viscomi C. Bier blocks: new tricks for an old dog. *ASRA News*. June 2003:4-5. http://www.asra.com/Newsletters/June_03.pdf. Accessed September 19, 2007.
55. Barry LA, Balliana SA, Galeppi AC. Intravenous regional anesthesia (Bier block). *Tech Reg Anesth Pain Manag*. 2006;10:123-131.

56. Ye L, Liu J, Zhu T. A useful modification of the Bier's block. *Int Anesth Res Soc J*. 2006;103(1):257.
57. Grande CM, Baskett PJF, Donchin Y, et al. Trauma anesthesia for disasters: anything, anytime, anywhere. *Crit Care Clin*. 1991;7(2):339-361.
58. Reuben SS, Steinberg RB, Klatt JL, et al. Intravenous regional anesthesia using lidocaine and clonidine. *Anesthesiology*. 1999;91(3):654-658.
59. Allen CW. *Local and Regional Anesthesia*. 2nd ed. Philadelphia, PA: W.B. Saunders; 1918:347-351.
60. Wilhelm TJ, Anemana S, Kyamanywa P, et al. Anaesthesia for elective inguinal hernia repair in rural Ghana: appeal for local anaesthesia in resource-poor countries. *Trop Doct*. 2006;36:147-149.
61. Amid PK, Shulman AG, Lichtenstein IL. Local anesthesia for inguinal hernia repair: step-by-step procedures. *Ann Surg*. 1994;220:735-737.
62. Sønderskov ML, Hallas P. The use of 'brutacaine' in Danish emergency departments. *Eur J Emerg Med*. 2013;20(5):370-372.
63. Brown JC, Klein EJ. The "superhero cape burrito": a simple and comfortable method of short-term procedural restraint. *J Emerg Med*. 2011;41(1):74-76.
64. King MH, ed. *Primary Anesthesia*. Oxford, UK: Oxford University Press; 1986:137.
65. Godoy D, Iserson KV. Single fascia iliaca compartment block for post-hip fracture pain relief. *J Emerg Med*. 2007;32(3):257-262.
66. Dochez E, van Geffen GJ, Bruhn J, et al. Prehospital administered fascia iliaca compartment block by emergency medical service nurses, a feasibility study. *Scand J Trauma Resus Emerg Med*. 2014;22:38.
67. Neubrand TL, Roswell K, Deakyne S, Kocher K, Wathen J. Fascia iliaca compartment nerve block versus systemic pain control for acute femur fractures in the pediatric emergency department. *Ped Emerg Care*. 2014;30(7):469-473.
68. Kennedy JA. A technic [*sic*] and device for application of ice anesthesia for amputation of extremities. *US Nav Med Bull*. 1943;41:226-230.
69. Bancroft FW, Fuller AG, Ruggiero WF. Improved methods in extremity amputations for diabetic gangrene. *Ann Surg*. April 1942;115(4):621-627.
70. Crossman LW, Ruggiero WF, Hurley V, et al. Reduced temperatures in surgery: II. amputations for peripheral vascular diseases. *Arch Surg*. 1942;44:139-156.
71. Van Blarcom C. Nursing care in ice anesthesia. *Am J Nurs*. 1943;9:799-800.
72. Husum H, Ang SC, Fosse E. *War Surgery: Field Manual*. Penang, Malaysia: Third World Network; 1995:684.
73. Brunton L, Lazo J, Parker K, et al, eds. *Goodman & Gilman's The Pharmacological Basis of Therapeutics*. 11th ed. New York, NY: McGraw-Hill; 2006:382.
74. Greene NM. Distribution of local anesthetic solutions within the subarachnoid space. *Anesth Analg*. 1985;64:715-730.
75. Covino BG, Scott DB, Lambert DH. *Handbook of Spinal Anaesthesia and Analgesia*. Philadelphia, PA: W.B. Saunders; 1994:84.
76. Barash PG, Cullen BF, Stoelting RK. *Clinical Anesthesia*. 4th ed. Philadephia, PA: Lippincott Williams & Wilkins; 2001:268.
77. Casey WF. Spinal anesthesia: a practical guide. *Pract Proced*. 2000;(12):2. http://www.nda.ox.ac.uk/wfsa/htmL/u12/u1208_01.htm. Accessed September 13, 2006.
78. Williams D. Practical techniques in developing countries. *Pract Proced*. 1998;9(8):1. http://www.nda.ox.ac.uk/wfsa/htmL/u09/u09_024.htm. Accessed September 13, 2006.
79. King MH, ed. *Primary Anaesthesia*. Oxford, UK: Oxford University Press; 1986:50.
80. Malhotra N, Jangra A. A simple and cheap alternative to spring loaded syringes for the identification of epidural space. *Trop Doct*. 2008;38:100.
81. Craven R. Ketamine. *Anaesthesia*. 2007;62(suppl 1):48-53.
82. Iserson KV. An hypnotic suggestion: review of hypnosis for clinical emergency care. *J Emerg Med*. 2014;46(4):588-596.
83. Marmer MJ. Present applications of hypnosis in anesthesiology. *West J Surg Obstet Gynecol*. 1961;69:260-263.
84. Flagg PJ. Anaesthesia in Europe on the Western battlefront. *Int Clinic*. 1918;3:210-228.
85. Faymonville ME, Meurisse M, Fissette J. Hypnosedation: a valuable alternative to traditional anesthetic techniques. *Acta Chir Belg*. 1999;99:141-146.
86. Faymonville ME, Mambourg PH, Joris J, et al. Psychological approaches during conscious sedation: hypnosis versus stress reducing strategies: a prospective randomized study. *Pain*. 1997;73:361-367.

16 | Sedation and General Anesthesia

INTRODUCTION

The following vignette provides an excellent picture of typical operating room (OR, theatre) anesthesia in a resource-poor venue[1]:

> John, an anaesthetic clinical officer, is administering a general anaesthetic [and] performs a rapid sequence induction with thiopental and suxamethonium and intubates using his own laryngoscope and a tracheal tube that has been used dozens of times before ... John carries all his own equipment with him, along with a supply of drugs for the day—anything left in theatre will disappear by tomorrow. Normal saline is running in through an 18G cannula that the patient's family were asked to buy from the local pharmacy.
>
> John administers 50 mg of pethidine—this may be the last analgesic the patient receives until the unpredictable visit of the night matron to the ward in 9 h time—and turns up the OMV [Oxford Miniature Vaporizer] to deliver 2% halothane. The inspired concentration must be estimated clinically because the halothane "expired" 8 months ago and the clinical effect is unpredictable. The EMO [Epstein-Macintosh-Oxford] vaporiser and a bottle of ether are on stand-by behind the anaesthetic machine, as we are down to our last bottle of halothane.... The modern anaesthesia monitor, looking out of place in these surroundings, was purchased, along with eight others, by the European project. The screen has a psychedelic tinge to it and I suspect it is on its last legs. The capnograph trace is flat, as the last remaining moisture trap has been "borrowed" for use in ICU, where it will be circulated around the four beds. The ECG trace is true, but periodically interrupted as the long out-of-date electrodes require a small drop of thiopental to improve their conductivity. The oximetry probe is a paediatric one and roughly taped with grubby Elastoplast around the man's little finger.
>
> John ventilates the patient using the Oxford Inflating Bellows as part of a draw-over system, aiming to keep him deeply anaesthetised and apnoeic using a high concentration of halothane. There are no muscle relaxants apart from suxamethonium. Emergency drugs, atropine and adrenaline, are drawn up on a redundant Boyle's machine, which acts as a trolley and equipment store. A lone size H oxygen cylinder is deep in dust in the corner and has been empty for several years.
>
> John requests a nasogastric tube, so I head to the locked anaesthetic store room where 10 or so years of unsorted donations to the department have piled up. After 15 min, I find one at the bottom of a box of out-of-date NG feed. I can tell by the look on his face that John is torn between using this valued commodity for this patient or saving it for the next.

Anesthesia in Austere Circumstances

Anesthesia's three principal functions are to keep the patient alive through surgery, to make surgery painless, and to provide the best possible surgical conditions.

The purpose of this chapter and, in fact, this entire book is illustrated by two questions that Drs. Boulton and Cole posed in their series "Anaesthesia in Difficult Situations"[2]:

1. What would I do if had to give an anesthetic and operate on a patient in an isolated hospital 100 miles from the nearest outpost of civilization?
2. What would I take on an expedition to the Arctic ... or in the Himalayas ... or on a ship ... or to an area of devastation following an earthquake or nuclear holocaust?

This chapter and the next are for clinicians who may need to administer anesthesia in austere situations with limited supplies and equipment. These chapters highlight medications that can safely be used by non-anesthesiologists (e.g., ketamine), little-used anesthetics that are generally available in austere situations (e.g., intravenous [IV] ethanol [ETOH]), and anesthetics available in austere settings that are not familiar to younger anesthesiologists from industrialized nations (e.g., ether, halothane), as well as classic basic methods of delivering anesthesia (e.g., open-drop). Those trained in anesthesia obviously are more familiar with these medications and techniques than are other clinicians. The key to providing safe and effective anesthesia is to use equipment and techniques that employ the skills you already possess.

Standards and Shortages

Although international standards for anesthesia administration exist, shortages of trained anesthesiologists, equipment, and medications limit the extent to which these standards can be implemented.

Scarcity of Trained Anesthetists/Anesthesiologists

A worldwide shortage of trained anesthetists means that in developing countries, other practitioners, including physicians, dentists, nurse practitioners, physician assistants, and paramedics, may need to provide general anesthesia with limited additional training and with minimal supervision.

The basic rule of thumb is that "a practitioner faced with the necessity of giving an emergency anesthetic, perhaps for the first time since his student days, is well advised to stick to a technique which he has at least seen used at one time or another." If an experienced anesthetist must supervise or manage multiple inexperienced practitioners giving anesthesia, which may be the case in many situations, "the technique employed would have to be as simple as possible so that it could be quickly taught."[2]

Commonly, the clinician must be both the surgeon and the anesthetist. In these cases, the rule is to "use local and regional methods where you can. If you have to give a general anesthetic, secure the patient's airway and make sure that there is [an IV] running before you start. With a clear airway and [an IV line], most of your problems will be over. Induce and intubate the patient yourself, and don't operate until anesthesia is stable."[3] During the procedure, have an assistant monitor the patient by continually checking the blood pressure (BP) and the pulse using an esophageal or precordial stethoscope.[3,4] (See Chapter 5 for how to improvise these devices.)

One competent clinician, however, can both sedate patients and perform closed reduction of major joint dislocations and forearm fractures (shoulder dislocation, elbow dislocation, hip dislocation, and forearm fracture) safely without assistance. Optimally, the patient will have continuous monitoring during the procedure and until his vital signs and mentation stabilize near presedation levels.[5]

Medication Standards and Scarcity

The World Health Organization (WHO) lists what they consider to be the essential medications for anesthetic care, although cost and supply problems may limit the anesthetics and associated medications (Table 16-1) that are available for local, regional, and general anesthesia.

GENERAL ANESTHESIA GUIDELINES

Goals of General Anesthesia

Administering general anesthesia provides three benefits: (a) hypnosis, putting the patient to sleep; (b) analgesia, relieving pain; and (c) relaxation, easing the muscles sufficiently to perform the procedure, primarily in abdominal and some orthopedic cases.[6]

Safety

An anesthetist's primary goal is to anesthetize patients and have them recover without ill effects from the anesthesia. Whether this happens depends a great deal on the anesthetist's abilities and how carefully he follows the rules for safely anesthetizing patients (Table 16-2).

Essential Elements

Four of the five essential elements for general anesthesia may need to be improvised or omitted in austere situations: premedication, monitoring, induction medications, and oxygenation.

TABLE 16-1 Availability of Anesthetic and Related Medications in the Developing World

	Percentage of Anesthetists With Medications Available		
	Always (%)	Sometimes (%)	Never (%)
Nitrous oxide	—	3	92
Naloxone	9	16	60
Neuromuscular blocking agent	15	12	69
Neostigmine	16	6	69
Magnesium	19	38	39
Blood for transfusion	23	59	16
Labetalol	29	29	30
Hydralazine	30	34	30
Halothane	38	16	39
Spinal local anesthetic	39	28	30
Narcotic (IV/IM)	45	30	21
Vasopressor	45	21	28
Succinylcholine	54	23	19
Oxytocin	57	31	7
Thiopental	59	24	15
Oxygen	63	25	10
Ether	68	20	9
Intravenous fluid	68	27	2
Local block anesthetic	70	18	7
Epinephrine	74	18	3
Diazepam	81	17	—
Ergometrine	81	14	1
Atropine	84	6	6
Ketamine	92	3	4

Abbreviations: IM, intramuscular; IV, intravenous.
Data from Hodges et al.[7]

In addition, anesthetists may need to use alternative maintenance drugs (anesthetics) or delivery methods.

Premedication

Premedication provides mild sedation for the patient and counteracts some side effects, primarily excess salivation and increased vagal tone.

A wide variety of narcotics, benzodiazepines, phenothiazines, and other medications may be used for premedication. Try to use sedating anticholinergics (e.g., those with antihistamine activity) if the normal medication cannot be used. Premedications are usually administered parenterally, but many may be given orally.

Promethazine 50 mg (1 mg/kg) tablets, which also have anticholinergic activity, can be used in adults for nausea and very mild sedation. Give promethazine about 2 hours before anesthesia. This medication is particularly good if ketamine is used as a general anesthetic. Diazepam tablets,

TABLE 16-2 Ten Rules for Safely Anesthetizing Patients

1. Assess the patient carefully to be aware of any underlying medical condition or medication that might interfere with the anesthesia or surgery.
2. If possible, keep the patient NPO for ≥6 hours before the procedure. (Modify for infants and small children.) Small sips of water taken with a preanesthetic medication are acceptable. Also consider this course for procedures done under local or regional blocks, because you may have to switch to using general anesthesia during the procedure.
3. Use a tilting OR table, so that you can put the patient in a head-down position if there is a risk of emesis. During surgery, turning the patient on his or her side may not be an option.
4. Check available drugs and equipment before you start. The truism is: whatever you do not have available or that doesn't function properly will be what you need in a crisis.
5. Have suction instantly available. This is the most-often-neglected piece of equipment. Check that the parts are assembled, the equipment is turned on or ready to be quickly turned on, and the vacuum works. When you don't have suction available, it is almost certain that you will need it—quickly.
6. Keep the patient's airway clear. Use a nasal or an oral airway, as needed. If the patient doesn't need it, he or she will spit out an oral airway.
7. Be ready to control ventilation. No matter what anesthetic you use (including ketamine), you may need to assist ventilations with a BVM, with or without a controlled airway device such as an LMA or ET tube.
8. Have an IV running. This is not only therapeutic, but also an excellent precaution if something goes awry. In a crisis, it is far easier to begin administering medications or fluids through an established IV than to struggle to insert one.
9. Continually monitor the pulse, BP, and skin color (and the color of any blood from the surgical site). A precordial or esophageal stethoscope, a BP cuff that is used on a regular basis (q5min), and good observation are all that is required for basic monitoring.
10. Have an assistant in the room who can help in an emergency.

Abbreviations: BP, blood pressure; BVM, bag-valve-mask; ET, endotracheal; LMA, laryngeal mask airway; NPO, nothing by mouth; OR, operating room.
Data from King.[8]

10 to 20 mg (0.15 to 0.25 mg/kg), can be used as a tranquilizer before either regional or general anesthesia. Oral diazepam has a more rapid and reliable onset than does intramuscular (IM) diazepam.[9] Diphenhydramine (Benadryl) is cheap and almost always available. It can be given parenterally or orally, and is both sedating and anticholinergic.

Considered by many anesthesiologists to be the only essential preoperative medication, atropine 0.4 to 0.6 mg dries secretions and diminishes vagal tone on the heart. Atropine may be administered IM 30 to 40 minutes before induction or diluted and given IV immediately before anesthesia.[7] Atropine can also be administered orally in tablet form (0.5 mg in an adult) at least 20 minutes before the general anesthetic is administered. There is no harm if the patient takes it with a small amount (~20 mL) of water.[9]

Basic Monitoring

In austere situations, anesthesia with only the most basic monitoring (even more basic than what you're thinking) is the norm. Often the only monitoring is checking the pulse: either constantly with an esophageal or precordial stethoscope or at least every 5 minutes while taking a BP. You can also monitor the pulse by laying a finger just anterior to the tragus of the ear to feel the superficial temporal artery pulsate. Also, monitor the patient's skin color, capillary refill, and the color of any blood from the surgical site, because these require no apparatus. A wisp of cotton taped near the nostril is a useful indicator that the patient is still breathing.[7]

Esophageal stethoscopes are particularly important during thoracic procedures. Only one earpiece is needed, although a modified stethoscope can also be used. Precordial stethoscopes (that can also be placed over the back) are particularly important to use during procedures on babies. Likewise, only one earpiece is needed, but the bell should be securely taped to the patient before the procedure begins.

Induction

Both IV and inhalation agents are often used for induction. Ketamine needs no induction agent.

Benzodiazepines, although not often used for induction, can be used for this purpose. Diazepam, often the most readily available benzodiazepine, can be used as an IV induction agent, although it has a longer onset and longer duration (i.e., longer "hangover") than most other agents.[10] The newer benzodiazepines generally work faster and have shorter half-lives.

Laryngospasm Treatment

The most feared complication during induction is laryngospasm. The traditional method of breaking a laryngospasm is to use constant positive pressure with an anesthesia bag or a bag-valve-mask (BVM). This normally breaks the spasm. A more rapid alternative is to apply pressure to the "laryngospasm notch." Place the long finger of each hand into the most superior part of the depression behind the pinna of each ear. The fingertip should press against the ascending mandibular ramus anteriorly, the mastoid process posteriorly, and the base of the skull superiorly. Press very firmly inward toward the base of the skull while lifting the mandible to perform a "jaw thrust." This action generally converts laryngospasm to laryngeal stridor within one or two breaths and, in another few breaths, to unobstructed respiration. The technique is effective in infants, children, and adults. Alternatively, clinicians have had similar success by applying digital pressure anterior to the tragus.[11] If this is unsuccessful, spray the cords with lidocaine, and be prepared to do a cricothyrotomy (rarely needed).

Oxygen

In austere situations, oxygen is frequently unavailable, and so is considered a luxury. If oxygen is scarce, use it only to preoxygenate patients who will undergo brief apneic procedures, to induce and intubate small children,[12] and to supplement anesthesia at altitudes >9000 feet (2743 m). Also provide it for patients with laryngospasm, acute desaturation, significant anemia (Hgb <9 g/dL), or heart or lung disease, and to those in shock.[10]

Also consider using oxygen when (a) inducing anesthesia in a patient using ether and air; (b) giving anesthesia with >8% ether; (c) doing a Cesarean section (C-section), but only until the baby is delivered; (d) patients have any respiratory disease or considerable airway secretions; and (e) the preoperative BP has fallen by >30%.

Stages of Anesthesia

Theoretically, all patients may go through four stages (plus substages, or planes) of anesthesia, no matter which agent is used (Table 16-3). Ether is the anesthetic that shows all the classic stages, so the pattern with ether is described more fully in the "Ether" section in Chapter 17.

When administering anesthesia with basic equipment and few medications, tracking anesthetic stages can be a useful safeguard against over-medication.

Anesthetics vary widely in their effects, so use staging with the particular drug's effects in mind. Staging follows the oversimplified, but useful, pattern that anesthetics suppress the central nervous system from the top down as blood concentration increases. This progression (stages) can be observed in the patient's body movements, respiratory rhythm, oculomotor reflexes, and muscle tone. The following paragraphs describe the classic anesthetic stages.

Stage 1: Analgesia

There is suppression of the highest cerebral centers, with the patient gradually losing the sensation of pain. Patients remain conscious and rational, and have decreased pain perception. Muscle tone, breathing, and pulse are normal. Use Stage 1 anesthesia for obstetric analgesia and as a supplement to local anesthesia for minor procedures.

TABLE 16-3 Signs of General Anesthesia Stages and Planes (Levels of Stages)

Stage	Plane	Respiration	Response to Surgical Stimulus	Eye Signs	Cardiac
I. Analgesia		Voluntary control	Voluntary control	Voluntary movement	Adequate output
Consciousness Lost					
II. Excitement (Delirium)	1. Early	Irregular Coughing[a] Spasm	Actively purposeful[a]	Lash reflex goes[a] Variable movement Disconjugate gaze	Possibly arrhythmias
	2. Late	Phonation Breath holding[a]	Weakly purposeful[a]		
III. Surgical anesthesia	1. Light	Regular[a]	Absent	Lid reflex gone[a]	Adequate output[b]
	2. Moderate	Adequate		Eyes fixed[a]	
	3. Deep	Tracheal tug[c]		Pupil dilated[a]	Hypotension[b]
IV. Medullary paralysis		Absent[a]		Pupil of anoxia[a]	Good contraction[b]
Death					Cardiac arrest

[a]Applicable to all anesthetics.
[b]Applicable only to ether.
[c]Paradoxical respiration.
Adapted with permission from Boulton.[6]

Stage 2: Excitement (Delirium)

This stage begins when patients lose consciousness and become excited, struggle, and (possibly) become difficult to control. Patients retain their gag reflex and can protect their airway, although they breathe irregularly and may hold their breath. Their pupils generally dilate. Their abdominal muscles contract during expiration. They lose their eyelash reflex and have roving eye movements and dilated but reactive pupils. They retain reflex responses to any painful or irritating stimuli, including noxious anesthetic vapors.

Stage 3: Surgical Anesthesia

In this stage, patients no longer respond to painful stimuli. Muscular relaxation progressively increases, spontaneous respiration diminishes, and patients lose their protective gag reflex. Non-anesthesiologists need only recognize two planes: acceptable ("light") and too deep.[13]

Plane: Light Surgical Anesthesia

This is the optimal anesthetic level for most patients during surgery. Patients' breathing becomes regular again, although they will inspire deeply every 2 to 3 minutes. The eyes no longer move and, as the anesthesia level deepens, the pupils gradually dilate. The patient no longer moves and muscular tone decreases. The abdomen and chest move synchronously. An artificial airway or endotracheal (ET) tube may be inserted in this plane—but not earlier.

Plane: Deep Surgical Anesthesia (Too Deep)

In this anesthesia plane, patients' intercostal muscles become progressively paralyzed, eventually having paradoxical movement (moving in with inspiration). Sudden inspirations pull on the mediastinum and trachea, drawing it downward (the "tracheal tug"). Patients' pupils become progressively less reactive to light. Abdominal surgery is very difficult at this anesthesia level if the patient is not pharmacologically paralyzed.

Stage 4: Medullary Depression (Way Too Deep)

During stage 4, the brainstem's respiratory center becomes depressed, which causes patients to stop breathing and lose all muscle tone. Their pupils are fixed and dilated. The heart may (as with chloroform) or may not (as with ether) be dangerously depressed.[7] If a patient stays in this stage too long, his or her heart stops and the patient dies.[13]

ANESTHESIA IN SPECIAL CIRCUMSTANCES

Trauma Patients

In trauma patients, the elective anesthesia standard of "nothing-by-mouth (NPO) for six hours" is a fantasy. Assume that all trauma patients have full stomachs. Optimized trauma anesthesia consists of airway control, preventing aspiration, and being prepared to provide immediate anesthesia to hypovolemic, unstable patients.

Altitude and General Anesthesia

High altitude, arbitrarily considered to be above 3000 meters or 10,000 feet, and extreme cold may affect anesthesia delivery. Three types of individuals may present for anesthesia at high altitude: the unacclimatized newcomer, the acclimatized newcomer, and the resident native.

Patients

The unacclimatized newcomer who has been at altitudes above 3000 meters for less than 4 months is in an extremely unstable physiological state and initially may suffer from acute mountain sickness (e.g., high-altitude pulmonary edema, high-altitude cerebral edema).[14] This makes sedation and general anesthesia precarious, at best.

Acclimatized newcomers may also be in danger of pulmonary edema. They have probably acquired similar physiological characteristics to the natives, including polycythemia, hypervolemia, increased pulmonary blood volume, pulmonary hypertension, right ventricular hypertrophy, and increased diffusion capacity. Nevertheless, give oxygen to these patients during any emergency surgery and, if at all possible, return them to sea level for surgical treatment.[14]

Resident natives, who were born and live at altitude, are capable of exhaustive physical exercise despite their often plethoric, cyanotic, and barrel-chested appearance. After visiting lower altitudes for a few days, however, they too may get acute pulmonary edema on their return to altitude.[14]

Anesthetic Agents

The provision and the choice of anesthesia and analgesia at high altitudes depend on three factors: (a) the patient's pathophysiological state, (b) the decreased oxygen tension due to low barometric pressure, and (c) the peculiarities of inhalational agents. With some modifications, particularly the addition of oxygen, general inhalation anesthesia may be administered.[15]

When preparing to deliver general anesthesia above 3000 meters, try not to use any drug that depresses the respiratory center. If you must use such a drug, reduce the dose of premedication. The increase in respiratory tract secretions at high altitudes, especially when using ether, suggests using higher doses of atropine, even though that risks increasing preexisting tachycardia. Provide careful fluid replacement because of the increased risk of pulmonary edema.

During surgery, use oxygen supplementation, if available, on all anesthetized patients. To achieve an oxygen tension equivalent to that at sea level (150 mm Hg), 32% supplementation is required at 3000 meters and 42% at 5000 meters (16,500 feet). However, unsupplemented ether–air anesthesia has been successfully used at altitudes of 2500 to 3000 meters.[14] On the other hand, nerve blocks and anesthetic infiltration may be limited by the vasoconstriction accompanying hypothermia.[15]

Consider using IV ketamine, because at doses of 2.0 mg/kg it produces a dissociative anesthesia, while not depressing the hypoxic drive or interfering with the pharyngeal or laryngeal reflexes. Use supplemental oxygen when available, especially during recovery, for less-acclimatized individuals.[16,17] Avoid using N_2O.

Equipment

Both anesthetics and the associated equipment work progressively less well as the altitude increases. The practical limits for general inhalation anesthesia are not precisely known, but, whenever possible, surgery should not be performed at altitudes higher than 4000 meters (~13,000 feet).[18]

Extreme Cold and General Anesthesia

Use caution when giving general anesthesia—or doing surgery—in extremely cold environments. Aside from the obvious problem of IV fluids freezing if not properly insulated, vasoconstriction reduces the size of veins, which makes IV placement difficult and reduces the absorption of drugs injected subcutaneously. Increased static electricity and open-flame heating units may augment the explosive hazard of the inhalational agents. To humidify the extra-dry air, use an IV infusion set to deliver normal (0.9%) saline (NS) at 2 to 4 drops per minute through a very fine hypodermic needle inserted into the connector between a BVM and the patient's ET tube.[15]

PROCEDURAL SEDATION

What Is Sedation?

While sedation implies that patients have a depressed consciousness rather than being asleep, there is often little difference between procedural sedation and short-term general anesthesia, except that the former usually does not include the use of neuromuscular blockade (NMB) or invasive airways (e.g., ET tube or laryngeal mask airway [LMA]). The similarity between the two is highlighted in the American Society of Anesthesiologists (ASA)'s description of sedation levels (Table 16-4).

Uses

In the acute, outpatient setting, the most common reasons to sedate patients are for fracture reductions/treatments, joint relocations, laceration repairs, and lumbar punctures. The fewest complications occur with ketamine (0.7% of cases), propofol (0.8%), or morphine (2.9%). Most complications occur when the sedative is hydromorphone (9.7%), fentanyl (9.5%), midazolam (6.4%), or etomidate (6.2%).[20]

While pediatric procedures often require sedation, if a practitioner does not have the skills or the appropriate medications and equipment to sedate the child safely, "tie-and-cry" (see Fig. 15-7) with liberal use of local or regional anesthesia is a more prudent way to proceed.[21]

TABLE 16-4 American Society of Anesthesiologists' Sedation Levels

	Minimal Sedation	Moderate Sedation	Deep Sedation	General Anesthesia
Responsiveness	Normal response to verbal stimulation	Purposeful response to verbal or tactile stimulation	Purposeful response following repeated or painful stimulation	Unarousable even with painful stimulation
Airway	Unaffected	No intervention required	Intervention may be required	Intervention often required
Spontaneous ventilation	Unaffected	Adequate	May be inadequate	Frequently inadequate
Cardiovascular function	Unaffected	Usually maintained	Usually maintained	May be impaired

Data from Godwin.[19]

Predictors of Failed Pediatric Sedation

Five variables predict that sedation will probably fail in a child. In diminishing importance, they are: (a) upper respiratory infection (odds ratio [OR], 2.73), (b) obstructive sleep apnea/snoring (OR, 2.06), (c) ASA Class III (OR, 2.31), (d) obesity (OR, 1.95), and (e) older age (OR, 1.15).[22]

Medications

Various medications can be used for sedation, depending on their availability and the clinician's comfort level and experience using them. These include ketamine, narcotics, ETOH, benzodiazepines, and propofol (Table 16-5).

Ketamine

Ketamine is often used for sedation, especially in children, and is discussed in Chapter 17.

Narcotics

Using IV narcotics to a point short of anesthesia is a valuable technique to know when "extreme emergency" conditions are physically dangerous to both the patient and clinician.[2,6] An initial dose of 10 mg of diluted morphine or 50 mg of meperidine will give you an idea of the patient's reaction. However, at least 30 mg of morphine or 200 to 300 mg of meperidine may be required before adequate sedation is achieved, especially if local anesthesia is not used simultaneously.[7] Maintaining an adequate airway may become a problem when using this method.

Ethanol

Since ancient times, ETOH has been a known soporific.[25-27] Intravenous alcohol has been used successfully as an anesthetic induction agent for nearly a century.[28] In the 1960s, Dundee used an 8% (weight/volume) solution prepared by adding 110 mL of 95% ETOH to a 1-L bag of Hartmann's solution (similar to lactated Ringer solution). Its pH was about 6.4. Each otherwise healthy adult patient received just over 500 mL of the solution. Of those receiving a strong opiate (meperidine) and often pentobarbital as a premedication, 70% could be induced with ethanol–nitrous oxide and 60% had the surgery completed with only these medications. He found that the onset of sleep with ETOH induction was accompanied by a progressive fall in oxygenation (PaO_2) and that any post-ETOH delirium could be rapidly controlled by small IV doses of benzodiazepines.[29]

Benzodiazepines

Benzodiazepines can induce relaxation and cooperation, and often provide an amnestic response. Titrate doses (see Table 16-5) to patient tolerance depending on the patient's age and other illnesses, the use of additional medications, and the procedure's complexity. Significant respiratory depression can occur, but is more common if these medications are combined with opiates. The two most commonly used medications in this class are midazolam (best) and diazepam (most readily available worldwide).

Midazolam is short acting, with a short recovery period. A dose of 0.02 mg/kg to 0.1 mg/kg IV typically produces sedation in 2 to 3 minutes, with the clinical effects lasting from 10 to 30 minutes. In elderly or debilitated patients, use lower doses, because these patients may be more sedated and have longer recovery periods at lower doses. Repeat doses until the desired effect is achieved. Side effects include dose-related respiratory depression, especially in elderly patients, patients with chronic obstructive pulmonary disease (COPD), or patients who have taken alcohol, barbiturates, opioids, or other central nervous system depressants. Hypotension can be significant in hypovolemic and elderly patients. Midazolam has no analgesic activity. It crosses the placenta and enters breast milk.[30] In children aged 6 months to 7 years old, aerosolized buccal or intranasal midazolam (0.3 mg/kg aerosolized parenteral solution; 10 mg maximum dose) is an effective and useful alternative to oral midazolam for sedation, although they may not provide superior sedation. One-fourth of children are inadequately sedated when midazolam is administered through a route other than IV or IM.[31]

Diazepam is also used for conscious sedation. However, because of its long half-life, it may be difficult to titrate and may last longer than desired. Compared to midazolam, diazepam poses

TABLE 16-5 Agents Commonly Used for Conscious Sedation

Medication	Side Effects	Route	Total Dose[a]	Onset	Duration
			Barbiturates		
Methohexital[b]	Respiratory depression Hypotension	IV	0.75-1.00 mg/kg	45 s	5-10 min
		PR	20-30 mg/kg	8-10 min	45-60 min
Pentobarbital[b]	Respiratory depression Hypotension	IV	2.5 mg/kg	45 sec	15 min
		IM	2.5 mg/kg	10-15 min	NA
		PO/PR	2-6 mg/kg	15-60 min	1-4 hr
Thiopental[b]	Respiratory depression Hypotension	PR	25 mg/kg	10-15 min	1-2 hr
			Benzodiazepines		
Midazolam	Respiratory depression	IV (<5 year)	0.05-0.1 mg/kg; *then* titrate to 0.6 mg/kg	2-3 min	30-60 min
		IV (6-12 years)	0.025-0.05 mg/kg; *then* titrate to 0.4 mg/kg	2-3 min	30-60 min
		IM	0.1-0.15 mg/kg	2-20 min	1-2 hr
		PO	0.5-0.75 mg/kg	15-30 min	60-90 min
		PR	0.25-1 mg/kg	10-30 min	45-90 min
		Nasal	0.2-0.5 mg/kg	10-15 min	45-60 min
Diazepam	Respiratory depression	IV	0.15-0.2 mg/kg	1-5 min	
		PO	0.15-0.2 mg/kg	30 min	
		PR	0.2 mg/kg	3 min	
			Opioids		
Fentanyl	Respiratory depression	IV	2 mcg/kg	1-2 min	20-30 min
Morphine	Respiratory depression Hypotension Nausea Vomiting	IV	0.1-0.2 mg/kg	1-5 min	3-4 hr
		IM/SQ	0.1-0.2 mg/kg	30 min	4-5 hr
			Other Sedative Agents		
Chloral hydrate[b]	Prolonged sedation	PO/PR	25-100 mg/kg; *may repeat* 25-50 mg/kg after 30 min	15-30 min	1-2 hr
Ketamine	Post-emergence delirium	IV	0.5-2 mg/kg	1 min	15 min
		IM	4 mg/kg	3-5 min	15-30 min
		PO	5-10 mg/kg	30-40 min	2-4 hr
		PR	5-10 mg/kg	5-10 min	15-30 min
		Nasal	3-6 mg/kg	5-10 min	15-30 min

(Continued)

TABLE 16-5 Agents Commonly Used for Conscious Sedation (*Continued*)

Medication	Side Effects	Route	Total Dose[a]	Onset	Duration
Propofol	Respiratory depression Hypotension	IV over 20-30 sec;	0.5-1 mg/kg	30 sec	<5 min
		then repeat boluses, *or*	0.5 mg/kg prn	30 sec	5-15 min
		IV Drip	0.05-0.1 mg/kg/min	30 sec	5-15 min
Etomidate	Myoclonus Nausea Respiratory depression Adrenocortical suppression	IV	0.15-0.2 mg/kg	30 sec	5-15 min

Abbreviations: IM, intramuscular; IV, intravenous; NA, not available; PO, by mouth; PR, per rectum; SQ, subcutaneous.

[a]Doses should be administered in fractional boluses (e.g., one-quarter to one-half) and titrated to effect.

[b]Particularly useful for sedation during diagnostic imaging.

Data from Spitalnic et al,[23] Green et al,[24] and other sources.

greater risk for phlebitis, has less associated amnesia, and has erratic absorption if given IM. If no other sedative agent is available, it may be useful, especially if given orally about 30 minutes prior to a procedure.

Propofol

Propofol, because of its high cost, will often be unavailable in austere settings. If it is available, use it in increments of 0.5 mg/kg every 60 seconds IV until the desired effect is achieved and then to maintain that level of sedation. Because of its pharmacokinetics, oral administration will not sedate the patient. (Angela M. Plewa, PharmD. Personal communication, April 8, 2008.) Similarly scarce will be the popular ketamine–propofol combination (ketofol), which is a 1:1 mixture of ketamine 10 mg/mL and propofol 10 mg/mL titrated in 1- to 3-mL aliquots to attain deep or dissociative sedation.

INTRAVENOUS GENERAL ANESTHESIA

Introduction

One method of administering IV agents is to use a syringe attached to an in-line three-way stopcock. This allows frequent administration of anesthetic boluses, because a reservoir of additional anesthetic is in the IV bag or bottle. If supplies are limited and there has been no backward gross contamination from the patient (which is probably more common than realized), only the IV needle and the extension tubing flowing from the three-way stopcock to the patient need be changed between patients.[7] Narcotics, ketamine, and short-acting barbiturates can be used in this fashion.

How much to give? In resource-scarce situations in which patients do not receive a neuromuscular blockade, slight movements of the fingers or toes indicate a need for supplementary anesthetic injections.[32]

Neuromuscular Blockade

Do not even consider using a neuromuscular blocking agent unless you are highly proficient at obtaining, and have the equipment to control, an airway using several means (e.g., BVM, intubation, LMA, and cricothyrotomy).

If an NMB is to be used, it may be important, especially for those not experienced in giving general anesthesia, to know whether the patient is awake. During surgery, paralyzing a patient who is awake is not, to say the least, good medical practice. The "isolated arm test" can help to determine whether a patient is awake. Just before administering the NMB, inflate a BP cuff on one arm to about 30 mm Hg above the systolic pressure, effectively isolating that arm from blood flow. Ten minutes after giving the NMB, ask the patient to signal to you by squeezing your hand or moving his or her thumb. If the patient does it, he or she is not asleep. Then deflate the BP cuff and either put the patient to sleep or stop the procedure—or both.[33,34]

GENERAL INHALATION ANESTHETICS

Overview

This section is designed only for clinicians who are highly experienced in airway and critical care monitoring and management. Optimally, only clinicians experienced in delivering anesthetics will provide general anesthesia, although that may not be possible in resource-poor situations. The most common inhalation anesthetics used in resource-poor settings are discussed in Chapter 17.

Basic Pharmacology

Inhaled anesthetics pass through the lungs, enter the circulation, and produce anesthesia in the brain. Anesthetics that are more soluble in blood, such as ether, take longer to act (induction) and to wear off (emergence; recovery). Those, such as nitrous oxide, that are relatively insoluble in blood have much faster induction and emergence.

Shortages

Ether (most portable) and halothane (inexpensive) are the inhalation agents commonly used in Africa and other places where resources are limited. Other inhaled anesthetics commonly used by anesthesiologists in developed countries, including N_2O, are generally not available. As Boulton noted, "In all isolated situations, the most likely commodities to be in short supply are composed medical gases. Not only are cylinders heavy and bulky and difficult to transport in regions where communications are limited, but they provide relatively few 'anesthesia-hours' in proportion to their bulk in comparison with volatile agents vaporized in ambient air."[2]

Cost

Both logistics and cost affect the availability of anesthetic agents. The following are approximate costs for common anesthetics. Cost can vary greatly by region. Note that some of these agents are also available from chemical supply companies.[35,36]

Chloroform—$27.00 (100 mL)
Halothane—$50.00 (200 mL)
Ether—$5.00 (500 mL)
Procaine—(for injection) $1.66 (20 mg/2 mL)
Ketamine—$7.69 (500 mg/10 mL)

Anesthesia Machines

In austere circumstances, improvising even the most basic methods of delivering anesthetic gases is vital, because more modern anesthesia machines may not be available. The so-called "portable" anesthesia machines may not really be so portable in rough terrain. As Boulton and Cole pointed out, "If the only available transport is the flat-footed anesthetist himself, even such apparatus as the EMO [Epstein-Macintosh-Oxford] air-ether outfit, which weighs 25 lb (11 kg), or the 'Haloxair' halothane-air-oxygen apparatus [at] 13 lb (6 kg) may prove to be intolerably heavy. In such a circumstance, the anesthetist might well prefer [a very] simple apparatus or even a resuscitator bag and intravenous drugs alone."[2] A can of ether and a mask, of course, weigh much less than any of these, and do not take much backpack space.

Using Volatile Agents

Anesthetic gases can be used for both the induction and the maintenance phases of anesthesia. Alternatively, an IV induction agent or a faster-acting volatile agent (e.g., chloroform to induce ether) can be used, followed by an anesthetic gas for maintenance.[37] Intravenous inductions are done with the agents discussed in the "General Anesthesia Guidelines: Essential Elements" section above. Take great care not to cause respiratory depression from the synergistic action of the induction agent and the inhaled anesthetic.

Inhalational induction requires a seal between the face and the mask for the gas to be drawn through the vaporizer. If there is no seal, the patient will breathe room air around the mask and remain conscious. In adult anesthesia "it is relatively easy to coax a mask on the face and still keep the patient calm and cooperative."[38] Premedicating patients, especially anxious ones, assists the process.

Use in Closed Spaces

Using anesthetic gases is problematic in closed spaces, such as on a ship or in "closed down" conditions such as might occur after a nuclear, chemical, or biological attack or contamination. This situation becomes more dangerous when using open methods, such as open-drop ether. Try to eliminate as much of the ambient anesthetic as possible.[39]

Nitrous Oxide

Nitrous oxide (N_2O; laughing gas), in combination with oxygen, is a commonly used anesthetic gas in developed countries. It has a sweet, pleasant aroma (although to a patient, it appears odorless in the presence of the smell from the anesthesia mask) and, when inhaled, it is absorbed by the body and has a calming effect. Normal breathing eliminates N_2O from the body. Nitrous oxide has a rapid onset and recovery. It is a good analgesic supplement for halothane and reduces the incidence of awareness. It produces minimal cardiovascular and respiratory effects.

A World War I physician described the benefits of N_2O: "Nitrous oxide is particularly useful for multiple short procedures in mass casualty situations. Induction and emergence take a matter of seconds rather than minutes and most of the patients can walk out of the OR alone or with minimal assistance."[40]

The main problem with N_2O is that it will usually be unavailable in situations of scarcity, because it is expensive to produce and transport. Anesthesiologists familiar with disaster and austere environments believe that N_2O should not be used because of the logistical nightmare of supplying it, the possibility of errors when using it, the high cost, and its tendency to diffuse into air-containing spaces, such as pneumothoraces, the gut, middle ear, and ET tube cuff.[37,39]

To be effective, the patient must receive at least 50% N_2O. It is delivered to the patient through a rotameter (a clear tapered tube with a float inside that is pushed up by flow and pulled down by gravity) and is mixed with oxygen to produce an inspired mixture of not less than 30% O_2. A hypoxic gas mixture may result from using it with an oxygen concentrator. Nitrous oxide should not be used in draw-over circuits, and it should never be given to a patient with an untreated pneumothorax or who has been scuba diving within the previous 24 hours due to the potential for decompression sickness.[37] Some places may have cylinders of a 50% mixture of N_2O in oxygen, primarily used for self-administered outpatient analgesia.

RECTAL ANESTHESIA

Rectal anesthesia, sedation, or analgesia (see also Chapter 14) is relatively uncommon, although it is effective in children for "preinduction" sedation. This method of delivery requires less technical skill and equipment than IV or IM drug administration.

A major limitation of this method is the poor predictability of the clinical effects. This variability stems from anatomical properties of the patient's rectum, individual variance resulting in inconsistent anesthetic absorption, and elimination.[41] Using hydrophilic solutions and larger volumes with lower concentrations results in improved absorption by increasing the mucosal surface in contact with the drug.

In clinical practice, rectally administering anesthetic medications is more common for procedural sedation or for use as an anesthetic premedication, where a lighter stage is needed and the exact timing of medication onset is not as vital. To deliver rectal medication to children, use a lubricated tip of a small (14-Fr) suction catheter or nasogastric tube. A similar-sized urethral catheter also works, as does simply using a syringe and holding it there for 2 or 3 minutes. Medications for sedation and anesthesia that can be used rectally include the benzodiazepines, barbiturates, and ketamine. Ether, although not commonly administered by this method, is also an option.

Doses and Method

- *Midazolam* 1.0 mg/kg (preinduction): Administer at least 30 minutes, but no longer than 90 minutes, prior to anesthetic induction.[42]
- *Methohexitone* (Methohexital): Administer 15 mg/kg of 10% methohexitone for anesthetic induction or for short procedures.[43]
- *Ketamine* 10 mg/kg: This medication has a delayed onset. Ketamine occasionally causes respiratory distress and, at the recommended 10 mg/kg rectal dose, may result in prolonged postoperative sedation if used for brief procedures.[41,44]

ANESTHESIA FOR CESAREAN SECTIONS

A common, but somewhat dangerous, situation is for the surgeon doing the C-section also to administer the anesthetic. If this is the only option, use ketamine via one of the methods described in the following paragraphs. Other methods include local infiltration (described next), spinal anesthesia (discussed here and in Chapter 15), or epidural anesthesia for those having experience with the technique. In these cases, having a trained assistant to monitor and care for the patient throughout the operation is vital.

Local Infiltration

The main advantages of using local anesthesia infiltration in austere situations are that it is safe, inexpensive, and uses few resources. Especially for mothers in poor condition and those who are hypotensive, local anesthesia may provide the best safety margin, especially if adjunctive sedatives are not used. Epinephrine added to the anesthetic reduces local bleeding. However, using local infiltration requires significant operator experience, and even then, it may not be completely effective. It also takes time to administer.[45]

Technique

Determine the maximum safe anesthetic dose and, if not premixed, add 0.1 mL epinephrine 1:1000 to each 20 mL of anesthetic to make a 1:200,000 solution. If available, give oxygen to the mother until delivery. Using a 10-cm (4-inch) needle, infiltrate two long bands of skin on either side of the proposed incision line. Keep the needle parallel to the skin; remember that the abdominal wall is very thin at term—do not stick the needle into the uterus. Infiltrate the rectus sheath after incising the skin. To anesthetize the parietal peritoneum, inject 10 mL anesthetic under the linea alba. Then inject 5 mL more into the loose visceral peritoneum of the uterus where the incision will be made.

Collins provided some additional advice: "Reassure the patient and explain that after the local anesthetic has been given, she will still feel certain sensations of touch. She may experience discomfort if the head is well engaged in the pelvis. However, the anesthetic will prevent her feeling significant pain."[45] Giving additional sedatives or analgesics, while desirable from an anesthetic standpoint, may adversely affect the baby. It is optimal to give nothing until the cord is clamped, after which small doses of narcotic or sedative may be used.

Ketamine

Ketamine is contraindicated in pregnancy before term because it is oxytocic, and it is a US Food and Drug Administration fetal-risk category C drug. It is also relatively contraindicated in patients with eclampsia or preeclampsia. When the woman goes into labor, ketamine 10 mg to 20 mg IV can be used to provide analgesia. It can be repeated every 2 to 5 minutes, but do not administer >1 mg/kg in 30 minutes; the total dose should not exceed 100 mg.[16]

While ketamine may be used for vaginal delivery, only an experienced anesthetist who can adjust the dose according to the circumstances should use it.[46]

Ketamine is often used for C-sections because it has some unique advantages: (a) Patients in advanced labor have less discomfort than with spinal or epidural anesthesia. (b) Although ketamine crosses the placenta easily and concentrations in the fetus are the same or higher than those in the mother, its use results in less fetal and neonatal depression than with other anesthetics.[16-18] (c) Babies have good APGAR scores, even after periods of neonatal asphyxia—an important consideration when limited neonatal resuscitation equipment is available. This depends in part on the skill and speed of the surgeon.[47] However, be careful with the dose, because a dose above 2 mg/kg may cause both respiratory depression and chest wall rigidity in the newborn.[48] (d) Uterine contractility is unimpaired, so there is less danger of postpartum hemorrhage. (e) Ketamine supports maternal BP, which may be important in the face of significant hypotension.[16] This BP increase can be ameliorated for those with eclampsia by using hydralazine or similar medications.[49]

If the mother experiences an emergence reaction to the ketamine, do not administer sedatives (benzodiazepines) to block the reaction until the baby is delivered, because these also can cause respiratory depression in the newborn. In cases of fetal distress, avoid ketamine, because it causes the uterus to contract.[48]

Methods for Cesarean Section

The following two methods show how ketamine can be used successfully for C-sections.

Working in a remote Kenyan hospital, Dr. Veeken describes the successful use of a combination of local infiltration and a ketamine drip:

> No premedication is given. An intravenous line is set up; local anesthesia (lidocaine 0.5%) is injected in the midline from symphysis up to the umbilicus. The doctor then scrubs. Opening is performed under this local anesthesia only. It's impressive how well the women tolerate this. If necessary, more local anesthetic could be administered for the deeper layers, but we never do. Atropine 0.6 mg is given IV. Just before the opening of the uterus, a bolus of 75 mg ketamine is given IV. The child is quickly delivered. The uterus is closed during the effect of the ketamine; a bilateral tubal ligation can be performed. Usually the women start waking up while closing the abdomen, the local anesthesia still enables us to close the fascia and the skin. If necessary, diazepam is given IV during the closure. This method is very safe for both mother and child.... Although not very elegant, it is satisfactorily cheap, very easy to administer, and extremely safe. It is highly recommended for working under primitive circumstances.[50]

Dr. Zimmermann described the method used in Bangladesh for 8000 C-sections (with one avoidable anesthetic death): "Routine premedication is omitted.... If necessary, oxygen is administered via mask or nasal tube. For induction, 0.6 mg atropine plus 100 mg ketamine diluted to 5 cc is administered IV over about 60 seconds."[49] While ketamine is normally given as an mg/kg dose, a standard dose is used to avoid errors. It results in <2 mg/kg in virtually all these patients. This injection achieves an adequate surgical stage of anesthesia, and the patient continues to breathe spontaneously. For C-sections, administer oxygen if there is fetal distress. Maintenance anesthesia is achieved using a ketamine drip of 200 mg ketamine diluted in 200 mL NS or dextrose solution, resulting in 1 mg ketamine/1 mL fluid. This is run at 20 to 30 drops per minute, which is 1 to 1.5 mg/min. A benzodiazepine (diazepam 10 to 20 mg has been used successfully) can be added once the baby is delivered. It provides a sound sleep and decreases possible psychomimetic reactions. The ketamine drip is discontinued once the surgical incision is closed.[49]

ANESTHESIA DELIVERY SYSTEMS

Improvised Vaporizers

Vaporizers deliver safe concentrations of volatile anesthetic vapor into the anesthetic system going to the patient. The volatile agent enters the vaporizer in liquid form and comes out as a vapor. Vaporizers can be improvised.

The ideal vaporizer has a clear chamber so the amount of anesthetic is visible. Keeping the anesthetic temperature relatively constant is also important, because the liquid's temperature falls as it passes into vapor. This, in turn, lowers the output of the vaporizer. In improvised vaporizers, the equipment sits in a water bath, which transfers heat to the anesthetic to minimize any fall in temperature.[38]

The Coffee Jar Vaporizer

Boulton devised a very workable vaporizer for a draw-over system using two sizes of jars. To make the large vaporizer suitable for ether administration, he used a 135-g (118-mL; 4-oz) Maxwell House coffee jar (7.5-cm [3-inch] diameter, 13-cm [5-inch] tall). Other containers of *this size* can be used instead. The jar's size partially determines the anesthetic concentration. The smaller jar, which can be used for ether, halothane, or trichloroethane, has a 5-cm diameter and is 19-cm (7.5-inches) tall.

Put a piece of plastic tubing with a 1.25-cm (0.5-inch) diameter through one of two holes of that size that you have punched into the lid; the tube should just fit. Cut the end of this obliquely, so that fluid is less likely to be sucked through it. Cut a wide hole in the tube, in such a position that you can lift it above the lid to reduce the vapor concentration, if necessary (Fig. 16-1). Fix a piece of cotton at one edge of the other open hole in the lid. Each time the patient breathes, it will move, allowing you to monitor his ventilation. If available, add oxygen through a tube that fits loosely in the open hole.[6]

Fill the large jar by adding 150 mL—about 4-cm deep—of ether. Once the patient is induced, the vaporizer is ready to put in-line with whatever system you are using (a non-rebreathing valve and an Oxford bellows or a self-inflating bag, or attached directly to a tracheal tube). The initial 11% ether concentration falls to 8% in 5 minutes and remains relatively constant thereafter. Gently shaking the bottle for 1 minute doubles the concentration. The concentration can be halved by opening a T-piece closed by the finger cot (the cut finger from a surgical glove) and still further reduced by tightening the screw clamp. Using trichloroethane, a constant 1% concentration is obtained, which is halved by opening the T-piece. Halothane gives too high a concentration for use with the larger vaporizer.

Convert the apparatus to a "semi-one-way" system by snipping off the end of the finger cot, thus creating a simple valve that closes on inspiration and opens on expiration. As it vaporizes, the ether will get cold and the concentration will diminish. At that point, gently agitate the bottle for about a minute, or put it in a bath of warm water. When using trichloroethylene, no water bath is needed.

If using the smaller bottle, prepare it the same way, but with 50 mL of halothane. A constant 1% vapor concentration is obtained, which is halved by opening the T-piece or doubled by shaking the jar for 1 minute. Secure this bottle firmly to the table or another fixed structure—the vaporizer is dangerous if knocked over.[6,51]

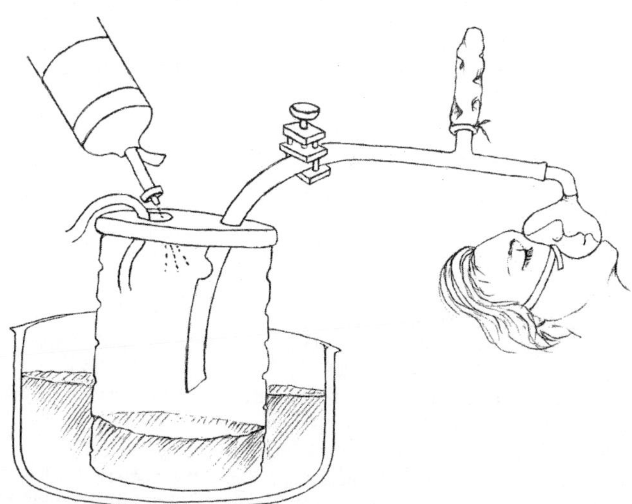

FIG. 16-1. Coffee jar vaporizer. *(Redrawn from Boulton.[6])*

Anesthesia (Plenum) Machines

Under normal circumstances, anesthesiologists in developed countries use plenum machines to deliver inhalational anesthetics. Boulton described the "frustrating experience of administering anesthesia with the 'rag and bottle' in a well-equipped OR while a typical modern anesthesia machine stood idle because of the lack of cylinders."[2]

POSTOPERATIVE RECOVERY

In situations with limited resources and few trained personnel, the safest place for an anesthetized patient to recover is in the OR. The key is ensuring that the patient is awake when he leaves the OR. Boulton notes that "if vigilance is relaxed when the drama of the operating room is over, death can still strike if the patient is left unsupervised."[52] To prevent this, leave the patient intubated until pharyngeal reflexes return.[53]

Postoperatively, place patients in the "recovery" position, lying on their side (see Fig. 8-1). As often as possible, check their airway, vital signs, blood loss, and temperature. The latter is important because, while many ORs in hot climates are now air-conditioned or cooled, patients run the risk of hyperpyrexia when they are transferred to a hot ward.[52]

REFERENCES

1. McCormick BA, Eltringham RJ. Anaesthesia equipment for resource-poor environments. *Anaesthesia.* 2007;62(suppl 1):54-60.
2. Boulton TB, Cole PV. Anaesthesia in difficult situations. What would I do if…? *Anaesthesia.* 1966;21(2):268-276.
3. King MH, ed. *Primary Anaesthesia.* Oxford, UK: Oxford University Press; 1986:4.
4. Husum H, Ang SC, Fosse E. *War Surgery: Field Manual.* Penang, Malaysia: Third World Network; 1995:66.
5. Vinson DR, Hoehn CL. Sedation-assisted orthopedic reduction in emergency medicine: the safety and success of a one physician/one nurse model. *West J Emerg Med.* 2013;14(1):47-54.
6. Boulton TB. Anaesthesia in difficult situations. 3. General anaesthesia-technique. *Anaesthesia.* 1966;21(4):513-545.
7. Hodges SC, Mijumbi C, Okello M, et al. Anesthesia services in the developing world: defining the problems. *Anaesthesia.* 2007;62:4-11.
8. King MH, ed. *Primary Anaesthesia.* Oxford, UK: Oxford University Press; 1986:11.
9. King MH, ed. *Primary Anaesthesia.* Oxford, UK: Oxford University Press; 1986:76.
10. King MH, ed. *Primary Anaesthesia.* Oxford, UK: Oxford University Press; 1986:70-71.
11. Shinjo T, Inoue S, Egawa J, Kawaguchi M, Furuya H. Two cases in which the effectiveness of "laryngospasm notch" pressure against laryngospasm was confirmed by imaging examinations. *J Anesth.* 2013;27(5):761-763.
12. Hodges SC, Walker IA, Bosenberg AT. Pediatric anaesthesia in developing countries. *Anaesthesia.* 2007;62(suppl 1):26-31.
13. King MH, ed. *Primary Anesthesia.* Oxford, UK: Oxford University Press; 1986:85-89.
14. Safar P. Anesthesia at high altitude. *Ann Surg.* 1956;144(5):835-840.
15. Boulton TB, Cole PV. Anaesthesia in difficult situations. (9) some solutions, new drugs and a conclusion. *Anaesthesia.* 1968;23(4):597-630.
16. Stevenson C. Ketamine: a review. *Update Anaesth.* 2005;20:25-29.
17. Tomlinson A. Ketamine. *Update Anaesth.* 1994;4(5):1-4.
18. Nunn JF. Anaesthesia at altitude. In: Ward MP, Milledge JS, West JB, eds. *High Altitude Medicine and Physiology.* 2nd ed. London, UK: Chapman & Hall Medical; 1995:523-526.
19. Godwin A. *Tough Cases of Sedation and Analgesia in the Critically Ill* (adapted from handout). ACEP Scientific Assembly, Seattle, WA, October 8, 2007.
20. Sacchetti A, Senula G, Strickland J, et al. Procedural sedation in the community ED: initial results of the ProSCED registry. *Acad Emerg Med.* 2007;14:41-46.
21. King MH, ed. *Primary Anesthesia.* Oxford, UK: Oxford University Press; 1986:137.
22. Grunwell JR, McCracken C, Fortenberry J, Stockwell J, Kamat P. Risk factors leading to failed procedural sedation in children outside the operating room. *Ped Emerg Care.* 2014;30(6):381-387.

23. Spitalnic S, Blazes C, Anderson AC. Conscious sedation: a primer for outpatient procedures. *Hosp Phys.* 2000;36(5):22-32.
24. Green SM, Krauss B. Procedural sedation and analgesia. In: Baren JM, Rothrock SG, Breenan JA, et al, eds. *Pediatric Emergency Medicine*. Philadelphia, PA: W.B. Saunders; 2008:1119-1137.
25. Wong SME, Fong E, Tauck DL, et al. Ethanol as a general anesthetic: actions in spinal cord. *Eur J Pharmacol.* 1997;329(2-3):121-127.
26. Armstrong-Davison MH. *The Evolution of Anaesthesia*. Altrincham, UK: John Sherratt; 1965.
27. Anon. *Civil War anesthesia*. http://home.nc.rr.com/fieldhospcsa/Anesthesia.htmL. Accessed April 6, 2008.
28. Constantin JD. General anaesthesia by the intravenous injection of ethyl alcohol. *Lancet.* 1929;1:1247.
29. Dundee JW, Isaac M, Clarke RSJ. Use of alcohol in anesthesia. *Anesth Analg.* 1969;48:665-669.
30. Waring JP, Baron TH, Hirota WK, et al. Guidelines for conscious sedation and monitoring during gastrointestinal endoscopy. *Gastrointest Endosc.* 2003;58(3):317-322.
31. Klein EJ, Brown JC, Kobayashi A, Osincup D, Seidel K. A randomized clinical trial comparing oral, aerosolized intranasal, and aerosolized buccal midazolam. *Ann Emerg Med.* 2011;58:323-329.
32. Ruben H, Knudsen EJ, Winkel E, et al. Anaesthesia in mass emergencies. *Lancet.* 1958; 1(7018):460-461.
33. King MH, ed. *Primary Anaesthesia*. Oxford, UK: Oxford University Press; 1986:18.
34. Motamed C, Kirov K, Lieutaud T, et al. The mechanism of pancuronium potentiation of mivacurium block: use of the isolated-arm technique. *Anesth Analg.* 2000;91:732-735.
35. Sid Patanwala, PharmD, BCPS, Clinical Assistant Professor, *The University of Arizona College of Pharmacy*, Tucson, AZ. Personal communication, April 9, 2008.
36. Other sources, including Epocrates (www.epocrates.com), PEPID (www.pepid.com), and on-line pharmacies.
37. Fenton P. Using volatile anaesthetic agents. *Update Anaesth.* 1995;5(5):1-3. www.nda.ox.ac.uk/wfsa/htmL/u05/u05_009.htm. Accessed September 13, 2006.
38. Simpson S, Wilson IH. Draw-over anaesthesia review. *Update Anaesth.* 2002;15(6):1-10. www.nda.ox.ac.uk/wfsa/htmL/u15/u1506_01.htm. Accessed September 14, 2006.
39. Grande CM, Baskett PJF, Donchin Y, et al. Trauma anesthesia for disasters: anything, anytime, anywhere. *Crit Care Clin.* 1991;7(2):339-361.
40. Flagg PJ. Anaesthesia in Europe on the Western battlefront. *Int Clinics.* 1918;3:210-228.
41. Jantzen JP, Diehl P. Die rektale medikamentenverabreichung: grundlagen und anwendung in der anaesthesie. [Rectal administration of drugs: fundamentals and applications in anaesthesia.] *Anaesthesist.* 1991;40(5):251-261.
42. Spear RM, Yaster M, Berkowitz ID, et al. Pre-induction of anesthesia in children with rectally administered midazolam. *Anesthesiology.* 1991;74(4):670-674.
43. Kotiniemi LH, Ryhanen PT. Behavioural changes and children's memories after intravenous, inhalation and rectal induction of anaesthesia. *Paediatr Anaesth.* 1996;6(3):201-207.
44. Tanaka M, Sato M, Saito A, et al. Reevaluation of rectal ketamine premedication in children: comparison with rectal midazolam. *Anesthesiology.* 2000;93(5):1217-1224.
45. Collins C, Gurung A. Anaesthesia for Caesarian section. *Update Anaesth.* 1998;9(3):1-6. www.nda.ox.ac.uk/wfsa/htmL/u09/u09_006.htm. Accessed September 13, 2006.
46. World Health Organization. *Model Prescribing Information: Drugs Used in Anesthesia*. Geneva, Switzerland: WHO; 1989:18-20. http://apps.who.int/medicinedocs/en/d/Jh2929e/. Accessed September 9, 2015.
47. Ketcham DW. Where there is no anaesthesiologist: the many uses of ketamine. *Trop Doct.* 1990;20:163-166.
48. Craven R. Ketamine. *Anaesthesia.* 2007;62(suppl 1):48-53.
49. Zimmermann H. Ketamine drip anaesthesia for Caesarean section: report on 200 cases from a rural hospital in Zimbabwe. *Trop Doct.* 1988;18:60-61.
50. Veeken H. Ketamine drip anaesthesia for Caesarean section. *Trop Doct.* 1989;19(1):47.
51. King MH, ed. *Primary Anaesthesia*. Oxford, UK: Oxford University Press; 1986:83-84.
52. Boulton TB, Cole P. Anaesthesia in difficult situations. (5) General and local complications. *Anaesthesia.* 1967;22(3):435-464.
53. King MH, ed. *Primary Anaesthesia*. Oxford, UK: Oxford University Press; 1986:19.

17 Anesthesia: Ketamine, Ether, and Halothane

WHY THIS CHAPTER?

A group of anesthesiologists familiar with international disaster relief operations wrote, "There is a danger of the modern practitioner becoming an 'anesthetic dinosaur,' unable to survive except in a sophisticated technological environment."[1] Inexperience with ketamine, ether, and halothane, the anesthetics commonly used in developing countries, may come to haunt those trying to deliver inhalational anesthesia in austere circumstances. Ketamine is an easy and safe anesthetic to give, even by non-anesthetists; ether is extremely safe, portable, and deliverable by improvised means. Modern anesthetists often aren't familiar with halothane. Therefore, a description of these three anesthetics will help clinicians deliver safe anesthesia.

KETAMINE

Ketamine merits a detailed discussion because of its wide spectrum of safe uses (e.g., for sedation, regional and general anesthesia, analgesia, and psychiatry) and its availability throughout the world, even in areas with resource scarcities. (A discussion of ketamine use for Caesarian sections is in Chapter 16.)

"Ketamine is remarkably safe and is certainly the safest anesthetic if you are inexperienced."[2] Not surprisingly, in some hospitals without a trained anesthetist, up to 90% of the operations are done under ketamine.[3]

Ketamine is unique, producing hypnosis (sleep), analgesia (pain relief), and amnesia (short-term memory loss).[4] Patients given ketamine rapidly go into a trance-like "dissociative" state, becoming detached from their surroundings. Patients' eyes are wide open, and they have a slow nystagmus, preserve their corneal and light reflexes, and make reflexive movements.[5,6] A major benefit of using ketamine is that, unless high doses are used or smaller doses are given rapidly, the patient's airway remains open and he or she breathes spontaneously.[2,5] Even if transient apnea occurs, brief bag-valve-mask (BVM) ventilation suffices until spontaneous respirations return. Another major benefit is that patients maintain their blood pressure (BP), even in shock.[7] Laryngeal spasm is an extremely rare complication and can be easily treated with pressure in the "laryngospasm notch" (see Chapter 16).[2]

Pharmacology

Being water and lipid soluble, ketamine can be administered intravenously (IV), intramuscularly (IM), orally, rectally, subcutaneously, transnasally, transdermally, and via an epidural block. Ketamine has a slower onset than other IV anesthetic agents after an IV bolus (1-5 minutes), and its duration of action depends on the route of administration (20-30 minutes for IM; 10-15 minutes for IV).[6]

Ketamine comes in three concentrations: 10 mg/mL, 50 mg/mL, and 100 mg/mL. If only one strength is to be kept in a hospital, the 50-mg/mL ampoule is the best compromise, because it can be used for IM injections or may be diluted down to 10 mg/mL for IV use. Protect the medication from light when stored. Table 17-1 lists ketamine's physiological effects.

Do not mix barbiturates or diazepam in the same syringe or infusion as ketamine, because they are chemically incompatible. Other cerebral depressant medications prolong ketamine's effects and delay recovery.[5,8] Patients who receive repeated sedations, such as for dressing changes, often develop tolerance to ketamine and require progressively higher doses. Stop ketamine administration for 3 days to allow patients to regain their normal response.[6]

Common Uses

Ketamine has a wide variety of uses. A frequent medication for procedural sedation in medical settings (Table 17-2), ketamine is also an excellent analgesic (see Chapter 14) and antidepressant

TABLE 17-1 Ketamine's Physiological Effects

System	Effects			
Cardiovascular system	⇑ Heart rate	⇑ BP	⇑ CVP	⇑ CO_2
	Baroreceptors: Normal function	Dysrhythmias: Rare		
Respiratory system	Bronchodilation	⇑ Respiratory rate	Preservation of airway reflexes	
Central nervous system	⇑ Cerebral blood flow	⇑ Metabolic rate	⇑ Intraocular pressure	
Autonomic system	Nausea and vomiting	⇑ Salivation		
Genitourinary system	⇑ Uterine tone			
Other	Emergence delirium/dreams/hallucinations			

Abbreviations: BP, blood pressure; CVP, central venous pressure; CO_2, carbon dioxide.

Data from Stevenson.[5]

(see Chapter 38), and a drug to use during rescues, such as for an amputation on a trapped patient.[5,9] The continued presence of a gag reflex under ketamine anesthesia makes operations inside the mouth problematic, although teeth can be wired for stabilization using ketamine. Bronchoscopy cannot be done under ketamine unless neuromuscular blockers are used.

Ketamine is the ideal anesthetic for elderly, poor-risk, and dehydrated patients. It sustains rather than decreases the BP, and provides bronchodilation and decreases bronchospasm in chronic obstructive pulmonary disease (COPD) and asthma patients. For that reason, it is often used to intubate and treat patients in status asthmaticus.

Ketamine can be used as an anesthetic premedication (orally or parenterally) for anesthesia induction prior to administration of inhalational anesthetics, or for both induction and maintenance of anesthesia. It is of particular value for patients in shock, for children requiring frequent repeated anesthetic, for procedures with the patient in a prone (face-down) position that without intubation might make controlling the airway difficult, for emergency surgery when a patient has recently eaten, for surgery on patients who may be difficult to intubate, and when other anesthetics, equipment, or techniques are not available.[5,8] It may also help severe asthmatic children who are unresponsive to other therapies. An optimal dose seems to be a 2- to 3-mg/kg bolus, followed by a 2- to 3-mg/kg/hr infusion.[10]

Advantages

Anesthesia persists for up to 15 minutes after a single IV injection and is characterized by profound analgesia. (See also Chapter 14.) Ketamine also produces retrograde amnesia. Children receiving an IM injection, for example, will not recall getting the injection when they awaken.

Apnea is unusual unless ketamine is administered rapidly IV or another respiratory depressant drug, such as an opioid, is given. If only ketamine has been administered, the apnea lasts only a short time (up to 1 minute) and can easily be managed with a BVM. After a slow IV induction, breathing is well maintained and may even increase slightly.[4]

TABLE 17-2 Common Procedures/Surgeries Using Ketamine Sedation

Fracture reduction	Joint relocation	Dressing changes
Abscess drainage	Burn debridement	Head/neck surgery
Dilation and curettage	Cesarean sections	Endoscopy
Foreign body removal	Laceration repair (children)	Cast changes
Radiotherapy	Chest tube placement	Bone marrow aspiration

Airway reflexes and skeletal muscle tone are relatively well preserved, but salivary and tracheobronchial secretions increase. Despite the retention of protective reflexes, normal airway care must be maintained to prevent obstruction or aspiration.[4] Laryngospasm occurs in about 1 in 500 cases after ketamine administration, although this is far less than the nearly 9 per 500 incidence with other agents.[7]

Ketamine stimulates the cardiovascular system, increasing the heart's workload slightly while maintaining systemic vascular resistance. Because it does not induce hypotension, the patient does not have to remain supine. Its sympathomimetic effects are of particular value in patients who are shocked, severely dehydrated, or severely anemic.[8] Ketamine raises the BP (in patients with an intact sympathetic response) by about 25% (systolic pressure increases by ~20 to 30 mm Hg) and the heart rate increases by ~20%. In the majority of patients, the BP rises steadily over 3 to 5 minutes and then returns to normal 10 to 20 minutes after injection, although there is wide individual variation that is related neither to dose nor to preexisting hypertension. Benzodiazepine premedication, such as with diazepam, reduces this rise in BP; additional small doses may control the pressure during the sedation.[4] This is particularly important if ketamine must be given to patients with uncontrolled hypertension, increased intracranial pressure, thyrotoxicosis, congestive heart failure, or eclampsia.

Disadvantages

The main problem with ketamine anesthesia is that there is no muscle relaxation. For abdominal operations or procedures on large joints (e.g., hip), a neuromuscular blocking agent and a controlled airway may be needed, requiring considerably more anesthetic prowess and eliminating one of the great benefits of using ketamine.

Preserved muscle tone may make airway control, if needed, more difficult. Unless other medications are given, the use of a laryngeal mask airway (LMA) or oral intubation will be extremely difficult.[5] Ketamine does raise intraocular pressure, although only for a few minutes after administration. Eye movements may continue throughout surgery, making it unsuitable for patients with perforating eye injuries or for ophthalmic surgery where a nonmoving eye is required.[4]

Patients receiving ketamine may have a prolonged recovery time, sometimes accompanied by nausea and vomiting. Hallucinations can occur during recovery (although less commonly noticed in children), but they are avoided if ketamine is used solely as an induction agent and is followed by a conventional inhalational anesthetic. Their incidence may also be greatly reduced by administering diazepam both as a premedication and after the procedure.[8]

Contraindications

Ketamine is contraindicated in a number of conditions (Table 17-3). In contrast to prior dogma, it is no longer contraindicated in patients with head trauma or in children 3 to 12 months old. When relative contraindications exist, balance the need to use ketamine with the risks involved.

Monitoring During Use

Despite its safety record, patients should be carefully monitored during ketamine anesthesia. Secretions can cause obstruction and, although airway reflexes are usually preserved, laryngospasm and aspiration can occur. If there is no monitoring equipment, using your palm to check their breathing pattern and palpating the rate and quality of the patient's pulse are usually sufficient.[5]

Judging depth of anesthesia under ketamine can be difficult, because there are few obvious signs. Spontaneous movement and eye opening may occur during adequate anesthesia, but are more common during subanesthetic doses.[5]

Premedicating Patients—Sedation

When ketamine is used for sedation, do not pretreat patients with anticholinergics. In children, premedication with benzodiazepines is unnecessary, although they should be available to treat the rare extreme emergence reaction. In adults, midazolam 0.03 mg/kg IV may be useful. Pretreating patients with odansetron may slightly reduce emesis.[11]

TABLE 17-3 Contraindications to Ketamine

Absolute Contraindications	Relative Contraindications	
Hypersensitivity to ketamine	Known or suspected cardiovascular disease, including heart failure, hypertension, and angina	Intracerebral mass, abnormality, or hemorrhage
Open eye procedures	Active pulmonary infection or disease, including upper respiratory infection and asthma	Acute porphyria
Age <3 months	Major procedures stimulating posterior pharynx (e.g., endoscopy)	History of airway instability, tracheal surgery, or tracheal stenosis
Liver failure	Preeclampsia	Glaucoma or acute globe rupture
Psychiatric disorders (e.g., schizophrenia, acute psychoses)	History of cerebrovascular accident	Thyroid disorder or taking thyroid medications

Data from Stevenson,[5] Craven,[6] Green et al,[11] and Cohen et al.[12]

Pretreating Patients—Anesthesia

When using ketamine for anesthesia, pretreat patients to decrease salivation, either with atropine or scopolamine 20 mcg/kg (to a maximum dose of 0.5 mg [500 mcg]) given IM or IV 30 minutes before ketamine administration, or with 10 to 20 mcg/kg (to maximum 0.5 mg) of either medication given IV at the time of induction.[4,13] Alternatively, glycopyrrolate, which may be a better choice due to its lower psychotropic and chronotropic effect, may be administered IV at 0.01 mg/kg (to a maximum 0.2 mg).[5,6]

Clonidine or diazepam may also be useful premedications before ketamine anesthesia. Oral clonidine (5 mcg/kg) reduces the hypertensive response. To reduce the dose of ketamine needed, give diazepam 0.15 mg/kg orally in adults, or promethazine 0.5 mg/kg orally in children, 1 hour prior to ketamine administration. Alternatively, give diazepam 0.1 mg/kg IV on induction.[4,5] To diminish any unpleasant hallucinations and decrease muscle tone, which is particularly important in abdominal surgeries, give diazepam 0.22 mg/kg IV just before induction or orally 1 hour before induction.[13] The downside is that, especially in infants, the routine administration of benzodiazepine reduces ketamine's safety margin, and so should be avoided. A better method to prevent hallucinations is to treat patients with small doses of IV diazepam during recovery.[6]

Ketamine as an Anesthetic Premedication

Ketamine can be used to premedicate children before anesthesia with other agents. Oral ketamine 8 mg/kg is effective, although recovery from anesthesia is longer than normal. Intranasal ketamine can be used both as a premedicant and as an analgesic. In children, 3 mg/kg diluted to 2 mL with NS (give 1 mL per nostril) produces analgesia and sedation, but not anesthesia. (For best effect, use an atomizer. Improvised atomizers are described in Chapter 14.) This allows mask-inhalation anesthesia induction and does not cause prolonged recovery.[5] Ketamine has also been used orally or rectally as a form of premedication/sedative, but its effect is unpredictable.[4]

Intramuscular Administration

Intramuscular (IM) ketamine can be used in analgesic/sedative doses or for anesthesia induction and maintenance (Table 17-4). The retrograde amnesia means that the child generally will not remember receiving the injection. IM doses last longer and wear off more slowly than do IV doses.[14] When IM ketamine is used for sedation, no separate IV line is necessary.[11]

For pediatric sedation, use 2 mg/kg IM. It takes about 5 minutes until the child is ready for the procedure.[6] To induce surgical-level anesthesia, administer 5 to 10 mg/kg ketamine + 20 mcg/kg

TABLE 17-4 Intramuscular Ketamine Administration Sequence

Step	Alternatives
Advance premedication	Atropine: 20 mcg/kg IM 30 min pre-op Diazepam: 0.15 mg/kg orally 1 hr pre-op (adults) Promethazine: 0.5 mg/kg orally 1 hr pre-op (children) No premedication
Premedication at surgery	Atropine 10-20 mcg/kg IV prior to ketamine *-or-* No premedication
Induction	1-2 mg/kg IV
Maintenance	IV boluses 0.5 mg/kg *-or-* IV drip 1-2 mg/min

Data from Tomlinson[4] and other sources.

atropine, mixed in the same syringe, by deep IM injection. The child will be asleep in 3 to 5 minutes and anesthesia will last about 25 minutes.[6,8] Anesthesia can be prolonged by using additional IV or IM doses of ketamine. If the IM route is used, administer additional doses of 3 to 5 mg/kg ketamine or 25% to 50% of the initial dose, as required. The need for supplementary doses is primarily determined by the patient's moving in response to surgical stimuli.[4,6,8]

Ketamine's effective dose seems to vary with a child's nutritional status or the amount of alcohol an adult normally consumes. In malnourished children, always use less than the normal dose; in alcoholics, the dose should be higher. Experience shows that if a patient shows no signs of anesthesia after receiving three times the normal dose, a different agent should be used.[4,15]

If ketamine is scarce, consider giving it IV or with a neuromuscular blocker. King notes that "while 12 mg/kg IM ketamine (~840 mg for a 70-kg patient) provides an adult patient with about an hour of anesthesia; the same result comes from using about 280 mg IV. Only about half that much is needed if a muscle relaxant is used simultaneously."[16]

Intravenous Administration

Intravenous Pharmacodynamics

When there is an option, administer ketamine IV, because it causes less emesis.[11] The action of IV ketamine is faster than IM, but slower than other IV anesthetics. For example, within 3 to 5 minutes after an IM injection of 6 to 8 mg/kg ketamine (mixed with atropine), the patient will be ready for surgery, yet the patient should be ready in only 1 to 3 minutes following an IV injection of 1 to 2 mg/kg (mixed with atropine).[9] Therefore, an IV dose of ketamine should not be given until the clinician is ready to start the procedure.

Induction

Induce a child with 1.5 to 2 mg/kg or an adult with 1.0 mg/kg ketamine by slow IV injection over 30 to 60 seconds; there appears to be no benefit to titrating it to effect with small boluses.[11] More rapid administration may result in respiratory depression or apnea, as well as an enhanced pressor response. A dose of 2 mg/kg produces surgical anesthesia within 1 to 3 minutes that should last from 10 to 15 minutes.[4,5,8]

Maintenance Boluses

Maintenance anesthesia with ketamine can be achieved using IV boluses. Either give intermittent boluses of IV ketamine (0.5 mg/kg, or 50% of the original IV dose) every 15 to 20 minutes, or give boluses according to the patient's response to surgical stimuli—pupil size, heart rate,

BP, movement, and so forth.[5,6,8,9] During longer procedures, the clinician should note the time interval between induction and the first supplemental dose, so that he or she can begin to inject further increments slowly at the next appropriate time.[4]

Maintenance Infusion

Maintaining anesthesia using a ketamine drip (a) allows better control of the anesthetic depth than do the IM or bolus IV methods, (b) has a rapid induction and recovery, and (c) is less likely to cause a respiratory arrest than using IV boluses.[17] In circumstances in which non-anesthetists (and even nonmedical personnel) must give anesthesia, a ketamine drip permits a standardized protocol that most physicians and nurses can follow to administer anesthesia safely with minimal instruction.[18]

To use this method, make a ketamine solution of 1 mg/mL by dissolving 10 mL of ketamine containing 50 mg/mL in 500 mL of 5% dextrose or normal saline (0.9%, NS). For short procedures, mix smaller volumes, but keep it at 1 mg/mL for ease of administration. If the surgeon will also be giving the anesthetic (not unusual in the developing world), he or she should start the ketamine drip (using a 10 drop/mL infusion set) before beginning to scrub.

The method that King and others use for an average size adult is to start the drip at 1 to 2 drops/kg/min (non-micro drip IV chamber 15 drops/mL), which equals 1 to 2 mg/min ketamine, to maintain spontaneous ventilation. Some patients may need as much as 4 mg/min. Adjust the rate of infusion according to the depth of anesthesia achieved and required, as well as the size of the patient. "Continue the drip beyond the point at which the patient becomes unconscious, until surgical anesthesia is reached. This is easy to recognize, but difficult to describe. [The patient] develops a vacant stare, he does not respond to pain, but he still has his eyelash, corneal, and pharyngeal reflexes. Test his sensation of pain by pricking him with a pin. When surgical anesthesia has been reached, slow the drip to 60 to 80 drops/minute. This is about one drop/minute/kg body weight (4 mg/kg/hour)."[19]

In part, the nature of the surgery determines the required level of anesthesia, with minor procedures needing a smaller dose. The dose also depends on whether the patient has received a premedication. "If the patient is shocky, give him the smallest dose of ketamine that will keep him quiet. If he seems to react to the pain of the operation, increase the speed of the drip to 120 drops a minute. Stop operating until conditions are again satisfactory. Later, you may be able to slow the drip."[19] Generally, the ketamine will need to be discontinued 10 to 20 minutes before the end of the operation to avoid delayed emergence.[4-6]

Depth of Anesthesia

During ketamine anesthesia, spontaneous patient movement is common, which may bother both the surgeon and the anesthetist. However, these patients are still anesthetized and the movements should not deter surgery. Surgeons and anesthetists who have experience using ketamine should be able to differentiate between spontaneous ketamine movements occurring during full ketamine anesthesia and spontaneous movements because of "lightening" of anesthesia.[4]

Ketofol

The 1:1 mixture of 10 mg/mL ketamine and 10 mg/mL propofol in a single syringe (ketofol) is commonly used around the world for pediatric sedation. With this formulation, each milliliter of solution contains 5 mg ketamine and 5 mg propofol. Titrate 0.5 mg/kg of either component drug at 30-second to 1-minute intervals to achieve the required sedation. Generally, <3.0 mg/kg (avg. 0.8 mg/kg) of each drug is used. The sedation is generally viewed as smoother than with ketamine alone and the recovery time is shorter, at <15 minutes.[20]

With a Neuromuscular Blockade

Ketamine infusion may be administered with a neuromuscular blockade (NMB) and intubation. This combination provides the muscle relaxation needed for abdominal and some large joint operations.

Dobson describes his procedure: "Use atropine and preoxygenate. Induce anesthesia with a fast-running ketamine infusion containing 1 mg/mL (average adult dose 50 to 100 mL). Give succinylcholine and intubate. Maintain anesthesia with ketamine 1 to 2 mg/min (more if no premedication given). After breathing returns, give a non-depolarizing relaxant. At the end of surgery, reverse muscle relaxant and extubate."[21]

Oral Administration

While the IV ketamine preparation is effective orally, a separate oral elixir is also available. Oral bioavailability is 16% to 20%, so the adult oral dose is 500 mg of ketamine plus 5 mg diazepam. For children, the oral dose is 15 mg/kg. One problem with oral administration is that the parenteral preparation tastes very bitter. Having the patient drink pure fruit juice or cola just before taking the medication or mixing the medication with juice or cola helps hide the taste. After oral administration, it takes 15 to 30 minutes to achieve sedation/anesthesia. Sedation begins earlier than anesthesia, but responses may be unpredictable and the onset may take longer.[5,6]

Complications

Complications with ketamine involve the airway and ventilation, gastrointestinal (GI) upset, psychiatric symptoms, unusual motor movements, and a series of relatively minor problems.

Administering ketamine too rapidly or in too large a dose can result in transient respiratory depression that may necessitate BVM or, rarely, mechanical ventilatory support.[8] Excess secretions may also lead to aspiration. Though rare (~0.3% of pediatric cases), laryngospasm does occur and must be aggressively managed.[13] This can be treated with constant positive pressure from a BVM or by using pressure in the "laryngospasm notch," as described in Chapter 16.

Nausea, vomiting, and hallucinations may accompany recovery. In patients with schizophrenia, ketamine may reactivate psychoses, but there are no long-term psychiatric sequelae in nonschizophrenic patients.[6]

Tonic and clonic movements resembling seizures occur in some patients. These do not usually indicate a light plane of anesthesia or the need to give additional anesthetic. Although a slight increase in ketamine dose may be tried, further increases may increase the movements. At that point, benzodiazepines or analgesics may help, although this risks respiratory depression.[6] Occasionally, patients under ketamine anesthesia become rigid. This can be a serious event and requires an NMB and intubation.

Other infrequent reactions include anorexia, pain and exanthems at the injection site, transient generalized erythema and morbilliform rashes, laryngospasm and other forms of airway obstruction, and transient postoperative diplopia, nystagmus, and elevated intraocular pressure.[8]

Recovery

Return to consciousness is gradual. In contrast to the smooth induction of most anesthesia, 5% to 30% of patients may be agitated when recovering from ketamine. This occurs most often in adults, women, and those receiving large doses or rapid IV boluses.[6] A state called emergence delirium, during which the patient may be disorientated, restless, and crying, sometimes occurs. The incidence of this reaction is reduced if the patient is not unnecessarily disturbed during recovery and is allowed to recover in a quiet area. However, in some tragic cases, isolating the patient has resulted in unsupervised recovery with fatal airway obstruction.

Emergence reactions are unlikely to occur if diazepam is administered preoperatively (usually diazepam 0.15 mg/kg orally 1 hour preoperatively or 0.1 mg/kg IV on induction) and supplemented, if necessary, by an additional 5 to 10 mg IV at the end of the procedure.[4,8] Alternatively, promethazine can be used; this has the added advantage of an antiemetic effect. Promethazine may be given as an oral premedication (age 2 to 5 years, 15 to 20 mg by mouth [po]; 5 to 10 years, 20 to 25 mg po) or by IV at induction (25 to 50 mg IV in adults). It is not recommended for use in children <2 years old due to the risk of severe respiratory depression.[6] Haloperidol can also be used to treat these reactions.[22] Patients may continue to experience unpleasant dreams up to 24 hours after ketamine administration.[4]

Discharge

Because delayed serious adverse events after ketamine sedation have not been reported, there is no reason to require that a child return to pretreatment levels of verbalization, awareness, and purposeful neuromuscular activity before discharge. In addition, requiring a child to tolerate oral fluids before discharge might unnecessarily provoke emesis. Do not wait for children to ambulate without assistance because they can experience ataxia for hours. Allow them to leave with close family observation to prevent falls.[11]

As a General Anesthetic in Children

In the absence of facilities for the safe administration of inhalational anesthesia, "ketamine anesthesia is considered the standard of care for children" in many developing countries.[3] IM ketamine is ideal to use in children, especially those who require repeated painful procedures. Atropine can be mixed with ketamine for a single injection.[5] The IM route is particularly useful in small infants prior to insertion of an IV.

Ketamine as a sole anesthetic agent is less successful in small babies, and repeated doses may lead to apnea. It is no longer recommended for sedation in children <3 months old, because they have markedly increased associated respiratory problems. If it must be used for general anesthesia in neonates, respirations can be tenuous, so always insert an airway and use a precordial stethoscope for continuous monitoring. In babies, do not use ketamine with neuromuscular blockers. Give IM atropine 15 to 30 minutes before the procedure, except in hot climates where hyperthermia may become an issue.[23] In small children, anesthesia with ketamine as the sole agent for prolonged surgery may lead to delayed recovery, especially if combined with opioids.[3]

ETHER

Pharmacology

Ether (diethyl ether) is a colorless, highly volatile, and flammable liquid that was first used as an anesthetic in the mid-19th century. It should be stored at temperatures >25°C (>77°F) in tightly sealed dark bottles or cans. These protect the ether from light, which may decompose it. Ether is a poor anesthetic at altitudes over 2000 meters (6000 feet), although it has been used at altitudes up to 3500 meters (~11,000 feet).[24]

Availability

Ether is probably the most widely used inhalational anesthetic in the world.[25] Where the supply of medical-grade ether is limited, industrial-grade ether can be used instead.[26] Industrial ether is the same as anesthetic ether, only much less expensive. But, because it comes in drums, it must be poured into dark bottles or sealed cans for use.[27] Common types of ether for anesthesia, many of which can be found in industrial settings, include trifluoroethyl vinyl, ethyl vinyl, divinyl, diethyl, and dichloro-difluoroethyl methyl.[28] Of these, ethyl vinyl is the safest and most potent; it also has the most rapid onset of anesthesia and the shortest recovery time. Divinyl ether is the least potent agent for surgical anesthesia and the most likely to produce respiratory arrest.[29]

Production

Ether (divinyl and ethyl/diethyl ether) can easily be produced locally because ethanol and sulfuric acid are available nearly everywhere.[30] However, non-chemists should try to produce ether only in the most desperate situations, and then only after consulting a reputable organic chemistry text and, if possible, a real chemist.

The substances involved in ether production are highly volatile; the risk of explosion is very real. Essentially, the process is to dehydrate ethyl alcohol with sulfuric acid. Here's how: (a) Obtain ethyl alcohol (i.e., drinking alcohol), because other alcohols will not produce diethyl ether and will be very dangerous. (b) Obtain sulfuric acid, which can often be taken from a lead-acid battery. If necessary, make sulfuric acid by burning sulfur and saltpeter (potassium nitrite) together, although this may prove more difficult than finding it premade. The sulfuric acid is reusable and catalyzes the process. (c) Heat the ethanol-sulfuric acid mixture in a glass distillation chamber, such as from any basic chemistry laboratory. This produces ether vapor, which condenses to liquid. It has to be maintained within a certain temperature range for the reaction to occur. The process is essentially a continuous one with repeated addition of further alcohol.[31]

Advantages

The main advantage of using open-drop ether rather than a closed anesthesia system is that it has proved to be very safe, especially in unskilled hands, with a wide margin between satisfactory anesthesia and a lethal overdose.[24,30,32,33] Dr. Paluel J. Flagg, who authored *The Art of Anaesthesia*, described ether as "fool proof," providing "perfect oxygenation."[34] Illustrating his comment that "the simplest apparatus is required," the only thing needed to give ether anesthesia is a vaporizer and mask—or just the ether and a makeshift mask, and therefore it is useful wherever a general anesthetic is needed. Ether is considered one of the anesthetics of choice for major operations requiring intubation and for high-risk cases (using a low dose), the best method for maintaining anesthesia in young children when the vapor method is not available, and the volatile agent of choice when general anesthesia is needed but no oxygen is available.[33,34]

Unlike many modern anesthetics, ether provides intrinsic analgesia, so it does not require the simultaneous use of N_2O. It also provides intrinsic neuromuscular relaxation, is a bronchodilator, rarely potentiates the dysrhythmic effect of sympathomimetic agents, causes little uterine relaxation, stimulates blood flow (helpful in shocky patients), and stimulates respiration (useful if no oxygen is available). Even if the patient receives enough ether to depress respirations, cardiac function remains good, and so ether has a wide safety margin.

The classic slow changes of anesthesia depth—the "stages" (see Table 16-3) with their attendant physical signs—are easily observed, suggesting that when one does not have the necessary monitoring equipment and needs to use an inhalation anesthetic, ether is the best choice.[24,30,33,35-37]

Disadvantages and Side Effects

Disadvantages associated with using ether are that it has an unpleasant smell (that both the patient and the staff notice), and slow induction and recovery times. In addition, the vapor irritates the bronchial tree, which bothers many patients, and often is accompanied by postoperative nausea, vomiting, and drowsiness.[27,30] It helps to get the patient accustomed to the ether smell before anesthesia begins.[38] Keep patients warm, because they easily lose body heat during ether anesthesia.

Laryngeal spasm is common during induction and when the anesthesia is too light. Stop surgery and deepen the anesthesia; add oxygen, if available, until the patient breathes normally.[24] Administer atropine to prevent excess secretion production.

Patients may vomit during ether induction, usually during the delirium stage when anesthesia is light. Because laryngeal reflexes persist at this stage, tilt the table head down, turn the patient on his side, and clean out the mouth and pharynx. As long as the patient's breathing, pulse, and color are normal, the patient probably has not aspirated and it is safe to continue anesthesia. If apnea develops, consider whether the patient has received too much ether, has an airway obstruction, is breath holding, or is in cardiopulmonary arrest. Treat the problem.[24]

Nausea and vomiting after ether anesthetic are due to a central emetic effect caused by prolonged deep-stage anesthesia or by gastritis from ether dissolving in the patient's saliva. Premedicate the patient with atropine or give ether through an endotracheal (ET) tube to lessen the chance of this occurring.[24] Try not to premedicate patients with morphine.

Ether also potentiates non-depolarizing neuromuscular blocking agents and may cause myocardial depression in patients on beta-blockers. Transient postoperative effects include liver function impairment and leukocytosis.[37] Operating room staff, including the surgeon and anesthetist, may complain about the ether smell and claim that it gives them headaches or makes them sleepy. Some symptoms improve over time; others may require efficient "scavenging" (i.e., redirecting excess ether). For example, if using a non-rebreathing valve, fit an exhaust tube to the valve and vent the exhaust gases to the floor.[24,33] Also, if the end of the scavenging tube is placed on the floor (away from any possible sources of ignition), then the heavy ether vapor will remain at floor level.[27] When using open-drop ether, the best choice is to have air circulating in the room.

Contraindications and Risks

While there are no absolute contraindications to using ether, it is best avoided in patients with moderate or severe preeclampsia, with liver or renal failure, with increased cerebrospinal fluid pressure, or who have pheochromocytoma.[33,37]

Ether is highly flammable in air and explosive when mixed with oxygen or N_2O. It is not explosive when mixed with air.[24] "Under clinical conditions, it is difficult to ignite and almost impossible to explode air-ether mixtures." That is because ether vapor at a 2% or 3% concentration in air will not burn. As soon as it escapes from the vaporizer circuit or beyond the ether mask, it is diluted beyond the limit of flammability. Even if it is not diluted, it only burns slowly. But, if as little as 1 L/min of oxygen or N_2O is added, ether becomes explosive. The risk of flames and explosions is greatest close to the expiratory valve.[39]

The safe distance between ether vapor and potential heat or spark sources is unknown, but the ether vapor "zone of risk" may be up to 100 cm (~40 inches). Ether vapor is heavier than room air, so the floor up to a height of 50 cm must be clear of any electrical appliances, sockets, and plugs. Electrical sockets and switches situated within 1 meter of the floor should be spark-proof. No potential source of combustion or sparking should be allowed within 30 cm of an expiratory valve emitting ether vapor.[26,30,37]

Particularly in a very dry atmosphere, such as in hot-dry or very cold climates, make all anesthetic equipment conductive, including all surgical booties and stretcher wheels, so that any electric charges go to ground.[24,37] In tropical countries, the high humidity (above 50%) offers added protection against static electricity build-up.[30]

Ether Anesthesia Stages

Being able to identify the stages of ether anesthesia (Fig. 17-1) makes the induction, maintenance, and emergence much more elegant. Identifying these stages is relatively easy, because they were developed for use specifically with ether.

Ether anesthesia is given in one of three ways:

1. Using ether without any adjuvant drugs. This requires enough medication to reach deep ("too deep") Stage 3 to provide the muscle relaxation required for intra-abdominal surgery.
2. Using ether with 10% to 20% of the normal NMB dose. Moderately deep Stage 3 can be achieved. Patients usually resume breathing spontaneously without the need to reverse the NMB.

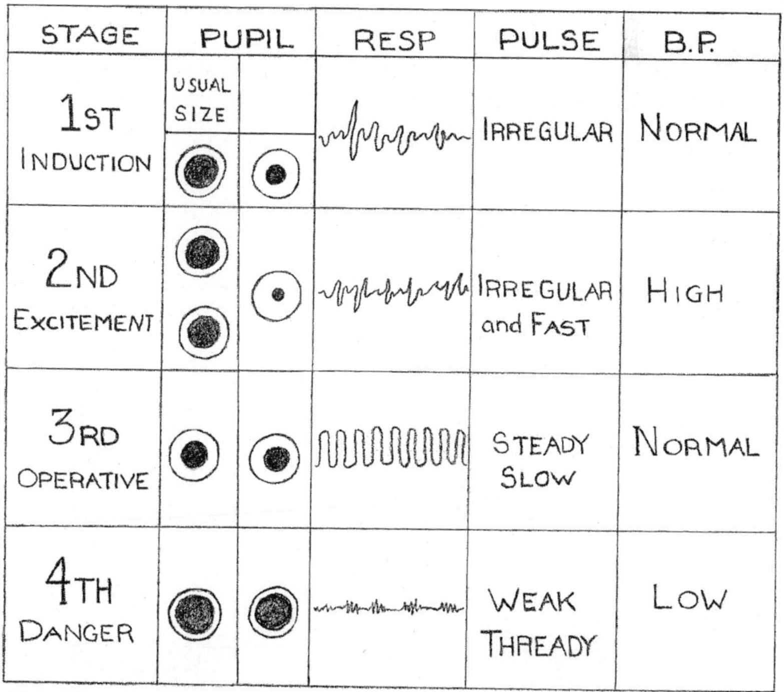

STAGE	PUPIL		RESP	PULSE	B.P.
1ST INDUCTION	USUAL SIZE			IRREGULAR	NORMAL
2ND EXCITEMENT				IRREGULAR and FAST	HIGH
3RD OPERATIVE				STEADY SLOW	NORMAL
4TH DANGER				WEAK THREADY	LOW

FIG. 17-1. Ether anesthesia stages.

3. Using ether with 50% of the normal NMB dose. Light ether anesthesia can be maintained, but patients may need NMB reversal to resume normal breathing.[30]

The second and third methods require both an NMB and controlled ventilation, which usually will not be available in austere situations.

Stage 1 anesthesia is useful for obstetrics and minor painful procedures. It can be self-administered. Give the patient a face mask delivering 2% to 3% ether and ask the patient to take deep breaths when he or she has pain. Tie the mask to their wrist; if they drop the mask, ether administration ceases.

Titrating ether's effects on spontaneously breathing patients is vital to be able to get them to and keep them at the right level. When you touch the patient's eyelash and the lid no longer contracts when touched, the patient is unconscious and is ready for surgery.[35] If the patient struggles and is difficult to control, holds his or her breath or moves slightly as a surgical incision is made, or moves his or her eyes about, the anesthesia is too light. Re-induce the patient steadily. Don't give the patient a sudden high concentration of ether or he or she may start to cough.[24,35]

If the patient's pupils become steadily larger, his or her chest falls on inspiration, and a "tracheal tug" develops (the patient's diaphragm contracts causing a "tug" on his trachea), the patient is too deeply anesthetized.[24,35] An overdose leads to severe medullary depression, with respiratory failure. Promptly stop ether administration and assist the patient's breathing; spontaneous respiration usually resumes quickly.[37]

Open-Drop Ether Anesthesia

The first method of administering inhalational anesthesia, now a relic of bygone days, is very safe and requires the least amount of equipment to administer.

When working in a major disaster or in other settings where resources are extremely limited, those giving general anesthesia may "have to confine themselves to the simplest possible method … that meant 'rag and bottle' with ether as the main volatile agent."[40] A benefit of ether anesthesia is that it is effective for most patients and most surgical procedures, except craniotomy and thoracotomy, just by dripping it on a gauze mask. "Without an anesthesia machine or ketamine, open-mask [open-drop] ether may be the safest way to administer anesthesia."[41]

When giving open-drop ether, premedicate the patient with atropine or scopolamine to reduce salivary and bronchial secretions. While the open-mask technique is very wasteful of ether, it only requires a dropping bottle and a "Schimmelbusch mask," which is simply a few thicknesses of gauze held in a wire frame (Fig. 17-2). An alternative is to use a Yankauer-Gwathmey mask, which looks like and can be improvised from a kitchen strainer (Fig. 17-3). Unfortunately, a smooth ether anesthetic is difficult to give with an open mask, especially in a large adult.[41]

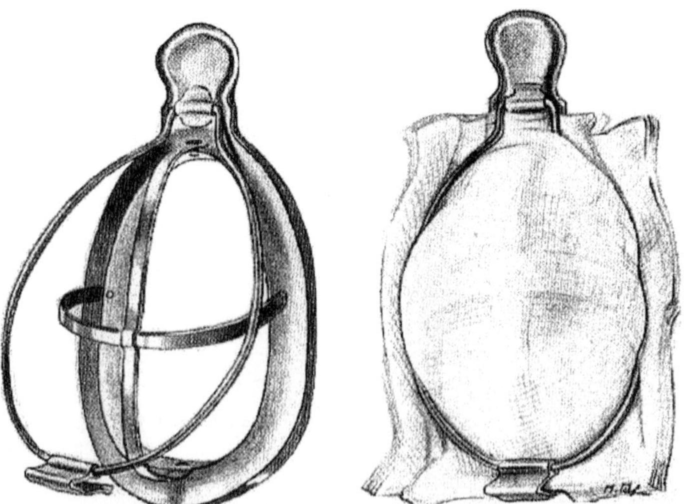

FIG. 17-2. Schimmelbusch mask. *(Source: Unknown original source. Illustration from 1894.[42])*

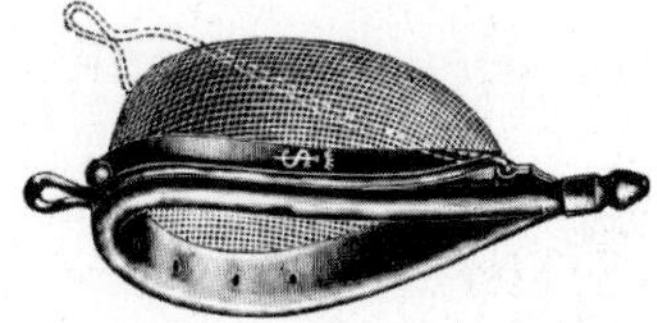

FIG. 17-3. The Yankauer-Gwathmey drop and vapor mask—similar to a kitchen strainer. *(Reproduced from Flagg.[34])*

Because diethyl ether is a weak anesthetic with a slow uptake, induction may be tedious and prolonged in a robust patient because it is difficult to reach >14% concentration. All the patient's inspired air must pass through the mask.

Open-Drop Equipment

Dropper

According to Flagg, "An emergency drop bottle may be provided by making a single pinhole in the centre of the lead cap in a can of ether, which has not been opened. If the can is now grasped in the palm of the hand, the rise in temperature resulting will cause the ether to spray out when the can is inverted. A drop may then be secured by controlling the spray with the finger tip."[34]

To improvise a "dropping bottle," use "any clean glass bottle with a rubber stopper. The goal is a device that will give large drops. Two tubes should pass through the stopper; one is for ether to come out and the other for air to enter the bottle" (Fig. 17-4). An alternative is to cut two slits in the bottle's stopper, inserting a cloth (the proverbial "rag") through one opening and leaving the other slit open to allow air to pass into the bottle. If the ether is in a can with a rubber top, "put a safety pin horizontally through the rubber stopper. The ether then drips from the pin."[43] (See Fig. 17-5.)

Improvised Mask

Administer open-drop ether by dripping it onto a piece of cloth held over the patient's face with a wire frame. The metal frame facilitates airflow and prevents the ether from coming in direct contact with the eyes and skin, which could cause serious burns. Cover the rest of the patient's face and eyes with gauze to protect them and, if available, apply petroleum jelly to exposed skin.

Make an improvised mask (preferably two) by stretching gauze over a small kitchen sieve, a large coffee strainer, a tea strainer (often an excellent infant mask), or a piece of screen that has

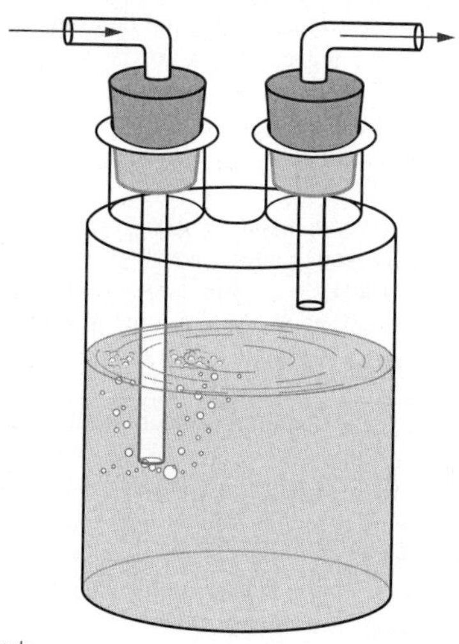

FIG. 17-4. Wolff (Woulff) bottle.

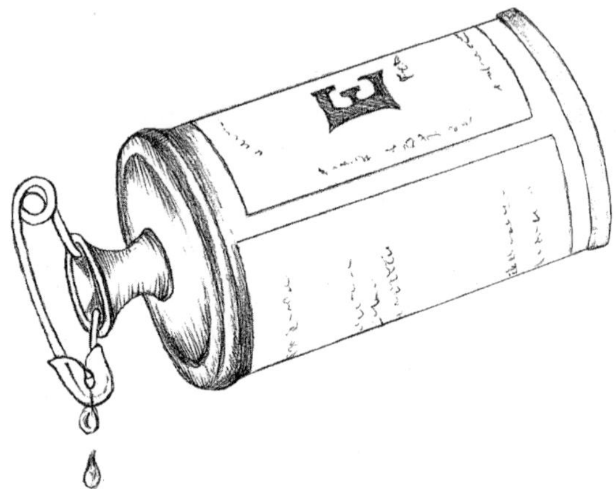

FIG. 17-5. Safety-pin-through-ether-can drip delivery system. Drawn from original photograph. *(Adapted from De Lee.[43])*

been bent and sewed into the desired shape. The ideal mask just fits over the patient's mouth and nose and should look like the classic Schimmelbusch mask (shown in Fig. 17-2). Place 10 to 12 layers of gauze (depending on the size of their mesh) over the masks. Have extra gauze; it may need to be changed frequently because, when the ether evaporates, a "frost" forms on the gauze that interferes with its effectiveness. You should be able to see light through the full thickness of the gauze; otherwise, sufficient air will not pass through it. Stockinette bandage, more closely woven than gauze, provides an excellent evaporating surface when forced down over the wire frame.[24,34,44] Do not place the mask directly on the patient's face; use cotton padding around the edges. Otherwise, the metal mask may get very cold and burn the patient.

Open-Drop Induction

The first part of giving the anesthetic is to induce the patient, or make the patient unconscious. To do this, the patient must receive as much ether as he or she can tolerate, which depends on how well the patient is breathing and his or her reaction to the ether. Ether is irritating, so too much will make the patient cough, gag, and hold his or her breath. Thus, induction with ether alone often takes 20 minutes.[24]

Either parenteral or inhalational agents can be used to smooth and speed inductions with ether, provided that the dose is small enough so that it does not depress respiration. Ketamine (1 mg/kg IV or IM) or a benzodiazepine (e.g., diazepam 0.1 to 0.2 mg/kg IV) eliminates slow induction.[24,30] An alternative is to drop 3 mL of halothane slowly onto the mask from a glass or nylon syringe. (Some disposable plastic syringes dissolve if used with these liquids.)[24] Then, immediately begin the ether maintenance. Don't let the surgeon start until the patient is at the surgical stage of anesthesia.

Take a thick piece of cotton or several layers of gauze, and cut a hole for the patient's nose and mouth. Hold the mask above the gauze, and drop ether onto it, 12 drops/min for 2 minutes, then 1 drop/second until the patient loses consciousness—usually within 5 minutes. Drop ether sparingly at first to accustom the patient to the irritating vapor. Dropping a little essence of orange, wintergreen, or some pungent essential oil on the mask before giving ether may mask the disagreeable odor.

When using ether alone, the tricks of a smooth induction are to have the patient breathe more frequently and more deeply than normal and to control the ether drops to avoid any respiratory spasm. Flagg found that one of the best methods was "to ask the patient to count slowly and loudly. This requires a certain attention and decidedly increases the tidal volume. In addition to this, the patient will give evidences of disturbed cerebration, which will indicate the progress of the induction. Most patients cannot count *slowly* and *loudly* for more than one hundred. We increase the drop as rapidly as we can and 'let up' if the patient catches his breath. If this method is pursued, the patient will rapidly develop a tolerance, and by the time he has ceased to count he will be accepting without spasm an amount of ether which almost or entirely saturates the mask."[34] The patient is then anesthetized.

Never place the mask directly on the face of a conscious patient, or he or she will feel suffocated. Wait until the eyelash reflex has gone, and then put on the mask. As soon as the patient begins to tolerate the ether, drop it on faster. Keep the stream of ether drops moving steadily over the mask to avoid freezing. Listen to every breath and make adjustments for any airway problem. Don't pour it on so fast that it makes the patient cough. If the patient does cough or hold his or her breath, give him a breath of air. You may have given him or her too much ether too quickly, given it irregularly, or have a poor fit between the mask and face. As things settle down, adjust the rate to provide the required depth of anesthesia. Give a few breaths of air and continue more slowly. Deep levels of surgical anesthesia cannot be achieved with this technique in less than 20 to 30 minutes.[24,37]

Ether is a weak anesthetic, so a patient must breathe a high concentration of vapor. In adults, it is useful to increase the ether concentration by using the "ether chimney." Improvised by prisoners of war (POWs) during World War II, the ether chimney is a metal column that sits over the mask, increasing the vapor concentration close to the face, which in turn increases the inspired concentration of ether. You won't need this for a child.

Construct an ether chimney using two cans that fit into one another (Fig. 17-6). Place one can over the patient's mouth and nose. Three (not more) layers of gauze go between the cans, and the second can fits into the first, holding the gauze. For use during long operations, make some side holes in the lower can to increase the air flow; tape them up during shorter operations.[24,35]

Open-Drop Maintenance

Keeping patients at the right anesthetic stage is a difficult art that must be individualized to the patient and the circumstances. "Most anesthetists like to err on the side of being just-too deep. If the patient becomes too light, regaining control will not be easy."[24] According to Flagg, "Maintenance is best controlled by a constant drop, which may be increased or diminished according to a demand for a high or low level of anesthesia. If the anesthetist becomes weary or loses interest during this stage, he will very likely change the drop into a spray or pour method. This will surely result in an uneven anesthesia."[34] Table 17-5 presents a rough guide to open-drop ether use.

When the mask becomes so cold that it is covered with frost, change it for a fresh one. To diminish the amount of ether escaping into the atmosphere and affecting the anesthetist and

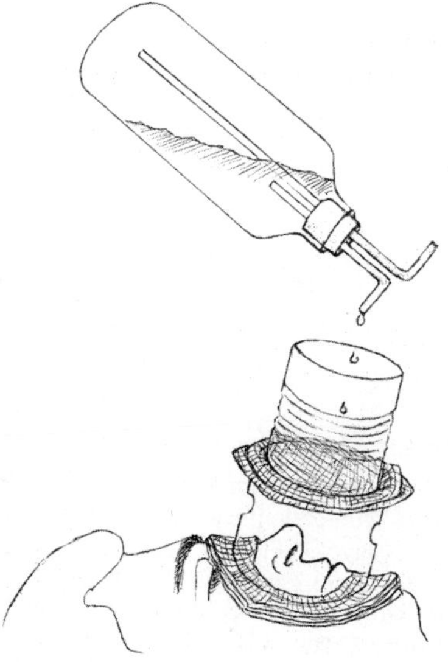

FIG. 17-6. Ether chimney.

TABLE 17-5 Guide to Ether Maintenance Dosing

Ether (drops/min)	Time (min)
12	1st min
24	2nd min
48	3rd min
96	4th-15th min
50	15th-30th min
20-30	After 30 min

Adapted with permission from The Remote, Austere, Wilderness and Third World Medicine Discussion Board Moderators.[38]

surgical team, put two layers of gauze over the mask after pouring the ether. Replace it with fresh (non-etherized) gauze each time that additional ether is poured.[24]

During long operations, if oxygen is available and all the precautions are in place to avoid an explosion (see the previous text), feed a small oxygen tube under the mask with a flow of from 2 to 5 L/min.

Recovery

To avoid a prolonged recovery, discontinue ether administration about 20 minutes prior to closure. After a long operation (with more saturation of the tissues), stop giving ether 15 minutes before the last stitch. If conditions allow, assist ventilation to promote ether washout and make recovery faster and to help decrease the incidence of nausea/vomiting.[30] Put the patient in the recovery position (on his side); do not send him or her back to the ward until it is safe to leave him or her alone: The patient should be able to talk, be breathing quietly and easily, and have warm hands and a good pulse.[24,33]

Special Situations: Pediatrics and Obstetrics/Gynecology

Pediatrics

Open-drop ether administration is one of the safest inhalation methods for children, especially if you lack specialized pediatric equipment. The anesthetic stages in children are the same as in adults. Take care not to administer more ether than necessary. An additional sign in babies is that they relax their grip as they become anesthetized.[24]

In febrile children, exposure to ether increases the risk of potentially fatal seizures. If seizures occur, immediately stop ether administration and lower the child's body temperature by sponging the child with tepid water. Administer small doses of a benzodiazepine or thiopental until convulsions cease.[37]

Obstetrics/Gynecology

Use ether during pregnancy only when the need outweighs any possible risk to the fetus. However, at term, ether is especially useful for C-sections because the baby tolerates it and the uterus contracts well.[33] Use low concentrations (no more than 4%) in obstetric procedures to avoid loss of uterine tone, excessive postpartum hemorrhage, and neonatal respiratory depression.[37]

Intravenous Ether Anesthesia

Intravenously administered ether is an excellent anesthetic, especially for procedures not needing profound relaxation, such as intra-abdominal surgery. Using this method, both adults and children can be anesthetized to Stage 3, Plane 1 anesthesia—in which there is a normal or increased rate and depth of respirations (see Table 16-3). Intravenous ether anesthesia at this stage has been successfully used for head and neck surgeries, including bronchoscopy, laryngoscopy, tonsillectomy, and oral surgery. Not only are the necessary tools for this anesthetic technique readily available, but they are also inexpensive.[45]

Begin by preparing a 5% ether solution. Dissolve 50 mL diethyl ether in 1 L 5% glucose solution (D_5W). Cool the mixture to about 4°C (40°F) in a refrigerator to facilitate dissolving the ether. Shake the mixture vigorously for about 1 minute to mix it thoroughly, which is necessary to obtain good anesthesia. Keep the solution at 4°C until it is used. Shake it again before use to obtain thorough mixing.[45]

To anesthetize the patient, attach the bottle with the ether solution to a D_5W IV using a three-way stopcock or Y-tubing. After inducing the patient into a light sleep with an IV induction agent, open the ether solution to its maximum flow (with a "macro drip"); increase the flow by raising the bottle or by using a pressure cuff on the bag. Keep the ether solution flowing "wide open" during induction. By the time 100 to 400 mL of the solution is administered over the first 5 to 10 minutes, the patient is usually well anesthetized. The patient reaches a surgical level of anesthesia in about 10 minutes. As the operation progresses, control the flow rate to maintain Stage 3, Plane I anesthesia. If available, administer oxygen continuously.[45]

The patient usually sleeps quietly. Jaw relaxation is adequate for oral surgery or endoscopy without the need to use a neuromuscular blocker. If necessary, use an airway. Should there be unwanted motion of the extremities or the head, give a small additional dose of the IV induction medication. Prolonged postanesthesia nausea and vomiting is rare.[45]

HALOTHANE

Halothane vies with ether as the most commonly used volatile inhalational anesthetic agent worldwide. Its use is limited by the need for an anesthetic machine and monitoring equipment during surgery, and by its relatively high cost.[36,37]

Pharmacology

Halothane is a colorless, volatile, nonirritant liquid with a sweet odor. It is neither flammable nor explosive. In anesthetic doses, it depresses both cerebral function and sympathetic activity and it produces little, if any, preliminary excitement.[37] Halothane should be stored <25°C (<77°F) in tightly closed, amber-colored glass containers to protect it from ultraviolet light. It contains thymol as a stabilizing agent.[27,37] Ideally, only those with anesthesia experience will use halothane, because it is used most frequently with various anesthesia machines, which will be unfamiliar to non-anesthesiologists.[30]

Advantages

Induction with halothane is smooth and rapid, and surgical anesthesia can be produced in 2 to 5 minutes. It is well tolerated and nonirritating, with a low dose needed for maintenance. It does not cause excess salivary or bronchial secretions. Patients have a rapid recovery with a low incidence of postanesthesia nausea and vomiting. There is a predictable, dose-related depression of respiration and cardiac function. While it can be used for virtually all general anesthesia, it has a special role for inhalation induction, especially in upper airway problems such as partial obstruction or in patients with status asthmaticus who need to be ventilated.[27,37]

Disadvantages

Halothane's poor analgesic properties necessitate deep planes of anesthesia before surgery can be tolerated. For this reason, it is generally not suitable as a sole agent without an analgesic supplement, for example, N_2O, opiates, trichloroethylene, local anesthetic blocks, or other analgesics. It provides no postoperative analgesia and causes uterine relaxation and hemorrhage, particularly if >0.5% halothane is used.[27]

Halothane-induced cardiovascular depression may cause bradycardia, hypotension, and a reduction in cardiac output. These effects may be marked in children, who should receive atropine either as premedication or by IV at induction. Always give supplemental oxygen with halothane.[27] Little margin exists between the doses needed to produce respiratory depression and vasomotor depression. Overdoses result in death from cardiovascular depression.

Halothane also sensitizes the heart to epinephrine and predisposes the patient to developing arrhythmias, most commonly in patients who are retaining CO_2 or who are in pain. Such patients can usually be managed by supporting the ventilation, reducing the amount of halothane, and providing additional analgesics. If these are not effective, IV lidocaine or propranolol (avoid in asthmatics) usually works.[27,37]

Using epinephrine during halothane administration (such as in a local anesthetic) increases the risk of ventricular dysrhythmias. If possible, avoid epinephrine; if epinephrine must be used, monitor the pulse closely and support ventilation. The total epinephrine dose should never be more than 20 mL of a 5 mcg/mL (1:200,000) solution in 10 minutes or 30 mL in 1 hour. (Do not use higher concentrations.)[27,37]

"Halothane hepatitis" occurs on rare occasions and is almost unheard of in children.[27] Halothane is, therefore, contraindicated in patients with a history of unexplained jaundice following previous halothane exposures. If it does occur, fever typically develops 2 or 3 days after anesthesia and is accompanied by anorexia, nausea, and vomiting. In more severe cases, this is followed by transient jaundice or, rarely, fatal hepatic necrosis. Allow at least 3 months to elapse between each reexposure to halothane. Repeated and frequent administration increases the risk of liver damage.[27,37]

Halothane also increases intracranial pressure and, with succinylcholine (suxamethonium), may increase the risk of malignant hyperthermia.[27,37]

Method

Always give halothane through a calibrated vaporizer. It is not suitable for open-drop anesthesia, although a few drops applied to a face mask may smooth the subsequent administration of ether. The maintenance dose is 1% to 2% for spontaneously breathing patients and 0.5% to 1% during controlled ventilation. Overdoses may occur easily with higher doses. If draw-over machines or inhalers are used, supplemental oxygen or assisted ventilation may be necessary to maintain full oxygenation, even when air is used as the carrier gas.[27,37]

If halothane is used alone (rather than with another induction agent), start a flow of gas containing at least 30% oxygen. Gradually introduce halothane and increase the concentration every few breaths until the inspired gases contain 2% to 3% halothane (adults) or 1.5% to 2% (children).[37] This method is well tolerated by all patients, and Stage 2 effects are minimized.[27]

Monitor the pulse and BP throughout anesthesia, and if hypotension develops, reduce the inspired halothane concentration—or stop administering the anesthesia. Premedicating patients with atropine reduces the risk of hypotension and bradycardia.[37]

Recovery time is relatively short, but varies with the concentrations of halothane used and the length of surgery. If ketamine is used for induction, recovery may be prolonged. Patients commonly shiver during recovery, but this can be controlled with warm blankets and, if this is insufficient, by administering a benzodiazepine or a small (~12.5 mg) dose of IV meperidine.[37]

Obstetrics

Use halothane during pregnancy only when the need outweighs any possible risk to the fetus. Employ low concentrations (no more than 0.5%) for Cesarean sections or for evacuating retained products of conception or the placenta, because a loss of uterine tone may result in excessive hemorrhage.[27,37]

REFERENCES

1. Grande CM, Baskett PJF, Donchin Y, et al. Trauma anesthesia for disasters: anything, anytime, anywhere. *Crit Care Clin.* 1991;7(2):339-361.
2. King MH, ed. *Primary Anaesthesia.* Oxford, UK: Oxford University Press; 1986:60.
3. Hodges SC, Walker IA, Bosenberg AT. Pediatric anaesthesia in developing countries. *Anaesthesia.* 2007;62(suppl 1):26-31.
4. Tomlinson A. Ketamine. *Update Anaesth.* 1994;4(5):1-4.
5. Stevenson C. Ketamine: a review. *Update Anaesth.* 2005;20:25-29.
6. Craven R. Ketamine. *Anaesthesia.* 2007;62(suppl 1):48-53.
7. Grant IS, Nimmo WS, Clements JA. Pharmacokinetics and analgesic effects of IM and oral ketamine. *Br J Anaesth.* 1981;53:805-809.
8. World Health Organization. *Model Prescribing Information: Drugs Used in Anesthesia.* Geneva, Switzerland: WHO; 1989:18-20. http://apps.who.int/medicinedocs/en/d/Jh2929e/. Accessed September 9, 2015.

9. Dobson MB. *Anaesthesia at the District Hospital.* 2nd ed. Geneva, Switzerland: WHO; 2000:73.
10. Jat KR, Chawla D. Ketamine for management of acute exacerbations of asthma in children. *Cochrane Database Syst Rev.* 2012;(11):CD009293. http://www.update-software.com/BCP/WileyPDF/EN/CD009293.pdf. Accessed September 9, 2015.
11. Green SM, Roback MG, Kennedy RM, Krauss B. Clinical practice guideline for emergency department ketamine dissociative sedation. 2011 update. *Ann Emerg Med.* 2011;57(5):449-461.
12. Cohen L, Athaide V, Wickham ME, et al. The effect of ketamine on intracranial and cerebral perfusion pressure and health outcomes: a systematic review. *Ann Emerg Med.* 2015 Jan;65(1):43-51.
13. Ketcham DW. Where there is no anaesthesiologist: the many uses of ketamine. *Trop Doct.* 1990;20:163-166.
14. Dobson MB. *Anaesthesia at the District Hospital.* 2nd ed. Geneva, Switzerland: WHO; 2000:53.
15. King MH, ed. *Primary Anaesthesia.* Oxford, UK: Oxford University Press; 1986:60-61.
16. King MH, ed. *Primary Anaesthesia.* Oxford, UK: Oxford University Press; 1986:5.
17. King MH, ed. *Primary Anaesthesia.* Oxford, UK: Oxford University Press; 1986:64.
18. Zimmermann H. Ketamine drip anaesthesia for Caesarean section: report on 200 cases from a rural hospital in Zimbabwe. *Trop Doct.* 1988;18:60-61.
19. King MH, ed. *Primary Anaesthesia.* Oxford, UK: Oxford University Press; 1986:63.
20. Andolfatto G, Willman E. A prospective case series of pediatric procedural sedation and analgesia in the emergency department using single-syringe ketamine–propofol combination (Ketofol). *Acad Emerg Med.* 2010;17(2):194-201.
21. Dobson MB. *Anaesthesia at the District Hospital.* 2nd ed. Geneva, Switzerland: WHO; 2000:74.
22. King MH, ed. *Primary Anaesthesia.* Oxford, UK: Oxford University Press; 1986:60-62.
23. King MH, ed. *Primary Anaesthesia.* Oxford, UK: Oxford University Press; 1986:64-65.
24. King MH, ed. *Primary Anaesthesia.* Oxford, UK: Oxford University Press; 1986:85-89.
25. Dobson MB. *Anaesthesia at the District Hospital.* 2nd ed. Geneva, Switzerland: WHO; 2000:79.
26. Simpson S, Wilson IH. Draw-over anaesthesia review. *Update Anaesth.* 2002;15(6):1-10. www.nda.ox.ac.uk/wfsa/htmL/u15/u1506_01.htm. Accessed September 14, 2006.
27. Fenton P. Using volatile anaesthetic agents. *Update Anaesth.* 1995;5(5):1-3. www.nda.ox.ac.uk/wfsa/htmL/u05/u05_009.htm. Accessed September 13, 2006.
28. Hunter AR. Inhalational anaesthetic agents: the relationship between chemical structure and pharmacological action. *Br J Anaesth.* 1962;34:224-228.
29. Mörch ET, Aycrigg JB, Berger MS. The anesthetic effects of ethyl vinyl ether, divinyl ether, and diethyl ether on mice. *J Pharmacol Exp Ther.* 1956;117:184-189.
30. Rahardjo E. Ether, the anesthetic from 19th through 21st century. *Int Cong Ser.* 2002;1242:51-55.
31. The Remote, Austere, Wilderness and Third World Medicine Discussion Board Moderators. *Survival and Austere Medicine: An Introduction.* 2nd ed. 2005:100. www.endtimesreport.com/Survival_Medicine.pdf. Accessed June 30, 2007.
32. Phillip HM. Comments. In: Soper RL, ed. Anesthesia for major disasters. *Proc Royal Soc Med.* 1958;52:239-246.
33. Fenton P. Using volatile anaesthetic agents. *Update Anaesth.* 1995;5:9-12.
34. Flagg PJ. *The Art of Anaesthesia.* 3rd ed. Philadelphia: J.B. Lippincott Company; 1922:123, Fig. 65.
35. Boulton TB. Anaesthesia in difficult situations. 3. General anaesthesia-technique. *Anaesthesia.* 1966;21(4):513-545.
36. Simpson S, Wilson IH. Drawover anaesthesia review. *Update Anaesth.* 2002;15:13-18.
37. World Health Organization. *Model Prescribing Information. Drugs Used in Anesthesia.* Geneva, Switzerland: WHO; 1989:22-24.
38. The Remote, Austere, Wilderness and Third World Medicine Discussion Board Moderators. *Survival and Austere Medicine: An Introduction.* 2nd ed. 2005:105-107. www.endtimesreport.com/Survival_Medicine.pdf. Accessed June 30, 2007.
39. Boulton TB, Cole PV. Anaesthesia in difficult situations. What would I do if…? *Anaesthesia.* 1966;21(2):268-276.
40. Woolmer R. Comments. In: Soper RL., ed. Anaesthesia for major disasters. *Proc Royal Soc Med.* 1958;52:239-246.
41. King MH, ed. *Primary Anaesthesia.* Oxford, UK: Oxford University Press; 1986:88.
42. Unknown original source. Illustration from 1894. www.johnpowell.net/pages/handout/schimm12.jpg. Accessed August 18, 2008.
43. De Lee JB. *Obstetrics for Nurses.* Philadelphia, PA: W.B. Saunders; 1919:137.
44. Olson LM. *Improvised Equipment in the Home Care of the Sick.* Philadelphia, PA: W.B. Saunders; 1928:69.
45. Butt H, Ochs I, Lyons J, et al. Using intravenous ether anesthesia. *Anesth Analg.* 1965;44(2):186-189.

18 Transfusion

In austere situations, there may be no blood available for transfusion. If blood is available, there is a greater risk that it could be contaminated and infect the patient than under optimal circumstances. In addition, the methods to rapidly rewarm blood to avoid the complications of hypothermic transfusion may not be available.

DANGERS IN BLOOD SUPPLY

Blood can easily transmit human immunodeficiency virus (HIV), hepatitis B virus (HBV), hepatitis C virus (HCV), Chagas disease, malaria, and other diseases. Only about 66% of developed countries and 46% of least-developed countries screen blood for HIV, although there is about a 90% seroconversion rate following the transfusion of blood infected with HIV. Even where (often, for-profit private) blood banks purport to screen for HIV, many either don't screen or use insensitive tests. Government oversight is sparse.[1,2]

AVOIDING BLOOD TRANSFUSION

Use non-blood substitutes, if possible. They are much safer, easier to use, and can be less costly than using blood. Substitutes include crystalloids, synthetic colloids (e.g., Dextran), and noninfectious plasma derivatives. For all but crystalloids, however, both cost and availability may be a problem.

To avoid a transfusion, especially in the operative patient: (a) restrict preoperative diagnostic phlebotomy, (b) use meticulous intraoperative surgical hemostasis, (c) use blood/cell salvage, (d) employ hemodilution, (e) use pharmaceutical hemostasis agents, (f) maintain normothermia, and (g) position patients to minimize blood loss and hypertension. Postoperatively, (a) use blood/cell salvage, (b) tolerate anemia (as described later in this chapter), (c) optimize fluid and volume management, and (d) restrict diagnostic phlebotomy. The units of blood potentially saved by not doing a transfusion with each strategy are shown in Table 18-1.[3]

DECIDING WHEN TO TRANSFUSE

The decision to transfuse blood depends on the patient's clinical condition and their ability to compensate for reduced tissue oxygenation. Patients with evidence of severe cardiac or respiratory disease or with preexisting anemia have a limited ability to compensate.[4] In critically ill, non-bleeding adult patients <55 years old and without evidence of an acute myocardial infarction

TABLE 18-1 Blood Conservation Methods in the Surgical Patient

Preoperative Options	Units of Blood Conserved
Tolerance of anemia (reduce transfusion trigger)	1-2
Increase preoperative red blood cell mass	2
Preoperative autologous donation	1-2
Intraoperative Options	
Meticulous hemostasis and operative technique	1 or more
Acute normovolemic hemodilution	1-2
Blood salvage	1 or more
Postoperative Options	
Restricted phlebotomy	1
Blood salvage	1

or unstable angina, keeping the hemoglobin (Hgb) >7.0 g/dL, rather than >10 g/dL, does not change mortality rates.[5] The mortality increases dramatically, however, when the Hgb drops lower than 5 to 6 g/dL, especially in postoperative patients.[6]

Severe Anemia

When the blood supply is scarce or dangerous, clinicians must tolerate levels of anemia in their patients that would be unacceptable under optimal conditions. The World Health Organization (WHO) defines very severe anemia in a child as Hgb <4 g/dL (40 g/L) or a hematocrit (Hct; packed-cell volume) <12%. If the blood supply is routinely tested for HIV and HBV, transfuse these children with 10 mL/kg packed red blood cells (PRBCs). If the blood supply may be tainted, wait to transfuse until the Hgb is <3 g/dL (30 g/L) or the Hct is <10%.[7] Also limit the amount transfused. Critically ill children in modern intensive care units do as well when transfusions keep their Hgb >7 g/dL as they do when kept at the more common Hgb level of 9.5 g/dL.[8]

In adults, clinicians generally use an arbitrary Hgb level of 10.0 g/dL to indicate that a transfusion is necessary. But patients can tolerate lower Hgb levels than previously believed.[6] Except for patients with ischemic cardiovascular disease, keeping critically ill patients' Hgb levels between 7.0 and 9.0 g/dL is as safe as keeping them between 10.0 and 12.0 g/dL.[3,9]

Acute Bleeding: Is a Massive Transfusion Required?

The primary method to avoid the need for transfusing patients with acute hemorrhage is to stop the bleeding as soon as possible. Frequently, this is not possible and transfusion will be required. The question in these settings is: Does the patient require a "massive transfusion" (MT)? An MT means transfusing three units of packed red blood cells (PRBCs) per hour or five units PRBCs per 3 hours, and signifies uncontrolled hemorrhage, which requires a special transfusion protocol.[10] (Note that the old, retrospective definition of MT, ≥10 PRBCs per 24 hours, is only useful for research.)

In most settings, two simple methods can determine whether a patient will require an MT: the Shock Index (SI) and the Assessment of Blood Consumption (ABC) Score, both of which are described below. In early hemorrhage, both the SI and the ABC Score are more helpful than inferior vena cava (IVC) measurements using ultrasound. The sensitivity of the dynamic IVC measures (collapsibility index and IVC end expiratory diameter) for detecting early blood loss is only around 80%.[11]

Shock Index

Particularly useful in prehospital and other resource-poor settings, the SI (heart rate [HR]/systolic blood pressure [SBP]) helps indicate a need for MT in "relatively normotensive" blunt trauma patients with SBP ≥90 mm Hg.[12] As the SI increases >0.9, the probability of needing an MT increases incrementally; with an SI >1.4, 57% of patients need an MT. The SI's sensitivity is equivalent to measuring the base deficit or lactate.[13] Be careful with elderly patients: The need for MT may occur at much lower SIs. Their vital signs may not demonstrate the seriousness of their injury, as in the following examples.[14]

<70 years old: HR ≥130/min and SBP <90 mm Hg (SI = 1.4)
≥70 years old may need a MT if: HR >90/min and SBP <110 mm Hg (SI = 0.8)

Assessment of Blood Consumption Score

ABC score is another method to determine need for MT. However, it requires using ultrasound for a FAST Exam. The four components of the ABC each receive 1 point if they are positive. The components are as follows:

1. Penetrating mechanism of injury
2. SBP ≤90 mm Hg
3. HR ≥120/min
4. Positive FAST examination

The ABC Score correctly classified patients as to whether they would need an MT if their score was 2 (82%), 3 (91%), or 4 (89%).[15]

TRANSFUSING BLOOD

Carrying O-Negative Blood in the Field

While relatively costly, both civilian and military medical units have shown that it can be safe and effective to carry and administer O-negative blood in the prehospital setting. The civilian units carry blood in special cold boxes (LifeBox50 Transport Containers; FareTec Inc, Painesville, Ohio, US), and the PRBCs are returned to the blood bank three times a week. In one large metropolitan civilian area, the EMS carried two units of "O-negative" PRBCs, of which they administered 26% to patients. Of the non-transfused units, they returned 98% to the blood bank in useable condition. The cost of providing PRBCs for civilian prehospital use was $500 to $700 for each unit transfused.[16] In the laboratory, studies have showed that PRBCs can survive parachute jumps and mechanical agitation over 12 hours at 48°C (118°F) without significant changes in chemistry or morphology.[17]

"Damage Control" Transfusion

When an MT is indicated due to major trauma with continuing blood loss (or a severe head injury), use a transfusion protocol that not only promptly replaces erythrocytes, but also promptly treats coagulopathy. Use PRBCs, fresh-frozen plasma (FFP) and platelets immediately, in a 1:1:1 ratio. If platelets are unavailable, use PRBCs and FFP in a 1:1 ratio. Do not wait for abnormal laboratory test results. To be able to quickly implement this protocol, discuss it with the blood bank in advance, so that they are responsive to your needs.

Using this protocol increases 6-hour, 24-hour, and 30-day survival. The mortality at 24 hours and at 30 days was no different than with using a ratio of 1:1:2 (platelets, FFP, PRBCs).[18,19] That is unsurprising, because both higher FFP:PRBC ratios and higher platelet:PRBC ratios improve survival at 24 hours and at 30 days.[20]

Whole Blood in Trauma Resuscitations

Most blood banks no longer have whole blood available for immediate transfusion, because this practice reduces the availability of blood components, while the unused whole blood units become outdated. The use of a "walking blood bank," that is, donors available when called, provides this resource (see the "Walking Blood Bank" section in this chapter). The benefits of using fresh whole blood include increased volume, plasma's coagulation factors, platelets, and the presence of circulating antibacterial substances.[21]

How to Determine Adequate Blood Replacement

If a patient has been adequately transfused after acute blood loss (assuming that the bleeding has ceased), the skin will become warm, dry, and, if the patient is Caucasian, pink. The nose will again be warm, and the capillary refill will be brisk (immediate). This is in contrast to the skin being cold, damp, and white, and having a delayed (not "brisk") capillary refill when acutely anemic. These clinical results of transfusion may be delayed, especially if the blood loss was severe or prolonged. A urine output of ≥1 mL/kg/hour is also an excellent sign of adequate blood replacement.[22]

HOW TO TRANSFUSE AUTOLOGOUS BLOOD

Acute Normovolemic Hemodilution

The easiest method for decreasing red cell loss during surgery in relatively normovolemic adults is to use acute normovolemic hemodilution (ANH), also known as acute isovolemic hemodilution. This is when the patient's blood is removed (to keep for later transfusion) and replaced with 500 mL to 1 L crystalloid (or occasionally colloid) immediately before surgery. This dilutes the blood volume and results in a smaller decrease in Hct for the same volume of blood loss.[1] Because this process reduces the loss of RBC mass during surgery, it can be used for urgent or elective procedures to decrease the requirement for preoperative blood donation and the use of banked blood.[23]

This technique provides fresh whole blood for use in the operating room (OR) and is safe (uses the patient's own blood), convenient for the patient, simple to perform, and inexpensive. Use ANH if the surgical blood loss is anticipated to be >15 mL/kg and the patient has a Hgb

≥10 g/dL before surgery. For nonemergent surgery, give iron to patients with a lower Hgb to raise their Hgb level before the operation. Patients excluded from this procedure are those with sickle cell disease, severe cardiac disease, bacteremia, liver disease, or bleeding disorders.[24] At the conclusion of surgery or if there is an indication that a transfusion is necessary during the procedure, transfuse the collected blood into the patient.[3] It is especially useful for hospitals with limited or no blood bank facilities.[25-27]

Acute Normovolemic Hemodilution Procedure

At the onset of surgery in a stable patient who is not hemorrhaging, use a 14-gauge intravenous (IV) catheter in an antecubital vein to remove either 2 L of blood or enough blood so the Hct is 28%, whichever comes first. Drain the blood into a sterile container with anticoagulant (generally 64 mL CPD [citrate-phosphate-dextrose] or the equivalent/500 mL blood).

The volume to be removed (V) is determined using the formula[25]:

$$V = EBV \times [(H^1 - H^2) \div H^{avg}]$$

where: EBV (patient's estimated blood volume) = body weight (kg) × 70 mL/kg
H^1 = patient's initial Hct
H^2 = patient's target Hct after hemodilution
H^{avg} = the average Hct = $(H^1 + H^2) \div 2$
Example: 70 kg patient; Initial Hct = 35%; Target Hct = 28%
Volume to remove = (70 kg × 70 mL/kg) × [(.35 – .28) ÷ {(.35 + .28)/2}] = 1,089 mL

As the first liter of blood is removed, it is simultaneously replaced with an equal volume of colloid solution, if available, and then with crystalloid in a 2:1 ratio. (Up to a 3:1 ratio can be used if only one unit is removed.)[27] If colloid is not available, use crystalloid for all replacements. If there is only one IV line, alternate the blood collection and the infusion of replacement fluids. If there are two IV lines, they occur simultaneously.[24] Immediately label all blood units with the patient's identifying information.

Obtain Hct levels and vital signs immediately before hemodilution, after the removal of each 500 mL of blood, and at the end of the hemodilution procedure. Patients should receive hemodiluted blood intraoperatively to maintain their Hct >25%. Transfuse all hemodiluted blood before discharging the patient from the recovery area.[25]

Unlike preoperative autologous blood donations (described subsequently), ANH requires minimal preoperative preparation and produces negligible patient inconvenience. The procedure can be used for some patients requiring unplanned operations—including Cesarean sections. Probably most important in austere situations is that the blood does not require a blood bank: it is stored at room temperature at the patient's bedside and administered only to that patient. This also reduces the human errors inherent in the process of giving the correct blood to the patient.[24,25]

Blood/Cell Salvage—Autotransfusion

Blood or cell salvage is when shed blood is collected from a wound or body cavity and then reinfused into the same patient. The general rule is to use this technique if the patient seems likely to lose <20% blood volume,[1] although this technique works well to supplement allogenic (another patient's) or presurgically donated blood.

This technique is often used for patients presenting with a ruptured ectopic pregnancy, which is a common cause of massive intraperitoneal hemorrhage. Many of these women present in hypovolemic shock, because considerable time often elapses between the ectopic rupture and the patient's arrival at the hospital. Part of the high mortality associated with ectopic pregnancies in both developed and least-developed countries is due to the scarcity of blood available for transfusion. Using blood salvage and autotransfusion often leads to a normal recovery.[28] The techniques are also used for hemothoraces from penetrating chest injuries and for blunt abdominal injuries with hepatic or splenic bleeding.[29]

What Blood to Use?

Use autologous transfusion only if blood can be removed from a cavity (usually the chest or abdomen) where it has been for <24 hours, although some clinicians try to limit it to 12 hours or less.

Blood from sterile cavities, such as the chest or abdomen, without visceral injuries or evidence of overt hemolysis is preferred.[1] Contraindications to salvage include blood contaminated with bowel contents, bacteria, fat, amniotic fluid, urine, malignant cells, and irrigation fluids.[4,24] Blood from contaminated abdominal wounds can be used, but with an increased risk of systemic infection.[30] The patient's condition determines when the blood is reinfused, although the units should be used within a few hours to limit the chance of bacterial growth. If possible, wait to transfuse until bleeding has been surgically controlled.

Technique: Abdomen

Draining the blood from abdominal bleeding, usually due to a ruptured ectopic pregnancy or blunt abdominal trauma, is often called pre-incision needle drainage, but it can also be performed through a tiny opening in the peritoneum once it is exposed. To do this, make a small peritoneal incision while "tenting" the peritoneum to avoid spillage. If the intraperitoneal blood appears fresh and is the normal color, collect it in small containers. If the hospital has a blood bank, send the first aliquot of blood for type and cross-match, in case additional blood is needed.

Multiple variations of the following two methods have been described. The first method is to collect the blood by scooping it (or letting it drain) into a sterile bowl and then pouring it through gauze into another sterile container. A person wearing sterile gloves then uses 50-mL syringes to infuse the blood into a transfusion bag. The syringe may need to be rinsed with normal saline 0.9% (NS) occasionally to prevent the plunger from sticking.[31]

The second method, faster and more elegant, to use for ruptured ectopic pregnancies (as well as hemothoraces), is to position the patient so that the fluid is dependent. With a hemoperitoneum, that will usually be in a feet-down (i.e., reverse Trendelenburg) position with the patient turned slightly to the right side. After prepping the area, introduce a 15-gauge needle into the right iliac fossa. Connect it to a standard blood set and blood collection bag with anticoagulant. Gently manipulate the needle, allowing the blood to flow freely into the bag. Another method to increase flow is to lavage the abdomen with NS, although this results in lowering the Hct of the collected blood. The blood is transfused using a filter to avoid clots.[32,33] The bowel is rarely injured when using the percutaneous needle because, like draining ascites, the bowel normally floats away from the needle. Of course, performing the process under ultrasound guidance may be even safer.[28]

After removing most of the fresh blood, enlarge the peritoneal incision and clamp the bleeding site. At that point, some clinicians scoop (not suck) blood from the abdomen into sterile containers[1]; others use gentle suction (<40 mm Hg).[28]

Technique: Chest

When there is bleeding into the chest cavity, blood is commonly drained out through a chest tube using gravity. Blood then drains through a funnel lined with several layers of gauze and into a sterile glass bottle containing anticoagulant such as CPDA-1 (citrate-phosphate-dextrose-adenine) (Fig. 18-1). The bottle can then be inverted and infused directly through an IV with a 200-μm filter.[29]

Filtration/Anticoagulation

Gauze is frequently used to filter the blood. No less than three, and preferably eight, layers of sterile gauze should be used to screen out small clots and tissue fragments that could cause pulmonary emboli or disseminated intravascular coagulation, before putting the blood into sterile bags or bottles with anticoagulant (if available).[1,4,28]

For each 500 mL of blood, add 60 mL of 3.8% sodium citrate (3.8 g/L) or 12 mL of citric acid monohydrate–trisodium citrate dihydrate–glucose solution. If clots appear, re-filter the blood. Reinfuse this blood immediately; do not store for later use.[33] If anticoagulant is not available, prepare acid-citrate-dextrose (ACD) by mixing 2 g sodium citrate and 3 g dextrose in enough sterile water to make a total volume of 120 mL, which is sufficient for 1 unit of blood.[28]

An alternate formula for preparing ACD is to combine 8 g citric acid monohydrate, 22 g trisodium citrate dihydrate, and 24.5 g dextrose monohydrate, mix, and add it to 1000 mL distilled water to make the ACD solution. Then place 75 mL of the ACD solution in a 500-mL blood bottle and autoclave it. Alternatively, separate the dry ACD mixture into 4-g portions and wrap

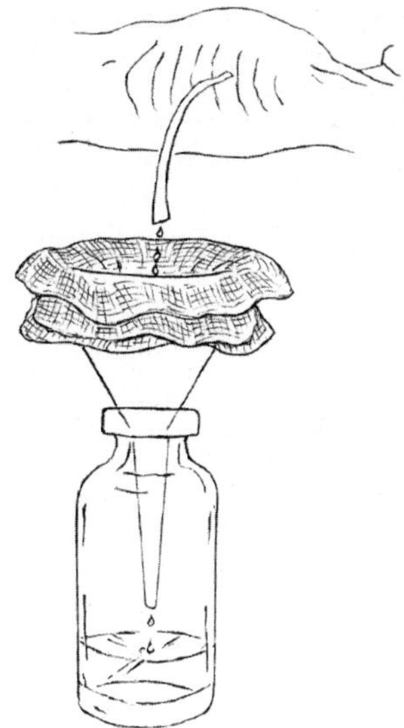

FIG. 18-1. Improvised cell salvage from a chest tube.

them in waxed paper. A 4-g packet is the amount necessary for one 500-mL blood bottle. Each time blood bottles are made up, empty the contents of one packet into the bottle, add 75 mL of distilled water, and autoclave the bottle.[34]

In some cases, especially in dire emergencies, cell salvage may be used either without anticoagulants or with alternative anticoagulants, such as heparin.[29,35] Blood that flows freely and has been in contact with serosal surfaces (e.g., peritoneum, pericardium, and pleura) usually lacks fibrinogen and may not need an extra anticoagulant. In these cases, clinicians have successfully either used heparin anticoagulation or not used anticoagulants without encountering any complications. If CPDA-1 is in short supply, a half-dose (30 mL/500 mL blood) can also be used.[29]

Advantages

Cell salvage has been shown to be safe, simple to use, and culturally acceptable. The method poses no risk of either transfusion reactions from mismatches or the transmission of blood-borne diseases. The blood is immediately available, because there is no need to do a type and cross-match. The method is so simple that it can be done in resource-poor settings without elaborate equipment or the electricity needed for blood refrigeration. In cultures that fear or ban blood donation or receiving blood from others, this method may overcome some of their concerns.

Disadvantages/Complications

The potential complications from autotransfusion include infection, embolism, and coagulopathies. However, the procedure's lifesaving potential far outweighs the risks. The chance of infection from the transfusion is markedly lessened by using sterile equipment and by discarding blood from a contaminated source, such as an abdomen with a ruptured bowel or tubo-ovarian abscess. Transfuse blood as soon as possible to avoid the proliferation of any bacteria that are present. Coagulopathy is more common when this technique is used with ruptured ectopic pregnancies (due to trophoblastic products) than with other abdominal or chest injuries. Yet, few complications have been reported. Some of these complications, including renal failure from transfusing hemolyzed blood, have led some clinicians to limit its use to bleeding sites that are no more than 3 hours old.[29]

Preoperative Autologous Blood Donation

Preoperative autologous blood donation (PABD) is one of the safest methods of obtaining blood for anticipated surgical blood loss. The method can be used anywhere a blood bank exists.

Ideally, 4 to 5 weeks before an elective operation, the patient donates blood for use during surgery.

However, PABD is expensive, because it requires that there be a functioning blood bank in which to store the blood. The procedure is also prone to some human error, because the correct patient's blood must be identified and administered. Moreover, because patients can donate only a limited amount of blood, that amount may be insufficient to replace the blood lost in surgery.[1]

TYPING BLOOD

Blood typing and Rh testing require special chemicals that are normally available only in a blood bank. Cross-matching is used to test whether a specific unit of blood is compatible with the patient. Cross-matching tests RBCs from the donor unit against the recipient's plasma/serum. The principle is that if the patient's serum contains antibodies against the antigens present on the donor's RBCs, agglutination occurs. Agglutination indicates that the donor unit is incompatible for that specific patient. If no agglutination occurs, the unit can be transfused into that patient.

Obtaining Samples

When drawing blood for either ANH or cell salvage, if a blood bank is available, send the first aliquot to them, in case additional banked blood is needed. In an emergency, blood can be scooped off the patient or out of an open wound. Just be sure that it is that patient's blood.

Emergency Cross-Matching

While emergency blood cross-matching is not optimal, if no other option exists, it is better than transfusing without any testing. These techniques may be used in austere situations when blood for transfusion is obtained from a "walking blood bank" (see the next section). Unlike the simple method, the more complex method requires a centrifuge, a magnifying lens or microscope, a pipette or syringe, and time.

Simple Method (White Tile)

The white tile method[30] uses a drop of the donor blood mixed with the recipient's serum. Put this mixture on a white ceramic tile and examine it after 4 minutes (a hand lens may be useful). If no agglutination occurs, the blood is acceptable for transfusion into that recipient.

Complex Method

1. Put 10 mL of the donor's blood in a tube and centrifuge it for 5 minutes at 3000 rpm. The serum and cells should separate. Use a pipette or syringe to remove the serum.
2. Add two drops of 0.9% NaCl (NS) to the tube.
3. Mix the donor's cells with the NS, using a wooden stick, and fill the tube with NS.
4. Centrifuge for 1 minute at 3000 rpm. Use the pipette or syringe to remove the NS.
5. Add two drops of the patient's serum to the donor cells.
6. Set the mixture aside for 5 minutes at 20°C to 25°C (68°F to 77°F).
7. Spin the mixture again for 1 minute at 3000 rpm.
8. Using magnification, examine the sediment. No agglutination indicates that the donor blood may be used for transfusion. Agglutination occurs from an antibody–antigen reaction, indicating that this donor blood should not be used for this patient.[36]

WALKING BLOOD BANK

The term walking blood bank (WBB), also called "blood on the hoof,"[37] refers to obtaining blood for transfusion from donors who are present or who can be called upon when the blood is needed. It may also provide coagulation factors when blood components are unavailable.[38]

The US Navy has used the WBB since transfusions became a part of medical therapy,[39] and it has been part of the emergency medical plan for most military units, including the Allied invasion at Normandy during World War II.[40] WBB also has been described for use in neonatal ICUs, rural hospitals, post-disaster settings, remote settings such as Antarctic bases, and aboard ships.[38,41,42] Furthermore, it should be included in blood services in resource-poor regions where culture, finances, or poor management leads to scarcity of transfusable blood.[43] Because a WBB is a community effort, it helps to involve religious leaders when generating potential donor lists for pretesting. Blood from a WBB donor is not stored, but rather transfused immediately. Retain samples (frozen, if possible) for "look-back" testing for blood-borne pathogens.

In planning for a disaster, if the use of a WBB involving a defined group of people as donors is probable, prescreen those donors (discussed in next section) and prepare a potential donor list. Practice the WBB procedures, including quickly locating the donors, in advance.[30,44]

Donors

Prescreening

In ideal situations, donors have been prescreened for a history of high-risk behaviors (e.g., sexual practices, parenteral drug abuse, or recent tattoos), blood-borne diseases, or prior rejection as a blood donor. Their blood should also have been typed and screened for laboratory evidence of anemia, hepatitis, dyscrasias, and Hgb variants, such as sickle cell trait, thalassemia minor, or glucose-6-phosphate dehydrogenase deficiency.[44] If possible, most individuals identified as potential donors for disaster situations should be blood type O (universal) donors. (Forty-six percent of the US population has type O blood, although it is rarer in other populations.) For the donor list to be used during community blood shortages, the entire spectrum of blood types should be included. Donors should wear or carry information about their blood types.[36] Whenever possible, their blood should be screened again when donated.

Emergency (No Prescreened/Identified Donors)

In situations where a WBB must be used unexpectedly, attempt to determine potential donors' blood types with local testing. If this is not possible, use information from the donor, military dog tags, or other records, but realize that this information is often incorrect. Even under the best circumstances, information about blood type printed on dog tags is wrong from 2% to 11% of the time.[40,45]

Try to select donors who have previously (ideally, recently) donated blood to a blood bank; they will have been tested for the appropriate infectious diseases. Even among this group, screen out all donors with a history of high-risk behavior.

Blood Storage

Whenever possible, collect the blood using standard blood collection bags that have a 600-mL capacity and that contain 63 mL of CPD or CPDA-1 anticoagulant. If enough blood is drawn so that the bag is almost full, it will contain 450 mL of blood. Label each bag clearly with the blood type and donor identification information.

The longer that warm blood is kept without being cooled or transfused, the greater the risk of bacterial growth and of the loss of clotting factors. Blood units should be kept at room temperature for no longer than 24 hours—and preferably for <6 hours. After 24 hours, destroy any warm whole-blood units: It is no longer safe to administer them—even in emergency situations. (Under normal circumstances, hospitals destroy blood units if they exceed 10°C [50°] for 30 minutes.)

If absolutely necessary, blood collected from WBB donors can be kept in a refrigerator or on wet ice for up to 3 weeks. While the RBCs remain viable, platelets may become inactive in whole blood stored cold (1°C to 10°C) for >24 hours, thus losing one of the main benefits of fresh whole blood.[30]

Advantages

The WBB is a source of fresh whole blood when replacement is absolutely necessary to preserve life and limb. For example, the US military used fresh whole blood in Iraq.[45] When standard blood component therapy is unavailable, the use of fresh whole blood can be lifesaving. Because whole blood contains clotting factors, it is effective for treating dilutional coagulopathy associated with massive blood loss and fluid resuscitation.[30]

Disadvantages

Critics of the WBB argue that planning for the use of blood in this manner constitutes an endorsement of substandard practice.[44] In some situations, donor performance may be impaired after donation, especially at high altitudes (where blood donation should be avoided if at all possible) and in battlefield circumstances. Women donors who are still menstruating should be on supplemental iron before and after donation.[30]

BLOOD BANK

Operating a blood bank requires an abundance of resources that are often not available. These include a constant source of power, laboratory and blood collection equipment, skilled personnel, and a ready supply of blood donors.

Blood should ideally be refrigerated and kept at from 3°C to 6°C (37°F to 43°F); it must not be frozen. Blood undergoes considerable deterioration if the storage temperature fluctuates greatly. Use an ordinary refrigerator capable of maintaining the required temperature. (The refrigerator needs alarms that detect temperature variations and a source of backup power.) Refrigeration can also be achieved by melting ice, because ice melts at 4°C, which is ideal for blood storage. The melting ice method is most often used when transporting blood, but it can also be used for longer periods if there is a constant and assured ice source. In well-insulated containers, ice can maintain the necessary 4°C for up to 72 hours.[46]

Even if a blood bank is available, there is often a problem getting sufficient blood donations to meet the need. One method of maintaining a stocked blood bank, if such facilities are available, is to try to make donating a unit of blood a requirement for having any minor surgery.[47]

In poorly nourished populations, blood may have Hgb contents much lower than those seen in well-nourished populations. That is of particular concern at many rural hospitals around the world, where they use a relative's fresh whole blood for transfusion.[48]

BLOOD WARMING

Because hypothermia is a major complication associated with blood transfusions, do everything possible to prevent it, especially during MTs.

In-Line Warming

A simple, slow method of blood warming is to add extra lengths of IV tubing between the PRBC units and the patient. Clinicians often place a coil of IV tubing into a bucket containing warm water of varying temperatures (Fig. 18-2). However, the slow passage of the cells through the tubing can damage erythrocytes if the water temperature is >40°C (104°F). Commercial in-line

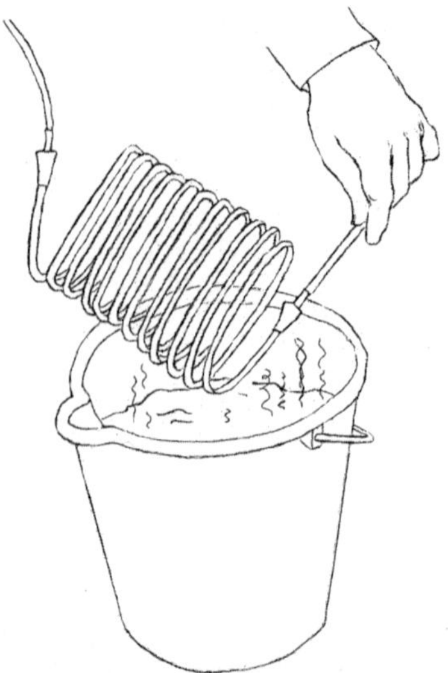

FIG. 18-2. Coiled IV tubing in bucket of water for "in-line" warming.

warmers are also available, although they are very expensive and can be used for only one IV line in one patient at a time.

Pre-Warming Method

One of the most common blood warming methods, used throughout the world, is to simply lay the PRBC bag (often of variable quantity) in a pan of tap water at about room temperature for 10 to 15 minutes. While the temperature reached using this method is unpredictable, this process will not harm the red cells and may provide some patient benefit.

Rapid Admixture Blood Warming

Patients needing rapid blood transfusions benefit tremendously if the blood is warmed to 37°C from the 4°C temperature that is the standard for banked blood. Clinicians' ability to warm blood units is hampered by the time constraints of needing to infuse blood quickly, the frequent need to infuse blood simultaneously through multiple IV lines, and the cost of blood-warming equipment.[49] The following method of "rapid admixture blood warming" is a rapid, safe, easy-to-use, and inexpensive method for warming blood that has been used at the University Medical Center Level 1 Trauma Center (Tucson, Ariz.) for >20 years with great success and no complications (Fig. 18-3). This method also dilutes the unit, leading to faster infusions and fewer complications. It achieves the four goals of PRBC warming for rapid transfusions:

1. Bring the unit to body temperature (37°C).
2. Be rapid.
3. Be safe.
4. Be inexpensive.

Rapid admixture blood warming involves combining 250 mL of 70°C (158°F) NS with a standard unit of packed RBCs (or erythrocytes, the common unit of "blood" transfused) using one of the two ports on the bag. Standard "plasma transfer set" male–male adapter tubing links the two bags. When the ~30-second mixing, performed manually, is complete, the blood unit is at 35°C to 37°C.

Note: If the plasma transfer set cannot be obtained (it is not sold in all countries), a slightly more cumbersome method is to use standard "Y" blood infusion IV tubing (Fig. 18-4). After shutting off flow to the patient, spike the 250-mL 70°C NS bag with one arm of the "Y" and the blood unit with the other arm. Transfer the NS into the PRBC bag and close the "Y" arm to the empty saline bag. Then open the IV tubing to the patient so that the warm PRBCs can be administered.

Concerns about RBC safety led to measurements of survival times for warmed cells: They survived longer than normal in a human subject. This method also dilutes the unit, leading to

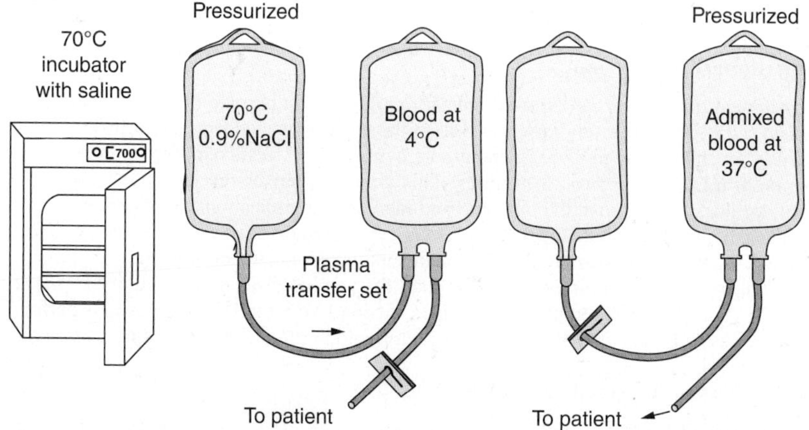

FIG. 18-3. Rapid admixture blood warming using a plasma transfer set.

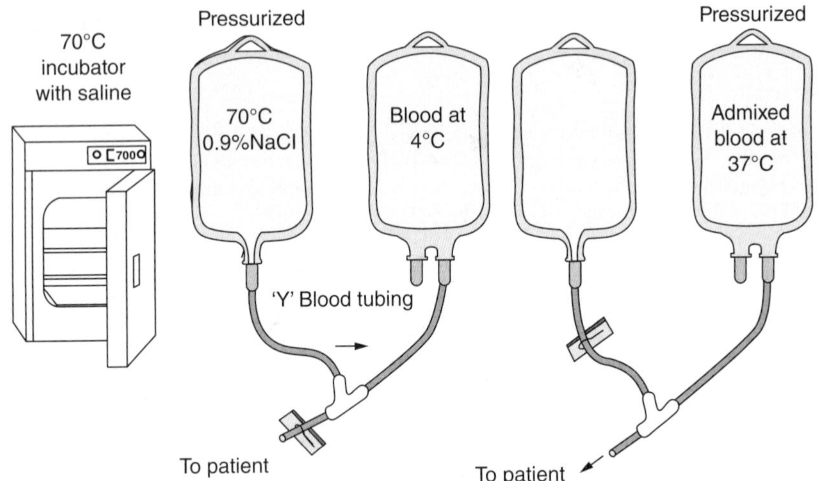

FIG. 18-4. Rapid admixture blood warming using the "Y-Tubing" from a standard blood administration set.[50]

faster infusions and fewer complications. To avoid infection after warming the blood to body temperature, the transfusions are completed within 30 minutes after warming.[51,52]

The only piece of capital equipment needed is a standard 70°C laboratory incubator in which to preheat the saline bags. Only one incubator is needed for an emergency department (ED), OR, or ICU; if they are in close proximity, only one is needed for all of them. (The initial warming oven at University Medical Center lasted nearly 20 years!) The cost of tubing is minimal. Because the method utilizes standard nursing procedures, minimal time is needed to teach the procedure. Standard IV equipment is used, so all of a patient's lines can have warmed blood using this method. ***Caution all personnel involved in this technique that they must never use the 70°C NS for direct infusion***.

Rapid admixture blood warming is so inexpensive, simple, safe, and fast that it should be the primary method used for blood warming in most parts of the world.[53-55]

ALTERNATIVES TO STANDARD TRANSFUSION

Blood will usually be infused intravenously. However, it can also be administered intraosseously and, to treat severe chronic anemia in children, intraperitoneally, using the technique described in Chapter 12.[56]

Intraperitoneal Transfusion

Intraperitoneal transfusion can be used only for children with chronic anemia, because it takes from 4 to 6 days to completely raise the Hgb to the levels expected from the infusion. It can be safely used in children up to 4 years old, although most are <3 years old. The optimal volume to infuse is 20 mL/kg over 5 to 15 minutes. This generally raises the Hgb by 4 g/dL. Giving >35 mL/kg does not improve the outcome and increases complications. This technique is safe, fast, and easily performed by nurses. It has fewer complications than venous cutdowns and does not require the skills necessary to place IV catheters in very small children.[56]

Transient dyspnea occurs in some cases when the volume distends the abdomen. (Limit the infusion to 20 mL/kg to lessen the risk of this occurring.) Very rarely, if the bowel is perforated, some rectal blood is seen, but this does not develop into peritonitis and needs no treatment.[56]

Person-to-Person "Direct" Transfusion

In this method, blood flows directly (or with a brief interlude in an in-line syringe) from one person to another. Use direct transfusion only in the most critical situations when there is no

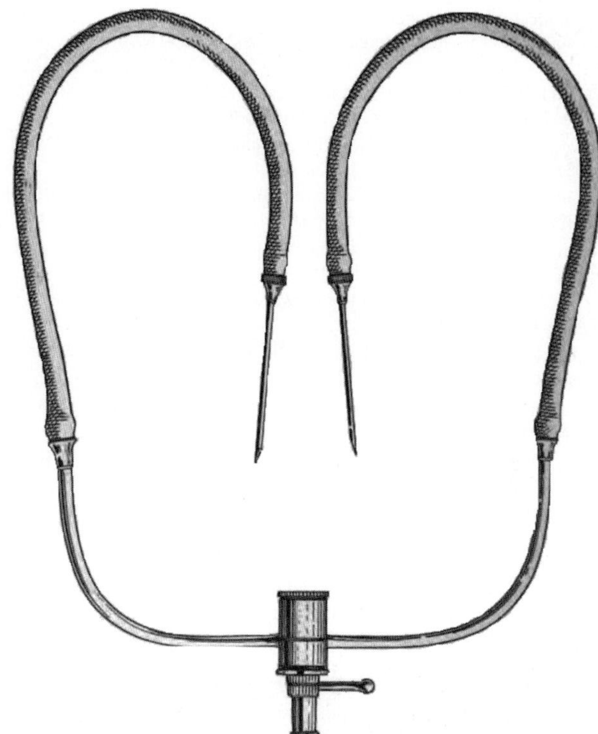

FIG. 18-5. Bernheim's direct transfusion device. *(Reproduced from Bernheim.[57])*

other option. If the amount of blood being taken from donors cannot be measured, carefully monitor their vital signs and physical condition to avoid over-phlebotomizing them.

In venous–venous transfusion, the venous tourniquet is removed from the recipient's arm when the IV needle (or, if a cutdown, the cannula) is placed in the recipient's vein. The tourniquet remains on the donor's arm until the procedure is complete. In 1917, Bernheim described his device for direct venous–venous transfusion: a glass syringe connected to a two-armed, double-needle IV tube. It had a revolving plug, the precursor to the three-way stopcock (Fig. 18-5). Used with IV needles and a three-way stopcock, the amount of blood delivered can be measured, and most health professionals should be able to place the lines. The blood transfused is measured by counting how many syringes of blood are infused. Problems with clotting may occur, however.

The advantage of direct transfusion is that it immediately provides a patient with whole blood using minimal equipment. The disadvantages are that probably no more than 2 units of blood (~1 L) can be removed acutely from one individual. Except in transfusions from adults to children, this often may not be enough. In desperate circumstances, taking blood from one member of the group may weaken him/her at a critical time, further endangering the group. Also, even if you "know" the donor, you cannot be absolutely certain without testing that the person does not have HBV, HCV, malaria, HIV, or another blood-borne disease. The potential donor may not even know they have it.

REFERENCES

1. Wake DJ, Cutting WA. Blood transfusion in developing countries: problems, priorities and practicalities. *Trop Doct*. 1998;28(1):4-8.
2. Knight RJ. Anaesthesia in a difficult situation in South Vietnam. *Anaesthesia*. 1969;24(3):317-342.
3. Goodnough LT. America's blood supply in the aftermath of September 11, 2001. Testimony to the House Committee on Energy and Commerce, September 10, 2002. http://energycommerce.house.gov/107/hearings/09102002Hearing705/Goodnough1167.htm. Accessed September 26, 2006.

4. Cherian MN. Clinical use of blood: WHO information of interest to anaesthesiologists. *Indian J. Anaesth*. 2002;46(2):149-150. http://medind.nic.in/iad/t02/i2/iadt02i2p149.pdf. Accessed September 9, 2015.
5. Hébert PC, Wells G, Blajchman MA, et al. A multicenter, randomized, controlled clinical trial of transfusion requirements in critical care. *N Engl J Med*. 1999;340(6):409-417.
6. Carson JL, Noveck H, Berlin JA, et al. Mortality and morbidity in patients with very low postoperative Hb levels who decline blood transfusion. *Transfusion*. 2002;42:812-818.
7. World Health Organization. *Management of Severe Malnutrition: A Manual for Physicians and Other Senior Health Workers*. Geneva, Switzerland: WHO; 1999:18.
8. Lacroix J, Hérbert PC, Hutchison JS, et al. Transfusion strategies for patients in pediatric intensive care units. *N Engl J Med*. 2007;356(16):1609-1619.
9. Hébert PC, Yetisir E, Martin C, et al. Is a low transfusion threshold safe in patients with cardiovascular disease? *Crit Care Med*. 2001;29:227-234.
10. Savage SA, Zarzaur BL, Croce MA, Fabian TC. Redefining massive transfusion when every second counts. *J Trauma Acute Care Surg*. 2013;74(2):396-402.
11. Juhl-Olsen P, Vistisen ST, Christiansen LK, et al. Ultrasound of the inferior vena cava does not predict hemodynamic response to early hemorrhage. *J Emerg Med*. 2013;45(4):592-597.
12. Vandromme MJ, Griffin RL, Kerby JD, et al. Identifying risk for massive transfusion in the relatively normotensive patient: utility of the prehospital shock index. *J Trauma*. 2011;70:384-390.
13. Shackelford SA, Colton K, Stansbury LG, et al. Early identification of uncontrolled hemorrhage after trauma: current status and future direction. *J Trauma Acute Care Surg*. 2014;77(3 suppl 2):S222-227.
14. Rady MY, Rivers EP, Martin GB, et al. Continuous central venous oximetry and shock index in the emergency department: use in the evaluation of clinical shock. *Am J Emerg Med*. 1992;10(6):538-541.
15. Cotton BA, Dossett LA, Haut ER, et al. Multicenter validation of a simplified score to predict massive transfusion in trauma. *J Trauma Injury Infection Crit Care*. 2010;69(1):S33-S39.
16. Bodnar D, Rashford S, Williams S. The feasibility of civilian prehospital trauma teams carrying and administering packed red blood cells. *Emerg Med J*. 2014;31(2):93-95.
17. Boscarino C, Tien H, Acker J, et al. Feasibility and transport of packed red blood cells into Special Forces operational conditions. *J Trauma Acute Care Surg*. 2014;76(4):1013-1019.
18. Holcomb JB, Wade CE, Michalek JE, et al. Increased plasma and platelet to red blood cell ratios improves outcome in 466 massively transfused civilian trauma patients. *Ann Surg*. 2008;248(3): 447-458.
19. Holcomb JB, Tilley BC, Baraniuk S, et al. Transfusion of plasma, platelets, and red blood cells in a 1:1:1 vs a 1:1:2 ratio and mortality in patients with severe trauma: the PROPPR randomized clinical trial. *JAMA*. 2015;313(5):471-482.
20. Perkins JG, Andrew CP, Spinella PC, et al. An evaluation of the impact of apheresis platelets used in the setting of massively transfused trauma patients. *J Trauma Injury Infection Crit Care*. 2009;66(4):S77-S85.
21. Iserson KV. Whole blood in trauma resuscitations. *Am J Emerg Med*. 1985;3(4):358-359.
22. King M. *Primary Surgery, Vol. 2: Trauma*. Oxford, UK: Oxford University Press; 1987:18.
23. Begovic M, Kozlicic A. Transfusion therapy during war and peace in Sarajevo. *Prehosp Disaster Med*. 1994;9(suppl 2):S16-S19.
24. Manda W, Buffy G. Experience of autologous blood transfusion at a district general hospital in Zambia. *Trop Doct*. 1994;24(3):108-111.
25. Monk TG, Goodnough LT, Birkmeyer JD, et al. Acute normovolemic hemodilution is a cost-effective alternative to preoperative autologous blood donation by patients undergoing radical retropubic prostatectomy. *Transfusion*. 1995;35:559-565.
26. Goodnough LT, Monk TG, Brecher ME. Acute normovolemic hemodilution should replace the preoperative donation of autologous blood as a method of autologous-blood procurement. *Transfusion*. 1998; 38(5):473-476.
27. Berege ZA, Jacombs B, Matasha MR, et al. Acute isovolaemic haemodilution: the best option for autologous blood transfusion in Africa? *Trop Doct*. 1995;25(4):152-155.
28. Poeschl U. Emergency autologous blood transfusion in ruptured ectopic pregnancy. *Update Anaesth*. 1992;2(2):1. www.nda.ox.ac.uk/wfsa/html/u02/u02_003.htm. Accessed September 14, 2006.
29. Baldan M, Giannou CP, Rizzardi G, et al. Autotransfusion from haemothorax after penetrating chest trauma: a simple, life-saving procedure. *Trop Doct*. 2006;36:21-22.
30. US Army. *Emergency War Surgery*. 3rd Rev. Washington, DC: Borden Institute, Walter Reed Army Medical Center; 2004:7.09-12.

31. Barss P. Blood bags for autotransfusion (letter). *Trop Doct*. 1985;15(2):67.
32. Price ME, Kernbey W. Collecting blood for autotransfusion in ectopic pregnancy. *Trop Doct*. 1985;15(2):67-68.
33. Dobson MB. *Anaesthesia at the District Hospital*. 2nd ed. Geneva, Switzerland: World Health Organization; 2000:42.
34. Monson MH, Mertens PE. A system for making hospital solutions in the Third World. *Trop Doct*. 1988;18:54-59.
35. Mattox KL, Walker LE, Beall AC, et al. Blood availability for the trauma patient: autotransfusion. *J Trauma*. 1975;15(8):663-669.
36. Husum H, Ang SC, Fosse E. *War Surgery: Field Manual*. Penang, Malaysia: Third World Network; 1995:707.
37. Grande CM, Baskett PJF, Donchin Y, et al. Trauma anesthesia for disasters: anything, anytime, anywhere. *Crit Care Clin*. 1991;7(2):339-361.
38. Lin G, Lavon H, Gelfond R, Abargel A, Merin O. Hard times call for creative solutions: medical improvisations at the Israel Defense Forces field hospital in Haiti. *Am J Disaster Med*. 2010;5(3):188-92.
39. Hrezo RJ, Clark J. The walking blood bank: an alternative blood supply in military mass casualties. *Disaster Manag Response*. 2003;1(1):19-22.
40. Heaton LD, Boyd Coates J Jr, Carter BN, et al. *Surgery in World War II: Activities of Surgical Consultants, Vol. II*. Washington, DC: US Army Medical Department; 1964:71-78.
41. Kakaiya RM, Morrison FS, Halbrook JC, et al. Problems with a walking donor transfusion program. *Transfusion*. 1978;19:577-580.
42. Benziger M, Benziger J, Canfield TM. Blood banking in the small hospital. *Surg Clin North Am*. 1979;50:471-482.
43. American Association of Blood Banks. American Association of Blood Banks Inter-organizational Task Force on Domestic Disasters and Acts of Terrorism Report and Recommendations, January 31, 2002. Cited in: Hrezo RJ, Clark J. The walking blood bank: an alternative blood supply in military mass casualties. *Disaster Manag Response*. 2003;1(1):19-22.
44. Pandolf KB, Burr RE, eds. *Medical Aspects of Harsh Environments, Vol. 2*. Falls Church, VA: Office of the Surgeon General US Army; 2002:903.
45. Holcomb JB. The 2004 Fitts Lecture: current perspective on combat casualty care. *J Trauma*. 2005;59(4):990-1002.
46. Pandolf KB, Burr RE, eds. *Medical Aspects of Harsh Environments, Vol. 2*. Falls Church, VA: Office of the Surgeon General US Army; 2002:77.
47. King M, Bewes P, Cairns J, et al, eds. *Primary Surgery, Vol. 1: Non-Trauma*. Oxford, UK: Oxford Medical Publishers; 1990:610.
48. Mock CN, Denno D, Adzotor ES. Paediatric trauma in the rural developing world: low cost measures to improve outcome. *Injury*. 1993;24(5):291-296.
49. Iserson KV, Huestis D. Blood warming techniques: current applications and techniques. *Transfusion*. 1991;31(6):558-571.
50. Iserson KV. Rapid admixture blood warming: fast, safe & inexpensive. *BMH Med J*. 2014;1(3):40-46.
51. Wilson EB, Knauf MA, Iserson KV. Red cell tolerance of admixture with heated saline. *Transfusion*. 1988;28(2):170-172.
52. Wilson EB, Knauf MA, Donohoe K, et al. Red blood cell survival following admixture with heated saline—evaluation of a new blood warming method for rapid transfusion. *J Trauma*. 1988;28:1274-1277.
53. Iserson KV, Knauf MA, Anhalt D. Rapid admixture blood warming—technical advances. *Crit Care Med*. 1990;18(10):1138-1141.
54. Iserson KV. Rapid high volume fluid infusions. In: Roberts J, Hedges J, eds. *Clinical Procedures in Emergency Medicine*. 2nd ed. Philadelphia, PA: W.B. Saunders; 1991:301-307.
55. Cohn SM, Stack GE. In vitro comparison of heated saline-blood admixture with a heat exchanger for rapid warming of red blood cells. *J Trauma*. 1993;35(5):688-691.
56. van Bemmel JAG, de Vries HR. Intraperitoneal blood transfusions. *Trop Doct*. 1988;18(2):89-91.
57. Bernheim BM. *Blood Transfusion, Hemorrhage and the Anaemias*. Philadelphia, PA: Lippincott; 1917:126.

19 | Radiology/Imaging

NON-IMAGE DIAGNOSES

In situations without imaging capacity, clinicians need to rely on the history, physical examination, observation with repeat examinations, and, in some cases, exploratory surgery.

ESSENTIALS

The World Health Organization (WHO) lists what they consider the essential diagnostic imaging equipment worldwide (Table 19-1).[1] This varies with the four levels of hospital capabilities (see Table 5-1).

VIEWING X-RAYS

Limited Imaging Situations—The Hot Light

Even if radiology is available, it may be intermittent or deliver poor quality images. Film, rather than digital images, may be the norm.

To help illuminate dark areas of the film, make a "hot light." Using a lamp with a 25-watt regular lightbulb, take off the shade and slip a tin can with both ends cut out over the shade's support wires. The can should fit tightly so the wires support the can. If this is not the case, cut the can lengthwise and wind tape around it so that it sits securely on the shade supports. Then take a piece of heavy cardboard, aluminum foil, or thin metal and cut a hole with a 2- to 3-inch diameter in the center. Lay this on top of the can and tape it in place. If using cardboard, be careful that it doesn't get too hot and burn. When you need to see a dark area on the film, turn on the light and hold the film over it—but not too close or it will begin to burn. Do not bother trying to use flashlights (too diffuse a beam) or penlights (too narrow a beam).

TABLE 19-1 WHO Imaging Essentials

	Facility Level			
Resources/Capabilities	Basic	GP	Specialist	Tertiary
Plain radiography	D	D	E	E
Portable plain radiography	I	D	D	E
Ultrasound for trauma (pleural cavity/abdomen for hemoperitoneum; fluid/heart for pericardial effusion)	I	D	D	D
Computerized axial tomography (CT scan)	I	D	D	D
Contrast radiography (barium, Gastrografin)	I	I	D	D
Angiography	I	I	D	D
Image intensification/fluoroscopy	I	I	D	D
Magnetic resonance imaging (MRI)	I	I	D	D
Nuclear medicine imaging	I	I	D	D

Abbreviations: D, desirable; E, essential; GP, general practitioners' hospital; I, irrelevant.

Adapted with permission from Mock et al.[1]

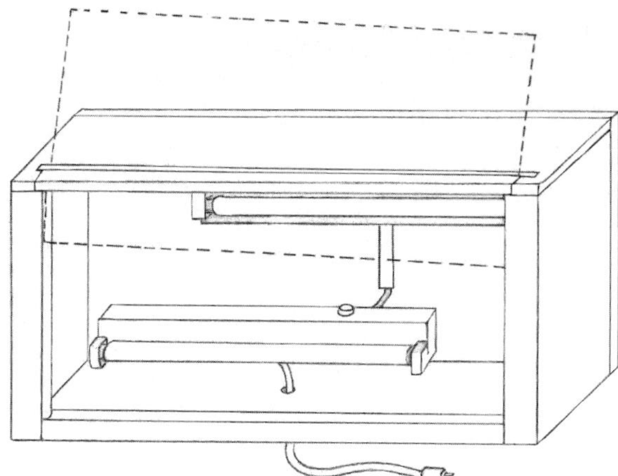

FIG. 19-1. A locally made radiographic viewing box. *(Reproduced with permission from Iserson and Timeb.[2])*

Light Boxes

Light boxes to view radiological images may be scarce. Make light boxes or read the film without one. Methods to view films without a light box include the following:

- Hold the radiograph up to a light source, such as a lamp or ceiling light. If you just want to get a general look at an x-ray, perhaps to make sure it is the right one, then basic background lighting should be sufficient. A more detailed examination, however, will require a stronger light source.
- Place the radiograph against a brightly lit window. Tape the film in place if it will be needed for some time, such as in the operating room or when teaching. Similar to a light box, this method backlights the radiograph so that you can see the contrast.

A view box can quickly (3 hours) and inexpensively (~$63 US) be made from locally available materials, as we did in Kintampo Municipal (District) Hospital in rural Ghana (Figs. 19-1 and 19-2). Our view box is a wooden case containing fluorescent bulbs with a translucent plastic viewing screen. The bulbs are the same as those used in the hospital's ceiling lights. The plastic, available locally, slides into grooves cut in the sides of the box, and can easily be lifted out to change the bulbs. Radiographs rest on a lip at the bottom of the box, and are held in place with both the top wooden slat that anchors the plastic sheet and two wires strung across the front of the box to eye bolts in the sides. The activation switch on the electrical socket is used to turn the light box on and off. Our light box design accommodates two full-size radiographs simultaneously. The light box can be set on a desk or shelf or, as at our hospital, mounted on the wall using standard brackets.[2]

Makeshift X-Ray Markers

Film Markers

Which is the right side? Normally, films are labeled with either "right" or "left" markers. (On chest and abdominal films, except with *situs inversus*, it should be obvious.) These metallic markers are small and easily lost. Bend a paper clip into an "L" (easier) or an "R" (if you are talented) and tape it on the film as you would with a standard marker.

Foreign-Body Markers

Localizing foreign bodies in soft tissues can be challenging.

Radiopaque markers used to localize embedded foreign bodies on radiographs include ball bearings, metallic pellets for air rifles (BBs), lead markers for radiographs (especially the "O"), hypodermic needles placed at right angles to a puncture, electrocardiogram (ECG) or electroencephalogram (EEG) leads, or paperclips. Use Vitamin E capsules as markers for magnetic resonance imaging (MRI) and computed tomography (CT) scans because they are visible but do not cause scatter.

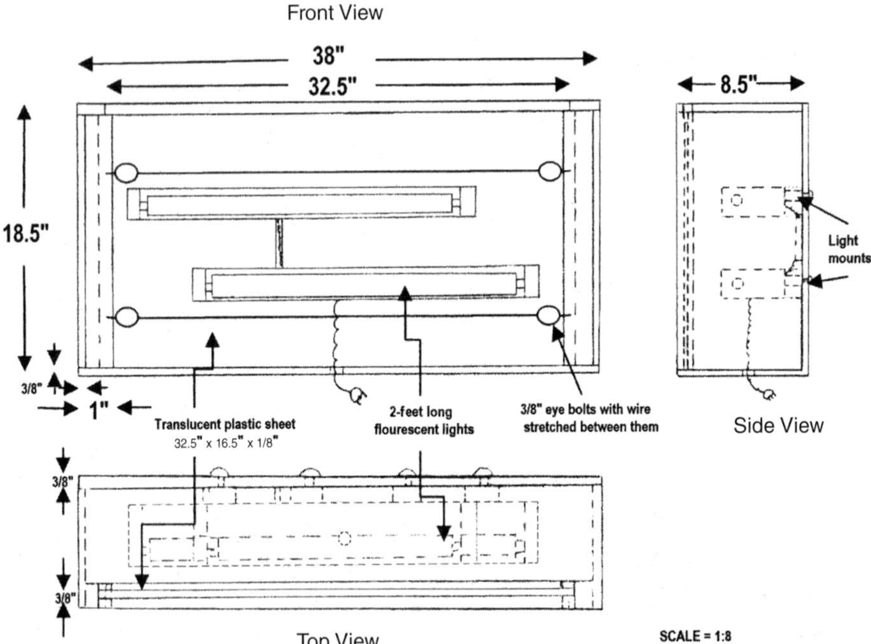

FIG. 19-2. Technical drawing for viewing box. *(Reproduced with permission from Iserson and Timeb.[2])*

Make a simple but highly effective marker from two paperclips, with one wire of each opened to about 45 degrees and pointed toward the wound. Tape them over and around the wound using clear adhesive tape. Use more for large wounds. With plain radiographs, obtain at least two views to better localize any foreign body. When using paperclip markers for a CT scan, unbend them to minimize scatter at the end of the marker nearest the wound. Once the site is determined, mark it with methylene blue or another skin marker before removing the paperclips.[3]

One variation on the paperclip foreign-body marker is to use a "forward arrow" (Fig. 19-3) pointing to penetrating wounds that enter anterior to the anterior axillary line (the front of the body) and a "backward arrow" pointing to those that enter posterior to that line (back of the body). This helps with localizing the penetrating foreign body's, usually a bullet's, trajectory.[4] Of course, everyone has to know what the different markers mean.

DETECTING PNEUMOTHORACES ON SUPINE CHEST RADIOGRAPHS

When neither ultrasound nor CT is available, use oblique views to detect occult pneumothoraces in supine patients, even when they cannot be seen by standard AP radiographs (Fig. 19-4).[5]

ESTIMATING THE SIZE OF A PNEUMOTHORAX

The treatment of pneumothoraces depends on their size. Rather than inserting a chest tube (and using many resources), it is possible to manage patients without dyspnea who are <50 years old and have a "small," first-time unilateral spontaneous pneumothorax solely with observation.[6] But, how can you tell that it is "small"?

To avoid using the complex, and often inaccurate, formulas and nomograms to calculate pneumothorax size, the British Thoracic Society suggests the use of a simple method that works well in clinical practice: A "small" spontaneous pneumothorax is determined when the average interparietal distance (AID) is <2 cm. The AID is an average of the distance between the parietal and visceral pleura at three points: the lung apex, and one-third and three-fourths of the way down

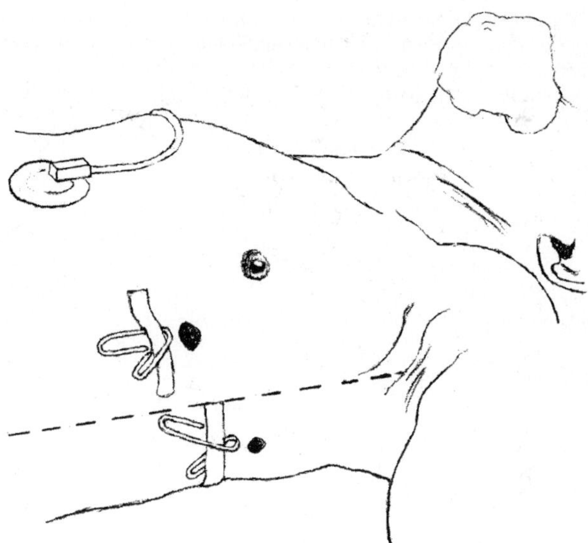

FIG. 19-3. "Forward"/anterior and "backward"/posterior paper clip arrow markers.

the lung. Other recommendations state that the distance between the apex of the chest to the cupula of the lung should be <3 cm to be considered "small."[7]

CONTRAST STUDIES

Contrast Esophagrams

If necessary, use barium for contrast esophagrams, because aspirating small amounts of barium causes no problems. Keep the patient sitting upright to reduce the aspiration risk. To reduce the amount of contrast used, patients can swallow a barium-soaked cotton ball rather than the liquid. However, if a foreign body must be extracted, the procedure can be more difficult after contrast has been used. These studies can be done with a portable x-ray machine.

Use water-soluble contrast (e.g., Gastrografin) if perforation is suspected, because it causes less mediastinal inflammation if extravasated. (Any iodine-containing contrast diluted with water can also be used.) However, if aspirated, it causes a severe chemical pneumonitis. Do not use it

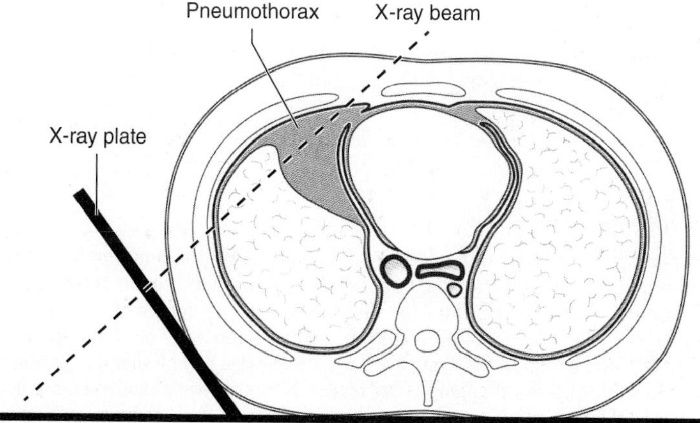

FIG. 19-4. Oblique supine technique for detecting pneumothorax.

in cases of complete esophageal obstruction. To test for a perforation, have the patient swallow progressively larger amounts of contrast, up to about 50 mL. If the result is negative, repeat the procedure with half-strength and then full-strength barium. If fluoroscopy is available, use it. It is easy to miss a perforation using portable radiographs, because you can take only one film for each swallow.

Gas Contrast

Air and carbon dioxide are effective, inexpensive, and readily available contrast agents for the stomach or colon. Inject air directly into these areas using a nasogastric (NG) tube or an enema tube. Children's effervescent tablets also produce gas if swallowed. Air injected through an NG tube usually provides sufficient contrast to make the diagnosis of a tracheoesophageal fistula in infants. It avoids introducing barium which has a real and dangerous risk of aspiration.[8]

Computed Tomography Contrast

Oral Contrast

The typical oral contrast material used for abdominal CT studies is expensive and is not well tolerated by many patients. Whole milk (4%), which is much less expensive, works well as a substitute contrast agent for abdominal CT studies. It seems to work better than using 2% milk, water, or no oral contrast agent. Whole milk functions as well as does barium suspension for gastrointestinal distention, mural visualization, and bowel loop and pancreas-duodenum discrimination.[9] In addition, patients are much more willing to drink the milk and they have fewer subsequent gastrointestinal effects.[10]

Intravenous Contrast

When a patient urgently needs a CT scan with intravenous (IV) contrast and there is a delay in obtaining venous access, give the contrast through an intraosseous (IO) line. The pressure needed to infuse dye through a proximal humeral IO line is less than at other sites, although awake patients experience considerable pain. Decrease the pain by slowly administering 2 mL of 2% lidocaine, followed, if necessary, by an additional flush of 2 mL 2% lidocaine before dye injection.[11]

Magnetic Resonance Imaging Contrast

Several positive oral contrast agents for MRI can be improvised. These include pediatric formula and homemade oil emulsions.[12] If you have an MRI, however, you probably don't need to improvise.

STEREOSCOPIC IMAGING

"Poor Man's CT"/Tomogram

When CT scanning is not available, plain radiographs can provide a "poor man's CT scan" of complex structures using stereoscopic imaging. Used until the mid-1980s in the United States, the technique clarifies difficult-to-read films and can localize lesions within a space, such as bullets or cavitary lesions in a chest or skull. Stereoscopic imaging was commonly used for facial bone (such as Water's views), PA chest, and complex fracture radiographs.

Taking Stereoscopic Films

Take stereoscopic films by first taking one film 5 degrees lateral from midline and then another film 5 degrees lateral from midline in the opposite direction, while keeping the part of the body (head, chest, or limb) being filmed still (Fig. 19-5). Alternatively, for each film, move the x-ray head to either side of midline, 10% of the distance between the x-ray head and the x-ray plate. The x-ray heads must be kept in the same horizontal plane. Be certain that the patient does not change position while you are changing x-ray plates. Note that some modern x-ray heads cannot be adjusted to shoot films at these angles, although it can be done with all portable machines.

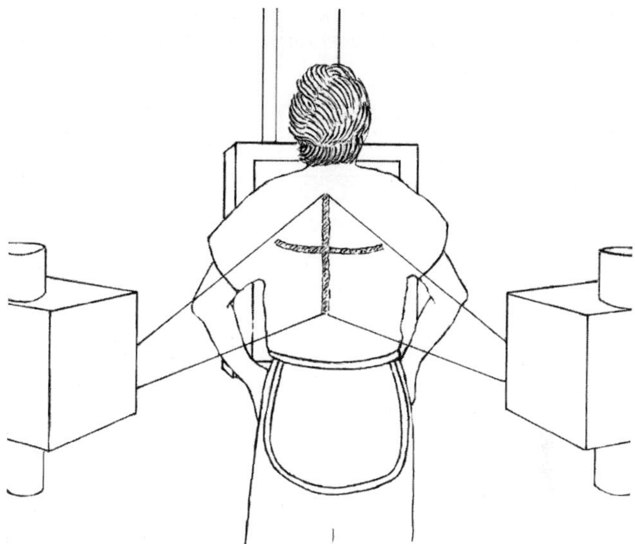

FIG. 19-5. X-ray positions to take a stereoscopic radiograph.

The tube motion must be in the direction of the grid lines if a grid is used to reduce x-ray scatter. (X-ray technicians will understand this.) The grid is usually along the long axis of the table and built into the x-ray table's Bucky cassette holder. It is also built into wall units, usually with a vertical orientation. The cassette may be placed against the patient (without a grid), although there will be more scatter and lower contrast than with a grid.

If only digital radiography is available, use the same technique to take the films and put them up side by side, using the "compare" feature available with most digital radiographic readers. The films may need to be rotated to make them line up correctly.

Viewing the Images

Reading stereoscopic radiographs requires either a stereoscopic viewer, rare in austere medical situations, or a little practice in crossing one's eyes to form a 3D image between the two slightly different films. Practice this eye-crossing technique using the old postcard-type images from a stereopticon or the images in Fig. 19-6. Just slightly cross your eyes until the two images merge

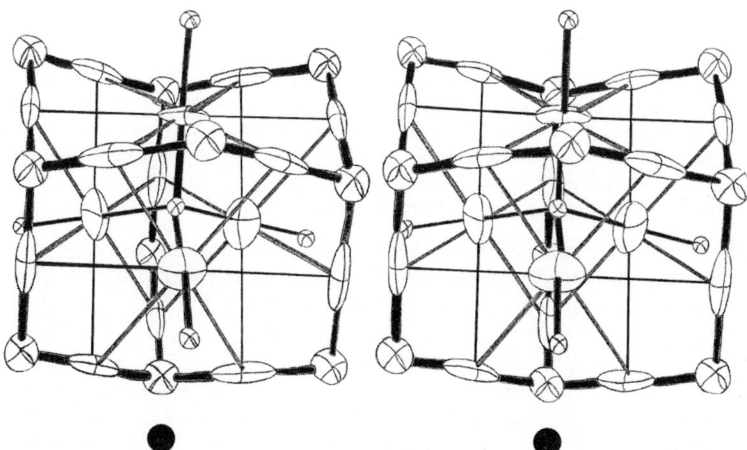

FIG. 19-6. Stereoscopic diamond. *(Source: Anon.[13])*

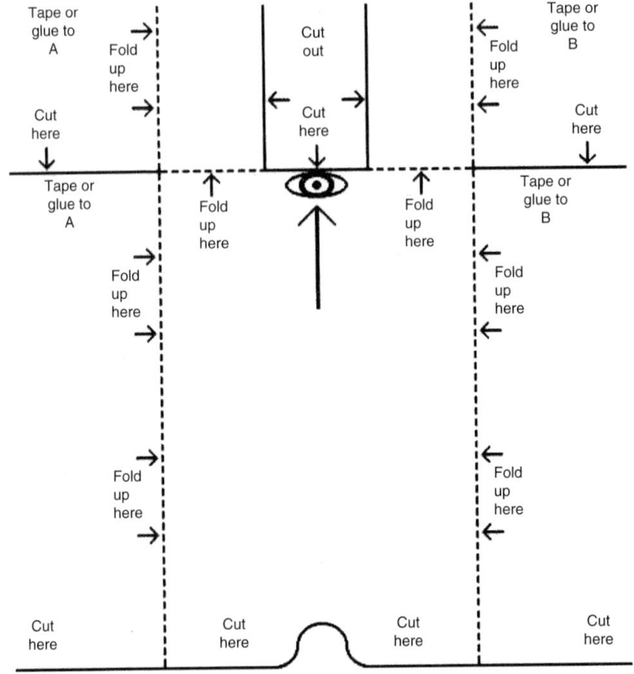

FIG. 19-7. Homemade stereoscopic viewer. *(From Samuel.[15])*

in the middle, giving a 3D picture. This is also how it is done with radiographs. Some people find it easier to merge specific points, such as the black dots below the figures, and then look at the image. A fun way to practice this technique is with stereoscopic photos, which can be found in antique stores and online.

For those who can't cross their eyes to see the stereoscopic image, Dr E.B. Morton devised a simple stereoscopic viewer using cardboard[14]:

> The simplest stereoscope for X-ray negatives or prints may be improvised in a few minutes. Take a piece of cardboard about 6 inches by 8 inches, and cut a rectangular opening in the middle, say 2 inches by 1½ inches. The two plates or prints are set upright side by side in a good light and from four to six feet from the observer. The card is held at arm's length, more or less, until the observer's right eye sees only the left hand plate, the left eye being closed, while the left eye sees only the right hand plate when the right eye is closed. Now open both eyes, concentrating attention on the edges of the opening in the card; in a few seconds or less the two images will coalesce, giving a perfect stereoscopic effect. At first it may be a little difficult to secure this, and there may be some ocular fatigue from the use of the muscles in an unaccustomed way, but this very soon disappears, and it is worth while learning how to use a device that can be made in a moment from a piece of dark paper if nothing better is at hand.

To make a similar viewer, enlarge the template in Fig. 19-7 to fit a letter-sized sheet of paper and cut it as indicated. The sides fold up so that it ends up looking like a trough with a hole at one end (marked with an eye) through which you view the images (Fig. 19-8). Use it in the same manner as described by Dr. Morton.

ULTRASOUND

Ultrasound has become the standard imaging modality in many austere situations. While clinicians now perform a wide variety of ultrasound examinations—the E-FAST and gallbladder being the most common—only the less common, but easily performed examinations to diagnose

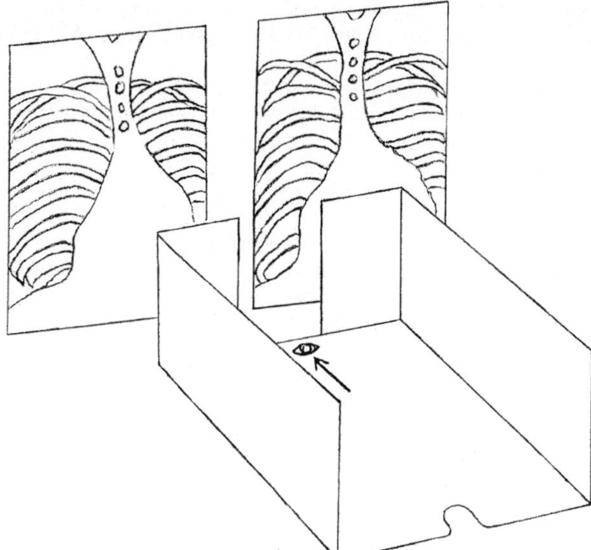

FIG. 19-8. Method to use homemade stereoscopic viewer.

fractures and neonatal intracranial bleeding are described here. Eye examinations are discussed in Chapter 30.

Tele-Ultrasonography

Ultrasound is the optimal imaging technology for austere environments. It has multiple clinical applications and can easily be operated by the clinician. In addition, its low cost, in comparison to other imaging hardware, and portability are ideal for remote areas. The machine uses batteries that can be recharged with solar energy, it does not require chemicals or film, and it immediately produces images of multiple body areas.[16]

Experts can guide remote ultrasound examinations using cameras to watch the operator, and images can be remotely interpreted using off-the-shelf, easily available technology. Images from remote sites (mountains, airplanes in flight, rural homes) can be obtained on handheld ultrasound machines and streamed to a standard free Internet service, such as Skype, using a smart phone. Experts can guide inexperienced operators who wear head-mounted webcams.[17]

Ultrasound Gels

In austere situations, “disposable” often means unavailable. That is frequently the case with ultrasound gel. Substitutes include ECG jelly, liquid soap, any water-soluble gel (e.g., K-Y Jelly), vegetable oil, and a water bath (extremities only). All provide images comparable to those produced using commercial gels. Vegetable oil, however, is not water soluble and stains everything it touches. While ordinary soap or water can be used as ultrasound gel, do not use petroleum-based materials, such as Vaseline, because they reportedly damage transducer heads.

An easy and inexpensive option is to make cornstarch-based ultrasound gel. Cornstarch, also known as corn flour, is available throughout the world, and the result is at least comparable to commercial gel. The method is as follows[18]:

1. Combine 1 part corn starch to 10 parts water (e.g., ¼-cup corn starch to 2½-cups water fills approximately two gel bottles).
2. Heat this mixture over medium heat for 3 to 5 minutes while stirring constantly so that it doesn’t clump.
3. The mixture begins to thicken and takes on a smooth, translucent appearance (like milk) about the time it begins to boil.

4. Turn off the heat and pour it into a clean container, such as an old commercial ultrasound gel bottle, a small soda bottle, or a baby bottle. Note that homemade gel does not have the same bacteriostatic quality as commercial ultrasound gel.
5. Allow the mixture to cool into gel form. This often takes several hours at room temperature.
6. Use the gel within 72 hours for best results. After that, the components may begin to separate, although it often is useable for a week.

Probe Protectors

A nonsterile very thin plastic bag, large condom, or rubber glove can be used to protect the transducer (probe) head when it is being used in the vagina or mouth. Put contact gel into the bag or glove before inserting the probe. If using a glove, put it on, put gel in the palm, grab the probe with the palm, and invert the glove around the probe. Then put additional gel outside the plastic for a good seal. Wrap tape around the proximal part of the cover to hold it in place. When a sterile probe cover is needed to help guide procedures done under aseptic condition, such as paracentesis, central line placement, and bladder aspiration, put a second sterile glove over the first before placing the gel. The glove, of course, will not fit very well. Then remove the top glove and tape it.

Neonatal Ultrasound of the Head

Use cranial ultrasound in infants to check for bleeding. Cranial ultrasonography can easily identify a subependymal hemorrhage or intraventricular blood. Also use it to identify posthemorrhagic ventricular dilation and midline shifts. Evaluation of arterial flow, especially in the neck, and intraparenchymal lesions is operator dependent.

Use a 7.5 MHz probe for premature infants <32 weeks of gestation or <1500 g, and a 5.0 to 3.0 MHz probe for older infants with an open fontanelle. With enough gel on the head and probe and with the child restrained, place the probe over and perpendicular to the anterior fontanelle in the coronal plane (across the head) and slowly angle it forward and backward to see the entire brain. The structures, especially those that are blood filled, should be easy to see. Repeat the process with the probe oriented in the sagittal plane (front to back), and slowly angle it from side to side to see the lateral ventricles and temporal lobe.

Water-Bath Ultrasound Technique in Children

Water-bath technique can be used for a painless ultrasound examination of superficial extremity structures and pathology, including shallow skin ulcers, subcutaneous masses, vascular malformations, osteomyelitis, foreign bodies, vascular malformation, trauma, and soft-tissue masses. Immerse the affected hand or foot in a disposable bedpan filled halfway with lukewarm tap water. With the skin just below the water, scan using a high-resolution linear transducer placed adjacent to, but not touching, the skin surface. This method results in a better quality image and a larger field of view than with the standard technique.[19]

Orthopedic Ultrasound

Although bone is a natural obstacle to high-frequency sound transmission, the large difference in acoustic impedance between soft tissue and bone results in a strong acoustic interface. This leads to an almost total reflection of sound energy from the bone, providing an excellent way to examine patients for fractures.[20]

Selecting the correct patients for examination is the key to using ultrasound for fracture diagnosis (Fig. 19-9). In patients exhibiting signs and symptoms of a fracture, clinicians with minimal training can diagnose many fractures using ultrasound, even those that they cannot see on radiographs. In patients with a medium-to-low probability of fracture, they are able to successfully rule out the presence of long-bone fractures.[21]

In children, ultrasound is most reliable for the detection of simple femoral (94%), humeral diaphyseal (90%), radial (89%), and ulnar (89%) fractures. Ultrasound can also show stress fractures that have been missed on plain radiographs and can help monitor the formation of callus in long-bone fractures.[22]

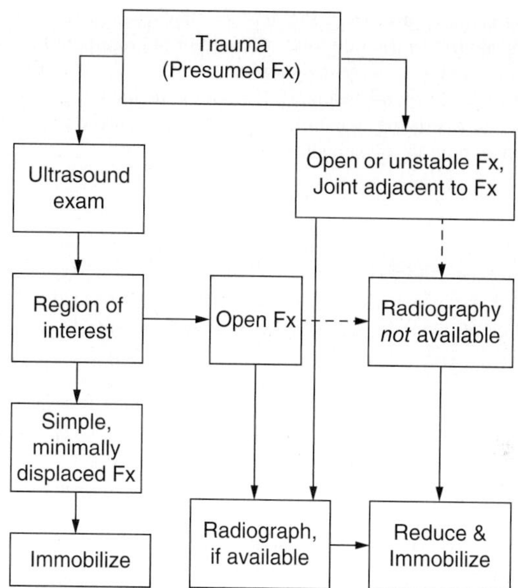

FIG. 19-9. Algorithm for use of ultrasound in fracture diagnosis. *(Abbreviation: Fx, fracture.)*

The ultrasound examination for fracture, which generally takes <5 minutes to complete, is usually performed with a high-frequency linear probe (10 to 5 MHz). Physicians can become proficient in administering the examination with only an hour-long standardized formal training session and a practice session on a live normal model.[21] Although, demonstrating on a child with a femur fracture, I taught rural Zambian nurses to successfully recognize fractures with ultrasound in 5 minutes. Some inexperienced examiners use pictorial reference cards to locate both ultrasound equipment controls and where to place the probe for various examinations.[23]

Method

The most common examination is of a long bone. Especially for those not completely familiar with the technique, a useful way to begin is to examine the unaffected extremity and to adjust the depth and maximize visualization of the cortical interface during this part of the examination. The cortical interface appears as an unbroken, hyperechoic line. Using sufficient gel, place the transducer transversely (across) the extremity just proximal to the patella or elbow. Identify the femur or humerus, and rotate the transducer 90 degrees so that it lies along the long axis of the bone. Slide it up the extremity (Fig. 19-10). Either the smooth shaft or an obvious

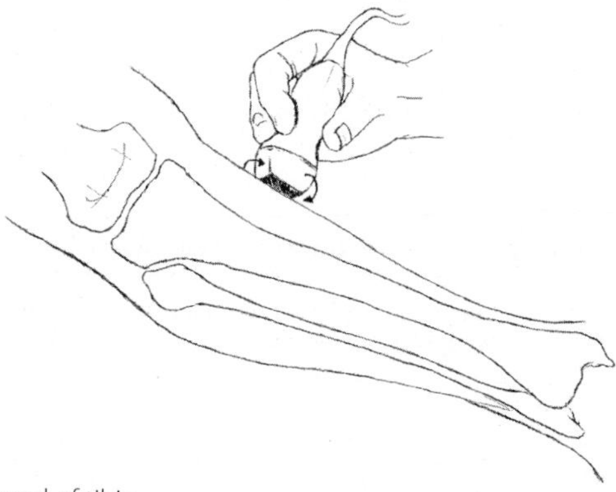

FIG. 19-10. Ultrasound of tibia.

discontinuity will be seen. Approaching the femoral neck, angle and rotate the transducer slightly and continue scanning to the midpoint of the inguinal ligament to visualize the femoral neck, head, and pelvic acetabulum. Near the shoulder, scan just distal to the acromial process of the scapula to visualize the humeral head.[21,24] If significant bleeding around the fracture has occurred, there may be an overlying hematoma that appears acutely as a hyperechoic area; the hematoma appears hypoechoic in the subacute stage.[20]

REFERENCES

1. Mock C, Lormand JD, Goosen J, et al. *Guidelines for Essential Trauma Care*. Geneva, Switzerland: World Health Organization; 2004:54.
2. Iserson KV, Timeb JM. X-ray view box: on-site manufacture. *Trop Doct*. 2011(July);41(3):144-145.
3. Gahhos F, Arons MS. Soft-tissue foreign body removal: management and presentation of a new technique. *J Trauma*. 1984;24(4):340-341.
4. Peterson B, Shapiro MB, Crandall M, et al. Trauma clip-art: early experience with an improved radio-opaque marker system for delineating the path of penetrating injuries. *J Trauma*. 2005;58(5):1078-1081.
5. Matsumoto S, Kishikawa M, Hayakawa K, et al. A method to detect occult pneumothorax with chest radiography. *Ann Emer Med*. 2011;57(4):378-381.
6. Henry M, Arnold T, Harvey J. BTS guidelines for the management of spontaneous pneumothorax. *Thorax*. 2003;58(suppl 2):ii39-ii52.
7. Baumann MH, Strange C, Heffner JE, et al. Management of spontaneous pneumothorax. In: American College of Chest Physicians' Delphi consensus statement. *Chest*. 2001;119:590-602.
8. Seear MD. *Manual of Tropical Pediatrics*. Cambridge, UK: Cambridge University Press; 2000:143.
9. Thompson SE, Raptopoulos V, Sheiman RL, et al. Abdominal helical CT: milk as a low-attenuation oral contrast agent. *Radiology*. 1999;211:870-875.
10. Koo CW, Shah-Patel LR, Jeanne W, et al. Cost-effectiveness and patient tolerance of low-attenuation oral contrast material: milk vs VoLumen. *AJR Am J Roentgenol*. 2008;190:1307-1313.
11. Knuth TE, Paxton JH, Myers D. Intraosseous injection of iodinated computed tomography contrast agent in an adult blunt trauma patient. *Ann Emerg Med*. 2011;57(4):382-386.
12. Balllinger JR. Positive versus negative GI contrast agents. www.mritutor.org/mritutor/ponocon.htm. Accessed June 1, 2007.
13. Anon. Crystallographic topology 101: introduction to critical nets. www.ornl.gov/sci/ortep/topology/diamond.gif. Accessed August 4, 2008.
14. Morton ER. *A Text-Book of Radiology*. New York, NY: EB Treat; 1915:129.
15. Samuel D. Stereoscopy. en.wikipedia.org/wiki/Stereoscopy. Accessed August 9, 2008.
16. Nelson BP, Melnick ER, Li J. Portable ultrasound for remote environments, part II: current indications. *J Emerg Med*. 2011;40(3):313-321.
17. McBeth PB, Crawford I, Blaivas M, et al. Simple, almost anywhere, with almost anyone: remote low-cost telementored resuscitative lung ultrasound. *J Trauma Acute Care Surg*. 2011;71(6):1528-1535.
18. Binkowski A, Riguzzi C, Price D, Fahimi J. Evaluation of a cornstarch-based ultrasound gel alternative for low-resource settings. *J Emerg Med*. 2014;47(1):e5-e9.
19. Krishnamurthy R, Yoo JH, Thapa M, Callahan MJ. Water-bath method for sonographic evaluation of superficial structures of the extremities in children. *Ped Rad*. 2013;43(1):41-47.
20. Wang CL, Shieh JY, Want TG, et al. Sonographic detection of occult fractures in the foot and ankle. *J Clin Ultrasound*. 1999;27(8):421-425.
21. Marshburn TH, Legome E, Sargsyan A, et al. Goal-directed ultrasound in the detection of long-bone fractures. *J Trauma*. 2004;57:329-332.
22. Hübner U, Schlicht W, Outzen S, Barthel M, Halsband H. Ultrasound in the diagnosis of fractures in children. *J Bone Joint Surg Brit*. 2000;82(8):1170-1173.
23. Tayal VS, Antoniazzi J, Pariyadath M, et al. Prospective use of ultrasound imaging to detect bony hand injuries in adults. *J Ultrasound Med*. 2007;26:1143-1148.
24. Dulchavsky S, Henry SE, Moed BR, et al. Advanced ultrasonic diagnosis of extremity trauma: the FASTER examination. *J Trauma*. 2002;53:28-32.

20 | Laboratory

LABORATORY SERVICES

Clinical laboratory tests have relatively less utility in resource-poor settings, but lives can be saved if a few simple tests are available, such as those for urine pregnancy and, in endemic/high-prevalence areas, for human immunodeficiency virus (HIV), malaria, and tuberculosis (TB) screening. This chapter discusses how to improvise various materials, equipment, and tests when clinicians need laboratory tests and the normal procedure for doing them is unavailable.

ESSENTIALS

Table 20-1 lists essential laboratory tests worldwide, which differ depending on the facility's capabilities (described in Table 5-1).

EQUIPMENT AND MATERIALS

Water

Use filtered rainwater rather than distilled water to make laboratory reagents, such as stains. Collect uncontaminated rainwater in rooftop tanks.[1] Distilled water is best for use in autoclaves and in pressure cookers used as sterilizers. If available, also use distilled water to produce intravenous (IV) fluids.

Distillation involves boiling clean water and collecting the steam, which then condenses back to water. The water from condensed vapor does not contain salt and other impurities. In austere situations, improvising distillation systems saves many lives, as is seen in the following story from a World War II prison camp[2]:

> Some six weeks before the outbreak [dysentary] I had constructed, as a precaution, a small plant for distilling water for intravenous saline. It was a very primitive affair, the condenser

TABLE 20-1 Laboratory Testing Essentials

Resources/Capabilities	Facility Level			
	Basic	GP	Specialist	Tertiary
HIV[a]	E	E	E	E
Urine pregnancy	E	E	E	E
Hemoglobin/hematocrit	D	E	E	E
Malaria[a]	D	E	E	E
Urinalysis	D	E	E	E
Glucose	I	E	E	E
Gram stain	I	D	E	E
Tuberculosis[a]	I	D	E	E
Sickle cell prep	I	D	E	E
Bacterial cultures	I	D	D	D
Electrolytes (Na, K, Cl, CO_2, BUN, creatinine)	I	D	D	D
Arterial blood gas measurements	I	D	D	D
Serum lactate	I	I	D	D

Abbreviations: BUN, blood urea nitrogen; D, desirable; E, essential; GP, general practitioners' hospital; HIV, human immunodeficiency virus; I, irrelevant.

[a]In endemic/high-prevalence areas.

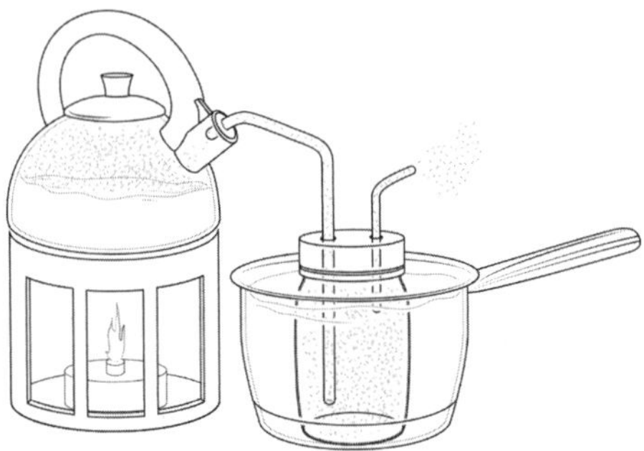

FIG. 20-1. Water distiller.

> being a coiled rubber tube inside a hollow bamboo in which cold water was circulated. The boiler was a 4-gallon kerosene can. Within 24 hours of the outbreak we were able to give intravenous saline. The plant was producing 40 pints daily, and eventually double that figure. The giving IV bottle was a jam-jar connected to a needle by a rubber tube.

Obtain small amounts of distilled water by heating water in a kettle and running rubber tubing from the spout through a hole in the lid of a collecting jar (Fig. 20-1). Use another small tube as a vent in the jar's lid. Seal all joints with adhesive tape, clay, or glue. Immerse the collecting jar in a pan of cool water so the steam will condense quickly.[3] Voilà, distilled water!

An alternative method of distilling small amounts of water is to fill a large pot one-half to three-quarters full of water. Invert the lid and suspend a heat-resistant cup from a cradle made from wires (coat hangers may be used) attached to the lid's handle. The cup should hang right-side up without dangling in the water when the lid is upside-down. This takes about 5 minutes to set up. As the water boils and steam collects on the lid, it drips down the handle into the cup.[4] If only a little water is used, watch the pot more closely (Fig. 20-2).

Power

In austere situations, the electrical supply is often intermittent, if available at all. Obtain suitable AC current for instruments from rechargeable batteries using a solar or DC/AC inverter.

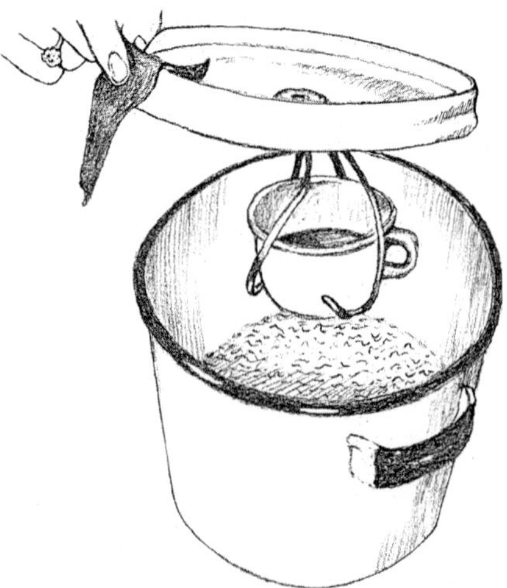

FIG. 20-2. Alternative water distillation method (for small amounts).

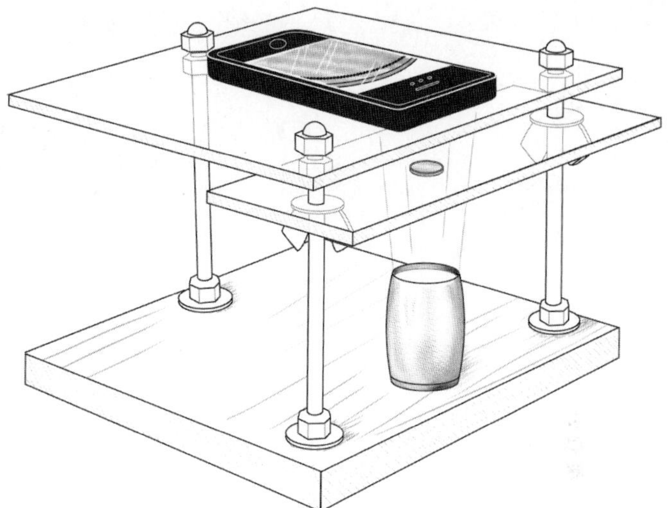

FIG. 20-3. Improvised microscope, using a smart phone stand with specimen stage below and a light source. *(Adapted from Yoshinok.[5])*

Microscope From a Smart Phone

For about $10 and with common tools in less than a half hour you can make a stand that will transform your smart phone into a powerful digital microscope with magnification levels as high as 175 to 375 power (Fig. 20-3). The materials required are 3 carriage bolts (4½ inches × 5/16 inches); 9 nuts (5/16 inches); 3 wing nuts (5/16 inches); 5 washers (5/16 inches); ¾ inches × 7 inches × 7 inches plywood for the base; ⅛ inches × 7 inches × 7 inches plexiglass for the camera stage; ⅛ inches × 3 inches × 7 inches plexiglass for the specimen stage; scrap plexiglass (~ 2 inches × 4 inches) for a specimen slide (optional but useful); a laser pointer focus lens (use two for increased magnification); and an LED click light (necessary only for viewing backlit specimens). The tools needed are: a drill, assorted bits, a ruler, and pliers. Video instructions, detailed photos of each step, and answers to some common questions can be found at: http://www.instructables.com/id/10-Smartphone-to-digital-microscope-conversion/?ALLSTEPS.

To use the microscope, place the phone (with camera or video activated) on the top piece of plexiglass. Put the specimen on a separate piece of plexiglass and slide it onto the viewing platform, just beneath where the camera sits. Bring the object into focus by turning the wing nuts on either side of the stage. Then observe the specimen and take a picture or video, if necessary. Zoom in using the camera's tools. Generally, this only requires laying your fingers on the image and spreading them apart. Use the focus lenses from one or two laser pointers for magnification, and use an inexpensive LED light to backlight specimens.

Microscope—Old Type

If using a standard microscope, when the electricity fails, use a mirror and sunlight or a battery-operated light as your light source.

Filters

If you need to filter solutions, including stains, use a flowerpot with a hole in the bottom. Loosely plug the hole with cotton, fill the pot with several inches of clean sand, and pour in the liquid. Collect the filtered solution in a jar placed under the pot (put it up on a stand). Replace the sand frequently.

Fire-Fighting Equipment

To put out small laboratory fires, keep buckets of sand available. Water may not be readily available (or appropriate for all laboratory fires), and fire extinguishers are expensive and need regular maintenance.

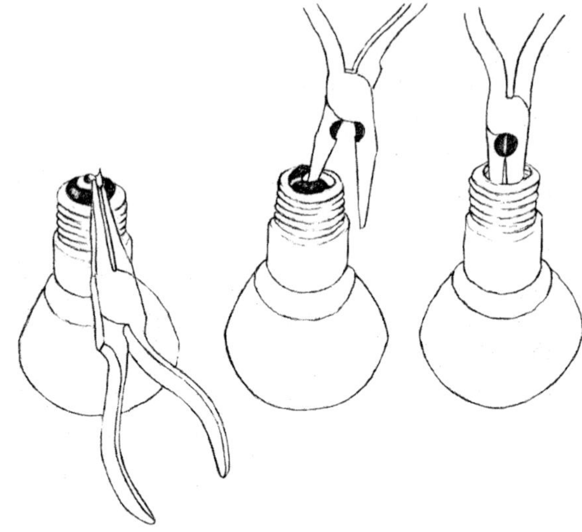

FIG. 20-4. Flask from a floodlight bulb. Remove button (left), remove porcelain base (center), and break inner filament holder (right).

Lab Burner

Speaking of fires, fashion a simple laboratory burner from an empty shoe polish container. Make a hole in the lid and fill the container with denatured or wood alcohol. If desired, solder a small piece of tin can to the lid to hold a cloth or cotton wick.

Refrigeration

If needed for samples and reagents, improvise refrigeration using the methods and equipment discussed in Chapter 5.

Flasks

Make laboratory flasks from "dead" light bulbs. Spotlight-type bulbs are the best, because they have flat "bottoms." If regular lightbulbs are used, an egg carton can serve as a holder. When modifying the bulbs, wear gloves and eye protection, and cover the bulb's glass with a cloth.

With either type of bulb, first use a pair of needle-nose pliers to pull off the little black button that holds the bulb's electrical contact (Fig. 20-4, left). Doing so leaves a hole in the bulb's porcelain base. Put one of the pliers' jaws into that hole, and gently work it around until the porcelain cracks (Fig. 20-4, center). Remove the pieces. The hole (with the filament) becomes visible.

After gently breaking off any protruding glass pieces in the hole, sharply tap the glass piece holding the filament (Fig. 20-4, right) to break it, and it will fall into the bulb. Turn the bulb over and dump the pieces out. A thin metal disc may remain in the bulb. Grab it with the pliers, bend it in two, and remove it. Then bend down any sharp edges on the metal (screw part) that remains on the bulb, rinse it out, and begin using it (Fig. 20-5).

This whole process takes about 5 minutes. Use a known amount of liquid to measure the flask's volume and mark it on the outside at convenient increments (e.g., 50 mL, 100 mL).

Test Tube Holder

To hold test tubes over a burner, fashion a test tube holder by bending a wire hanger or similar material (Fig. 20-6). Use pliers (rather than just your fingers) to do the bending.[6]

Scales

Tiny Scale

To measure small quantities or objects, build a scale using a jar lid and a heavy rubber band (Fig. 20-7). Insert a nail in an upright piece of wood. Make four holes that are equidistant around

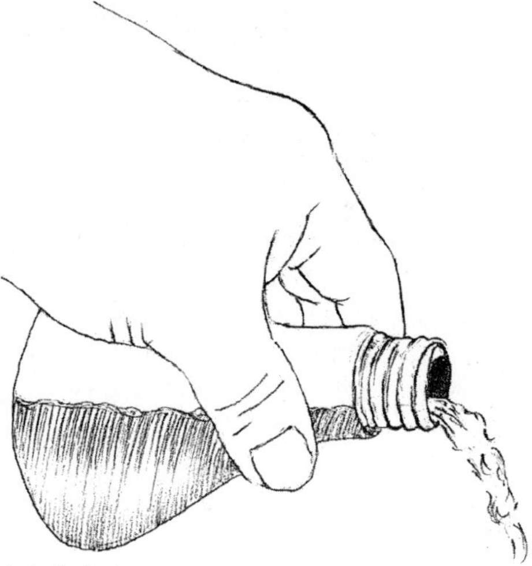

FIG. 20-5. Finished lightbulb flask.

the lid, attach a wire to each, and tie or twist all the ends together. (Sutures or fishing line may also be used in place of wire.) Use a paper clip (unwound to an "S" shape) to join the wires and the rubber band.[7] Now that the scale has been assembled, it must be calibrated. Attach a piece of tape that you can write on to the upright wood, and mark the gradations as you add small known weights. (Small quantities of water can also be used.) Once the scale is calibrated, either keep the original set of weights or find small stones (mark each stone with its weight) that can be used to recalibrate this scale. Change the rubber band and recalibrate the scale daily.

Heavy-Duty Scale

Used for heavier weights, this scale holds larger items and measures in kilograms. Attach a heavy spring from a chair or automobile cushion to a solid wooden base. Affix two upright posts on opposite sides (Fig. 20-8). These steady the structure and can be marked with incremental measurements when the scale is calibrated. Affix a metal pan to the top of the spring, either by soldering it to the spring or by passing wires through the pan onto the spring. Calibrate the scale by putting objects of known weights on it and marking the slat as the spring is depressed.[7] Known quantities of water (1 kg = 1 L = 2.2 lb) work well. Use the top of the pan as the point to mark.

"Steelyard" Scale

Several types of "steelyard" scales can easily be made. Make the long beam from either wood or metal; use pieces of metal pipe for the sliding counterweights. Fasten the beam and the pan together with wire. For support, place the entire balance on a stiff piece of wire that goes either through or around the beam (Fig. 20-9). As with the other scales, use known weights to calibrate this scale.[8]

Bubble Wrap as Laboratory Test Tubes and Petri Dishes

In resource-limited regions, the sterile gas-filled compartments in "bubble wrap" packing material can be used as an inexpensive alternative to glass test tubes and culture dishes; 1 square foot

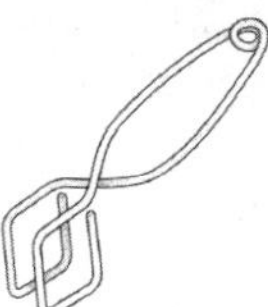

FIG. 20-6. Test tube holder.

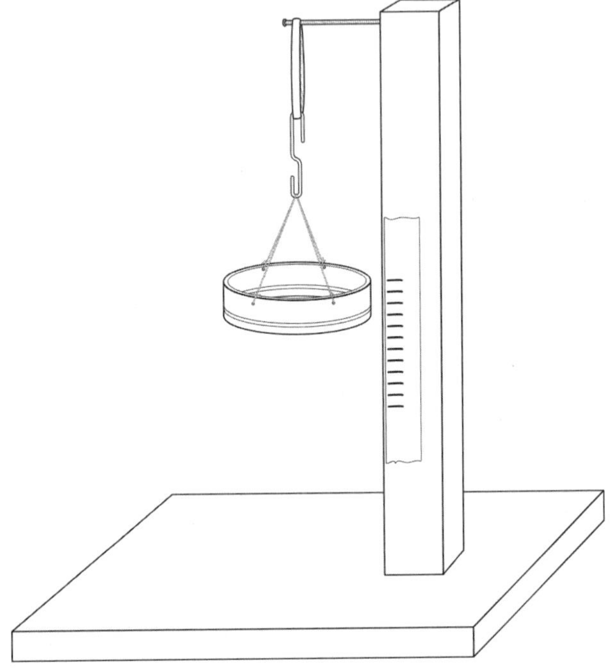

FIG. 20-7. Tiny scale.

contains from 100 to 500 bubbles and costs about 6 cents. The bubbles can be used to store reagents, perform bioanalysis, and culture and store microorganisms. Using a syringe with a needle or a pipette tip, inject the samples into the bubbles and seal the hole with fingernail hardener. Because they are transparent in the visible spectrum, also use the bubbles as "cuvettes" for absorbance and fluorescence measurements. Of note, the bubbles are also gas permeable and chemically inert to most aqueous samples.[9]

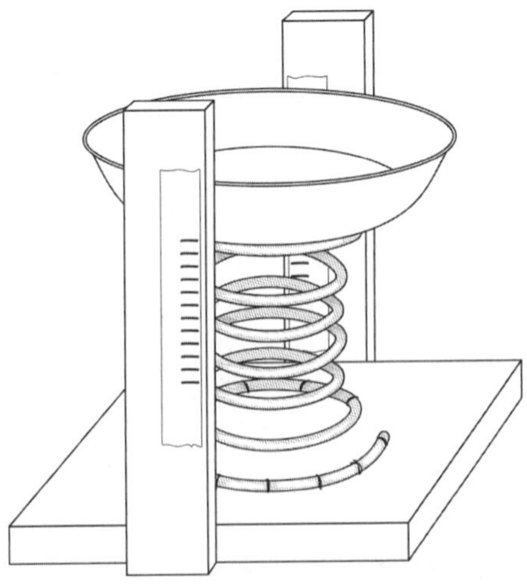

FIG. 20-8. Heavy-duty scale.

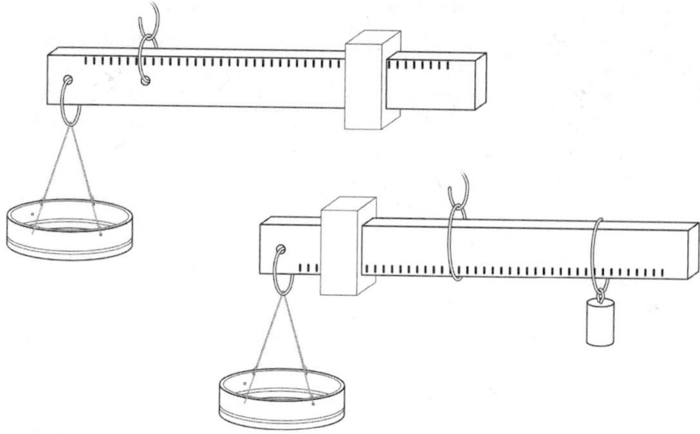

FIG. 20-9. "Steelyard" scales.

Incubator and Culture Media

Making media for bacteriology is a complex process; so, if you really need to grow cultures, buy the prepackaged powder.

To build an incubator, get a 20-gallon glass aquarium or any container having the same volume (Fig. 20-10). A cardboard box will do in a pinch, but it may not last long. Turn the container on its side with the open end facing front. Tape a piece of heavy plastic sheeting to the top, draping it down so that it covers the open end. The sheeting is the incubator's "door." A bacteriology incubator is normally kept at body temperature, 98.6°F (37°C). Tape a standard thermometer inside the container so that you can easily read it. Set a standard incandescent lamp enclosed in a can or small pail inside the incubator with the electrical cord going out the "door" to a plug. Begin with a 40-W bulb and assess the temperature after 12 to 24 hours. If it needs to be warmer, use a higher-wattage bulb. It will probably not be exactly 98.6°F, but if it is a little cooler, that will still work. To be more accurate, use a higher-watt bulb with a dimmer switch to modulate the emitted heat.[10]

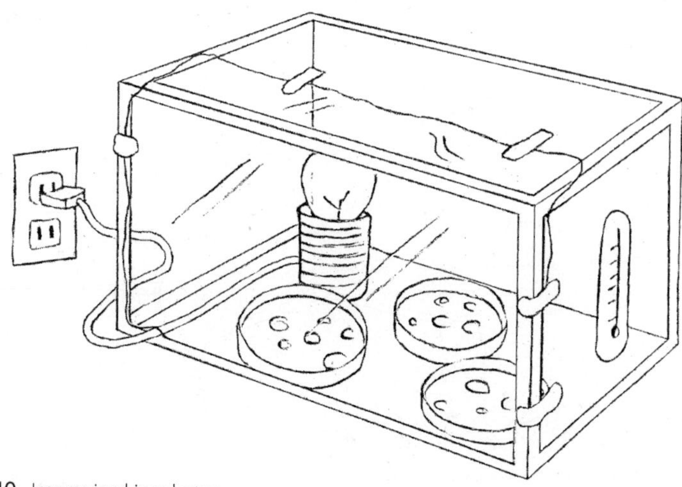

FIG. 20-10. Improvised incubator.

Centrifuge

Centrifuges separate liquid suspensions into their component parts, such as consolidating urine sediment or separating blood cells from serum. They are useful for laboratory work.

If possible, procure a real centrifuge. The difficultly with building a centrifuge is getting it balanced correctly. If it is not balanced, not only does it make a lot of noise, but it will also self-destruct. Although improvised machines often will not produce the rotational speeds needed for some tests, even the simplest centrifuge can cause significant damage if the tubes break or fly out of the machine while it is spinning. Given those caveats, relatively simple and workable centrifuges can be made, if necessary.

Hand-Drill Centrifuge

A hand-powered centrifuge can be built using a wooden spoon, a hand drill, plastic test tubes, small eye-screws (with 0.5-inch eyes), and cotter pins (Fig. 20-11). It is very rudimentary, but can be used to spin urine, small aliquots of blood, and similar specimens.[11]

1. Cut two 1-inch pieces off the end of the spoon handle. These are the "stoppers."
2. Check to be certain that the spoon's handle fits securely into the drill—where a bit would go. If it is too big, shave it down until it fits.
3. At this point, if you have an extra piece of wood with a wide base, drill a hole into it with a little larger diameter than the spoon handle. This can serve as a stand while completing the rest of the construction and also later when working with fluid-filled tubes.
4. Link the two pairs of eye-screws by opening one of each pair, inserting the other, and closing it again.
5. Drill tiny guide holes in the top of the stoppers and twist an eye-screw from each pair into that hole.
6. Drill little holes through the plastic test tubes, 0.5 inch from the top. They must be exactly opposite to each other at the widest part of the tube (180 degrees apart).
7. Insert the stoppers into the test tubes, and mark where the test tube holes meet the stopper.
8. Drill a small hole very carefully through each stopper from the mark on one side to the mark on the other side.
9. Put the stoppers into the test tubes and insert the locking pins. If they fit, remove them for the moment.

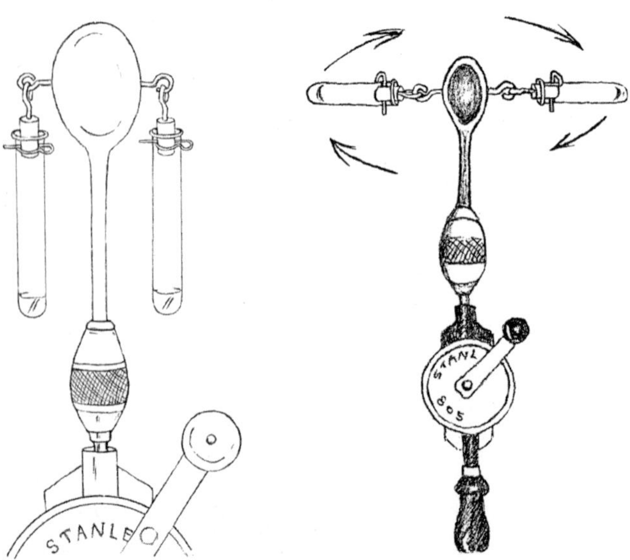

FIG. 20-11. Hand-drill centrifuge: close-up (left) and in operation (right).

10. Screw the other eye-screw from each pair into opposite sides of the widest part of the spoon.
11. Reinsert the stoppers into the tubes, insert the cotter pins through the holes, and bend one side of each cotter pin so that it forms a locking pin for the test tubes.
12. If a vice is available, use it to secure the drill handle. This makes the centrifuge much easier to use. If no vice is available, steady the drill base on a hard surface before operating your centrifuge.
13. Gently rotate the drill handle.
14. *Caution*: Significant centrifugal force is created. Wear goggles, and if the centrifuge can be operated inside a container (put it in a large cardboard box and make holes to stick your hands through), it would be best. Note that this is dangerous enough with a hand drill. *Do not use a power drill.*
15. If the system works, add water to the test tubes and try it again.
16. Still okay? Then add your test materials.
17. If you have slightly larger amounts of material, use two identical small plastic screw-top jars in place of the test tubes. Drill holes in their lids the same size as the test tube stoppers. When using jars, put the stoppers through these holes; the cotter pins go underneath the lids.

CONVERSION FACTORS

Table 20-2 contains a variety of conversion factors needed when working in different locales.

TABLE 20-2 Conversion Factors

Unit A	Symbol	Conversion Factor	Unit B	Symbol
1 unit A multiplied by the conversion factor = 1 unit B				
Celsius	°C	Multiply by 1.8, then add 32	Fahrenheit	°F
centimeter	cm	2.54	inch	in
		0.1	millimeter	mm
		30	foot	ft
centimeter square	cm^2	6.5	square inch	sq in
cubic foot water	cu ft H_2O	62.3	pound	lb
cubic meter	m^3	0.03	cubic foot	cu ft
cup	c	2	pint	pt
dram	dr	8	ounce	oz
Fahrenheit	°F	First subtract 32, then multiply by 0.555	Celsius	°C
foot	ft	0.33	centimeter	cm
		3.3	meter	m
gallon	gal	31.5	barrel	bb
gallon water (UK)	gal H_2O (UK)	10	pound	lb
gallon water (US)	gal H_2O (US)	8.33	pound	lb
grain	gr	480	ounce	oz
		5760	pound	lb
gram	g	28	ounce	oz
hectar	ha	0.4	acre	ac *or* A
inch	in	0.4	centimeter	cm

(Continued)

TABLE 20-2 Conversion Factors (*Continued*)

Unit A	Symbol	Conversion Factor	Unit B	Symbol
1 unit A multiplied by the conversion factor = 1 unit B				
inches cubic	in^3	277	gallon	gal
kilogram	kg	0.45	pound	lb
kilometer	km	1.6	mile	mi
kilometer square	km^2	2.6	square mile	sq mi
liter	L	0.24	cup	c
		3.8	gallon	gal
		0.95	quart	qt
meter	m	0.9	yard	yd
microliter	µL	10^6	liter	L
milliliter	mL	103	liter	L
		30	ounce (fluid)	fl oz
		15	tablespoon	Tbsp
		5	teaspoon	tsp
millimeter	mm	10	centimeter	cm
ounce	oz	12	pound	lb
peck	pk	4	bushel	bu
pint	pt	2	quart	qt
pound	lb	2.2	kilogram	kg
quart	qt	1.05	liter	L
		8	peck	pk
		4	gallon	gal
teaspoon	tsp	3	tablespoon	Tbsp
yard	yd	1.1	meter	m

SPUTUM

Diagnoses Without a Laboratory

If laboratory tests (or imaging) are not available, the evaluation of sputum volume, stratification, color, consistency, and odor can help make the diagnosis.

Volume

A person normally produces ≤20 mL of sputum daily. An increase in volume to ≥100 mL/24 hours occurs in pulmonary edema, bronchiectasis, chronic bronchitis, advanced pulmonary tuberculosis (TB), lung abscess, asthma, pulmonary gangrene, and extrapulmonary lesions (e.g., amoebic liver abscess bursting into the lung). Observing daily sputum volume is a good indicator of deterioration or improvement of lung conditions. Sudden cessation of sputum is highly suggestive of bronchial plugging.[12]

Stratification

Sputum from many patients with lung infections separates into three layers when left standing in a tall narrow container; the top layer is frothy, the middle is faintly turbid, and the bottom layer consists of tissue debris. Such layering occurs in bronchiectasis, lung abscess, and gangrene of the lung.[12]

Color and Consistency

Various disease processes and organisms will produce characteristic changes in the color and consistency of sputum.[12] This can assist clinicians in making a diagnosis.

Type (color, consistency) of Sputum	Diagnosis
Tenacious sputum	Asthma
"Rusty" sputum	Lobar pneumonia, mitral stenosis
Blood-streaked sputum	Early pulmonary TB
Mucopurulent or purulent sputum	Bronchopneumonia, bronchiectasis
Greenish sputum	*Bacillus pyocyaneus* infection
Black sputum	Anthracosis
Red frothy sputum	Hemoptysis with alkaline reaction to litmus
Nummular (coin-like) sputum	Fibrocaseous TB
Chocolate-colored sputum	Amoebic abscess

Odor

A putrid odor is associated with bronchiectasis and lung abscess.[12]

Tuberculosis Testing

The laboratory examination for TB should begin with an acid-fast stain (read by someone who is not colorblind). If that is negative, concentrate the sputum and stain the concentrate using the acid-fast method. Without sophisticated laboratories, that is the most that can be done.

Concentrating Sputum

Using concentrated sputum to test for TB greatly improves the sensitivity of staining for the organism. In austere situations, a centrifuge may not be available to perform the typical concentration technique used in laboratories. If an initial stain for TB is negative, use the following overnight sedimentation technique. This procedure increases the sensitivity of direct TB smears as much as standard centrifugation techniques.[13]

Collect three sputum samples. While these have traditionally been obtained on successive days, they are just as likely to contain the organism if collected at different times on the same day.[14] Put the sample in a flask and add twice that volume of a solution containing 3% ammonium sulfate and 1% sodium hydroxide. Shake the mixture by hand and let it stand overnight (≥12 hours) at room temperature. After sedimentation occurs, decant the supernatant fluids and make smears from the sediment. The sensitivity of the smears against the culture is 58% for the direct method and 81% for the concentration method.[15]

Using a similar method, add 5% sodium hypochlorite (bleach) to an equal quantity of the sputum, agitate by hand for 10 minutes, and then add four times the amount of distilled water and let stand overnight. As an example, add 1 mL 5% sodium hypochlorite to 1 mL sputum. After 10 minutes, add 8 mL distilled water and let it stand for ≥12 hours. This method is statistically equivalent to the classic concentration and centrifugation methods—and much cheaper and easier to do.[16]

BLOOD

Decreasing Hemolysis in Blood Samples

Using butterfly needles for phlebotomy rather than IV catheters is the most effective strategy to reduce the rate of hemolysis in blood samples.[17]

Hemoglobin Measurement

The World Health Organization–sponsored, commercially available colorimetric determination kits are accurate for estimating hemoglobin (Hgb) levels, particularly in neonates and young infants.[18] No special skills are necessary except for the ability to obtain a drop of blood. Normal color vision and color interpretation are also important.

The kits, containing 200 to 1000 test strips, include a small card with six shades of red representing Hgb levels of 4, 6, 8, 10, 12, and 14 g/dL. The results indicate whether the patient is anemic and can be used to decide whether the patient needs a blood transfusion, formal blood count, or referral. Results cannot be used to identify minor changes in Hgb during treatment.

To use the kit, place a drop of blood on the test strip (~2¢ US each). Wait for 30 seconds and immediately compare the strip to the hemoglobin color scale that accompanies each kit. The comparison must be made in bright light. Training nonprofessionals to use the kit takes about 30 minutes.[19] One benefit of this kit is that it also screens out sickle cell anemia, because these patients always have grave anemia; an Hgb level above 8 g/dL (Hct 24%) excludes the disease.[20]

Coagulation Tests

While more sophisticated coagulation tests will not be available in resource-poor settings, health care workers can easily do a bedside clotting time, which is vital to determine which patients need snake (Crotalid) antivenin after envenomations. Bleeding time tests, while easily done, are less useful.

Clotting Time

Put 1 to 2 mL of blood into a new, never-washed test tube and let it sit for 20 minutes. At 20 minutes, tip the tube upside down once. If no clot is seen, the test is positive (they are not clotting sufficiently). If *any* clot is present, even a very small one, the test is negative.[21] In some remote settings, the syringe in which a 5-mL blood sample was drawn is used in place of a test tube. It is laid on a desk or taped to the wall. In other cases, the blood is injected into an empty ceftriaxone bottle and set on a flat surface. The test time is when any clot forms. Failure to clot after 20 minutes is positive. Studies show that these three methods produce congruent results, and, when used with clinical findings, they can be used to guide therapy.[22]

Bleeding Time

Doing a bedside bleeding time may have some utility for (a) determining the cause for ongoing bleeding; (b) explaining previous bleeding episodes; and (c) diagnosing hereditary bleeding disorders, especially von Willebrand disease.[23] However, without standardization, the results must be interpreted cautiously.

To perform the test, seat the patient with his or her elbow slightly flexed and his or her forearm resting on a steady support with the volar surface exposed. Place a sphygmomanometer above the antecubital fossa and clean the forearm with alcohol, letting it air dry. Inflate the cuff to 40 mm Hg and wait for 30 seconds. Holding a sterile #11 scalpel blade at right angles to the skin, make two 1-mm deep punctures about 1.5 cm from each other, parallel to the antecubital crease, and about 5 cm distal to the antecubital fossa. Avoid cutting superficial veins. Begin timing immediately after making the incisions. Blot the incisions with filter paper every 30 seconds until blood no longer stains the filter paper. Do not blot the wound edges. The bleeding time is the average of the time it takes for each of the two cuts to stop bleeding. A normal value is <11 minutes.[24]

Rapid Malaria Diagnosis

The Giemsa stain is the gold standard for diagnosing malaria on blood smears. The classical staining procedure requires between 30 and 45 minutes. Reduce the time by making a 1:10 or 1:5 dilution of Giemsa from a standard solution (Merck, Darmstadt, Germany), stain the slide, and read it after 5 or 10 minutes. This method produces the same quality results as the standard method, with both thick and thin smears, and even with very low levels of parasitemia.[25]

TABLE 20-3 Urine Color and Associated Pathology

Color	Substance	Pathology
Yellow foam	Bilirubin	Obstruction of bile duct system or severe hepatocellular damage
Greenish foam	Biliverdin	Increased red cell destruction or liver pathology produces bilirubin oxidation product
Reddish	Hemoglobin, porphyrins	Renal or bladder bleeding, pernicious or hemolytic anemia, lead or barbiturate poisoning, congenital porphyria
Light red to red-brown	Hemoglobin	Renal or bladder bleeding, malaria, paroxysmal hemoglobinuria, transfusion reaction
Orange	Pyridium	Iatrogenic (urinary analgesic)
Smoky red to brown	Blood	Renal or bladder bleeding, acute nephritis, kidney infarction
Dark or smoky	Phenol	Phenol poisoning
Brown to black	Melanin	Leukemia, malignant melanoma, ochronosis, liver carcinoma
Blue	Methylene blue	Iatrogenic
Milky	Chyle	Filariasis

Data from Kothare.[12]

URINE

Color

Normal urine varies from yellow to amber, depending on its concentration. Edible dyes, including those in medications, and certain illnesses can change its color (Table 20-3).

Urinalysis

Urine is easily tested with multifunction sticks. These can test for the presence of protein, glucose, ketones, nitrites, bilirubin, urobilinogen, red blood cells (RBCs) or free Hgb, white blood cells (WBCs), leukocyte esterase, pH, and specific gravity, depending on the stick used. The strips must also not have deteriorated due to moisture or temperature.

Cloudy urine can be due to a variety of reasons. Usually, it is due to the presence of blood (generally pink or red), crystals, or infection. If signs and symptoms of infection are present, do the three-glass test to improve the chance of localizing the infection. During a single void, collect the first 5 mL in one container. Collect nearly all the rest of the urine in a second container. In the third container, collect the last 5 mL or so. If the first container is very cloudy, but the urine clears in the second and third containers, the infection is probably urethral. If the second and third containers are cloudier than the first, the infection probably resides in the bladder or kidney. If the third container is the cloudiest, the prostate is probably the culprit.

Rather than spinning urine, with or without a Gram stain, an easier method to determine the presence of infection in a good urine sample is to look for ≥1 bacterium/HPF (high-powered field). That correlates well with >100,000 organisms/mL if the same specimen is cultured.

Taste

Even the ancients knew that urine that tastes like sugar indicates diabetes mellitus. Go ahead—taste it. That's real austere medicine. (I prefer to use the test strips.) In Guyana in the 1960s, US physicians screened for diabetes by leaving patient's urine containers open. If they attracted flies, it signaled sugar in the urine. (Ronald Goodsite, MD, Tucson, Ariz. Personal communication, July 10, 2014.)

Protein

If a urine dipstick to measure protein is not available, another way to check for proteinuria is to fill a test tube three-quarters full with a clean-catch specimen and heat the top half of the tube over a low flame. Use metal tongs to hold the tube, and rotate the tube while heating it so that the glass does not shatter. If the urine turns cloudy and white, add a few drops of vinegar (2% acetic acid). If it stays cloudy or gets whiter, there is protein in the urine.[26] Protein can appear in the urine due to infection, bleeding, intrinsic renal disorders, or preeclampsia.

Using Whole Blood With Urine Pregnancy Strips

Most urine pregnancy test kits in the United States are approved for both urine and serum samples, but not for whole blood. However, it appears that whole blood works rather well on urine pregnancy strips, especially when you have no other option. One study looked at using whole blood to diagnose pregnancy using Urine Chorionic Gonadotropin (UCG) sticks. The results for whole blood pregnancy tests (425 patients) were: sensitivity, 95.8%; specificity, 100%; negative predictive value, 97.9%; and positive predictive value 100%. This suggests that all positive results are valid. However, if possible, confirm all tests with a urine qualitative test or a quantitative serum beta–HCG (human chorionic gonadotropin).

To use whole blood for this test, apply several drops of whole blood (instead of urine) into the pregnancy test cassette, and do not dilute the whole blood sample by adding water or saline. Wait at least 5 minutes for the blood to spread across the entire test strip.[27,28]

Gram Stain

Gram stains of urine specimens are done either on spun sediment or on bacteria from urine cultures. Gram-staining slides can provide a tentative identification of bacteria in urine, pus, sputum, cerebral spinal fluid (CSF), and bacterial cultures. Although not highly accurate for identifying species, a Gram stain enables the clinician to make an educated guess about the appropriate antibiotic to use if that information is combined with knowledge of the clinical situation. The test requires several chemical solutions to prepare the slide and a microscope to view the end product.

The basic "sure-fire" technique is to make a slightly uneven smear from the specimen. Unless you are in a hurry, air-dry rather than heat-fix the slide. Wear gloves to avoid staining your hands rather than using forceps to handle—and often drop—the slide. Once the slide is dry, cover the slide with ammonium oxalate crystal violet and wash off the back (not the front) of the slide using a thin stream of water. While smears of pus are relatively durable, urine sediment is fragile and, if washed directly, it will go down the drain. Then, do the same with Gram's iodine solution. The amount of time the stains are on the slide (3 seconds to 3 minutes) does not matter—but they must be identical. Then, hold the slide with one end slanting down, and drip on the acetone-alcohol until the color draining from the slide sharply decreases. Immediately wash the back of the slide. Pour on the safranin and immediately wash it off. Dry the back of the slide and, if in a hurry, dry the front by waving the back of the slide over a Bunsen burner, alcohol lamp, or similar heat source. With uneven smears, WBCs in the thin areas will have pink nuclei, but they will be bluish or purple in the thicker areas. Note that the organisms may vary in color. That is usually because, unlike laboratory specimens grown at the same time, "bugs" from real specimens are at different stages in their life cycle, and hence will have different colors.[29]

Draw conclusions with care—accuracy depends on training and skill. Gram-positive bacteria may appear gram-negative if they are old, if the patient has been treated with antibiotics, or if you washed the stain off the slide. Artifacts, such as particles of crystal violet, may be misinterpreted as cocci or bacilli. Some material from the smear may have disappeared during staining if you did not fix it properly or if you made the smear too thick.

STOOL

Parasite Examination

The presence of parasites in stools is common, especially in austere situations. Microscopic examination for a wide variety of intestinal parasites is easier and more successful using the following technique than with other common methods.[30] Even with this method, however, experts will identify only about 38% of the patients who have parasites. Get other samples if you think the patient has an intestinal parasite.

1. Collect the stool in a container.
2. Mix it with an applicator stick until uniform or homogeneous.
3. Use the same applicator to place a thick circular stool smear over an area 1- to 1.5-cm diameter on a glass slide.
4. If the stool is dry, hard, or well formed, add a few drops of sterile saline so that it has the consistency of paste.
5. Before the specimen dries, add one to two drops of lacto-phenol cotton blue (LPCB) stain. This is one of the most commonly available laboratory stains in the world.
6. Examine the slide for ≥5 minutes.

Presence of Mucus

A stool with fresh or altered blood and plenty of mucus is passed in amoebic dysentery. It often has an acidic reaction to litmus paper. Fresh, watery stools with mucus flakes, an alkaline reaction to litmus paper, and an offensive odor accompany bacillary dysentery. "Rice water" and "pea-soup" stools are passed with cholera and typhoid, respectively. Increased mucus or mucus in tape-like form is often passed in mucous colitis. Large frothy stools are associated with pancreatic dysfunction, celiac disease, and tropical sprue.[12]

CEREBROSPINAL FLUID

A devastating and common disease, bacterial meningitis may be difficult to distinguish from viral meningitis and normal patients—especially with clear or bloody CSF. In austere situations, this differentiation is vital, both to conserve resources (antibiotics, hospital beds, personnel time) and to properly treat those patients who actually have bacterial meningitis.

Bacterial Meningitis Diagnosis

Urine test strips can help distinguish patients with bacterial meningitis from those with viral meningitis, or no meningitis, despite the CSF being clear or bloody. That is, they help make the decision to treat patients who might otherwise go untreated even though they have the disease.

Rapidly differentiate between bacterial and viral meningitis using three components of typical urine test strips, with a specificity of 100% and sensitivity of 97%. This test helps in making a rapid decision about whether to use antibiotics in patients with suspected meningitis. If adequate CSF is available, the reagent strip is dipped directly into a tube that will not be used for microbiologic tests. Otherwise, one to two drops of CSF are placed on the glucose, protein, and leucocytes portions of the strip. Wash off the strips after 60 seconds, and compare the color change against the standard on the test strip container. The presence of leukocytes is graded as negative, 10 to 25, 75, or 500/μL; protein as 30, 100, or 500 g/L; and glucose as <2.8, 2.8, or 5.5 mmol/L.

A diagnosis of viral meningitis is made if the glucose is from 2.8 to 5.5 mmol/L, protein is present, and the leukocyte count is from 10 to 75/μL. Patients with values lower than this do not have meningitis; those with higher values have bacterial meningitis.[31] This test, however, will not detect all patients with bacterial meningitis.[32] A positive urine nitrite strip test may also help to indicate which patients with turbid, bloody or, most importantly, clear CSF have bacterial meningitis. The test is negative in patients with CSF malaria.[33]

Protein Evaluation

Without urine test strips, the Pandy test is an alternative method of testing for CSF protein. Prepare Pandy solution by filling a bottle (~100 mL) one-quarter full with phenol and the other three-quarters with clean water. Shake the bottle and let it stand for 24 hours. The two fluids will partially separate, with phenol being at the bottom of the bottle and a phenol-water (Pandy) solution being at the top. Carefully decant a few drops of the top mixture (avoid including phenol from the bottom layer) into a test tube, and add a few drops of the CSF. If the mixture in the tube is cloudy against a dark background, it is positive for excess protein. It becomes positive with

25 to 35 mg/dL protein. While a weak positive may sometimes occur in young children (who may have up to 40 mg/dL protein), a strongly positive test is always abnormal.

Cerebral Spinal Fluid Turbidity

CSF turbidity, if present, is one way to identify patients with bacterial meningitis. Although this test may often be falsely negative, checking for CSF turbidity may be the only method of diagnosing meningitis. To have the best chance of identifying turbidity, use clean water to fill an identical tube to the tube with the CSF sample. Compare the two in good light, or at least with a strong light behind them. If the CSF is as clear as the water, there are probably <100 WBC/μL.[26] Note that when looking only for CSF turbidity, one misses a significant number of bacterial meningitis cases.

POINT-OF-CARE AND HOME TESTS

Home pregnancy tests and home blood glucose tests have become ubiquitous and are generally adequate for clinical use. They are often much less expensive than similar tests sold for professional use. The only caveat is that heat and humidity can make them inaccurate.[34]

RESTORING EQUIPMENT'S OPERATING TEMPERATURE

In austere environments, the limited temperature range in which point-of-care laboratory instruments function often cannot be constantly maintained. For example, the commonly used i-STAT1 Analyzer (Abbott Point of Care Inc., Abbott Park, IL) requires a working temperature from 61°F to 86°F (16°C to 30°C); cool it using either evaporation in a low-humidity situation or a cold pack in high humidity. For evaporative cooling, wrap the machine in a thin damp cloth. Likewise, set the machine on top of a chemical cold pack. Both methods should drop the temperature sufficiently in about 5 minutes. Repeat the process as necessary. Presumably, this would also work using warm packs in cold environments.

REFERENCES

1. Carter J, Materu S, Lema O. Basic laboratory services. In: Seear MD, ed. *Manual of Tropical Pediatrics*. Cambridge, UK: Cambridge University Press; 2000:423-446.
2. Pavillard SS. Medical experiences in Siam (Thailand). *COFEPOW*. www.cofepow.org.uk/pages/medical_experiences.htm. Accessed July 1, 2015.
3. *UNESCO Source Book for Science Teaching*. Paris, France: United Nations Educational, Scientific and Cultural Organization; 1956:35.
4. American Red Cross. *Food and Water in an Emergency*. ARC, 1997. (Redistributed by FEMA.)
5. Yoshinok. *$10 Smartphone to digital microscope conversion!* http://www.instructables.com/id/10-Smartphone-to-digital-microscope-conversion/?ALLSTEPS. Accessed July 23, 2014.
6. *UNESCO Source Book for Science Teaching*, 1956:37.
7. *UNESCO Source Book for Science Teaching*, 1956:31.
8. *UNESCO Source Book for Science Teaching*, 1956:32.
9. Bwambok DK, Christodouleas DC, Morin SA, et al. Adaptive use of bubble wrap for storing liquid samples and performing analytical assays. *Anal Chem*. August 2014;86(15):7478-7485.
10. Iovine J. Genetically altering *Escherichia coli*. *Scientific Amer*. 1994;270(6):108-111.
11. Arbur R. *A micro-centrifuge, cheap & easy*. http://www.microscopy-uk.org.uk/mag/artjul00/centrif.html. Accessed July 1, 2015.
12. Kothare SN. Clinical pathology without microscopy. *Trop Doct*. 1978;8(4):207-209.
13. Vasanthakumar R. Concentration sputum smear microscopy: a simple approach to better case detection in pulmonary tuberculosis. *Ind J Tub*. 1988;35:80-83.
14. Brown M, Varia H, Bassett P, et al. Prospective study of sputum induction, gastric washing, and bronchoalveolar lavage for the diagnosis of pulmonary tuberculosis in patients who are unable to expectorate. *Clin Infect Dis*. 2007;44(11):1415-1420.
15. Garay JE. Analysis of a simplified concentration sputum smear technique for pulmonary tuberculosis diagnosis in rural hospitals. *Trop Doct*. 2000;30:70-72.
16. Rasheed MU, Dechu T. An overnight sedimentation method: improving the diagnosis of tuberculosis when electrical centrifuge is not available. *Trop Doct*. 2008;38(2):78-79.

17. Wollowitz A, Bijur PE, Esses D, Gallagher EJ. Use of butterfly needles to draw blood is independently associated with marked reduction in hemolysis compared to intravenous catheter. *Acad Emerg Med.* 2013;20(11):1151-1155.
18. Van Rheenen PF, de Moor LTT. Diagnostic accuracy of the haemoglobin colour scale in neonates and young infants in resource-poor countries. *Trop Doct.* 2007;37:158-161.
19. Gosling R, Walraven G, Manneh F, et al. Training health workers to assess anaemia with the WHO haemoglobin colour scale. *Trop Med Int Health.* 2000;5(3):214-221.
20. Husum H, Ang SC, Fosse E. *War Surgery: Field Manual.* Penang, Malaysia: Third World Network; 1995:283.
21. Ghana Health Services. *Standard Treatment Guidelines—Ghana.* Accra, Ghana: GHS; 2010.
22. Punguyire D, Iserson KV, Stolz U, Apanga S. Bedside whole-blood clotting times: validity after snakebites. *J Emerg Med.* 2014;44(3):663-667.
23. Lind SE. The bleeding time does not predict surgical bleeding. *Blood.* 1991;77:2547-2552.
24. Mielke CH Jr., Kaneshiro MM, Maher IA, et al. The standardized normal Ivy bleeding time and its prolongation by aspirin. *Blood.* 1969;34:204-215.
25. Jager MM, Murk JL, Piqué RD, Hekker TAM, Vandenbroucke-Grauls CM. Five-minute Giemsa stain for rapid detection of malaria parasites in blood smears. *Trop Doct.* 2011;41(1):33-35.
26. Klein S, Miller S, Thomson F. *A Book for Midwives—Care for Pregnancy, Birth, and Women's Health.* Berkeley, CA: Hesperian Foundation; 2005:127.
27. Fromm C, Likourezos A, Haines L, et al. Substituting whole blood for urine in a bedside pregnancy test. *J Emerg Med.* September 2012;43(3):478-82.
28. Habbousche JP, Walker G. Novel use of a urine pregnancy test using whole blood. *Am J Emerg Med.* September 2011;29(7):840.e3-e4.
29. Lindsey D. *Simple Surgical Emergencies.* New York, NY: Arco Medical; 1983:199-201.
30. Parija SC, Bhattacharya S, Padhan P. Thick stool smear wet mount examination: a new approach in stool microscopy. *Trop Doct.* 2003;33(3):173.
31. Moosa AA, Quortorn HA, Ibrahim MD. Rapid diagnosis of bacterial meningitis with reagent strips. *Lancet.* 1995;1345:1290-1291.
32. Molyneux E, Walsh A. Caution in the use of reagent strips to diagnose acute bacterial meningitis. *Lancet.* 1996;348:1170-1171.
33. Maclennan C, Molyneux E, Green DA. Rapid diagnosis of bacterial meningitis using nitrite patch testing. *Trop Doct.* 2004;34(4):231-232.
34. US Food and Drug Administration, Center for Devices and Radiological Health. FDA offers tips about medical devices and hurricane disasters. www.fda.gov/MedicalDevices/Safety/EmergencySituations/ucm055987.htm. Accessed September 15, 2015.

21 | Patient Transport/Evacuations

MEDICAL TRANSPORT IN AUSTERE CIRCUMSTANCES

In austere circumstances, a functioning emergency medical system (EMS) may not exist or an existing system may not function as it should. In these circumstances, you may not be able to reach patients or they may not be able to get to you using normal methods, such as if the roads are impassible. This chapter discusses improvised methods to transport patients or medical personnel.

TRANSPORT THE PATIENT?

The first question is always whether to transport the patient. In resource-poor settings, this decision is a delicate balance between patient benefit and the appropriate use of available resources. It comes down to two vital questions: *Can* we transfer and *should* we transfer? The detailed parts of each question are listed in Table 21-1. All the parts must be answered "Yes" for a transfer to take place.

PREHOSPITAL FLUID THERAPY

Optimally, prehospital resuscitation should be goal directed, based on the presence or absence of prehospital hypotension. In severely injured blunt trauma patients without hypotension, a prehospital crystalloid volume >500 mL is associated with an increased risk of mortality and coagulopathy.[1] Obtaining prehospital intravenous (IV) lines are associated with longer EMS on-scene and prehospital times; the patients with prehospital IVs do not receive blood products any faster than those without them.[2]

IVs During Transport

If the patient has an IV line in place, keep it flowing during transport: Either put a pressure cuff (or a blood pressure (BP) cuff or an elastic bandage) around the bag or place the bag under the

TABLE 21-1 Elements of Patient Transfer Decisions

Can We Transfer?	
Yes	**No**
Higher level of care (facility/equipment/skills) reasonably available (time/distance)	No higher level of care reasonably available
Referral facility accepts transfer	Referral facility refuses transfer
Transfer method available	Transfer method unavailable
Transfer safe for personnel	Unacceptable danger to personnel
Should We Transfer?	
Yes	**No**
Patient benefit probable	Patient benefit uncertain
Patient will probably survive transfer	Patient will probably die during transfer
Resources used for transfer not needed immediately by other patients and can be replaced before other patients need them	Other current patients need the resources to be used for transfer, or resources can't be replaced before needed by other patients
Patient/surrogate wants/accepts need for transfer	Patient/surrogate does not want/accept need for transfer

patient to maintain pressure and flow. The danger of this practice is not paying attention to the now-hidden IV bag, which can result in letting the bag run dry, thus ruining the IV access port.

If the patient has an IV line but does not currently need fluids—or needs them only intermittently—use a saline lock and put the IV fluids through it in boluses, as necessary. That also works for works for stopping the fluids and later restarting them without having to restart an IV line. Improvised saline (or heparin) locks are described in Chapter 5.

TRANSPORTING PATIENTS WITHOUT LITTERS

If a litter is not readily available or cannot be improvised, rescuers can choose from a variety of methods to transport patients, including carrying or dragging the patient. Evacuation from a multistory hospital or other building is discussed below in this chapter.

One-Person Drags

Patients can be dragged head or feet first for short distances to remove them from a dangerous, time-critical situation or when they are in a confined space and no other method is practicable. If the time and circumstances allow, wrapping the patient in a sheet, blanket, or similar cloth makes it easier to drag them. This also provides more protection from any debris over which the patient may be dragged.

One-person drags are particularly useful when it is necessary to go under low obstructions. The downside is that there is no way to support the victim's head. Place the patient in a supine position. Cross the patient's wrists and tie them together with any available material (e.g., belt, rope, hose, or scarf), then kneel over the patient and lift the tied wrists over your head so they rest on the back of your neck (Fig. 21-1). When crawling forward, raise your neck just high enough so that the patient's head does not bump against the ground.

One-Person Carries

Most people can carry a person in their arms for a short distance, as long as they are relatively small and lightweight compared to the rescuer.

Larger patients can be transported more easily across the rescuer's back (Fig. 21-2). If the person is standing or can be lifted into a standing position, the rescuer drapes the patient's arms over his shoulders and holds the wrists with one hand (pack-strap carry). Once upright, the rescuer should lean slightly forward so the patient's feet are just off the ground and then begin to move.

To get an adult on your back takes extra effort if a patient is supine and no one is available to help the patient stand. With the patient supine, lie on your side alongside the uninjured or less-injured side. Position your shoulder next to the patient's armpit, and pull his far leg over your own, holding it there if necessary. Grasp the patient's far arm at the wrist and bring it over your upper shoulder as you roll and pull the patient onto your back. Get up to your knees, using your free arm for balance and support. Hold both the patient's wrists close against your chest with your

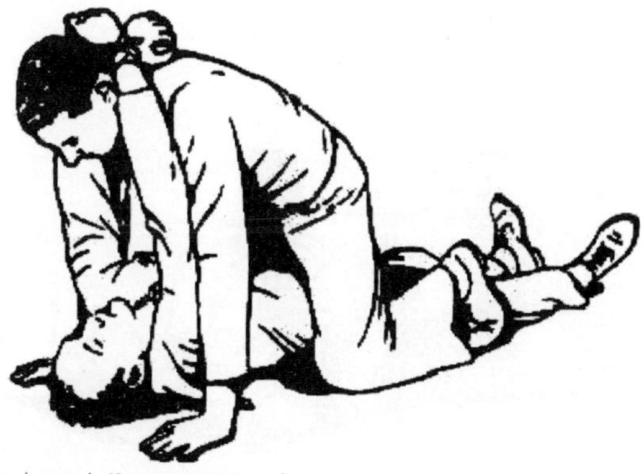

FIG. 21-1. Tied-hand crawl. *(Source: US Navy.[3])*

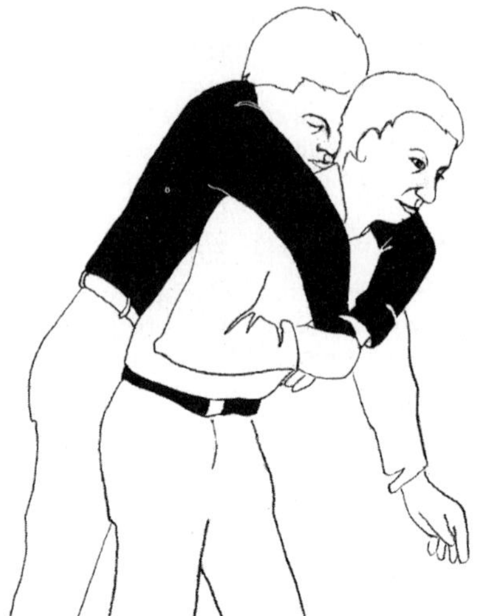

FIG. 21-2. Pack-strap carry. *(Adapted from Community Emergency Response Team.[4])*

other hand. Lean forward as you rise to your feet, and keep both of your shoulders under the patient's armpits.[3] If this carry is to be used for more than a short distance, tie the patient's wrists together with any available material to secure a better handhold on the arms.

Two-Person Carries

It is much easier for two people to carry a patient, especially for long distances.

The most basic two-person carry has both rescuers squatting on the same side of the patient, with one at chest level and the other at the thighs. The person at the chest passes both arms under the patient while the other rescuer puts one arm under the knees and his other arm over the pelvis, gripping his partner's wrist. They then pull the patient toward their own chests and move forward (Fig. 21-3).

Another method that can be used for longer distances starts with rescuer A squatting at the victim's head. Then rescuer B lifts the patient to a sitting position by pulling on the patient's arms, if necessary. Rescuer A grasps the patient from behind around the midsection, holding his own wrist with the other hand for security. Rescuer B then squats between the patient's legs and grasps the knees. This rescuer can face toward or away from the patient (Fig. 21-4); for longer distances, the rescuers should face in the same direction and walk forward. Both rescuers then stand while holding the patient. This carry, as well as some of the others, can be used for bedbound patients by first moving them to a sitting position in the bed and then having the two rescuers sit on either side of the patient to begin their lift.[5]

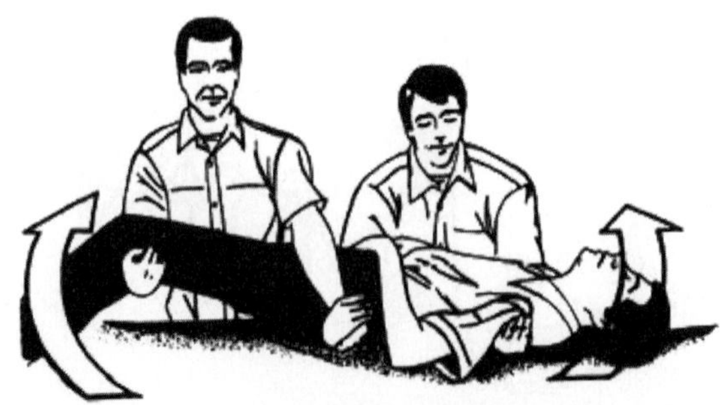

FIG. 21-3. Two-person carry, side view. *(Adapted from US Navy.[3])*

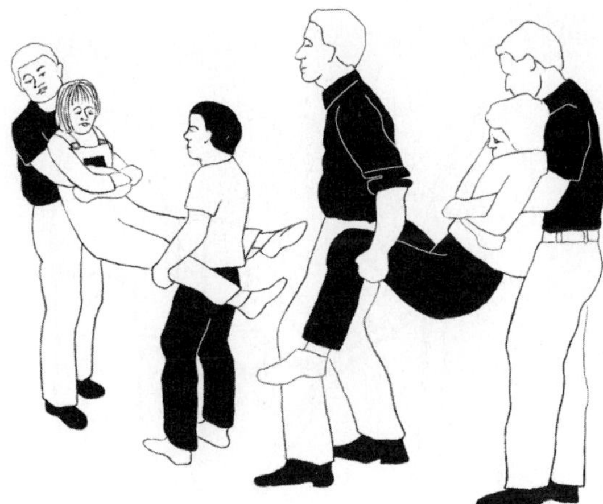

FIG. 21-4. Two-person carry, anterior-posterior view. *(Adapted from Community Emergency Response Team.[4])*

The two-person chair carry is more useful over longer distances. The two rescuers squat on either side of the patient and slide their arms under the patient's back and thighs. Although Fig. 21-5 shows the two rescuers holding onto the patient's side, it is more secure if they hold onto each other's arms in the back and grab each other's wrists under the thighs. They then stand and begin walking forward.

Chair Carry

Two rescuers can also sit a patient in a chair, with one grasping the back of the chair and the other the bottom of the chair's front legs. Starting from a squatting position, they tilt the chair backward and stand, both facing in the same direction (Fig. 21-6). The rear person (the more strenuous position) must also support the patient's head and shoulders. A key to success is finding a sturdy chair that is not too heavy.

LITTERS

Litters can be used either as the only means of transporting patients or to get them to another form of transportation. They often are used as the patient's "bed" while in transit. When no litter

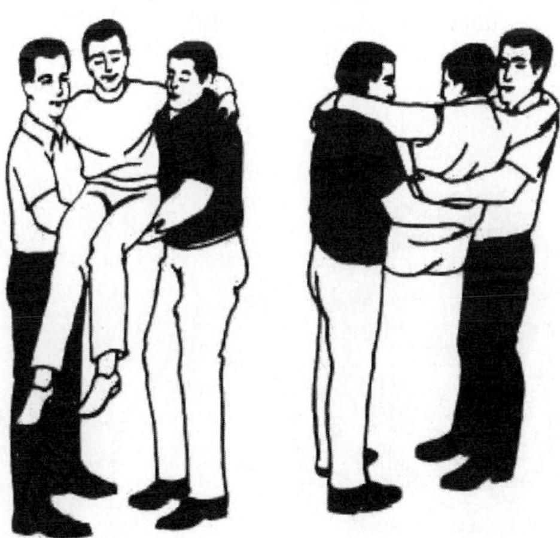

FIG. 21-5. Two-person chair carry. *(Source: US Navy.[3])*

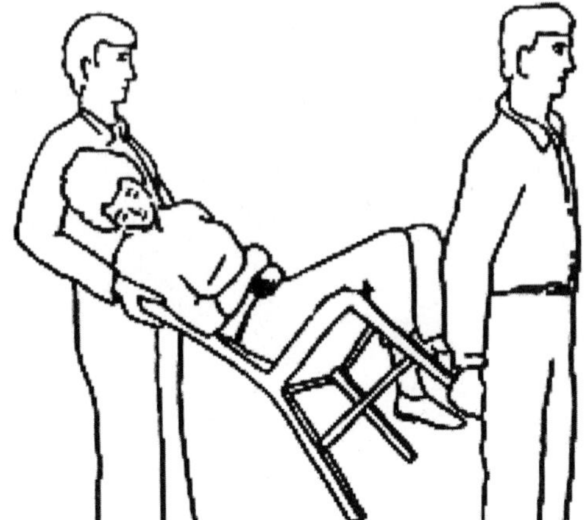

FIG. 21-6. Carry using chair. *(Adapted from Community Emergency Response Team.[4])*

is available, improvise one from available materials. This is an emergency measure; always use standard litters when available.

When using any type of litter, designate a team leader to keep those carrying the litter synchronized. Once the team is squatting in position and holding the litter, it is customary for the leader to announce, "Ready to lift on the count of three: One, two, three, lift." Once they are standing, the leader should say, "Ready to move on the count of three: One, two, three, move." The team begins moving. The leader gives the same directions for "Ready to stop" and "Ready to lower."

Be kind to the patient if using a rigid litter—pad it. Use any available soft material, such as clothing or sleeping bags. For a head or neck rest (assuming the person does not need to be in a cervical collar), use a roll of toilet paper. Stand on it to squash it. It is the right size and softness for a head/neck support. If it is too thick, unroll some of it.[6]

Improvised Litters

Litter Without Poles

If material for poles is not available, roll a blanket, sheet, poncho, cloth sack, or similar item from both sides toward the center so that the rolls can be gripped for carrying a patient. Bunch up a blanket lengthwise next to the patient. Push one side under the patient; the patient may need to be "log rolled" to get the blanket underneath. Roll the edges as close as possible to the patient. All rescuers should squat facing the patient, three on each side. They each grasp a rolled-up portion of the blanket, and the team leader instructs the team to lift in unison (Fig. 21-7). They stand and begin walking.

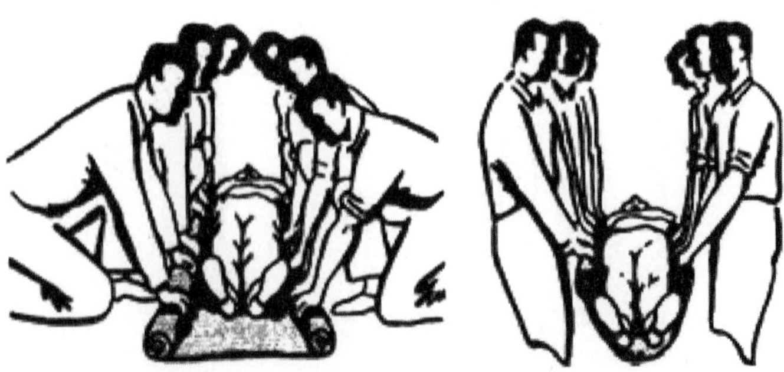

FIG. 21-7. Blanket/sheet litter. *(Source: US Navy.[3])*

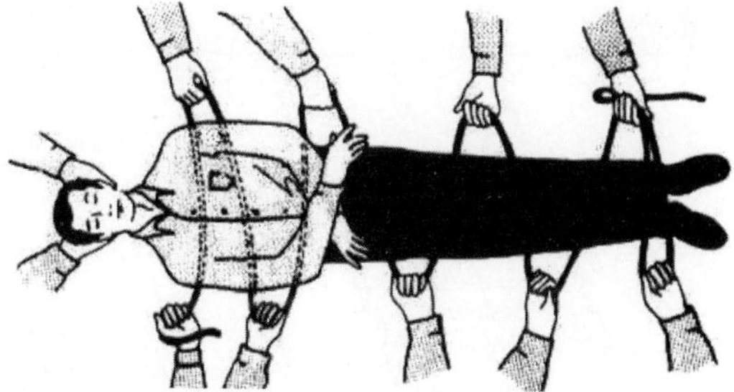

FIG. 21-8. Rope litter. *(Source: US Navy.[3])*

Rescuers should pull out sideways on the blanket as they lift; this avoids straining their backs and prevents the blanket from sagging too much in the middle. This type of litter is useful for carrying a patient only for limited periods, because it is much more tiring than using one with poles. At least six people are needed to safely move an adult patient.

Rope Litter

Make a rope litter by passing a strong rope back and forth beneath the patient, with the loops extending past the patient's body. Rescuers on each side use these loops and each end of the rope as handholds to carry the patient (Fig. 21-8). Another rescuer supports the patient's head. These litters are useful only over relatively short distances.

Flat-Surfaced Objects

Most flat objects that are not too heavy can be used as a litter. These include doors, slabs of wood or light metal, benches, ladders, and cots. This type of rigid stretcher is excellent for patients with suspected spinal injuries. An ingenious litter can be fashioned from two chairs by tying or wiring them together with one back overlapping the other.[7] The two back legs serve as handles (Fig. 21-9). Some backpack frames can be linked together in a similar manner to form a stretcher.

Blanket and Poles

To improvise a stretcher using a blanket and two poles, lay one pole lengthwise across the middle of the blanket. Then, fold the blanket over the pole. Place the second pole across the middle of the folded blanket. Fold the free edges of the blanket over the second pole so the edge is almost at the first pole. The patient's weight on the litter will keep the blanket from unfolding when carried (Fig. 21-10). Poles can be fashioned from strong tree branches, tent poles, skis, pipes, and so forth.

Shirt/Jacket Litter

Use two long-sleeved shirts or jackets. Button the shirts or jackets and turn them inside out, leaving the sleeves inside. Pass the poles through the sleeves. Two to four shirts or jackets will often be needed to make an adequate litter (Fig. 21-11).

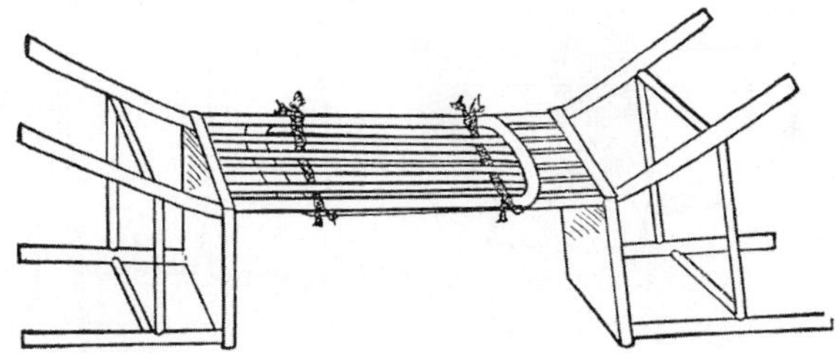

FIG. 21-9. Two-chair litter. *(Reproduced from Olson.[7])*

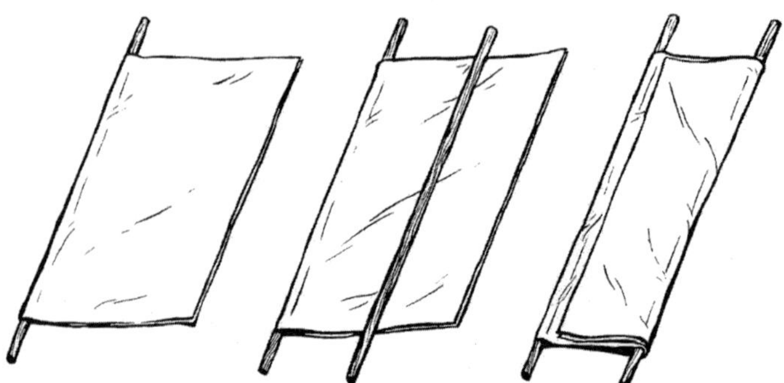

FIG. 21-10. Blanket litter. *(Source: US Army.[8])*

Sleeping Bag/Cloth Sack Litter

A sleeping bag may also be used as a litter. Zip it up completely and make a small hole at each of the two corners away from the opening. Put carrying poles through the bag's wide opening and then through the new holes. The patient lies on top of the sleeping bag. Gunny sacks, grain bags, or similar containers made of cloth may also be used in this manner, although two or more will be needed, depending on the height of the patient.

Standard Litters Not Used in Hospitals

Military Collapsible Litter

The US military's standard collapsible litter (Fig. 21-12) will probably be available in large-scale emergencies when organizations, including hospitals, begin using their disaster resources. The collapsible litter is commonly used in conjunction with military transport vehicles, including fixed-wing aircraft. It folds lengthwise and has a cotton cover to hold the patient. There are four wooden handles for carrying it and four metal stirrups (one bolted near the end of each pole) to support the litter when it is placed on the ground. Two spreader bars (one near each end of the litter) are extended crosswise at the stirrups to hold the cover taut when the litter is open. Two straps secure the litter when it is closed. Most also have straps to secure the patient.

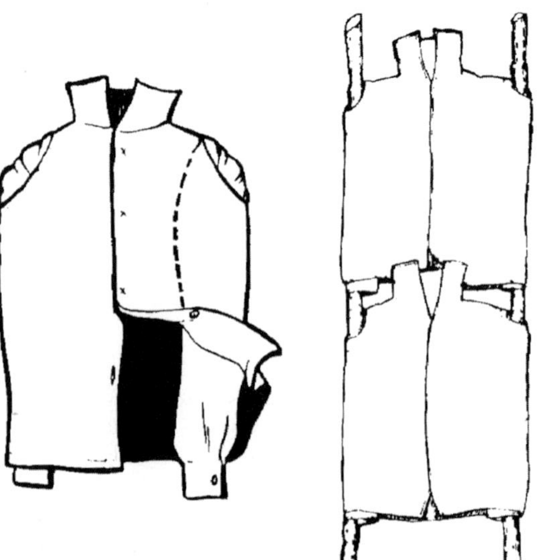

FIG. 21-11. Shirt/jacket litter. *(Source: US Army.[9])*

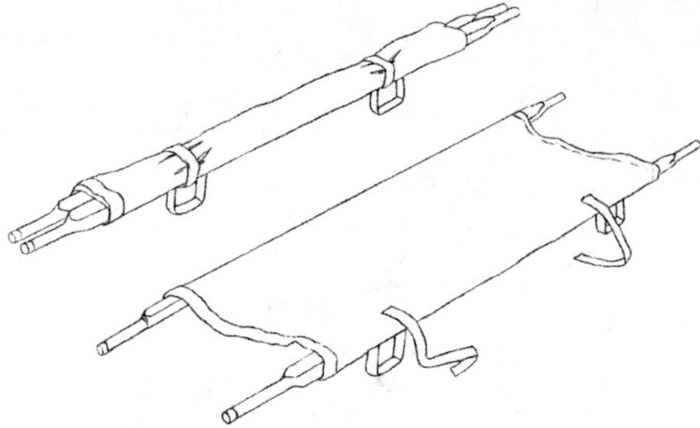

FIG. 21-12. Standard litter, closed and open. *(Source: US Army.[10])*

The litter weighs 15 pounds and is 90 inches long by 22.88 inches wide. The patient area is 72 inches long and 22.88 inches wide.

Stokes Litter

The Stokes litter provides maximum security for the patient when the litter is tilted, such as during ground-to-helicopter, ship-to-ship, or vertical-ground transfers. Its steel or aluminum tubular frame supports wire mesh netting on which the patient lies—first pad the basket with blankets or other material. If it doesn't come with patient straps, they can be improvised using webbing or rope secured to the end of one side rail and passed back and forth over the patient—first toward the head and then back toward the feet, forming a crisscross pattern. It may also have carabineers and cables for attaching to helicopter long lines or ship-to-ship transfer cables. Some baskets are fitted with handles so they can also be used as a litter. A search and rescue improvisation is to attach a large wheel to the underside to assist in moving the patient long distances. The standard basket is 84 inches long, 23 inches wide, and, without attachments, weighs 3.5 pounds.

Specialized Litters

Litter With Skis

Many types of litters can be fitted with skis. The formal type is known as an Ahkio. This Alaskan sled is particularly useful when evacuating patients through deep snow.

Litter for Paralyzed Patients

An improvised method of making prolonged litter extrications more tolerable for paralyzed or immobile patients is to use two stretchers. The first stretcher has a hole for the patient's face and a hole for urine output when the patient is in the face-down position (Fig. 21-13). The second stretcher has a hole for stool output, for use when the patient is in the face-up position. Turn the patient every 2 to 4 hours, by first sandwiching the patient between the two stretchers and then flipping them over. This also prevents the patient from developing pressure sores or autonomic dysreflexia from a distended bladder.[11]

VERTICAL TRANSPORT

Vertical Intra-Hospital Transport

Hospitals are rarely forced to evacuate their non-ambulatory patients. When they must, vertical evacuations from multilevel facilities represent a major logistical hurdle. The options often employed include lowering patients out of windows or moving them down stairways.

Lowering Patients

In some circumstances, such as when normal hospital exits are blocked, patients may need to be lowered out of the windows to safety. For this risky maneuver, get the most experienced people to help, such as fire department and rescue personnel.

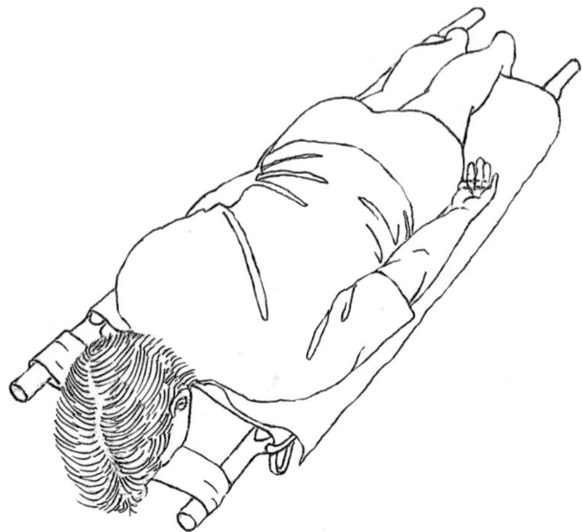

FIG. 21-13. Litter modified for face-down position.

The basic technique, without normal litters and ropes, involves securing the patient as well as possible into sheet slings and using additional sheets as "ropes." Anchor bed-sheet ropes to hospital beds, or the rigid "standpipes" in stairwells can be used to belay the patients.

Down the Stairs

It may be necessary to move non-ambulatory patients down the stairs when the elevators do not work. This has traditionally been an extremely slow process involving fire department stretchers and many teams of strong people.[5,12]

However, the following method, which can be used in nearly any situation, including in non–health care facilities for less-than-fully ambulatory individuals, is much faster, takes only a few people of normal strength to operate, and requires no specialized equipment.[13]

1. Check the entire length of the stairwell to be certain that it is clear and that an exit is available at the bottom. For safety, station someone at the bottom of the stairway to ensure that the exit stays open and to warn the team if it doesn't.
2. Place patient mattresses end-to-end on the stairs. Cover each flight of stairs (the stairs between a flat landing) with mattresses by putting a mattress even with the top stair and having mattresses extend to the landing. Push all the mattresses against the wall side of the stairway so there is a narrow area for personnel to walk.
3. Repeat the process for the entire length of stairs to be traversed.
4. Prepare the patients to be transported by wrapping them with two sheets (Figs. 21-14 and 21-15), leaving their faces uncovered. Tie both sheets individually at the head and foot ends with square knots. Wrapping the patient in two sheets provides extra support and allows the two rescuers at the head end to each hold a different sheet (for safety). The rescuer at the foot end holds both sheets.
5. To get the patient off the bed, turn the mattress 90 degrees on the bed, with the foot end on the floor. Using the sheet for control and one or two people holding the sheets on each end, slide the patient off the mattress and onto the floor. With most smooth hospital floors, two health care workers can then easily slide most normal-sized patients to the head of the stairs.
6. Once at the stairs, lift the patient's foot, using the sheets, onto the end of the mattress at the top of the stairs. The person holding that (foot) end begins walking down the stairs, sliding the patient. The person holding the head end of the sheet follows, simultaneously holding onto the stairway handrail and slowing the patient's slide as necessary. If available, it often helps to have a third person hold the top (head) person's belt to steady him (Fig. 21-16).
7. Once at the landing, slide the patient to the next set of mattresses and repeat the process, continuing to the bottom of the stairs.
8. Once each team clears a landing, the next patient can be started down the mattress ramp from the flight above.

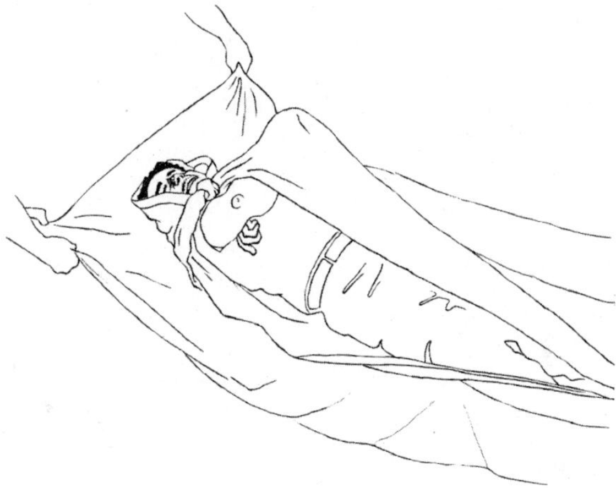

FIG. 21-14. Tying patient into sheets.

NON-AMBULANCE TRANSPORTATION

In the United States, mortality may be higher for gunshot wound patients transported by EMS when compared to private vehicle transport.[14] For emergency patient transport in resource-poor areas, potential solutions include motorcycle ambulance programs, collaboration with taxi and river boat services, police or fire department vehicles, and cooperation from owners of private vehicles. In many low-income countries, <1% of the population has access to conventional emergency transport (e.g., ambulances). In some countries, the population in rural households must travel distances >15 km for public transport.[15]

Any type of vehicle or transport method can be used to get health care workers and equipment to patients, and to get patients to initial or better-equipped health care facilities. For example, in Kenya, current methods of emergency transportation include canoes, bicycles with trailers,

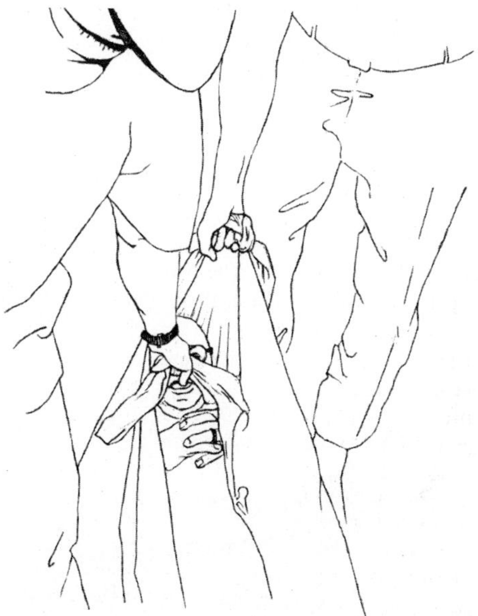

FIG. 21-15. Carrying patient.

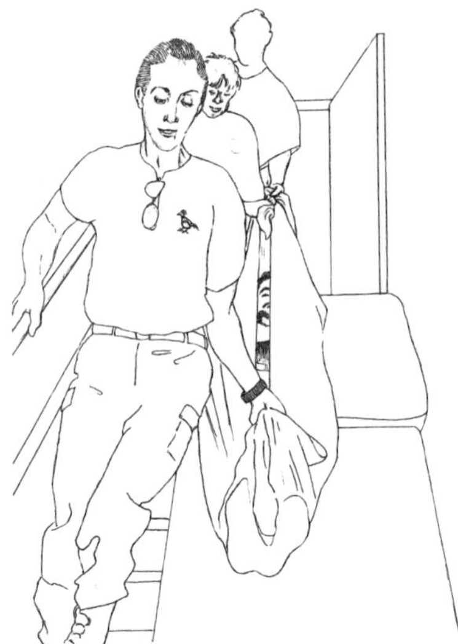

FIG. 21-16. Sliding patient down mattresses.

tricycles with platforms, tractors with trailers, reconditioned public vehicles, and ox carts (Charles O. Otieno, MD. Personal written communication, June 22, 2008). Bicycle EMS services have been used in many locales for special events involving large numbers of people, for wilderness search and rescue operations, and for disaster response.[16]

Domesticated Animals

Riding

Any domesticated animal can be used to transport either health care workers or patients, and they are especially good in rugged terrain.[17] However, experience has demonstrated that (a) a patient's fear can make using a pack animal dangerous, (b) some individual animals that are typically used for transport (including horses or donkeys) may not have the calm temperament needed to carry patients, (c) having experienced handlers available for the animals helps greatly, (d) patients may need to be removed from the animals when going over especially difficult terrain, and (e) putting a safety strap around the patient is useful.

Travois

A travois (Fig. 21-17) is a crude sled lashed to a horse or similar animal. The animal drags the travois along the ground. A travois may also be lashed between two animals in single file and carried level. A travois is made from two long poles fastened together by two crossbars and a litter bed fastened to the poles and crossbars.[18] The patient is secured on the litter bed. If only one animal pulls the travois, the bearers should lift up the end from the ground when going uphill, fording streams, or crossing obstacles.

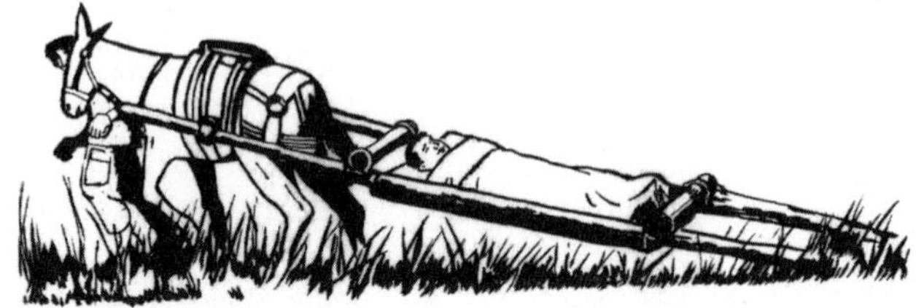

FIG. 21-17. Travois with one animal.

Motorized Vehicles

Factors that complicate emergency medical transport include (a) Travel times: these can range from 10 minutes to more than 1 day to reach a healthcare facility. One study reported a 9% increase in mortality for every 30 minutes of vehicular travel; (b) Wait times: searching for transport or waiting up to 2 days for transport to arrive; (c) Transport options: a complete lack of transportation due to weather conditions or impassable roads, inability to pay, unreliable public transport services, and full vehicle occupancy. Some forms of transport (motorcycle ambulances, such as the "Uhuru" and "eRanger") were effective because they were particularly compatible with the local terrain.[19]

Community Sidecar Ambulance

Intermediate means of transport help poor communities serve difficult-to-reach areas. One example is the motorized community ambulances, such as the Uhuru, which many Sub-Saharan countries use. The Uhuru is a specially designed sidecar attached to a low-capacity motorcycle. Easily constructed, it is a simple, multipurpose, all-terrain motorcycle ambulance that can often traverse otherwise impassable village roads. It costs 10 times less to use than conventional transport vehicles and has low maintenance costs.[20]

All-Terrain Vehicle

All-terrain vehicles (ATVs) equipped with advanced life-support supplies have been used to decrease response times at mass gatherings.[21] Golf carts, motorcycles, snowmobiles, mopeds, motorized bicycles, and similar vehicles also can be equipped for medical purposes.

Flat-bed trucks are particularly useful for transporting morbidly obese patients who cannot fit into a standard ambulance or on a standard ambulance stretcher. The "stretcher" can be the patient's own mattress or a large canvas sheet. Trucks can also be used to transport multiple casualties, although one must take care to see that there is adequate light, ventilation, and protection from the elements (if an open-bed truck).

Trains

For the past two centuries, trains have been used to transport large numbers of casualties. For trains not specially configured to transport casualties, seat ambulatory patients in normal passenger cars, in box cars (provided there is adequate light and ventilation, perhaps with doors fully or partially open), on flat cars (although there is no protection from the elements), or on top of passenger or box cars (if there is no other space and the risk of injury or death from falling off the train is less than from leaving patients behind).

Litters can be placed over the backs of the seats in passenger cars and firmly tied down, put in passenger cars after the seats have been removed (or in box cars, again providing there is adequate ventilation), or put on flat cars, exposed to the elements. To stack litters in a car, make improvised fittings using strapping, ropes, or wood (like bunk beds). Firmly affix them to the train compartment wall, because the load on them—due to the patient's weight compounded by the train's movements—will be significant.

Ships/Boats

Use rafts, canoes, inflatables, jet skis, and similar small boats for rescues and to transport both medical personnel to patients and patients to medical facilities.

Small ships, such as ferries and military landing craft, may be requisitioned either to transport patients or for use as medical facilities. Ships are self-contained units, and so can often provide food, shelter, air-conditioning, and other amenities that are lacking in a devastated locale.

Hospital ships are set up to care for patients. The primary issue will be getting to them, or getting them to you.

Those responsible for medical care aboard a ship must know the ship's exact capabilities and limitations, as well as what situations will trigger medical evacuation of patients off the ship. The ship's captain must also be aware of these, especially if the ship is to travel beyond the reach of air transportation or to areas where on-shore hospitals offer limited care.[22] Plans must be in place to evacuate patients under specific circumstances.

Medical Evacuation at Sea

Consider medical evacuation at sea only after predetermined medical criteria are met, telemedicine consults have been fully exploited, and the risks of evacuation are outweighed by the patient's needs. Improvised transfers can be accomplished by using a smaller boat to carry the patient from one ship to another, but this can be very dangerous. The best way to transfer a patient to a medical facility is from a ship docked at the pier.[23]

AEROMEDICAL TRANSPORT

Air transport is often the optimal method to deliver advanced medical supplies, and to transfer patients for initial treatment during medical emergencies or to tertiary care centers, especially when the patient is far from medical facilities or, even, civilization. Yet, aeromedical transport is a costly, often scarce commodity, so practitioners must use it wisely.

Two general types of aircraft are used for aeromedical transport: fixed-wing planes and helicopters. Each is discussed separately.

General Problems

Major adverse events occur in about 12% of aeromedical evacuations. These are often because of high altitude, rushed patient assessments, hurried evacuation of unstable patients, a patient's long immobilization during flight, health care worker fatigue, the difficulty of in-flight evaluation and treatment, and the unpredictable availability and length of evacuation.[24,25]

Special problems arise when arranging for international nonmilitary air transport. The cost, which may be $100,000 or more for a transoceanic air ambulance, must be paid or guaranteed by an insurance agency in advance. Other problems may include communicating with the transferring and accepting physicians, obtaining visas, and obtaining transportation for the patient at both ends of the flight.[25]

In all aeromedical transport, preparation lessens the chance for untoward events. This includes completing all the paperwork before taking the patient to the plane and carefully envisioning any medical problems that may occur en route. The medical preparation should include placing any tube or doing any procedure that may become necessary during the flight. If possible, have sufficient battery power and oxygen, medications, functioning IV lines, and any other equipment you may need—even if the trip is delayed.

Specific Problems

The major problems in air transport stem from the decreased barometric pressure at altitude and transporting contaminated patients. In addition, the noisy environment may interfere with the ability to hear monitors, use stethoscopes, and communicate with the patient, other staff, and the aircraft's crew.

Decreased Barometric Pressure

The diameter of a gas bubble in liquid (such as blood) or in tissues doubles at 5000 feet above sea level, doubles again at 8000 feet, and once again at 18,000 feet. Cabin pressure in most passenger planes is maintained at 5000 to 8000 feet; on military aircraft, cabin pressure is between 8000 and 10,000 feet. Not all aircraft can increase their internal pressure to simulate sea level. At a cabin altitude of 8000 feet, a normal person's oxygen saturation drops to 90%: Correct this by using 2 L/min of oxygen to raise saturation levels to between 98% and 100%. During the flight, the lowest possible "cabin altitude" should be maintained; if necessary, that may mean flying at a lower altitude, which will increase both the flight time and fuel consumption.

Maintaining the lower cabin altitude (ask the aircrew if this can be done) is most important when transporting patients who have penetrating eye injuries with intraocular air, free air in any body cavity, or severe pulmonary disease. It may also be necessary if gas expansion would cause a tension pneumothorax, surgical wound dehiscence, intracranial hemorrhage, or irreversible ocular damage. Patients at greatest risk for this are those who have had recent surgery or have head or chest trauma. Unfortunately, problems related to gas expansion can be difficult to diagnose and treat aboard an aircraft.

It is vital to maintain a constant ground-level cabin pressure throughout the flight when transporting patients with decompression sickness or arterial gas embolism. If there is no aircraft that can maintain this, the cabin altitude should not exceed 800 feet (242 m), especially with helicopter evacuations. These patients must also be on 100% oxygen (by aviator's mask, if available).[26]

Before they are transported in any aircraft without ground-level (1 atmosphere) cabin pressure, prepare patients by[24]

- Inserting a chest tube with a Heimlich valve or collection system, even for small, asymptomatic pneumothoraces.
- Venting ostomy collection bags to prevent excess gas from dislodging the bag from the stoma wafer. Use a straight pin to put two holes in the bag above the wafer ring.
- Using rigid splints rather than air splints, because the air within them expands at altitude and they would need to be readjusted frequently.
- Doing fasciotomies or escharotomies if they could conceivably be necessary in flight.
- Bivalving casts if the cast is over a surgical wound site. This "window" permits tissue expansion and emergency access.
- Adjusting ventilator settings in neurosurgical patients to meet the increased oxygen demand at altitude.

Situations Requiring Decontamination

Aeromedical transport may be limited or delayed in environments contaminated with radiological, biochemical, or infectious agents. These situations may limit or delay air resources due to (a) the time needed to decontaminate aircraft after the flight, (b) the availability (or lack) of an aircrew that is not contaminated and is willing to fly, (c) the need to batch similarly exposed patients, and (d) the ability to isolate patients on the aircraft.[24] Prior to transport, decontaminate any patients with external contamination. During the flight, isolate any patient with a communicable disease.

Fixed-Wing Aircraft

Military Aircraft

When large numbers of patients require transport, military planes generally are used. In such situations, prioritizing patients is a concern. Load the sickest ones first; they should be off-loaded first as well. Plan for cabin temperatures ranging from 15°C (59°F) to 25°C (77°F) in the winter, and from 20°C (68°F) to 35°C (95°F) in the summer.

Safety

Safety is a major concern when using military fixed-wing aircraft. Unlike commercial passenger planes, which are normally entered through a controlled point in the terminal (even for litter patients), military planes usually sit on the tarmac without an obvious approach path.

A "circle of safety" exists around the aircraft. It is an imaginary circle 10 feet from the plane's nose, wings, and tail (Fig. 21-18). Vehicles and people must not enter the safety circle unless instructed to do so by the flight crew. Vehicles within that area (such as those carrying patients) must have a spotter when in motion and use chocks when parked.

When entering the aircraft, use a flashlight, preferably one with a low light intensity and a red or blue filter, to avoid compromising the aircrew's night vision.

On an aircraft equipped with webbing along the sides (primarily military), tie a bandana or cravat through the webbing and around the patient's forehead to provide support when sitting for long periods.

Other safety caveats are as follows: (a) do not run near any aircraft; (b) do not walk under the wings or propellers, even when the engines are not running; and (c) wear eye protection near the aircraft, especially when the propellers are in motion.

Passenger Airlines

The most common situations involving passenger airlines are using them to transport patients and confronting medical emergencies during a flight.

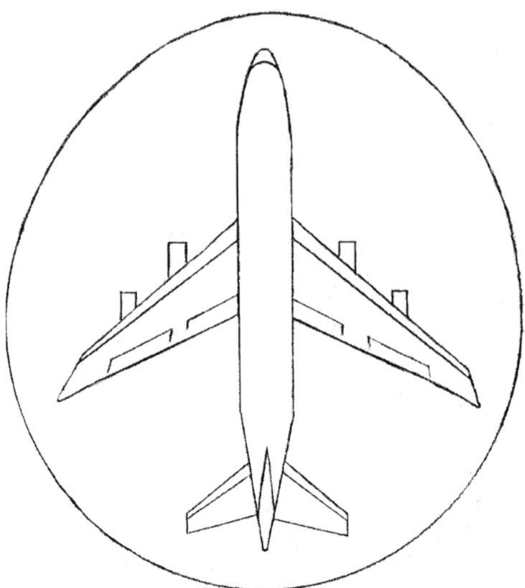

FIG. 21-18. Circle of safety around aircraft. *(Redrawn from Cocks and Liew.[27])*

Transporting Patients

Transporting patients via a regularly scheduled commercial passenger airliner is cheaper and, usually, more readily available than is an air ambulance. If the patient can sit, simply purchase a seat for him or her and for the medical attendant(s). Airlines may get a bit nervous, however, about accommodating medical equipment; check with them in advance.

Getting a stretcher-bound patient onto a commercial aircraft may be difficult, because the aisles are too narrow to accommodate standard ambulance stretchers. Take patients aboard using a soft (scoop) stretcher or an improvised stretcher. Then place the stretcher in the back of the plane across several seats; the medical team sits across the aisle. Some airlines permit stretcher patients only in the first-class cabin. Some airlines specifically prohibit access to the aircraft's electrical systems. This requires operating any equipment on battery power, which may be difficult on long flights. The airlines generally do allow hanging IV solutions from overhead bins, as well as taping flow sheets and other medical information to them.[25]

Treat hypoxia with supplemental oxygen. Bring extra oxygen in case of delays in air travel or another unexpected need for additional oxygen. Aircrews prefer not to provide oxygen from their own medical supplies.

Even on commercial aircraft, airframe vibrations may interfere with monitoring devices, and the high ambient noise level can interfere with using a stethoscope or communicating with the patient, other team members, or the aircraft crew.[25]

Medical Emergencies During a Flight

Few locations are more isolated than the small tube of an airliner 35,000 feet above the ground, with limited space and medical equipment. Fortunately, medical emergencies on board aircraft are relatively rare: About one in-flight medical emergency occurs every 604 flights.[28] The goal when providing in-flight medical assistance on commercial airline flights is to stabilize the patient's condition until the aircraft lands. The most common in-flight emergencies on commercial aircraft are syncope or presyncope (37.4% of cases), respiratory symptoms (12.1%), nausea or vomiting (9.5%), cardiac symptoms (7.7%), and seizures (5.8%).[28] Alcohol consumption and more stressful flying conditions have increased the need to restrain passengers for disruptive and violent behavior.[29] While this may seem like a medical emergency, it is best to let restraint experts, such as police, security personnel, an air marshal, or a psychiatric worker, intervene. Health care professionals can be useful if sedation is necessary.

A general approach to in-flight emergencies on commercial aircraft is in Table 21-2. Note that the option to ask for advice from ground-based health care providers is now commonly available.

TABLE 21-2 General Approach to Managing In-flight Medical Incidents

Approach the nearest flight crew member.
Identify yourself and your training/expertise.
Treat the patient in a seat if possible, using the aisle blocks flight crew mobility.
Document your findings and any treatments administered.
Communicate and coordinate with flight crew and ground resources.
Do not attempt to practice beyond your expertise.
Request access to the emergency medical kit. (You may have to show your professional license.)
Use a translator if necessary.

Adapted from Chandra and Conry.[30]

Many commercial airlines have links to physicians with experience in on-board medical emergencies.

Treatment options include providing oxygen and using the patient's medications, medications (labeled) from other passengers, or the medications and supplies in the plane's emergency medical kit. Some air carriers may have insufficient oxygen aboard to treat ill passengers, because the Federal Aviation Administration's standards for the minimum medical equipment for US commercial aircraft does not define the amount of oxygen for medical use that must be available.[31,32] One treatment option is to request that the pilot reduce the plane's altitude to increase cabin pressure. That may alleviate altitude-related chest pain, dyspnea, and abdominal pain by resolving relative hypoxia and decreasing the expansion of gas that results from the decreased pressure at altitude.[33] The final option is to ask that the plane be diverted to the closest airport, if possible.

Ask the captain to land at the closest airfield if a passenger (a) has chest pain, shortness of breath, or severe abdominal pain that does not improve with basic interventions; (b) is persistently unresponsive; (c) has cardiac arrest that has responded to initial treatment; or (d) has an acute coronary syndrome, severe dyspnea, stroke, refractory seizure, or severe agitation.[33] Note that if a patient does not respond to cardiopulmonary resuscitation (CPR), initial attempts at defibrillation (many planes, especially those flying internationally, are now equipped with automatic external defibrillators [AEDs]), and the administration of cardiac drugs (e.g., epinephrine, atropine), he or she will not survive, so diverting the plane will not be helpful.

In-flight medical incidents are stressful. There is not much light, it is hard to lie someone flat, the seats are cramped, and it is noisy. Hearing anything through a stethoscope is nearly impossible. Personal experience demonstrates that resuscitation in a plane's narrow aisle can be challenging. The widest space is near the galley; if possible, get patients who need to be supine to that area. There may even be enough room to spread out the plane's medical kit and, if necessary, to position the AED. Use a pillow under your knees—a plane's floor has paint-thin carpeting. Also, ask the flight attendant to help steady you during landing if you absolutely must stay with the patient. On miniscule regional planes or in small private planes, there may be no place to position a patient supine except near the exit.

Helicopters

Working With a Medical/Rescue Helicopter

Helicopters are often used in austere medical environments both to transport health care professionals to patients and to extract patients who need a higher level of medical care. When extracting patients, the health care provider may need to prepare and direct ground operations. This is outside the training for most health care workers, so they need to be aware of how (a) to set up a landing zone (LZ) and (b) to work safely around a helicopter.

Special Situations

When the helicopter used to transport patients is neither medically configured nor staffed (most commonly military helicopters in disasters), patients do not receive medical care during the flight.[24] Patients may be dangled in a basket (horizontally) or in a restraint device (vertically) at the end of a "long-line" attached to the helicopter. When patients will experience any of these exciting/scary excursions, tell them what will occur. Then, secure them tightly into the basket or follow the crew's instructions about using the vertical restraint device. Be careful to let the long-line touch the ground before touching it yourself, to avoid getting hit by a static electricity charge; it's not pleasant.

Establishing a Landing Zone

It may be necessary to establish an LZ before you can evacuate a patient from a difficult environment. While action movies often show helicopters hovering or doing one-skid landings to offload people (and skilled pilots can do that in emergencies), loading a patient normally requires a stable platform—the LZ. There are five major considerations in locating an LZ[34]:

1. *Surroundings.* Ideally, it should be free from overhead wires, trees, poles, structures, or anything else that could damage the aircraft.
2. *Size.* An LZ should be 100 feet by 100 feet to permit safe landing and lift-off. Pace off an "X" of 50 steps in each direction from a central point. Assuming that an adult's pace is about 2.5 feet, this provides the needed space. The center of the "X" is the landing spot.
3. *Slope.* Find a relatively flat site. If the slope is >15 degrees, there is a chance that the aircraft could roll over.
4. *Surface.* Dust or snow will reduce the pilot's visibility. Some surfaces may not support the craft. Clear the LZ of debris. Any loose debris can be blown up into the air and, if struck by a rotor blade, can seriously damage the blade.
5. *Access.* Place the LZ at least 200 feet away from the medical facility, so that rotor wash will not damage the facility. But, remember that you need easy access for patients, personnel, stretchers, and equipment.

Other considerations for the LZ are as follows[35]:

- If the LZ will be used multiple times, find a way to prevent unauthorized people from entering it.
- Mark the LZ's corners to identify it for the pilot. Do not use material (e.g., cones, cloth) that can blow around; fluorescent surveyor's tape is excellent. At night, use red- or yellow-colored lights or strobe lights (not flares) to mark the LZ perimeter.
- Protect the pilot's night vision by not using bright white lights.
- If the LZ must be on a highway or in an area where vehicles are present, use their headlights to illuminate the LZ.

Wind conditions are extremely important for helicopter operations, so be prepared to signal the wind direction, especially if the pilot asks that you do so. Several methods may be appropriate, including using flares, hand signals, ribbons, and kicking dirt into the air (Fig. 21-19).[36]

Safety

Safety is a huge concern when working around a helicopter. Horrific accidents have occurred when people have violated these rules.

1. Do not approach the craft until instructed to do so by the flight crew. If you must approach the craft for a "hot on-load" or "hot off-load," approach only from the front, between 3 o'clock and 9 o'clock (Fig. 21-20).
2. Danger can come from the main rotor blades or the tail rotors. The tail rotor, which can be as low as shoulder height, is difficult to see when it is spinning. Stay away from the rotors!
3. Wear eye and, preferably, ear protection. Secure any loose items that the blades could pick up (clothing, supplies, equipment).
4. Do not radio the helicopter during the last 30 seconds of the landing, except to warn of an immediate hazard. If there is an immediate hazard, radio "Abort Landing" or "Wave-Off." Repeat the message until you see them lifting or hovering. If you have no radio, use the hand signal shown in Fig. 21-21.

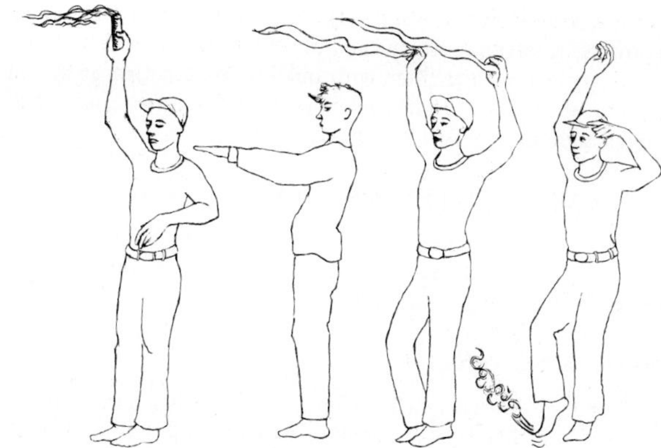

FIG. 21-19. Methods of signaling wind direction.

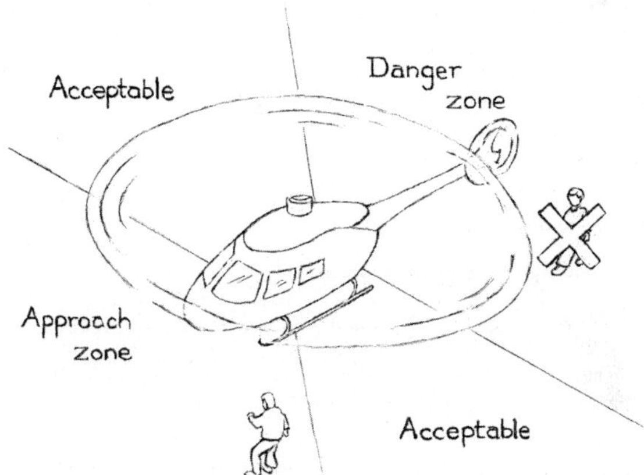

FIG. 21-20. Safe and dangerous zones around a helicopter.

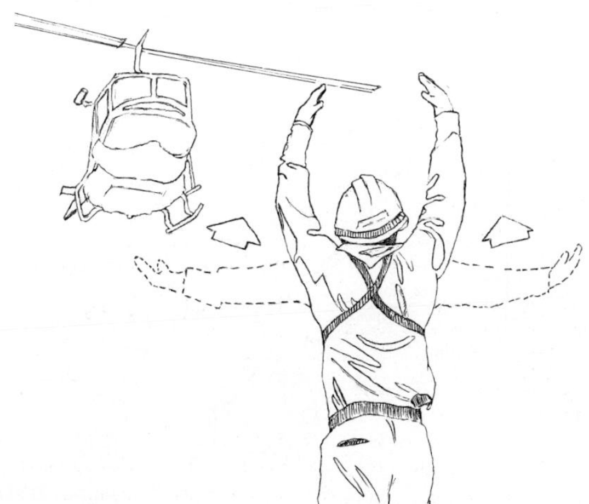

FIG. 21-21. "Abort-landing" hand signal.

Prepare patients for safe helicopter transport. Insulate the patient from cold—especially when under the spinning rotors. If traveling over water, put the patient in a survival vest that does not need inflating. Secure patients to the litter with quick-release straps, if possible. Secure any oxygen or IV tubing so it cannot become entangled with aircrafts' equipment. Most patients should receive supplementary oxygen, if it is available.[23]

HOSPITAL/HEALTH CARE FACILITY EVACUATION

A major part of disaster planning is preparing for the evacuation of hospitals and other health care facilities. Facilities should be assessed in advance for their ability to survive disasters and to safely shelter-in-place their patients and staff.[37]

Should/Must Patients Be Evacuated?

A major question, either after a disaster strikes (Fig. 21-22) or when one is expected (Fig. 21-23), is whether to evacuate or to shelter-in-place. Making this decision is difficult and its implementation can be costly. Who makes this decision may be as important as how to make the decision. (See Appendix 1 for "triggers" that force decisions and how to identify the decision makers.) The decision of whether to order an evacuation relies on the infrastructure assessment, which includes knowing how long the hospital can maintain a safe, clean environment without city water during hot months and how long the facility can maintain essential backup power with only the current on-site fuel supply (Table 21-3).

If the critical infrastructure still functions (or it is assumed that it will function after the event), the hospital's ability to shelter-in-place will depend largely on whether the supply of critical consumable resources can meet the needs of patients and staff without relying on outside supplies.

How Long Will It Take to Safely Evacuate?

If the decision to evacuate the facility is made, how long will it take? Table 21-4 lists factors to consider. The most important of these are the number of patients, the mix of patient acuity, available staff, exit routes within the hospital, patient transportation requirements, available transportation resources (personnel, vehicles and equipment), road and traffic conditions, and the locations of the receiving care sites.

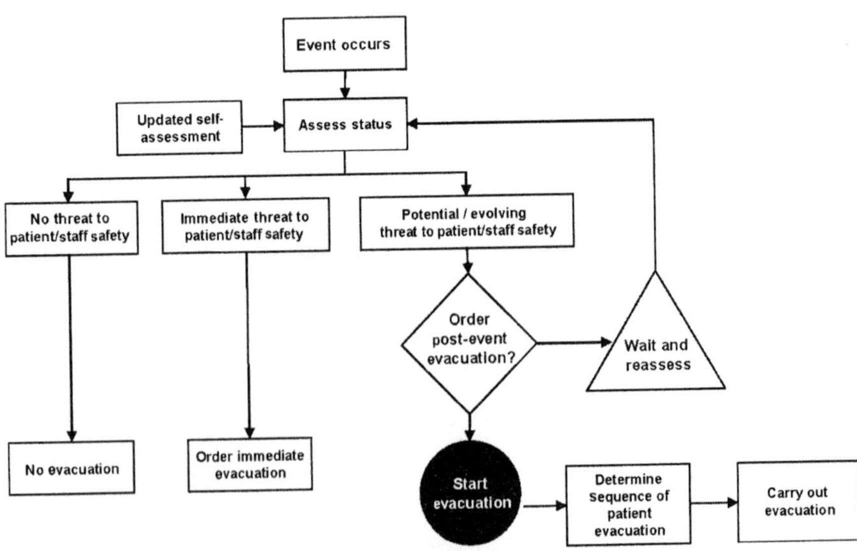

FIG. 21-22. No-advanced-warning-event evacuation decisions. *(Reproduced with permission from Zane et al.[38])*

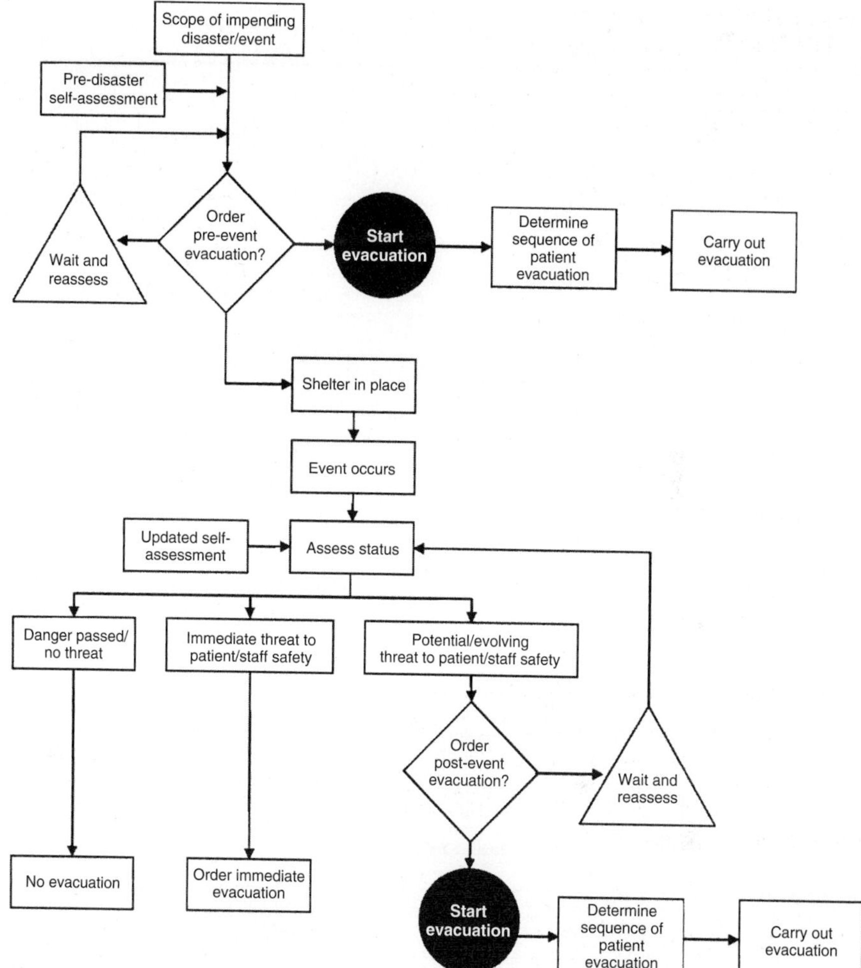

FIG. 21-23. Advanced-warning-event evacuation decisions. *(Reproduced with permission from Zane et al.[38])*

Time is the major issue in hospital evacuations: the time needed both to empty the building and to transport the patients safely. In planning, one must distinguish between an orderly, planned evacuation that maximizes safety for patients and staff and a "drop everything and go" evacuation, such as during a major fire. In emergencies posing an immediate danger, you may need to abandon optimal procedures for safely moving patients in favor of just getting everyone out as fast as possible.

The time to empty the building includes the time required to move patients from their location inside the hospital (e.g., rooms, operating room, emergency department, clinics) to an ambulatory area in which they can be assessed and discharged or to an area for non-ambulatory patients from which they can be loaded into ambulances and other vehicles for transport. One factor that determines how elegantly and quickly this can be done is whether the facility has a means of tracking patients and generating patient discharge summaries. In addition, evacuation time depends on whether elevators are operational (or staff have practiced using the evacuation method described in the "Vertical Intra-Hospital Transport" section earlier in this chapter) and how quickly additional staff can arrive to help with the evacuation.

Evacuation time also depends on the time needed to transport patients from the assembly/staging areas to receiving hospitals or other appropriate health care facilities.

TABLE 21-3 Pre-disaster Evacuation Decision Factors

Factor	Issues to Consider	Implication
	Event Characteristics	
• Arrival	• When is the event expected to "hit" the hospital? The metropolitan area? • How variable is the time the event is expected to "hit"?	• The amount of time until the event "hits," combined with the anticipated time to evacuate patients, determines how long an evacuation decision can be deferred.
• Magnitude	• What is the expected strength of the event? • How likely is the event to gain or lose strength before it reaches the hospital? The metropolitan area?	• The magnitude of the event forewarns of the potential damage to a facility and utilities, which could cut off the supply of key resources, or otherwise limit the ability to shelter-in-place and care for patients.
• Area impacted	• How large a geographic area will be affected by the event? • How many vulnerable health care facilities are in this geographic area?	• Competition for resources needed to evacuate patients (especially vehicles) increases when several facilities evacuate simultaneously.
• Duration	• How long is the event expected to last? • How variable is the expected duration of the event?	• The duration of the event will affect how long hospitals have to shelter-in-place or operate using backup, alternative, or less predictable sources of key resources.
	Anticipated Effect on Key Resources	
• Water source	• Is the main city water supply in jeopardy? Already nonfunctional? • Is there a backup water supply (a well, nearby building with intact water mains)? If not, how soon will city water return?	• Water loss of unknown duration (more than 1-2 days) is almost always cause for evacuation.
• Heat source	• Is the heat source in jeopardy (steam, water for boilers, etc.)? Already nonfunctional? • Is there a backup (intact nearby building that still has power/heat)? • If not, will the building become too cold for patient safety before adequate heat returns?	• Loss of heat, especially during a northern winter, is almost always a cause for evacuation—often within 12 hours.
• Electricity	• Is power in jeopardy? Just for the hospital or for a wider area? • Are backup generators functional? How long can they run without refueling? Is refueling possible (e.g., intake not under water)? • Can some sections/wings be shut down to reduce fuel consumption and stretch fuel supplies?	• Loss of electricity endangers ventilated patients, among others, and may affect the sequence in which patients are evacuated.

(*Continued*)

TABLE 21-3 Pre-disaster Evacuation Decision Factors (*Continued*)

Factor	Issues to Consider	Implication
• Building's structural integrity	• Is the building obviously/visibly unsafe? All of it or only portions (e.g., can people be consolidated in safer sections)? • Was there a water tower on the roof, and is it intact? • Is a building engineer needed to determine structural integrity/safety?	• Earthquakes or explosions may cause rooftop water towers to fall, flooding the building. • Safety/integrity may not be obvious to untrained occupants.
Anticipated Effect on the Surrounding Environment and Community		
• Road conditions	• Are major routes from the hospital to potential receiving care sites closed? • Is traffic at gridlock on major routes from the hospital to potential receiving care sites? • Are access routes to the hospital cut off?	• There may be a limited window of opportunity to carry out a ground-based evacuation. • Increased use of helicopters to evacuate patients may be required. • Staff may not be able to get to the hospital to relieve existing staff or assist in the evacuation.
• Community/ building security	• Have any nearby areas experienced increases in disorder or looting? • Are local law enforcement agencies understaffed due to self-evacuations or significant additional responsibilities? • Are additional private security officers available to secure the hospital?	• If patient and staff safety cannot be assured, evacuation will be necessary.
• Evacuation status of nearby health care facilities	• Are other hospitals or health care facilities evacuating or planning to evacuate, or have they decided to shelter-in-place?	• If other hospitals or health care facilities are evacuating: – the competition for ambulances, wheelchair vans, and buses may be substantially increased. – the hospital may be asked to accept additional patients. – patients may have to be relocated to facilities further away than anticipated.
• State/ county/local evacuation orders	• Have evacuation orders been issued in areas that are closer to the event? • Have any public or private statements been issued regarding the possibility of an evacuation order? • Have any other incidents occurred that increase the likelihood that an evacuation order will be issued?	• You may have no choice but to evacuate.
• Availability of local emergency response agencies	• Are local emergency response agencies understaffed (or otherwise unavailable) due to self-evacuations or additional responsibilities?	• Unavailability of local fire agencies increases the risk of sheltering-in-place.

Adapted from Zane et al.[39]

TABLE 21-4 Factors Affecting Facility Evacuation Time

Evacuation-Relevant Resources	Implications
People	
• If a mandatory city-wide evacuation order is issued, what percentage of your staff is likely to leave with their families (and not report for work)?	High % = more vulnerable
• Has additional trained staff been identified/located to assist, if necessary, with the evacuation?	No = more vulnerable
Patient Census and Mix	
• How many patients are in the ICU (including adult, pediatric, and neonatal ICUs) and other units (e.g, burn units) with special evacuation needs (e.g, patient must be accompanied by two health care professionals)?	The more ICU and special care patients, the more limited the options for where they can be taken.
• Typical census of adult and pediatric patients.	
• Typical census of patients with special evacuation needs (e.g., psychiatric patients, bariatric patients, patients from correctional facilities).	
Patient Transportation Needs	
• What percentage of patients could self-evacuate (e.g., be taken home or evacuated by family/friends)?	The higher the percentage, the more vulnerable.
• What percentage of patients are ambulatory (e.g., could be evacuated by bus)?	
• What percentage can sit up but not walk (e.g., could be evacuated in wheelchair vans)?	
• What percentage requires medical attention at the BLS level during transport?	
• What percentage requires life support equipment (e.g., could only be evacuated in an ALS ambulance or medevac helicopter)?	
Evacuation Transportation	
• Does the hospital have an *exclusive* contract with transportation providers to supply vehicles, or is it dependent on public/private vehicles that must also provide services to other hospitals?	No exclusive contract = more vulnerable
• Has the hospital established relationships with state and regional emergency management agencies and developed coordinated plans for sharing transportation resources?	No = more vulnerable
• How long would it take to get all patients out of the hospital and on the road to another location (assuming the hospital is full, roads are not damaged/blocked, and appropriate vehicles and staff are available)?	Hours = time until evacuation

(Continued)

TABLE 21-4 Factors Affecting Facility Evacuation Time (*Continued*)

Evacuation-Relevant Resources	Implications
• Does the hospital plan specify an off-site "assembly point" where patients could be moved without vehicles and from which transportation/loading into vehicles would be faster?	No off-site "assembly point" specified = more vulnerable
• How long would this two-stage evacuation take?	Hours = time until evacuation
• How quickly could all the patients be moved out of the building (e.g., in case of a fire)?	Minutes = time until evacuation

Abbreviations: BLS, basic life support; ALS, advanced life support; ICU, intensive care unit.

Adapted from Zane et al.[40]

When Can the Facility Be Reopened?

Subsequent decisions about whether, how, and when to move back into a damaged and evacuated health care facility are complex and involve many people. A US government publication, *Hospital Assessment and Recovery Guide*, describes the process and provides detailed checklists.[41] It is available online at http://www.ahrq.gov/prep/hosprecovery/hosprecovery.pdf.

REFERENCES

1. Brown JB, Cohen MJ, Minei JP, et al. Goal directed resuscitation in the prehospital setting: a propensity adjusted analysis. *J Trauma Acute Care Surg*. 2013;74:1207-1214.
2. Engels PT, Passos E, Beckett AN, Doyle JD, Tien HC. IV access in bleeding trauma patients: a performance review. *Injury*. 2014;45(1):77-82.
3. US Navy. *Hospital Corpsman 1 & C—Advanced Navy Nursing Manual for Hospital Training Purposes.* http://tpub.com/content/medical/10669-c/. Accessed May 27, 2008.
4. Community Emergency Response Team. *Unit 5: Light Search and Rescue Operations*. US Citizen Corps.
5. Alvarez AR, Russell MT. Emergency evacuation: removal of the critically ill patient. *Focus Crit Care*. 1987;14(6):18-22.
6. Dick T. Handy padding in a pinch. *JEMS*. July 2008:38.
7. Olson LM. *Improvised Equipment in the Home Care of the Sick*. Philadelphia, PA: W.B. Saunders; 1928:104.
8. US Dept. of the Army. *Medical Evacuation in a Theater of Operations: Tactics, Techniques, and Procedures. Field Manual 8-10-6, Chapter 9: Litter Evacuation*. Washington, DC. October 31, 1991:9-5.
9. US Dept. of the Army. *Medical Evacuation in a Theater of Operations: Tactics, Techniques, and Procedures. Field Manual 8-10-6, Chapter 9: Litter Evacuation*. Washington, DC. October 31, 1991:9-6.
10. US Dept. of the Army. *Medical Evacuation in a Theater of Operations: Tactics, Techniques, and Procedures. Field Manual 8-10-6, Chapter 9: Litter Evacuation*. Washington, DC. October 31, 1991:9-1.
11. Husum H, Ang SC, Fosse E. *War Surgery: Field Manual*. Penang, Malaysia: Third World Network; 1995:311.
12. Manion P, Golden IJ. Vertical evacuation drill of an intensive care unit: design, implementation, and evaluation. *Disaster Manag Response*. 2004;2(1):14-19.
13. Iserson KV. Vertical hospital evacuations: a new method. *S Med J*. 2013;106(1):37-42.
14. Zafar SN, Haider AH, Stevens KA, et al. Increased mortality associated with EMS transport of gunshot wound victims when compared to private vehicle transport. *Injury*. 2014;45(9):1320-1326.
15. Wilson A, Hillman S, Rosato M, et al. A systematic review and thematic synthesis of qualitative studies on maternal emergency transport in low-and middle-income countries. *Int J Gyn Ob*. 2013;122(3):192-201.
16. Gorham JF, Kramer TS. The utilization of bicycles in the delivery of EMS: a preliminary report. *Prehosp Disaster Med*. 1997;12(2):173-179.
17. Pandolf KB, Burr RE, eds. *Medical Aspects of Harsh Environments*. Vol 2. Falls Church, VA: Office of the Surgeon General US Army; 2002:866-867.

18. US Dept. of the Army. *Medical Evacuation in a Theater of Operations: Tactics, Techniques, and Procedures. Field Manual 8-10-6, Chapter 9: Litter Evacuation.* Washington, DC. October 31, 1991:9-15, 9-16.
19. Wilson A, Hillman S, Rosato M, et al. A systematic review and thematic synthesis of qualitative studies on maternal emergency transport in low-and middle-income countries. *Int J Gyn Ob.* 2013;122(3):192-201.
20. Riders for Health. The Gambia update report – April 2009: bringing freedom to the rural Gambia. www.globalgiving.org/pfil/1245/Riders_for_Health_report_on_Kankurang_Uhuru_April_2009.pdf. Accessed July 1, 2015.
21. Ounanian LL, Salinas C, Shear CL, et al. Medical care at the 1982 US Festival. *Ann Emerg Med.* 1986;15(5):520-527.
22. Pandolf KB, Burr RE, eds. *Medical Aspects of Harsh Environments.* Vol 2. Falls Church, VA: Office of the Surgeon General US Army; 2002:889.
23. Pandolf KB, Burr RE, eds. *Medical Aspects of Harsh Environments*. Vol 2. Falls Church, VA: Office of the Surgeon General US Army; 2002:898-899.
24. US Army. Aeromedical evacuation. *Emergency War Surgery*. 3rd rev. Washington, DC: Borden Institute, Walter Reed Army Medical Center; 2004:4.1-4.9.
25. Teichman PG, Donchin Y, Kot RJ. International aeromedical evacuation. *N Engl J Med.* 2007;356: 262-270.
26. Pandolf KB, Burr RE, eds. *Medical Aspects of Harsh Environments*. Vol 2. Falls Church, VA: Office of the Surgeon General US Army; 2002:946.
27. Cocks R, Liew M. Commercial aviation in-flight emergencies and the physician. *Emerg Med Australas.* 2007;19:1-8.
28. Peterson DC, Martin-Gill C, Guyette FX, et al. Outcomes of medical emergencies on commercial airline flights. *New Engl J Med.* 2013;368(22):2075-2083.
29. Tonks A. Cabin fever. *BMJ.* 2008;336:584-586.
30. Chandra A, Conry S. In-flight medical emergencies. *West J Emerg Med.* 2013;14(5):499-504.
31. Federal Aviation Administration. Policy AC 121-33B—Emergency Medical Equipment. 2006 http://www.faa.gov/regulations_policies/advisory_circulars/index.cfm/go/document.information/documentID/22516. Accessed July 1, 2015.
32. Christian Martin-Gill C, Peterson DC, Yealy DM. Medical emergencies on commercial airline flights. *New Engl J Med.* 2013;369(9):877.
33. Gendreau A, DeJohn C. Responding to medical events during commercial airline flights. *N Engl J Med.* 2002;346(14):1067-1073.
34. Stoffel R, LaValla P. *Personnel Safety in Helicopter Operations: Heli-Rescue Manual.* Olympia, WA: Emergency Response Institute; 1988:43-57.
35. Batchelor S. *Aircraft Safety for NDMS Response Teams.* FEMA: NDMS Response Teams Training Program; 2003.
36. Setnicka TJ. *Wilderness Search and Rescue*. Boston, MA: Appalachian Mountain Club; 1980:410.
37. Zane R, Biddinger P, Hassol A, et al. *Hospital Evacuation Decision Guide*. Rockville, MD: Agency for Healthcare Research and Quality; 2010:18-20. www.ahrq.gov/prep/hospevacguide/hospevac.pdf. Accessed September 11, 2010.
38. Zane R, Biddinger P, Hassol A, et al. *Hospital Evacuation Decision Guide*. Rockville, MD: Agency for Healthcare Research and Quality; 2010:45. www.ahrq.gov/prep/hospevacguide/hospevac.pdf. Accessed September 11, 2010.
39. Zane R, Biddinger P, Hassol A, et al. *Hospital Evacuation Decision Guide*. Rockville, MD: Agency for Healthcare Research and Quality; 2010:39-41. www.ahrq.gov/prep/hospevacguide/hospevac.pdf. Accessed September 11, 2010.
40. Zane R, Biddinger P, Hassol A, et al. *Hospital Evacuation Decision Guide*. Rockville, MD: Agency for Healthcare Research and Quality; 2010:29-31. www.ahrq.gov/prep/hospevacguide/hospevac.pdf. Accessed September 11, 2010.
41. Zane R, Biddinger P, Gerteis J, et al. *Hospital Evacuation Recovery Guide*. Rockville, MD: Agency for Healthcare Research and Quality; 2010. www.ahrq.gov/prep/hosprecovery/hosprecovery.pdf. Accessed September 11, 2010.

IV | SURGICAL INTERVENTIONS

22 | Surgical Equipment

In austere situations, surgical instruments may need to be manufactured. Physician prisoners of war (POW) in World War II camps made surgical appliances from scrap materials using common items, including forks and spoons. With these rudimentary instruments, they performed thousands of successful operations.[1,2]

A relatively simple method for obtaining basic surgical equipment is to recycle instruments that are labeled as "single-use" or "disposable." The most common of these are disposable suture and suture-removal kits. Made completely of metal, they can be easily sterilized and safely reused.

WOUND GLUES

While cyanoacrylate (e.g., "Superglue"), either the medical or the household variety, is the most commonly available glue to use for closing wounds, others can also be used. The problems with nonmedical cyanoacrylates are that they may not hold the tissue well, may irritate the tissues, and may even have some toxic properties. Among those that have been used are wood glue, panel adhesive, hobby cement, and various native substances. One caution: When using glue to close a wound, tell the patient that he or she should avoid putting an antibiotic ointment on the wound. Most have a petroleum base that will dissolve the glue.

Cyanoacrylate

Availability

Cyanoacrylate, which comes in a wide variety of commercial brands for medical and nonmedical use, is a methacrylate resin that bonds surfaces almost instantly. Nonmedical cyanoacrylate is not approved for medical use, although the medical literature shows that it has been used without difficulty in multiple situations. (Remember, the techniques in this book are primarily for austere medical circumstances; if approved compounds are available, use them.)

Uses

Cyanoacrylates have been used successfully as a wound adhesive, for emergency dental repairs, and to treat corneal ulcerations and perforations, urinary and esophagobronchial fistulas, variceal bleeding, and esophagogastric varices (obliteration). They have also been used to repair peripheral nerves and for therapeutic embolism of vascular abnormalities.[3,4] During the Vietnam War, both liquid and spray forms of *n*-butyl cyanoacrylate were successfully used to control bleeding from penetrating wounds of the liver, retroperitoneum, kidney, pancreas, and vascular anastomoses after standard surgical treatment failed.[5,6] Simple lacerations that are closed with tissue adhesive not only show no difference in cosmesis compared to those that are closed with sutures, but also have reduced pain scores and shorter procedure times.[7]

Nonmedical superglues effectively close wounds in a similar manner to medical tissue adhesives. However, they are not sterile, which is likely to have little impact. One benefit of the medical form, which is 2-octyl cyanoacrylate (2-OC), is that it forms a bond about four times stronger than does butyl cyanoacrylate.

Advantages/Disadvantages

The advantages of using cyanoacrylate are: (a) it is easy to obtain; (b) it can be applied rapidly; (c) it requires little technical knowledge; (d) a small amount can be used for many patients; (e) it can be used on many parts of the body (e.g., skin, oral, intra-abdominal); and (f) it is bactericidal against gram-positive (including multi-resistant strains of *Staphylococcus aureus*) and, to a lesser extent, gram-negative organisms.[8] Cyanoacrylate can also bolster thin edges of flaps or lacerations so that they can be primarily closed. This is particularly useful in the elderly and for those on chronic steroids.[9] It can also protect skin that surrounds fistulas when other modalities are not available.[10]

The primary disadvantages to using cyanoacrylate on wounds are dehiscence and contamination of other body parts.

Dehiscence

Because of cyanoacrylate's lower tensile strength compared to sutures, wounds dehisce more readily than when closed with sutures. Lower the incidence of dehiscence by (a) not using it for wound closure over areas under tension, such as joints; and (b) using it only in areas and for wounds where a 5-0 suture would be appropriate.[11]

Contamination of Other Areas

Prevention

When using cyanoacrylate to close wounds around the eyes or the mouth, don't let it get onto the lids or lips: It can seal them shut for hours. The easiest way to avoid this is to position the patient so that any extra cement will run away from, rather than toward, the patient's eye or mouth. This may require having the patient turn his or her head away from the wound, lie on his or her side, sit up, or, if the wound is above the eye, lie in a Trendelenburg position.

Keep cyanoacrylate away from sensitive areas in two other ways: by using petroleum jelly (e.g., Vaseline) or an adhesive plastic drape. Petroleum jelly can be used to make a barrier around the wound to protect other tissues and sensitive areas (such as on the eyelids) from the adhesive.

If you have an adhesive drape (e.g., Tegaderm), fold it in half and cut a half-circle in the middle to make a hole. When opened, it forms a circular area that can be placed over the wound to be closed. The rest of the drape protects the surrounding areas. The edges of the drape closest to the wound must firmly adhere to the skin to make a successful barrier to the adhesive.

Treatment

There are several treatment modalities if cyanoacrylate does get on an unwanted area during wound closure, or if someone tries to remove the cap with their teeth or accidentally squirts a cyanoacrylate tube at home.

To remove cyanoacrylate, most commonly from the eye or an eyelid, use a petroleum-based product such as ophthalmic bacitracin, erythromycin ointment, or mineral oil. The alternative is to wait (usually less than a day) and the lids will open without treatment.

Table 22-1 is a modified version of a list of complications seen with cyanoacrylate's use on wounds. It was compiled by Dr. Loren Yamamoto from Kapiulani Medical Center in Hawaii.

STAPLES

Staples are a great way to rapidly close wounds. They can be used quickly for multiple patients on a variety of body parts. However, they cannot be improvised. The best suggestion, if you know that you will be in an austere medical situation, is to take staple guns and the staples with you. They are lightweight and relatively inexpensive. (Airlines may not permit you to have them in your carry-on luggage.)

TABLE 22-1 Cyanoacrylate Wound Adhesive, Complications and Solutions

Complication	Solution/Prevention
Latex glove stuck to wound	Use vinyl gloves that can be removed with gentle tension.
Gauze stuck to wound	Use damp gauze rather than dry gauze.
Cyanoacrylate hardens inside wound	Maintain pressure on wound edges to prevent this.
Hematoma formation	Ensure hemostasis before using glue.
Adhesive applied over sutures	This makes suture removal difficult; don't do it.

Data from Yamamoto.[12]

To avoid using scarce resources to sedate a child while stapling a small laceration, use two people and two staple guns. Fire both at the same time; the child has a brief moment of pain, starts crying, and it is all over.

Other methods to bind wound edges together are the ordinary clips used to clamp paper pages together and safety pins—primarily to provide some closure to large gaping wounds. When passing the safety pin through the wound, engage enough tissue so that the wound doesn't gape.[13] Consider carrying several sizes of pins (see Appendix 2), from ¾- to 3-inches, to accommodate different wounds.

Nature's staples (i.e., ant or other insect pincers) are used in remote areas of the world to close wounds. Do not try this at home! If a native healer with experience wants to use them, they will probably work well.

BINDING/TAPING

Use nearly any tape to close a wound. There is no magical quality to medical tapes. Other than cleaning and debriding the wound, this procedure requires no technical expertise and is amazingly fast, painless, and virtually cost free. Use duct tape (originally "Duck tape"), as well as any adhesive tape. Cut it lengthwise into strips if you want to be able to see part of the wound (Fig. 5-25).

Tapes do not stick well on areas that are hairy (shave the area, if necessary), wet or prone to perspiring, or under tension, such as joints. As with medical tape, you may need to use benzoin, cyanoacrylate, or another adhesive to help it stick. Alternatively, wrap a bandage around it, or use additional tape.

SUTURE MATERIALS

Many items can be used as suture materials. Some are used routinely (e.g., nylon fishing line) around the world. Others must be improvised from available materials. The key is to use common sense, but don't be "picky."

Bulk Suture Material

Purchase monofilament (suture material) in rolls. If used with ordinary sewing needles, the suture materials for a single operation cost almost nothing. Purchasing prepackaged monofilament suture material costs 20,000% more than buying it in reels.[14]

Fishing Line

Often sold as "colorless fishing nylon," fishing line is about $^1/_{30}$th to $^1/_{500}$th the cost of suture material sold in bulk. (Nylon carpet thread is very similar.) It can be precut to length and sterilized on the tray with other surgical instruments.[15] It retains its strength after autoclaving, and, if translucent (uncolored) line is used, it is inert and nonallergenic once autoclaved. It provides comparable results to commercial nylon suture.[16] If employing improvised needles made from hypodermic needles (for a method to make these, see the "Suture Needles" section below in this chapter), use the correct size line (Table 22-2).

Natural Materials

Hair Tying (With Glue) for Scalp Wound Closure

Scalp lacerations <10 cm long in patients with long hair (≥3 cm) near the wound can be closed by either tying or twisting hair on opposing sides of the wound. To tie the hair, twist a few strands together on each side of the laceration. Tie them and immediately secure them with benzoin, Nobecutane wound dressing, or a similar adhesive to prevent slippage. These knots will need to be cut out of the hair after the wound heals.

An alternative is to take several strands of hair from each side of the wound, pull them across the laceration to the opposite sides, and twist them around each other—once. Immediately put a drop of cyanoacrylate at the juncture. These will not have to be removed, because the cyanoacrylate will gradually wear off. Instruct patients not to wash their hair or put petroleum hair products near the wound for 48 hours. This technique is extremely fast, cost-effective, and can be done with virtually no technical skills or equipment.[18,19]

TABLE 22-2 Fishing Line Approximating Standard Nonabsorbable Suture Sizes and Appropriate Improvised Needle Sizes

Nonabsorbable Suture Size, USP (Metric)	Diameter Limits, in mm	Fishing Line Size by Breaking Strength, in Pounds (Approximate Diameter, mm)	Uses	Minimum Improvised Syringe Needle Gauge (Inner Diameter, mm)
7-0 (0.5)	0.045-0.60	N/A	Corneas, blood vessels	N/A
6-0 (0.7)	0.070-0.099	N/A	Face, eyelids, blood vessels	31 (0.114 mm)
5-0 (1)	0.100-0.149	1 lb (0.12-0.14 mm)	Face, neck, blood vessels, plastic closures	29 (0.165 mm)
4-0 (1.5)	0.150-0.199	2-4 lb (0.15-0.20 mm)	General use—neck, hands, limbs, tendons, scalp	26 (0.241 mm)
3-0 (2)	0.200-0.249	6 lb (0.23-0.26 mm)	Limbs, trunk, scalp, bowel, over joints	24 (0.292 mm)
2-0 (3)	0.300-0.339	8-10 lb (0.30-0.33 mm)	Trunk, fascia, viscera	22 (0.394 mm)
0 (3.5)	0.350-0.399	12-14 lb (0.35-0.39 mm)	Very heavy suture—abdominal wall closure; fascia; muscle; suturing drains, tubes, and lines; bone	22 (0.394 mm)
1 (4)	0.400-0.499	15-20 lb (0.40-0.48 mm)		20 (0.584 mm)
2 (5)	0.500-0.599	25-30 lb (0.50-0.58 mm)		18 (0.838 mm)
3 and 4 (6)	0.600-0.699	N/A		18 (0.838 mm)
5 (7)	0.700-0.799	50 lb (0.70-0.77 mm)		18 (0.838 mm)

Data from Pereira and Cotton.[17]

Chicken Egg Membrane

A fresh chicken egg membrane can be used to close wounds and reduce bleeding. The membrane contains types I, V, and X collagen, retains albumen, prevents penetration of bacteria, and is essential for the egg's formation. This low-cost dressing has been used as a skin-graft donor-site dressing to relieve pain, protect the wound, and promote healing.[20] One patient used a chicken egg membrane to close a full-thickness lip laceration, stop its profuse bleeding, and allow it to heal. He removed the membrane 3 days later and did well with no other therapy.[21]

Horsehair Sutures

Black or brown hairs from the tail of a horse make excellent sutures for skin wounds. They should be washed first with soap and water and then with alcohol. When needed, they are easily sterilized in boiling water or in steam. They are not as strong as silk.[22]

Other Nontraditional Materials

Dental Floss

Frequently cited as a suture alternative, most dental floss approximates a size 0 or 00 suture. It also may be made of many different fibers (e.g., silk, nylon, or Teflon) and can be a single strand or braided.[23] This should only be used as suture material as a last resort.

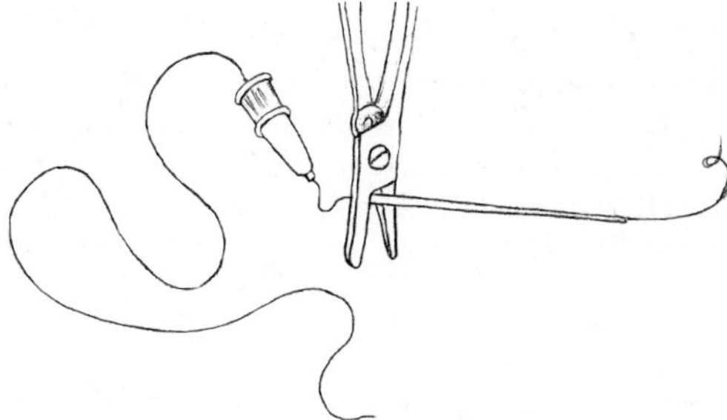

FIG. 22-1. Improvised swaged suture.

Stainless Steel Wire

Wire is often used for surgical sutures. Nonsurgical stainless steel wire can easily be sterilized and used in a similar fashion. To swag it onto a needle requires using a large-gauge hypodermic needle (Fig. 22-1).

Cotton Thread

Cotton and linen threads have long been used as the standard surgical suture. Both are easily sterilized and do not irritate the skin. If using colored thread, choose one with a color-fast dye, or else boil it long enough to extract as much of the dye as possible.[24] In austere circumstances, "use ordinary sewing cotton, No. 30, white, for the heavier work on the abdominal wall, and No. 40 or No. 50, black, for finer work on intestine or delicate tissues."[25]

Disinfecting/Sterilizing Alternative Suture Materials

Rather than sterilization, high-level disinfection is most practical for the majority of alternative suture material. Disinfecton methods include boiling them in water or soaking them in alcohol (medicinal, drinking), hydrogen peroxide, bleach, surgical or regular soapy water, or lemon juice. Some residual substances (alcohol, bleach, lemon juice) on the suture may be painful if no local anesthetic is available.

To sterilize suture materials, wrap them in foil and either use an autoclaving method (see Chapter 6) or put them in or near the coals from a fire. How well that works without destroying the suture material will vary. Wire sutures can be flame-sterilized.

Infection

While infection arising from alternative suture materials depends on the material used, it is primarily a function of wound cleaning and debridement.

Visualizing Sutures

Tan-colored suture, such as plain gut, may be difficult to see, even with good lighting. A solution is to dye the suture by pulling it between two sterile cotton-tipped applicators soaked in 2% gentian violet solution in 10% alcohol. The suture will be useable within 15 seconds. Gentian violet is a potent, fast-drying dye; take care not to touch it to anything else.[26]

SUTURE NEEDLES

A wide variety of needles with eyes to pass the suture through can be used. Use tailors' round needles in soft tissues and triangular sharpened leather (cutting) needles for fascia, tendons, etc.[27]

Suture needles can be fashioned from the appropriate-size hypodermic needles (see Table 22-2). Use a file to score the needle as close as possible to its hub and break it off. Make a loop of a fine wire (e.g., one strand of a thin braided electrical wire) and insert the two ends into the cut end of the needle. Use pliers to crimp this end and to bend the needle into a shallow arc; keep the needle's beveled end inside the arc. After sterilizing the needle, thread the suture material through the loop.[28] In a similar manner, bend the end of a large standard suture needle to 90 degrees about one-third of the distance from the tip to use in tight spaces when smaller needles are unavailable.[29]

Another method to convert a hypodermic needle into a suture needle is to pass the suture through the needle from the sharp end. Once it appears at the needle's hub, hold the suture in place and break off the hub by repeatedly bending it (Fig. 22-1). Then pull the suture through the needle so that only a small amount remains within the needle. Crimp the "hub" end of the needle to fix the suture in place. Because all this can be done under sterile conditions at the patient's bedside, the "swaged" suture can be used immediately.[30] Alternatively, prepare several in advance, wrap the suture around a piece of cardboard, and autoclave them en masse.[31] Note that it may not be possible to use the newer safety needles (those designed to prevent personnel from being inadvertently stuck) for some of the improvised techniques involving needles described in this book.

If the available suture material is insufficient for use with a swaged needle, insert the piece of suture into the sharp end of an injection needle. Pass the needle through the tissue while holding on to the free end. Retrieve the suture's needle end and tie the two ends together. If necessary, repeat this process with multiple suture pieces for each suture. Physicians in some parts of the world (such as Córdoba, Argentina) preferentially use this method for most of their wound repairs and minor surgeries.

NEEDLE HOLDERS

Use small needle-nosed pliers, locking pliers, or similar tools as needle holders. They can be sterilized in an autoclave, although any rubber handle(s) may need to be removed first. While any of these can be used in austere circumstances, the best result will be obtained when they fit the clinician's hand and are as similar to regular needle holders as possible. These tools may work better than the straight hemostat that is often used.

SCALPELS

In desperate circumstances, perform surgery with any clean, preferably sterile, sharp object. This could include the lid from a can partially folded over to form a non-sharp handle or a piece of glass. Nearly any piece of metal can be sharpened to act as a knife. (For an example, see how well prisoners make "homemade" knives.) To hone the blade, not just the tip, to surgical sharpness takes special metal, tools, and expertise.

The best option, if this is the route you must take, is to start with a cutting knife and sharpen it as well as possible. In extreme circumstances, these may even become the routine surgical instruments, as happened periodically during World War II. Dr. J. Markowitz, the surgeon at Chungkai jungle hospital camp in Thailand, crowded with 7000 POWs, performed 1200 operations using "a carpenter's saw and a few butcher knives, sharpened and re-sharpened."[2]

A frequent situation is to have a scalpel blade, but no handle. (In most places around the world, they are still packaged separately.) In those cases, clamp the base of the blade with a straight clamp, such as a needle holder, and use the clamp as a handle. For increased stability, insert one jaw of the clamp through the hole in the blade. Alternatively, clamp the blade with needle-nosed pliers or similar tools; these are often found on universal tools (e.g., Leatherman, Victorinox, SOG, Gerber). Even easier, improvise a scalpel handle by bending the cover of a scalpel blade back to expose the blade. Then bend the wrapper around the proximal blade to form a (short) handle (Fig. 22-2).[32]

Surgical-grade scalpels with blades of various sizes can be easily made using a razor blade (disposable multiblade, single flat blade, or other), cyanoacrylate (i.e., Superglue or Dermabond), and a flat piece of metal to use as a handle. The handle must be flat for the blade to adhere. The flat handles of eating utensils (spoons seem to be the easiest handles to hold) or the back of a butter or similar knife may work best. Use old-fashioned flat razor blades, if available. They are very inexpensive (~1¢ US/blade) and make excellent scalpels, even for delicate intraocular ophthalmic surgery. The best way to make a surgical knife is to hold pieces of the blade with a razor blade breaker, no longer common in industrialized countries, but sold and used internationally. Carbon steel blades work better than stainless steel blades but, to retain their

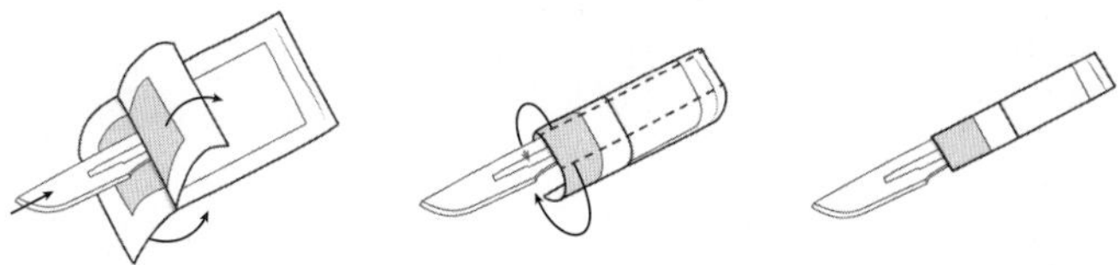

FIG. 22-2. Making a scalpel handle for a blade from the packaging.

sharpness, they must be chemically sterilized rather than steam-autoclaved or boiled. One razor blade provides up to six surgical knives, three blades from each edge (Fig. 22-3).[33]

To use multiblade disposable razors, carefully separate the blade from its holder by using a tool to bend one end, which will make the blades pop out (Fig. 22-4). Then put a few drops of cyanoacrylate on both the blade and the utensil/holder. Experience shows that you may need to wait about 10 minutes before the larger blades are firmly fixed. Be sure that the blade extends over the side of the handle and that the blade is parallel to the other side for better control of the scalpel.

Reusing scalpels is, of course, an option. Cleaning, sterilizing, and reusing equipment is discussed in Chapter 6.

SKIN HOOKS

Skin hooks are the best way to handle wound tissue with the least amount of trauma. They are also excellent for retrieving and stabilizing torn tendons during repair.[34] Small instruments, they are frequently unavailable when needed, but can be easily improvised (Fig. 22-5).

A straight hemostat or a small-gauge needle bent at the tip and attached to a 1- to 10-cc syringe (depending on the size of the clinician's hand) makes an excellent skin hook. Using a hemostat, fashion a double skin hook by clamping the hubs of two bent needles; to have more space between the ends, cross two needles, and clamp them where they cross.[35] Use a 30-gauge needle when handling fine tissues, such as during shave excisions and biopsies.[36] A skin hook can also be made by unbending a safety pin so that the two "limbs" on each side of the spring form a straight line; put a small bend in the tip and sterilize it.[37]

MAYO SAFETY PIN

Used to hold and organize any surgical instruments with finger holes during sterilization and storage, these pins can be fashioned from heavy wire, such as a clothes hanger (Fig. 22-6).

SPONGES/LAP PADS/GAUZE SUBSTITUTES

The way to increase the number of useable gauze bandages may be to reuse them, as was done in a POW camp during World War II. As the physician-prisoners wrote, "Due to the scarcity of surgical gauze it was necessary to save and wash bandages and dressings for use over and over again."[1] An acceptable alternative is to cut up and sterilize toilet paper or, even better, paper towels to use as swabs.[38]

While gauze is often called a "sponge," especially when folded, if gauze is in short supply, actual sponges can be used instead. Cellulose surgical sponges are excellent as absorbent dressings over draining wounds or fistulas, either in place of gauze or as wound and graft dressings.

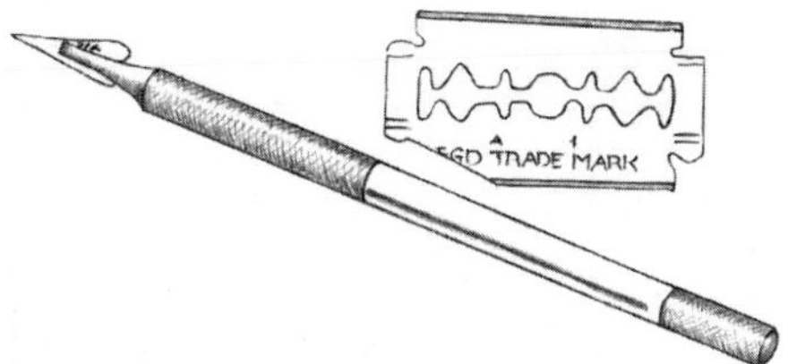

FIG. 22-3. Scalpel made from razor blade.

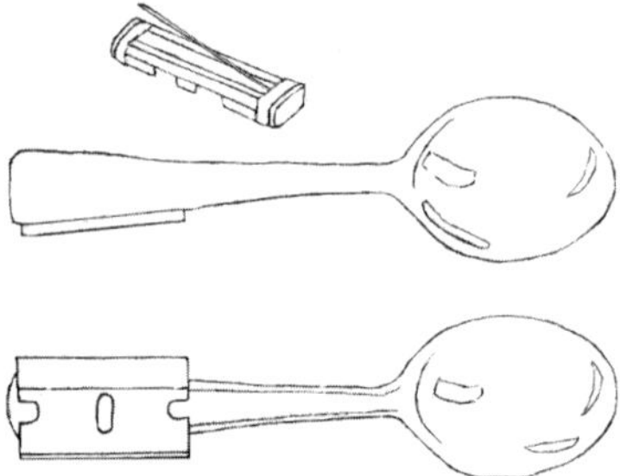

FIG. 22-4. Disposable razor blades fashioned into scalpel.

Sponges can be made by cutting 1-cm cubes from long strips of cellulose, which is widely available, often as packaging material. Another alternative is to cut up an old polyurethane foam mattress or cushion. The sponges should be sterilized before use. Do not discard them after use, but rather, wash and re-sterilize them. They often can be used three or four times.[38-40]

To make laparotomy pads, fold linen sheets into several layers, sew them to the size you want, and then sterilize them. If thick gauze is at a premium, sew enough pieces of 20 cm by 25 cm gauze together to make a 5-mm layer. Attach a tape to one end so that it can be clamped with a hemostat and won't disappear in the wound. Lap pads are a convenient and economical way of washing and reusing gauze.[38]

CAUTERY

Disposable microcautery units, although intended for one-time use, may be used for multiple surgeries—up to 20 ophthalmic surgeries, for example. Note that chemical or steam sterilization ruins the instrument. Once it has been used, hold the contaminated handle with a sterile towel and clean the tip with alcohol-soaked cotton.[41]

Fashion a makeshift cautery from a platinum-tipped hollow metal tube attached by a hose to an atomizer bottle of benzene. To use it, first heat the tip over an alcohol lamp and keep it hot by infusing the tip with benzene.[41]

SUCKER

Quickly assemble a microsurgical sucker by cutting a small wedge from the end of suction tubing and inserting the tubing end into the barrel of a 5-mL syringe. Attach an intravenous (IV) catheter (without the needle) to the syringe's Luer lock connection. Use as small a size as needed and begin sucking.[42]

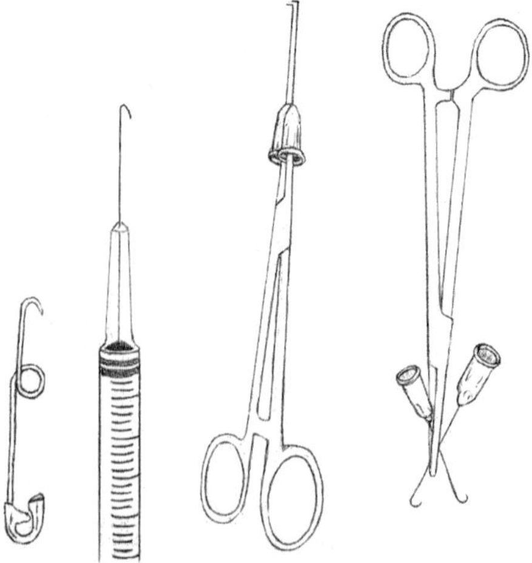

FIG. 22-5. Improvised skin hooks.

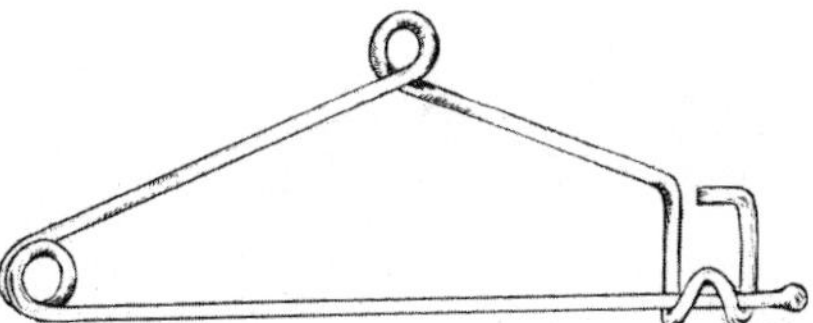

FIG. 22-6. Mayo safety pin.

PETROLEUM JELLY GAUZE

To make sterile "petroleum jelly" gauze for wound dressings, spread petroleum jelly onto layers of ordinary gauze. Place them in a watertight can and autoclave them.[43]

RETRACTORS

Self-retaining retractors are excellent tools to have when working alone or with inexperienced assistants. These retractors can make doing an open peritoneal lavage, for example, much faster. Bend stiff metal rods into the form shown in Fig. 22-7. Use 3-mm rods for minor surgery and heavier rods for major wounds.[27] To work on more delicate tissues, fashion them from lighter material, such as paper clips.

Unscrubbed "Off Table" Surgical Retraction

When a small surgical field, cramped conditions, or a scarcity of sterile gowns makes it difficult to have assistants help with retraction during surgery, use remote retraction. Tie a sterile gauze or an abdominal pad to a handheld retractor (Fig. 22-8) and hand it to an assistant standing outside the sterile field. The surgeon places the retractor while the assistant pulls.[44]

TWEEZERS

Tweezers, or "pickups," for surgical procedures can easily be fashioned from pieces of the metal strapping used to secure boxes to pallets. These straps come in various widths and can be cut to any length. Fold them with a slight bulge in the end to avoid having them break at the fold after repeated use (Fig. 22-9). File down the ends to as sharp a point as you need.[45] Alternatively, two pieces can be riveted together, although that takes more effort. These instruments can be autoclaved repeatedly.

Tiny foreign bodies in the skin, such as a thorn, can be removed using the hinge of a pair of metal eyeglasses. Haywood Hall, MD, president of PACEMD, explains that you simply close one of the "temples," the long part extending to the ears, as you would when storing the glasses. Then place the hinged area over the foreign body and open the glasses as you would to wear them. The hinge area closes around the foreign body like a pair of tweezers would. (Personal communication, February 6, 2007.)

IMPROVISED CURETTES FROM CLAMPS

Fashion curettes, such as those needed for uterine curettage or to extract a placenta, by dismantling and reshaping a sponge holder. Separate the two halves of the sponge holder and sharpen the end, forming the curette.[44]

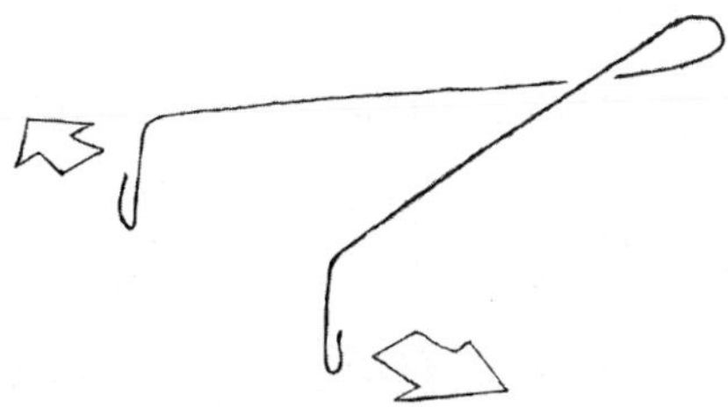

FIG. 22-7. Lightweight self-retaining retractor.

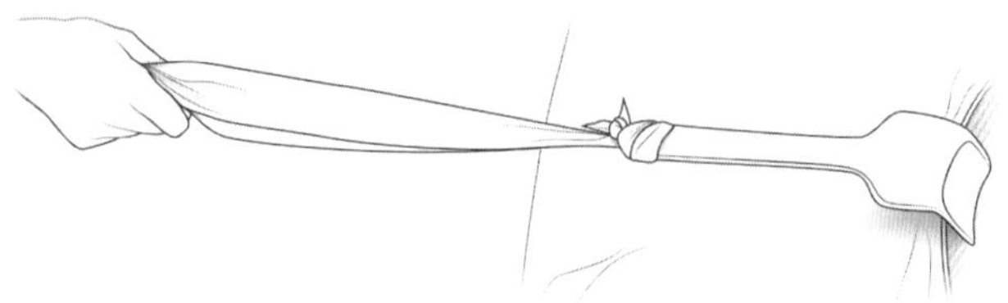

FIG. 22-8. A lap pad is tied to a Fritsch retractor for remote assistance.

WOUND BOLSTERS—URINARY CATHETER OR NASOGASTRIC TUBE

Bolsters distribute suture tension over skin and subcutaneous tissue when wounds do not close easily (usually laparotomy incisions). To make wound bolsters, cut two equal lengths of urine catheter or nasogastric tubing that match the incision length. Place them parallel and equidistant from the edge on each side of the incision, securing them with percutaneous vertical mattress sutures (Fig. 22-10). Place sufficient vertical mattress sutures along the tubing, both to hold the tubing in place and to provide maximum distribution of wound closure tension. Remove the bolsters several days in advance of the other sutures to minimize reversible cutaneous indentations and epithelialized suture tracts.[46]

MARKING SURGICAL SITES

Marking vital skin landmarks to guide incisions and key sutures avoids losing them when local *anesthesia alters topography*. If commercially available sterile ink marking pens are unavailable, use nonsterile markers before creating a sterile field. Clinicians can use ballpoint or felt tip pens, hypodermic needles, an artist's brush, or a cotton-tipped applicator stick to scratch the skin or to use ink. A variety of instruments can be used with a pre-inked marking pad saturated with gentian violet. Once a sterile field is established, a way to mark additional points or lines is to place an applicator stick or a clean surgical instrument (such as the rounded edge of a curette) in the wound and use the blood to draw new marks. The blood dries quickly and clearly delineates the new lines.[47]

STERILE DRAPES

Sterile drapes can easily be fashioned from sheets that have been autoclaved. An alternative that disinfects rather than sterilizes is to hang them in sunlight. (See Chapter 6, "Dressings and Other Textiles," for more information.)

For small procedures, such as lacerations and lumbar punctures in neonates, use the inside of a sterile glove package.

SURGICAL TABLE

Nearly any surface can be and has been used as a surgical table. Surgeons once routinely cleared the kitchen or dining room table for operations done in homes.[48] During World War II, POW surgeons performed an emergency appendectomy using a ship's "hatch cover as operating table and a mosquito bar for protection against insects."[1] Disaster teams use cot-like stretchers placed on rigid metal sawhorses.[49]

COTTON-TIPPED APPLICATORS

For safety and to assist with surgical procedures when fingers may be too bulky and cumbersome, use cotton-tipped applicators (e.g., Q-tips) to stabilize tissues, apply counter-traction,

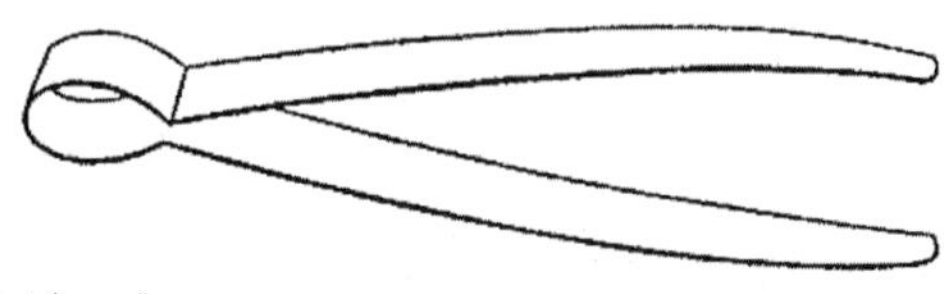

FIG. 22-9. Surgical "pickups."

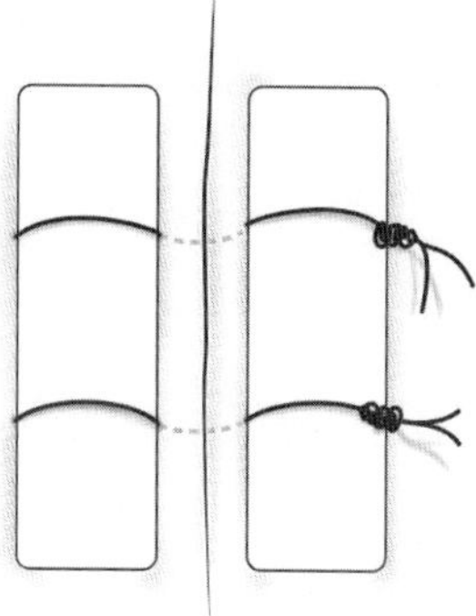

FIG. 22-10. Using tubing as wound bolsters.

improve visualization, and provide local pressure and hemostasis. When using cautery, roll a dry cotton-tipped applicator over the operative field to identify the offending vessel.[50]

DISPOSAL OF SMALL SURGICAL WASTE

One way to minimize exposure to infectious surgical waste after suturing or other small procedures is to enclose it in the clinician's glove. When the procedure is completed, collect the non-sharp surgical waste (e.g., gauze, cotton balls, disposable drapes) in the palm of one hand and make a fist around the material. Use the other hand to pull off and invert the glove over the waste; then, holding the waste within that glove, pull off and invert the second glove over the first. The waste material is now enclosed in two gloves. Not only does this protect others (an inverted glove effectively contains infectious agents for several hours), but it also reduces the time spent cleaning up after procedures.[51]

PROTECTION FROM INJECTION BACKSPRAY

Backspray from injecting or irrigating wounds poses a significant blood-borne pathogen risk to the provider. In addition to personal protective equipment, a barrier to this spray is helpful. Make one using a surgical mask with an attached face shield. After cutting the ties off the mask, center the small opening between the clear eye shield and the mask over the wound. Inject through this opening and the mask will block the spray (Fig. 22-11).[52]

PROTECTION AGAINST "SHARPS"

Suture needles frequently injure health care personnel. To minimize the risk of accidental injury, put a small thin magnet on the corner of surgical/suture trays before they are sterilized. When not in use, place the needle on the magnet. An added benefit is that the needle does not get lost on the tray between uses.[53]

To help prevent needle sticks when suturing, use the cap from an 18-gauge needle, rather than a finger, to buttress the other side of a wound when passing a needle through the skin. Even better and safer, use a small syringe barrel with the plunger removed (Fig. 22-12).[54,55] Alternatively, bolster the skin with the back end of a pair of tweezers (pick-ups) or a hemostat.

NEEDLE SAFETY

A sharps container may not be readily available when you have finished using a needle. To avoid sticking yourself or colleagues with the needle, turn the needle around on the needle driver so that the needle's pointed end faces the handle and is locked between the instrument's jaws.[56] Another option is to lay the shot glass often found on a surgical tray on its side and put needles into the glass.

Safely recap plain injection needles by laying the cap on a flat surface and, without touching the cap, guiding the needle into it. Alternatively, wedge the needle cap into a forceps, with the opening facing up. Put the needle in and snap it into place (Fig. 22-13).[57]

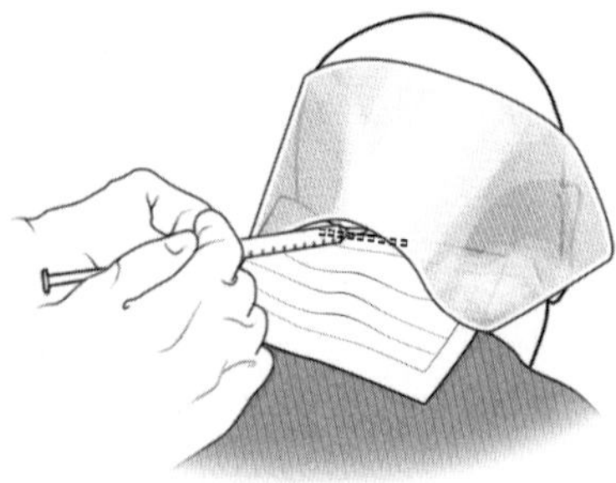

FIG. 22-11. Mask on patient used to limit spray from local injection.

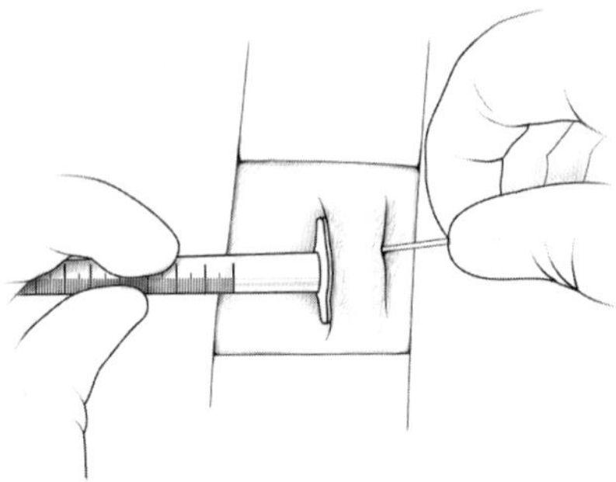

FIG. 22-12: Use a small syringe barrel with the plunger removed to keep fingers away from needle point.

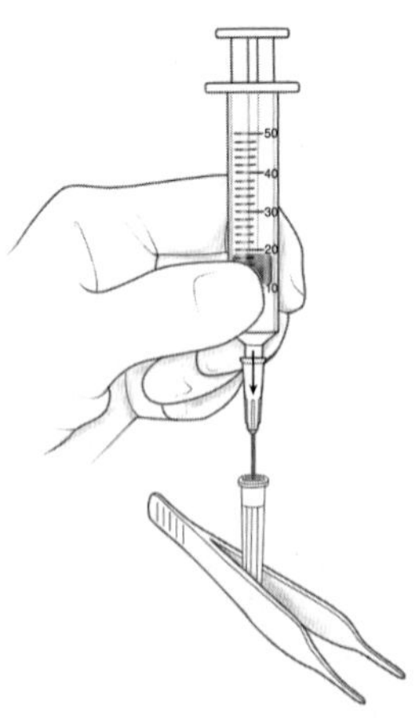

FIG. 22-13. Safely recapping an injection needle.

REFERENCES

1. Report from Lt. Col. John R. Mamerow to American Prisoner of War Information Bureau, April 12, 1945. Supplied by the US Army Medical Department Museum, Ft. Sam Houston, TX, used with permission.
2. Markowitz J. *I Was a Knife, Fork and Spoon Surgeon*. COFEPOW. http://www.cofepow.org.uk/pages/medical_knifeformspoon.html. Accessed September 14, 2006.
3. Lerner R, Binur NS. Current status of surgical adhesives. *J Surg Res*. 1990;48:165-181.
4. Leggat PA, Smith DR, Kedjarune U. Surgical applications of cyanoacrylate adhesives: a review of toxicity. *ANZ J Surg*. 2007;77:209-213.
5. Husum H, Ang SC, Fosse E. *War Surgery: Field Manual*. Penang, Malaysia: Third World Network; 1995:70.
6. Collins JA, James PM, Levitsky SA, et al. Cyanoacrylate adhesives as topical hemostatic aids. II. Clinical use in seven combat casualties. *Surgery*. 1969;65(2):260-263.
7. Farion KJ, Russel KF, Osmond MH, et al. Tissue adhesives for traumatic lacerations in children and adults. *Cochrane Database Syst Rev*. 2002;(3):CD003326.
8. Davis KP, Derlet RW. Cyanoacrylate glues for wilderness and remote travel medical care. *Wild Environ Med*. 2013;24(1):67-74.
9. Bain M, Peterson EA, Murphy RX. Dermabond®-assisted primary closure of atrophic skin. Presented at American Society of Plastic Surgeons Annual Meeting, October 28, 2007. In: Evans J. Cutaneous adhesive effectively helps close wounds on thin skin. *ACEP News*. 2008;27(5):6.
10. Chintamani SV, Mehrotra M, Kulshreshtha P, et al. 'Superglue': a novel approach in the management of faecal fistulae. *Trop Doct*. 2007;37:147-148.
11. Farion KJ, Osmond MH, Harling I, et al. Tissue adhesives for traumatic lacerations: a systematic review of randomized controlled trials. *Acad Emerg Med*. 2003;10:110-118.
12. Yamamoto LG. Preventing adverse events and outcomes encountered using Dermabond. *Am J Emerg Med*. 2000;18(4):512-517.
13. Tactical Medical Solutions. *Improvised Medicine, Part II: The Safety Pin*. (video) tacmedsolutions.com. Accessed July 1, 2015.
14. King M, Bewes P, Cairns J, et al, eds. *Primary Surgery, Vol. 1: Non-trauma*. Oxford, UK: Oxford Medical Publishing; 1990:43.
15. Bewes P. Abdominal closure. *Trop Doct*. 2000;30:39-41.
16. Freudenberg S, Nyonde M, Mkony C, et al. Fishing line suture: cost-saving alternative for atraumatic intracutaneous skin closure—randomized clinical trial in Rwanda. *World J Surg*. 2004;28:421-424.
17. Periera EAC, Cotton MH. Using fishing line for suturing. *Trop Doct*. 2006;36:155-156.
18. Officer C. Scalp lacerations in children. *Aust Fam Physician*. 1981;10(12):970.
19. Ong ME, Coyle D, Lim SH, et al. Cost-effectiveness of hair apposition technique compared with standard suturing in scalp lacerations. *Ann Emerg Med*. 2005;46:237-242.
20. Yang JY, Chuang SS, Yang WG, et al. Egg membrane as a new biological dressing in split-thickness skin graft donor sites: a preliminary clinical evaluation. *Chang Gung Med J*. 2003;26:153-159.
21. Zadik Y. Self-treatment of full-thickness traumatic lip laceration with chicken egg shell membrane. *Wild Environ Med*. 2007;18:230-231.
22. Foote EM. *A Text-book of Minor Surgery*. New York, NY: Appleton; 1912:693.
23. Dorfer C, Book M, Staehle HJ. *Schweiz Monatsschr Zahnmed*. [Microscopic studies of the structures of different dental floss types; German.] 1993;103(9):1092-1102.
24. Foote EM. *A Text-book of Minor Surgery*. New York, NY: Appleton; 1912:694.
25. Perrill CV. Surgery, simplified and improvised. *Christian Nurse (Mysore)*. 1969;224:8-12.
26. Albertini JG. Surgical pearl: gentian violet-dyed sutures improve intraoperative visualization. *J Am Acad Derm*. 2001;45(3):453-455.
27. Husum H, Ang SC, Fosse E. *War Surgery: Field Manual*. Penang, Malaysia: Third World Network; 1995:71.
28. Remis R. Improvisation of medical equipment in developing countries. *Trop Doct*. 1983;13:89.
29. Hartman CL, Boyce SM, Huang CC. Surgical pearl: the "fishhook" needle technique: a solution to the large needle, small space dilemma. *J Am Acad Derm*. 2005;53(1):144-146.
30. Freudenberg S, Samel S, Sturm J, et al. The improvised atraumatic suture: a cost-reducing technique, not only for the tropics? *Trop Doct*. 2001;31(3):166-167.
31. Van Oosterwyk, Hodges AA. Atraumatic sutures can be made locally. *Trop Doct*. 2004;34:95-96.

32. Tactical Medical Solutions. *Improvised Medicine, Part I: The Mini Scalpel Handle.* (video) tacmedsolutions.com. Accessed July 1, 2015.
33. Schwab L. *Primary Eye Care in Developing Nations.* Oxford, UK: Oxford University Press; 1987: 141-142.
34. Morris RJ, Martin DL. The use of skin hooks and hypodermic needles in tendon surgery. *J Hand Surg Br.* 1993;18(1):33-34.
35. Peled IJ. Improvised double skin hooks. *Ann Plastic Surg.* 1982;9(6):516.
36. King DF, King LA. The 30-gauge needle: a versatile surgical instrument. *J Am Acad Dermatol.* 1986; 142:280.
37. Fischl RA. An improvised skin hook. *Br J Plastic Surg.* 1966;19:391.
38. King M, Bewes P, Cairns J, et al, eds. *Primary Surgery, Vol. 1: Non-trauma.* Oxford, UK: Oxford Medical Publishing; 1990:10.
39. Schwab L. *Primary Eye Care in Developing Nations.* Oxford, UK: Oxford University Press; 1987:147.
40. Weston PM. Simple resources for essential surgery. *Trop Doct.* 1986;16(1):25-30.
41. Schwab L. *Primary Eye Care in Developing Nations.* Oxford, UK: Oxford University Press; 1987:143.
42. Batchelor AGG. An improvised microsurgical sucker. *Br J Plast Surg.* 1984;37:406.
43. King M. *Primary Surgery, Vol. 2: Trauma.* Oxford, UK: Oxford University Press; 1987:81.
44. Lin G, Lavon H, Gelfond R, Abargel A, Merin O. Hard times call for creative solutions: medical improvisations at the Israel Defense Forces field hospital in Haiti. *Am J Disas Med.* 2009;5(3):188-192.
45. *UNESCO Source Book for Science Teaching.* Paris, France: United Nations Educational, Scientific and Cultural Organization; 1956:37.
46. Salasche SJ, Williams WL, Caradonna SA, Skidmore RA. Surgical pearl: the red rubber Robinson bolster in cutaneous surgery. *J Am Acad Derm.* 1999;41(1):78-80.
47. Adams BB, Gloster H. Surgical pearl: a unique surgical marker. *J Am Acad Derm.* 1999;41(3): 464-465.
48. Olson LM. *Improvised Equipment in the Home Care of the Sick.* Philadelphia, PA: W.B. Saunders; 1928.
49. Owens PJ, Forgione A, Briggs S. Challenges of international disaster relief: use of a deployable rapid assembly shelter and surgical hospital. *Disaster Manag Response.* 2005;3(1):11-16.
50. Orengo I, Salasche SJ. Surgical pearl: the cotton-tipped applicator—the ever-ready, multipurpose superstar. *J Am Acad Derm.* 1994;31(4):658-660.
51. Kimyai-Asadi A, Jih MH, Goldberg LH, Friedman PM. Surgical pearl: a rapid sanitary technique for surgical waste disposal. *J Am Acad Derm.* 2004;50(4):642-643.
52. Freed J, Smith J. Surgical pearl: a novel technique to contain the backspray from intralesional injections. *J Am Acad Derm.* 2006;54(1):151.
53. Ali SO, Vogel PS. Surgical pearl: simple method for controlling surgical sharps. *J Am Acad Derm.* 2006;54(5):878-879.
54. Nelson BP. Making straight needles a little safer: a technique to keep fingers from harm's way. *J Emerg Med.* 2008;34:195-197.
55. Bauer S, Tauferner D, Carlson D. Improving straight needle safety: an alternate method. *J Emerg Med.* 2011;41(1):e19-e20.
56. Dixon BK. Preventive practices can blunt suture needle sticks. *ACEP News.* 2008;27(5):6.
57. Katz KH, Maloney ME. Surgical pearl: safely recapping needles during surgery. *J Am Acad Derm.* 2002;46(2):294-295.

23 Surgery: Non-Trauma and Environmental Injuries

AUSTERE SURGICAL SITUATIONS

According to RS Bransford, a Western surgeon working in a Sub-Saharan hospital, "The OR [operating room] is only marginally clean. You can see through the cloth you put on your operating table. Most in the OR, including their doctors, are marginally safe with regard to sterile technique." (Personal communication, January 21, 2007.)

In 2007, *Anaesthesia* published [2007;62(suppl 1):54-60] the following composite description of an OR in a very poor country, written by Drs. BA McCormick and RJ Eltringham, anesthesiologists with considerable developing-world experience:

> The general theatre has a cement floor painted red and polished, with pale green-washed walls. The windows are open because of the stifling heat and flies hover overhead, occasionally coming to rest on the surgeon's mask or even the patient himself. The patient lies on an archaic-looking operating table. One end is supported on a trolley that prevents its faulty tilt mechanism from allowing it to collapse to the floor. The surgeon is calmly rejecting numerous drapes that are riddled with holes and can serve no purpose in maintaining a sterile field. Normal saline is running in through an 18G cannula that the patient's family were asked to buy from the local pharmacy; the best we could offer from the department stores was a 22G. The surgeon is keen to start operating as the procedure was delayed for 2 h waiting for supplies of sterile and nonsterile rubber gloves to arrive. Shortages of all consumables have been a major problem since additional financial support to the hospital and medical school from a European government programme was withdrawn 6 months ago. It appears that the infrastructure for procurement, storage and delivery of essential items dwindled during this time of plenty, when supplies were 'parachuted in' via alternative routes.
>
> John administers 50 mg of pethidine—this may be the last analgesic the patient receives until the unpredictable visit of the night matron to the ward in 9 h time. The surgeon asks for some antibiotics to be given and we enquire whether he would like chloramphenicol, gentamicin or both, as this is all the pharmacy can currently supply to us. The ex-pat surgeon nods at his lockable trolley, packed with privately procured goods for use in this theatre only. A sense of irony hits me as I reach past his iPod and speakers for a vial of cefotaxime, taking care not to interrupt the tones of Steve Harley and Cockney Rebel.

Essential Surgical and Trauma Care

The surgeons who run the international "Primary Trauma Care" course, which is taught in many developing countries, take issue with using the normal Advanced Trauma Life Support (ATLS) methods in those regions. They wrote that "the reality of trauma management in developing countries is, however, substantially different. The reasons for these differences are multifactorial, but they include geographical factors, relative lack of resources, funding, manpower and education. . . . The [ATLS] so-called 'golden hour' must be extended into the 'silver day' or the 'bronze week.'" They also note that the goals of transferring a stabilized patient on a firm stretcher for definitive care and of treating people in intensive care for complications from trauma are "often unrealistic in the developing world with minimal resources."[1]

The World Health Organization (WHO) lists what they consider essential to treat abdominal (Table 23-1) and chest (Table 23-2) injuries worldwide, varying with four levels of hospital capabilities (described in Chapter 5).

TABLE 23-1 WHO Essentials to Treat Abdominal Injuries

Resources	Facility Level			
	Basic	GP	Specialist	Tertiary Care
Clinical assessment	E	E	E	E
Diagnostic peritoneal lavage	I	D	E	E
Ultrasonography (pleural cavity for air and fluid; abdomen for fluid; heart for pericardial effusion)	I	D	D	D
Skills and equipment for intermediate laparotomy	I	PR	E	E
Skills and equipment for advanced laparotomy	I	I	E	E
CT	I	I	D	D

Abbreviations: CT, computerized axial tomography; D, desirable; E, essential resources; GP, general practitioner's hospital; I, irrelevant; PR, possibly required.

Adapted with permission from Mock et al.[2]

Should You Operate?

Clinicians may find themselves in situations in which they must perform a critical procedure with which they are not completely comfortable. In these situations, "time is the critical factor. Basic life-saving surgery can be done with simple standard equipment under intravenous (IV) ketamine anesthesia. The procedures must not be delayed and should be done by the surgeon at hand on dying patients or dying limbs when the alternative to nonintervention may be death."[4] The surgeon should also not be deterred when surgery is required urgently, but a trained anesthetist is unavailable.[5]

The following guidelines, while primarily for surgeons, also apply to clinicians doing other invasive procedures on patients, such as placing drainage tubes, intubating or placing a surgical airway, and placing central or intraosseous (IO) vascular access lines. The real skill of a medical practitioner is making the decision about when to do a procedure; nearly anyone can be taught to actually do the procedures. These questions, adapted from King and colleagues, can help you make the decision[6]:

1. What happens if you don't do the procedure?
2. How difficult is the procedure? Will you be able to do it?
3. How safe is the procedure in your hands? What disasters may occur? Can you deal with them?

TABLE 23-2 WHO Essentials to Treat Chest Injuries

Resources	Facility Level			
	Basic	GP	Specialist	Tertiary Care
Adequate pain control for chest injuries/rib fractures	D	E	E	E
Respiratory therapy for chest injuries/rib fractures	I	E	E	E
Rib block or intrapleural block	I	PR	E	E
Skills and equipment for intermediate thoracotomy	I	I	D	E
Autotransfusion from chest tubes	I	D	D	D
Epidural anesthesia for pain control	I	I	D	D
Skills and equipment for advanced thoracotomy	I	I	I	D

Abbreviations: D, desirable; E, essential resources; GP, general practitioner's hospital; I, irrelevant; PR, possibly required.

Adapted with permission from Mock et al.[3]

4. Do you have the necessary equipment and staff to do the procedure?
5. Are you inclined to do procedures too readily—or not readily enough?

Improvised Surgery

If surgery will be performed in austere circumstances, the clinician must understand that "this is minimum-level surgery and you have to improvise.... Select an assistant for the surgery. Instruct him on the need to keep everything sterile, and not to touch anything without your explicit permission. His main function is to provide manual retraction in the wound."[7]

Surgical Location

Surgery can be and has been performed in many settings. If there are several locations to choose from, consider factors such as lighting, space where equipment is located, temperature, and ventilation in relation to the type of surgery, assistants, etc. Operating outdoors provides light from the sun; in addition, it may actually lessen the chance of infection. If operations are being performed with non-vented volatile anesthetics (e.g., open-drop ether), fresh air quickly dilutes the gases so that the surgical team is not affected.

A concern with operating outside, however, is the ambient temperature. This may be a significant factor with young or elderly patients who cannot easily regulate their body temperatures. It may also affect patients with extensive burns, whose body cavities are open for a prolonged period, or who have suffered significant trauma. A rule-of-thumb is that basic lifesaving surgery with severe bleeding should not last >1 hour to prevent hypothermia.[8] Insects, inclement weather, and the onset of darkness also may limit the ability to operate in the open.

Cleanliness

Patients who survive a thoracotomy done in the emergency department (ED) have the same or lower incidence of infection than patients whose thoracotomies were done in the OR. Sterility is important, but it is the time the patient is open that matters most in terms of infection.

Even so, it is harder to maintain total sterility when operating outside the OR; you will have to be prepared for minimal sterility.

"Scrubbing Up"

Surgery may need to be done bare-handed. If so, it is best if the surgeon does not have an open wound on the hand or arm, to avoid either contracting or transmitting an infection. This, of course, may not be possible. Try to scrub with ordinary soap and water for 10 minutes prior to surgery.[9,10]

In less-austere circumstances, clean tap water (not sterile water, as has been required in some countries) is more than adequate for scrubbing before surgery. Rather than using special soaps and sterile brushes, gently rub the hands and forearms under tap water with a standard disinfecting soap (e.g., 7.5% povidone iodine or chlorhexidine gluconate). Using a quick-drying alcohol-based disinfectant scrub as the final step may be helpful. The faucets should be kept clean, and the water's chloride level should be >0.1 ppm.[11]

Using nonsterile gloves out of a box for wound repair (not surgery) in immunocompetent patients has an equivalent risk of wound infection as does using sterile gloves. The caveats are that the clinician must wash his or her hands before—and, for safety, after—the repair and that the box of gloves must be kept dry between uses. Damp glove boxes may become contaminated with fungus. While comfort in austere circumstances is not a huge issue, some clinicians may find working with poorly fitting nonsterile gloves to be awkward.[12]

Telesurgery

Modern telecommunication allows clinicians who have never done a procedure to do it under audio, and sometimes even video, guidance from more experienced clinicians at a remote location. This technology is still not used as frequently as it might be. On occasion, however, the use of telemedicine in austere situations has expended resources that could have been used more productively elsewhere; this situation must be avoided.[13,14] See Chapter 3 for a further discussion of telemedicine.

ABDOMEN

Bowel obstructions are common and it is tempting to see if they will respond to time and non-operative measures. However, waiting >3 days to operate increases these patients' morbidity and postoperative hospitalization.[15]

Cholecystitis and Appendicitis

When imaging, laboratory, and surgical resources are limited, practicing "elegant" medicine involves using only those resources that are absolutely necessary. That means making diagnoses on history and physical examination alone.

Cholecystitis

Clinical findings may help you decide who needs further evaluation or intervention in patients with suspected cholecystitis. Table 23-3 ranks them in order of their helpfulness in making a correct diagnosis.[16] If the patient has a Murphy's sign (and still has a gallbladder), this is the person who should get the ultrasound rather than laboratory tests. Confusing for many clinicians, the tenderness of Murphy's sign may actually be located in the epigastrium, rather than further laterally. In the absence of evidence for acute cholecystitis, unrelieved emesis or pain, biliary obstruction, or perforation, treat the patient with analgesics and have the patient return if symptoms do not resolve.

Appendicitis

Right-lower-quadrant pain is a very strong predictor of appendicitis in adults, with a likelihood ratio of having appendicitis of 7.3 to 8.5. It is also an excellent predictor in older children. Independently, fever, anorexia, nausea, and vomiting are poor predictors of appendicitis in both adults and children. Rebound and the psoas sign have an intermediate reliability in both groups.

The MANTRELS scoring system, also known as the Alvarado Score, helps determine if a child has appendicitis. Table 23-4 lists the factors (MANTRELS is a mnemonic for these) and their values for this simple score. While it uses a white blood cell count and a differential as two of its parameters, the other six factors come from the clinical history and physical examination. The system provides between a 3.8 and 5.0 positive likelihood ratio that the child will have appendicitis if the score is ≥7, and between a 0.09 and 0.40 likelihood ratio that no appendicitis exists if the score is <7.[17] In a pediatric and adult Nepalese population, the score's sensitivity for a diagnosis of "sure appendicitis" was 94%, the specificity was 91%, the positive predictive value was 96%, and it had a negative predictive value of 87%.[18] When a leukocyte count is unavailable, omit it from the MANTRELS score. In that case, the scores will range from 0 to 9, with scores <4 reportedly having a very low risk of appendicitis. However, this modified test is less sensitive in excluding appendicitis (72%) than is clinical judgment.[19]

While appendectomy, rather than antibiotics, remains the treatment of choice,[20] if surgery is not an immediate option, treat presumed appendicitis with antibiotics alone.[21] Delaying surgery for most adult patients with presumed appendicitis does not significantly alter their morbidity or mortality, but does slightly increase their postoperative hospital stay. The highest risks when using this treatment course are in women and the elderly, who may have other serious intra-abdominal pathology that the antibiotics may mask and not treat.[22]

TABLE 23-3 Clinical Findings in Cholecystitis

Factor	LR	Sensitivity	Specificity
Murphy's sign	2.8	0.65	0.87
Emesis	1.5	0.71	0.53
Fever	1.5	0.35	0.80
RUQ tenderness	1.6	0.77	0.54
Rebound	1.0	0.30	0.68

Abbreviations: LR, likelihood ratio; RUQ, right upper quadrant.

TABLE 23-4 The MANTRELS (Alvarado) Appendicitis Score

Symptom	Score
Migration of pain to the right lower quadrant	1
Anorexia	1
Nausea/Vomiting	1
Tenderness in the right lower quadrant	2
Rebound pain	1
Elevation of temperature (≥37.3°C)	1
Leukocytosis (WBC >10,000/μL)	2
Shift of WBC count to the left (>75% neutrophils)	1
Maximum Score	10

Abdominal Procedures

Laparoscopy

An 18-gauge spinal needle can be used to establish pneumoperitoneum prior to laparoscopy if the normal needle is not available. After draining the bladder, make a 1-cm transverse incision in the midline just below the umbilicus. Grasp and elevate the lower abdominal wall, and introduce the spinal needle at 45 degrees to the horizontal plane, aiming toward the hollow of the sacrum. There is a distinct "give" when the needle passes through the linea alba. Remove the stylet and attach a syringe, aspirating to check that the needle has not entered either a vessel or the bowel. Inject 5 mL of saline and then attempt to withdraw it. Free flow and an inability to withdraw the saline suggest proper needle placement. Then attach the gas supply to the spinal needle and establish a pneumoperitoneum.[23]

Cystoscopes, available in most rural locations, can be successfully used both for diagnostic laparoscopy and to perform simple laparoscopic surgery. The method is to pass the scope through a small abdominal incision that is tightened around the scope with a purse string suture or a towel clip (Fig. 23-1). For example, to do an appendectomy, insert the instrument through a small (~3-cm) incision at McBurney's point. Then produce a pneumoperitoneum with an inflation bulb with a valve, such as from a sphygmomanometer, attached to the scope's proximal inflation port. Use the working port to take biopsies or do surgery.

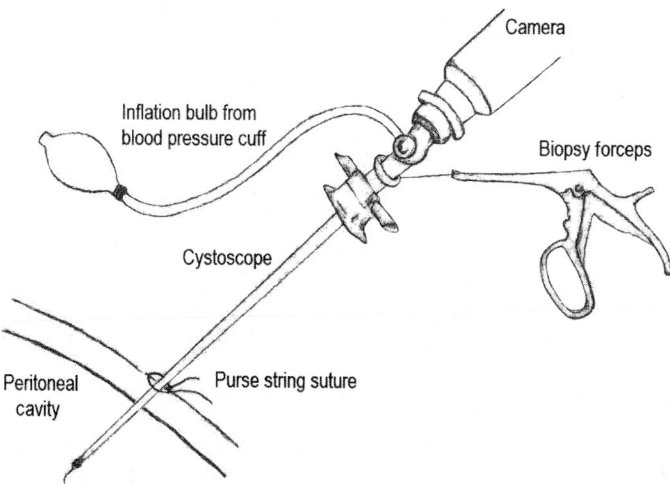

FIG. 23-1. Cystoscope used for diagnostic laparoscopy. This figure shows a camera attached.

During an appendectomy, an alligator forceps (flexible grasper) holds the tip of the appendix; bring it and the cystoscope out through the incision. The normal dissection of the appendix occurs and the wound is closed. This procedure also has been used diagnostically for infertility assessments, ascites diagnoses, evaluations of probably stomach carcinoma, liver biopsies, abdominal mass evaluations, and acute abdomen evaluations.[24,25]

Urobag Zipper Laparostomy

To avoid repeating laparotomies on patients with gross intraperitoneal sepsis, the laparotomy incision is often left open, with a zippered laparostomy bag attached. An excellent inexpensive alternative exists to these high-cost commercial devices—the improvised zipper bag.[26,27] Construct one using the commonly available Urobag and a handbag or suitcase zipper. Choose a zipper length appropriate for the incision size and sterilize it in an autoclave. Immediately before attaching it to the abdominal wall, cut the Urobag to exactly fit the incision. Then, attach the zipper to the bag with a running, nonabsorbable suture (e.g., silk, polypropylene). Fix the bag to the rectus sheath on either side and at the angles using nonabsorbable sutures. Suture it to the fascia when the sheath is not available or is retracted. Periodically remove and resuture the bag at the bedside, using local anesthesia.

Chewing Gum for Postoperative Ileus

After abdominal surgery, if patients are allowed to chew gum beginning on their first postoperative day, they may nearly halve the time until they begin taking oral sustenance. In one group of post-laparoscopic colectomy patients, bowel motility was stimulated when they chewed the gum three times a day.[28]

ENVIRONMENTAL INJURIES

Heat-Related Illness

All heat-related illness is treated with rehydration (oral, unless there is a diminished level of consciousness or trouble swallowing), removal from heat sources, and, in the case of life-threatening hyperthermia, rapid reduction in body temperature. Unless the patient has severe hyperthermia, he or she will live.

Moving patients into the shade (passive cooling) can externally decrease the ambient temperature; however, this is most effective when temperatures are <20°C (<68°F). Place the patient on an insulating barrier such as a sleeping pad or a sleeping bag to reduce heat conduction from the ground. Optimize air circulation (convection) by loosening or removing clothing.

Oral and IV hydration are equally effective in replenishing water deficiencies. Use whatever method is safe and available. Use the patient's blood pressure, heart rate, urine color, and urine output to guide the patient's response to fluids.

Hyperthermia

The treatment for acute, severe hyperthermia, such as might be found in heat stroke, can be done with minimal equipment. First, remove the heat source and quickly cool the patient. Delay cooling efforts only when you need to treat airway and breathing problems. If the patient is in cardiovascular collapse, begin cooling first before treating the cardiac problem. In a hyperthermic individual with an altered mental state, initiate cooling immediately, even if no thermometer is available.

To cool the patient, remove most or all his or her clothing and cover with a thin sheet of cloth. An alternative is to wrap the patient in wet towels or douse their loose clothes with any available liquid and generate as much breeze over the cloth as possible. Use a fan, if available, or do it by hand (conductive/evaporative cooling). The idea is to evaporate the water in the cloth, which cools as the water evaporates. This can lower the patient's temperature 0.04° C/min to 0.08°C/min. A helicopter's downdraft may drop the temperature about 0.10°C/min. Be careful not to continue cooling too long; the target active cooling temperature is about 39°C.

Cold-water immersion therapy, when available, is the optimal field treatment to cool heat stroke patients. It lowers body temperature by about 0.20°C/min. To do this, remove the patient's clothes and equipment, then immerse the trunk and extremities in a cold-water bath or another convenient body of water. Protect the patient's airway. If a body of water is not available, repeatedly douse the person with cold water or ice or snow if available. Shivering is not an immediate problem in heat stroke patients.

Chemical cold packs or ice packs have minimal benefit in heat reduction unless they cover the entire body. Medications do not help in heat stroke.[29]

Cold Injuries

Hypothermia

Hypothermia is a significant problem for infants and small children, the elderly, those with prolonged cold exposure, and major trauma and burn patients.[30] "Hypothermia secondary to hemorrhagic shock is as bad a problem now (2004 Iraq war) as it was in 1918."[31]

The easiest way to treat hypothermia is to prevent it. Use insulation to protect patients when they are being transported or otherwise are at risk of hypothermia. Good insulation includes paper, such as newspapers or paper bags. Even better is corrugated cardboard, such as from boxes, because it has an air layer sandwiched between the paper sheets.

The first step in treating these patients is to remove any wet clothing and dry the patient. Use layered material to insulate the patient from the cold, including sleeping bags, plastic sheets, blankets, bubble-wrap, and foam pads. Then begin passive or active rewarming. Both can be done in most resource-poor environments.

Passive and Active External Rewarming

There are many passive rewarming techniques. If core temperature is >90°F (32°C), for example, remove any wet clothing, cover the patient in insulating material, and, if possible, warm the room to >72°F (22°C).[32] Further "field expedient" (US Army term) rewarming techniques include placing patients in cardboard boxes and administering warm fluids. The fluids are often warmed by "placing a lightbulb in a cardboard box to warm IV fluids up to 40°C, the innovative use of the meals-ready-to-eat (MREs) warming units for warming a liter of Ringer lactate to 44°C, a hand-held hair dryer and a cardboard box unit that can be placed over casualties in a bed, which allows efficient warming when bed huggers are not available, and, finally, a radiator that was pulled off the wall and stuck under a sheet next to the casualty."[31]

Another method for passive rewarming is to put hypothermic patients into body bags, leaving their face free and cutting holes for the arms. The arm openings are used for IV lines and monitoring cables, if available. Use tape to seal the openings around the extremities to prevent the egress of warmed air.

Active external rewarming should be limited to putting the person in a sleeping bag or other insulated container along with a warm person, and applying insulated hot water bags or bottles to their axillae and groin. Insulate the hot water bags with mittens or cloth. Additional active external rewarming drops the patient's core temperature ("afterdrop" or "rewarming shock") because it transfers blood from the core to the suddenly dilated periphery.

Warming the head is as effective as, but often less comfortable than, warming the torso and produces no differences in shivering heat production, afterdrop, or rate of rewarming. In field conditions, warming the head may be preferable if: (a) exposing the patient's torso to the cold is contraindicated, such as when it is already wrapped in insulation; (b) excessive movement is contraindicated; or (c) if the torso is otherwise inaccessible due to other emergency interventions.[33]

Active Core Rewarming

Use active core rewarming for moderate-to-severe hypothermia with core temperatures <90°F (32°C). The effects of these techniques are additive, so they should be used simultaneously whenever possible. Depending on your situation, all can be done in austere environments.

Deliver warm, up to 45°C (113°F), humidified oxygen. It must be humidified to warm sufficiently. This technique works better when using an endotracheal tube rather than using a mask, but the difference is not enough to warrant intubating the patient.

Infuse crystalloid warmed to 40°C to 42°C (104°F to 108°F). Insert a peritoneal lavage catheter (see the "Diagnostic Peritoneal Lavage" section in Chapter 24), and infuse isotonic dialysate (1.5% dextrose with potassium) at 40°C to 45°C (104°F to 113°F). Alternatively, use normal saline or lactated Ringer's as the dialysate. Infuse 10 to 20 mL/kg; retain it for 20 to 30 minutes and then aspirate it.[34]

Irrigate through a nasogastric or rectal tube, using crystalloid no warmer than 45°C (113°F). Infuse ≤300-mL aliquots in an adult; aspirate and replace that volume every 15 minutes. Don't bother irrigating a urethral catheter; there is not enough surface area to make much difference. Warmed fluid can also be lavaged through large-bore thoracostomy tubes, with one placed anteriorly (second or third interspace, mid-clavicular line) and the other posteriorly on the same side (fifth or sixth interspace, posterior axillary line). Run 40°C to 42°C (104°F to 107.6°F) crystalloid into the anterior tube, and drain it out of the posterior tube. If only one tube is used, use 200- to 300-mL aliquots.[34]

Frostbite

As with hypothermia, it is far better to prevent than to treat frostbite. If frostbite or any of its precursors, such as "frostnip," occur, remove any jewelry and make a decision whether to thaw the body part immediately. If there is a possibility it could refreeze, keep it frozen until it can be kept thawed. If it thaws spontaneously, prevent the area from being refrozen, because that will worsen the injury. Do not purposefully keep tissue frozen, because that can result in greater tissue damage and morbidity.

Administer fluids, ibuprofen/nonsteroidal anti-inflammatory drugs (NSAIDS), and pain control, if possible.

If the proper equipment and methods are available and definitive care is >2 hours away, attempt to rapidly rewarm the affected part using a water bath at 37°C to 39°C (98.6°F to 102.2°F). If a thermometer is not available, ensure a safe water temperature by placing an uninjured hand in the water for at least 30 seconds to confirm that the water temperature is tolerable and will not cause burn injury. Continually, but carefully, warm the water to maintain the target temperature. Circulate the water around the injured part without letting the skin touch the hot sides of the container.[35] Because the nose and ears are often involved, soaking or carefully using chemical warmers over a thin cloth, rather than immersion, may be required. Administer analgesics during rewarming and as needed afterward. Using anti-inflammatory medications such as ibuprofen 12 mg/kg/day and topical *Aloe vera* may decrease tissue loss.[36]

Rewarming is complete when the involved part takes on a red/purple appearance and becomes soft and pliable to the touch. This takes about 30 minutes, depending on the extent and depth of the injury. Once rewarming is complete, let the body part air dry or gently blot it dry with a soft cloth. Then dress the part with bulky, clean, and dry dressings, if available, applying dressings between the toes and fingers. Do not routinely debride blisters until definitive care is available, and, if possible, elevate the extremity above the level of the heart to decrease dependent edema. Boots (or inner boots) may need to be worn continuously to compress swelling. If at all possible, the patient should not use a frozen or thawed extremity for walking, climbing, or other maneuvers until definitive care is reached. However, each case requires assessing the risks and benefits. Boots that are removed may not be able to be replaced if walking or climbing is absolutely necessary in order to self-evacuate.[35]

High-Altitude Illness

High-altitude illness can affect anyone ascending to ≥8000 feet (~2500 m), especially if he or she has not taken time to acclimatize en route. Its occurrence cannot be predicted, and it can affect people who have been to that altitude previously without symptoms. When disasters occur at high altitudes, rescuers who are flown in to help are at particular risk, with high-altitude pulmonary edema (HAPE) occurring in ~16% of rescuers flown directly from sea level to 14,500 feet.[37]

The appropriate acetazolamide dosage for prophylaxis against acute mountain sickness (AMS) remains uncertain, as does the comparative effectiveness of dexamethasone with high doses of acetazolamide. Current recommendations to prevent AMS or high-altitude cerebral edema (HACE) are acetazolamide 125 to 250 mg twice per day (bid). During early acclimatization, acetazolamide reduces the ability to exercise hard and increases fatigue, especially in older individuals.[38] If acetazolamide produces unacceptable side effects or is contraindicated, use dexamethasone 4 mg two or three times per day. To prevent HAPE, use nifedipine 30-mg slow-release formulation bid. If this is not available or cannot be tolerated, use a phosphodiesterase-5 inhibitor (e.g., tadalafil 10 mg bid) or dexamethasone 8 mg bid. Inhaled salmeterol (125 mcg bid) is less effective than the other options.

The diagnosis of high-altitude illness is clinical. AMS is diagnosed when victims have a headache accompanied by other nonspecific symptoms. HACE victims have AMS symptoms plus altered mental status and ataxia. HAPE victims have inappropriate dyspnea progressing to frank pulmonary edema. The treatment of HACE and severe AMS is to descend as soon as possible or to use a hyperbaric bag and administer oxygen (2-4 L/min) and dexamethasone 8 mg initially, followed by 4 mg/6 hr (IV, intramuscular [IM], by mouth [PO]). For HAPE, use descent and oxygen plus slow-release nifedipine 60 to 80 mg/24 hr divided into several doses.[39]

REFERENCES

1. Wilkinson D, McDougall R. Primary trauma care. *Anaesthesia*. 2007;62(suppl 1):61-64.
2. Mock C, Lormand JD, Goosen J, et al. *Guidelines for Essential Trauma Care*. Geneva, Switzerland: World Health Organization; 2004:35.
3. Mock C, Lormand JD, Goosen J, et al. *Guidelines for Essential Trauma Care*. Geneva, Switzerland: World Health Organization; 2004:33.
4. Husum H, Ang SC, Fosse E. *War Surgery: Field Manual*. Penang, Malaysia: Third World Network; 1995:39.
5. Ketcham DW. Where there is no anesthesiologist: the many uses of ketamine. *Trop Doct*. 1990;20: 163-166.
6. King M, Bewes P, Cairns J, et al, eds. *Primary Surgery, Vol. 1: Non-Trauma*. Oxford, UK: Oxford Medical Publishing; 1990:8.
7. Husum H, Ang SC, Fosse E. *War Surgery: Field Manual*. Penang, Malaysia: Third World Network; 1995:66.
8. Husum H, Ang SC, Fosse E. *War Surgery: Field Manual*. Penang, Malaysia: Third World Network; 1995:130.
9. King M, Bewes P, Cairns J, et al, eds. *Primary Surgery, Vol. 1: Non-Trauma*. Oxford, UK: Oxford Medical Publishing; 1990:11.
10. Husum H, Ang SC, Fosse E. *War Surgery: Field Manual*. Penang, Malaysia: Third World Network; 1995:172.
11. Furukawa K, Tajiri T, Suzuki H, Norose Y. Are sterile water and brushes necessary for hand washing before surgery in Japan? *J Nihon Med Sch*. 2005;72(3):149-154.
12. Perelman VS, Francis GJ, Rutledge T, et al. Sterile versus nonsterile gloves for repair of uncomplicated lacerations in the emergency department: a randomized controlled trial. *Ann Emerg Med*. 2004;43: 362-370.
13. Houtchens BA, Clemmer TP, Holloway HC, et al. Telemedicine and international disaster response: medical consultation to Armenia and Russia via a Telemedicine Spacebridge. *Prehosp Disaster Med*. 1993;8:57-66.
14. Iserson KV. Ethics of clinical telemedicine. In: Chadwick R, Meslin EM, eds. *The Sage Handbook of Health Care Ethics: Core and Emerging Issues*. Los Angeles, CA: Sage Publications; 2011:379-391.
15. Keenan JE, Turley RS, McCoy CC, et al. Trials of nonoperative management exceeding 3 days are associated with increased morbidity in patients undergoing surgery for uncomplicated adhesive small bowel obstruction. *J Trauma Acute Care Surg*. 2014;76(6):1367-1372.
16. Trowbridge RL, Ruttconski NK, Shojania KG. Does this patient have acute cholecystitis? *JAMA*. 2003;289:80-86.
17. Bundy DG, Byerley JS, Liles EA, et al. Does this child have appendicitis? *JAMA*. 2007;298(4):438-451.
18. Mahato IP, Karn NK, Lewis OD, et al. Effect of the Alvarado score on the diagnostic accuracy of right iliac fossa pain in an emergency. *Trop Doct*. 2011;41(1):11-14.
19. Meltzer AC, Baumann BM, Chen EH, et al. Poor sensitivity of a modified Alvarado score in adults with suspected appendicitis. *Ann Emerg Med*. 2013;62(2):126-131.
20. Varadhan KK, Humes DJ, Neal KR, Lobo DN. Antibiotic therapy versus appendectomy for acute appendicitis: a meta-analysis. *World J Surg*. 2010;34(2):199-209.
21. Søreide K. Should antibiotic treatment replace appendectomy for acute appendicitis? *Nat Clin Pract Gastroenterol Hepatol*. 2007;4(11):584-585.
22. Ingraham AM, Cohen ME, Bilimoria KY, et al. Effect of delay to operation on outcomes in adults with acute appendicitis. *Arch Surg*. 2010;145(9):886-892.
23. Bako AU, Iliyasu Z. The use of spinal needle for insufflation in diagnostic laparoscopy: clinical experience in a tropical setting. *Trop Doct*. 2000;30(4):246-247.

24. Gnanaraj J. Minimally invasive appendicectomy using the cystoscope. *Trop Doct.* 2008;38(1):14-15.
25. Gnanaraj J. Diagnostic laparoscopies in rural areas: a different use for the cystoscope. *Trop Doct.* 2010;40:156.
26. Chintamani SV. Urobag zipper laparostomy in intraperitoneal sepsis. *Trop Doct.* 2003;33(2):123-124.
27. Personal written communication from Prof. Singhal V. Chintamani, MS, FRCS(Edin.), FRCS(Glasg.), FICS, FIAMS, Dept. of Surgery, Vardhman Mahavir Medical College, New Delhi, India. Received July 17, 2008.
28. Asao T, Kuwano H, Nakamura J, et al. Gum chewing enhances early recovery from postoperative ileus after laparoscopic colectomy. *J Am Coll Surg.* July 2002;195(1):30-32.
29. Lipman GS, Eifling KP, Ellis MA, et al. Wilderness Medical Society practice guidelines for the prevention and treatment of heat-related illness. *Wild Environ Med.* 2013;24(4):351-361.
30. Husum H, Ang SC, Fosse E. *War Surgery: Field Manual.* Penang, Malaysia: Third World Network; 1995:276.
31. Holcomb JB. The 2004 Fitts Lecture: current perspective on combat casualty care. *J Trauma.* 2005;59(4):990-1002.
32. Suner S. *Accidental hypothermia.* NDMS Response Team Training Program, September 2003.
33. Sran BJK, McDonald GK, Steinman AM, Gardiner PF, Giesbrecht GG. Comparison of heat donation through the head or torso on mild hypothermia rewarming. *Wild Environ Med.* 2014;25(1):4-13.
34. Danzl DF. Accidental hypothermia. In: Auerbach PS, ed. *Wilderness Medicine.* 5th ed. Philadelphia, PA: Mosby; 2007:125-160.
35. McIntosh SE, Hamonko M, Freer L, et al. Wilderness Medical Society practice guidelines for the prevention and treatment of frostbite. *Wild Environ Med.* 2011;22(2):156-166.
36. Heggers JP, Robson MC, Manavalen K, et al. Experimental and clinical observations on frostbite. *Ann Emerg Med.* 1987;16:1056-1062.
37. Xu T, Wang Z, Li T, et al. Tibetan plateau earthquake: altitude challenges to medical rescue work. *Emerg Med J.* 2013;30(3):232-235.
38. Bradwell AR, Myers SD, Beazley M, et al. Exercise limitation of acetazolamide at altitude (3459 m). *Wild Environ Med.* 2014;25(3):272-277.
39. Bärtsch P, Swenson ER. Acute high-altitude illnesses. *New Engl J Med.* 2013;368(24):2294-2302.

24 | Surgery: Trauma

PRIORITIZING PATIENTS FOR THE OPERATING ROOM

As with all medical care under austere circumstances, priority for the operating room (OR) should be given to patients with the best chance of benefiting. For example, when prioritizing multiple patients with penetrating abdominal injuries, keep these statistics in mind[1]:

- If operating <3 hours after the injury, there is a 10% mortality rate.
- If operating >10 hours after the injury, there is a 50% mortality rate.
- Stable patients with abdominal wounds should be prepared for surgery, but can wait up to 4 hours post-injury for surgery.

For patients in shock, assume that these unstable patients have ongoing abdominal bleeding. A laparotomy is the only effective basic life support. Control external bleeding, administer volume and transfuse (type O or type-specific), and perform a laparotomy without further examination.

Patients who arrive >10 hours after injury have a high risk of complications from surgery, which does not increase much with a further delay. Provide basic fluid and airway support; give broad-spectrum antibiotics, if available; and, at surgery, concentrate on establishing a diversion stoma and effective drainage.

RAKING AND SWEEPING FOR UNDETECTED WOUNDS

Combat medics and many prehospital providers use the "rake and sweep" method to detect injuries when they cannot remove clothing due to combat, extreme cold, constricted or dangerous environments, etc. Form the hand into a rake/claw and firmly pass it over the patient, beneath as many layers of clothing as possible. The fingers may catch in and identify penetrating injuries. Using clean gloves (or hands), again pass the open hand over the body and as close to the skin as possible to identify blood. Use a combination for best effect.

NECK

Penetrating neck injuries are commonly treated using an ever-changing set of rules that often depend on the resources available. In austere circumstances, with limited evaluation and monitoring resources, exploration may often be the safest treatment, especially for Zone 2 injuries (Fig. 24-1), if any doubt exists regarding injury to deep structures.

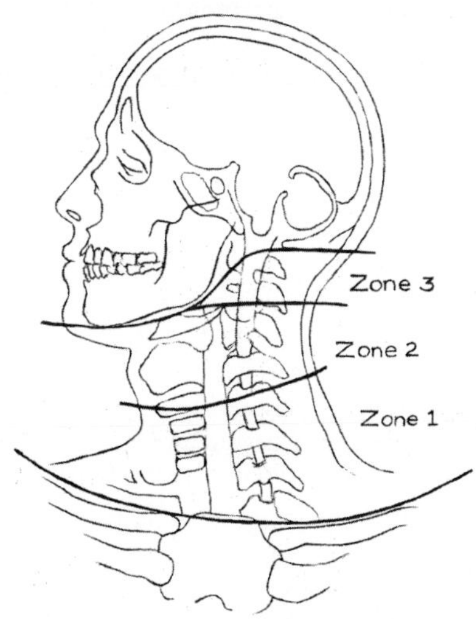

FIG. 24-1. Neck injury zones.

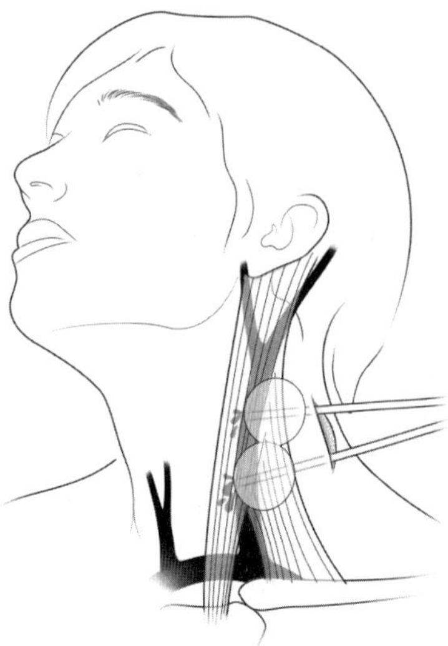

FIG. 24-2. Two Foley balloons applied to jugular vein wound. *(Adapted from Weppner.[3])*

When faced with severe hemorrhage from neck or facial injuries that cannot be stopped any other way, Dr Husum and colleagues advise that "the internal jugular vein or the carotid artery on one side may be ligated for lifesaving reasons: The brain is well drained through the other side. Some neurological problems may follow ligature of a bleeding carotid artery, but in most cases the blood supply from one carotid artery is sufficient."[2]

The US military medical community has found that inserting Foley catheters to tamponade arterial or venous bleeding for wounds in any zone of the neck or in the maxillofacial area buys sufficient time to get patients to a higher level of care. It is far superior to direct pressure on these wounds.

First, place a hemostat on the distal end of an 18-French Foley catheter. Then, use a finger directed along the wound track to place the catheter at the estimated or palpated source of bleeding; inflate the Foley balloon with sterile water until the bleeding stops or there is moderate resistance. If this technique fails to stop the hemorrhage, place a second catheter into the wound and inflate it to provide more proximal control (Fig. 24-2). With Zone I injuries of the supraclavicular fossa, insert the catheter as far as possible past the defect in the vessel, inflate the balloon, and firmly pull back on it to compress the injured vessel onto the first rib and clavicle (Fig. 24-3). Secure it with a hemostat. If bleeding continues at any site after Foley placement, supplement it with direct pressure to the wound. Foley catheter treatment for these wounds significantly reduced mortality when compared with direct pressure techniques.[3]

ABDOMEN

Abdominal Procedures

Emergency Laparotomy

In critical, austere situations, a decision to open an abdomen may be lifesaving—or lethal. In their book, *War Surgery*, Dr. Husum and colleagues list the reasons (Table 24-1) to perform laparotomies under these circumstances, suggest widening the scope of who can do them, and detail ways of shortening the procedure.

Diagnostic Peritoneal Lavage

An excellent technique that has all but disappeared in developed countries with the advent of ultrasound and computed tomography (CT) scans, diagnostic peritoneal lavage (DPL) requires few resources and is a good tool to diagnose intraperitoneal bleeding, perforations, and infections.

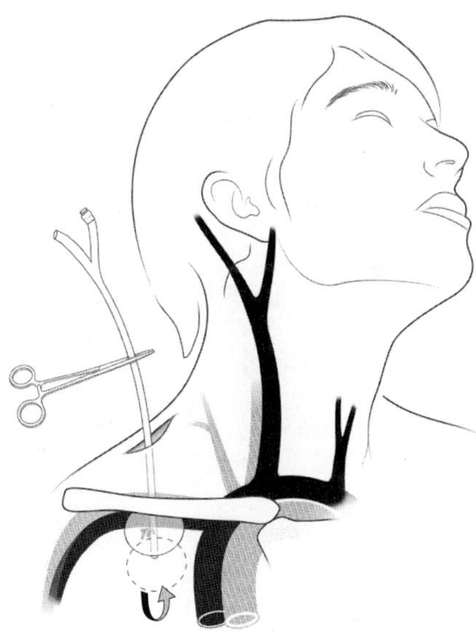

FIG. 24-3. Wound to subclavian vein controlled with Foley balloons. *(Adapted from Weppner.[3])*

This relatively simple and fast procedure helps a clinician decide whether to do exploratory laparotomy after blunt abdominal injuries. It can be done using local infiltration or low-dose ketamine anesthesia.

The abdomen is entered 2 cm inferior or superior to the umbilicus. (Go above the umbilicus if a pelvic fracture is suspected.) The technique can be done through an incision or by using the

TABLE 24-1 Emergency Laparotomy

Reasons and Methods
Done on dying patients, or on unstable patients before prolonged evacuation.
Can be lifesaving.
Should be done immediately, to be effective.
Uses a few simple surgical instruments.
Is performed in the field.
Use intermittent intravenous (IV) ketamine anesthesia.
The operator should be anyone ("paramedic") trained in the procedure.
Procedures to Shorten Emergency Laparotomy
Pack tears of abdominal organs with dry gauze.
Then pack the bleeding quadrants with large, dry gauze packs, 40 cm × 40 cm.
Consider leaving vascular clamps until the second-look laparotomy without tying ligatures.
Tie the intestines proximal and distal to intestinal wounds with ribbon gauze.
Consider closing the midline incision with towel clamps.
Distended abdomen: Suture plastic infusion bags to the abdominal wall fascia to close the midline incision temporarily.

Data from Husum et al.[4]

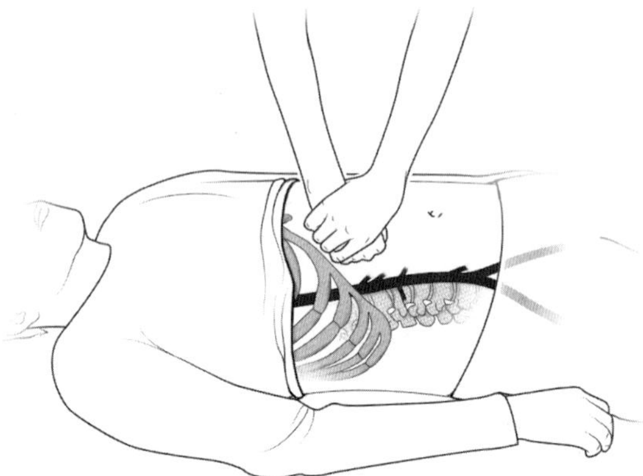

FIG. 24-4. Bimanual external aortic compression. *(Adapted from Douma et al.[6])*

Seldinger (catheter-through-needle) technique. Using the Seldinger technique, insert the needle into abdomen and pass a catheter through the needle into the peritoneal space. This method may be hazardous in patients with prior abdominal surgery due to adhesions and the possibility of bowel perforation. This method is much faster and has, in reality, proved to be as safe as the open method.[5]

The more common technique is to make a small midline incision through the abdominal wall. The reason this method fails is that the midline cannot be identified. Experience shows that by using a self-retaining retractor, the midline is much easier to find and the procedure is easily and quickly done by one clinician. When the peritoneum is identified, make a small hole and insert a soft catheter, such as sterile intravenous (IV) tubing in which additional side holes have been cut distally.

Once the catheter is in the peritoneum, immediately aspirate to check for ≥10 mL of gross blood, which indicates a "positive" lavage and the need for a laparotomy. Otherwise, tie a purse-string suture around the tube and close the incision tightly. Instill 1 L of normal saline; once it is instilled, let it drain from the abdomen using gravity by putting the IV bag or bottle on the floor.

A diagnostic lavage requires 250 mL to return out of the abdomen. A positive result is not being able to read newspaper-sized print through the tubing. (Don't assess the IV container's clarity, because it may vary with the amount of fluid in the bag or bottle.) If laboratory testing is available, a positive lavage will have >100,000/mL red blood cells (RBCs) in blunt trauma patients or >10,000/mL RBCs for penetrating trauma patients, a white blood cell count >500/mL, elevated amylase (>175 IU), elevated bilirubin, food particles, or a high bacterial count in the effluent.

Manual External Aortic Compression

Applying external compression to the abdominal aorta may provide time to use other modalities to treat victims of traumatic hemorrhage, postpartum bleeding, and some cardiac conditions. (It has been used to increase cardiac afterload after severe cyanosis in a 3-month-old with Tetralogy of Fallot). To do this, the clinician applies maximal bimanual force to the patient's epigastrium to compress the abdominal aorta by pressing the right fist (bolstered by his left hand) between the xiphoid and umbilicus (Fig. 24-4). Experience shows that, to be effective, the clinician must be considerably larger than the patient.

CHEST

Open Chest Wounds

Chest wounds can be open or closed. Open, or "sucking," chest wounds should be covered with what amounts to a one-way valve. To do this, tape three sides of an airtight dressing over the hole in the chest. Many things fit that description, but some commonly used materials include plastic food wrap, aluminum foil or aluminum foil packaging, and meal-ready-to-eat (MRE, a military food container) packaging. If the patient has increased difficulty breathing or diminished pulses or blood pressure (BP), remove the dressing.

Pneumothorax

Needle Decompression

The common teaching is that a tension pneumothorax is easily treated with simple 14-gauge-needle thoracentesis.[7] Maybe that is true in children and thin adults, but it is not true in other cases. Failure rates with 5-cm needles range from 25% to 50%, and are up to 77% with a 3.2-cm needle. Failure is attributed to excessive chest wall thickness, user error, catheter malfunction, and obstruction.[8]

Needle thoracostomy is most successful in children and younger men because of their smaller chest-wall size. Whether the standard 14-gauge over-the-needle catheter (5-cm long needle; 4.5-cm long catheter) relieves a pneumothorax in adult patients depends on their position, gender, and age. If the chest puncture is in the second intercostal space at the mid-clavicular line, the catheter won't reach the pleural cavity in one-half to three-fourths of women and in one-fifth to one-third of men in the arms-down position, which is the typical position of patients needing chest decompression. Even if the catheter does reach the pleural space, it can easily pop out when the patient is moved. If the catheter is placed with the patient's arms raised, it pops out as soon as they lower their arms.[9]

For optimal pleural space decompression with a needle, consider that the chest wall thickness at the fourth intercostal space/anterior axillary line is significantly thinner than at the traditional entry site—the second interspace in the mid-clavicular line. In addition, there is a much better chance of actually decompressing the chest when using an 8-cm rather than a 5-cm catheter (7.6 cm = 3 inches). For maximum success, insert the 8-cm needle at a 90-degree angle to the chest wall at the fourth intercostal space/anterior axillary line. This technique has a similar injury rate to that of a 5-cm needle.[8]

Mini-Thoracotomy

Pneumothoraces in critical trauma patients can be treated initially without a chest tube when there is no tube, if there are questions about the sterility of the surroundings, or when cramped quarters (helicopter, ambulance, etc.) do not permit easy manipulation of the tube. The following "simple thoracostomy" technique is both preferable to using a needle thoracostomy and safe and effective for intubated and ventilated trauma patients who have evidence of decreased breath sounds, subcutaneous emphysema, serial rib fractures with chest wall instability, or a penetrating chest wound.

The technique is to thoroughly clean the chest wall at the fifth intercostal space between the anterior and mid-axillary lines and make a 5-cm incision, bluntly dissecting down to, and entering, the pleural cavity. (This can also be done at the mid-clavicular line if access to the side presents a problem.) Cover the incision with a sterile gauze dressing that should be taped down on only three sides. Any air in the pleural space naturally exits as the intrapleural pressure rises with ventilation, while no air enters the chest.[10] A chest tube is inserted when the patient arrives at the hospital or at another facility that can easily and safely insert one.[11]

Pneumothorax Aspiration

Rather than inserting a chest tube (with many resources used), observation alone is adequate treatment for healthy young patients who present with a small (<20% of the hemithorax) primary spontaneous pneumothorax. The intrinsic reabsorption rate of intrapleural air is about 1% to 2% of the total lung volume per day. Administering 100% oxygen increases the reabsorption rate three- to fourfold (~5%/day). For those with <20% collapse, simply observe for 6 hours and repeat imaging.

If the collapse is >20% but <40%, aspirate the air. (Determining the percent of collapse for a pneumothorax is always an approximation; see Chapter 19 for reasonably accurate methods to assess it.) Do this under local anesthesia through the second intercostal space in the mid-clavicular line using a 16-gauge cannula, a three-way stopcock, and a 50-mL syringe. Repeat imaging in

6 hours. If, after 6 hours, the collapse is still >20%, either repeat the protocol once or insert a chest tube. If, at any point, the patient becomes dyspneic or the lung collapse significantly increases in size, insert a chest tube. Have the patient return for a reassessment in 1 week.[12]

Heimlich Valve

Use

One-way (Heimlich) valves attached to chest tubes or needle thoracostomies are commonly used to treat pneumothoraces. A contraindication to using them is the drainage of large volumes of fluid or viscous secretions, which may cause the flutter valve to malfunction.[13] It handles smaller or less viscous amounts of fluid without difficulty.[14]

For example, British physicians involved in the Falkland Islands (Malvinas) War wrote, "All penetrating wounds of the chest were treated with intercostal drainage with, in many cases, relief of respiratory embarrassment by the drainage of substantial volumes of blood. Heimlich valves were used to provide a one-way seal to these drains and these often became blocked if blood was draining. The only solution was to change the valves frequently."[15]

Even with this caveat, Heimlich valves have been jury-rigged to collect chest drainage using urine (standard and leg) collection bags, sterile gloves, colostomy bags, and similar containers. To attach the valve to urine collection bags may require cutting off the bag's standard adapter for attaching it to the urethral catheter and inserting the Heimlich valve's universal adapter.[16] Other connection adaptations are the same as with a chest tube and are discussed below.

Containers attached to a Heimlich valve must be vented with a hole in the proximal (or least dependent) part of the bag. The patient and caregivers must be warned never to seal that hole and to remove the drainage system (but not the Heimlich valve) if breathing difficulties ensue. Also, they must keep the collecting container upright so that the fluid does not drain out.[17]

Makeshift Heimlich Valves

The standard Heimlich valve is a small (about 3-cm-diameter by 10-cm-long) plastic cylinder, with a rubber one-way valve in the center, and universal adapters ("Christmas tree adapters") on either end. Similar flutter valves can easily be improvised and, if fluid drainage is required, may actually work better than commercial devices.

Fashion a flutter valve by tying a condom or the finger from a medical glove to a standard or makeshift chest tube or needle thoracostomy (Fig. 24-5). For ease, tie it on before inserting the needle or put the needle through the fingertip end of the glove's finger, leaving the glove intact or cutting it at the finger's base.[18]

Adjust the hole in the glove to vary the pressure required for air to exit. If fluid is draining from a chest tube, a large hole is useful. (If using a chest tube, use only the glove's finger.) This results in significant "PEEP" (positive end-expiratory pressure) and so should be used with caution. If the entire glove is used and the patient experiences difficulty breathing, one solution is to cut the glove so that only the finger portion remains.

If draining fluid through improvised flutter valves, incorporate them into the drainage system by putting the valve, along with the end of the chest tube, into the drainage bag.

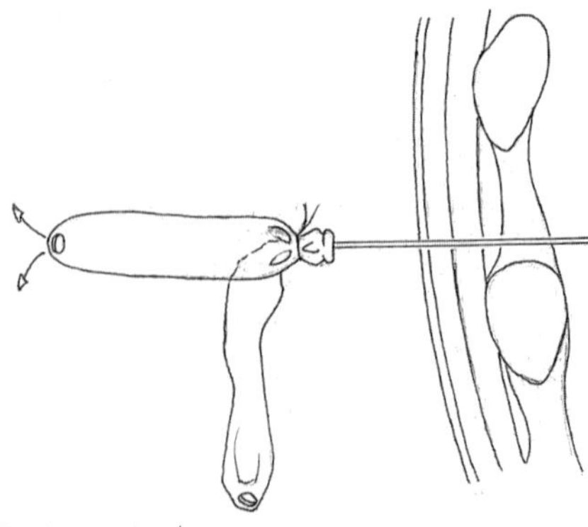

FIG. 24-5. Heimlich valve, improvised.

Chest Tube

In resource-poor situations, problems with chest tube drainage include not having an appropriate tube, lacking a connection to the drainage system, and not having a drainage system to begin with—especially one that doesn't break easily.[19] Not all these problems can be solved.

The purpose of the drainage system for chest tubes is to collect fluid and to prevent air from leaking back into the pleural space. A sterile water bottle, IV tubing, and an IV bag can serve as a chest tube drainage system with an underwater seal.

Thoracostomy Tube

Chest Tube Placement for Auscultation After a Chest Injury

If imaging is not available to confirm the pneumothorax, some physical findings may help confirm the diagnosis.

1. "Dull drum sound and weak stethoscopic lung sounds: Hemothorax ⇒ insert chest tube!
2. Hyper-resonant drum sound and weak stethoscope lung sounds: Pneumothorax ⇒ insert chest tube!
3. Hyper-resonant drum sound at top level, dull drum sound at the lung base and weak stethoscopic lung sounds: Combined hemopneumothorax ⇒ insert chest tube!"[20]
4. Also, increasing difficulty bagging an intubated patient with a patent endotracheal tube (ETT) ⇒ insert chest tubes bilaterally, if necessary!

Bougies for Seldinger-Type Insertion

Use bougies to guide thoracostomy tubes into morbidly obese patients or other patients with thick soft tissue around the entry site. Because the typical adult chest tube is 51 cm and a bougie is either 60 or 70 cm long, it is easily long enough to use for this technique. Use a sterilized bougie, because it will be entering the pleural space.

Improvised Chest Tube

The chest tube is made of plastic or rubber and has multiple perforations at one end to prevent clogging. If a standard chest tube is unavailable, use any semirigid large-sized catheter or tubing to improvise one. Cut multiple holes in the end that will be inserted into the patient.[21] Any clean (preferably sterile) hollow tube works well as a chest tube, although the connections to a drainage system or Heimlich valve should be considered in advance. Note, however, that most nonopaque tubes will not be easily seen on chest radiographs. Some forms of tubing that have been used are as follows:

- Stiff plastic water tubes of appropriate diameter. Trim the tube end and add some side holes.[22]
- A urethral catheter can be used, especially as a pediatric chest tube. The big problem with using catheters is that both the pressure of the chest wall and of any suction applied to them will collapse the tube.
- Endotracheal tubes work well as chest tubes. They do not kink like a urethral catheter and, with a bigger diameter, drain much better. I have used ETTs for chest tubes on wilderness search and rescue (SAR) cases and they worked very well—and were also useful in a SAR medical kit, because they can be used for more than one purpose. ETTs can be attached to a Heimlich valve or to standard chest tube drainage. Unlike other alternative tubes, these will be visible on chest radiographs, because they intentionally have a radiopaque stripe.
- A piece of hollow metal tubing, such as a tent pole, could also be used in a dire emergency. While not pretty, it can keep a thoracostomy incision open, thus relieving a tension pneumothorax. If the patient is being ventilated, that is all that is required.

Chest Tube Position

There is no uniformly correct placement site for a chest tube. Place it where it will be easiest to use, where access is available depending on the patient's position (e.g., a patient trapped so only the back is accessible), and in a place where it will make the patient more comfortable and provide the best subsequent cosmesis.

Chest tubes can be placed in the anterior, mid-, or posterior axillary lines. They can be placed in the second intercostal space at the mid-clavicular line, which may be more accessible. However, in patients with significant breast tissue, have an assistant push the breast down (caudally) to get the least amount of interposed tissue. (This is also useful when placing a subclavian line in this area.) Chest tubes can also be placed posteriorly. With the patient sitting, insert the tube at the second interspace just medial to the medial border of the scapula. Note that the chest is 3 to 7 cm thick at this point, so it is not a particularly easy procedure.[23]

Connections

Think about how to connect the tubes while assembling your improvised thoracic drainage system. Don't assume that an appropriate tube connector will be available, even in well-stocked facilities.

Some connectors that are easily fashioned from readily available equipment or techniques are as follows:

- *Glove fingers:* Cut a finger from a glove and also cut off the fingertip. Put each end over a tube end and tie or tape them tightly and close together.
- *Distensible (rubber) tubing:* Cut a relatively short piece of distensible tubing that has a smaller or equal size to the tubing being attached. Use a hemostat to pull an end over each of the tubes being connected. Reinforce this with tape, sutures, or cyanoacrylate.
- *Highly adhesive tape:* Put the tubing ends as close together as possible and wrap with electrician, duct, medical rubberized, or a similar very adhesive tape.
- *Syringe barrel:* Cut off both the flange and the Luer lock ends of a plastic syringe barrel that approximates the inside, or outside, diameters of the tubes to be connected. Put the tubes over or inside the barrel (or one inside; the other outside) and tape them in place.
- *Cut tubing:* Tubing can often be forced into a slightly larger tube if a "V"-shaped cut is made in the larger tubing end. At least one of the tubes should be stiff, such as is the typical chest tube.

Drainage System (Plastic Bottles/Bags)

The fundamental idea of a chest tube drainage system is for the air to leave the thorax (chest) without any air being able to reenter the chest via the system. Figure 24-6 shows the simplest arrangement, which can be made from virtually any bottle and tubing. A tube that extends beneath the water in the container is connected to the patient's chest tube. The hydrostatic pressure of the water keeps air in the bottle from returning up the tube. A patient with a pneumothorax expels (bubbles) air out, but it cannot return. The vent in the bottle keeps the pressure within the bottle from rising as new air enters from the patient. If the patient has fluid in his chest (e.g., blood, empyema), this system can still be used. However, the bottle will need to be emptied periodically.

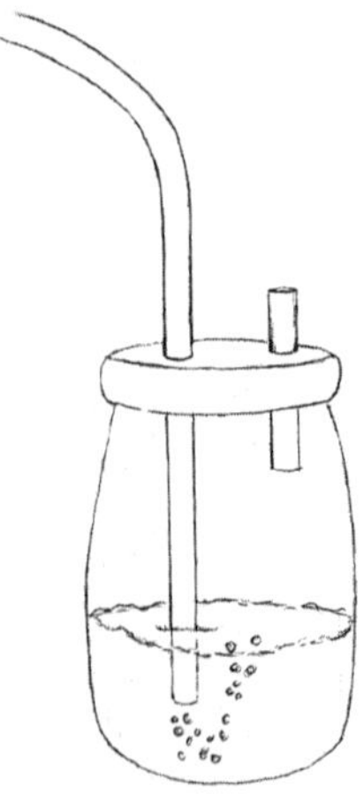

FIG. 24-6. One-bottle chest drainage system.

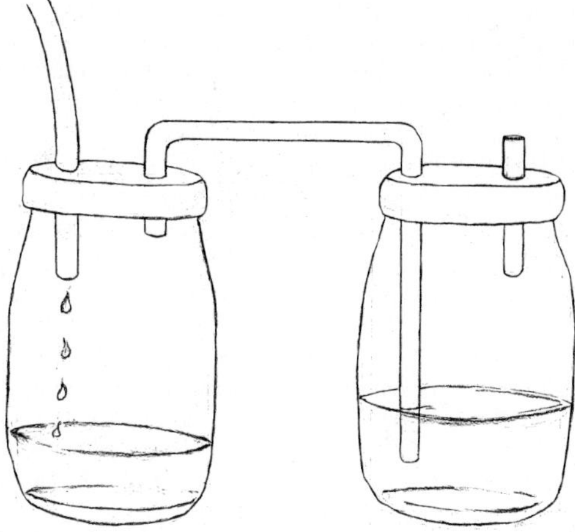

FIG. 24-7. Two-bottle chest drainage system.

Figure 24-7 illustrates a two-bottle system. The system pressure is maintained in the second bottle, whereas the first is used solely to collect fluids from the chest. This system has the same connections as the one-bottle system. Note that either system can be open to the air or attached to suction. Many types of plastic or glass bottles can be used for these systems.

A US Navy physician constructed a two-bottle chest tube drainage system from an empty 1-L plastic sterile-water bottle, a 1-L IV bag, two IV tubing sets, and a 24-Fr chest tube.[24] This system collects and measures the fluid that drains out of the tube. To reproduce this system, empty a plastic sterile-water bottle and put one hole in the cap and another in the bottle's neck; each hole should barely allow passage of the IV tubing (Fig. 24-8). Cut the patient (IV–catheter attachment) end off one (the "first") IV tubing set, and insert this cut end into the hole in the top of the empty bottle. The other (IV bag-spike) end of this tube should fit into the end of the 24-Fr chest tube. Next, take the other (the "second") IV tubing set and cut off the spike end between the filter and the reservoir. Position the fluid-filled IV bag with its ports up and the saline bag down, and insert the cut-off spike from the second IV tubing set into one port in the IV bag. This is now the system's air vent. Open the other port (cut or remove the rubber cap), and insert the cut end of the second IV tubing so that it is well beneath the level of the saline in the bag. Then place the other end of the second

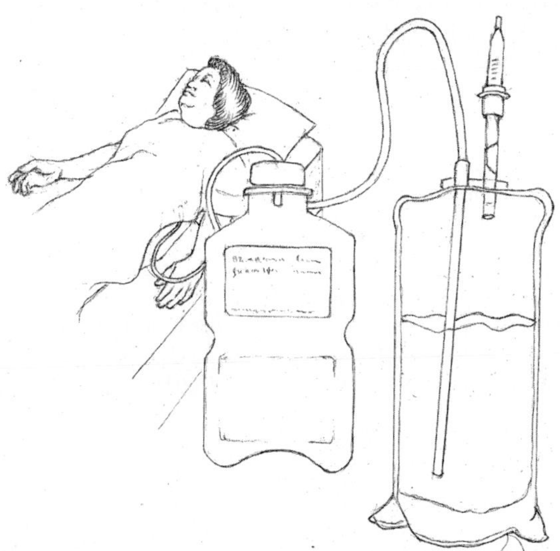

FIG. 24-8. Chest tube drainage with water bottle and saline bag.

IV line through the hole in the neck of the empty bottle. Use cyanoacrylate, any other cement, or duct tape to seal the tubes in position. Keep the IV bag inverted to provide a water seal for the system. To dispose of any accumulated fluid, clamp the chest tube, unscrew the cap from the water bottle, and empty it out. Then screw the cap back on and unclamp the chest tube.

Alternative to Chest Tube Suction

Instead of using chest tube suction, use a soap solution in place of water in the collecting bottle, give the patient analgesia, and then have him or her blow up a child's balloon or surgeon's glove. The positive respiratory pressure inflates his or her lungs and promotes chest drainage.[22]

Drainage Bag

Chest drainage systems, either with chest tubes or flutter valves, must often allow the patient some mobility, especially for outpatient treatment. A variety of disposable, inexpensive alternatives have been used. The most common is an "urosac" or "UroBag," which usually has graduated markings to measure output and a method of draining it without separating the chest tube, and may include its own one-way flutter valve that prevents backflow into the tube.[25-27] They often can hang the bags from a thong around a patient's neck.

Improvised Median Sternotomy

As just one example of improvisation in the face of necessity, one surgeon who lacked the standard tools did a median sternotomy with a heavy pair of scissors ("trauma shears"), saving the patient's life. This patient, who had suffered a stab wound and had a positive cardiac FAST (focused assessment with sonography for trauma) examination, dropped his or her pressure abruptly, precipitating this response. His cardiac laceration and tamponade were quickly repaired.[28]

INJURIES

Vital Signs After Trauma

When trauma patients arrive at a hospital with a normal systolic BP, reports from prehospital personnel that the patient was hypotensive before arrival are often downplayed. That is a mistake. Patients for whom trained ambulance personnel report prehospital hypotension are more than three times as likely to need an operation to repair damaged organs as are those reported as being normotensive. Their mortality is also more than twice as high.[29]

Predicting the Need for Massive Transfusion

Clinicians can quickly assess the need for a massive transfusion/ongoing hemorrhage without laboratory tests using two simple protocols: the Shock Index (SI) or the Assessment of Blood Consumption (ABC) Score. See the "Acute Bleeding: Is a Massive Transfusion Required?" section in Chapter 18.

Gunshot Wounds to Extremities

Low-velocity gunshot wounds to the legs are part of the "urban war" being waged between gangs around the world. Rather than tying up resources observing or studying them, patients who present hemodynamically stable with no associated fractures and with a normal ankle-brachial index (ABI) (≥0.90) can be discharged after a short observation period.[30]

Without a sphygmomanometer (or a Doppler for a true ABI), the best method is to compare the circulation in both limbs. Assess capillary refill. It will be either "brisk" or "impaired," meaning possible vascular compromise. Also, carefully check neurological status; damage to the nerve associated with an artery is often an early sign of vascular injury.[31]

High-velocity and large-projectile wounds, as well as blast injuries, will often require the use of tourniquets.

Tourniquets

Tourniquet Use and Dangers

Placing a tourniquet can be lifesaving; it also can cost the patient his or her limb. In civilian settings, tourniquets should be used to control a hemorrhaging extremity only if direct pressure is not adequate or possible (e.g., multiple injuries, inaccessible wounds, multiple victims). Tourniquets can be left in place for up to 2 hours "warm ischemic time,"[32,33] and longer if the limb is cool. However, if tourniquets are left on for ≥6 hours, the limb will probably need to be amputated.

Tourniquets may be overlooked when they are hidden under clothing, a jumble of bandages, or the other clutter surrounding a badly injured patient. Make it clear to any subsequent health care provider that your patient has a tourniquet. Place a large "T," using a marker, lipstick, or the patient's blood, on their forehead, as well as the time that the tourniquet was placed.

Tourniquet Attributes

To be effective, a tourniquet must be designed so that it may be placed easily and quickly. The device must also be compact and light enough to be carried, simple to use, and rugged. Although upper-extremity wounds may not require tourniquets as often as lower-extremity wounds, it is vital that clinicians be able to use any premade tourniquet on both upper and lower extremities. Single-arm operation, while optional, permits a person who has a wounded upper extremity to, if still alert, apply the device without assistance.[34]

Combat Use

An Israeli Defense Force (IDF) review of prehospital tourniquet use on soldiers in combat and on civilians after terrorist attacks found that there was no indication to use a tourniquet in about half the tourniquets placed by physicians, medics, or fellow soldiers (Table 24-2). They attributed this to "the stressful situation and the relatively little prior experience of most medical care providers" with tourniquet use.

They also found that 94% of tourniquets applied to the upper extremity were effective; only 71% applied to the lower limb were effective. The "Spanish Windlass," also known as the "Improvised" or "Russian" tourniquet, was the most effective type of tourniquet to use on a lower extremity. There was a relatively low incidence of complications (5.5%), primarily neurological. No deaths resulted from uncontrolled limb hemorrhage, although in Vietnam, it caused about 10% of all deaths and 60% of preventable deaths.[35]

The standard procedure for tourniquet use in the IDF is to (a) place it as distally as possible, but at least 5 cm proximal to (above the) injury; (b) place it above as few joints as possible; (c) place it on exposed skin to avoid slipping; (d) place a second tourniquet above the first if the first one fails to work—leaving the first, ineffective, tourniquet in place; and (e) convert it to a pressure dressing as soon as possible.[35]

"Russian" Tourniquet

A "Russian" tourniquet is the typical first-aid model, with a nonelastic cloth tied around the limb. It has been used on battlefields since at least 1674 and is often the only one available for use when needed. A short stick is placed over the knot and tied into the bandage (Fig. 24-9). It is then twisted to wind the cloth until tight and then tied in place.

TABLE 24-2 Indications for Tourniquet Application

Cannot stop bleeding with direct pressure or injury does not allow direct pressure
Amputation
Bleeding from multiple locations
Protruding foreign body (not seen in their study)
Need for immediate airway/breathing management
Injury under fire in combat
Injury in total darkness
Mass casualty event

Data from Lakstein et al.[35]

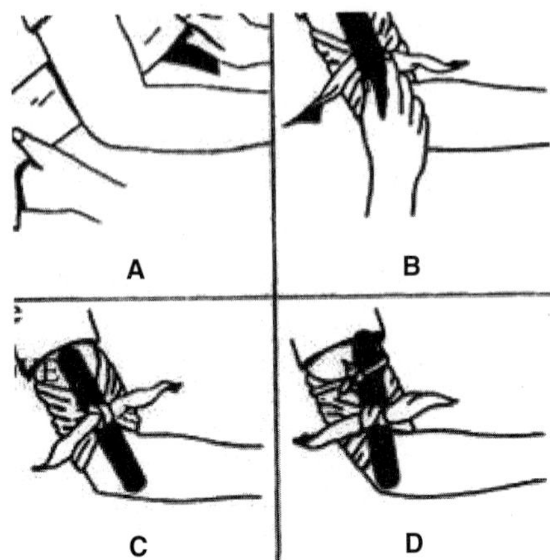

FIG. 24-9. "Russian" tourniquet application. *(Source: US Navy.[36])*

Tests show that this tourniquet, when placed correctly, eliminates the palpable pulse in an extremity 70% of the time and Doppler pulses in 30% of cases. It takes about 32 seconds to apply. In simulated winter conditions, it eliminates 80% of palpable and 50% of Doppler pulses, but takes nearly 39 seconds to apply. While it causes the most pain in simulated patients, this is probably not a huge issue when a tourniquet is needed.[37]

Other Good Tourniquets

The only tourniquet that always (100% success) stops bleeding from the upper and lower extremities is the manual BP cuff used for Bier blocks.[34] As with Bier blocks, a standard manual BP cuff will work successfully if adhesive tape or another secure tie is placed around the cuff after it is inflated so that it won't "pop" off. A clamp is often needed on the tubing to the inflation device and manometer so that they don't leak.

In one test, 0.5-inch-diameter latex tubing, readily available in most health care facilities, was found to be the lightest, least-expensive, fastest to apply, and easiest-to-learn tourniquet. First used in the 1870s, it was very popular in World War II. Under ideal conditions, wrapping the tubing tightly around the extremity and clamping the ends together eliminated the palpable pulse 100% of the time and the Doppler pulse in 90% of cases. It took <24 seconds to apply. The results were similar in simulated winter conditions. Medics prefer using this tourniquet rather than many others that are available. While it is relatively difficult to secure, a heavy clamp will do the trick.[37]

Improvised Tourniquets

While a multitude of devices are often recommended for use as tourniquets, most do not work well, if at all. Belts, wires, and similar materials were shown to rarely function as tourniquets and some caused major problems. If nothing else is available, women's stockings reportedly do make adequate tourniquets.[35]

Civilian Use of Tourniquets

While the tourniquet has been shown to be very useful in military situations, it is rarely used in the civilian world. When it is, it is generally used for penetrating trauma from firearms and stabbings (although these low-velocity injuries rarely require tourniquets), from blast injuries (terrorist or accidental/industrial), that occurs in remote/wilderness environments, and from industrial accidents. Other suggested nonmilitary indications for tourniquet use, adapted from Lee and colleagues, include[38]:

1. Extreme life-threatening limb hemorrhage or limb amputation/mangled limb with multiple bleeding points. The tourniquet can be used until the airway and any other immediate, life-threatening problems are treated. Its use can then be reassessed.

TABLE 24-3 Algorithm for Civilian Tourniquet Use

Apply direct pressure over a dressing ± limb elevation
⇩
Pack wound
⇩
Apply direct pressure using the windlass technique[a]
⇩
Apply indirect pressure
⇩
Apply a tourniquet
⇩
Use topical hemostatic agent (at any time)

[a]The windlass technique involves increasing the pressure directly on the wound. A dressing directly on the wound is cinched down using a circumferential bandage that has a knot directly over the wound. The entire bandage is cinched tight using a dowel, pen, eating utensil, or similar device and secured in place. Unlike a tourniquet, it is not above, but rather on top of the wound. Also, it is not meant to stop distal flow, only to staunch the flow from the wound.

Data from Lee et al.[38]

2. Multiple casualties and a lack of resources to adequately staunch hemorrhage in all patients.
3. The point of significant hemorrhage is not accessible for compression or clamping.
4. Any other reason that life-threatening limb hemorrhage cannot be controlled.

The algorithm shown in Table 24-3 should be used for assessing the need for tourniquets in civilian injuries.

REFERENCES

1. Husum H, Ang SC, Fosse E. *War Surgery: Field Manual*. Penang, Malaysia: Third World Network; 1995:356.
2. Husum H, Ang SC, Fosse E. *War Surgery: Field Manual*. Penang, Malaysia: Third World Network; 1995:304.
3. Weppner J. Improved mortality from penetrating neck and maxillofacial trauma using Foley catheter balloon tamponade in combat. *J Trauma Acute Care Surg*. 2013;75:220-224.
4. Husum H, Ang SC, Fosse E. *War Surgery: Field Manual*. Penang, Malaysia: Third World Network; 1995:155,157.
5. Velmahos GC, Demetriades D, Stewart M, et al. Open versus closed diagnostic peritoneal lavage: a comparison of safety, rapidity, efficacy. *J R Coll Surg Edinb*. 1998;43:235-238.
6. Douma M, Smith KE, Brindley PG. Temporization of penetrating abdominal-pelvic trauma with manual external aortic compression: a novel case report. *Ann Emerg Med*. 2014;64:79-81.
7. Holcomb JB. The 2004 Fitts Lecture: current perspective on combat casualty care. *J Trauma*. 2005;59(4): 990-1002.
8. Chang SJ, Ross SW, Kiefer DJ, et al. Evaluation of 8.0-cm needle at the fourth anterior axillary line for needle chest decompression of tension pneumothorax. *J Trauma Acute Care Surg*. 2014;76:1029-1034.
9. Zengerink I, Brink PR, Laupland KB, et al. Needle thoracostomy in the treatment of a tension pneumothorax in trauma patients: what size needle? *J Trauma*. 2008;64(1):111-114.
10. Deakin CD, Davies G, Wilson A. Simple thoracostomy avoids chest drain insertion in prehospital trauma. *J Trauma*. 1995;39:373-374.
11. Massarutti D, Trillo G, Berlot G, et al. Simple thoracostomy in prehospital trauma management is safe and effective: a 2-year experience by helicopter emergency medical crews. *Eur J Emerg Med*. 2006;13: 276-280.
12. Chan SS. The role of simple aspiration in the management of primary spontaneous pneumothorax. *J Emerg Med*. 2008;34(2):131-138.

13. Crocker HL, Ruffin RE. Patient-induced complications of a Heimlich flutter valve. *Chest.* 1998;113:838-839.
14. Sasse S, Nguyen T, Teixeira LR, et al. The utility of daily therapeutic thoracentesis for the treatment of early empyema. *Chest.* 1999;116(6):1703-1708.
15. Williams JG, Riley TRD, Moody RA. Resuscitation experience in the Falkland Island campaign. *Br Med J.* 1983;286:775-777.
16. Reis ND, Dolev E, eds. *Manual of Disaster Medicine: Civilian and Military.* Berlin, Germany: Springer-Verlag; 1989:444-445.
17. Mariani PJ, Sharma S. Iatrogenic tension pneumothorax complicating outpatient Heimlich valve chest drainage. *J Emerg Med.* 1994;12(4):477-479.
18. Crawshaw CC. Glove and cannula approach is easier. *BMJ.* 1995;311:1507.
19. Thompson DT. An improved and simpler system for drainage of the pleural cavity both in emergency and post-operative conditions. *Cent Afr J Med.* 1981;27(6):104-110.
20. Husum H, Ang SC, Fosse E. *War Surgery: Field Manual.* Penang, Malaysia: Third World Network; 1995:107.
21. Hughey MJ. Operational medicine: health care in military settings. US Navy, NAVMED P-5139. January 1, 2001.
22. Husum H, Ang SC, Fosse E. *War Surgery: Field Manual.* Penang, Malaysia: Third World Network; 1995:70.
23. Aslam PA, Eastridge CE, Hughes FA. Insertion of apical chest tube. *Surg Gynecol Obstet.* 1970;130: 1097-1098.
24. Vinson ED. Improvised chest tube drain for decompression of an acute tension pneumothorax. *Mil Med.* 2004;169(5)403-405.
25. Adegboye VO, Adebo OA, Brimmo AI. Postoperative closed chest drainage without an underwater seal: a preliminary report. *Afr J Med Med Sci.* 1997;26:1-3.
26. Graham ANJ, Cosgrove AP, Givvons JRP, et al. Randomised clinical trial of chest drainage systems. *Thorax.* 1992;47:461-462.
27. Joshi JM. Intercostal tube drainage of pleura: urosac as chest drainage bag. *J Assoc Physicians India.* 1996;44(6):381-382.
28. Personal experience with Dr. D.J. Green, University of Arizona Medical Center, Tucson, January 1, 2008.
29. Lipsky AM, Gausche-Hill M, Henneman PL, et al. Prehospital hypotension is a predictor of the need for an emergent, therapeutic operation in trauma patients with normal systolic blood pressure in the emergency department. *J Trauma.* November 2006;61(5):1228-1233.
30. Sadjadi J, Bullard K, Twomey P, et al. Expedited treatment of lower extremity gunshot wounds. *J Am Coll Surg.* 2007;205(3):S67.
31. Husum H, Ang SC, Fosse E. *War Surgery: Field Manual.* Penang, Malaysia: Third World Network; 1995:115.
32. Ostman B, Michaelson K, Rahme H, Hillered L. Tourniquet-induced ischemia and reperfusion in human skeletal muscle. *Clin Orthop Relat Res.* 2004;418:260-265.
33. Klenerman L. Tourniquet time—how long? *Hand.* 1980;12(3):231-234.
34. Calkins MD. Evaluation of possible battlefield tourniquet systems for the far-forward setting. *Mil Med.* 2000;165(5):379-384.
35. Lakstein D, Blumenfeld A, Sokolov T, et al. Tourniquets for hemorrhage control on the battlefield: a 4-year accumulated experience. *J Trauma.* 2003;54(5):S221-S225.
36. US Navy. *Hospital Corpsman 1 & C Advanced Navy Nursing Manual for Hospital Training Purposes.* http://tpub.com/content/medical/10669-c/. Accessed May 27, 2008.
37. King RB, Filips D, Blitz S, et al. Evaluation of possible tourniquet systems for use in the Canadian Forces. *J Trauma.* 2006;60(5):1061-1071.
38. Lee C, Porter M, Hodgetts TJ. Tourniquet use in the civilian prehospital setting. *Emerg Med J.* 2007;24:584-587.

25 | Wounds and Burns

WOUND CARE

Essentials

The World Health Organization (WHO) lists what it considers to be the essentials for wound care worldwide (Table 25-1), varying with four levels of hospital capabilities (described in Table 5-1).

Hemostasis

Wound Tourniquets

Optimal wound care requires an inspection for deep structure injury and foreign bodies. A dry field, without bleeding, is usually necessary. For wounds on a finger or toe, the best method is to apply a large venous tourniquet tightened around the base of the finger or toe and secured with a large clamp (Fig. 25-1). No one will forget that they have a hemostat attached to their hand. The old "rubber band" tourniquets are generally not a good idea, because they are easy to inadvertently leave on after the procedure is complete.

Make another type of digital tourniquet by cutting the finger off a surgical glove and putting it on the finger to be sutured—or putting the entire glove on the patient's hand. Then cut a small hole at the top and roll the rubber down to the finger or toe's base and, voilà, a dry field in which to explore and suture the laceration or remove part of the toenail (Fig. 25-2). It is safer if you leave the entire glove on the hand so that no one forgets the tourniquet is there. The cut-off glove finger alone works well on a toe, especially the hallux of an ingrown nail needs to be removed.

Pyramid Dressing

While large pressure dressings, tourniquets, and vessel ligation can all stop bleeding from a wound, an elegant and easily improvised pyramid dressing can often stop significant bleeding using fewer resources. Once you identify a briskly bleeding area—often from a relatively small wound—occlude it with finger pressure. Then replace the finger with a tightly folded "nugget" of gauze held firmly on the spot. If the positioning is correct, the bleeding should cease. Then place several layers of progressively larger, or less-folded, pieces of gauze on top (Fig. 25-3). This "focuses" the pressure on the bleeding point. Then place a very light-pressure dressing over this gauze pyramid; it works because it conforms to the equation: Pressure = Force/Area.[2]

Epinephrine (Adrenaline) Spray and Epinephrine/KY Jelly Mixture

Both epinephrine spray and epinephrine combined with KY jelly (water-based, water-soluble lubricant, primarily methyl cellulose and carboxymethyl cellulose) help to quickly achieve

TABLE 25-1 WHO Wound Treatment Essentials

Resources/Capabilities	Facility Level			
	Basic	GP	Specialist	Tertiary
Assess wounds for potential death and disability	E	E	E	E
Nonoperative management: clean and dress	E	E	E	E
Tetanus prophylaxis (toxoid, antiserum)	D	E	E	E
Minor surgical—cleaning and suturing	PR	E	E	E
Major surgical—debridement and repair	I	PR	E	E

Abbreviations: D, desirable resources; E, essential; GP, general practitioners' hospital; I, irrelevant; PR, possibly required.

From Mock et al.[1]

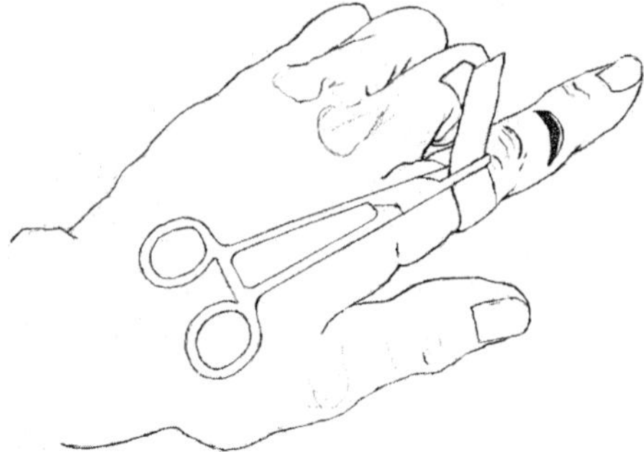

FIG. 25-1. Safe method of applying tourniquet to finger.

hemostasis. This is particularly useful for patients requiring larger split skin graft harvests or burn wound debridement, or in other cases with significant topical blood loss. Using a typical alternative, thrombin, is more costly, slower, and often not available.[3,4]

To make the epinephrine/K-Y jelly mixture, mix 1 mL of 1:1000 epinephrine with a newly opened tube of 50 mg K-Y jelly from Johnson and Johnson, Arlington, TX. Make a saline-epinephrine spray by combining 400 mL normal saline (NS) with 1 mL of 1:1000 epinephrine. With this formula, the final concentration of saline-epinephrine spray is 1:400,000; the final concentration for the KY jelly-epinephrine mixture is 1:50,000.[5]

Topical Hemostasis From Surgical Instruments and Epinephrine

Obtain local hemostasis by applying pressure to the edge of small wounds using a surgical instrument (e.g., needle driver, hemostat, skin hook, scissor's finger ring). Use the inside (finger) ring of a scissors or hemostat to apply pressure around the rim of annular wounds.

Alternative Wound Treatments

Honey

Honey has been used to treat wounds, scalds, ulcers, and burns at least as far back as ancient Egypt. It is readily available, inexpensive, and easy to apply. Honey has antibacterial and anti-inflammatory activity, has a deodorant effect, aids debridement, and provides a moist healing

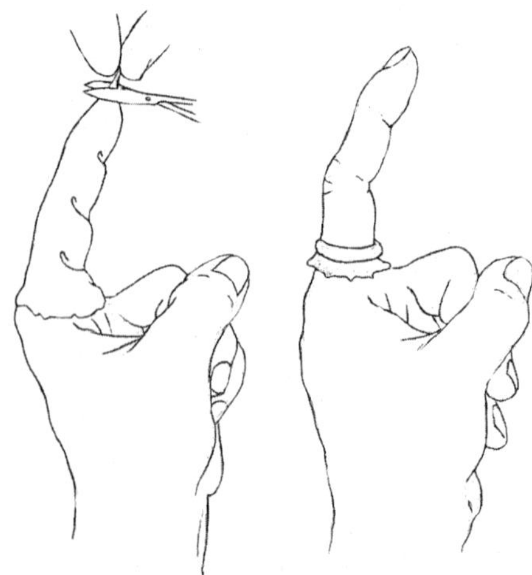

FIG. 25-2. A finger tourniquet made by rolling a glove's finger or finger cot down the digit.

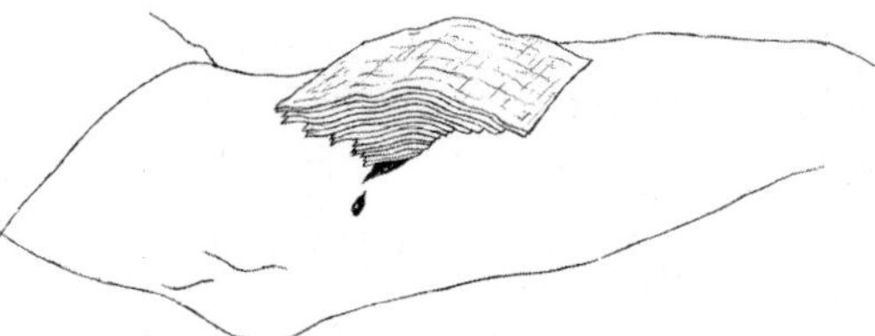

FIG. 25-3. Pyramid of gauze over bleeding point.

environment. It also creates a non-adherent interface between the wound and the dressing.[6-10] While multiple randomized controlled trials suggest that it is often inferior to standard therapy, when it is the only option, use it.[11]

Dressing wounds, burns, and skin ulcers with unprocessed natural honey (under bandages) may work in place of antibiotics or even in some organisms that are resistant to antibiotics (such as with some cases of methicillin-resistant and vancomycin-resistant *Staphylococcus aureus*).[12] Theoretically, honey works by depriving microbes of water and by frequently releasing low levels of hydrogen peroxide into wounds. While natural honey may have batch-to-batch variability in its bactericidal activity, the main difference between natural and medical-grade honey is the cost. In austere situations, use whatever honey is available. It works.

If using honey on wounds or burns, first clean the site. Apply 15 to 30 mL pure, unprocessed, undiluted honey and bandage the area. One drawback is that honey attracts insects. Bandaging helps reduce this problem. Change the dressing daily.[13,14]

Sugar Paste

Pharmaceutical sugar paste, a similar treatment to honey for wounds and abscesses, was developed at Northwick Park Hospital (UK). Available in both thin and thick consistencies, sugar paste supposedly is very effective on large abscesses. How well it works is unclear, but the basic ingredients are inexpensive and readily available. The originators specify that the sugars used are "pharmaceutical grade" and that the paste should be made under sterile conditions, although that is unnecessary if the paste is used immediately.[15]

Formulae for Thick and Thin Sugar Pastes[15]

Material	Thin Paste	Thick Paste
Fine granulated sugar	1200 g	1200 g
Powdered sugar	1800 g	1800 g
Polyethylene glycol 400	1416 mL	686 mL
Hydrogen peroxide 30%	23.1 mL	19 mL

THIN SUGAR PASTE

Use thin sugar paste for small abscesses. Prepare it by mixing 23.1 mL 30% hydrogen peroxide (final concentration 15% volume to weight [v/w]) with 1416 mL polyethylene glycol 400. Mix 1200 g fine granulated sugar with 1800 g additive-free powdered sugar. Combine the two mixtures in a heavy blender until smooth. Store it in sterile screw-capped bottles. The mixture is stable for 6 months at 4°C (39°F). Apply to the wound with a syringe and catheter.[15]

THICK SUGAR PASTE

Use thick paste for large open wounds. Prepare it by mixing 19 mL 30% hydrogen peroxide (final concentration 15% v/w) with 686 mL polyethylene glycol 400. Mix 1200 g fine granulated sugar with 1800 g additive-free powdered sugar. Combine the two mixtures in a heavy blender until smooth. Store the paste in sterile screw-capped bottles. If prepared under sterile conditions, the mixture is stable for 6 months at 4°C. Apply by molding like clay into wounds.[15]

Vacuum Wound Dressings

Poorly healing wounds pose a problem for clinicians and patients. A highly successful and inexpensive treatment employs a topical vacuum that can be fashioned from materials readily available in resource-limited settings.

After cleaning the wound and packing it with sugar, place a piece of gauze in the wound. Insert a sterile 14-Fr nasogastric (NG) tube into a sterile (autoclaved, if possible) sanitary napkin, and place this over the wound. Use cellophane paper tacked down with adhesive tape to seal the edges and make the wound airtight. (Clear plastic wrap can also be used.) Apply intermittent (15 min/hr) suction to the NG tube. In place of a suction machine, a glass intravenous (IV) bottle with a vacuum can be a low-cost suction device.

Normally, change these dressings daily or every 2 days if cellophane adhesive is used; it does not stay firmly attached to the skin longer than this and the vacuum is lost.[16]

Debridement—Basic Methods

Dead tissue in wounds is a nidus for infections. Remove it with a scalpel. For those not used to debriding wounds, follow this principle: If it bleeds or blanches, it is living tissue; if it does not, debride it.

If there is a question about which tissue is nonviable, use a delayed primary closure (described in the "Wound Closure" section below in this chapter). This is especially important in vital areas where excess debridement may cause cosmetic problems or compromise function. No worries: In 3 to 5 days, the viable tissues will clearly demarcate from the nonviable tissues.

Those uncomfortable doing sharp debridement can rely (at least partly) on wet-to-dry dressings. Put thin dressings moistened with 0.9% NS on the wounds. When they dry, remove them along with the necrotic tissue. Change the dressing three to four times a day.[17]

Maggot Therapy for Wound Debridement

Maggot therapy is a relatively rapid and effective debridement method, particularly for large necrotic wounds. Also known as biodebridement, biosurgery, maggot debridement therapy (MDT), and larval therapy, the technique is useful for debriding necrotic tissue, and also for eliminating and preventing biofilm formation,[18] disinfecting the wound (gram-positive antibiotic activity), and promoting wound healing.[19]

MDT generally has been used on lower extremities in patients with chronic ulcers, chronic osteomyelitis, and other pus-producing infections; most of these patients have diabetes, peripheral arterial disease, or both. The majority of patients achieve debridement of >90% of the necrotic tissue in 2 to 10 days. Most wounds then heal with follow-up moist wound care.[20] In some cases, this therapy avoids amputations.

Ideally, purchase sterile, medical-grade maggots, because they are unlikely to cause an infection or to introduce a species that eats live, as well as dead, tissue. These are usually larvae of the *Lucilia sericata* (sometimes called *Phaenicia sericata*), a green bottle blowfly. However, when medical-grade is unavailable, clinicians have had success using "wild" maggots, that is, those that arrive with the patient (see "Wild Maggots" section, below).

For successful MDT, provide the maggots with oxygen, moisture/dampness, and substrate/dead tissue. Avoid using topical antiseptics and surfactant agents on the wound, but use systemic antibiotics as needed. Each maggot consumes about 0.3 grams of necrotic tissue per day.

Method

1. Administer required tetanus immunization.
2. Inform the patient and family of the process. (Most tolerate the procedure well, especially because it may be the last option to avoid amputation.)
3. Surround ("picture frame") the wound with an adhesive protective covering (e.g., hydrocolloid, ostomy dressing, or the local equivalent).
4. Apply skin cement to adhesive protective covering to keep ostomy appliances in place.
5. Place maggots in the wound. Depending on the size and depth of the wound, use from 50 to 1000 maggots (5 to 10 larvae/cm^2 necrotic tissue) that are 24 to 48 hours old.
6. Apply a piece of nylon mesh/"chiffon" directly on the wound, overlapping onto the adhesive dressing. (Chiffon is usually included with medical-grade maggots.)

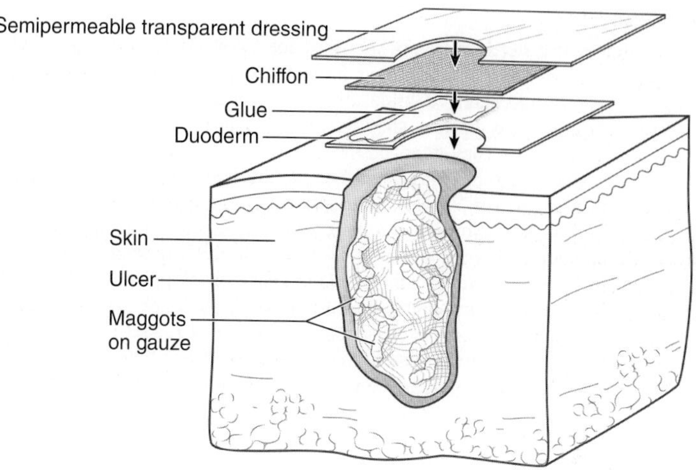

FIG. 25-4. Maggot debridement therapy (MDT) dressing.

7. Use tape or transparent film (e.g., Opsite, Tegaderm) to further secure the nylon mesh/chiffon edges to the adhesive protective covering/hydrocolloid dressing. For improved adherence, extend the tape out onto the skin (Fig. 25-4).
8. Cover the leg (usually it is the leg or foot) with knee-high pantyhose.
9. Secure the pantyhose around the top with tape to contain any "escaped" maggots.
10. Apply surgical pads, two thin layers of gauze, or a highly absorbent incontinence pad to the dressing to absorb wound exudate.
11. Be extremely careful that excessive dressings neither suffocate nor squash the maggots.
12. Replace the gauze as often as every hour at the start; this is when the most fluid will be expelled from wound. If the fluid is not absorbed, maggots drown, because they are aerobic. Later, the amount expelled will decrease. Some blood may be seen, but there should never be any frank bleeding.
13. Patients and family can replace gauze and bandage at home when it becomes saturated.
14. Leave for 1 to 2 days.
15. Do this 2 to 5 times weekly until at least 90% of the necrotic tissue is debrided.
16. At the end of each period, remove the maggots with a jet of sterile NS. If necessary, remove them with forceps, or use other methods (discussed below).
17. Patients completing MDT can often be grafted or treated with normal wound dressings. (Personal communication, Mario Llurie, RN, CWCS, Wound Specialist, University Medical Center, Tucson, Ariz., July 25, 2014; and Katherine Mehaffey, BSN, RN, CWS, CWOCN; Wound, Ostomy, and Continence Nursing Service, University Medical Center, Tucson, Ariz., January 14, 2015.)

Side Effects[18]

- Wound pain (very common); use of analgesics is recommended
- Wound bleeding (common)
- Tingling sensation, itching, skin reactions

Contraindications

- Allergy to soy, eggs, or disinfectants—all used to produce commercial/medical-grade larvae[20]
- Psychological aversion to MDT[20]
- Need for urgent surgical intervention[20]
- Patients receiving anticoagulants or with wounds at risk of hemorrhage[18]
- Wounds near exposed large blood vessels[18]
- Wounds near body cavities or internal organs[18]
- Tissue with inadequate perfusion[18]
- Wounds with *Pseudomonas* infection[18]
- Rapidly progressing infections or the risk of sepsis[18]

Using Wild Maggots

While it is optimal to use sterile maggots approved for medical use, the Israeli Defense Force used wild maggots by necessity during their humanitarian deployment after the Haiti earthquake. Unable to sedate and safely debride all infected necrotic wounds, especially those in complex anatomical areas like the feet, they left maggots in place when patients arrived with them already in their wounds. They wrapped the wounds so that larvae could not crawl out and then opened the dressings after 2 days: Two of five patients had much cleaner wounds, and these were redressed with maggots for 2 more days, after which the patients had clean wounds. Two other patients showed no improvement and underwent below-knee amputations. One patient's maggot treatment was aborted when he could not stand the tickling sensation.[21] Note that wild maggots in a patient's wound will contain larvae at every development stage, including eggs, which firmly attach to the tissue and cannot be washed out immediately. Using them for debridement may still be a reasonable option, because removing them will require several washings over days as the maggot eggs age and release their hold on tissues. (Mario Llurie, RN, CWCS, Wound Specialist, University Medical Center, Tucson, Ariz. Personal communication, July 25, 2014.)

Killing Maggots in Wounds

Two methods exist for eliminating maggots from open wounds, either after MDT or in those presenting with wild maggots: wound cleaners and suction. The best cleaning agent is Dakin solution (sodium hypochlorite), followed by isopropyl alcohol, Betadine, and hydrogen peroxide. Make full-strength Dakin solution by adding half a teaspoon of baking soda and 95 mL (3 oz) bleach to 32 oz (4 cups) of sterile water or boiled tap water.[22] However, no treatment resulted in 100% maggot mortality, and some of these agents will be painful.[23]

The second method is to use suction. To do this, apply suction with a Yankauer (large) tip directly to the wound containing maggots. Remove the superficial maggots and wait for additional larvae to emerge from deeper within the wound, then remove them the same way. Place all components in a biohazard disposal container, making disposal of the larvae simple, rapid, and clean.[24] Repeat this procedure over several days to allow time for deep or immature larvae to emerge.

Wound Cleansing

Irrigate wounds with soap and water, especially if disinfectants are scarce or nonexistent. Then use a disinfectant, if available. Even for open fractures, irrigating wounds with hand soap is at least as effective as irrigation with an antibiotic solution.[25]

Wound irrigation under pressure can be beneficial. Irrigate uncontaminated wounds with potable tap water or NS using a pressure of 8 to 13 psi (lb/in^2). Filtered (if necessary), boiled, then cooled water is an alternative if suitable tap water or NS is not available.[26] While higher irrigation pressures have a theoretical disadvantage, the bottom line is to use whatever means are available to thoroughly irrigate wounds, especially when subsequent treatment may be difficult or not available. The exact amount of irrigation fluid to use is unclear and depends on the size, depth, and cleanliness of the wound. A general rule is "the more, the better." It must be at least enough to remove any visible foreign material. Complex wounds may need to be irrigated with ≥9 L.[27]

An IV bag connected to a 19-gauge needle pressurized to 400 mm Hg with a blood pressure (BP) cuff (and kept at that pressure, even when the volume in the bag diminishes) generates from 6 to 10 psi. A 35- or a 65-mL syringe with a 19-gauge needle generates about 35 psi and 27.5 psi, respectively.[28] Easily make an improvised splash guard/irrigator with the nipple end of a baby bottle and a syringe. Attach a catheter or needle to the syringe and you have a perfect manually operated system (Figs. 25-5 and 25-6). Other types of sealed bags under mechanical pressure should provide equivalent pressure, while commonly used and recommended irrigation methods produce inadequate pressure. These include a bulb syringe (0.05 psi), gravity flow from a fluid-filled bag, manual pressure on an IV bag (5 psi), or any plastic bag or bottle (2 psi) punctured with a needle.[28]

Although using water directly from a faucet has been suggested as "pressure irrigation," its success depends on whether the water is potable (generally not in austere circumstances) and on the water pressure/flow rate (usually insufficient). If the water is suitable, increase the pressure generated onto the wound by decreasing the size of the outlet. Do this by tying the finger from a rubber glove with a small hole to the end of the spigot.

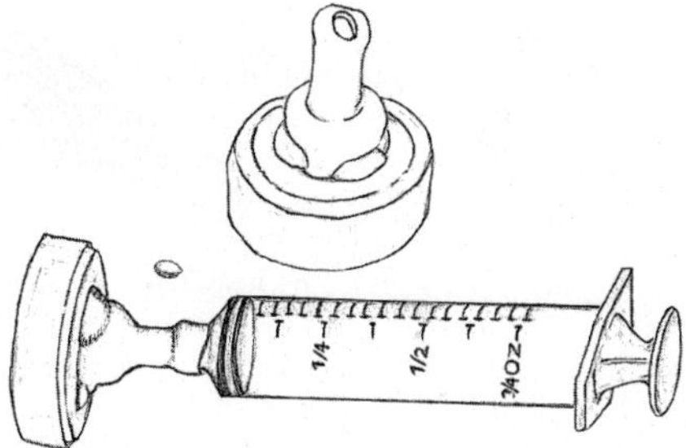

FIG. 25-5. Wound irrigator with splashguard.

If no irrigation methods exist or they are impractical, copiously cleanse the wound with dressing material or a swab using potable tap water, sterile NS, or boiled and cooled water. This is an especially effective technique in wounds >3 hours old. Irrigation does not replace the debridement of devitalized tissue from a wound.

Cleaning extensive areas of road rash is a common and uniquely difficult problem. Analgesia is usually required to help patients tolerate a thorough cleaning, which is necessary to reduce scarring and lessen the chance of infection from foreign bodies. Dr. Larry Raney, former Director of Emergency Services at the Medical University of South Carolina, devised an improvised pressure washer for large areas of road rash. The only problem is that it requires a jet insufflation device such as is occasionally used with a needle cricothyrotomy. So, if you have one, put it to good use. Take a 21-gauge needle and a 16-gauge IV catheter with the inner needle removed. Insert the 21-gauge needle into a 16-gauge IV cannula so that the needle is in the center of the catheter, with the tip fully inside and below the tip of the catheter. Attach the needle-jet insufflation device to the inner 21-gauge needle and IV tubing to the 16-gauge catheter (Fig. 25-7). Tape the needle, catheter, and tubing together (firm enough to hold the unit like a pencil). Placing one piece of tape at the juncture and another a few inches up is enough. Turn on the IV and jet-insufflator and begin irrigating. A large area takes about 1 hour to clean. (Written communication, August 3, 2007.)

Cleansing Solutions

The most commonly used antiseptic products in clinical practice today include povidone iodine, chlorhexidine, alcohol, acetate, hydrogen peroxide, boric acid, silver nitrate, silver sulfadiazine, and sodium hypochlorite. Antiseptics usually target all pathogenic bacteria in a wound, and there is little microbial resistance to them. Where available, using 1% povidone-iodine solution prior to suturing reduces the incidence of wound infection.[30] In resource-poor situations, alcohol and hypertonic saline may be the best choices. Note that neither hydrogen peroxide nor modified Dakin solution is acceptable as a wound cleanser.

ALCOHOLS

Alcohols denature the protein of bacterial cells, producing excellent antibacterial activity against most gram-positive and gram-negative organisms, the tubercle bacillus, and many fungi and viruses, including cytomegalovirus and human immunodeficiency virus. They are not, however, sporicidal. Alcohols are extremely safe skin antiseptics. They are most effective at concentrations between 70% and 92% by weight, and most effective on clean skin. Immersing or scrubbing the skin with alcohol for 1 minute is as effective as 4 to 7 minutes with other antiseptics;

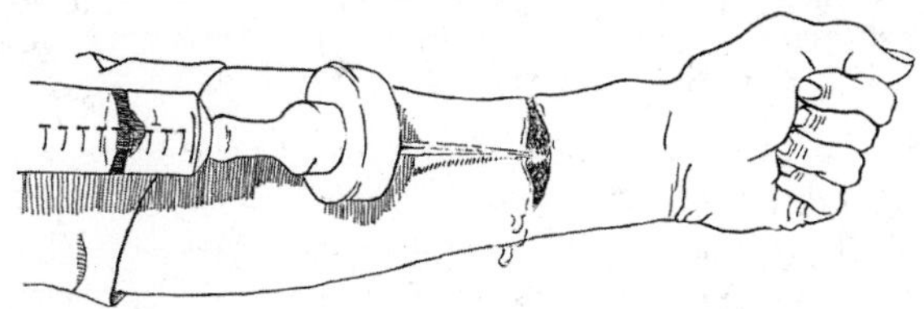

FIG. 25-6. Improvised wound irrigator in use.

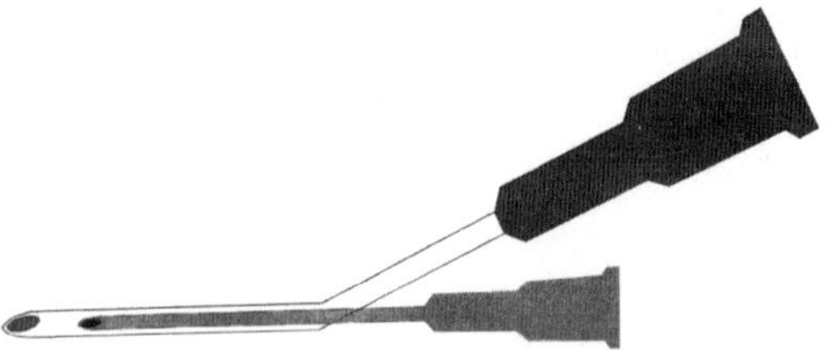

FIG. 25-7. Improvised road rash irrigator. *(Image contributed by Laurence H. Raney, MD.[29])*

washing with alcohol for 3 minutes is as effective as 20 minutes scrubbing with other antiseptics. After an alcohol scrub, bacterial counts continue to decrease for several hours after gloving. The three types of alcohol suitable for skin use are ethyl (ethanol), normal propyl (*n*-propyl), and isopropyl.[31]

Hypertonic Saline

Sir Almroth Wright and his colleagues (including Sir Alexander Flemming) had good success using hypertonic salt solution as a wound antiseptic.[32] Ulcerating wounds, after being cleaned and dressed with gauze soaked in hypertonic saline (changed two to three times per day if very dirty), showed significant improvement. Wounds lost their odor, edema, and most of their necrotic material. At 2 weeks, there was no bacterial growth. The optimal solution strength is 1.5 osmol/L.[33]

Foreign Bodies

Foreign bodies in open wounds may be difficult to visualize. Even if you can visualize the bottom of a wound, 7% of glass particles seen on x-ray will be missed. For deeper wounds, the missed-glass rate is 21%.[34] If available, use high-resolution ultrasound, which can detect nonradiopaque foreign bodies ≥1 mm by 2 mm in size more than 95% of the time.[35]

Removing Metallic Foreign Bodies

Although the dramatic extraction of bullets or other metal fragments seems to be a part of every war movie, the reality is that you should leave most of them in the body. The worldwide experience with these injuries is that it is usually far worse to operate to remove these fragments than to leave them in situ. Migrating bullets or fragments are rare occurrences, and lead poisoning from retained bullet and shotgun fragments usually does not occur.

The International Red Cross recommends that clinicians should remove a metallic foreign body only if it[36]

- Causes a localized infection, such as an abscess or non-healing fistula.
- Disturbs function, such as when it is located within a joint or in a body area that is subjected to repeated pressure (e.g., sole of foot, palm back, sacrum, or subcutaneously over the elbow).
- Can easily be retrieved and is an obvious source of pain.
- Causes documented (blood levels >40 mcg/dL in an adult or >10 mcg/dL in a child, positive ethylenediaminetetraacetic acid (EDTA) challenge test, or bone marrow evaluation) lead poisoning. Even then, treat the lead level before removing the offending fragments.
- Has lodged in the spinal cord and there is clear evidence that it is causing cord compression. Only do this if an experienced surgeon is available.
- Is in the anterior chamber of the eye and both an experienced surgeon and the proper equipment are available.

Difficult Ring Removal

Tungsten, Ceramic, and Natural Stone Ring Removal

Ring cutters will not work on tungsten carbide, ceramic, or natural stone (onyx/jade) rings. Since these hard substances have very little flexibility, use a pair of locking pliers (e.g., Vise-Grip) to break them. Adjust the plier's jaws to clamp lightly over the ring's circumference.

Then release it and adjust the tightening screw slightly (~1/4 turn) and clamp down on the ring. Repeat this process until a crack is heard and the ring pieces fall away. It sometimes helps to move the pliers around the ring for each clamping. Once it breaks, handle the pieces carefully, because the ends may be very sharp.

Other Ring Removal Methods

Wind thread, floss, the elastic from an oxygen mask, or a similar material around the finger and then slide the ring over the thread to avoid cutting or bruising the finger. Even easier: Spray a little glass cleaner (e.g., Windex) on the stuck ring and it will slip right off. Soap or another lubricant may work, although it may still be very painful to remove the ring, and can damage the tissues of the finger. If the swelling is too bad, it does not work at all!

Kelly Clamp to Remove Ring

If nothing else works, very slowly force the ring off using the jaws of a large Kelly clamp to apply pressure on both sides of the ring simultaneously. While applying continuous pressure, rock the clamp from side to side very slowly as the edema is compressed. Do not relax the pressure or the procedure will need to be restarted. Have someone else hold the patient's hand steady during what is often a long (~20 minutes) procedure. Unlike the other methods, digital anesthesia is vital to success.[37]

Marking the Skin

It may be necessary to mark a patient's skin to determine the spread of cellulitis or the swelling after an envenomation, to denote the proper side of the body or limb for invasive procedures, to designate incision points for complex plastic surgical procedures, or to help localize a foreign body. Apply skin marks with normal ballpoint or felt-tip pens, or by using methylene blue, gentian violet, or self-made dyes applied with a toothpick or the wooden end of a swab. One formula for skin-marking dye is to add 1.3 g basic fuchsin dye, 5.6 mL acetone, and 11 mL alcohol to 100 mL distilled water. (Add alcohol to further dilute it.) The benefit of this self-made dye is that it will remain visible on the skin after five scrubs with Betadine, as might occur preoperatively. It does not stand up that well to repeated scrubs with povidone iodine.[38]

If a dye is used, the cap from an 18-gauge or similar-sized needle works well as an inkwell for a toothpick "pen." Use a pipette to transfer dye into the needle cap. One benefit is that, even when the cap is lying on its side, the dye does not run out due to surface tension.[39]

Gloves, Sutures, Needles, and Glue

For a discussion of these, see Chapter 22.

Wound Closure

Materials Cost

The cost of materials may vary greatly in resource-poor situations. Table 25-2 lists cost differences among the three most common types of wound closure, as well as their complication rates. Consider cost when choosing wound closure methods, especially when large numbers of patients need attention.

Undermining

Undermine wound edges to relax tissue tension. Clinicians generally use sharp scissors or, occasionally, a #11 or #15 scalpel blade to bloodlessly separate the skin from the underlying stroma. When none of those instruments were available in Guyana, we used small hemostats to successfully perform the same procedure.

Delayed Closure

Not every wound needs to be closed; not every wound that needs closure should be closed immediately. Do not increase the risk of infection, especially in areas in which infections can become life- or limb-threatening, such as the palm or sole, by immediately closing a dirty wound.

TABLE 25-2 Cost for Wound Closure Materials and Frequency of Complications

	Sutures	Adhesive Tape	Glues
Complication: Dehiscence	1.6%	2.0%	4.0%
Complication: Infection	1.9%	1.6%	0.7%
Cost of materials*	$15	$3	$24
Labor (time)	8.6 min	3.7 min	4.0 min

*Per unit needed to treat wound.
Data from Zempsky et al.[40]

DELAYED PRIMARY CLOSURE

Delayed primary closure markedly reduces the infection rate, morbidity, and resources needed to treat contaminated wounds, including most war injuries. To use this technique, thoroughly clean and debride the wound, and then dress it with fine mesh gauze, or an equivalent dressing, to separate the wound edges and permit the wound to drain. Apply a bulky dressing.

Have the patient return in 3 to 4 days, or earlier if he or she has pain, drainage, or fever. At that time, clean and debride the wound. If there is no infection, close the wound in the same manner as in a primary wound closure. If the wound appears infected or if any necrotic tissue was excised, wait to do a secondary closure at 7 to 10 days. For particularly contaminated wounds, a more aggressive approach is to examine and clean the wound daily for 3 to 5 days. If there is no sign of infection at that point, close the wound.[41-44]

Clinicians often think that dog and cat bites require delayed primary closure. Yet they have equivalent (6% to 8%) infection rates whether they are treated with primary or delayed closure. Neither needs antibiotics unless they are on the hand; human bites do better with antibiotics, if they are available.[45,46]

SECONDARY CLOSURE

At 7 to 10 days, if a wound appears clean and granulation tissue is present, it can be safely closed. Sharply debride wound edges that have an inadequate blood supply to heal directly. Use a tourniquet to control bleeding, and undermine the wound so it is not under tension. Gently scrape the granulation tissue off the wound surface. Remove the tourniquet and close the wound with simple sutures. If the edges cannot easily be opposed, a graft will be necessary.[47]

Healing by Secondary Intention

Healing by secondary intention means letting the wound heal on its own, without any type of formal closure. This simple method is particularly useful for treating both small lacerations and wounds with a high risk of infection due to the type or location of injury. It can also be used for patients who will be unavailable for delayed closure. This method still requires irrigation and, where necessary, debridement, and results in scar formation followed by contracture that reduces the wound size. In some cases, it has the same cosmetic result as primary closure.[48] The disadvantage is that the wound takes longer to heal than when it is formally closed.

Suture Techniques

Improvised sutures and needles are discussed in Chapter 22.

Conserving Sutures

To conserve as much suture material as possible, use instrument, rather than hand, ties.

Removing Subcuticular Sutures

To remove a subcuticular suture that has become hung up, insert the sterile hook of a small crochet needle or the bent tip of a blunt hypodermic needle into the wound margin and pull out the suture where it is caught.[49]

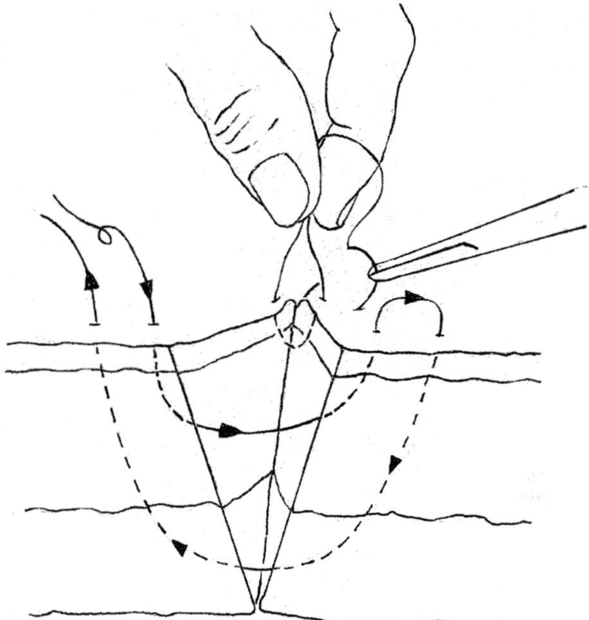

FIG. 25-8. "Near-near, far-far" method for placing a vertical mattress suture.

Vertical Mattress Sutures

For vertical mattress sutures, use the easy near-near, far-far technique. Put your first suture in like a simple interrupted stitch. Lift the two suture ends, everting the wound edges (Fig. 25-8). Place your next stitch in the same plane as the first, but farther from the wound edges. Voilà! A perfect vertical mattress suture, if you do not tie it too tightly.

Single-Layer Closures

Time can be saved, less suture material can be used and a reduced incidence of dehiscence achieved by closing abdominal incisions with a single layer of monofilament suture (nylon, Prolene, stainless-steel wire). This layer should include the fascia and all layers excluding the skin. Use a continuous non-locking one-layer suture with "big bites and slack suturing." For cosmetic reasons, close the skin as a separate layer.[50]

Friable Skin

Teflon pledgets (small pieces) have long been used in the operating room to prevent sutures from tearing through friable tissue. This can also be applied to outpatient wounds, especially in pretibial lacerations and flaps in elderly patients. If standard pledgets are not available, place sterile wound-closure tapes (e.g., Steri-Strips, sterilized nylon or cloth tape) either across the wound where you plan to put sutures or parallel to both sides of the wound edges and sew through them.[51,52]

Operative Wound Drainage and Irrigation

For larger wounds, including those after fasciotomy and debridement, use any piece of sterilized rubber (e.g., bicycle tube), cloth/canvas, or synthetic rope as a drain.[53]

Clinicians usually improvise constant wound or joint irrigation systems, although commercial systems exist. A simple method is to cut additional holes in the end of a sterile tube, such as a small multiport urethral catheter. Insert it into the joint or wound as it is being closed. Attach one end to the irrigation solution and the other to the drainage bag. Use this system to irrigate with NS or antibiotic solution.[54]

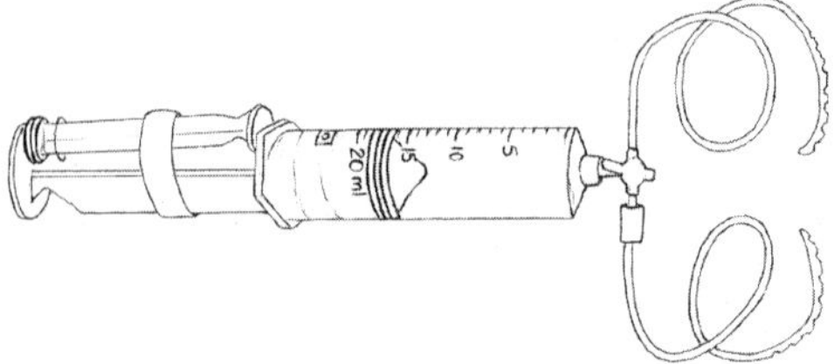

FIG. 25-9. Wound suction device.

While it is best to avoid drains in simple wounds, only one's imagination and the equipment on hand limits the variety of innovative wound drains that can be made. For small wounds, cut off the IV and make multiple small holes on the side of the distal (patient) end of the tube for a butterfly IV or in an infant feeding tube. The easiest way is to fold the tube and use a scalpel. Insert the tube into the wound through a separate stab incision. Sew the wound tightly to obtain an airtight closure, and connect the tube to the end of a 20- or 50-mL syringe (the size depends on the wound size and the expected drainage). One way to obtain suction is pull out the plunger of the syringe and tape the plunger of a 10-mL syringe (or smaller, if less suction is desired) to the large syringe. Interpose the smaller syringe between the flange on the barrel and the flange on the plunger. Although Figure 25-9 shows the suction applied with the drains outside the wound, this is only so the device can be better seen. The catheters must be sewed into the wound before the suction is applied.[55]

Vacuum suction can also be fashioned by attaching a large syringe to the Luer lock of a tubing inserted into a wound and pulling the plunger out to form a vacuum. The plunger is kept in that position by passing a K-wire or sterilized nail through the syringe's plastic plunger as close as possible to the syringe barrel.[56]

Vacuum blood collection tubes make an excellent suction drain for small wounds. Remove the Luer lock connector for a butterfly (scalp vein) needle. A 10-mL tube produces about 75 mm Hg of negative pressure. Cut several holes about 1 cm apart in the butterfly needle's tubing and cut off the IV/syringe connector. Cut the tubing to the needed length, and insert it into the wound as it is being closed. Then insert the needle into the collection tube to start the suction. Tape the tube to the adjacent skin. The tube needs to be changed frequently, but can be done by the patient.[57,58]

Surgical Drains

Fashion a wound drain from a condom or from a non-powdered, sterile glove. First, cut the appropriate-length finger from the glove, and then make two or three V-shaped cuts along the side (Fig. 25-10).[59]

T-Tube Substitute

Surgeons usually leave a T-tube in place after exploring a common bile duct. When a standard T-tube is not available, one can be fashioned from a 16-gauge nasogastric (NG) tube or other similar tubing. After the fenestrated section of tubing is removed, cut off a short section (long enough to act as the portion within the bile duct) and then split it lengthwise. Cut a small hole on the convex side of that piece, and push the end of the remaining long piece of tubing into the hole. Sew it together using 2-0 atraumatic nylon or Prolene sutures. (Alternatively, cyanoacrylate might work well.) The resulting T-tube is a little stiffer than normal, although no problems were found when using it. Note that the "logical" improvised T-tube, made by simply splitting the end of the tube and spreading it into a "T" shape, may cause problems, because the ends tend to slide out of the common duct.[60]

Draining Hematomas

Drain hematomas without incision and drainage (I&D) using simple equipment. Large hematomas often cause discomfort by exerting excessive pressure on the overlying dermal and subdermal capillaries. Because of the clots that are usually present, they may be difficult to aspirate, so a modified liposuction method is used.

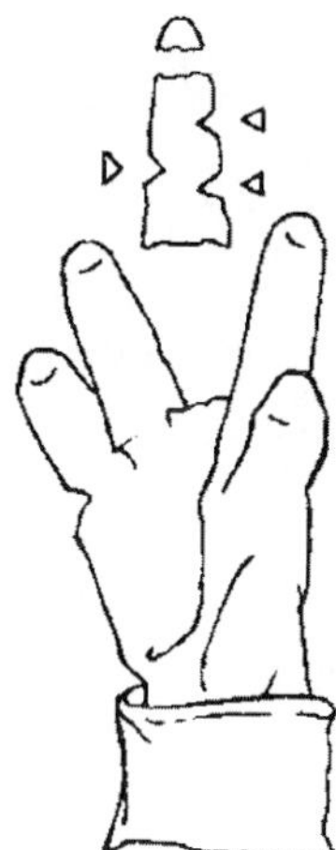

FIG. 25-10. Surgical drain from a glove.

When I&D is not possible, try this method using only three instruments: a 50-mL syringe, a 10-mL syringe, and a 16-gauge needle IV. Attach the needle to the 50-mL syringe, and advance it into the hematoma at an oblique angle, or "Z-track." Use the sharp angle to prevent subsequent leakage when the catheter is withdrawn. Withdraw the syringe plunger so that the 10-mL syringe can be inserted on the outside of the syringe between the 50-mL syringe plunger and barrel. (This employs the same technique seen in Fig. 25-9.) This maintains suction without the need to use a vacuum suction device. Move the needle back and forth in the hematoma to break up any clots, and then aspirate them into the syringe. If the syringe fills, empty it and then reattach it to the needle and continue the procedure. Place a simple dressing over the needle hole. This technique has been used successfully even with patients who are on therapeutic levels of warfarin. While it may not be possible to evacuate the entire hematoma, no significant reaccumulation occurs.[61]

Treating Abscesses

Incision and Drainage

When incising an abscess, avoid recurrence and reaccumulation by either making an "X" incision through the abscess roof or removing an oval piece of skin from the abscess roof. If using multiple small strips of cloth/gauze to pack an abscess or similar lesion (including packing in the nose), tie the ends together to make one long strip. This minimizes the chance of leaving a piece of gauze behind when the packing is removed.

After thorough debridement, consider closing the abscess cavity with sutures. Superficial abscesses requiring drainage were found to need many fewer resources if, after draining and irrigating, the abscess cavity was obliterated using interrupted vertical mattress skin sutures. Place a wound drain, if necessary. This treatment results in improved outcome, shorter-than-normal healing time, and less pain. If the patient is hospitalized, this treatment also results in a shorter length of hospitalization and less need for nursing assistance.[62]

Ingrown Toenail Treatment

In some cases, the often messy and labor-intensive surgical approach to ingrown toenails can be replaced by a noninvasive nail edge separation technique using dental floss. This method reportedly produces no pain during or after the procedure and no secondary infection. If at an early stage, insert a string of dental floss or heavy suture obliquely under the unanesthetized ingrown nail's corner and push it proximally (Fig. 25-11) to separate the spicule from the toe. This procedure immediately relieves the pain, and patients can resume normal activities. Leave the string in place. As the splinted spicule grows out, the patient or clinician can replace the string if it

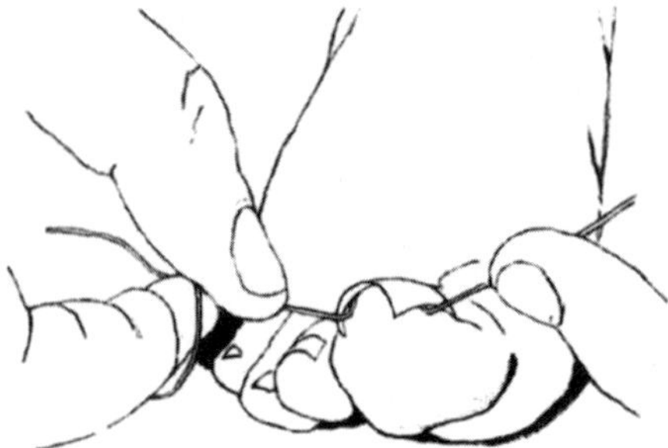

FIG. 25-11. Inserting dental floss under an ingrown nail.

comes off or gets dirty. Otherwise, simply wait until the lateral anterior tip of the nail grows out and can be cut.[63]

Moist Occlusive Dressings for Cellulitis and Small Abscesses

Widely used before antibiotics became available, locally warming infected skin with moist occlusive dressings can often augment or supplant antibiotic treatment. For example, nurses commonly apply warm moist dressings after an IV has infiltrated. Its benefit relies on the leukotactic effect and the vasodilation produced by locally warming the skin.

To use the technique, select a towel, washcloth, or similar material of a size that will cover the affected area. Soak it under the hot water tap or in a pan of hot (~49°C [120°F]), not boiling, water. Wring out the cloth and apply over the affected area of skin. Quickly cover the cloth and surrounding areas with a plastic bag, plastic sheeting (such as sandwich wrap), or other impermeable material. Leave it on for 20 minutes. Repeat every 2 to 3 hours while awake, until the area is healed.

Localizing Lesions for Excision

Once a local anesthetic has infiltrated the injection site, it can be difficult to localize small subcutaneous lumps for removal. Impaling the lesion exactly in its center with a 30-gauge needle prior to injection helps to localize the lesion and guide the incision, despite the fact that after anesthetizing the lesion, the lump often cannot be palpated. This technique causes the patient little discomfort and does not rupture even tiny cysts, which can be removed intact.[64]

BURNS

Developing countries have a major problem with burned patients. Most of the world's burn injuries, and 98% of the fire-related deaths, occur in developing countries. In part, this is due to exposure to open fires for cooking, heating, and other household tasks. Children in developing regions usually suffer burns from hot water and other liquids such as soup, from direct contact with flames, and from electrocution. Aside from the infections common after major burns, patients often suffer from anemia, malnutrition, persistent hypothermia, and tetanus.[65]

Among the vital clinical issues in treating burns are (a) the burns distract patients from sensing other injuries that may be more serious, (b) the burn injury may not be obvious (e.g., electrical and respiratory burns), and (c) the burns may indicate child or spousal abuse.

Essentials

The WHO lists (Table 25-3) the essential resources for burn care worldwide, varying with four levels of hospital capabilities (described in Chapter 5).

Transferring Patients

Consider transferring patients to higher levels of care or getting outside assistance (e.g., telemedical) if they have partial-thickness burns >10% body surface area (BSA), full-thickness burns,

TABLE 25-3 WHO Burn Treatment Essentials

Resources/Capabilities	Facility Level			
	Basic	GP	Specialist	Tertiary
Ability to assess depth and extent of wound	E	E	E	E
Sterile dressings[a]	D	E	E	E
Topical antibiotic dressings	D	E	E	E
Physiotherapy and splints to prevent contractures in burn wounds	I	E	E	E
Ability to debride wounds	I	PR	E	E
Ability to perform escharotomies	I	PR	E	E
Skin graft capability	I	PR	E	E
Reconstructive surgery	I	I	D	E
Early excision and grafting	I	I	D	D
Clean dressings[a]	E	I[a]	I[a]	I[a]

Abbreviations: D, desirable resources; E, essential; GP, general practitioners' hospital; I, irrelevant; PR, possibly required.

[a]Sterile dressings supersede clean dressings.

Adapted with permission from Mock et al.[1]

electrical or chemical burns, or burns that involve the hands, feet, genitalia, perineum, or major joints. Also, transfer burn patients showing evidence of inhalation injury, any preexisting significant medical disease, or other trauma.[66]

Estimating Burn Size

Burns involving <15% BSA in adults and <10% BSA in children are considered "minor"; more extensive burns are "major." Major burns also include first-degree burns to the perineum and genitals, as well as inhalation burns. The BSA calculation normally considers only burns that are second-degree (partial thickness), third-degree (full thickness), and fourth-degree (full thickness plus underlying structures).

A common method that (generally, over-) estimates the percentage of BSA burned is to use the area of the patient's palm as 1% BSA. However, the actual area of the palm alone is only 0.6% BSA in adult males and 0.56% BSA in females. The area of the palm plus the palmar surface of the fingers (not including the thumb) averages 1.2% of the individual's BSA in males and 1.15% BSA in females. For overweight individuals, the palm alone approximates 0.5% BSA and the palm plus fingers is 1% BSA.[67] For most individuals, the calculation should be made using the area of two palms (without fingers) ≈ 1% BSA.

Burn Size Estimate—Children

Inaccurate overestimation of burn size remains a problem in children. Two common reasons are that clinicians include initial erythema in the acute burn area assessment[68] and they use multiple methods to assess burn area. However, in clinical practice, an error of 2% to 3% total body surface area (TBSA), especially in the case of a burn >15% TBSA, is unlikely to be of clinical significance.[69]

Photographing Wounds for "Tele-estimates" of Size

When not in a burn center, get help in assessing burns by sending photographs of the patient to burn specialists. This way, distant burn experts can reliably assess the extent and severity of burn wounds. It can also improve the patient's treatment and help ensure a timely transfer.[70]

Tar/Bitumen Burns

Commonly seen, tar burns pose a particular problem because they may continue to burn for some time. Tar is difficult to remove from the skin. There are two treatment options—use the one that requires the fewest resources. In all cases, cool the tar immediately to reduce continued burning. To do this, immerse the extremity in ice water for a short period so that the tar hardens (but do not make the patient hypothermic). After that, there is a choice: to remove the tar or not.

British burn surgeons report excellent results with leaving the tar in place if it is in a low-risk area of the body. The tar comes off as the skin desquamates. If tar is in a high-risk area, you may want to remove it with a solvent, such as mineral or baby oil, alcohol, ether, acetone, kerosene, or gasoline. Many of these may cause further damage to the skin. Neosporin ointment or cream is an antibiotic dissolved in a petroleum base, so this will generally remove tar over a 12-hour period. Polysorbate (Tween 80) or De-Solv-It also are frequently available and work well without reported side effects.[71] However, British surgeons found that removing the tar did not change either the need for surgery or the time to heal.[72]

Controlling Pain

Non-opioid and mild opioid analgesics often are all that is necessary for pain control when treating burns. If the patient needs a stronger analgesic, especially during extensive dressing changes on partial-thickness burns, ketamine works well (see Chapter 17).

Alternatives to pharmacologic analgesics are available. Clinicians and patients willing to try hypnosis or distraction (see Chapter 15) will find them useful.

Basic Monitoring and Treatment

Urine Output

Evidence supports using hourly urine output (described in "Fluid Therapy," later in this chapter) to guide fluid therapy in burn resuscitation.[73]

Temperature

Hypothermia can be deadly in burn patients, especially if they were treated with saline wraps in a cool environment. Prevent thermal (cold) stress by keeping the environment as warm as possible, preferably from 80°F to 85°F (17°C to 29°C).[74]

Electrocardiogram Leads

Electrocardiogram (ECG) leads can be placed using noninvasive methods, including with small hypodermic needles, as shown in Fig. 10-2.

Nasogastric Tubes

Decompressing the stomach early is vital in patients with major burns. The ileus they develop can lead to aspiration and respiratory distress, if not corrected.

Secure NG tubes in patients with facial burns by passing a large suture through the thin area between the anterior nasal septum and the skin (columella). When doing this, leave both suture ends long enough to make a knot below the nose and then wrap them around the NG tube and tie another knot. Leave some distance between where you tie a secure knot and the nose to prevent pressure necrosis on the columella. Use the remainder of the suture to tie the NG tube tightly.

A less-invasive alternative is to use a 3-cm-long piece of rubber tubing with ≥1 cm internal diameter (ID). Cut an "X" through opposing sides of the tubing (Fig. 25-12) and a small hole at each end. Pass an NG tube through the "X." The friction should keep it in place; if not, use a suture to tie the NG tube to the small tubing. Fix the rubber tubing to the patient with a tie or thin tubing passed through the two holes at its ends. A second X-shaped hole can be made in the rubber tube to accommodate a second NG tube, an oxygen tube, or a nasal monitor (i.e., CO_2).[75]

Infection

"Experience in 'need-based' countries has shown that patients treated in a large, airy ward with good cross ventilation are less likely to get infected than those treated in a small air-conditioned room.

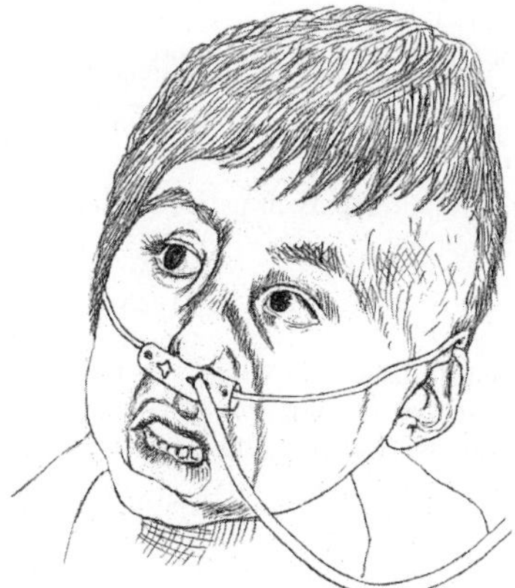

FIG. 25-12. Method of securing nasogastric tube in burn patient.

However, fly-proofing the ward with nets on the doors and windows and ensuring that the distance between two beds is at least 5 feet are simple, but important, requisites which should not be ignored."[76]

Burn patients often develop a rim of erythematous tissue at their wound margins. If it extends beyond this and the patient shows signs of infection, treat for beta-hemolytic streptococcal cellulitis.

Nutrition

As soon as any ileus resolves, provide high-caloric nutrition orally or via an NG tube. See Chapter 36 for feeding information.

Burn Depth

If the patient is conscious, even if nonverbal (e.g., a small child), his or her reaction to a pinprick can often differentiate between second-degree and third-degree burns. Using a sterile hypodermic needle, first touch a nonburned area. The adult patient should feel the touch as being sharp; a child should give an appropriate response for his or her age. A similar reaction results if the burn is second degree (partial). In full-thickness (third-degree or fourth-degree) burns, the nerves are dead and there should be no reaction to the pinprick.

All burns, or all parts of burns, are not always easy to categorize. A good rule is that any burn that remains unhealed after 3 weeks should be considered a full-thickness burn and should be treated by excision of the eschar (if still present) and skin grafting.[76]

Fluid Therapy

Pediatric Burn Treatment

Do not give too much fluid to burn patients. Over-resuscitation with fluids leads to third spacing and significant edema, manifested by abdominal and extremity compartment syndromes, airway edema, and respiratory distress. Children receiving >180 mL/kg of fluid during resuscitation may develop airway edema, which presents with stridor, hoarseness, drooling, gagging, retractions, and a brassy cough. Carefully monitor hourly urine output and adjust infusion rates so that the urine output is 1 to 2 mL/kg/hr (0.5-1.0 mL/kg/hr in larger children). Also, children need glucose-containing maintenance fluids that are best given as a continuous and constant-rate infusion of 5% dextrose in one-half NS.[77]

The American Burn Association's *Practice Guidelines for Burn Resuscitation* say that, based on the quality of available evidence,[73]

- Adults and children with burns >20% BSA should undergo formal fluid resuscitation using estimates based on body size and surface area burned.
- Common formulas used to initiate resuscitation estimate a crystalloid (usually lactated Ringer's) need of 2 to 4 mL/kg body weight/% BSA burned during the first 24 hours. Half is given over the first 8 hours after the burn, and the remainder over the next 16 hours.

- All formulas are an estimate. Fluid resuscitation, regardless of solution type or estimated need, should be titrated to maintain a urine output of approximately 0.5 to 1.0 mL/kg/hr in adults and 1.0 to 1.5 mL/kg/hr in children.
- Administer glucose-containing maintenance fluids to children in addition to their calculated fluid requirements caused by injury.
- Anticipate increased volume requirements in patients with full-thickness injuries, inhalation injuries, and delays in resuscitation.

Options

The addition of colloid-containing fluid following burn injury, especially after the first 12 to 24 hours postburn, may decrease overall fluid requirements.

Consider oral resuscitation for awake, alert patients with moderately sized burns.

Deficit on Arrival

Fluid loss and the calculations for fluid replacement begin at the time of burn, not when the patient arrives for medical care. In Zimbabwe, for example, the average delay in getting to medical treatment is 6 hours; in many regions or circumstances, it will be much longer. After 6 hours, the fluid deficit is already about 6/8 × 2 mL/kg/%BSA burned. The "6/8" signifies the 6 hours that have passed in the initial 8-hour fluid resuscitation period. With that level of delay, one recommendation is to initially administer 2 mL/kg/hr Ringer's lactate until the fluid deficit is corrected.[78]

The keys are (a) to administer the least amount of fluid necessary to maintain adequate organ perfusion and (b) to titrate the volume infused continually to avoid both under- and over-resuscitation.[79]

Fluid Replacement Formulas

Standard Regimen

All standard burn resuscitation formulas from burn centers in the United States use lactated Ringer's solution. Although lactated Ringer's is the most popular choice of crystalloid to use, there is no good evidence to support its use over 0.9% NS or other similar isotonic crystalloid solutions.

The standard burn formulas all give one-half the calculated amount of IV fluid over the first 8 hours post-burn; give the balance over hours 9 to 24.

Parkland (Baxter-Shires) Formula[80]

- 4 mL × kg body weight × %BSA burned. Give half the total calculated volume in the first 8 hours post-burn. Give the balance over hours 9 through 24.

Modified Brooke Formula

The Modified Brooke formula is "often quoted, [but] it is rarely correctly applied."[78] Use this only for replacement fluids.

- 2 mL × kg body weight × %BSA burned. Give half the total calculated volume in the first 8 hours post-burn. Give the balance over hours 9 through 24.

Children's Formulas

Children require more fluids than do adults with similar-sized burns, in part due to their higher BSA-to-weight ratio. They need maintenance fluid in addition to the resuscitation fluid. An estimate is that children require 6 mL/kg/%BSA burned in the first 24 hours.[81]

Shriners-Cincinnati (Older Children) Formula

- 4 mL/kg/%BSA burned + 1500 mL/m^2 total BSA
- For younger children, they add 50 mEq $NaHCO_3$ to the solution for the first 8 hours and change to 5% albumin in lactated Ringer's for the third 8-hour period.

Galveston Formula

- 5 L/m^2 %BSA burned + 2 L/m^2 total BSA

Special Cases

Patients who have deeper burns, those who had a delay in resuscitation, and those with inhalation injuries may need more fluid than is specified in these formulas.

Fluid Creep

In what has been termed "fluid creep," most seriously burned patients receive more, rather than less, fluid than is required, often more than 5 to 7 mL/kg/%BSA burned over the first 24 hours.[82,83] This results in serious complications. Decrease fluid administration when urine output exceeds the target goal.

Burn Patient Hydration—Oral

In burned patients with no contraindications such as an abdominal injury or intestinal obstruction, give oral salt and sodium bicarbonate solutions, such as Moyer's solution (3 g NaCl plus 1.5 g $NaHCO_3$ in 1 L of water).[84] Alternatively, use WHO's oral replacement therapy formula (20 g glucose, 3.5 g sodium chloride, 3 g sodium citrate, and 1.5 g potassium chloride in 1 L of clean water). The traditional mixture of one fistful of sugar, three pinches of common salt, and half a lemon in 1 L of clean water may also be used, especially during what may be a long transport to the nearest hospital.[76] These solutions are adequate for adults with burns of up to 15% BSA and have been successfully used to treat burns of up to 30% BSA.

Burn Dressings

General Principles

In resource-poor environments that lack both the materials and the personnel to do intensive burn dressing changes, treating significant burns open ("exposure method") may be the best course; use the saline method on deep burns. Treat outpatient burns, especially those on the extremities, with occlusive dressings, while those on the hands and feet can be encased in plastic bags. Use special dressings when transferring patients to burn centers.

Plastic Wrap Dressings[85]

Polyvinylchloride film, the thin, clear sheeting frequently used to wrap food, is an excellent short-term dressing for burns and to put over skin graft donor sites. It is inexpensive, pliable, easy to apply and readily available. The film is also permeable to oxygen, carbon dioxide, and water vapor, and does not cause hypothermia, as saline dressings might. A common use is to demonstrate wound healing during rounds so that adherent dressings need not be removed. It is also useful when transferring patients to burn centers, since the receiving physicians can more accurately estimate the size and depth of the burns without ointments or creams obscuring the lesions.[86]

Use standard rolled sheets and, taking care to touch only the edges, lay the plastic over the burned areas and adjacent skin to provide adequate margins. The plastic adheres to itself and decreases the patient's pain by blocking air flow to first- and second-degree burns and other open wounds. Sheets, blankets, and clothing may be placed over wrapped areas without causing discomfort.

On arrival at the burn center, the plastic wrap is simply unwrapped or cut off. The wrap does not adhere to the burns, so the patient has no pain from this procedure. Because of concern about bacterial growth beneath the plastic, it has generally been used only for short-term dressings. However, prehospital providers in Australia and New Zealand routinely use store-bought plastic wrap for burns, and they have found the bacterial (fomite) risk is extremely low.[87]

Treating Burned Hands or Feet

In resource-poor settings, enclose significant burns of the hands or feet in a clear plastic bag. (While this violates the rule to use plastic occlusive dressings only for short periods of time, it has proven to be effective and safe.) The bag must be large enough for the patient to easily move his hand or foot; do not use a synthetic glove.

Wrap gauze around the wrist or ankle and secure it with tape. Cover the hand or foot, or fill the bag, with an antiseptic such as silver sulfadiazine, if available. Place the hand or foot in the bag and use another bandage to secure the bag to the wrist or ankle over the initial gauze dressing. This forms a watertight "sweat band" to prevent the generally large amount of burn exudate from dripping down the patient's forearm or leg.

Encourage the patient to actively use his or her hand or foot immediately, but also try to keep it elevated to reduce the inevitable swelling. Change the bag every 24 hours: wash the hand or foot thoroughly with soap and water, and replace the antiseptic, as necessary. Observe the vascular supply to the extremity to assess the need to do escharotomies, especially of the fingers or toes.[74,88]

Occlusive Dressings

Because of the normally inadequate materials, personnel, or understanding, do not use occulsive dressings for inpatient burn treatment in resource-poor environments. As Dr. King wrote, "Done badly, this method is a disaster, and too easily converts a partial thickness burn into a full thickness one."[89] That is due to applying too little dressing over too small an area with infrequent dressing changes.

If applying occlusive dressings on outpatients, cover the burned area with silver sulfadiazine or an alternative or with petroleum jelly gauze, followed by a thick (≥2.5 cm) dressing to occlude the wound and absorb exudate. The bandaging should extend 10 cm beyond the burned area. For partial-thickness burns, the dressings can remain in place for 10 days if there are no signs of infection (exudate seeping through bandages, swelling, increasing pain, fever, regional lymphadenitis, or decreased perfusion distal to the burn). Little children can have plaster splints applied to keep them from removing the dressing. In full-thickness burns, change the dressing at least every 4 days or when any of the signs or symptoms noted earlier occurs. If using 0.5% silver nitrate, change the dressing daily.[90]

Exposure (Open) Method

Best used for partial-thickness burns, this method requires little nursing involvement. Clean the burned areas after providing adequate sedation and analgesia. Do not break intact blisters. Place the patient on sterile sheets in a warm (40°C [104°F]) room with ≥40% humidity. Make a cradle over him to keep a top sterile sheet off the burns (Fig. 25-13). (Other methods to improvise bed cradles to support top sheets are shown in Figs. 5-4 and 5-5.) Use topical antibiotics, if available.[91]

Saline Treatment Method

The saline method of burn treatment keeps the burned area constantly wet with half-strength NS until it heals. Boiled sea water may also be used.[92] This method is very useful for full-thickness burns.

Use a relatively thin layer of gauze and keep it constantly moist, not wet, by periodically dripping the saline onto it from a container. Change the gauze only once a day; this is best done in a bath or under a shower. Because the burns are mainly full thickness, dressing changes are not too painful, but give analgesics (generally paracetamol/acetaminophen) as necessary.

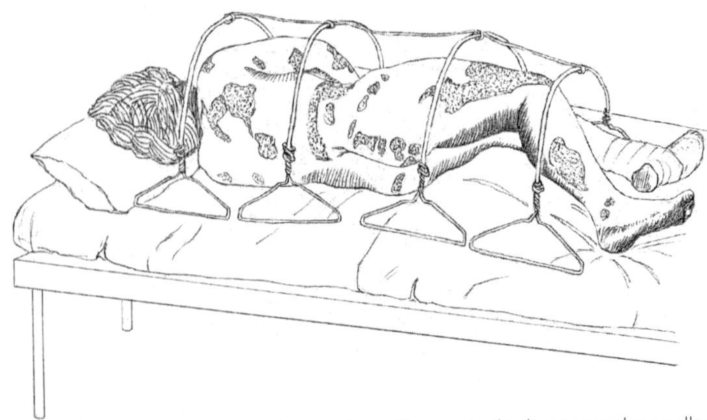

FIG. 25-13. Improvised cradle over a burn patient. Place a sterile sheet over the cradle.

Extremity wounds can also be treated this way, generally by dipping the extremity in the NS.

Saline treatment is an excellent—and the least expensive—method of treating burns; however, it is time consuming. It is best done in a tiled burn-treatment room that also has a bath or shower. Family or friends can assist in this treatment.

An obvious danger with this method, especially if treating a large surface area, is hypothermia. This occurs if the room is cool or if, even in a warm room, there is a draft. (Evaporation quickly cools the body.)

Some clinicians use Eusol rather than NS if there is any sign of *Pseudomonas*, with the typical smell and green-blue staining of dressings. In those cases, also use 0.5% silver nitrate (or silver sulfadiazine).[93]

Debridement

Using either the saline or exposure methods, debridement can be accomplished by "simple bathing or showering once or twice a day with 'soap and water' … [which] not only reduces pressure on the nurses but is more humane, less painful and far less costly. It also allows the active involvement of a relative or friend who can help with the bathing and feeding of the patient."[76]

Escharotomy

The two indications for an escharotomy are difficulty breathing and a pulseless extremity. Breathing problems stem from circumferential burns around the neck or chest. Assess pulseless extremities by the lack of an audible Doppler pulse (if available) or of a palpable pulse if there is no Doppler. If using a Doppler, listen for pulses in the palm, not at the wrist. The decision to perform an escharotomy is clinical and, if the life or extremity is to be saved, the procedure must be done immediately. Note that progressive edema can develop rapidly, especially in the face of fluid over-hydration.

The stiff eschar of a deep circumferential limb burn may cause a compartment syndrome when edema accumulates under it. Wide eschars on the chest, neck, and abdomen may restrict breathing.

"Escharotomy may be done bed-side without anesthesia as the eschar itself is insensible. One or more longitudinal incisions are made through the eschar into bleeding subcutaneous tissue. The soft tissue pressure will widen the incisions and confirm that the escharotomy was necessary."[94] Using a scalpel, incise the burned area into the underlying subcutaneous fat. When you have gone through the eschar (correctly), the tissue "pops" apart. For a thoracic escharotomy, begin the incision high in the mid-clavicular line (Fig. 25-14). Continue the incision along the anterior axillary lines down to the level of the costal margin. Extend the incision across the epigastrium as needed. For an extremity escharotomy, make the incision through the eschar along the mid-medial or mid-lateral joint line.[95]

Skin Grafts

Many burns and escharotomy sites eventually require grafting. Small, full-thickness burns should immediately be excised and grafted.[74] Thin partial-thickness skin grafts are the best

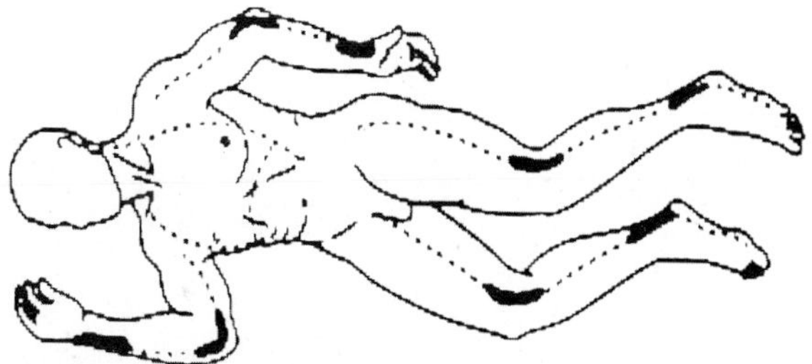

FIG. 25-14. Escharotomy sites. The dashed lines indicate the preferred sites for escharotomy incisions. The bold lines indicate the importance of extending the incision over involved major joints. *(Source: US Army.[95])*

dressing possible—they stimulate healing and help prevent wound infection. Improvise equipment to take partial thickness grafts when the normal equipment is not available.

Grafting Procedure

To take a graft, infuse the subcutaneous area (hypodermoclysis) with saline solution containing 1:1,000,000 dilution of epinephrine. This smoothes the site and reduces bleeding. This infusion is essential when taking grafts from the scalp and is helpful at other locations.

While obtaining the graft, get hemostasis by applying warm gauze soaked in a 1:100,000 epinephrine solution. Once the graft is taken, dress the site with fine-mesh petroleum jelly gauze. Apply a heat lamp until the gauze is dry, and leave the site open.

For a post-traumatic immediate or delayed graft, use viable skin from an amputated extremity to avoid the morbidity associated with a donor site. The retrieved skin can be wrapped in saline-soaked gauze, refrigerated, and transplanted a few days later when the wound is clean.[21]

Obtaining Partial-Thickness Grafts

Take free-hand split-thickness skin grafts with an ordinary scalpel. Even better is to use a razor blade with a needle holder handle or a barber's razor. These can take grafts of any thickness.[53]

An easy way to perform this procedure is to first anesthetize the skin with a field block around the site. Hold uniform tension on the skin using two wooden blocks. Then make parallel incisions the length of the grafts and slightly closer together than the scalpel blade's length. Initially, hold the blade at a 20-degree angle to the skin. After the first 0.5 cm of the graft is cut, hold the blade parallel to the skin and cut with a sawing motion.[96] Hold the free edge of the graft with a skin hook (Fig. 25-15).

Graft Preparation and Dressings

When a skin mesher is not available for skin grafting, hand meshing can work as well. Use a #15 surgical blade to make a 1:15 expansion graft; a #20 blade works well to make a 1:3 expansion graft.[97]

Cover skin grafts and donor areas with a piece of sponge, which acts as an absorbent dressing. Put a layer of non-adherent petroleum jelly-impregnated gauze over the site, and then suture the sponge or the foam pad from a standard disposable scrub brush without detergent onto the site using long sutures that cross over the sponge like it was a package (Fig. 25-16). The grafts themselves need not be sutured. Petroleum jelly dressings can be easily made; do not add antibiotic if they will be used on grafts.[98,99]

Immobilize graft sites on extremities for 4 to 5 days and do not inspect them earlier unless there are indications of infection.

Rehabilitation

Early physical therapy reduces the incidence of post-burn contractures and subsequent limited function.

Various devices have been fabricated using inexpensive and readily available materials such as wood, cane, coat hanger wire, foam, rubber bands, clothespins, and plaster. The devices

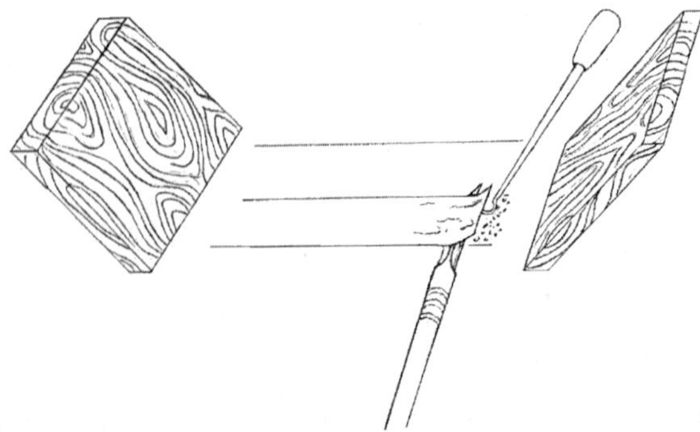

FIG. 25-15. Obtaining split-thickness grafts with scalpel.

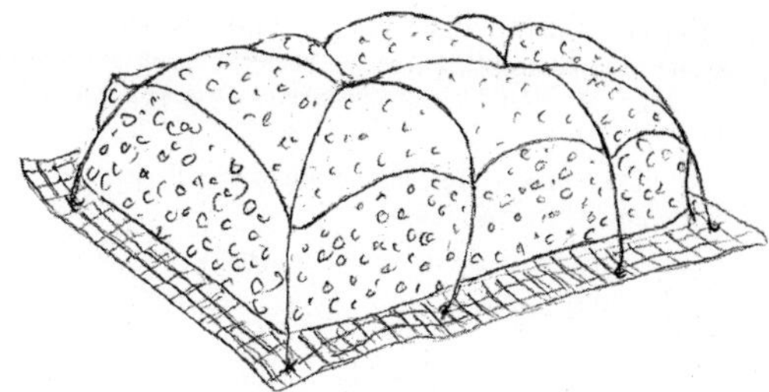

FIG. 25-16. Absorbent sponge dressing over graft or graft site.

include hand (static and dynamic), elbow, knee, and mouth splints, as well as axillary pads. Underwear elastic, spandex material, and animal-leather sheets are used to fabricate inserts and pressure garments such as gloves, sleeves, and face masks. Make airplane splints (for arms/shoulders) with plaster and wood. Achieve appropriate positioning of the burn patient in the emergent and acute recovery phases with homemade cane "IV" poles, pieces of wood, and foam.[100]

Lethal Burns

When health care resources are scarce, a decision must be made about the treatment of extensive serious burns. With limited resources and experience, it may be rare to save the lives of patients with 50%, or even 30%, BSA deep burns, due to "pseudomonas infection, anemia, lack of extra nutrition and patient exhaustion."[93] A physician group wrote: "Under these circumstances, it seems reasonable to utilize the limited resources of a 'need based' country like India to concentrate on saving the lives of those with burns of less than 50% of body surface area."[76]

If a decision is made not to aggressively treat such patients, they still should receive the maximum comfort care possible.

REFERENCES

1. Mock C, Lormand JD, Goosen J, et al. *Guidelines for Essential Trauma Care*. Geneva, Switzerland: World Health Organization; 2004:44.
2. Shokrollahi K, Sharma H, Gakhar H. A technique for temporary control of hemorrhage. *J Emerg Med*. 2008;34(3):319-320.
3. Groenewold MD, Gribnau AJ, Ubbink DT. Topical haemostatic agents for skin wounds: a systematic review. *BMC Surg*. 2011;11(1):15.
4. Howe N, Cherpelis B. Obtaining rapid and effective hemostasis: part I. Update and review of topical hemostatic agents. *J Am Acad Derm*. 2013;69(5):659.e1-e659.e17.
5. Netscher DT, Carlyle T, Thornby J, et al. Hemostasis at skin graft donor sites: evaluation of topical agents. *Ann Plast Surg*. 1996;36(1):7-10.
6. Molan PC. The evidence supporting the use of honey as a wound dressing. *Int J Low Extrem Wounds*. 2006;5(1):40-54.
7. Anon. Medicinal use of honey: sticky solution. *The Economist*. 2007;383(8526):90.
8. Efem SE. Clinical observations on the wound healing properties of honey. *Br J Surg*. 1988;75(7): 679-681.
9. Molan PC. Potential of honey in the treatment of wounds and burns. *Am J Clin Dermatol*. 2001;2(1): 13-19.
10. Cooper RA, Molan PC, Harding KG. The sensitivity to honey of Gram-positive cocci of clinical significance isolated from wounds. *J Appl Microbiol*. 2002;93(5):857-863.
11. Vandamme L, Heyneman A, Hoeksema H, Verbelen J, Monstrey S. Honey in modern wound care: a systematic review. *Burns*. 2013;39(8):1514-1525.
12. Kwakman PHS, Van den Akker PC, Güçlü A, et al. Medical-grade honey kills antibiotic-resistant bacteria in vitro and eradicates skin colonization. *Clin Infect Dis*. 2008;46:1677-1682.
13. Subrahmanyam M. Honey dressing versus boiled potato peel in the treatment of burns: a prospective randomized study. *Burns*. 1996;22(6):491-493.

14. Ndayisaba, G, Bazira L, Habonimana E, et al. Evolution clinique et bacteriologique des plaies traitees par le meil. Analyse d' une serie 40 cas. [Clinical and bacteriological outcome of wounds treated with honey: an analysis of a series of 40 cases.] *Revue de Chirugie Orthopedique et Reparatrice de Lappareil Moteur*. 1993;79(2):111-113.
15. Tanner AG, Owen ER, Seal DV. Successful treatment of chronically infected wounds with sugar paste. *Eur J Clin Microbiol Infect Dis*. 1988;7(4):524-525.
16. Gnanaraj J. Low-cost topical negative pressure wound dressing system. *Trop Doct*. 2010;40:208-209.
17. Husum H, Ang SC, Fosse E. *War Surgery: Field Manual*. Penang, Malaysia: Third World Network; 1995:579.
18. Medical Corps International Forum. http://www.mci-forum.com/category/experiences/555-care_lexicon_a_series_to_collect.html. Accessed July 26, 2014.
19. Sherman RA, Hall MJR, Thomas S. Medicinal maggots: an ancient remedy for some contemporary afflictions. *Ann Rev Entomol*. 2000;45(1):55-81.
20. Campbell N, Campbell D. Retrospective, quality improvement review of maggot debridement therapy outcomes in a foot and leg ulcer clinic. *Ostomy Wound Manag*. 2014;60(7):16-25.
21. Lin G, Lavon H, Gelfond R, Abargel A, Merin O. Hard times call for creative solutions: medical improvisations at the Israel Defense forces field hospital in Haiti. *Am J Disaster Med*. 2010;3:188-192.
22. University of Virginia Health System. How to make Dakin's solution. www.virginia.edu/uvaprint/HSC/pdf/09024.pdf. Accessed February 14, 2015.
23. McIntosh MD, Merritt RW, Kolar RE, Kimbirauskas RK. Effectiveness of wound cleansing treatments on maggot (Diptera, Calliphoridae) mortality. *Forensic Sci Int*. 2011;210(1):12-15.
24. Elder JW, Grover CA. Wound debridement: lessons learned of when and how to remove "wild" maggots. *J Emerg Med*. 2013;45(4):585-587.
25. Anglen JO. Comparison of soap and antibiotic solutions for irrigation of lower-limb open fracture wounds: a prospective, randomized study. *J Bone Joint Surg Am*. 2005;87:1415-1422.
26. Fernandez R, Griffiths R, Ussia C. Effectiveness of solutions, techniques and pressure in wound cleansing. *JBI Reports*. 2004:2(7):231-270.
27. Svoboda SJ, Bice TG, Gooden HA, et al. Comparison of bulb syringe and pulsed lavage irrigation with use of a bioluminescent musculoskeletal wound model. *J Bone Joint Surg Am*. 2006;88(10):2167-2174.
28. Singer AJ, Hollander JE, Buramanian S, et al. Pressure dynamics of various irrigation techniques commonly used in the emergency department. *Ann Emerg Med*. 1994;24(1):36-40.
29. The original illustration, now modified, was produced by Laurence H. Raney, MD, former Director of Emergency Medicine, Medical Univ. of South Carolina. Used with permission.
30. Drosou A, Falabella A, Kirsner RS. Antiseptics on wounds: an area of controversy. *Wounds*. 2003;15(5):149-166.
31. Laufman H. Current use of skin and wound cleansers and antiseptics. *Am J Surg*. 1989;157(3):359-365.
32. Wright A. The question as to how septic war wounds should be treated. *Lancet*. 1916;II:503. Cited in: Cope Z. The treatment of wounds through the ages. *Medical Hist*. 1958;2(03):163-174.
33. Mangete EDO, West D, Blankson CD. Hypertonic saline solution for wound dressing. *Lancet*. 1992;340(8831):1351.
34. Avner JR, Baker MD. Lacerations involving glass: the role of routine roentgenograms. *Am J Dis Child*. 1992;146(5):600-602.
35. Schlager D, Sanders AB, Wiggins D, et al. Ultrasound for the detection of foreign bodies. *Ann Emerg Med*. 1991;20(2):189-191.
36. Baldan M, Giannou CP, Sasin V, et al. Metallic foreign bodies after war injuries: should we remove them? The ICRC Experience. *East C Afr J Surg*. 2004;9(1):31-34.
37. Janson P. Ring removal. *J Emerg Med*. 2014;47(1):83-85.
38. Ayhan M, Silistreli O, Aytug Z, et al. Skin marking in plastic surgery. *Plast Reconstr Surg*. 2005;115(5):1450-1451.
39. Shimzu H, Keyaama A, Saito T. A novel use of the needle plastic cap as a gentian violet container. *Plast Reconstr Surg*. 2005;115(5):1453.
40. Zempsky WT, Zehrer CL, Lyle CT, et al. Economic comparison of methods of wound closure: wound closure strips vs. sutures and wound adhesives. *Int Wound J*. 2005;2(3):272-278.
41. Hepburn HH. Delayed primary suture of wounds. *Br Med J*. 1919;1(3033):181-183.
42. Dimrick AR. Delayed wound closure: indications and techniques. *Ann Emerg Med*. 1998;17(12):1303-1304.
43. Verrier ED, Bossart KJ, Heer FW. Reduction of infection rates in abdominal incisions by delayed wound closure techniques. *Am J Surg*. 1979;138(1):22-28.

44. Tobin GR. An improved method of delayed primary closure. An aggressive management approach to unfavorable wounds. *Surg Clin North Am*. 1984;64(4):659-666.
45. Maimaris C, Quinton DN. Dog-bite lacerations: a controlled trial of primary wound closure. *Arch Emerg Med*. 1988;5:156-161.
46. Medeiros I, Saconato H. Antibiotic prophylaxis for mammalian bites. *Cochrane Database Syst Rev*. 2001;(2):CD001738.
47. King M. *Primary Surgery, Vol. 2: Trauma*. Oxford, UK: Oxford University Press; 1987:27.
48. Quinn JQ, Cummings S, Callaham M, et al. Suturing versus conservative management of lacerations of the hand: randomized controlled trial. *BMJ*. 2002;325:299-305.
49. Perrill CV. Surgery, simplified and improvised. *Christian Nurse (Mysore)*. 1969;224:8-12.
50. Bewes P. Abdominal closure. *Trop Doct*. 2000;30:39-41.
51. Silk J. A new approach to the management of pretibial lacerations. *Injury*. 2001;32:373-376.
52. Davis M, Nakhdjevani A, Lidder S. Suture/Steri-Strip combination for the management of lacerations in thin-skinned individuals. *J Emerg Med*. 2011;40(3):322-323.
53. Husum H, Ang SC, Fosse E. *War Surgery: Field Manual*. Penang, Malaysia: Third World Network; 1995:71.
54. Copeland S. A simplified wound irrigation technique. *Injury*. 1979;(1):81.
55. Kamath JB, Kamath RK, Bansal H. An improvised two in one syringe suction drain for surgeries of the extremities. *Indian J Plast Surg*. 2005;38(2):173-174.
56. Singh A, Singh G. Syringe suction drain-II. *Br J Plast Surg*. 2003;56(3):313.
57. Peled IJ, Wexler MR. An improvised suction drain. *J Dermatol Surg Oncol*. 1982;8(1):18-19.
58. Riordan AT, Connor CD, Glaser DA. Surgical pearl: use of the vacutainer as a closed, active, surgical drain. *J Am Acad Derm*. 2003;48(6):933-934.
59. Peterson S, Chilukuri S, Goldberg L, Joseph AK. Surgical pearl: use of sterile glove finger as a surgical drain. *J Am Acad Derm*. 2003;49(5):902-903.
60. Adotey JM. Improvisation of a T-tube. *Trop Doct*. 1997;27(1):62.
61. Chami G, Chami B, Hatley E, et al. Simple technique for evacuation of traumatic subcutaneous haematomas under tension. *BMC Emerg Med*. 2005;5:11.
62. Abraham N, Doudle M, Carson P. Open versus closed surgical treatment of abscesses: a controlled clinical trial. *ANZ J Surg*. 1997;67(4):173-176.
63. Woo SH, Kim IH. Surgical pearl: nail edge separation with dental floss for ingrown toenails. *J Am Acad Derm*. 2004;50(6):939-940.
64. Larrabee R. Localizing lesions. *Postgrad Med*. www.postgradmed.com/pearls.htm. Accessed September 23, 2007.
65. Uba AF, Edino ST, Yakubu AA. Paediatric burns: management problems in a teaching hospital in northwestern Nigeria. *Trop Doct*. 2007;37:114-115.
66. Hartstein B, Gausche-Hill M, Cancio LC. Burn injuries in children and the use of biological dressings. *Ped Emerg Care*. 2013;29(8):939-948.
67. Lee J-Y, Choi J-W, Kim H. Determination of hand surface area by sex and body shape using alginate. *J Physiol Anthropol*. 2007;26:475-483.
68. Hettiaratchy S, Papini R. Initial management of a major burn: II – assessment and resuscitation. *BMJ*. 2004;329:101-103.
69. Chan QE, Barzi F, Cheney L, Harvey JG, Holland AJ. Burn size estimation in children: still a problem. *Emerg Med Australas*. 2012;24(2):181-186.
70. Kiser M, Beijer G, Mjuweni S, et al. Photographic assessment of burn wounds: a simple strategy in a resource-poor setting. *Burns*. 2013;39(1):155-161.
71. Stratta RJ, Saffle JR, Kravitz M, et al. Management of tar and asphalt injuries. *Am J Surg*. 1983;146:766-769.
72. James NK, Moss ALH. Review of burns caused by bitumen and the problems of its removal. *Burns*. 1990;16(3):214-216.
73. Pham TN, Cancio LC, Gibran NS. American Burn Association Practice Guidelines burn shock resuscitation. *J Burn Care Res*. 2008;29(1):257-266.
74. Latarjet J. A simple guide to burn treatment. *Burns*. 1995;21(3):221-225.
75. Horng SY, Lin T-W, Chen MT. A simple device for nasal tube fixation in facial burns patients. *Br J Plast Surg*. 1993;46:173-174.
76. Antia NH, Baver BM, Arora S. Management of burns. *Trop Doct*. 1999;29:7-11.
77. Hartstein B, Gausche-Hill M, Cancio LC. Burn injuries in children and the use of biological dressings. *Ped Emerg Care*. 2013;29(8):939-948.

78. Cotton MH. Management of burns. *Trop Doct*. 2000;30(2):124-125.
79. Shires T. Consensus Development Conference. Supportive therapy in burn care: concluding remarks by the chairman. *J Trauma*. 1979;19:935-936.
80. Baxter CR, Shires T. Physiological response to crystalloid resuscitation of severe burns. *Ann NY Acad Sci*. 1968;150(3):874-894.
81. Graves TA, Cioffi WG, McManus WF, et al. Fluid resuscitation of infants and children with massive thermal injury. *J Trauma*. 1988;28:1656-1659.
82. Cancio LC, Chavez S, Alvarado-Ortega M, et al. Predicting increased fluid requirements during the resuscitation of thermally injured patients. *J Trauma*. 2004;56:404-413.
83. Saffle JR. The phenomenon of "fluid creep" in acute burn resuscitation. *J Burn Care Res*. 2007;28: 382-395.
84. King M. *Primary Surgery, Vol. 2: Trauma*. Oxford, UK: Oxford University Press; 1987:9.
85. Wilson G, French G. Plasticised polyvinylchloride as a temporary dressing for burns. *Br Med J*. 1987;294:556-557.
86. Wilson G, French G. Plasticized polyvinylchloride as a temporary dressing for burns. *BMJ (Clin Res Ed.)* 1987;294(6571):556.
87. Liao AY, Andresen D, Martin HC, Harvey JG, Holland AJ. The infection risk of plastic wrap as an acute burns dressing. *Burns*. 2014;40(3):443-445.
88. King M. *Primary Surgery, Vol. 2: Trauma*. Oxford, UK: Oxford University Press; 1987:90.
89. King M. *Primary Surgery, Vol. 2: Trauma*. Oxford, UK: Oxford University Press; 1987:72.
90. King M. *Primary Surgery, Vol. 2: Trauma*. Oxford, UK: Oxford University Press; 1987:77.
91. King M. *Primary Surgery, Vol. 2: Trauma*. Oxford, UK: Oxford University Press; 1987:75.
92. Fösel S, Rocha E. Seawater and fresh water for treating first and second degree burns. *Trop Doct*. 1984;14(3):113-114.
93. James J. Burns management. *Trop Doct*. 2002;32:124.
94. Husum H, Ang SC, Fosse E. *War Surgery: Field Manual*. Penang, Malaysia: Third World Network; 1995:565.
95. US Army. *Emergency War Surgery*. 3rd rev. Washington, DC: Borden Institute, Walter Reed Army Medical Center; 2004:28.1.
96. Chowfin A. A method of taking Thiersch grafts using a scalpel blade. *Trop Doct*. 1995;25(1):37.
97. Salathiel MJ, Nkk N. Burn care with limited resources in Zimbabwe. *Burns*. 2006;33(1):S73.
98. Weston PM. Simple resources for essential surgery. *Trop Doct*. 1986;16(1):25-30.
99. Salasche SJ, Egan CA, Gerwels JW. Surgical pearl: use of a sponge bolster instead of a tie-over bolster as a less invasive method of securing full-thickness skin grafts. *J Am Acad Derm*. 1998;39(6): 1000-1001.
100. Serghiou M, Huang T. Burn rehabilitation made thrifty and affordable. *Burns*. 2006;33(1):S98.

26 Dental: Diagnosis, Equipment, Blocks, and Treatment

"Love conquers everything except poverty and toothaches." Mae West, *Irish Times*

Unlike much of the rest of this book, which assumes health care professionals already have the skills and knowledge to provide treatment, but not their normal equipment, this section describes dental diagnoses and basic treatments in considerably more detail. Treating dental emergencies is a critical skill, especially in situations of resource scarcity. Yet, even though dental emergencies are common, painful, and may occur with little or no warning, non-dentists rarely have in-depth knowledge about their treatment options.

BASIC DENTAL ANATOMY

Describing Teeth

When annotating the patient's medical record or communicating with another health care provider, such as a dentist, use a picture in the medical record. When communicating with another provider by phone or radio, describe the type and position of the tooth.

Teeth are either baby or adult teeth.

They are either maxillary or mandibular, and are on either the right or the left side of midline. Midline is the space between the front two teeth (incisors).

There are four types of teeth (Fig. 26-1).

Those with *one* root are:

- Incisors
- Canines
- Premolars

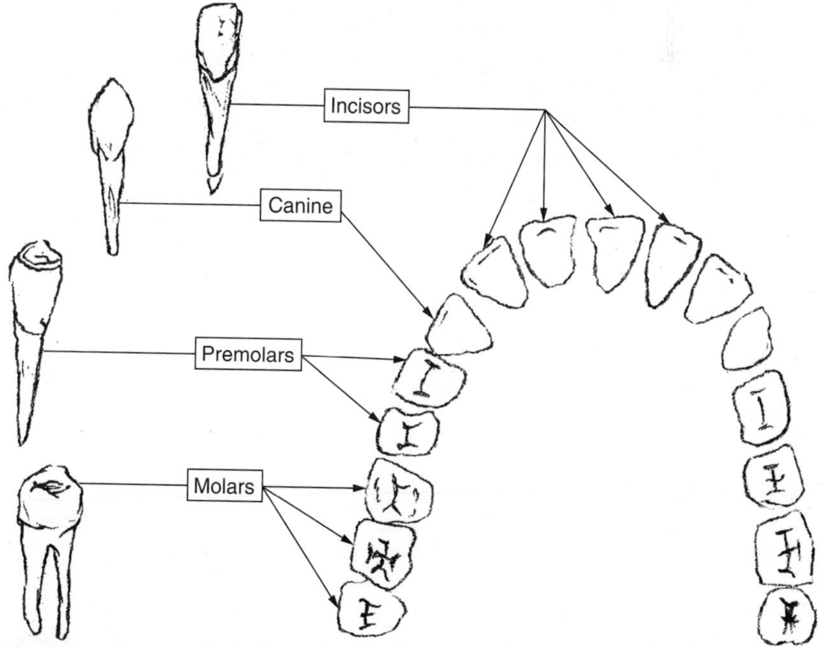

FIG. 26-1. Types of teeth.

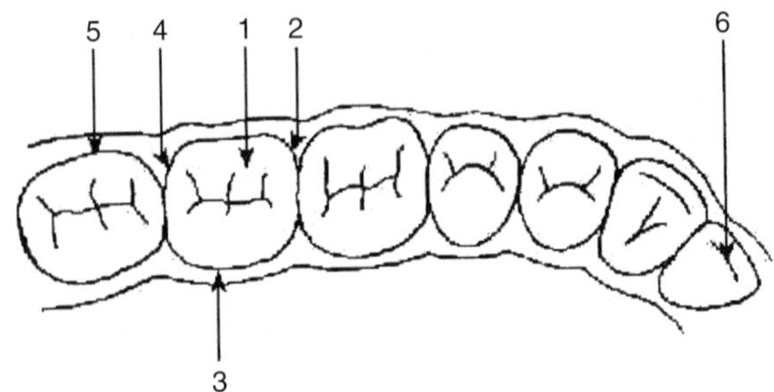

FIG. 26-2. Tooth surfaces. *(Redrawn from Frencken et al.[1])*

One type has *two* or more roots:

- Molars

Tooth Surfaces

The following names describe the surfaces of the teeth. The number corresponds to those in Fig. 26-2.

1. *Occlusal surface:* The chewing surface of molars and premolars.
2. *Mesial surface:* The surface nearest the midline of the body (medial).
3. *Lingual surface:* The surface nearest to the tongue in the lower jaw; it is called the palatal surface in the upper jaw.
4. *Distal surface:* The surface furthest from the midline.
5. *Buccal surface:* The surface nearest to the lips and cheek.
6. *Incisal edge:* The incisors and canines have a cutting edge instead of an occlusal surface.
7. *Proximal surfaces* (not shown): Surfaces that are close together, that is, the mesial surface of one tooth may touch the distal surface of the next tooth.

A Tooth's Three Layers

Tooth problems may involve any of the tooth's three layers or their supporting structures (Fig. 26-3).

CROWN

The part of the tooth above the gum line is the crown. Covered with hard enamel, the crown protects the other layers. Do not confuse the term "crown" as part of the tooth with the dentist's "crown" (also known as a "cap"), which is a dentist-made covering for a tooth.

DENTIN

Softer than enamel but about the same density as bone, dentin is a yellowish substance that lies under the enamel and surrounds the tooth's pulp cavity.

PULP CAVITY

The "heart" of the tooth, the pulp cavity contains nerves and blood vessels. Generally, it extends from the gum line to the end of the root. The vessels and nerves then continue into the alveolar bone of the mandible or maxilla.

Tooth Attachments

Every tooth has tight attachments to the bone and gums. These are the periodontal ligaments. They must be severed below the gum line when removing a tooth.

PREVENTION/CLEANING

The primary culprit in dental pathology is plaque: the soft, white or yellow layer that sticks to the teeth. Consisting primarily of bacteria, plaque also contains dried saliva, blood cells, and food particles. It accumulates at the base of the teeth, in the grooves of the tooth's occlusal

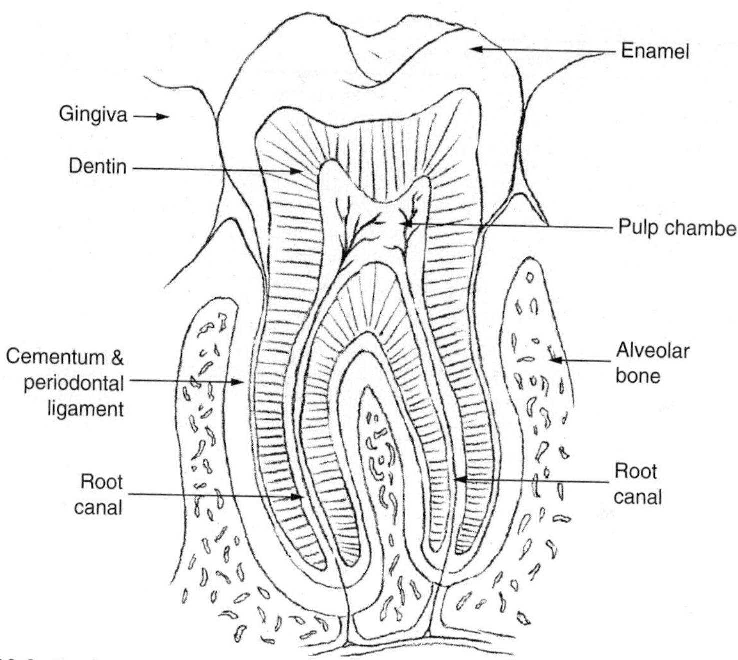

FIG. 26-3. Tooth anatomy.

surfaces, and in the spaces between the teeth. The simplest way to remove plaque from tooth surfaces when it is still sticky is to wipe it off with a cloth. A common alternative method is to thoroughly chew a green twig from a nonpoisonous plant until it becomes soft and fibrous. Use the twig's end to brush the teeth and gums. Eventually, this sticky, mineralized deposit (calculus) hardens and requires formal removal. At that point, it must be scraped off with a thin, bent metal tool. Dentists use a "scaler" or "dental pick." Alternatively, practitioners can use a small blunt needle to make a suitable instrument. First, cut off and sand the sharp end of the needle. Then, bend the end and attach it to a small syringe, which becomes a handle.

PAIN WITHOUT TRAUMA

Oral Lesions

Many types of lesions can cause pain and swelling in the mouth and face.[2,3] Table 26-1 provides a brief overview of the presentation, diagnosis, and treatment of various causes of mouth and jaw pain.

Mucosal Diseases and Facial Swelling

The most common painful oral lesions are aphthous ulcers (canker sores), traumatic ulcerations, and cold sores (*Herpes labialis*). While suitable treatment is "tincture of time," they may heal faster with less pain if they are covered, at least for several hours, with any lip balm or salve such as petroleum jelly—until they are licked off. An equally effective and possibly longer-lasting covering is cyanoacrylate (e.g., commercial Super Glue and multiple brands for medical wound closure).[4] (See below for more details on how to use it.)

Patients with multiple intraoral lesions, including mucositis in immunocompromised (e.g., cancer, AIDS) patients, may be helped by taking a mouthful of "magic mouthwash" every 2 to 3 hours, swishing it around in their mouths, and spitting it out. Make the solution using any of a dozen formulations. The most common basic elements are a 1:1:1 combination of (by volume) diphenhydramine (e.g., Benadryl) elixir, viscous lidocaine 2%, and a liquid antacid. Other common ingredients are tetracycline or erythromycin (that may be helpful with bacterial infections in the mouth) or, especially for cancer and immunocompromised patients, a steroid such as

TABLE 26-1 Diagnosis and Treatment of Mouth and Jaw Pain

Presentation	Diagnosis	Definition	Complications	Treatment
Pain, erythema, and swelling.	Cellulitis	Diffuse soft tissue bacterial infection	Regional spread	Antibiotics and root canal or extraction
Jaw hurts when touched. Teeth do not fit together properly or difficulty opening mouth. Recent trauma.	Mandible fracture	Mandible broken; may communicate using mouth (open fracture)	Malocclusion, infection, continued pain	Soft diet, wire jaw (stabilization)
Swelling under or behind jaw, worsens when hungry or smells food.	Salivary gland infection or obstruction	Usually stone in salivary duct; occasionally tumor	Infection, abscess, continued pain	Increase salivation: suck on tart candy, stone, etc. Antibiotics, if infected
Non-tender swelling in front of ear or on neck.	Branchial cleft cyst	Residual from embryological development	Infection (rare)	Surgery, if desired
Tender swelling in front of both ears with fever.	Mumps	Viral infection involving parotid glands	Orchitis in older males	Isolate from nonimmunized individuals, provide support
Swelling present for a long time. It is firm and does not seem to get better.	Tumor	Cancer	Local tissue destruction and metastatic disease	Biopsy. Excision, radiation, or chemotherapy, as indicated
Gums between teeth have died and are no longer pointed. Foul odor from mouth due to pus and blood around teeth.	Necrotizing ulcerative gingivitis (Trench mouth, Vincent's angina or stomatitis)	Infection from mouth flora due to poor oral hygiene and life situation	Pain and decreased oral intake, continued gum deterioration and tooth loss	Clean/debride area. Gentle daily brushing; qh warm salt H_2O or bid 1.5% H_2O_2 or 0.12% chlorhexidine rinses. Improve diet. Antibiotics if thorough teeth cleaning not available
Sore or small abscess near root of bad tooth.	Gum bubble	Extension of periapical abscess through a fistula	Cellulitis	Incision/drainage and root canal or extraction
Pain and clicking sound from in front of ear when moving jaw, including when chewing.	Temporomandibular joint (TMJ) pain	Degeneration of the TMJ from trauma, arthritis, etc.	Continued pain, decreased oral intake, sleeplessness, depression	Analgesics, bite guard, local injections, soft diet. Surgery only as last resort

Data from Dickson[2] and Douglass and Douglass.[3]

dexamethasone or hydrocortisone, or nystatin. One common formula uses 4 parts nystatin suspension 100,000 units/mL, 3.5 parts diphenhydramine elixir, and 1 part lidocaine viscous 2%. If the solution is made with a substance such as Kaopectate or sucralfate (Carafate), the ingredients will adhere to surfaces, and so it can be applied directly to the intraoral lesions.

If standard oral agents are not available, treat oral candidiasis (thrush), a very common oral lesion, by having the patient suck on a vaginal anti-yeast suppository or apply a vaginal anti-yeast cream to the lesion four times a day (qid).

Gum Inflammation and Pain

Painful gums can result from poor oral hygiene, infections, inflammation over an erupting tooth, or dental appliances such as orthodontics.

To avoid or treat inflamed gums resulting from poor oral hygiene, patients gently brush their teeth and gums and floss with dental floss or a substitute. They also can rinse their mouth with warm saltwater (0.5 tsp table salt in 4 oz of warm potable water) or a solution containing one part potable water and one part 3% hydrogen peroxide (H_2O_2) several times a day.[5]

More serious, and much more painful, is necrotizing ulcerative gingivitis, also known as trench mouth, Vincent angina or stomatitis, or necrotizing ulcerative periodontitis. This serious but treatable disease of the gums and deeper tissues usually begins abruptly; the patient may be febrile. The gums are very painful and bleeding, with punched-out ulcers covered with a gray pseudomembrane. Patients have extremely foul breath, pain on talking or swallowing, and may have lymphadenopathy. Treatment consists of gently debriding the area over several days. Wipe the gums with cotton or other absorbent cloth soaked in 3% H_2O_2. Use one part H_2O_2 to five parts water in children. Then scrape off the larger pieces of tartar. Have the patient gently brush their teeth and gums daily with a soft brush and rinse every waking hour with warm saltwater or twice a day with 1.5% H_2O_2 or 0.12% chlorhexidine. For the pain, use nonsteroidal analgesics and, if available, local anesthetic on the gums—after drying them. Encourage patients to avoid spicy foods and to improve their diet. They may need to be on a liquid or soft diet for a while. They should drink lots of liquids, take supplemental vitamin C, and avoid smoking and chewing betel nuts or tobacco. If thorough cleaning and debridement is not available, give oral penicillin VK 500 mg, erythromycin 250 mg, or tetracycline 250 mg q6hr until 72 hours after the symptoms resolve.

Pericoronitis occurs when inflammation develops around a partially erupted (usually molar) tooth. A flap of gingival tissue remains over the tooth, which traps food particles and is irritated by chewing. Local swelling may cause enough irritation to make it difficult to fully open the jaw. To treat this, gently irrigate the area under the flap. Have the patient rinse his or her mouth with warm saltwater for 10 minutes every 2 hours while awake. If no dentist will be available within a few days, excise the flap over the tooth.

If orthodontic appliances are causing pain, use a blunt object, such as a tongue depressor or pencil eraser, to bend the wire away from the gum. If it cannot be bent, cover it with wax (candle or dental) or a tiny piece of cloth or cotton. Paradoxically, chewing (preferably sugarless) gum reduces the general pain caused by orthodontic appliances.

Toothache

Most cases in which non-dentists will need to provide emergency dental treatment will be for toothaches. While teeth can be transiently painful for a number of reasons, constant, often excruciating, pain in a tooth constitutes a toothache. Generally, toothaches are caused by fractures or decay (caries; causes cavities) that extends into the tooth's central area (pulp). A tooth in which the pulp is no longer healthy often has a history of persistent, often severe and throbbing, pain after eating hot or cold food. Cold stimulus causes prolonged pain, but the tooth is generally not sensitive to palpation.

Diagnosis

To locate the painful tooth, have the patient point to it or gently tap on teeth in the affected area with an instrument until the patient experiences discomfort. When a tooth is tender to percussion, it is likely that there is a periapical abscess. The affected tooth can also be located by touching it with the corner of an ice cube. A normal tooth will briefly feel the cold stimulus; a diseased, but salvageable, tooth with some healthy pulp may have slightly more prolonged pain after withdrawal of the ice and is not usually sensitive to percussion. Treat them as described in the subsequent paragraphs. Be sure to check adjacent teeth for their relative sensitivity to percussion and cold. An unsalvageable tooth generally has no sensation to percussion or to a cold stimulus.

Table 26-2 provides a method of diagnosing about 90% of non-trauma-related toothaches. However, for the clinician faced with a patient's sore tooth, this table may not help in differentiating between an abscess and pulpitis. (Pulpitis is inflammation of the pulp, or center, of the tooth that contains vessels and nerves). To make this differentiation easier, remember the mnemonic *PAIN* to indicate that pain on **P**ercussion (the tap test on the tooth) = **A**bscess (periodontal or periapical), while pain with **I**ce (test the tooth by touching ice to it) = **N**erve pain (pulpitis).

Treatment

First, try to treat a toothache conservatively. Have the patient rinse vigorously with warm water. Then clean out the tooth defect and insert an analgesic gauze or filling. (See the "Filling Cavities" section in Chapter 27.) Clean the tooth using dental floss, a toothbrush, a toothpick, or a similar narrow and relatively blunt tool. If an abscess is present, treat accordingly.[6] (See the "Dental Abscesses" section discussed next.)

Using small tweezers, a hemostat, or a similar instrument, put a very small piece of cotton or other cloth soaked in local anesthetic, such as oil of cloves (long-acting) or benzocaine, into the cavity or over the fracture site. Use a paste of oil of cloves and zinc oxide, if available. When using oil of cloves rather than the less-potent commercial products containing eugenol, avoid using too much or letting it drip onto the gums or mouth tissues, because it causes mucosal burns. This provides immediate, but temporary, pain relief.

Cover this anesthetic dressing with a temporary soft putty-like filling material that can be molded to the cavity. To use wax from a candle, melt some wax, let it cool until it is pliable, and then place it over the affected area. An alternative is to use cyanoacrylate glue.

If this does not work, open the pulp chamber (center of tooth) to drain the tooth. As a last resort, extraction may be necessary (see the "Extractions" section in Chapter 27).

Dental Abscesses

Dental (periapical and periodontal) abscesses occur adjacent to the affected teeth. These abscesses often cause swelling of the cheek, the mouth, or the neck. The adjacent tooth will generally be very tender to gentle percussion. The patient with a periapical abscess may also have increased pain when recumbent, have a bad taste in his or her mouth, or say that the tooth feels "longer" than adjacent teeth. In addition, he or she may have a gumboil (an abscess under the gum at the end of a sinus tract extending from the periapical abscess). The abscess may also develop into facial cellulitis with significant swelling. Periodontal abscesses may be more localized than periapical abscesses and usually result from chronic gingival disease, rather than from caries.

Treat periodontal abscesses by having the patient rinse the abscessed area with warm salt water for 10 minutes every 2 hours while awake. This may provide some immediate relief and can help the abscess drain spontaneously. Apply ice to the face. Nonsteroidal analgesics may decrease the pain; opioids may be required.

If no dental care will be readily available and the abscess is pointing, drain it using a scalpel, needle, or fishhook that has been thoroughly cleaned. Be sure to remove the barb before using a fishhook. Subsequent warm saltwater rinsing, although initially painful, will help the drained abscess resolve more quickly.

If the tooth is loose due to the abscess or, if not, as a last resort after more conservative treatment has failed, extract the tooth (see the "Extractions" section in Chapter 27). Because the tooth acts like any infected foreign body (such as a splinter), the infection is best treated by removing the tooth as soon as possible once it is determined that the tooth cannot be salvaged. (Daniel Kemmedson, DMD. Personal written communication, June 5, 2008.) If extraction is not possible, treat the patient with antibiotics, if available, to cover mouth flora (usually penicillin); have the patient use warm moist soaks over the affected area and warm water rinses in the mouth.

Antibiotics

Because antibiotics may be scarce, it is worthwhile to consider whether they are necessary for dental lesions.[7] While antibiotics may not make a difference in most outcomes, "without good

TABLE 26-2 Differential Diagnosis of Toothache

Presentation	Diagnosis	Definition	Complications	Treatment
Pain after eating or drinking Caries: present Cold test: negative Tap test: negative Biting pain: negative	Caries (cavity)	Hole in tooth enamel	Pulpitis	Clean hole, filling (temporary)
Pain after eating or drinking Caries: present; previously filled Cold test: negative Tap test: negative Biting pain: negative	Lost or broken filling	Caries, previously filled, with lost or broken filling	Pulpitis	Clean hole, filling (temporary)
Pain on eating hot, cold, or sweet food Caries: present Cold test: positive/negative Tap test: negative Biting pain: negative	Reversible pulpitis	Inflammation of tooth pulp	Periapical abscess, cellulitis	Filling
Spontaneous, persistent, poorly localized pain Caries: present Cold test: persistent Tap test: negative Biting pain: negative	Irreversible pulpitis	Inflammation of tooth pulp	Periapical abscess, cellulitis	Root canal, extraction
Severe, constant, localized pain and swelling—even when trying to sleep; recent toothache; tooth may feel slightly loose Caries: present Cold test: negative Tap test: positive Biting pain: positive	Periapical dental abscess	Localized bacterial infection	Cellulitis	Incision/drainage and root canal or extraction
Moderate to severe, constant, localized pain; recent toothache Caries: absent Cold test: negative Tap test: positive Biting pain: positive	Periodontal dental abscess	Localized bacterial infection	Cellulitis	Incision/drainage and root canal or extraction
Difficulty in or pain on opening mouth; constant, localized pain and swelling over back tooth; recent toothache Caries: present or absent Cold test: negative Tap test: positive Biting pain: positive	Dental abscess around molar	Localized bacterial infection around back tooth	Cellulitis	Incision/drainage and root canal or extraction

(Continued)

TABLE 26-2 Differential Diagnosis of Toothache (*Continued*)

Presentation	Diagnosis	Definition	Complications	Treatment
Steady pain, erythema, bad taste, and swelling, probably from a back molar; difficulty opening mouth; patient 16 to 24 years old	Pericoronitis	Inflamed gum over partially erupted tooth	Cellulitis	Irrigation, antibiotics if cellulitis also present
Pain when breathing cold air; recent trauma	Tooth fracture	Cracked or broken tooth	Pulpitis and sequelae	Filling, with or without root canal, extraction
Pain in tooth when scuba/hard-hat diving or in airplane	Barotrauma	Pain from pressure change in space under filling, abscess, or sinus	Disruption of filling; inability to continue dive or flight	Analgesics, drainage (medications for sinus; repair for fillings)

Cold test: Touch the tooth with the corner of an ice cube. Tap test: Tap the tooth gently with the oral mirror or a similar tool. Biting pain: Pain when biting on a tongue depressor or similar object.

Data from Dickson,[2] Douglass and Douglass,[3] and Shiller.[6]

radiographic and pulpal evaluation or good follow-up, and [given] the potential of serious deep-space infection risk, antibiotics should probably be prescribed for at-risk patients."[8] So, prescribing antibiotics will depend on both the specific circumstances and the availability of the medication. If used, options for antibiotics for dental infections include penicillin VK 500 mg po qid, erythromycin 500 mg po qid, and clindamycin 300 mg po three times a day (tid).

Lost Filling or Lost Crown (Cap)

If a dentist-formed crown, otherwise known as a "cap," is lost, gently clean out the hole where the filling resided. Do not try to replace the cap unless the patient is in so much pain that there is no other choice or if dental care will not be available in a timely manner. Save the cap for a dentist to use at a later time. The danger in replacing the cap is that it could come off again and the patient might aspirate it. In the meantime, cover the exposed pulp with softened candle wax, cyanoacrylate, or a commercial temporary tooth filling material.

If a non-dentist must replace a cap, gently clean out any residual cement from inside the cap with a very small knife, paperclip, the filament from a light bulb, or similar tool. Then place a thin layer of dental filling, denture adhesive, cyanoacrylate, or a thick mixture of flour and water inside the crown. Having the patient gently bite down on the replaced cap helps position it correctly. Remove any excess material. Advise the patient not to use that tooth when eating; the cap will most likely come off.

Cavities

If a tooth has a cavity but is not abscessed, try to put in a temporary filling. (A permanent filling requires the skill and equipment that only a dentist can provide.) This decreases the chance of further tooth decay, prevents an abscess from forming, decreases the patient's pain, and may ultimately save the tooth.[9]

Do not put a filling in an abscessed tooth! It will only make the pain and swelling worse. If the tooth has an abscess and you are in a situation with few resources and no dentist, pull the tooth. (Even if you break the tooth, it will allow the abscess to drain, improving the patient's condition.[9])

Chapter 27 provides detailed information on how to do fillings and extractions.

DENTAL INSTRUMENTS AND EQUIPMENT

If dental instruments (hand tools) are available, great! If not, they can often be fashioned from many different items or replaced by available tools. For example, Native healers fashion knives and dental extractors from beaten iron nails.[10] I used electrician's tools to remove several molars in the Arctic.[11]

General Equipment

Before beginning any dental procedure, three things are necessary: the patient in the correct position, adequate light, and a way to dry and isolate the tooth.

Chair

A key element of successful dental work is to not be bending over. Raise the patient's mouth to a level where you can work comfortably. The patient is most comfortable if his or her head, back, and neck are supported. One method of putting the patient in the proper position for dental work is to use a regular office-type chair, back it up to a desk or table, and place the patient's head on several pillows on that surface.[6] Modify a chair with two side posts by securely attaching two pieces of wood or metal and tying a cloth between them (Fig. 26-4). Have the patient rest his or her head on the cloth. You can also use a low chair with a back. If the chair is too low for you to work comfortably, have the patient sit on books.

Headlamp/Light Source

A headlamp is standard equipment for all surgical procedures in austere situations. If you do not have a headlamp, use any available light source, including a lamp, laryngoscope, or fiber-optic light. To direct the light so that it illuminates the part of the patient's mouth you are working on, use a hand mirror or have someone hold the light source (or a mirror) in the best position. To work in the sunlight, position the patient toward the sun. (In some cases, you may want to cover his or her eyes.) If indoors, position the patient to face the window.

Secretion Barriers

To isolate a tooth from mouth secretions, position cotton rolls or 2×2 gauze squares inside the lip next to the tooth and between the tongue and the tooth. If working on a maxillary tooth, place the gauze or cloth roll over Stensen duct (opening of the parotid salivary gland).

Dental Drill

Dental drills should only be used by trained dentists.

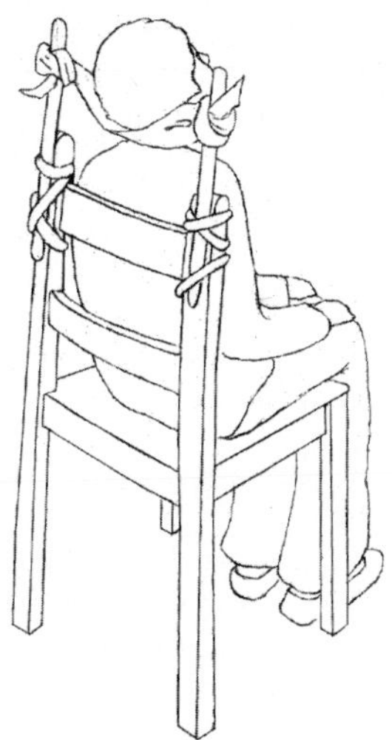

FIG. 26-4. Improvised dental/ENT chair.

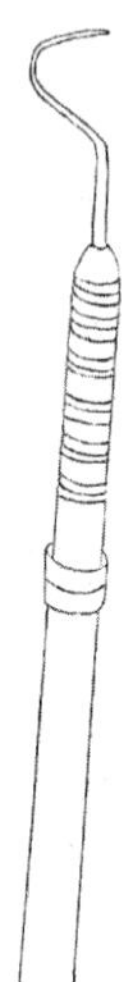

FIG. 26-5. Dental probe (explorer).

Mirror

Use a mirror to reflect light onto the field of operation, to view the cavity indirectly, and to retract the cheek or tongue as necessary. Fashion a mouth mirror by first taping the edges of a small piece of broken mirror (to protect the patient from the sharp edges) and then gluing it onto the end of a short piece of a coat hanger or other relatively stiff metal wire.

Needed to Fill Cavities

Besides a headlamp and a mirror, a standard set of instruments to apply a temporary filling includes the following items:

Probe (Explorer)

Use a probe (Fig. 26-5) to identify where soft carious dentin is present. Take care not to penetrate very small caries (this may destroy the tooth's surface) or obvious deep cavities (this may damage the pulp). A probe can be fashioned from a small (23- or 25-gauge) needle that has the tip filed off and is bent on the end. Use a small syringe or wooden dowel (e.g., Q-tip, cotton swab) as a handle.

Cotton Pledgets/Absorptive Gauze

Use cotton pledgets or any small pieces of absorptive gauze to soak up any saliva and keep the work area dry.

Mixing Block and Tool (Cement Spatula)

If a polymer with two components, generally a liquid and a powder, is used, these have to be mixed. A piece of glass or a rigid plastic sheet will work as a mixing block. Use a piece of wood as a spatula.

Tweezers (Pickups)

Use a tweezers to place materials in the mouth. This is more elegant than using your fingers, which are what you must use if tweezers, hemostats, or similar devices are not available.

Dental Hatchet

This tool widens the entrance to a cavity so there is better access for the excavator. It is also used to remove the thin, unsupported carious enamel that remains after carious dentin has been removed. A thin piece of rigid metal, such as a large-gauge (12- or 14-gauge) needle with its point filed off, should be used. It helps to bend the tip.

Spoon (Spoon Excavator)

Use a spoon excavator to remove soft carious dentin. A needle that fits into the caries can be used instead. File down the sharp tip to make it easier to use.

Filling Tool (Filling Instrument)

If a dental filling tool to put the filling material into the cavity and smooth it over is not available, use a small thin piece of metal. If using cyanoacrylate, the top of the tube often works well.

Sterilizing Dental Equipment

Failing to sterilize dental equipment between patients can lead to transmission of serious diseases, such as hepatitis and human immunodeficiency virus (HIV). Before sterilization, clean the instruments of any visible grime. Neither chemical sterilization nor boiling effectively sterilizes dental equipment. In austere environments, use dry-heat ovens with an uninterrupted cycle, including a holding time of 60 minutes at 160°C (320°F).[12] Whenever possible, autoclaving should be used to sterilize dental instruments.

CYANOACRYLATE FOR DENTAL EMERGENCIES

Cyanoacrylate (e.g., Super Glue) as a surgical adhesive is discussed more thoroughly in the "Wound Glues" section in Chapter 22.

To use any cyanoacrylate properly, all surfaces must be dry. Use gauze, tissue paper, or cloth to dry the affected tooth and to keep saliva away from it during the process. Use the top of the cyanoacrylate tube or a small piece of metal to keep pressure on the tooth for the few seconds it is drying. Try not to use your fingertip, because that will result in it being stuck in the patient's mouth for a while. After the glue sets, immediately have the patient salivate and wet the entire area.

Try to keep the glue off the gums if this is not necessary for the procedure. Glue near the gums can irritate them; excess glue can form a rough edge that also irritates the tongue. Correct the latter by carefully filing the edge or by covering the area with a small amount of additional glue.

Using the glue may result in an abnormal bite after repairing dentures or teeth. People notice even the smallest change in their dental occlusion. File down excess glue. See the method for optimizing the patient's bite using carbon paper in Step 6 of the "How to Fill a Tooth: Procedural Steps" section in Chapter 27. Even if the fit is not perfect, do whatever you can to improve the situation. As a non-dentist, you are using these techniques only to buy time until the patient can see a dentist.

If cyanoacrylate is used, warn the patient not to put too much pressure on the tooth and to try not to bite with it. These dental repairs generally last days to weeks, but eventually the procedures must be redone. Of course, if the patient can see a dentist, that is optimal.

Cyanoacrylate adhesives can be used for many dental problems. These include protecting or repairing oral soft tissues, repairing dentures and teeth, and even protecting hypersensitive teeth.

Oral Soft Tissues

People have applied cyanoacrylate to aphthous lesions (canker sores) for many years to reduce the pain. One need only apply the glue to the lesion. It remains until the moisture of the lip and natural turnover of skin make it peel off. Of course, anything that covers the lesion (such as a lip balm) will lessen the discomfort. In 1999, the US Food and Drug Administration approved a cyanoacrylate (Colgate Orabase Soothe-N-Seal Liquid Protectant) for over-the-counter use in the treatment of aphthous ulcers, mouth sores, and traumatic ulcerations. This formulation has much less tensile strength than do the standard medical formulations and will slough off in only 6 to 10 hours: It may have to be replaced if continued coverage is needed.[13]

Cyanoacrylate is also useful for repairing abrasions and lacerations to the lip and oral mucosa.[14,15] Perhaps because of its occasionally unpleasant taste, some people have tried to develop flavored products. Cyanoacrylate has been used for wound closure in oral surgery; it compares favorably with sutures, showing normal healing of incisions and immediate hemostasis.

It has also been useful in relieving the pain when dressing donor sites and mucosal ulcerations, while helping them to heal quickly.[15]

Orthodontic Appliances

Cyanoacrylate can also be used to re-bond loose orthodontic brackets, although care must be taken to be sure they remain in the correct position.[16]

Denture Repair

Use cyanoacrylate to temporarily glue a tooth or part of a tooth back into a denture (dental prosthesis). The glue may not be strong enough to repair a denture that breaks in half, however, depending on the denture material.[17] If the denture is made of acrylic, it can be repaired using cyanoacrylate adhesive. In the developing world, acrylic is still widely used for dental prostheses because of its relatively low cost.

When doing these repairs, the dentures must be properly aligned. If done incorrectly so that the dentures no longer fit well, the adhesive can be very difficult to remove.[18]

Dental Trauma

As noted above, cyanoacrylate can be used to repair tooth fractures, to glue on pieces of fractured teeth, and to attach temporary dental splints.[19]

Filling Cavities

Cyanoacrylate is very effective in filling holes for root canals. It also controls micro-leakage of oral fluid at the tooth–filling interface, and so is effective, at least temporarily, for filling a cavity.[20,21]

Gluing Avulsed Teeth

When avulsed teeth have been temporarily glued in to keep them in position, it is best to use cyanoacrylate as part of a splinting process, as described above in Chapter 27. One patient was found to have repeatedly used cyanoacrylate over a year to retain an avulsed second upper incisor.[22] Another man, who had four adjacent maxillary teeth fractured in a baseball game, glued them to each other and repeatedly glued the group back onto adjacent teeth over a period of a year until seen by a dentist (and, since he was lost to follow-up due to a lack of insurance, probably after that). His technique was to first carefully dry the crowns and roots that were broken, and next glue them together with nonmedical cyanoacrylate while in the correct position in his mouth. The four teeth were also bonded together. (Having used a larger amount of glue than necessary, it adhered to his palate but separated "after a few hours.") He then removed the four-tooth piece and "shaped it with a file," reinserting it into position and gluing it to the adjacent teeth. He removed the four-tooth piece every 4 to 6 weeks, cleaned it, filed it as necessary to improve the fit, and re-glued it to adjacent teeth. While he initially used the liquid cyanoacrylate, he eventually switched to the gel, which worked better. The patient's lack of pain during the initial procedure was attributed to the pulp (and nerves) being dead.[23]

Hypersensitive Teeth

Cyanoacrylate is more effective than some standard methods for treating hypersensitive teeth. After drying the hypersensitive area, apply cyanoacrylate and allow it to dry. Patients then rinse their mouths thoroughly with lukewarm water. For approximately half of all patients, the treatment lasts about 3 months; it can then be repeated.[24]

ANESTHESIA AND ANALGESIA

Analgesics

Oral analgesics that are effective for most dental problems include acetaminophen 650 to 1000 mg q6hr and nonsteroidal anti-inflammatory drugs (NSAIDs), such as ibuprofen 400 to 800 mg q6hr. For severe pain, combine these drugs with opioids, such as 5 mg codeine.[25]

Local Anesthetics for Dental Blocks

Use standard local anesthetics for dental blocks, with or without epinephrine. Two easy methods are available to dose children with local anesthetics. The first is Clark's rule, which says that the maximum dose of any local anesthetic = (weight of child in lb/150) × max adult dose (in mg) calculated for that child. For example, the dose of lidocaine without epinephrine for a child weighing 50 lb would be: (50 lb/150) × (2.0 mg/lb × 50 lb) = $^{1}/_{3}$ × 100 mg = 33 mg.

An even simpler method is to use 1.8 cc of 2% lidocaine/20 lb. The volume of a normal dental anesthetic "carpule" used in dental syringes is 1.8 cc.

Blocking Individual Teeth

Supraperiosteal Infiltration

Use supraperiosteal infiltration to block individual teeth. If topical benzocaine (20%) is available, first apply it to the injection site using a cotton swab. Then retract the lip and shake it to get access and provide some mechanical anesthesia (or useful distraction). Using a 25-, 27-, or 30-gauge needle (or the smallest gauge available), enter at the junction of the lip and the gum directly over and parallel to the long axis of the affected tooth. Advance the needle 3 to 4 mm and inject 0.5 cc of 2% lidocaine with 1:100,000 epinephrine or 0.5% bupivacaine (Marcaine) with 1:100,000 epinephrine (adults). Repeat the procedure, as needed. When blocking a mandibular tooth, more anesthetic will be needed because the mandibular bone is denser than the maxilla.[26] (The maximum dose of bupivacaine for intraoral injection is 90 mg. The maximum intraoral dose of lidocaine with epinephrine or articaine with epinephrine is 500 mg.)

Infraorbital Nerve Block

While an infraorbital nerve block is actually a regional block for the upper (maxillary) incisors, the upper lip, and the side of the nose, the procedure is a simple extension of supraperiosteal infiltration (Fig. 26-6). It often has to be performed bilaterally, especially for lacerations involving the middle third of the upper lip.[27] The needle inserted over the upper canine tooth need only advance about 2 cm, so that the needle tip is over the most prominent part of the cheek (malar eminence) (Fig. 26-7). Experience shows that injecting 2 to 3 cc of 2% lidocaine with or without epinephrine works nearly 100% of the time.

Mental Nerve Block

This blocks the chin, lower lip, and buccal mucosa from midline to the second premolar, and uses the same technique as with supraperiosteal infiltration. Insert the needle at the juncture of the

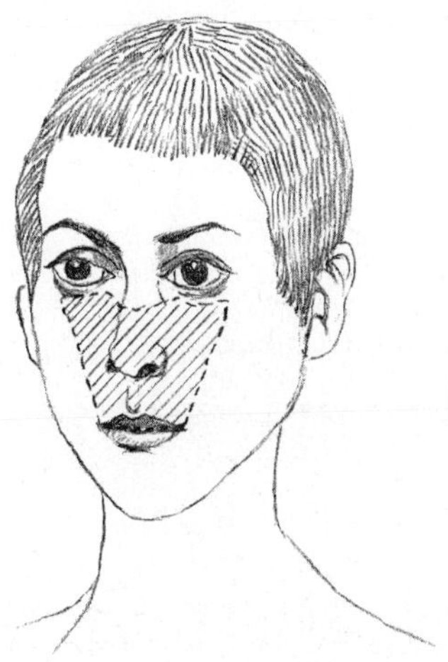

FIG. 26-6. Areas anesthetized with bilateral infraorbital block.

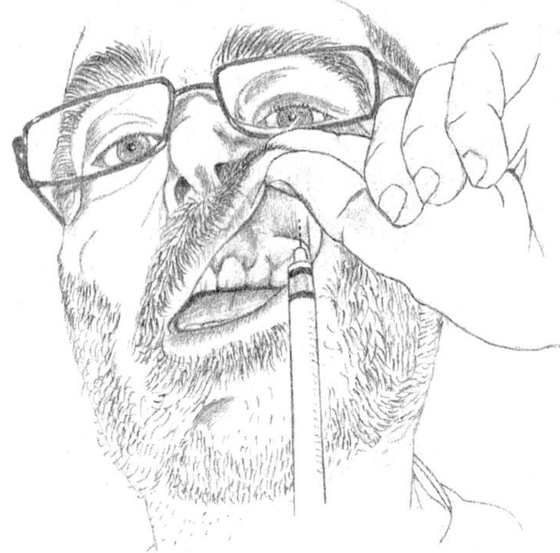

FIG. 26-7. Infraorbital block technique.

gum and lip in line with the lateral nare. For lesions toward the mid-third of the face, do the block bilaterally.

Regional Blocks

Inferior Alveolar Nerve Block

This blocks all mandibular teeth on the side injected and, if done correctly, can also block the side of the tongue.

Procedure

Direct the needle through the mouth from the opposite side to the side to be blocked. The operator's thumb (shown as the index finger in the figure) is placed in the coronoid notch of the mandible, and the index finger is on the mandible external to the mouth (Fig. 26-8). The coronoid notch can be located by passing the thumb over the lower molars until it contacts the mandibular ramus. The notch is the hole that the thumb tip naturally falls into when doing this.

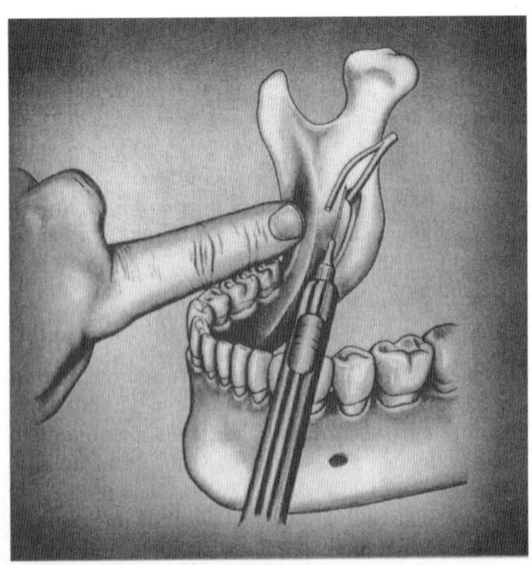

FIG. 26-8. Inferior alveolar block.

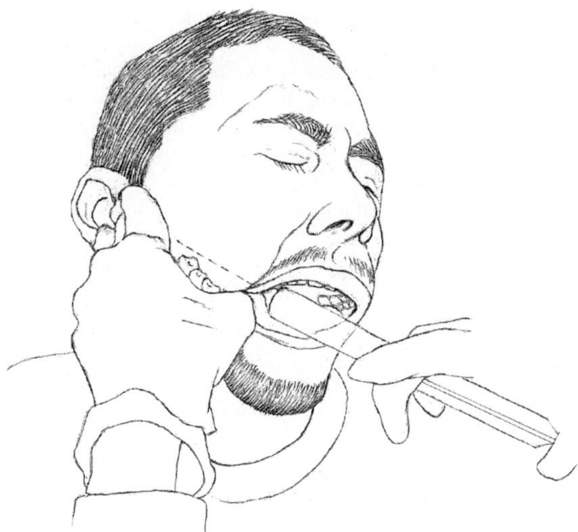

FIG. 26-9. Gow-Gates block.

Direct a 25- or 27-gauge needle toward the mucosa on the medial border of the mandibular ramus. Generally, this should be just next to (just medial to) the tip of the thumb in the coronoid notch. This should place the needle 6 to 10 mm above the mandibular molars. Insert the needle about 25 mm (1 inch) and, after a negative aspiration, inject ~0.5 to 1.5 cc of local anesthetic, such as bupivacaine. Continue to aspirate, and inject ~0.5 to 1.0 cc on removal from the injection site to anesthetize the lingual branch (side of the tongue).

Inject another 0.5 to 1.0 cc of anesthetic into the mandibular coronoid notch (where the thumb was, just distal to the last molar) to perform a long buccal nerve block. This anesthetizes the buccal surface of the mandibular molars and adjacent gum.

Gow-Gates Technique: Alternative to Inferior Alveolar Block

The Gow-Gates mandibular block is another technique for mandibular anesthesia, especially when the standard inferior alveolar nerve block fails to supply adequate anesthetic effect. It anesthetizes the inferior alveolar, lingual nerve, and the long buccal nerve with one injection.[28]

Perform the Gow-Gates block by inserting the needle higher than with a standard alveolar block. The technique will anesthetize the mandibular teeth to the midline, the buccal tissues and bone, the floor of the mouth and tongue to the midline, lingual tissues and bone, the body of the mandible, and the skin over the zygoma.

TECHNIQUE

Insert a 25- or 27-gauge needle distal to the last (second or third) molar on the medial surface of the mandibular ramus. Guide the needle on an imaginary line from the intertragic notch (ear) to the corner of the mouth (Fig. 26-9). Use a thumb in the coronoid notch and the index finger over the head of the condyle. (Find the head of the condyle at the temporomandibular joint by having the patient open and close his mouth to feel it move.) The needle is aiming for the head of the mandibular condyle. Keep the barrel of the needle approximately over the mandibular premolars on the same side, and insert the needle using the landmarks of the tragus and second molar. Keep the needle parallel with the imaginary line from the corner of the mouth to the intertragic notch, and advance the needle slowly until bone is contacted. This will be the head of the condyle. Insert the needle to the same depth as for the inferior alveolar nerve block—about 25 mm in an adult. If bone is not contacted, slightly withdraw the needle and reinsert it.

Once the needle contacts bone, withdraw it about 1 mm and aspirate. Positive aspiration for this injection occurs less often than with similar blocks (< 2% of the time), but aspiration is still necessary. If positive, the needle is probably in the internal maxillary artery, inferior to the target.

In that case, withdraw the needle, get new anesthetic solution, and redirect the needle superiorly to the previous injection site.

If the aspiration is negative, slowly deposit ~2 to 3 cc of local anesthetic. After the needle is withdrawn, have the patient keep his mouth open for a few minutes for the anesthetic to properly diffuse and until he reports signs of inferior alveolar anesthesia.[28] To help the patient keep his mouth open, have him bite down on the syringe you just used. Onset of anesthesia may take longer because the nerve is denser at this point and the area of deposition is somewhat farther from the nerve. The patient's tongue and lower lip should be numb. Check all areas for anesthesia before proceeding with treatment.[29]

REFERENCES

1. Frencken J, Phantumvanit P, Pilot T, et al. *Manual for the Atraumatic Restorative Treatment Approach to Control Dental Caries*. Geneva, Switzerland: WHO; 1997. http://www.researchgate.net/profile/Yupin_Songpaisan/publication/228553340_Manual_for_the_Atraumatic_Restaurative_Treatment_approach_to_control_dental_caries/links/02e7e51f0ef4f102d1000000.pdf. Accessed September 25, 2015.
2. Dickson M. *Where There Is No Dentist*. Berkeley, CA: Hesperian Foundation; 2006:80-83.
3. Douglass AB, Douglass JM. Common dental emergencies. *Am Fam Physician*. 2003;67(3):511-516.
4. Jasmin JR, Muller-Giamarchi M, Jonesco-Benaiche N. Local treatment of minor aphthous ulceration in children. *ASDC J Dent Child*. 1993;60:26-28.
5. Barsky NH, Londeree K. First aid procedures for dental emergencies. *J Sch Health*. 1982;52(1):43-45.
6. Shiller WR. *Emergency Dental Treatment by Medical Officers on Isolated Duty*. Groton, CT: US Naval Submarine Medical Center, Report MR005.19-6024.01; 1968.
7. Runyon MS, Brennan MT, Batts JJ, et al. Efficacy of penicillin for dental pain without overt infection. *Acad Emerg Med*. 2004;11(12):1268-1271.
8. Benko K. Acute dental emergencies. Presented at ACEP Scientific Assembly, Seattle, WA. October 10, 2007.
9. Dickson M. *Where There Is No Dentist*. Berkeley, CA: Hesperian Foundation; 2006:143-151.
10. Ellis J, Arubaku W. Complications from traditional tooth extraction in South-western Uganda. *Trop Doct*. 2005;35:245-246.
11. Iserson KV. Dental extractions using improvised equipment. *Wild Environ Med*. 2013;24:384-389.
12. Jamani J, Rababah T, Qsous R, et al. Testing of several methods of sterilization in dental practice. *Eastern Mediterranean Health J*. 1995;1(1):80-86.
13. Hille LM, Linklater DR. Use of 2-octyl cyanoacrylate for the repair of a fractured molar tooth. *Ann Emerg Med*. 2006;47(5):424-426.
14. de Blanco LP. Lip suture with isobutyl cyanoacrylate. *Endod Dent Traumatol*. 1994;10:15-18.
15. Perez M, Fernandez I, Marquez D, et al. Use of N-butyl-2-cyanoacrylate in oral surgery: biological and clinical evaluation. *Artif Organs*. 2000;24(3):241-243.
16. Bishara SE, VonWald L, Laffoon JF, et al. Effect of using a new cyanoacrylate adhesive on the shear bond strength of orthodontic brackets. *Angle Orthod*. 2001;71:466-469.
17. Gordon J. Coping with dental emergencies, broken dentures and crowns (caps) that fall out. www.howstuffowrks.com/dental12.htm. Accessed December 29, 2006.
18. Clancy JM, Dixon DL. Cyanoacrylate home denture repair: the problem and a solution. *J Prosthet Dent*. 1989;62:487-489.
19. Leggat PA, Kedjarune U, Smith DR. Toxicity of cyanoacrylate adhesives and their occupational impacts for dental staff. *Ind Health*. 2004;42:207-211.
20. Barkhordar RA, Javid B, Abbasi J, et al. Cyanoacrylate as a retrofilling material. *Oral Surg Oral Med Oral Pathol*. 1988;65:468-473.
21. Lage-Marques JL, Conti R, Antoniazzi JH. The use of Histoacryl in endodontics. *Braz Dent J*. 1993;3:95-98.
22. Leyland JT. Amateur dentistry and the anesthesiologist. *Anesthesiology*. 2004;101(4):1051.
23. Winkler S, Wood R, Facchiano AM, et al. Esthetics and super glue: a case report. *J Oral Implant*. 2003;29(6):286-288.
24. Javid B, Barkhordar RA, Bhinda SV. Cyanoacrylate—a new treatment for hypersensitive dentin and cemenum. *J Am Dent Assoc*. 1987;114:486.

25. Anon. Fractured and avulsed teeth. *Merck Manual Professional.* http://www.merck.com/mmpe/sec08/ch096/ch096a.html. Accessed March 22, 2008.
26. Benko K, Turturro M, Mattis J, et al. Dental skills lab. Presented at ACEP Scientific Assembly, Seattle, WA. October 10, 2007. http://meetings.acep.org/NR/rdonlyres/BE685599-3E36-4089-A1C8-E5684AA9CF2D/0/WE183.pdf. Accessed March 31, 2008.
27. Allen CW. *Local and Regional Anesthesia.* 2nd ed. Philadelphia, PA: W.B. Saunders; 1918:513.
28. Meechan JG. How to overcome failed local anaesthesia. *Br Dent J.* 1999;186(1):15-20.
29. Dental Learning Network. Injection techniques: other mandibular nerve block anesthetic techniques. *Local Anesthetic Review.* http://www.dentallearning.org/course/fde0010/c12/p03.htm. Accessed March 22, 2008.

27 Dental: Fillings, Extractions, and Trauma

Non-dental health care providers fear few things more than having to do dental procedures. The most common dental problems that non-dentists face in austere environments are filling cavities, extracting teeth, and managing oral trauma. The information in this chapter will help you manage these cases, even with limited or no formal dental equipment or training. (See also Chapter 26 for basic information about nerve blocks and how to improvise some of the equipment you will need.)

FILLING CAVITIES

Depending on the materials used, a temporary filling will last from only a few weeks to a few months. A dentist should replace this temporary filling as soon as practicable with a permanent filling. In the meantime, the temporary filling helps the patient to feel more comfortable.[1]

Never put a filling in an abscessed tooth. You are probably safe filling the cavity if:

- There is no swelling of the face or gums near the bad tooth.
- The tooth hurts only occasionally—such as when eating or if breathing cold air.
- The tooth is not tender to percussion.

Filling Materials and Equipment

The basic filling material for cavities is usually zinc oxide powder and oil of cloves liquid (eugenol). These materials come in a wide variety of brands, but are usually readily available. Intermediate restorative material (IRM) may be available; it provides more durable fillings. Often much easier to obtain is cyanoacrylate, which works well as a temporary filling, although it may not last as long as traditional materials.

While dentists routinely use drills to help fill teeth, these will usually not be available in austere circumstances. In addition, a dental drill is not a tool that the inexperienced practitioner should use. Instead, non-dentists can use dental hand tools, which are easy to use. If there are none available, they can be improvised or purchased at a relatively low cost. Hand tools are also less painful for the patient than a low-speed drill, such as a foot-pedal-powered drill, which may be available in remote or austere settings. Dental tools should be sterilized after each use.

Chapter 26 lists dental equipment you will need to fill a tooth and suggests ways to improvise these items.

How to Fill a Tooth: Procedural Steps

1. The initial task is to isolate the tooth so you can keep the cavity dry. A dry cavity allows you to see what you are doing and, more importantly, strengthens the bond with the cement you are using. To keep the tooth and cavity dry, put cotton or other absorbent cloth between the cheek and gums. When working on a lower (mandibular) tooth, put some under the tongue. Change the cloth whenever it becomes wet, and wipe the cavity itself while you work. Leave a piece of cloth inside the cavity if you mix the filler (unnecessary if using cyanoacrylate). Using continuous suction in the mouth helps reduce the saliva; give the suction to the patient to hold in the hand opposite the side on which you are working.
2. Then remove some of the decay from the cavity. As you remove the pieces, put them on a piece of cloth or cotton gauze that sits on the patient's chest. Removing them as you go prevents the patient from swallowing them. Scrape the walls and the edge of the cavity to remove all decay from the cavity's edge. This prevents later enlargement of the defect when germs and food lodge in the space between the cement and the cavity. If the edge is thin and

weak, dentists can break it with the end of their instrument, which will result in stronger sides to hold the cement; non-dentists need not do that. Use the spoon tool (or a large-bore needle) to lift out soft decay from inside the cavity, but do not try to remove decay at the cavity's bottom; it may be covering a nerve. There is no problem leaving some decay at the bottom of the cavity if you cover it with filling material so it stops growing. Enlarge the cavity just enough to give the cement a suitable bonding area. Use a mirror to carefully examine the cavity's edges for additional decay. Put some cotton or cloth inside the cavity, and leave it there while you mix the cement.

3. If using cement that needs mixing, such as commercial dental filling material, mix the cement on a piece of smooth glass or plastic. To mix zinc oxide powder and eugenol, place some zinc oxide powder on the glass and, a distance away from it, a few drops of eugenol liquid. Use a mixing tool, such as a piece of a tongue depressor or a coffee stirrer, and add a small amount of the powder to the liquid, mixing them together. Continue adding small amounts of the powder until the cement mixture becomes thick. It helps to practice with the cement in advance to hone the mixing technique, determine the time it takes for the cement to harden, and see how best to manipulate it. Using this cement is much easier when it is thick and not too sticky. To test for "stickiness," roll some between your fingers; if it sticks to the fingers, it is not ready. Add more powder and then try it again.
4. Once the filler is prepared or you are ready to use the cyanoacrylate, remove any cotton or cloth from the cavity and make certain that the cavity is dry. Then press (or drip, in the case of cyanoacrylate) some filling material into the cavity. Keeping the area dry with cotton or absorbent cloth around the tooth, put a small ball of cement on the end of a filling tool (or a small, thin flat screwdriver) and spread it over the floor of the cavity, in particular into the corners. Add another ball of cement, pressing it against the cement already in the hole and against the sides of the cavity. The key is to pack the cavity completely and tightly to stop the growth of decay. Keep adding cement until the cavity is overfilled. Then, smooth the extra cement against the edge of the cavity. If a cavity goes down between two teeth, one other step is necessary: You need to take care that the cement does not squeeze and hurt the gum. Before you spread the cement, place something thin between the teeth. You can use the soft stem from a palm leaf, a toothpick, or a tooth from a comb, but be sure it has a rounded end to prevent damage to the gums.[2] If you are using cyanoacrylate, no filling tool is needed, but you must avoid leaving air bubbles in the cement.
5. Remove the extra cement before it gets too hard. Press the flat side of the filling tool against the cement and smooth it toward the edge of the cavity. As you smooth the cement, shape it to look like the top of a normal tooth. This way, the tooth above or below it can fit against the filling without breaking it. If you are using cyanoacrylate, work fast to smooth the filling, because it dries very quickly. Do not touch it with your finger or you may get stuck to the patient! After you take out the object you have placed between the teeth, smooth the cement. Remove any pieces of cement that stick out, are in the gum pocket, or are not smooth. These may injure the patient's gums and may break off, allowing food and bacteria to enter the cavity. Check carefully that no pieces of cement are in the gum pocket below the tooth.
6. After removing the cotton or cloth used to absorb saliva from around the tooth, ask the patient to gently bring his or her teeth together. (Too much pressure on the filling may break it.) The teeth should come together normally and not first hit against the filling. Always check to see if part of the filling is too high: (a) If the cement is still wet, you can see the smooth place where the opposite tooth bit into it. Scrape the cement away from this place. (b) If the cement is dry, have the patient bite on a piece of carbon paper. (If you have no carbon paper, darken some paper with a pencil.) If there is too much cement, the carbon paper will darken the cement. Scrape away that extra cement. The patient must not leave your clinic until the filled tooth fits properly against the other teeth.[3]
7. If the tooth hurts more after the filling is in place, there is probably an abscess. Extract the tooth now or, if there is too much swelling, extract it after treating the swelling.
8. After-care instructions: Ask the patient not to eat anything for 1 hour so that the cement has time to harden and the temporary filling does not break or loosen. The patient should try not to use that tooth for biting or chewing until there is a permanent filling, because the cement and sides of the cavity are weak.

EXTRACTIONS

Extract teeth only when absolutely necessary. However, extraction may represent the only possible care that can be delivered in austere circumstances.[4] The general reasons to extract a tooth are[5]:

- The patient has constant pain from the tooth.
- The tooth is loose and painful when moved.
- The tooth is already broken with an exposed nerve root.

General Extraction Techniques

In old movies, extractions appear to be a simple procedure. In reality, tooth extraction is painful and difficult to accomplish without breaking the tooth. A dental, preferably a regional, anesthetic block is required. (See the "Anesthesia and Analgesia" section in Chapter 26.)

The keys to successful extractions are patience and finesse. Do not try to yank the tooth out; this will only break it off. The basic principle is to first break the periodontal ligaments holding the tooth to the bone and then rock/lever the tooth out. Generally, the ligaments holding the tooth to the gum and jaw are loosened using a tiny sharp instrument inserted between the tooth and the gum all the way around the tooth. A number of techniques have proved successful most of the time, but the main requirement is not to hurry the procedure.

Slow gradual luxation (i.e., dislocation/rocking) of the tooth with either an elevator (screwdriver) or forceps (pliers) is crucial. The bone will expand and the inflammatory process in the periodontal ligament that follows luxation further loosens the tooth. The steps in a dental extraction are (a) position the patient, (b) administer anesthesia, (c) position yourself, (d) separate the tooth from alveolar bone, (e) apply leverage, (f) grasp the tooth, (g) luxation, (h) rest period, (i) extract the tooth, (j) hemostasis, (k) tooth inspection, and (l) post-extraction care.[6]

Michael A. Grossman, DDS, of Tucson, Ariz., says that one method is to push down and rotate or move the tooth in a figure-eight pattern, with movement in any direction lasting 8 seconds. (Personal communication, May 9, 2008.) Another experienced dentist, Dr. Manuel Bedoya, gently rocks the tooth outward and inward until he can lever it out. He has found that this technique of leveraging the tooth and rocking it back and forth is the easiest way to remove a tooth. Once the tooth rocks back and forth, he advises letting it "rest" for 20 to 30 minutes and then return to extract the tooth. During the rest period, enzymes are generated that further help to loosen the tooth. (Personal communication, December 23, 2007.)

If a tooth breaks, because it often does when being extracted by non-dentists or with makeshift extractors, pry out the remaining fragments using small metal instruments. Or, send the patient to a dentist later, because the key element, drainage, is accomplished when the tooth breaks.

Root fractures are particularly common in nonmobile molar teeth. However, most retained roots are not a problem, and experienced dental practitioners know that they will eventually come out on their own, will remain in place without causing a problem, or, especially if surrounded by infected tissue, will be the focus of an abscess that can be drained through the gum and the root removed.

Tools

Although commonly suggested, using regular pliers wrapped in gauze for extractions generally just pulverizes the tooth at the gum line—especially if the tooth is diseased. Use either a dental extractor (a pediatric universal extractor should work in most situations) or cut off the end of an awl, file it flat, and put a tiny notch on the side of the filed tip. A large-gauge needle with the sharp end filed down also works. Push it between the tooth to be extracted and the gum, breaking the ligaments. Then, carefully lever the tooth out of the socket. (Michael Grossman, DDS. Personal communication, December 22, 2006.)

Dental forceps are designed to fit the shape of the teeth, including their roots. The inexperienced operator will find it simpler to rely on one pair of universal forceps for the upper jaw and one pair for the lower jaw.[7] If channel-lock pliers or a bone rongeur that has jaws curved inward like dental pliers is available, use that. There is less chance of breaking off the enamel, especially if you pad the tool's ends with gauze or other suitable cloth. Dr. Bedoya adds that even a screwdriver, if used gently, can help to pry the tooth from the socket. (Personal communication, December 23, 2007.) (Also see the "Dental Instruments and Equipment" section in Chapter 26 for improvising dental tools.)

Experience shows that if you take your time, you can successfully use even electrician's tools to extract teeth. In a remote environment—on a rocking ship, I had to improvise not only appropriate dental tools, but also personal protective equipment (plastic bags and painters' masks), a functional suction machine, medications for a dental block (compounded epinephrine and lidocaine), a dental chair (a tall office chair covered in plastic), and dental consent forms and follow-up instructions in the patients' language.[6]

Extracting Abscessed Teeth

If the tooth is abscessed, try to extract it. Tooth extraction is the best way to drain an apical abscess when no facilities are available for root canal treatment. Removing a tooth is appropriate if it cannot be preserved, is loose and tender, or causes uncontrollable pain. In these circumstances, according to Barnett R. Rothstein, DMD, even if you must use pliers or a similar instrument that breaks the tooth, opening the abscess in this manner will allow it to drain, thus avoiding the severe complications (e.g., Ludwig's angina, airway compromise, sepsis) that might otherwise occur. (Personal communication, April 9, 2007.)

According to Dr. Manuel Bedoya, the abscess will still drain even if part of the tooth remains, and the rest of the tooth will eventually work its way out without complications. (Personal communication, December 23, 2007.) One benefit is that it is easy to extract loose teeth with periodontal laxity/destruction.

Positioning the Patient

The first step is to position the patient correctly. Patients needing a *lower* tooth extracted should be sitting *lower* than the clinician, because the extraction technique for the lower jaw is to push down and then to pull up on the tooth. Standing on a stable platform, such as a box, may be useful for the practitioner. Position patients who need an *upper* tooth removed *higher* than the clinician, because the extraction technique for the upper jaw is to push up and then pull down on the tooth. Sitting the patient on several cushions often accomplishes the necessary height adjustment.[8] It also helps to have a dental chair that prevents the patient from pulling his or her head back during the procedure. A dental chair can be fashioned from a straight-back chair, two broomsticks, tape, and some webbing (see the "Dental Instruments and Equipment" section in Chapter 26).

Tooth Extraction: Procedural Steps

1. Seat the patient in a chair with a high back that will support his or her head. After rinsing the mouth, swab the gum with 70% ethanol. Do a supraperiosteal or other dental block, as described in Chapter 26 under "Blocking Individual Teeth." Wait 5 minutes for the anesthetic to work, and then test to be sure the tooth is numb. If the patient still feels pain, give another injection.[9]
2. Position yourself to best work on the tooth you are extracting. Right-handed clinicians should stand behind and to the right of the patient when extracting lower right molar or premolar teeth. Face the patient, standing on the patient's right, when working on all other teeth.
3. The first step is to separate the gum from the tooth so that the gum does not tear when the tooth is removed. This is vital because torn gums bleed more and take longer to heal. Slide the end of the instrument along the side of the tooth and into the gum pocket alongside the tooth. At the deepest part of the pocket, you can feel the place where the gum attaches to the tooth. The attachments are strong, but thin. Push the dental instrument or blunted needle between these attachments and the tooth. Then separate the tooth from the gum by moving the tool back and forth. Do this on both the buccal (cheek) and the lingual (tongue) side of the tooth. Take care not to go too deep and to cut only the attachments to the tooth.[9]
4. Next, loosen the tooth. While a loose tooth may not break when you extract it, a strong one will if you do not loosen it first. While a dentist will use an elevator to loosen the tooth, you

may need to use a small flat screwdriver. Either tool can cause harm if not used carefully. The blade goes between the bad tooth and the good one in front of it. Put the face of the blade against the tooth you are removing and slide it down the side of the tooth, as far as possible under the gum. Turn the handle so that the blade moves the top of the bad tooth backward and loosens it. Rest your first finger on the adjacent tooth while you turn the handle. This will control it.[9] Now that you have loosened the tooth, waiting about 20 minutes will allow the tooth to loosen even more, according to Dr. Manuel Bedoya. (Personal communication, December 23, 2007.) You may want to get a cup of coffee or do any required paperwork for this patient.

5. You are now ready to remove the tooth. While supporting the gum and underlying bone with the thumb and finger of your nondominant hand, apply the forceps to either side of the crown, parallel with the long axis of the tooth. Push your grasping tool (extractor, pliers, etc.) as far toward the roots as possible. The idea is for the forceps to grasp the tooth's root under the gum. Your fingers will feel the bone expanding a little at a time as the tooth comes free. Rather than "pulling" the tooth, think about rocking it back and forth or levering it out.[7] To decide which way to move a tooth, think about how many roots it has. If a tooth has one root, you can turn it. If a tooth has two or three roots, you need to tip it back and forth. Take your time. If you hurry and squeeze your forceps too tightly, you can break a tooth. As Dr. Dickson wrote in *Where There Is No Dentist*, "Removing a tooth is like pulling a post out of the ground. When you move it back and forth a little more each time, it soon becomes loose enough to come out."[10] If the tooth does not begin to move, loosen the forceps, push them deeper, and repeat the rocking movements. Avoid excessive lateral force on a tooth, because this can lead to its fracture.[7] After you extract the tooth, examine its roots to be certain that you have not broken any part.
6. Stop the bleeding. Apply direct pressure by squeezing the sides of the socket for 1 to 2 minutes and covering it with cotton gauze or absorbent cloth. Have an adult patient bite firmly against it for 30 minutes; a child should continue biting for 2 hours.[10] After the patient has rinsed his or her mouth, inspect the cavity for bleeding. If the bleeding continues, if you have removed two or more teeth, or if the gums are torn or loose, suture the extraction site with absorbable (if available) mattress sutures across the cavity.[7,11]
7. Carefully inspect the extracted tooth to confirm its complete removal. A broken root is best removed by loosening the tissue between the root and the bone with a curved elevator. After completely removing the tooth, squeeze the sides of the socket together for a minute or two and place a dental roll over the socket. Instruct the patient to bite on it for a short while.
8. Instruct the patient to do the following:[7,11]
   - Not to rinse his or her mouth again for the first 24 hours: if he or she does, the blood clot may be washed out, leaving a dry socket. After 24 hours, he or she should rinse his or her mouth frequently with warm saltwater during the next few days.
   - To bite on cotton gauze or absorbent cloth if bleeding starts again.
   - To take acetaminophen or, if there has not been much bleeding, NSAIDs if needed for pain.
   - Not to explore the cavity with his or her finger.
   - To drink lots of cool fluids, if possible, using the opposite side of the mouth. He or she should not drink hot liquids like tea or coffee, because they promote bleeding.
   - To eat soft food that is easy to chew. He should try to chew food on the side opposite from where the tooth was removed.
   - To keep his or her mouth clean, especially the teeth near the extraction site.

Extraction Problem: Broken Tooth

Even when handled with care, extractions sometimes lead to a broken tooth. If you can see the root, try to remove it. If you leave a broken root inside the bone, it can become the nidus for an infection. However, small broken roots are better left inside the socket. They will loosen over the next week or so and will be easier to remove.[12]

If you do try to remove a tooth root, use one of the following techniques.

To remove a broken *upper* root[12]: Slide the blade of a straight elevator or thin flat screwdriver along the wall of the socket until it meets the broken root. Then

1. Force the blade between the root and the socket.
2. Move the root away from the socket wall.

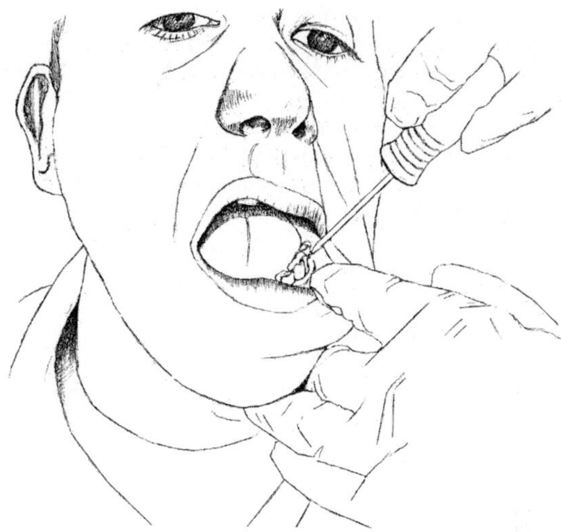

FIG. 27-1. Screwdriver used for tooth extraction.

3. Move the root further until it is loose.
4. Grab the loose root and pull it out.

To remove a broken *lower* root[12] (Fig. 27-1): Use a straight elevator (or a curved elevator if you have one). If the broken root is from a molar tooth, slide the blade into the socket beside the broken root.

1. Break away the bone between the root and the blade.
2. Force the blade between the root and the socket.
3. Move the root away from the socket wall.
4. Grab the loose root and pull it out.

If dental equipment is not available, this technique is recommended if you have a bright light to work under: Dry the socket with gauze, and then firmly wedge a 26-gauge needle into the root canal of the errant piece. "With gentle manipulation it is possible to retrieve the root fragment impaled onto the stainless steel needle."[13]

Post-Extraction Problems

Bleeding

Post-extraction bleeding usually occurs in the small vessels. If the patient presents with persistent bleeding after a tooth extraction, remove any clots extending out of the socket with gauze. Then take a small folded gauze pad or a regular tea bag saturated with lidocaine/epinephrine and either wrap it in a thin cloth or suture it to a gauze roll for stability (Fig. 27-2).[14] Then, place it

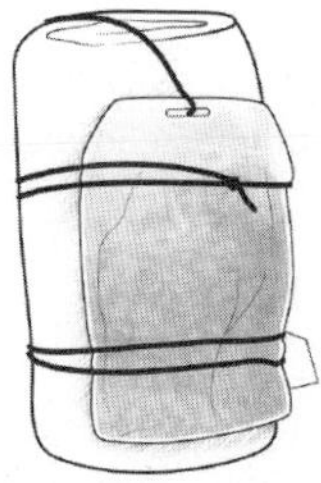

FIG. 27-2. Tea bag tied or sutured to a gauze roll.

over the socket, and have the patient gently bite on it for 1 hour. The tea contains a procoagulant as well as tannic acid, which helps relieve pain. Repeat this as necessary; it often takes two or three applications. Tell patients to wait at least 1 hour before checking the site so they do not disrupt clot formation. If bleeding continues, give a local anesthetic block, and then curette and irrigate the socket with normal saline to remove the existing clot and to freshen the bone. If this does not stop the bleeding, suture the area with gentle tension.[15] If bleeding is excessive, including in anticoagulated patients, drying the area as much as possible and then applying cyanoacrylate has been effective.[16]

Pain

If a patient presents with severe pain about 2 to 3 days after a tooth extraction, it is most probably due to alveolar osteitis, a "dry socket." A dry socket occurs most commonly after wisdom tooth extraction, in patients using oral contraceptives, and in smokers. It is due to losing the clot from the socket, with a subsequent growth of anaerobic organisms leading to a localized alveolitis. The pain can be localized to the tooth or extend throughout the dentition on that side. While it generally resolves spontaneously in about 2 weeks, the patient will be in so much pain that treatment should be instituted to resolve the problem.

Treatment

Block the tooth. Then gently rinse the socket with warm saline or potable water. Gently place a 1- to 2-inch piece of iodoform gauze or cloth soaked in eugenol, iodine or a saline/anesthetic solution (such as lidocaine 0.5%) in the socket. A piece of gauze with eugenol, oil of cloves, or a local substitute (damp, but not wet) can also be used, as can cyanoacrylate (not the best choice in this case). The patient should bite down on a piece of dry gauze, cotton, or cloth over the tooth dressing. Discard that cloth after 1 hour. Change the dressing gauze every 1 to 3 days until symptoms do not return when the gauze is left out for a few hours. This procedure eliminates the need for systemic analgesics. If the symptoms last a month, suspect osteomyelitis and evaluate the patient for long-term antibiotic treatment.

Root (Pulp) Extraction

Dentists use a thin, barbed wire to extract the pulp. While a thin wire like a filament will get down the canal, removing the pulp requires a hook or lateral projections to pull or scrape the soft tissue out. However, Daniel Kemmedson, DMD, suggests that making a very small bend on the bevel portion of a thin (25-, 27-, or 30-gauge) hypodermic needle might work. (Personal written communication, June 7, 2008.)

ORAL TRAUMA

Gum Lacerations

Many gum lacerations need no treatment other than keeping them clean. They can, of course, be sutured. Alternatively, apply cyanoacrylate directly to the wound.

Tooth Injuries: Spectrum

Multiple methods exist for describing injuries to teeth. The simplest that has clinical applicability is that teeth may be:

- Subluxed (loose, but without change in position)
- Luxated (loose and in a different position than normal)
- Fractured (missing a part of the tooth)
- Avulsed (missing)

Loose Teeth: General Approach

A common presenting complaint is that a patient's tooth is loose. Table 27-1 describes the symptoms, complications, and treatment for various causes of loose teeth. These are described in more detail in subsequent sections of this chapter.

TABLE 27-1 Loose Teeth: Presentation, Diagnosis, Complications, and Treatment

Presentation	Diagnosis	Definition	Complications	Treatment by Non-dentist
Tooth in good position, but loose.	Tooth subluxation	Loose tooth	Dead tooth (rare)	Mechanically soft diet until tooth is stable
Tooth appears taller, shorter, or out of alignment with adjacent teeth. Recent trauma.	Tooth luxation	Very loose tooth	Aspiration of tooth, pulpitis, dead tooth	Splinting, extraction
Tooth injured and now loose. No obvious injury.	Root fracture	Tooth root broken under the gum	Pulpitis, dead tooth	Extraction
Bone around a loose tooth, as well as the adjacent tooth, moves. May have had recent trauma.	Fracture of alveolar bone - *or* - Osteomyelitis	Broken bone around the tooth's roots - *or* - Infection inside the bone, probably from "trench mouth" (Vincent's angina or stomatitis)	Progressive infection, infection in sequestered bone, dead tooth	Stabilize tooth (fracture) or prolonged antibiotics, and drainage, if necessary
Missing tooth, recent trauma.	Tooth avulsion	Missing tooth	Ankylosis (tooth immobility due to direct attachment to bone), resorption of bone	Reimplantation and splinting

Data from Dickson[17] and other sources.

Subluxed: Loosened Tooth

If the tooth is minimally loose but in normal position, place the patient on a liquid or soft diet progressing slowly to a normal diet. Follow-up with a dentist is rarely required. If the teeth need to be stabilized, dental follow-up is recommended within 48 hours, if possible.

Luxation

A luxated or displaced tooth is shifted out of normal position but remains intact. Whether it is really intact may be unclear without radiographs, because the surrounding alveolar bone is normally fractured. Luxated teeth, usually the upper front teeth (incisors), may be either in normal position or loose (subluxed), pushed back, or partially or completely out of the socket. When communicating with a dentist, they are described as extrusive = coming out; intrusive = pushed inward; or lateral = to the side.

The treatment depends on the tooth's position. If the tooth appears longer than the others (extrusion), try to push it back firmly into the socket with steady, gentle pressure. You can get a better grip on the tooth if you use a piece of gauze to hold it. If the tooth seems to be pushed ahead of or behind the other teeth (lateral displacement), also try to firmly realign it. If it is loose, the patient can gently bite on a piece of gauze or cloth. Then splint the tooth in position, as described in the "Splinting/Wiring" section below in this chapter. If it seems shorter than surrounding teeth (intruded), it probably will not survive and there is little that can be done in adults without advanced dental equipment.[18] In children, intruded teeth are allowed to re-erupt.

Tooth Fractures

If a tooth breaks (generally it is the crown, which is the part of the tooth above the gum line), treatment is often necessary to reduce pain. Tooth fractures may initially seem to have significant bleeding, although much of this may be a mixture of saliva and blood. If the patient can bite down on a gauze or cloth, the bleeding generally stops. Although the following classifications seem obvious, if it is unclear how much damage was done to the tooth, watch it over several days. If it changes color or if signs of an abscess develop, extract it.

Classification of Tooth Fractures

Fractured Enamel

The most common dental injuries are those to the tooth's crown, involving the enamel and the enamel-dentin without pulp involvement. These usually involve a child or young adult's anterior maxillary incisors. About one in four children worldwide will have such an injury before age 18 years, with most occurring between the ages of 6 and 13 years.[4]

If only the tooth enamel is fractured, the tooth will not be sensitive to temperature or touch and there is a very small (<3%) chance of pulp necrosis. Although the tooth may later need filling, no treatment is required immediately. If no dental care is available, smooth any sharp edges with sandpaper, a small file, an emery board, or a hard stone.[4]

Reattaching the tooth fragment is the ideal treatment when the piece is available, because it can improve both the appearance of the tooth and its function. While dentists can use a variety of techniques to accomplish this reattachment, including the use of special preparations and cements, using a simple adhesive, such as cyanoacrylate, can restore 25% or more of the tooth's pre-injury strength. This method provides immediate cosmetic improvement and allows a dentist to provide more definitive care at a later time. Until the tooth fragment is reattached, keep it in sterile water, milk, or Hank's Balanced Salt Solution (HBSS) (see the formula in the "Preservation" section below in this chapter).[19,20] Gently dry both the tooth and the fragment before applying the cement. If the fragment is not reattached and the patient will see a dentist, immerse it in a preservative solution (see the "Avulsed Tooth" section below) and send the piece to the dentist with the patient. Place the patient on a liquid or soft diet until they can be seen by a dentist and tell him or her not to pick at the adhesive. The tooth or the cement may irritate the patient's tongue or lip. If this irregularity bothers the patient, it can be smoothed with a variety of instruments, as described in steps 5 and 6 in the section "How to Fill a Tooth: Procedural Steps" above in this chapter.

Dentin Fracture

If the dentin is fractured, it will usually be visible as a deep, golden yellow inside the tooth. The tooth will be very sensitive to percussion, temperature, and air. Pulp necrosis (dead tooth) occurs in 7% to 10% of these patients. After blocking the tooth, dry it and cover it with calcium hydroxide (CaOH) paste or cyanoacrylate. The CaOH paste will stay in place for about a week if the patient is on a soft/liquid diet. To apply cyanoacrylate, drop it onto the tooth and, with a metal tool or the top of the adhesive tube, rapidly try to smooth it. Have the patient keep his or her mouth open for a few minutes to let it dry. For CaOH paste, use a flat instrument, such as a knife blade (cover the cutting edge), ice pop (e.g., Popsicle) stick, or similar tool to place dental filling material or wax over the area. Have the patient bite down gently, and remove the excess material. He or she will have to avoid using that tooth to eat; the piece may come loose.

Pulp Exposed

A tooth's pulp space may be fractured with the tooth in place or with a piece missing. If the tooth remains in place and the root is broken, the tooth will move if you firmly grasp the alveolar bone (by holding the gum over the bone) and try to move the tooth. Of course, the bone does not move unless it is broken. If the pulp is exposed, a piece of the tooth is missing and blood will be visible coming from the pulp cavity. This is generally quite painful because the nerve is exposed also. But, if the nerve is concussed, it may not hurt. In that case, pulp necrosis (dead tooth) is likely.

Treatment

The first priority is to help control the pain and bleeding. Gently treat these teeth, either without anesthetic or after using one of the blocks discussed in Chapter 27. The specific block to use depends on which tooth is involved.

The basic principle is to dry the tooth and cover it using either standard dental materials or cyanoacrylate. If using standard dental materials, cover the tooth with a mixture of cotton fibers in a zinc oxide and eugenol paste. This paste should be very thick. Apply it over both the injured tooth and several adjacent teeth. If possible, leave the gum line clear so the patient can keep it clean. Caution the patient not to bite into food with these teeth until seen by a dentist.[21] If dental supplies are not available, use cyanoacrylate to stabilize the tooth.

Adequate pain control may require removing the tooth pulp from the chamber. If the tooth fracture has exposed the pulp space and a very tiny pulp removal tool is available, remove the pulp. A light bulb filament with a tiny drop of cyanoacrylate may suffice in a pinch. Whether or not the pulp can be removed, use a small piece of gauze or cotton to seal the hole and avoid contamination. Cover it with oil of cloves or zinc oxide. If only cyanoacrylate is available, use that to cover the hole.

An alternative is to gently wash the tooth and try to reattach it with cyanoacrylate. A splint is normally required to keep it in place (see the "Splinting/Wiring" section below in this chapter). Splint the tooth in place until a dentist can do a root canal or the tooth can be extracted. (Extracting this type of fractured tooth is very difficult, especially for the novice.) Occasionally, a tooth may split vertically and, after drying, may be able to be glued together with cyanoacrylate in situ. This, however, may be only temporary, because such teeth may have too much intrinsic damage to be retained.[22]

Fractured Bone

If the bone moves when you attempt to move the teeth after an injury, the alveolar bone is most likely fractured. Do not take those teeth out until the bone is healed. Otherwise, the bone will come out with the teeth and there will be a big hole in the patient's jaw. Instead, support the teeth in order to hold both sides of the bone steady. Stabilize the tooth with a splint (e.g., interdental wires) or use cyanoacrylate to attach it to the adjacent tooth. If more than the alveolar bone is fractured (a substantial maxillary or mandibular fracture), wiring may be the only option. See the "Splinting/Wiring" section and Fig. 27-3.

Avulsed Tooth

Avulsion means that the entire tooth has come out of the socket. If the tooth is out, the ligaments that hold the tooth, as well as the nerve and blood vessels for that tooth, have been completely torn.

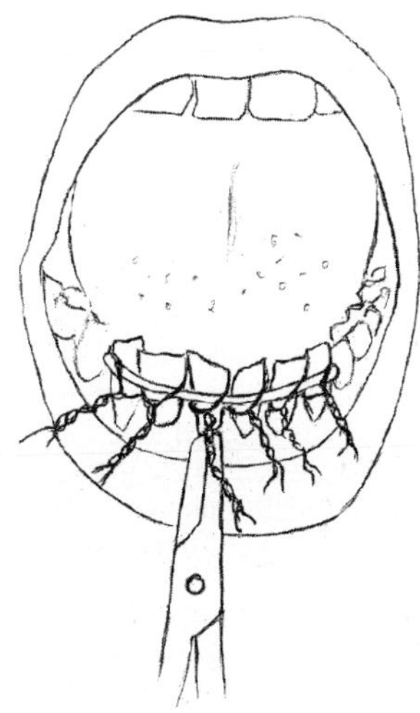

FIG. 27-3. Splint stabilized with wires.

Handle the tooth only by the enamel (crown), because the root structures can be damaged easily and this would prevent the tooth from being successfully reimplanted.

Preservation

If the tooth cannot be reimplanted immediately, store it for up to 4 hours in sterile saline, potable water, milk (better), or HBSS (best). The practice of placing the tooth between the patient's gum and lip is not as good. Use this method only if there is no risk of the patient aspirating the tooth. A chemist or pharmacist can compound HBSS in advance. To make a 100 mL solution, add to distilled water: 0.80 g NaCl, 0.04 g KCl, 0.014 g $CaCl_2$ anhydrous, 0.01 g $MgSO_4$-$7H_2O$, 0.01 g $MgCl_2$-$6H_2O$, 0.006 g Na_2HPO_4-$1H_2O$, 0.006 g KH_2PO_4, 0.1 g glucose, 0.035-g $NaHCO_3$, and usually, 20 mg phenol red.[23] Sterilize the solution, if necessary, by filtering rather than by heating it. For dental work, no sterilization is needed.

Treatment

If the tooth is whole, reimplant it within 30 minutes after the injury, if possible. Hold the tooth only by the crown (enamel) so as not to injure the periodontal ligament covering the root. Gently rinse it off with sterile saline, potable water, milk, HBSS, water from a green coconut, or cold running water for about 10 seconds. Do not scrub it or use any chemicals.[24,25] Gently rinse the socket with warm water to clean out any debris and clot. After doing a supraperiosteal, alveolar, or Gow-Gates block, push the tooth into the socket with firm, gentle, steady pressure; it often "snaps" into place. (See Chapter 26 for dental blocks.) Hold it in place for about 5 minutes. Then have the patient bite down lightly on a piece of gauze or cloth. If dental care is not readily available, stabilize the tooth by splinting or wiring it to adjacent teeth (see the "Splinting/Wiring" section in this chapter). The tooth may still darken and die months or years later. In that case, the option is to extract it or for a dentist to do a root canal.

Children

Deciduous teeth, also known as milk teeth, baby teeth, temporary teeth, and primary teeth, need not be reimplanted, because doing so typically leads to them becoming necrotic and, then, infected. They may also become fused to the bone (ankylosed) and not fall out, or they can fuse to the erupting adult teeth, thus interfering with the eruption of the permanent tooth.[26,27]

Splinting/Wiring

Stabilize teeth and surrounding boney structures with glue, glue and wire, splints, or interdental wiring.

Glue Only

To stabilize a tooth, cyanoacrylate or dental cement may be the easiest and best makeshift method. After drying the affected tooth and the adjacent teeth and gums, apply the adhesive to the teeth and to the gingiva below them. Apply the adhesive to both the mesial (closest to midline) and distal (away from midline) sides of the tooth so that it bonds to the adjacent teeth.

Glue or Wire and Splint

Simpler than using wires alone to stabilize teeth, an effective temporary method, suggested by Barnett R. Rothstein, DMD, is to combine adhesive and wire. (Personal communication, May 7, 2007.) Cut a piece of wire to the length necessary to cover multiple teeth. If used for loose or avulsed teeth, the wire need only cover four or five teeth; if used for a mandibular or maxillary fracture, cover as many teeth as possible. The wire can be the metal bridge from a surgical mask, a thin orthopedic wire; a small-gauge spinal needle with the ends clipped; a thin paperclip; or similar thin-gauge, malleable, but relatively rigid, wire. Bend the wire so it conforms to the convexity of the normal tooth configuration (Fig. 27-4).

Beginning with four teeth on either side of the fracture line—or all the teeth that will be used in the case of a loose or avulsed tooth—dry the teeth thoroughly. Hold the lip away from the teeth manually or by using gauze or absorbent cloth between the lip and gum. Put cyanoacrylate or dental cement on the anterior tooth and embed the wire in the glue. Be certain that

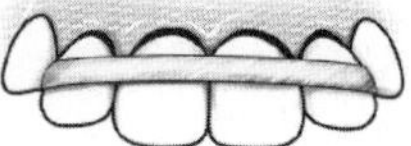

FIG. 27-4. Wire band across anterior teeth.

the teeth are aligned as well as possible. Continue the same process until the entire wire is cemented.[28]

A more secure alternative is to use wires or heavy nonabsorbable sutures around the teeth to secure the stabilizing wire (see Fig. 27-3).

These are only temporary fixes. The patient must be placed on a liquid or soft diet and be seen by a dental professional as soon as possible.

Makeshift Splints

WAX SPLINT

Another alternative to stabilize a loose tooth is to use beeswax. According to Dr. Dickson in *Where There Is No Dentist*, the method is to

> Soften some beeswax and form it into 2 thin rolls. Place 1 roll near the gums on the front side of five teeth: the loose tooth and the two teeth on each side of it. Press the wax firmly, but carefully, against these teeth. Do the same with the second roll of wax on the back side of the same teeth, again near the gums. It is good if the wax on the back side is touching the wax on the front side. This helps the wax hold the teeth more firmly. To do this, you can push the wax between the teeth with the end of your cotton tweezers.[29]

SPLINT FROM DENTAL FILLING MATERIAL

Cotton fibers can be mixed in with standard temporary filling mix to form a fibrous mix. This then can be molded to make a splint between the injured tooth and its healthy neighbors.[28]

Interdental Wires for Dental Stabilization

Interdental wire fixation simply means tying wires around stable and unstable teeth, and then affixing these to a heavy wire splint laid across the involved teeth (Fig. 27-3). Use this for unstable teeth or for fractures of the mandible or maxilla. Because extracting teeth when the alveolar bone is fractured can leave a big hole in the jaw, supporting the teeth with a splint until the bone heals is the optimal treatment.

Interdental wiring is much easier to do on anterior teeth than on others, especially with limited equipment. If dental equipment is not available, use a pair of scissors and small pliers to cut and manipulate the wire.

ALTERNATIVE TECHNIQUES

A basic method is to place a double strand of wire around several teeth (one to three teeth) and twist it tight. Place the wires so that, if possible, they do not touch the gums. Tuck the cut ends between the teeth.[4]

Another method for applying interdental wires is to use your thumb and finger to gently move the loose teeth and bone back into normal position.[30] Cut a wire to use as a splint. It should be long enough to lie across two strong teeth on each side of the loose tooth or teeth. The splint can be a thin orthopedic wire; heavy electrical wire with the insulation removed; a small-gauge spinal needle with the ends clipped; a thin paperclip; or thin-gauge, malleable, but relatively rigid wire. Curve the wire so that it fits the curve of the teeth. If using a needle, smooth the sharp end with a file or stone. Then tie each tooth to the splint wire using short pieces of 20-gauge ligature wire or, if that is not available, heavy surgical suture, dental floss, or nylon fishing line. Put one end of the ligature under the splint. Bring it around the back of one tooth and out to the front again over the needle. Use the end of a small instrument to hold down the ligature at the back of the teeth. Then twist or tie the ends together. Tighten the ligature around each of the six teeth. If using wire ligatures, cut the ends and bend them toward the teeth, so they will not cut the lip. If using wire ligatures, tighten them the next day, and then once each week. But be careful:

Only half a clockwise turn usually is needed ("Righty tighty; lefty loosey"). More, and the wire will break.

Patient Aftercare Instructions

Explain to the patient that it takes 4 weeks for the bone to heal. The wires must remain on the teeth for this time. To help the teeth to heal, ask the patient to use other teeth for chewing, to clean both the teeth and the wires with a soft brush frequently, to rinse with two cups warm saltwater every day, and to return to have the wires tightened every week.

After 4 weeks, cut and remove the ligatures. Ask the patient to watch those teeth. A dark tooth and gum bubble are signs that the tooth is dying. If those appear, the patient must return for the tooth to be extracted or be referred for specialized dental treatment.

Dental Wiring for Facial Fractures

To wire teeth to treat a maxillary or mandibular fracture, an adequate number of teeth must be included. With facial fractures, place wires on both upper and lower teeth and then tie them together for increased stability.

With a fracture of either bone, tie the wires around at least six teeth in the maxilla and the same number of mandibular teeth. Twist the wires to attach them to the teeth. Try to adjust the teeth so that they appear aligned. This will place the facial fracture segments in correct position. Tie the upper and lower wires together, tying the lateral ones together first, then others, crossing some ties over the fractured area. Tie them loosely at first, and then tighten them.[31] A specific contraindication for interdental wiring for facial fractures is poorly controlled seizures, because the patient could easily vomit and, without the ability to open their mouth, aspirate.

Wiring for mandibular/maxillary fractures should remain in place for 6 weeks. During that time, the patient will be on a liquid diet and should carry a wire cutter on a string around his or her neck in case there is a need to emergently cut the wires—such as if he or she has an airway problem.

REFERENCES

1. Dickson M. *Where There Is No Dentist*. Berkeley, CA: Hesperian Foundation; 2006:143-151.
2. Dickson M. *Where There Is No Dentist*. Berkeley, CA: Hesperian Foundation; 2006:148.
3. Dickson M. *Where There Is No Dentist*. Berkeley, CA: Hesperian Foundation; 2006:149.
4. Klein RM. Special issues in disaster care: field dentistry. NDMS Response Team Training Program. http://mediccom.org/public/tadmat/training.html. Accessed September 24, 2003.
5. Dickson M. *Where There Is No Dentist*. Berkeley, CA: Hesperian Foundation; 2006:153.
6. Iserson KV. Dental extractions using improvised equipment. *Wild Environ Med*. 2013;24:384-389.
7. World Health Organization. *Surgical Care at the District Hospital*. Geneva, Switzerland: WHO; 2003: 5-21, 5-22.
8. Dickson M. *Where There Is No Dentist*. Berkeley, CA: Hesperian Foundation; 2006:156.
9. Dickson M. *Where There Is No Dentist*. Berkeley, CA: Hesperian Foundation; 2006:157.
10. Dickson M. *Where There Is No Dentist*. Berkeley, CA: Hesperian Foundation; 2006:159-160.
11. Dickson M. *Where There Is No Dentist*. Berkeley, CA: Hesperian Foundation; 2006:163.
12. Dickson M. *Where There Is No Dentist*. Berkeley, CA: Hesperian Foundation; 2006:165.
13. Uppal N. Dental root fragment extraction using a hypodermic needle. *Trop Doct*. 2008;38(1):16.
14. Fisher W. Tricks of the trade: break room bonanza. *ACEP News*. 2013 May;32(5).
15. *Merck Manual Professional*. http://www.merck.com/mmpe/sec08/ch096/ch096d.html. Accessed March 22, 2008.
16. Al-Belasy FA, Amer MZ. Hemostatic effect of n-butyl-2-cyanoacrylate (histoacryl) glue in warfarin-treated patients undergoing oral surgery. *J Oral Maxillofac Surg*. 2003;61(12):1405-1409.
17. Dickson M. *Where There Is No Dentist*. Berkeley, CA: Hesperian Foundation; 2006:80-83.
18. Hubbell F. The agony of the teeth. *Wild Med Newsletter*. 2004;15(5):1-5.
19. Reis A, Loguercio AD. Tooth fragment reattachment: current treatment concepts. *Pract Proced Anesthet Dent*. 2004;16(10):739-740.
20. Terry DA. Adhesive reattachment of a tooth fragment: the biological restoration. *Pract Proced Anesthet Dent*. 2003;15(5):403-409.

21. Shiller WR. *Emergency Dental Treatment by Medical Officers on Isolated Duty*. Groton, CT: US Naval Submarine Medical Center, Report MR005.19-6024.01; 1968.
22. Hille LM, Linklater DR. Use of 2-octyl cyanoacrylate for the repair of a fractured molar tooth. *Ann Emerg Med*. 2006;47(5):424-426.
23. Dawson RMC, Elliott DC, Elliott WH, et al. *Data for Biochemical Research*. 3rd ed. Oxford, UK: Clarendon Press; 1986.
24. Gopikrishna V, Baweja PS, Venkateshbabu N, Thomas T, Kandaswamy D. Comparison of coconut water, propolis, HBSS, and milk on PDL cell survival. *J Endodontics*. 2008;34(5):587-589.
25. Flores MT, Andersson L, Andreasen JO, et al. Guidelines for the management of traumatic dental injuries. II. Avulsion of permanent teeth. *Dent Traumatol*. 2007;23(3):130-136.
26. Benko K. Acute dental emergencies. Presented at ACEP Scientific Assembly, Seattle, WA. October 10, 2007.
27. Anon. Fractured and avulsed teeth. *Merck Manual Professional*. http://www.merck.com/mmpe/sec08/ch096/ch096b.html. Accessed March 22, 2008.
28. Anon. Austere dental care. In: *Survival and Austere Medicine*. http://www.endtimesreport.com/Survival_Medicine.pdf. Accessed March 30, 2008.
29. Dickson M. *Where There Is No Dentist*. Berkeley, CA: Hesperian Foundation; 2006:98.
30. Dickson M. *Where There Is No Dentist*. Berkeley, CA: Hesperian Foundation; 2006:112.
31. Husum H, Ang SC, Fosse E. *War Surgery: Field Manual*. Penang, Malaysia: Third World Network; 1995:326.

28 | Otolaryngology (Ear, Nose, and Throat)

HEADREST

A headrest for head and neck surgery can be fashioned from foam packing material (Styrofoam) or a piece of foam cushion or mattress. Use a 25 cm × 25 cm × 10 cm piece and hollow out the middle so that it is only one-third of the original depth. This space is for the patient's head. The foam material will provide traction to keep it in place on the operating room (OR) table.[1] This headrest can also be used as a sleeping pillow if the individual needs, or wants, to be only on his or her back.

REGIONAL NERVE BLOCKS

Most of the regional nerve blocks useful for ear, nose, and throat (ENT) procedures are discussed in Chapter 26.

Paravertebral Block

To relieve most or all orofacial pain in adults, use a simple paravertebral block. This is an extremely safe procedure, because the injection is made with a 1.5-inch-long, 25-gauge needle. Inject 1.5 mL of 0.5% bupivacaine into the paravertebral musculature on both sides, 1 inch lateral to the seventh cervical spinous process. Bupivacaine provides good pain relief within 15 minutes for adults with toothache (odontalgia), mandibular fractures and dislocations, temporomandibular joint (TMJ) syndrome, ocular pain, facial pain from a variety of other causes, and headaches.[2,3]

EAR

Otoscope

If an otoscope is not available, use an ophthalmoscope to look through any type of speculum into the ear canal. Objects that can substitute for a speculum include a pen casing (cut the tapered point off a little and smooth it), a 1-cc syringe barrel with the end cut off and smoothed, a nasal speculum (be careful not to put it in too far), and similar objects. Note that many late-19th century otoscopes looked no different than modern nasal speculums. They used a direct or an indirect (head mirror) light source.[4]

Foreign-Body/Cerumen Removal

Knowing how to remove foreign bodies from an ear can save time and resources. There is no evidence to support choosing one method over another in most cases, and many different techniques are available. It is also useful to know which cases may need to go to the OR to have foreign bodies removed under sedation. The most difficult foreign bodies to remove are spherical objects, those in contact with the tympanic membrane (TM), and those that have been in the ear for >24 hours.[5] Most foreign bodies can be removed using irrigation, dissolution, suction, glue, or by other physical means. The removal of insects and metal objects requires special techniques.

Anesthesia

Current sedation techniques (see the "Procedural Sedation" section in Chapter 16) make it safe to administer sedation to both adults and children before undertaking what may be painful or prolonged attempts at foreign-body removal. Anesthetizing the ear can gain the patient's cooperation, although good anesthesia in the ear canal is difficult to achieve. Topical anesthetic can be dropped into the canal (if the foreign body is neither vegetable matter nor a button battery), although it usually has only a modest effect.

Irrigation

Irrigation is the least traumatic way to remove cerumen and smaller foreign bodies that are close to the TM. If the TM is not perforated, irrigate the ear with clean water at body temperature.

(Cold water produces emesis.) For earwax, it may help to put in a softening agent for a few days before attempting irrigation.

Use a small piece of tubing connected to a syringe; a plastic intravenous (IV) catheter or the tubing from a butterfly cannula—with the needle cut off—works well. An alternative is to use a bulb syringe or a turkey baster. With both, low-pressure volume, rather than a directed stream of water, works best. Other successful improvisations have included oral jet irrigators (this may have too high a pressure, depending on the state of the batteries),[6] a recreational water gun,[7] and mouthfuls of water instilled (by the patient's nurse-wife) through a cocktail straw.[8] Aim the fluid stream at the superior aspect of the ear and, if possible, pulse the fluid for best results. Alternatively, direct the stream along the wall of the ear canal and around the object, flushing it out.

Do not irrigate the ear to remove hygroscopic objects, such as vegetables, beans, and other food matter, because these may swell. Also, do not irrigate button batteries that are more common in noses than in ears, because it only accelerates the tissue necrosis. Also, avoid nasal and otic drops in these patients.

Dissolve

Styrofoam is a common foreign body found in the ear. It is often compressed and tightly impacted in the ear canal. The friable substance tends to fragment if grabbed with forceps. The best removal method is to instill acetone or ethyl chloride, both organic solvents. This results in rapid and near-complete dissolution of the Styrofoam without any patient discomfort.[9]

Suction

Quickly remove objects that are light and will move easily with suction. Use a small soft-rubber suction catheter (e.g., pediatric feeding tube), a standard metal suction tip (e.g., Frazier tip), or a specialized flexible tip. It takes 100 to 140 mm Hg (or higher) negative pressure to attach an object, so using your mouth to suck on a tube will not work.

Mechanical Removal

Mechanically removing an object involves grabbing the object and pulling it out of the ear. Most commonly done with cerumen, it also works for other compressible objects when using tiny (alligator) forceps. Alligator forceps are best for grasping soft objects like cotton or paper, although they are rarely available in resource-poor settings.

To remove cerumen and small, visualized foreign bodies, fashion improvised cerumen spoons by bending the end of a paper clip into a very tiny "U" shape. Do not do this with your fingers—use pliers or a similar tool. This "spoon" can also be used for removing foreign bodies from the nose.[10] If the foreign body is at all irregularly shaped and is not made of organic material, grasp it with any available forceps or hemostat and remove.

Metallic objects, such as the appropriately feared button batteries, can sometimes be removed from the ear using a magnetized screwdriver.[11] (Borrow one from your maintenance staff.) Remove the batteries immediately to prevent corrosion or burns. A delay of only an hour or two, or a missed diagnosis of a battery in a nose or an ear, may lead to liquefactive necrosis extending deep into tissues. Do not crush the battery during removal. Avoid nasal and otic drops. These electrolyte-rich fluids enhance battery corrosion and leakage, the generation of an external current, and local injury. After removing the battery, irrigate the canal to remove any alkali residue.

Glue

If the object is dry and smooth, put a tiny amount of cyanoacrylate (Super Glue) on the wooden end of a tiny swab (e.g., Q-tip) and touch the object. It will dry in about 15 seconds and then both can be extracted. The danger is gluing the stick to the patient. If this happens, do not fret—remove it with acetone or simply wait several hours.[12]

Removing Insects

Insects are a special case of organic foreign body. They are the most frequent ear foreign body in adults. Generally, they are alive, and often panic the patient because of both the pain and the noise they generate.

Kill the insect before attempting to remove it. Quickly drop in any liquid that will not injure the ear canal (e.g., mineral or cooking oil, lidocaine, liquid soap, alcohol, etc.) to kill the insect—and to restore the patient to relative calm. Plain water or normal saline usually is ineffective. Most insects die in less than 3 minutes after dropping liquid into the ear.[13]

Improvised Ear Wick

Patients with edematous otitis externa need a method of getting the medication into the ear canal. This usually requires an ear wick. To improvise an ear wick, use thin ribbon gauze, impregnated at the bedside with antibiotic/anti-inflammatory ointment. This gauze can be removed by patients, is inexpensive, and requires fewer visits than when patients use standard ear wicks.[14]

Alternatives to Otic Medications

Acetic acid (10% vinegar) is an amazing, nontoxic, inexpensive, and widely used preventive and treatment for most cases of external otitis. Scuba divers routinely use it. Mix one part acetic acid (vinegar) with nine parts water. Instill enough to fill the ear canal as often as needed. The only side effect is a streak of white where it drips out of the ear. Simply wipe it off. *One caveat*: Diabetic patients and individuals whose ear canals have swollen shut need additional treatment; the latter can be treated with this medication if an ear wick is inserted. While patients with diabetes may be able to temporize with acetic acid, they should also have the appropriate antibiotics or antifungals instilled, if these are available. A mixture of 50% rubbing alcohol, 25% white vinegar, and 25% distilled water can also be used for external otitis. This should only be used four times a day (qid).[15]

Myringotomy

Clinicians may need to perform a myringotomy if the patient is in pain from otitis and no analgesic, decongestant, or antibiotic is available. If a myringotomy is necessary, nearly any local anesthetic drops will anesthetize the TM if you wait 10 minutes after instilling them. For example, use one spray of 10% lidocaine aerosol directed into the clear external meatus onto the tympanum.[16] Another option is to put in one drop (only!) of 10% phenol. If phenol is used, start the procedure immediately, because the anesthetic effect lasts only 10 minutes. (Phenol also can anesthetize other areas, such as pilonidal cysts.) To do the myringotomy, insert an 18-gauge needle into the anterior-inferior part of the TM. To take a culture, attach a tuberculin (TB) syringe. Avoid puncturing the membrane posteriorly. (David Merrell, MD. Personal communication, October 2006.)

NOSE

Nose Drops and Washes

Nose drops and washes are reasonably benign ways to make "stuffed up" patients feel better and, in some cases, to "clear the way" for other medications. If the commercial varieties are not available, there are a variety of recipes that patients can make at home.

- *Recipe #1:* Mix 1/2 teaspoon salt in 8 oz warm water, and store the solution in an empty spray bottle. Make a new solution after 2 days.[17,18]
- *Recipe #2:* Add 2 to 3 heaping teaspoons of table salt and 1 rounded teaspoon of baking soda to 1 quart of boiled tap or bottled water. Store it in a 1-quart glass jar. If the mixture is too strong, reduce the salt to 1 to 2 teaspoons. If the patient's nose is dry, add 1 tablespoon of corn syrup to the mix. Stir or shake before each use and store in the refrigerator; mix a fresh batch weekly.

For adults, use two to three times daily. Instill with a bulb, ear, or medical syringe. Warm the solution to body temperature and have patients stand over the sink or in the shower as they squirt toward the back of each nostril. Avoid contaminating the stock solution. For children, instill three drops as often as necessary in each nostril while they are supine with their head turned to one side. Have them blow their nose after 1 minute or, for younger children, use a suction bulb to remove mucous.[18]

Anesthesia

Using intranasal anesthetic gains a patient's cooperation for any manipulation. Obtain good intranasal anesthesia in several ways. Use 1 to 3 sprays of 10% lidocaine aerosol in

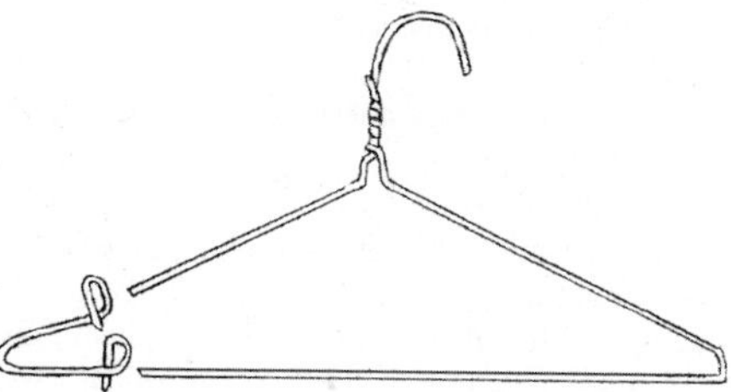

FIG. 28-1. Improvised nasal speculum.

the nose. Or spray the nose with 2 to 3 mL 4% lidocaine plus 1 drop (0.05 mL) of 1:1000 epinephrine. Then pack the nose with gauze soaked in the same solution.[16]

To anesthetize the entire nasal cavity, hyperextend the head and pour 20 mL of 1.25% lidocaine with 0.25 mL of 1:1000 epinephrine into each nostril; allow it to remain there for 3 minutes. (Before instilling the liquid, warn the patient to close his or her glottis by forming but not saying a "ggg" sound while the liquid is in his or her nose.) The patient then blows his or her nose.[16] A less traumatic method is to attach a standard face mask to a nebulizer containing the solution and have the patient breathe through the nose.[19] A variation is to connect wall oxygen to an atomizer using oxygen tubing with a lateral hole cut in it. Intermittently occluding the hole with a fingertip produces a spray of lidocaine from the atomizer nozzle. Held at the nostril, the nozzle can deliver 2% lidocaine throughout inspiration and produce dense anesthesia of the airway from the nose to the trachea in less than 5 minutes.[20]

Nasal Speculum

A nasal speculum provides an excellent view when examining the nose and is vital when doing procedures, including packing the nose for epistaxis or draining a septal hematoma. The problem is finding the right-size speculum when it is needed. There are at least two methods to improvise a speculum, depending on the available resources.

If disposable otoscope specula are available, simply snip off the end of one to get the size you need, put it on an otoscope, and you have a speculum adequate to examine the nose.[21]

For a speculum that approximates the standard instrument, snip the corner off a wire hanger and bend the ends to the size you need (Fig. 28-1). Note that the loops bend inward so that the handle can be oriented toward the cheek (Fig. 28-2). Be careful to bend the V-shaped "corner" of the wire so that it exerts less pressure than you might need if making this into a self-retaining retractor.

Epistaxis

Epistaxis is one of the most common complaints. It varies from a simple problem to a life-threatening event. Nasal bleeds are either anterior, posterior, or a combination of the two.

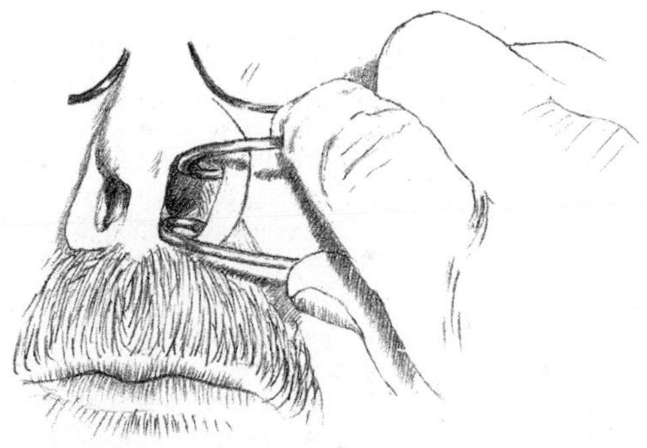

FIG. 28-2. Improvised nasal speculum in use.

While many clinicians use prepackaged materials to stop nasal bleeds, these are usually not available in austere situations.[22]

Adding a vasoconstrictor to an intranasal anesthetic stops up to 65% of anterior bleeds. A number of different, often readily available, anesthetics work well. Cocaine 4% is safe when used appropriately. Use a maximum of 200 mg (5 mL) or 2 to 3 mg/kg. Try to avoid using it in patients with coronary artery disease.[22] Lidocaine 4% plus phenylephrine has an effect equivalent to that of cocaine.[23] The maximum dose of lidocaine is 4 mg/kg. If using the injectable form, use up to 7 mg/kg lidocaine plus epinephrine. Tetracaine 1% plus 0.05% oxymetazoline (Afrin) works as well as lidocaine plus phenylephrine.[24] It also lasts longer, up to 60 minutes. The maximum adult dose of tetracaine is 50 mg.

Anterior Bleeds

Direct Pressure

The vast majority (90%) of nosebleeds arise from the mucosa in the anterior part of the septum (Little's area, Kiesselbach's plexus). Ask patients to blow their nose to remove any inadequate clots and then press their anterior nose continuously for 10 minutes. Show them how to press directly over the ala nasi (the soft part of the nose nearest the nares). Use a clock or a watch to time it or they will stop too early. This technique stops nearly all anterior bleeds. (Do not press over the nasal bones, as even experienced personnel often do.[24]) Alternatively, make a nasal pressure device by tightly taping two tongue depressors together at one end. To apply pressure, spread the non-taped end apart and place one tongue depressor on either side of the nares.

These techniques work even better if you first insert cotton or gauze with a small amount of oxymetazoline (Afrin), phenylephrine (Neo-Synephrine), or another vasoconstrictor into the anterior nose before applying the pressure. For patients with von Willebrand's disease or with other clotting problems, David Merrell, MD, says that packing fresh (uncooked) liver or bacon in the nose often helps because of the clotting factors they contain. (Personal communication, October 2006.)

Iced Lavage

If neither vasoconstrictors nor direct external pressure stops the bleeding, try an iced normal saline lavage of each nostril, with the patient leaning forward. This may help decrease or stop the bleeding and allow better assessment of bleeding sites. Have the patient seated during both the examination and the therapeutic procedures; this will lower his or her blood pressure.[25]

Packing

Anterior packing is almost a lost art among many clinicians. Lubricating a vaginal tampon and slipping it into the nose can make an improvised "prepackaged" anterior pack. (David Merrell, MD. Personal communication, October 2006.) As with anything else inserted into or through the nose, insert the tampon straight back along the floor of the nose.

If other measures do not stop the bleeding, an actual anterior pack may be required. For this, you need a cooperative patient, a petroleum gauze strip, a long forceps or hemostat, a nasal speculum, and a strong arm. Having a support behind the patient's head, even if only a wall, is helpful to stop the patient from continually backing away from you—the natural response. (See how to make a dental/ENT chair in Chapter 26 and Fig. 26-4.)

After anesthetizing and vasoconstricting the nasal cavity, sit the patient upright in a chair with a headrest. While lighting is not vital, using a headlight or a head mirror is useful. Sit facing the patient, and insert the nasal speculum with the handle pointing away from the nasal septum. It often helps to have an assistant hold the petroleum gauze so that you can easily pick it up at each step of the packing process. If the piece you have is not long enough to fill the nose, tie another piece onto the first one and continue. Never use more than one long continuous piece in each side; they will get lost in there.

Pick up one end of the ribbon gauze and insert it as far back as possible while not letting it drop into the nasopharynx. The most common error in doing anterior packs is that the gauze does not extend far enough back into the nose. Then, pick up the gauze at a point about twice the distance that the first portion went in. Try to push this back in the nose as far as the first piece went, layering the gauze (Fig. 28-3). Continue this process—forcefully—until absolutely no

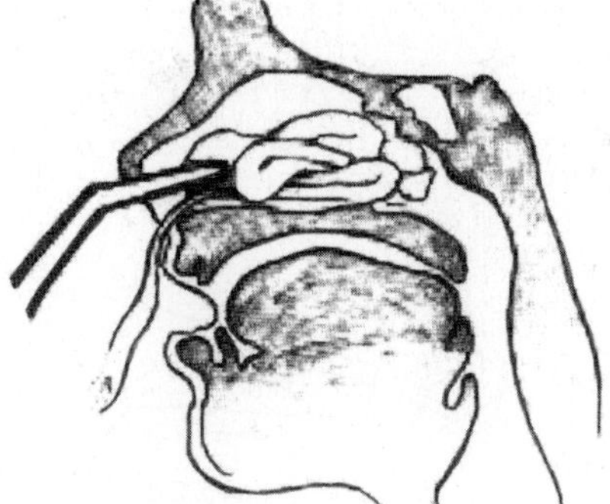

FIG. 28-3. Anterior nasal packing with petroleum gauze.

more gauze can fit into the nose. Cut off any remaining gauze. Have the patient return in 2 to 3 days to have the packing removed. Many of these patients will need analgesics.

Posterior Bleeds

Without a fancy balloon designed to stop posterior nasal bleeding, two options, aside from surgery, are available: a balloon-tipped urethral (Foley) catheter[26] and a posterior nasal pack.[27]

FOLEY CATHETER METHOD

1. If possible, anesthetize the nose and posterior pharynx.
2. If a flow-control roller clamp from an IV infusion set is available, slide it over a large (14-Fr) urethral (Foley) catheter with 30-mL balloon.
3. Trim the distal tip of the catheter; do not cut the balloon.
4. Slide the well-lubricated large catheter through the nares that is bleeding the most. Pass it along the floor of the nose until it is visible in the nasopharynx (~8 to 10 cm).
5. Fill the balloon with 15 to 30 cc of water.
6. Pull the balloon back until it firmly seats against the posterior nasal opening (choana).
7. If an IV roller clamp was placed on the catheter, put a gauze pad against the nares for protection and, while holding gentle traction on the catheter to apply pressure to the posterior bleeding site, slide the roller clamp to the nares and lock it in place.
8. Otherwise, pad the nose, pull the catheter tight against the back of the nose, and secure it with tape, a safety pin, or a nasogastric or umbilical clamp.
9. Pack the anterior nose, as in above section, around the catheter.
10. If significant bleeding continues, repeat the entire process on the other side. If bleeding persists, consider surgery.
11. Place the patient (irrespective of age or medical condition) on oxygen, because he or she is nearly always going to be hypoxic.

POSTERIOR NASAL GAUZE-PACK METHOD

1. Fold two 4 × 4 pieces of gauze or, if not available, a similar quantity of clean cloth into a small ball. Tie it securely at the middle of a very long piece of heavy thread or silk suture. Wrap the ties around the cloth several times in each direction. You will use these strings later to secure anterior nasal packing.
2. If possible, anesthetize the nose and posterior pharynx.
3. Pass a small-gauge urethral catheter or an infant feeding tube through the nares that is bleeding the most. When it is visualized in the posterior pharynx, grasp it with an instrument and pull it out through the mouth (Fig. 28-4).
4. Tie the free end of the heavy thread to the mouth end of the catheter (Fig. 28-5) and pull it out through the nose, bringing the thread with it through the nares. Cut the string where it connects to the catheter and discard the catheter.
5. Gently pull on the string and, with your other hand, guide the cloth pack tightly up into the nasopharynx until it lodges firmly against the posterior nasal opening (choana) (Fig. 28-6).

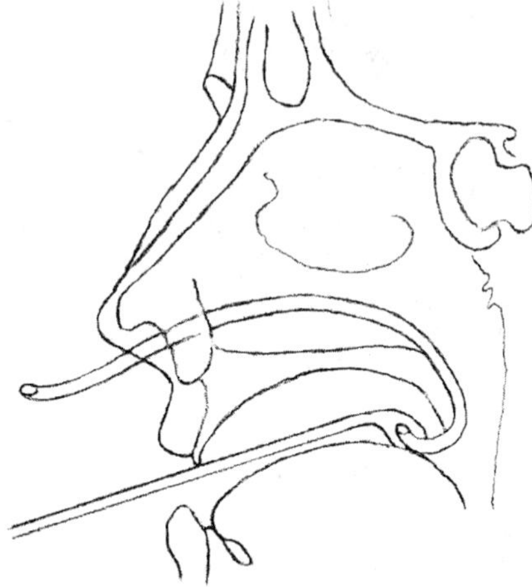

FIG. 28-4. Posterior pack, step 1: Pull catheter out through mouth.

6. Have your assistant hold traction on the thread while you pack the anterior nose (as described above).
7. Place a small piece of gauze or a cloth against the anterior nose and tightly tie the ends of the thread that is connected to the nasopharyngeal pack. This secures both the anterior and posterior nasal packs.
8. If significant bleeding continues, repeat the entire process on the other side. If it still continues, consider surgery.
9. Place the patient (of any age or medical condition) on oxygen, because he or she is nearly always going to be hypoxic.

Foreign-Body Removal

Foreign bodies in the nasal passages are common and occur almost exclusively in children. The danger of working on a nasal foreign body is that it might accidentally dislodge into the airway. Try to position the patient in a sitting or lateral position so that this is less likely. Vasoconstrictors are immensely helpful, including the otherwise little-used 4% cocaine solution, which is also an anesthetic. (Be careful of toxicity from using too much.) Alternatives include oxymetazoline

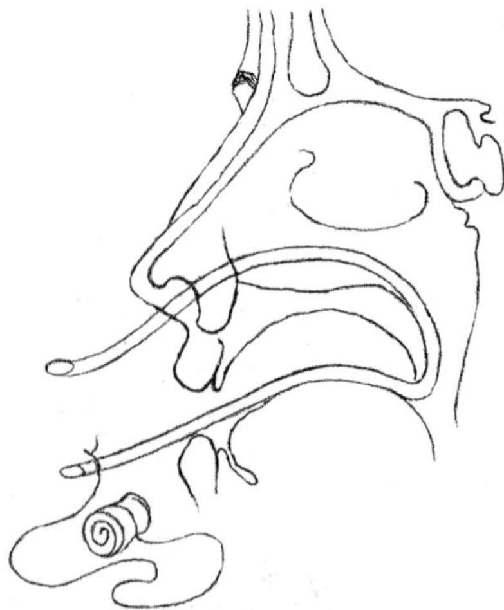

FIG. 28-5. Posterior pack, step 2: Tie gauze pack to catheter.

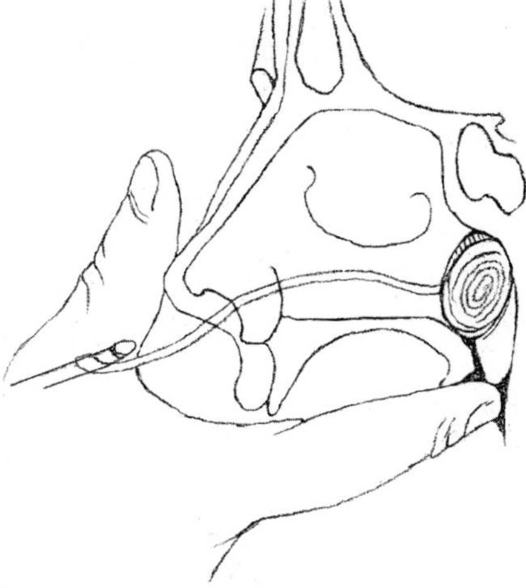

FIG. 28-6. Posterior pack, step 3: Push gauze pack firmly into nasopharynx.

(Afrin) or phenylephrine hydrochloride (Neo-Synephrine). Gain patient cooperation by using anesthetics, such as spraying 4% lidocaine (or cocaine). Anesthesia is the same as discussed above in the "Epistaxis" section.

Mechanical Removal

If a nasal foreign body is visualized, it can sometimes be retrieved by getting behind it using an ear curette, a right-angle ear hook, or the tip of a paper clip or calcium alginate swab (Calgiswab) whose metal-shaft has been bent to a 90-degree angle. Bend the paper clip by clamping the tip between the handle end of bandage scissors; the swab shaft is thin enough to easily bend by hand.[28]

Grasp small malleable objects close to the anterior nares with bayonet or alligator forceps. Retrieve harder objects with hemostats.

Retrieve magnetic metallic objects, such as the dreaded button battery, with a magnetic screwdriver or other tool, or by using metal forceps and a magnet. Place a magnet on the outside of the nose, and touch the forceps to the foreign body. Place the magnet against the nasal skin and slide toward the tip of the nose. The magnet often attracts the metallic object, which can then be painlessly removed.[29]

Suction

Suction may also work. However, the other methods usually work so well that suction is unnecessary. If it is used, turn the suction to 100 to 140 mm Hg, touch the foreign body with a thin rigid suction catheter (Frazier) tip, and withdraw the catheter and, hopefully, the foreign body with it. Rather than the rigid suction tip, attach a pediatric endotracheal (ET) tube to standard wall suction tubing, cutting it to ~5 to 7 cm in length. Drill a hole in the 15-mm adapter to control the suction, and attach a semirigid suction catheter onto the end of the ET tube (Fig. 28-7). Then use it as you would a Frazier tip.[30]

Glue

Although this method may also not be needed, it is good to know. Put a drop of cyanoacrylate glue on the end of a wooden or plastic applicator stick. Press it against the foreign body for approximately 1 minute and then remove it, trying not to also glue the stick to the patient's nasal mucosa. However, because the nasal mucosa is moister than the ear canal, if the patient is inadvertently glued to the stick, it comes off faster.

Catheter

One of the fastest and most reliable methods to remove a nasal foreign body is to pass a well-lubricated catheter with a balloon (urethral, vascular, or cardiac catheter) behind the foreign body.

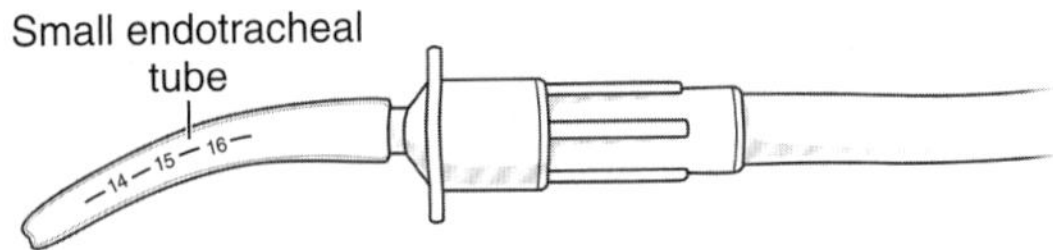

FIG. 28-7. Suction tip to extract foreign bodies.

A vascular catheter is stronger and stiffer than a pediatric urethral catheter, and may pass by the object more easily, although the urethral catheter nearly always is sufficient. Use the smallest diameter available. Do not try to visualize the foreign body or guide the catheter—just gently let it find its own passage around the object. Once the catheter enters the nasopharynx, inflate the balloon with 2 to 3 cc of air (not liquid that patients can aspirate if it breaks!). Remove the syringe used to inflate the balloon from the catheter before pulling it from the nasopharynx. This prevents the most common mistake with this technique: failing to maintain the balloon inflation during catheter removal.

Positive Pressure

Positive pressure behind the nasal object is also an effective removal method. If a child is cooperative, first ask the child to blow his or her nose while you, the parent, or the child occludes the other nostril. Sneezing, which can be stimulated with pepper, may also work.

If that does not work, a parent can forcefully do one or two breaths of mouth-to-mouth breathing on a child with the opposite nostril occluded. Calm the child in advance by telling him or her that the parent will be giving him or her "a big kiss." Have the child sit, stand, or, if supine, place them in the Trendelenburg position. Then have the parent firmly seal the child's open mouth with theirs, as in mouth-to-mouth resuscitation, and give a short, sharp puff of air. This usually blows the foreign body onto the parent's cheek. If it does not work the first time, reposition the parent and child and try again.[31] If the parent is not willing to do "the kiss," use a bag-valve-mask in a similar manner.[32]

Another easy method is to use air pressure from wall oxygen or an air outlet, if that is available. Connect a tubing (Christmas tree) adapter to the end of oxygen tubing. Spray phenylephrine in both nostrils and lay the child on his or her side, with the foreign body side down. Make sure the other side is unobstructed. Hold the child securely, with one person keeping control of the head. Turn the oxygen flow meter to 15 L/min or slightly higher. Quickly place the tubing connector into the nostril without a foreign body (Fig. 28-8A). Within several seconds, the offending object usually blasts out of the other nostril. (Do not stand in the line of fire.) It is postulated that, startled by the air blast, the child temporarily lifts his or her soft palate, forcing the air to flow out of the opposite nostril.[33] This technique also works using a stethoscope earpiece or the top of a medicine dropper. Attach it to an 8-Fr feeding tube that is bent at a right angle as close as possible to the rubber piece (Fig. 28-8B). Connect the other end of the tube to a standard oxygen outlet, adjusting the flow rate to 15 L/min (pressure equal to 100 to 160 mmHg). In patients ≤3 years old, use the same positioning as earlier. Children >3 years old can sit on the parent's lap with their arms controlled. Crimp the oxygen tubing, insert the device into the unaffected nostril, and uncrimp the tubing. In acute nasal foreign bodies, this method is successful >90% of the time with up to three attempts.[34] David Merrell, MD, suggests that if the patient is cooperative, have them say "K, K, K" to close the soft palate while doing this. (Written communication, September 3, 2008.)

MOUTH/PHARYNX

Anesthesia

Anesthetize the oral cavity, pharynx, larynx, and trachea using a standard nebulizer fitted with a mouthpiece to administer 4 mL of 4% lidocaine at 8 L/min oxygen flow over 3 minutes.[35]

To anesthetize the tonsil, apply topical anesthesia and then inject 1 mL of 1% lidocaine with 1:250,000 epinephrine above the tonsillar fossa, followed by 1 mL infiltration of both the posterior and the anterior pillar. Then inject 1 mL through the anterior pillar into the tonsillar bed to "float" the tonsil forward.[16]

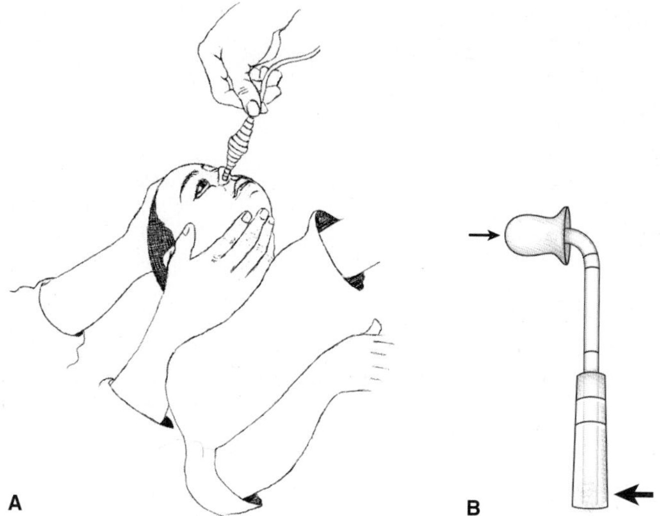

FIG. 28-8. (A) Christmas tree adapter for positive-pressure foreign-body removal. (B) Device to blow out nasal foreign body. The small arrow indicates the rubber piece that goes in an ear; the lower, larger arrow indicates the feeding tube.

Direct Laryngeal Examination

Direct laryngoscopy is a relatively easy way to examine the larynx and vocal cords. The only tools needed are a laryngoscope and topical local anesthetic for the oral mucosa, tongue, oropharynx, and larynx.

Topical anesthesia can be as simple as spraying lidocaine and then having the patient gargle with 4% lidocaine viscous to anesthetize the oral cavity and pharynx. Then spray the vocal cords under direct vision when the laryngoscope is inserted. An alternative method of anesthetizing the vocal cords, if that is necessary to remove a foreign body, is to spray or syringe 2 mL 4% lidocaine into the nose. Then insert a nasal airway coated with lidocaine ointment, apply cricoid pressure, and spray or inject 4 to 5 mL of 4% lidocaine down the tube directly at the larynx.[16]

If topical anesthetic is not available, use an oral block that includes the tongue, such as the Gow-Gates block (see the "Gow-Gates Technique: Alternative to Inferior Alveolar Block" section in Chapter 26).

Carefully explain the procedure to the patient: You need their full cooperation. Stand at the patient's head as you would when intubating. Have suction available, as well as long blunt (Magill) forceps if you suspect a foreign body. Lay the patient nearly flat, with their head on a level with your mid-chest. Then, carefully insert the laryngoscope into the patient's mouth, trying not to touch any non-anesthetized structures. Ask the patient to pant and then to say "E" so you can visualize vocal cord movement. Finally, evaluate the larynx and remove any foreign body.

Peritonsillar Abscess

After anesthetizing the mouth and pharynx, use a laryngoscope to provide exposure when draining a peritonsillar abscess. The patient should be sitting, and the laryngoscope handle should point down toward the patient's waist.

Possibly less intimidating to the patient than the laryngoscope, use the bottom half of a disposable, clear plastic gynecologic speculum with a light source attached to depress the tongue and illuminate the pharynx.[36] Another option is to tape a penlight to the proximal end of a tongue blade—this provides direct vision and allows the practitioner to have one hand free to do procedures.

Pharyngitis

Relieve sore throat pain with a variety of solutions, including warm saltwater gargles, a topical anesthetic, and lozenges. Although it is not often used, obtain good relief lasting several hours from gargling with a suspension of two crushed, regular-strength aspirin tablets dissolved in a small amount of warm water. Note that coated or buffered aspirin does not work; neither does acetaminophen.[37]

Oral Mucositis Analgesia

Patients on chemotherapy and radiation therapy often have intractable pain from oral mucositis. Ketamine provides effective analgesia if used as an oral rinse. To make a rinse, mix 0.2 mL ketamine 100 mg/mL (20 mg) with 5 mL of artificial saliva. Have the patient swish it around his or her mouth and expectorate after 1 minute. The artificial saliva (1% sodium carboxymethylcellulose and 3% sorbitol) helps local irrigation and mucosal retention. Repeat this every 3 hours as needed, for months if necessary.[38]

Foreign-Body Removal

Small high-powered magnetic balls, such as those found in toys, can be nearly impossible to remove when fixed on opposite sides of tissue, such as a lip (or nasal septum or ear). The easiest way to remove them is to apply magnetized instruments to both magnetic balls simultaneously. Instruments, such as forceps, become magnetized when they come near a magnet and become attracted to the magnet's opposite pole, instantly releasing the magnet from the tissue.[39]

TRAUMA

General Principle

As described by Sir Harold Gillies during World War I, patients with maxillofacial trauma die if their airways are not protected.[40] His method was to sit patients up or to put them on their side with their face down. If a patient with a severe maxillofacial injury has no neck injury or is awake and cooperative enough to protect their own spine, sit them up or put them in the "recovery" position.

Nasal Fractures

To reduce brisk bleeding from a nasal fracture, intermittently pack the nose with adrenaline-saline gauze.

Most nasal fractures do not need to be reduced immediately. Furthermore, when swelling exists, there is no good way of determining the proper orientation. If a nasal fracture does need reduction, stabilize the septum with metal scalpel handles or major artery forceps wrapped in gauze or with rubber tubes slipped over their blades. "Grasp the nose septum and wings: Mobilize the fragments by traction and careful twisting. Model the nose into normal configuration."[41] Then pack both sides of the nose for one week.

Midface Fractures

Midface fractures, if displaced backward, may occlude the airway. If this is suspected, simply grab the midface and pull it forward. If it is unstable, maintain manual traction on the nose to keep the segment forward.[42] If necessary (and if the patient is unconscious or chemically paralyzed), one or two fingers can be introduced behind the soft palate to pull it forward. If this works, use heavy sutures placed around stable anterior teeth as a handle to continue traction.

Lacerations

Tongue Lacerations

Close tongue lacerations using sutures or cyanoacrylate. Close any tongue laceration >1 cm long or that splits the tongue anteriorly. Also suture any laceration that is large enough to trap food particles. If suturing, anesthetize the tongue using a Gow-Gates block or an inferior alveolar block (see the section on blocks in Chapter 26); this may need to be done bilaterally. An alternative, if the laceration is small, is to apply gauze soaked in 4% lidocaine to the wound for 5 minutes.

Before suturing begins, have an assistant (or the patient, if cooperative) secure the tongue by holding the tip with gauze. An alternative is to place a suture, towel clamp, or safety pin vertically through the tip (as shown in Figs. 8-2 through 8-4). Irrigate the wound and close it with 4-0 or 5-0 absorbable sutures. (You do not want to have to take these stitches out!) Pass the suture through at least one-half of the tongue's thickness with each stitch. Tie the sutures loosely, because the tongue tends to swell. Tying the knots over an instrument or over the wooden end of a cotton swab lying on the laceration helps keep the sutures loose enough. Put four to six knots in each suture or they will unravel when the patient talks, eats, or just fiddles with the sutures. Applying cold (e.g., ice, Popsicles) to the tongue for the next day or so helps relieve the swelling and pain.

Cyanoacrylate may often work better and faster in cooperative patients. Grasp the tongue with gauze, and thoroughly dry any oral secretions. If available, use compressed air to further dry the tongue. Hold the wound edges together and apply three layers of cyanoacrylate; hold the tongue until the glue dries. Tell the patient not to manipulate the wound and to avoid drinking hot liquids for a week. If the wound needs additional support at 24 hours, remove the old glue and reapply it.[43]

Lip Lacerations

The most difficult part of treating lip lacerations is carefully approximating the vermillion border. Anesthetizing the lip with an infraorbital (upper lip) or mental (lower lip) nerve block makes it easier to do this because it does not distort the tissues. The infraorbital nerve block also anesthetizes the anterior maxillary teeth and the external anterior nose. The mental nerve block also numbs the chin. (For a description of both blocks, see Chapter 26.)

Gingival Mucosa

To close a laceration at the juncture of the upper lip and gingiva above the upper incisors, pass a 4-0 or 5-0 absorbable suture through one piece of the mucosa of the avulsed lip, completely around the adjacent tooth to the inside of the mouth and then out. When it is on the other side of the tooth, pass it through the avulsed tissue flap again and tie it. Repeat this process at the level of each tooth that abuts the laceration. Remove these sutures, even if absorbable, in 1 week. If the teeth are so tight that the sutures cannot be passed between them, insert them using a flossing action.[44]

Mandible

Mandibular Dislocations

Always attempt to reduce TMJ dislocations using standard methods and local or general anesthetics. In austere situations, patients may not present for some time after the dislocation occurs. Mandibular dislocations that have been out for >48 hours may be difficult to reduce. In difficult cases, try one of the following methods.

In difficult cases or when no anesthetic is available, gradually reduce a TMJ dislocation by first placing as many tongue depressors as possible, stacked one on top of the other, into the existing space on the side with the most prominent dislocation. Then insert new tongue depressors, one at a time, into the stack. The TMJ spasm should gradually relax enough for the joint to relocate.[45] If that doesn't work for non-traumatic dislocations, try the method below or place splints on the upper and lower teeth (see the "Splinting/Wiring" section in Chapter 27).

Used only for non-traumatic TMJ dislocations, the "syringe" technique entails placing a 5- or 10-mL syringe between the posterior molars on the dislocated side. Have the patient gently bite down on the syringe while rolling it back and forth along the posterior teeth. The originators reported a 97% success rate—most within 1 minute.[46]

Mandibular Fractures

If a mandible fracture is suspected, ask the patient if his or her teeth or, even better, his or her dentures fit like they used to. The absence of malocclusion virtually rules out a mandible fracture. A remarkably accurate test (96% sensitive, 65% specific) for mandibular fractures is to put a tongue blade between a patient's teeth (or have them do it) and ask him or her to bite down on it, bend it, and try to break it. People with normal mandibles are able to do it. Treat mandibular fractures with soft diets and splints, as described in Chapter 27.

REFERENCES

1. Schwab L. *Primary Eye Care in Developing Nations*. Oxford, UK: Oxford University Press; 1987:140.
2. Mellick LB, Mellick GA. Treatment of acute orofacial pain with lower cervical intramuscular bupivacaine injections: a 1-year retrospective review of 114 patients. *J Orofac Pain*. 2008;22(1):57-64.
3. Mellick LB, Mellick GA. Regional head and face pain relief following lower cervical intramuscular anesthetic injection. *Headache*. 2003;43:1109-1111.
4. Hamilton FH. *The Principles and Practice of Surgery*. 2nd ed. New York, NY: William Wood & Co.; 1879:590.
5. Schulze SL, Kerschner J, Beste D. Pediatric external auditory canal foreign bodies: a review of 698 cases. *Otolaryngol Head Neck Surg*. July 2002;127(1):73-78.
6. Aung T, Mulley GP. Removal of ear wax. *BMJ*. 2002;325(7354):27.
7. Keegan DA, Bannister SL. A novel method for the removal of ear cerumen. *CMAJ*. 2005;173(12):1496-1497.
8. Linden C. Novel methods for cerumen removal (letter). *CMAJ*. http://www.cmaj.ca/cgi/eletters/173/12/1496#3585. Accessed July 28, 2008.
9. White SJ, Broner S. The use of acetone to dissolve a Styrofoam impaction of the ear. *Ann Emerg Med*. 1994;23(3):580-582.
10. Ezechukwu CC. Removal of ear and nasal foreign bodies where there is no otorhinolaryngologist. *Trop Doct*. 2005;35:12-13.
11. Landry GL, Edmonson MB. Attractive method for battery removal. *JAMA*. 1986;256(24):3351.
12. Pride H, Schwab R. A new technique for removing foreign bodies of the external auditory canal. *Pediatr Emerg Care*. 1989;5(2):135-136.
13. Antonelli PJ, Ahmadi A, Prevatt A. Insecticidal activity of common reagents for insect foreign bodies of the ear. *Laryngoscope*. 2001;111:15-20.
14. Pond F, McCarty D, O'Leary S. Randomized trial on the treatment of oedematous acute otitis externa using ear wicks or ribbon gauze: clinical outcome and cost. *J Laryngol Otol*. 2002;116(6):415-419.
15. Waitzman AA. Otitis externa. *Emedicine*. http://emedicine.medscape.com/article/994550-overview#showall. Accessed September 26, 2015.
16. Boulton TB. Anesthesia in difficult situations. The use of local analgesia. *Anaesthesia*. 1967;22(1):101-133.
17. Anon. Using nasal sprays with children. University of Wisconsin Health Facts for You. http://www.uwhealth.org. Accessed September 23, 2007.
18. Ferguson BJ. Allergic rhinitis. *Postgrad Med*. 1997;101(5):117-131.
19. Bourke DL, Katz J, Tonneson A. Nebulized anesthesia for awake endotracheal intubation. *Anesthesiology*. 1985;63:690-691.
20. Davies PH, Benger JR. Foreign bodies in the nose and ear: a review of techniques for removal in the emergency department. *J Accid Emerg Med*. 2000;17:91-94.
21. Wells M. Create your own nasal speculae. *Postgrad Med*. http://www.postgradmed.com/pearls.htm. Accessed September 23, 2007.
22. Krempl GA, Noorily AD. Use of oxymetazoline in the management of epistaxis. *Ann Otol Rhinol Laryngol*. 1995;104(9 Pt 1):704-706.
23. Cara DM, Norris AM, Neale LJ. Pain during awake nasal intubation after topical cocaine or phenylephrine/lidocaine spray. *Anaesthesia*. 2003;58(8):777.
24. McGarry GW, Moulton C. The first aid management of epistaxis by accident and emergency department staff. *Arch Emerg Med*. 1993;10:298-300.
25. Aijaz Alvi A, Joyner-Triplett N. Iced saline lavage for acute epistaxis. *Postgrad Med*. www.postgradmed.com/pearls.htm. Accessed September 23, 2007.
26. Hartley C, Axon PR. The Foley catheter in epistaxis management—a scientific appraisal. *J Laryngol Otol*. 1994;108(5):399-402.
27. Reis ND, Dolev E, eds. *Manual of Disaster Medicine: Civilian and Military*. Berlin, Germany: Springer-Verlag; 1989:373.
28. Hendrick JG. Another solution for the foreign body in the nose problem. *Pediatrics*. 1988;82(3):395.
29. Brown L, Tomasi A, Salced G. An attractive approach to magnets adherent across the nasal septum. *Can J Emerg Med*. 2003;5(5):356-358.
30. McGuirk T. Tricks of the trade: an improvised, semi-rigid, nasal/aural suction catheter. *Emerg Med News*. 2009;31(9).

31. Botma M, Bader R, Kubba H. 'A parent's kiss': evaluating an unusual method for removing nasal foreign bodies in children. *J Laryngol Otol.* 2000;114:598-600.
32. Finkelstein JA. Oral Ambu-bag insufflation to remove unilateral nasal foreign bodies. *Am J Emerg Med.* 1996;14(1):57-58.
33. Navitsky RC, Beamsley A, McLaughlin S. Nasal positive-pressure technique for nasal foreign body removal in children. *Am J Emerg Med.* 2002;20(2):103-104.
34. de la O-Cavazos M, Ríos-Solís J, Montes-Tapia F, et al. A new positive-pressure device for nasal foreign body removal. *Ped Emerg Care.* 2014;(2):94-96.
35. Sutherland AD, Sole JP. Fiberoptic awake intubation: a method of topical anaesthesia and orotracheal intubation. *Can Anaesth Soc J.* 1986;33:502.
36. Anon. Light touch. *Emerg Med.* December 2007:12.
37. Voith MA. Soothing the sore throat. *Postgrad Med.* http://www.postgradmed.com/pearls.htm. Accessed September 23, 2007.
38. Slatkin NE, Rhiner M. Topical ketamine in the treatment of mucositis pain. *Pain Med.* 2003;4(3): 298-303.
39. Kondamudi NP, Gupta A, Kaur R. Magnet balls stuck to the frenulum of the lip. *J Emerg Med.* March 2014;46(3):345-347.
40. Bamji A. Sir Harold Gillies: surgical pioneer. *Trauma.* 2006;8:143-156.
41. Husum H, Ang SC, Fosse E. *War Surgery: Field Manual.* Penang, Malaysia: Third World Network; 1995:328.
42. Husum H, Ang SC, Fosse E. *War Surgery: Field Manual.* Penang, Malaysia: Third World Network; 1995:322.
43. Kazzi MG, Silverberg M. Pediatric tongue laceration repair using 2-octyl cyanoacrylate (Dermabond®). *J Emerg Med.* 2013;45(6):846-848.
44. Armstrong BD. Lacerations of the mouth. *Emerg Med Clin North Am.* 2000;8(3):471-480.
45. Technique used in very difficult cases by Dan Klemmedson, MD, DDS, Oral Surgeon, Tucson, AZ, at University Medical Center.
46. Gorchynski J, Karabidian E, Sanchez M. The "syringe" technique: a hands-free approach for the reduction of acute nontraumatic temporomandibular dislocations in the emergency department. *J Emerg Med.* 2014;47(6):676-681.

29 | Neurology/Neurosurgery

EVALUATION/DIAGNOSIS/TREATMENT

Lumbar Punctures

Lumbar punctures (LPs; spinal taps) can provide invaluable information, but only if the local culture allows them to be done and the laboratory can analyze the specimen accurately. In children ≤5 years old, consider using a short small-gauge hypodermic needle; a butterfly needle works well in infants. For children >5 years old, use a standard LP needle, if one is available. Otherwise, use a longer small-gauge hypodermic needle.

Lumbar puncture needles may need to be reused. While this is potentially dangerous, it may be safer to reuse these needles than to reuse hypodermic needles. The obturator allows large material to be cleaned out of the needle's core. After cleaning, steam autoclave the needles. If that is not possible, high-level disinfection by boiling has been recommended.[1] To do this:

1. Put the needles into a pan and cover them with 3 cm of potable water. Put the lid on the pan and bring the water to a boil. Once it begins to boil, keep it boiling for 15 minutes.
2. While holding the lid on the pan, pour out the water without letting the needles fall out. This is not as easy as it sounds; practice this before you boil the needles.
3. Leave the nearly dry needles in the covered pan until they are needed. Never put them anywhere else.

Finding the Midline for a Lumbar Puncture

In resource-poor settings, finding the midline with an ultrasound for an LP may hold the key to success, because there may be no one available to help with a failed LP. In adults, use a curvilinear low-frequency (5 to 2 MHz) transducer to image non-palpable bony landmarks, even if they are deeper than 9 cm. In children, use a linear high-frequency transducer. With a musculoskeletal "preset," adjust the depth (adults) to 10 to 12 cm and place the probe near the presumed midline with the marker cephalad. Slowly slide the transducer left or right until the facet joints are seen—they look like humps on the ultrasound screen. Then slide the probe caudad until the sacrum is seen as a horizontal hyperechoic line. Use this landmark to identify the L3 to L4 and L4 to L5 interspaces, marking their location on the skin. Then, rotate the transducer 90 degrees to locate the anatomic midline. Slide the probe cephalad and caudad, identifying and marking the spinous processes. Connect the skin markings from the midline and the interspace levels; they will cross at the ideal sites for needle entry. Follow standard LP technique.[2]

Psychogenic Disorders and Malingering

Patients with psychogenic neurological disorders may present with bizarre motor findings and neurological tests that indicate a functional (psychogenic) disorder. They usually will have normal muscle tone, no atrophy or fasciculations, and no ataxia, although they may try to simulate it. The following are a number of quick, easy tests that suggest a patient may be malingering—or not. In resource-poor settings, you will have to rely on these simple tests; in other settings, they can save clinicians time and effort.

The Hoover Crossed-Leg Test examines leg strength. A supine person who tries to lift his straight leg against gravity or resistance will push down (for leverage) with the other heel. To do the test, the examiner asks the patient to lift the affected leg while keeping one hand under the patient's other heel. No or little pressure on the examiner's hand while the person says he is trying to lift his leg signifies malingering—as long as both legs are not affected. A more effective modification is for the examiner to put a thumb over both ankles while doing the test (Fig. 29-1). This provides additional resistance to lifting the leg and also provides information on the relative strength exerted by each leg.

The Crossed-Hand Test (Fig. 29-2) is used to discover whether a complaint of unilateral hand numbness is valid. Have the patient cross his arms at the forearm level, turn the palms facing

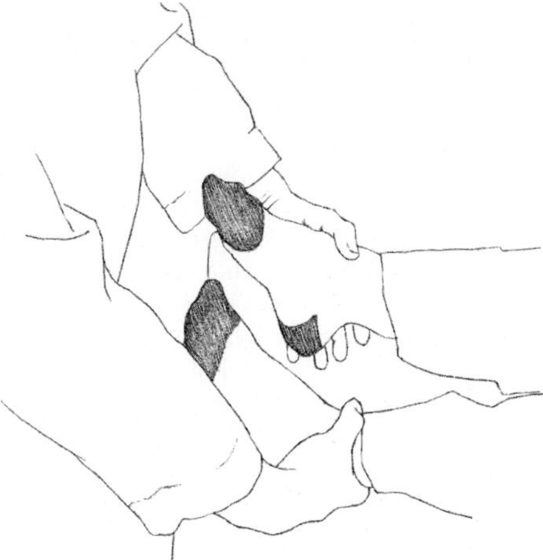

FIG. 29-1. Hoover crossed-leg test.

each other, and interlock the fingers. Then, if the patient is limber enough, he can bring his hands up in front of his face. With the patient watching, test the sensation in the fingers. Visual miscues due to the hand position will cause malingerers to pause before responding to sensation when the examiner touches each finger; they often identify the sensation incorrectly.

"Splitting the tuning fork" identifies patients with psychogenic sensory disturbance. These patients typically have a sharply demarcated loss of sensation to the midface. Use a tuning fork to test vibratory sensation on both sides of the forehead. These patients often complain that they lack vibratory sensation when tested on the affected side of the forehead, but will have intact vibratory sensation on the unaffected side. Of course, that is not possible, because the vibration is transmitted through the frontal bone to both sides.[3]

Use "optokinetic testing" for individuals who claim to be blind but are not. This test produces nystagmus in those who can see. To induce optokinetic nystagmus (vertical, horizontal, or rotational), have the patient look at moving visual stimuli, usually on a special rotating drum. If patients have nystagmus, it means they can see the drum. Improvising optokinetic testing equipment is easy: Make an optokinetic drum by attaching a paper with alternating black and white stripes around an empty soda can. Alternatively, use a black sheet of paper with multiple strips of white tape (~2 cm wide) attached so that there are alternating stripes of black and white.

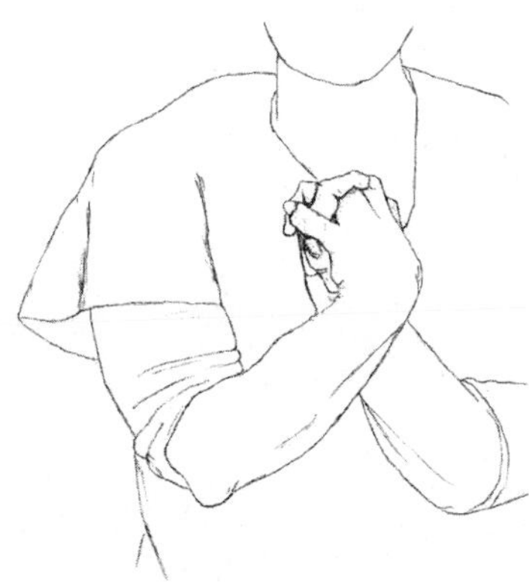

FIG. 29-2. Crossed-hand test.

Make a photocopy of this and wrap it around an empty soda can. Extend a straight piece of metal, such as a hanger, through the top and bottom parts of the can as a handle to rotate the drum. Another method of eliciting optokinetic nystagmus is to pass a vertically striped cloth (such as a striped tie) horizontally across the patient's visual field at about 5 to 10 cm/second. A measuring tape with large markings also works well. This reflex can be elicited starting at about 4 to 6 months of age and confirms cortical vision.[4]

Tunnel vision may be another manifestation of psychogenic visual disturbance. Patients may complain that they can see only a tiny part of the visual field in the center of vision, not unlike looking through a soda straw. To test whether such a complaint is legitimate, do the following: Make a small hole (about the diameter of a pencil) in a piece of paper. Have the patient close one eye and hold the paper with the hole positioned over his or her open eye. Move your face in front of the paper such that the patient can see only your nose, and then move back 3 to 6 feet from the patient and ask him or her what they see. If he or she says that they can see only your nose, they are feigning, because the degree of visual arc subtended has increased. In other words, they should see your whole face (at the very least). (Geoffrey Ahern, MD, PhD, University of Arizona, Tucson. Personal written communication, September 1, 2008.)

If the patient complains of being blind, but you do not think he or she is, leave some money on the floor and see how the patient reacts when he or she enters the room. (Joseph Miller, MD, PhD, University of Arizona, Tucson. Personal written communication, September 8, 2008.)

Monocular diplopia that does not correct using a pinhole device is almost always a functional problem.[5] And eyelids that flutter when a person is in "coma" means that they are completely awake. If you do not have time to wait for their spontaneous awakening, break two or three ammonia capsules and hold them under the patient's nose.

Use the sedative-hypnotic interview in Chapter 38 to easily assess suspected complex psychogenic complaints.

Neuropathies

An early sign of a peripheral neuropathy is the inability to feel vibration. If a low-pitched tuning fork is not available, use a pager or a cell phone (set on vibratory mode, or use a "women's vibrator" app) to see if a patient feels vibrations over bony prominences.[6]

If concerned about polyneuropathy in a patient, test the Achilles tendon reflex. Patients with normal Achilles reflexes rarely have a clinically significant polyneuropathy.[7]

Headaches

A large number of patients, especially when populations are under stress, will come in with the complaint of headache, often a "migraine." Historical and physical findings usually can differentiate their headaches from more serious problems.

For patients with non-migraine headaches, 20 mg IV metoclopramide plus 25 mg IV diphenhydramine provides better immediate (<1 hour) pain relief, decreases the likelihood of needing "rescue medications," and provides more sustained pain relief at 24 hours than does 30 mg IV ketorolac.[8] In some cases, peripheral nerve blocks also may be useful. The most commonly used blocks include the greater occipital, lesser occipital, supratrochlear, supraorbital, and auriculotemporal. If used, the block should produce cutaneous anesthesia and, hopefully, relieve an acute headache attack or terminate a headache cycle. Limit the adult local anesthetic dose per treatment session to <300 mg lidocaine or <175 mg bupivacaine. However, with the exception of using a greater occipital nerve block (often with corticosteroids) for cluster headaches, there is little consistent evidence about its effectiveness.[9]

If a migraine is diagnosed, and if medications are limited, try using a medication from Table 29-1. Even when other medications are available, 1 gram magnesium sulfate IV in 100 mL 0.9% normal saline given over 20 minutes has been shown to provide better relief than a combination of dexamethasone and metoclopramide.[10]

Abort cluster headaches, often considered the most painful type of headache, with oxygen by face mask, if it is available. Various medications, including corticosteroids, can suppress attacks during cluster periods. Two "street drugs," the ergot derivative lysergic acid diethylamide (LSD) and the related drug, psilocybin, have been the only medications to induce remission of a cluster period. In "sub-hallucinogenic doses," LSD aborted the cluster period after one dose; psilocybin generally took three doses.[15]

TABLE 29-1 Migraine Treatment, Selected Alternative Medications

Medication	Dose
	I. ABORTIVE AGENTS
	A. Oral or Sublingual
Acetaminophen	325-1300 mg
Acetaminophen/butalbital/caffeine	325-650 mg acetaminophen
Aspirin	325-1950 mg
Aspirin/butalbital/caffeine	325-650 mg aspirin
Dexamethasone	4-8 mg
Ergotamine tartrate (sublingual)	2 mg; then 1 q30min prn. Max 6 tabs/24 hr and 10 mg/week
Ergotamine tartrate/caffeine	2 tabs, then 1 q30min × 4, prn. Max 6 tabs/attack
Ergotamine tartrate/caffeine (suppository)	0.5-2 mg ergotamine; may repeat once after 1 hour
Ibuprofen	400-800 mg
Indomethacin	25-50 mg
Isometheptene/acetaminophen/ dichloralphenazone	325-975 mg acetaminophen
Ketorolac	10 mg
Naproxen	500-1000 mg
Sumatriptan	50-100 mg; may repeat in 2 hours. Max 200 mg/24 hr
	B. Parenteral
Butorphanol	2 mg IM or intranasally
Chlorpromazine	7.5-37.5 mg IV (slowly) or 25-50 mg IM
Dexamethasone	12-20 mg IV or IM, may follow with prednisone taper: 60 mg × 1 day; 40 mg × 1 day; 20 mg × 1 day
Dihydroergotamine	0.75-1 mg IV or SQ, or IV over 2-3 min (premedicate with 10 mg metoclopramide or prochlorperazine); may repeat qh to max 3 mg/24 hr and 6 mg/week 1 spray (0.5 mg) into each nostril; may repeat q15min. Max 3 mg/24 hr
Droperidol	2.5 mg IV or IM
Ergotamine/caffeine	1 rectal suppository; may repeat in 1 hour
Hydrocortisone	100-250 mg IV over 10 min; may follow with prednisone taper: 60 mg × 1 day; 40 mg × 1 day; 20 mg × 1 day
Ketamine	0.1-0.2 mg/kg IV
Ketorolac	30 mg IV or 60 mg IM
Magnesium sulfate	1-2 g IV over 10 to 30 min
Metoclopramide	10-20 mg IV
Oxygen	100% by mask at 8-10 L/min for 30 min
Prochlorperazine	5-10 mg IV

(*Continued*)

TABLE 29-1 Migraine Treatment, Selected Alternative Medications (*Continued*)

Medication	Dose
Sumatriptan	6 mg SQ; 5-20 mg intranasally; may repeat after 2 hours. Max 40 mg/24 hr
Zolmitriptan	5 mg intranasally; may repeat after 2 hours
	II. PROPHYLACTIC AGENTS
Amitriptyline	30-150 mg qhs
Candesartan	8-32 mg qd
Divalproex sodium	250-500 mg bid; extended-release 500 mg-1g qd
Lisinopril	5-40 mg qd
Metoprolol	50-100 mg bid; extended-release 100-200 mg qd
Nadolol	20-40 mg qd
Naproxen	250 mg bid or tid
Nortriptyline	10-150 mg qhs
Propranolol	160-240 mg/day divided bid, tid, or qid; extended-release 160-2400 mg qd
Timolol	10-15 mg bid or 20 mg qd
Topiramate	50 mg bid
Verapamil	80 mg tid or qid; extended-release 240 mg qd

Abbreviations: bid, twice a day; IM, intramuscular; IV, intravenous; qd, once a day; qhs, at bedtime every night; qid, four times a day; SQ, subcutaneous; tabs, tablets; tid, three times a day.

Data from Shah and Kelly,[11] Editors to Medical Letter,[12] Tintinalli,[13] and Rapoport.[14]

Stroke Syndrome ("Brain Attacks")

Predicting a Stroke After a Transient Ischemic Attack

If a patient with a transient ischemic attack (TIA) presents, how many resources must you devote to this patient? In other words, what is the chance of this patient developing a stroke in the next 7 days? Use a scoring system, such as the one below, to help determine the answer.

The 9-point ABCD3 Scale uses a score calculated on the basis of the patient's **A**ge, **B**lood pressure (BP), **C**linical features, **D**uration of symptoms, the presence of **D**iabetes, and **D**ual TIA symptoms (a TIA prompting medical attention plus at least one other TIA in the preceding 7 days). Assign points according to the list in Table 29-2, and then add them to get the ABCD3 score. Table 29-2 can also be used to calculate the shortened ABCD and ABCD2 scores, as described below.

The 6-point ABCD score (which does not include Diabetes or Dual TIA) has been validated. In one validation study of 274 consecutively enrolled patients with TIA (based on World Health Organization [WHO] standards), no patient with an ABCD score ≤3 had a stroke within 30 days. Of the patients suffering a stroke within 7 days, 20% had an ABCD score of 4, 40% scored 5, and 40% scored 6.[16]

Neither the 7-point ABCD2 score (without Dual TIA) nor the 9-point ABCD3 score has been thoroughly validated. Neither can identify all patients who will have a new stroke within two weeks or 30 days. However, an ABCD2 score <2 can identify patients at very low risk; an ABCD3 score <4 identifies even more patients at low risk. Those with an ABCD3 score ≥4 or an ABCD2 score ≥2 suggest a higher likelihood of stroke within 14 days.[17,18]

Stroke Diagnosis

Nearly one-third of patients presenting with a possible stroke have a different diagnosis. With limited imaging and consultation, rapid clinical differentiation becomes especially important. It saves resources and can guide therapy and diagnostic measures in the correct direction.

TABLE 29-2 ABCD3 Score to Predict Stroke Risk*

Age	≥60 years = 1 point <60 years = 0 points
Blood pressure	Systolic >140 mm Hg or diastolic >90 mm Hg = 1 point
Clinical features	Unilateral weakness = 2 points Speech disturbance without weakness = 1 point Other symptoms = 0 points
Duration of symptoms	≥60 min = 2 points 10-59 min = 1 point <10 min = 0 points
Diabetes mellitus	1 point
Dual TIA	2 points

Abbreviation: TIA, transient ischemic attack.

*Also used to calculate ABCD and ABCD2 scores.

The likelihood that the patient had an acute stroke increases dramatically if there is a definite history of focal neurological symptoms (odds ratio = 7.21), if you know the exact time that symptoms began (odds ratio = 2.59), or in the presence of any cardiovascular abnormality (systolic BP >150 mm Hg, atrial fibrillation, valvular heart disease, or absent peripheral pulses; odds ratio = 2.54).[19] On presentation, a stroke is more likely if the patient has facial paresis, arm drift, or abnormal speech (odds ratio = 5.5). If none of these symptoms are present, it is unlikely that the patient had a stroke (odds ratio = 0.39).[20]

TRAUMA

Head Injury

Determining True Coma/Level of Consciousness

Is the patient unconscious? Hysteria, psychological disease, drugs, or alcohol may all make patients seem unconscious when they are not. The following are simple, rapid methods to test for the level of consciousness (LOC) in these patients:

- *Sternal rub:* Use your knuckles and progressively increase pressure as you rub.
- *Ammonia capsules:* Break three or four and cup them in your hand. Place your cupped hand firmly over the patient's mouth and nose.
- *Supraorbital nerve pressure:* Similar to a sternal rub; be careful that your finger does not slip and injure the eye.
- *Jaw pull:* Place your second and third fingers behind the ascending ramus of the mandible and pull the patient's jaw forward.
- *Nose-hair tickle:* Use cotton strands (e.g., from a cotton swab) and gently stimulate the hair inside the nares.
- *Hand–face drop:* When the patient's hand is held over his or her face and dropped, the patient in psychogenic coma typically avoids letting the hand hit their face by making subtle movements to the side.[3]
- *Corneal reflex:* Use saline drops to get a response, rather than a wisp of cotton.
- *Rectal examination:* Part of the normal full examination for unconscious patients, this procedure may arouse the hysteric. When done in unconscious patients who are about to be chemically paralyzed for intubation, the absence of tone means they are paralyzed from a spinal injury.
- *Foley catheter:* (especially males) This stimulation will usually awaken any male who can be awakened by external stimuli.

Coma Scores

The simplest way to transmit information about the level of head injury is either to use a coma score that the receiver understands or to describe the patient's response to the score's elements.

TABLE 29-3 AVPU, ACDU, and SMA (TROLL) Coma Descriptions

AVPU Scale	ACDU Scale	SMS (TROLL)
A = Alert	A = Alert	Test responsiveness:
V = Responds to verbal stimuli	C = Confused	Obeys commands
P = Responds to painful stimuli	D = Drowsy	Localizes pain
U = Unresponsive	U = Unresponsive	Withdrawal from pain or Less responsive

Adapted from Green.[22]

Neurological consultants will want to know this critical information, especially when you ask for their advice or want to transfer head-injured patients to them. Do not assume that everyone uses the same scoring system. The best way to deliver or receive information about a patient is to ask for the specific brief neurological findings that the clinician found when determining any of the coma scores described next.

The most widely understood coma score is the Glasgow Coma Score (GCS; also known as the Glasgow Coma Scale), although its 13 levels are confusing, unreliable, unnecessarily complex, and were never designed to be used for acute care. If used, the 6-point motor component of the GCS provides the same results as the entire scale. If the entire GCS is used, note that patients ≥70 years old with a GCS score of 14 have a greater mortality than do those <70 years old with a GCS of 13.[21]

Two similar alternatives now commonly used in prehospital care are the AVPU scale and the ACDU scale (Table 29-3). These, as well as the Simplified Motor Scale (SMS), provide essentially the same prognostic information as the GCS, but are easier to use and describe to other clinicians. Steve Green, MD, has suggested that we change SMS to TROLL (**T**est **R**esponsiveness: **O**beys, **L**ocalizes, or **L**ess), because the name is both memorable and a mnemonic for the test elements.

Common Mistakes

Do not rely on the ophthalmoscopic examination to show evidence of acute rises in intracranial pressure. These changes appear only in chronic conditions, including retinal hemorrhages in infants with head injuries from child abuse.

In the midst of trauma resuscitation turmoil, be careful not to let easily salvageable head-injured patients die because (a) you confused a bad scalp laceration with an open skull fracture or (b) you did not control significant scalp bleeding. Control scalp hemorrhage by simply wrapping a tourniquet-type bandage around the head above the eye line. (Remember that all vessels to the scalp travel up from the neck.) When the bleeding slows, quickly use scalp clips, staples, or big sutures to stop the bleeding; then remove the tourniquet. Do a better closure later, if necessary.

Unsalvageable Head Injuries

Knowing which patients will not survive is the key to maximizing the use of limited resources to treat hordes of patients with multiple severe injuries. As the US military recognizes, "the prognosis of brain injuries is good in patients who respond to simple commands, are not deeply unconscious, and do not deteriorate. The prognosis is grave in patients who are rendered immediately comatose (particularly those sustaining penetrating injury) and remain unconscious for a long period of time."[23]

Similarly, Dr. Husum and colleagues, in their book *War Surgery*, write about patients who are "beyond salvation," saying that "bilateral dilated pupils that do not improve after a few hours in a comatose [head-injured] patient are a sign of major brain injury which normally will not respond to treatment. Operation in such cases is wasted."[24] In a similar vein, the US military writes that "a GCS <5 indicates a dismal prognosis despite aggressive comprehensive treatment, and the casualty should be considered expectant [comfort care provided, but not treatment]."[25]

Head Injury Decision Rules

In austere situations where computed tomographic (CT) scans are not readily available, it may be an extremely weighty and costly decision to send patients for a CT scan. The question is: How much chance of making an error is reasonable in your situation? In these environments, the best option may be to use the Canadian Rules (adult and child), because these will detect more patients who actually need neurosurgical intervention. Those at high risk (adult or child) have one of the listed findings:

Canadian Adult Rule (≥16 Years Old; GCS 13 to 15)

- GCS <15 within 2 hours after injury
- Suspected open or depressed skull fracture
- Any sign of basilar skull fracture (hemotympanum, raccoon eyes, otorrhea, rhinorrhea, Battle's sign)
- Two or more episodes of emesis
- >65 years old
- Moderate risk of brain injury on CT scan
- Retrograde amnesia ≥30 minutes
- Dangerous injury mechanism (pedestrian struck by motor vehicle, ejection from motor vehicle, fall from 3 feet/1 m or ≥5 stairs)

The Canadian Adult Rule has a sensitivity of 100% and a specificity of 38% for detecting any lesion requiring neurosurgical intervention, and a sensitivity of 87% and a specificity of 39% for detecting any clinically important CT abnormality.[26]

Canadian Child Rule

- Age <2 years
- GCS <15
- Mental status change
- Sensory deficit
- Palpable skull defect (A large or soft [boggy] scalp hematoma is associated with positive CT findings)[27]
- Any sign of basilar skull fracture (hemotympanum, raccoon eyes, otorrhea, rhinorrhea, Battle's sign)

The Canadian Child Rule has >95% sensitivity and ~49% specificity, with a negative predictive value of >99% and a positive predictive value of >11%.[28]

The Pecarn Pediatric Head Injury Rules

Designed to assess which children need CT scans after head injuries, these rules can identify high-risk patients.[29] Children with blunt head injury fall into two groups: those <2 years old and those 2 to 18 years old. The rules to determine whether the child has a clinically important traumatic brain injury (ciTBI) are:

<2 Years Old

The child is at *serious risk (4.4%)* for having a ciTBI if any one of the following are present:

1. GCS ≤14
2. Altered mental status
3. Palpable skull fracture

The child is at *moderate risk (0.9%)* for having a ciTBI if any one of the following are present:

1. Non-frontal scalp hematoma
2. LOC ≥5 seconds
3. Severe injury mechanism
   a. Pedestrian or bicyclist without helmet struck by motorized vehicle
   b. Fall >1 m or 3 feet
   c. Head struck by high-impact object
4. Abnormal activity per parents

2 To 18 Years Old

The child is at *serious risk (4.3%)* for having a ciTBI if any one of the following are present:

1. GCS ≤14
2. Altered mental status
3. Signs of a basilar skull fracture

The child is at *moderate risk (0.9%)* for having a ciTBI if any one of the following are present:

1. History of vomiting (Children with vomiting as the sole risk factor have only a 0.2% risk of ciTBI)
2. LOC
3. Severe injury mechanism
   a. Pedestrian or bicyclist without a helmet struck by motorized vehicle
   b. Fall >2 m or 5 feet
   c. Head struck by high-impact object
4. Severe headache

Optic Nerve Sheath Diameter Measurement

Use ultrasound to determine whether a patient has elevated intracranial pressure (ICP). The optic nerve sheath communicates pressure from the cerebrospinal fluid and is readily visible using portable ultrasound machines. First, have a responsive patient stare forward or open the unconscious patient's eyes to check pupil position. With the eyelid closed and the probe in line with the globe axis, position the screen marker along the nerve 3 mm from the posterior globe. At that point, once the nerve is centered with clear optic sheath margins, measure the optic nerve width. An optic nerve sheath diameter (ONSD) of ≥5.2 mm accurately predicts elevated ICP 83% of the time. The negative predictive value of ONSD <5.2 mm is 95.5%.[30] ONSD diameters >5 mm correlate with ICP elevations, with sensitivities up to 100% and specificities ranging from 63% to 95%.[31]

Concussions

Concussions are the most common closed head injury. Diagnose a concussion if there is

1. Observed and documented disorientation or confusion immediately after the event
2. Impaired balance within 1 day after injury
3. Slower reaction time or impaired verbal learning and memory within 2 days after injury

In most cases, cognitive deficits resolve within 1 week.[32]

Head Injury Diagnosis and Treatment in Austere Situations

Skull radiographs may still be valuable in head injury management if other imaging is not available. Locate radiopaque foreign bodies, usually bullets, using both posteroanterior (PA) and lateral or stereoscopic films (see Chapter 19). Also, finding a skull fracture is useful because (a) a patient with a simple skull fracture and no abnormal neurological signs may have up to a 1:30 chance of developing an intracranial hematoma; (b) if there are abnormal neurological signs with the fracture, the risk rises to 1:4; and (c) an intracranial hematoma nearly always will be on the side of, and at the site of, the fracture.[33]

Need for Intervention in Children with Head Injuries

Children ≤5 years old with nondepressed skull fractures and an initial normal neurologic examination result (GCS 15) do not develop neurologic deterioration. If child abuse is not an issue, discharge the child. Those with a GCS <15 are at major risk for serious neurologic dysfunction and death. Patients ≤18 years of age with isolated closed head trauma and a GCS score of 15 will not require neurosurgical intervention unless they have a depressed skull fracture.[34]

Isolated Subarachnoid Hemorrhage After Mild Head Trauma

In the absence of other significant trauma, manage patients with an isolated subarachnoid hemorrhage and a mild traumatic brain injury without routine follow-up imaging or intensive care unit admission.[35]

Treating Increased Intracranial Pressure

Basic treatment for head injuries or for other patients with increased ICP is to elevate the head of the bed 30 degrees to augment venous drainage. Also, ventilate patients with a controlled airway, when possible. To reduce edema and buy additional time, use an osmotic diuretic (3% saline, mannitol).

Use small repeat boluses of 3% hypertonic saline (HTS) to treat increased ICP and cerebral edema in children and adults. HTS administration decreases ICP more than mannitol or barbiturates, and the ICP continues to decrease in the second hour after therapy.[36] When given as 10 mL/kg of HTS over 1 hour, it also acutely reduces concussion pain in children.[37]

Burr Holes

Prior to Transfer

Consider trying to drain any extradural fluid collection before transferring a patient with a severe head injury and evidence of herniation. The length of the delay before decompression adversely affects prognosis. Poor outcome is associated with patients who have (a) intracranial hematomas and evidence of brainstem dysfunction on physical examination, (b) greater deterioration in physical examination, and (c) longer time to decompressing the hematoma. The duration of decerebration before surgery drastically affects outcome: Survival is 70% if <2 hours, 40% if 4 to 6 hours, and 0% if >6 hours. A delay of >4 hours before surgery in acute subdural hematoma changes the mortality from 30% to 90% regardless of other factors.

Clinicians must also consider that the time to craniotomy at a referral site includes the time spent at the first hospital, in transit, and preparing for the operating room (OR) at the receiving hospital. In Australia, because only 14% of these referred patients received a craniotomy in <4 hours, the Royal Australasian College of Surgeons now recommends that rural practitioners perform burr hole drainage for patients with herniating epidural hematomas if transfer is expected to take >2 hours. If you need to do this procedure, consider using a telemedicine neurosurgery consultation.[38]

In American Samoa, 3000 miles from the nearest neurosurgeon (at the time), Dr. Schecter and his general surgery colleagues reported that with neither CT scanner nor angiographic capability, they did exploratory burr holes for patients suffering closed head injuries. Their indications were either a depressed skull fracture or a closed head injury accompanied by lateralizing neurological signs, progressive deterioration, or coma. Of the 50 patients on whom they operated, 41 survived and 32 were neurologically normal.[39]

The Technique

Doing burr holes may be necessary to evacuate a hematoma or to elevate a seriously depressed skull fracture. If possible, place the patient in a supine position, with a shoulder roll under the side where the burr hole(s) will be placed. Turn the head so that the surgical side is up.

Landmarks will vary, depending on the purpose of the burr hole. For trauma, place the first burr hole next to (not over) a depressed skull fracture or a skull fracture line seen on x-ray. Without a localizing indicator, place the hole at a point that is three of the patient's fingerbreadths superior to the tragus (anterior ear). If a pupil is dilated, begin on that side. Note that in up to 5% of cases with a dilated pupil, the extra-axial hematoma will be on the contralateral side.[40]

DRILLING THE BURR HOLE

1. Shave and prep the area. For patients with penetrating injuries or scalp lacerations, rapidly shave the entire head. Infiltrate the area for the burr hole using a local anesthetic with epinephrine (see Fig. 15-2).
2. Make a 4- to 5-cm incision down to the bone. For a blind temporal burr hole, begin the incision at the superior zygoma, two of the patient's fingerbreadths anterior to the tragus. Angle it posteriorly, staying two fingerbreadths above the external ear (Fig. 29-3). If a scalp laceration is present, incorporate it into the incision.
3. Control bleeding with constant firm pressure on the wound edges.
4. Free the periosteum from the bone with the scalpel handle, and place dry gauze on the wound edges. Firmly place a self-retaining retractor to control bleeding.
5. Drill through the outer table of the skull. Once the inner table is reached, use a "conical" burr or work by hand.[41-44]

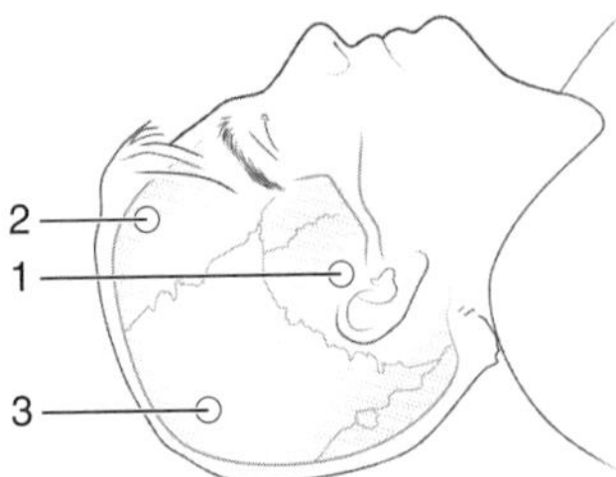

FIG. 29-3. Typical burr hole sites for acute trauma: (1) Temporal (Generally, the initial "blind" burr hole.) (2) Frontal. (3) Parietal.

Drills

A variety of drills have been used to make burr holes. Ancient people trephined using natural stones; some of their patients lived. In modern times, dental drills and ordinary burrs (8-12 mm) on a carpenter's drill may be used for trephination, but take care not to penetrate dura; the inner table of the skull bone is removed by "nibbling" at it with a rongeur.[45] Use bone wax to control bleeding.

Dr. T. R. Wiggin relates a case where improvising a drill saved a 6-year-old boy's life after he fell from a tree while collecting mangoes in Uganda. His initial GCS quickly dropped from 9 to 4, mandating surgery to save his life. With no neurosurgical or even orthopedic equipment available, the boy's father, a hospital technician, searched the carpentry workshop for a substitute burr or drill as the boy was being taken to the OR. His colleagues had been making new pit latrine covers and had left their tools, including a hole saw attached to a breast drill, "as good substitute as any for our needs." The hole saw consisted of an outer 3.8-cm cutter and a central 0.7-cm bit. An epidural hematoma was found and evacuated. By the time the child was back on the ward, he was awake and wanted a drink. By day 5, he was up and walking with no residual headache or neurological deficit. On day 7, his sutures were removed and he was discharged home. According to his father, he is again climbing mango trees.[46]

Acute Subdural/Epidural Hematomas

If dark blood immediately drains from the burr hole, there is an epidural hematoma. Rongeur enough bone to have good access to the area. Suction and wash out the clot with saline. Identify all bleeding points and control them with cautery or ligation. This may be difficult and requires persistence. Enlarge the burr hole with a rongeur, as needed.

If the dura is dark blue and bulging, there is a subdural hematoma. Rongeur enough bone to have good access to the area. Carefully open the dura and evacuate it with suction.

If the first burr hole has no sign of hematoma, look carefully under the dura; you may be close. Place gauze soaked in antibacterial solution in the burr hole and move on. Place a second hole in the frontal area, just anterior to the coronal suture and at least 3 cm lateral to the midline, approximately at the mid-pupillary line. Make the third and fourth burr holes in the posterior skull ~2 cm above the ear, and about 2 cm and 6 cm, respectively, behind the ear. If those are dry, repeat the process on the opposite side. As Dr. Husum and colleagues wrote, "If you are sure there is a hematoma inside his skull—do not stop making burr holes even if the patient seems to be dying in your hands: Identification and evacuation of a hematoma may still save him!"[47]

If an epidural hematoma is found, place a drain. Meticulously control any bleeding, place a hemostatic agent in the burr hole, and close the scalp.

Subacute/Chronic Subdural Hematomas

Subacute and chronic subdural hematomas (those >2 weeks old) can initially be asymptomatic, but may eventually progress in size and cause neurologic deficits. If more extensive surgical intervention is not possible, drainage through a single burr hole (sometimes with subsequent needle aspiration or re-exploration through the burr hole for a recurring hematoma) produces excellent results in >90% of patients. Patients who are appropriate for this procedure have a demonstrated subacute/chronic subdural hematoma with mass effect and a neurological deficit consistent with the hematoma's location or a severe headache.

Make a burr hole, then evacuate the hematoma and irrigate extensively with normal saline. Irrigate through a 10-Fr urethral catheter and continue until clear (usually 1 to 3 L). Then fill the defect with saline, pack the burr hole (use Gelfoam, if available) to prevent scalp blood from entering the space, and close the scalp.[48]

Although intracranial drains may not be necessary in many cases, if they are needed, an inexpensive substitute for commercial systems is to insert a pediatric feeding tube connected to an empty IV tube and bag. The tube drains to gravity; place the patients on antibiotics.[49]

Spinal Injury

Disc Injury

Although usually chronic, injuries to the intervertebral discs can also occur acutely. Pain is often severe, and, being neuropathic, may be unresponsive to normal analgesics, including narcotics. In austere situations, generic tricyclic antidepressants (e.g., amitriptyline) are often effective.

Trauma

To preserve their airway, place patients with facial injuries or who are not fully conscious in the lateral decubitus or "recovery" position. If a spinal injury is suspected, consider using the "trap squeeze" method to move them (described below). Also, place patients in the HAINES (High Arm IN Endangered Spine) modified recovery position (see Fig. 8-1), with the dependent arm (the one nearest the ground) extended above the head, before rolling them into the lateral decubitus position. When patients are on their side, flex their legs for support and rest the head on the dependent arm. This reduces lateral neck flexion to less than half of what it is when the dependent arm extends away from the body and the head droops down, as is normally the case. [50]

Spinal Immobilization Decisions

Standard field spinal immobilization guidelines are rapidly changing with the recognition that completely unstable spinal injuries that do not cause immediate, irreversible injuries are extremely rare.[51] Because spinal immobilization is not a benign procedure, use the NEXUS criteria (Table 29-4) or the Canadian C-Spine Rule to determine which patients to immobilize. As a prehospital faculty consensus statement stated, spinal immobilization is uncomfortable, takes time and delays initiation of specialist treatment in time-critical patients, raises intracranial pressure, increases aspiration risk and the risk of decubitus ulceration, potentially reduces airway opening and respiratory efficacy, and may increase mortality and morbidity.[52]

As the National Association of Emergency Medical Services Physicians wrote, "Full-spine immobilization, if it is not required, can be unnecessarily difficult, impractical, impossible, and even dangerous during prolonged evacuation, especially in severe environments or when using improvised equipment."[53] Likewise, the Wilderness Medical Society now says that if a patient has blunt trauma suspicious for spine injury, only immobilize the spine if they are severely injured—especially if they have a significant distracting injury, or have altered mental status, a neurological deficit, or significant spine pain or tenderness. Because neurologic deficits from penetrating assault are generally established and final on presentation, no immobilization is indicated in the civilian setting, where gunshot wounds are predominately of low velocity.[54]

Other spinal immobilization practices should also be modified. Use long spinal boards only for extrication, when necessary. Rather than carefully immobilizing a physically trapped patient with no indications for spinal immobilization, ask them to self-extricate and then, as with the upright patient, lay them supine for examination and, only if indicated, immobilize them.[52] Reevaluate patients with C-collars or on spine boards as soon as possible so that they can be removed before pressure ulcers develop.[55]

NEXUS C-SPINE RULE

The NEXUS C-Spine Rule (see Table 29-4) uses five very subjective criteria. If the patient meets all five criteria, he or she has a low probability of a clinically significant ("likely to result in any harm to patient") cervical spine (C-spine) injury. The NEXUS C-Spine Rule has a sensitivity of 99% and a negative predictive value of 99.8%.[56]

TABLE 29-4 NEXUS C-Spine Rule

1. No tenderness at the posterior midline of the cervical spine[a]
2. No focal neurological deficit[b]
3. A normal level of alertness[c]
4. No evidence of intoxication[d]
5. Absence of clinically apparent pain that might distract the patient from the pain of a cervical-spine injury[e]

[a]Midline posterior bony cervical-spine tenderness is present if the patient reports pain on palpation of the posterior midline neck from the nuchal ridge to the prominence of the first thoracic vertebra, or if the patient evinces pain with direct palpation of any cervical spinous process.

[b]A focal neurologic deficit is any focal neurologic finding on motor or sensory examination.

[c]An altered level of alertness can include any of the following: a GCS ≤14; disorientation to person, place, time, or events; an inability to remember three objects at 5 minutes; a delayed or inappropriate response to external stimuli; or other findings.

[d]Patients should be considered intoxicated if they have either of the following: a recent history provided by the patient or an observer of intoxication or intoxicating ingestion, or physical evidence of intoxication on examination (such as an odor of alcohol, slurred speech, ataxia, dysmetria, other cerebellar findings, or any behavior consistent with intoxication). Patients may also be considered intoxicated if tests of bodily secretions are positive for alcohol or drugs that affect the level of alertness.

[e]No precise definition of a painful distracting injury is possible. This category includes any condition thought by the clinician to be producing pain sufficient to distract the patient from a second (neck) injury. Such injuries may include, but are not limited to, any long-bone fracture; a visceral injury requiring surgical consultation; a large laceration, degloving injury, or crush injury; large burns; or any other injury causing acute functional impairment. Physicians may also classify any injury as distracting if it is thought to have the potential to impair the patient's ability to appreciate other injuries.

How to Immobilize the Spine

"Trap Squeeze" Technique

If patients need spinal immobilization, use the "trap-squeeze" technique while lifting and sliding them on and off a spine board, because it immobilizes the entire spine better than the log roll, especially in agitated patients. Grab the patient's trapezius muscles on either side of the head with your hands, firmly squeezing the head between the forearms. Keep the thumbs anterior to the trapezius muscle and the forearms approximately at ear level (Fig. 29-4).[54]

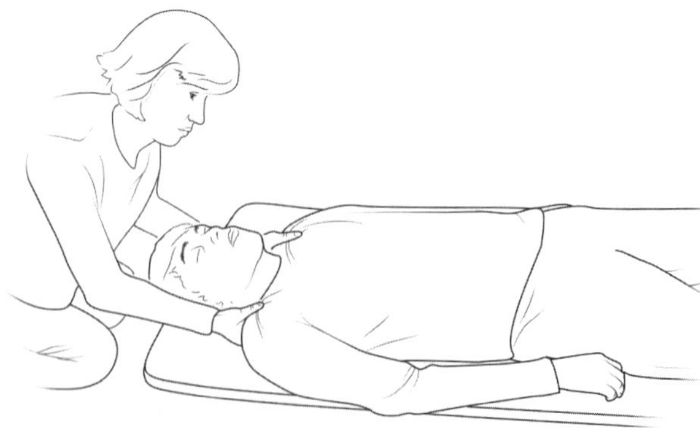

FIG. 29-4. "Trap squeeze" technique to stabilize a patient needing spinal immobilization.

C-Spine Immobilizers

If the patient needs C-spine immobilization, a number of improvised options are available. While only bilateral sandbags held together with tape over the forehead has been proven to immobilize the spine in the prehospital and emergency department setting,[57] in emergency situations, fashion cervical immobilization collars from a sleeping pad; the padded hip belt from a pack; any cloth, padding, or clothing; a tarp; or a tent flap. They may also be made from cotton and gauze and bandages (Schanz collar), newspapers, cardboard, blankets, plaster of Paris, or polyvinyl chloride (PVC) pipe.

Gauze (Schanz) Collar

To make a Schanz collar, wind a 5-inch-wide strip of cotton around the patient's neck several times. Over this, apply gauze to compress the cotton. Add additional layers of cotton and gauze, winding the gauze tighter as the collar's thickness increases. To get the desired effect, this collar should fill the entire submental space. As the collar loosens over time, apply additional cotton under the edges, with a tighter gauze bandage over it.[58] Although similar to a commercial "soft collar," a Schanz collar provides considerably more support.

Newspaper Collar

To fashion a useable c-collar from newspaper and socks, stack 10 open sheets of newspaper. Fold the stack in half along its longest dimension. Then fold it in thirds. The width should be appropriate for an adult. For a child, use seven sheets and fold them in half until the correct width for that child is found. Then slip a heavy sock over each end, pass the collar around the patient's neck, and secure it with tape, a scarf, a necktie, or bandage material.

Cardboard/Plastic Collar

The framework for this c-collar is made either from a corrugated cardboard box, such as that in which stores receive merchandise, or by cutting off the top of a plastic bucket. Cut an 18- × 6-inch piece, and cut an indentation in the middle of one long edge to accommodate the chin; cut two shallower pieces from the sides where the collar passes over the shoulders. Finally, cut a shallow indentation on the upper (chin) side at each end of the piece to accommodate the occiput.

If using cardboard, bend it at multiple sites along its length so that it will easily encircle the neck. Next, wrap the cardboard with cotton, socks, or other soft padding materials. Then slip it into a stockinet or long sock, or wrap it with a tight elastic or gauze bandage (Fig. 29-5). Secure it around the neck with additional bandaging, tape, a belt, or a similar item. The tightness of these ties determines how much stability the collar will have.[58]

Blanket Collars

Blanket rolls can easily be made and stored for use as cervical collars by patients who are supine, who are prone, or who must be kept on their sides. Blankets can also be used to make a collar

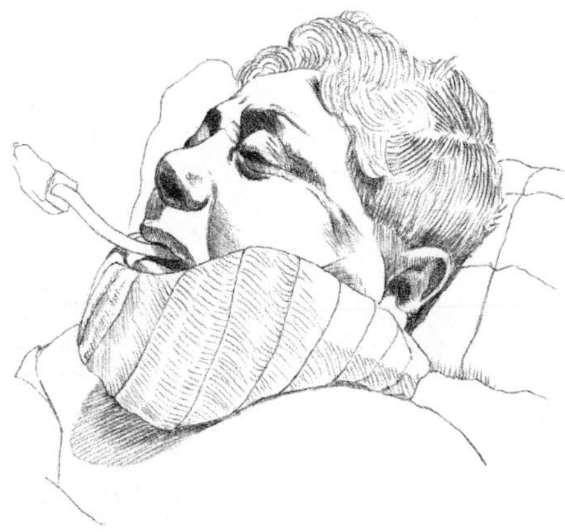

FIG. 29-5. Cervical collar from wrapped cardboard.

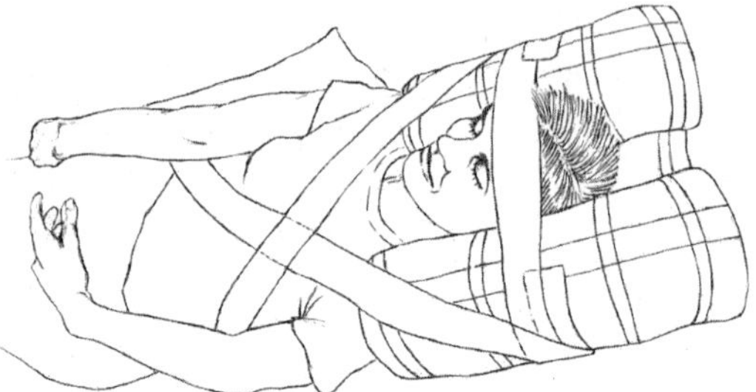

FIG. 29-6. Blanket roll as c-spine stabilizer for supine patient.

for a seated patient. First, fold a heavy blanket lengthwise once. Then tightly roll it toward the middle from both ends. When the two rolls meet, tape the entire package together for storage. Experience shows that it needs two layers of tape. When a collar is needed, cut the tape open as far as necessary.

For a cervical collar (patient supine, prone, or on his side), open the two rolls wide enough to accommodate the patient's head and position the back of the roll behind the head (Fig. 29-6). Then put tape around the package. This is often easiest if the patient is on a backboard. For a seated patient, unroll the package, but keep the blanket folded. Roll it tightly lengthwise and wrap it around the patient's neck, with the ends overlapping across his chest. Tightly tape the two ends of the blanket together (Fig. 29-7).[59]

Plaster of Paris Collar

Plaster of Paris has long been used as a c-collar. Place it over virtually any type of padding as a primary collar, or use it to hold other materials (such as clothing being used as a c-collar) in place.[60] A c-collar made totally of plaster is heavy, so it is not generally used in ambulatory patients.

The cast must extend the entire length of the c-spine. It must have a broad weight-bearing base over the shoulders and support the jaw and occiput. Unless the patient is already in cervical traction, someone must maintain traction while the plaster is applied and until it sets. To apply it, put thick padding over the shoulders, jaw, and occiput. Next apply two broad plaster slabs—one anteriorly and the other posteriorly. Then apply the plaster around the neck to secure these slabs.[61] The problem with this collar is that once applied, it is difficult to adjust. "After the first day, or two, a certain amount of play will develop from compression of the padding material."[58]

Polyvinyl Chloride Pipe Collars

Make more durable cervical collars from pieces of a large plastic (PVC) drain pipe. Although these collars take some time to make, PVC pipe is ubiquitous and the collars last a long time.

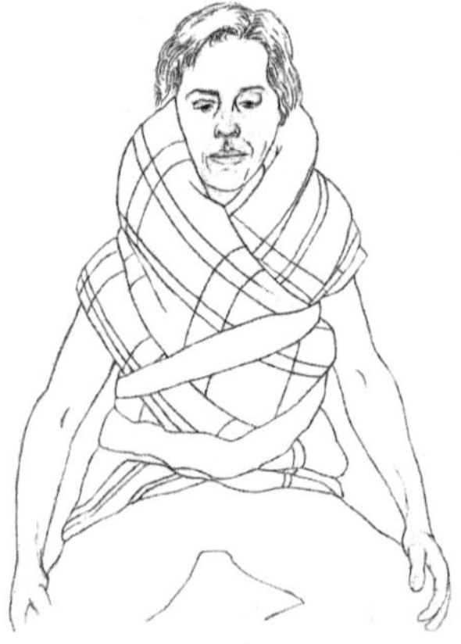

FIG. 29-7. Blanket roll stabilizing c-spine in seated patient.

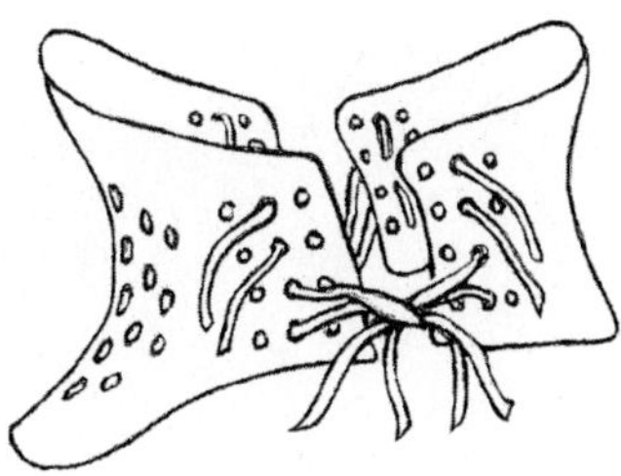

FIG. 29-8. C-collar from PVC pipe.

Use a piece of pipe that has an internal diameter of the neck(s) you want to stabilize, and saw the piece in half. Drill 0.25- to 0.5-inch holes in it so air can pass through to the neck for comfort. Drill smaller holes along the edges that fit together, and use lacing to close the two halves around the neck (Fig. 29-8). Making multiple rows of holes for lacing material allows this collar to be used on various sized patients.

Shape the collar so that it will fit better around the neck, chin, and occiput by placing it in boiling water or by using a welding torch or other low-intensity flame to soften it. If a flame is used, take care not to burn the plastic.[62] (See Chapter 30 for more information on making medical equipment using PVC pipe.)

SAM Splint As a C-Collar

The SAM splint, when molded into a cervical collar, is as effective as the Philadelphia collar at limiting movement of the cervical spine.[63]

Thoracic and Lumbar Spine

A number of makeshift litters are described in Chapter 21. However, many are not rigid enough to provide optimal support for suspected thoracic or lumbosacral spine injuries. Ideally, patients with a suspected thoracic spine injury should be immobilized from head to pelvis, with their hips adjusted for comfort. Patients with potential lumbar-pelvic injuries should have their thoracic spine, pelvis, and hips (in a position of comfort) splinted. This generally requires using a backboard, which can be made from a flat door, a piece of wood or metal (usually too heavy), or another strong flat object.

Removing the Immobilizer

In austere medical situations when the patient cannot be imaged, you will need to make a decision at some point to remove the collar—or to leave it on long term. Remove spinal immobilization (without imaging) if the patient meets the same rules used for initially applying c-spine immobilization (earlier).

Traction

Reasons for Use

Cervical spine injury with neurological signs indicates the need for cervical traction.[64] For unstable c-spines, surgery or braces are generally used rather than traction. However, in austere circumstances, traction may be the only option and progress nearly always needs to be followed using radiographs. That is the only way to determine if there is sufficient weight pulling in the correct direction.

Halter Traction

Halter or sling traction is the easiest and least-invasive traction method; use it not only for unstable c-spines and subluxations, but also for cervical disc pain. If used for disc pain, apply it intermittently as an outpatient or use it in the patient's home. When using this method, do not exceed 5 kg of weight (which may not be sufficient in spinal injuries). If used for spinal injury, attempt to replace it with a more formal traction method within 24 hours.[65]

Make halter traction equipment easily and inexpensively from local resources. The basic parts of the system are the pulleys, cord, head harness, and weights.[66] Pulleys are made from small

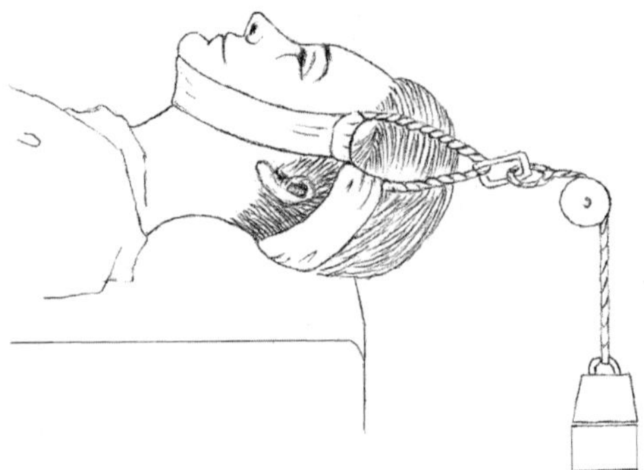

FIG. 29-9. Improvised halter.

pipes grooved to allow passage of the cord. These can be taken from orthopedic traction devices and attached to the end of the bed or stretcher. Any cotton or nylon rope is suitable, as long as it is strong enough to hold the weights and fits in the pulley grooves.

Pad the head harness with a soft cloth. Use cow leather and sandal buckles to make it. It could also be made from jeans or khaki clothing material, or from canvas (Fig. 29-9). Remember, the hole between the two strips must be wide enough to slip over the head.

Fashion weights from 5-L heavy-plastic bags (irrigation bags), large jars, or plastic bottles. Calibrate them in kilograms by water weight: Add 1 L of water at a time and mark them at each level (1 L water = 1 kg). Make hooks from 0.25-inch metal rods shaped into an S.

Cervical Traction Management

These rules apply to most cases where cervical traction is being applied for acute trauma.[67,68]

1. Traction is strictly neutral—the patient's neck should be neither in flexion nor in extension.
2. Apply counter-traction by elevating the head of the bed about 4 cm for each kilogram of weight applied (as with femoral traction).
3. Traction weight for adults (larger individuals may need more): C1, use 2.5 to 5 kg; C2, 3 to 5 kg; C3, 4 to 7 kg; C4, 5 to 10 kg; C5 & C6, 7 to 15 kg.
4. Increase the weight stepwise, adding 2 kg every 4 to 6 hours. Use lateral c-spine radiographs at each step. The spinal deformity will gradually reduce under traction.
5. Analgesia prevents muscle spasms and makes the traction more effective.
6. Most c-spine fractures are in the correct position within 24 hours. The traction weights are then gradually reduced under radiographic control.
7. Displaced neck fractures >1 week old may require several days to reduce.
8. Displaced neck fractures >3 weeks old may not respond to traction. Stabilize them in a cast or a collar.

REFERENCES

1. King M, King F, Martodipoero S. *Primary Child Care: A Manual for Health Workers.* Oxford, UK Oxford University Press; 1978:173.
2. Nagdev A, Riguzzi C, Frenkel O, Mantuani D. How to perform an ultrasound-assisted lumbar puncture. *ACEP Now.* 2014;33(7):20-21.
3. Shah SM, Kelly KM. *Emergency Neurology: Principles and Practice.* Cambridge, UK: Cambridge University Press; 1999:11.
4. Yamashiroya VK. Neurologic examination. *Case-Based Pediatrics for Medical Students and Residents.* Chapter XVIII.1. www.hawaii.edu/medicine/pediatrics/pedtext/s18c01.html. Accessed November 15, 2006.
5. Shah SM, Kelly KM. *Emergency Neurology: Principles and Practice.* Cambridge, UK: Cambridge University Press; 1999:289.
6. Mechaber A. Vibrating pager tests nerves. *Postgrad Med.* http://www.postgradmed.com/pearls.htm. Accessed September 23, 2007.

7. Shah SM, Kelly KM. *Emergency Neurology: Principles and Practice*. Cambridge, UK: Cambridge University Press; 1999:270.
8. Gavaghan LS, Disch J. *Metoclopramide plus diphenhydramine is preferred over ketorolac in the treatment of non-migraine and non-cluster benign headaches*. www.medscape.com/viewarticle/826531. Accessed July 17, 2014.
9. Blumenfeld A, Ashkenazi A, Napchan U, et al. Expert consensus recommendations for the performance of peripheral nerve blocks for headaches–a narrative review. *J Headache Pain*. 2013;53(3):437-446.
10. Shahrami A, Assarzadegan F, Hatamabadi HR. Comparison of therapeutic effects of magnesium sulfate vs. dexamethasone/metoclopramide on alleviating acute migraine headache. *J Emerg Med*. 2015;48(1):69-76.
11. Shah SM, Kelly KM. *Emergency Neurology: Principles and Practice*. Cambridge, UK: Cambridge University Press; 1999:113.
12. Editors of the Medical Letter. Drugs for migraine. *Treatment Guidelines From the Medical Letter*. 2011;9(102):7-12.
13. Tintinalli J. *Tintinalli's Emergency Medicine*. Philadelphia, PA: McGraw-Hill; 2011, Table 227-4, Headache and facial pain (Access Emergency Medicine).
14. Rapoport AM. Acute and prophylactic treatments for migraine: present and future. *Neurol Sci*. 2008;29:S110-S122.
15. Sewell RA, Halpern JH, Pope HG Jr. Response of cluster headache to psilocybin and LSD. *Neurology*. 2006;66:1920-1922.
16. Sciolla R, Melis F. SINPAC Group. Rapid identification of high-risk transient ischemic attacks: prospective validation of the ABCD score. *Stroke*. 2008;39(2):297-302.
17. Johansson E, Bjellerup J, Wester P. Prediction of recurrent stroke with ABCD2 and ABCD3 scores in patients with symptomatic 50-99% carotid stenosis. *BMC Neurology*. 2014;14(1):223.
18. Kiyohara T, Kamouchi M, Kumai Y, et al. ABCD3 and ABCD3-I scores are superior to ABCD2 score in the prediction of short-and long-term risks of stroke after transient ischemic attack. *Stroke*. 2014;45(2):418-425.
19. Hand PJ, Kwan J, Lindley RI, et al. Distinguishing between stroke and mimic at the bedside: the brain attack study. *Stroke*. 2006;37:769-775.
20. Goldstein LB, Simel DL. Is this patient having a stroke? *JAMA*. 2005;293:2391-2402.
21. Caterino JM, Raubenolt A, Cudnik MT. Modification of Glasgow Coma Scale criteria for injured elders. *Acad Emerg Med*. 2011;18:1014-1021.
22. Green SM. Cheerio, laddie! Bidding farewell to the Glasgow Coma Scale. *Ann Emerg Med*. 2011;58(5):427-430.
23. US Army. *Emergency War Surgery*. 3rd rev. Washington, DC: Borden Institute, Walter Reed Army Medical Center; 2004:15.1.
24. Husum H, Ang SC, Fosse E. *War Surgery: Field Manual*. Penang, Malaysia: Third World Network; 1995:296.
25. US Army. *Emergency War Surgery*. 3rd rev. Washington, DC: Borden Institute, Walter Reed Army Medical Center; 2004:15.5.
26. Smits M, Dippel DW, de Haan GG, et al. External validation of the Canadian CT Head Rule and the New Orleans Criteria for CT scanning in patients with minor head injury. *JAMA*. 2005;294:1519-1525.
27. Knapp S, Davies F. What is the significance of a 'boggy' (soft) scalp haematoma in head-injured children? *Emerg Med J*. 2014;31:78-79.
28. Atabaki SM, Stiell IG, Bazarian JJ, et al. A clinical decision rule for cranial computed tomography in minor pediatric head trauma. *Arch Pediatr Adolesc Med*. 2008;162(5):439-445.
29. Kuppermann N, Holmes JF, Dayan PS, et al. Identification of children at very low risk of clinically-important brain injuries after head trauma: a prospective cohort study. *Lancet*. 2009;374(9696):1160-1170.
30. Frumin E, Schlang J, Wiechmann W, et al. Prospective analysis of single operator sonographic optic nerve sheath diameter measurement for diagnosis of elevated intracranial pressure. *West J Emerg Med*. 2014;15(2):217.
31. Tayal VS, Neulander M, Norton HJ, et al. Emergency department sonographic measurement of optic nerve sheath diameter to detect findings of increased intracranial pressure in adult head injury patients. *Ann Emerg Med*. 2007;49:508-514.
32. Carney N, Ghajar J, Jagoda A, et al. Concussion guidelines step 1: systematic review of prevalent indicators. *Neurosurgery*. 2014;75:S3-S15.
33. Worrell J. Head injury management (with no CT scanner). *Trop Doct*. 2000;30:120-123.

34. Hassan SF, Cohn SM, Admire J, et al. Natural history and clinical implications of nondepressed skull fracture in young children. *J Trauma Acute Care Surg*. 2014;77:166-169.
35. Quigley MR, Chew BG, Swartz CE, Wilberger JE. The clinical significance of isolated traumatic subarachnoid hemorrhage. *J Trauma Acute Care Surg*. 2013;74:581-584.
36. Colton K, Yang S, Hu PF. Intracranial pressure response after pharmacologic treatment of intracranial hypertension. *J Trauma Acute Care Surg*. 2014;77:47-53.
37. Lumba-Brown A, Harley J, Lucio S, Vaida F, Hilfiker M. Hypertonic saline as a therapy for pediatric concussive pain: a randomized controlled trial of symptom treatment in the emergency department. *Ped Emerg Care*. 2014;30(3):139-145.
38. Nelson JA. Local skull trephination before transfer is associated with favorable outcomes in cerebral herniation from epidural hematoma. *Acad Emerg Med*. 2011;18(1):78-85.
39. Schecter WP, Peper E, Tauatoo V. Can general surgery improve the outcome of the head-injury victim in rural America? a review of the experience in American Samoa. *Arch Surg*. 1985;120:1163-1166.
40. Ortler M, Langmayr JJ, Stockinger A, et al. Prognose nach epiduralem Hämatom: ist die notfallmässige Bohrlochtrepanation beim Schädel-Hirn-Trauma heute noch zeitgemäss? [Prognosis of epidural hematoma: is emergency burr hole trepanation in craniocerebral trauma still justified today?]. *Unfallchirurg*. 1993;96(12):628-631.
41. Woodruff M: Emergency bedside craniotomy (burr holes). In: Shah K, Mason C, eds. *Essential Emergency Procedures*. Philadelphia: Lippincott Williams & Wilkins; 2008:153-156.
42. Husum H, Ang SC, Fosse E: *War Surgery: Field Manual*. Penang, Malaysia: Third World Network; 1995:300-301.
43. Donovan DJ, Moquin RR, Ecklund JM. Cranial burr holes and emergency craniotomy: review of indications and technique. *Mil Med*. 2006;171(1):12-19.
44. Head trauma. In: Greenberg MS: *Handbook of Neurosurgery*, 6th ed. New York: Thieme; 2006:646.
45. Husum H, Ang SC, Fosse E. *War Surgery: Field Manual*. Penang, Malaysia: Third World Network; 1995:71.
46. Wiggin TR. Emergency craniotomy using improvised instruments. *Trop Doct*. 2001;31(3):174.
47. Husum H, Ang SC, Fosse E. *War Surgery: Field Manual*. Penang, Malaysia: Third World Network; 1995:301.
48. Benzel EC, Bridges Jr RM, Hadden TA, Orrison WW. The single burr hole technique for the evacuation of non-acute subdural hematomas. *J Trauma*. 1994;36(2):190-194.
49. Clarke HA, St. John MA. Use of a paediatric feeding tube in the drainage of chronic subdural haematoma—an inexpensive and simple technique. *Trop Doct*. 1990;20(3):135.
50. Gunn BD, Eizenberg N, Silberstein M, et al. How should an unconscious person with a suspected neck injury be positioned? *Prehosp Disaster Med*. 1995;10(4):239-244.
51. Hauswald M. A re-conceptualisation of acute spinal care. *Emerg Med J*. 2013;30:720-723.
52. Conner D, Greave, I, Porter K, Bloch M. Pre-hospital spinal immobilization: an initial consensus statement. *J Paramedic Practice*. 2014;6(5):242-246.
53. Rural Affairs Committee, National Association of Emergency Medical Services Physicians. Clinical guidelines for delayed or prolonged transport. III. Spine injury. *Prehosp Disaster Med*. 1993;8(4):369-371.
54. Quinn RH, Williams J, Bennett BL, et al. Wilderness Medical Society practice guidelines for spine immobilization in the austere environment: 2014 Update. *Wild Environ Med*. 2014;25(4):S105-S117.
55. Ham W, Schoonhoven L, Schuurmans MJ, Leenen LP. Pressure ulcers from spinal immobilization in trauma patients: a systematic review. *J Trauma Acute Care Surg*. 2014;76(4):1131-1141.
56. Hoffman JR, Mower WR, Wolfson AB, et al. Validity of a set of clinical criteria to rule out injury to the cervical spine in patients with blunt trauma. *N Engl J Med*. 2000;343:94-99.
57. Markenson D, Ferguson JD, Chameides L, et al. Part 13: First aid: 2010 American Heart Association guidelines for cardiopulmonary resuscitation and emergency cardiovascular care. *Circulation*. 2010;122(suppl 3):S768-S786.
58. Weisenburg TH, ed. *Manual of Neuro-Surgery*. Washington, DC: Department of the Army; 1919:267-268.
59. Dick T. Sweet rolls: stuff you can do with blankets. *JEMS*. 2001;26(5):81.
60. Taylor HL, Ogilvy C, Albee FH. *Orthopedics for Practitioners*. New York, NY: Appleton; 1909:475-476.
61. Husum H, Ang SC, Fosse E. *War Surgery: Field Manual*. Penang, Malaysia: Third World Network; 1995:316.

62. Platt A, Carter N. *Making Health-Care Equipment: Ideas for Local Design and Production*. London, UK: Intermediate Technology Publications; 1990:58.
63. McGrath T, Murphy C. Comparison of a SAM splint-molded cervical collar with a Philadelphia cervical collar. *Wild Environ Med*. 2009;20(2):166-168.
64. Husum H, Ang SC, Fosse E. *War Surgery: Field Manual*. Penang, Malaysia: Third World Network; 1995:314-315.
65. Husum H, Ang SC, Fosse E. *War Surgery: Field Manual*. Penang, Malaysia: Third World Network; 1995:310.
66. Iyor FT. A simple design for cervical traction kit. *Trop Doct*. 2002;32:216-217.
67. King M. (ed.). *Primary Surgery, Vol. 2: Trauma*. Oxford, UK: Oxford University Press; 1987:152-153.
68. Husum H, Ang SC, Fosse E. *War Surgery: Field Manual*. Penang, Malaysia: Third World Network; 1995:315.

30 | Ophthalmology

As with most medical areas, ophthalmology generally divides into diagnosis and treatment, although these frequently overlap. For clarity, that is how this chapter is divided.

DIAGNOSTIC EXAMINATION AND EQUIPMENT

Visual Acuity Testing

Testing visual acuity is, by far, the most important diagnostic test on the eyes; yet, it is frequently overlooked. Even with penetrating or apparently corneal-occluding injuries (e.g., alkali burns), test visual acuity in this order: light perception, movement, counting fingers, and reading/identifying at distance. Testing takes only a short time—just seconds if stopped at counting fingers—but provides invaluable information to a consulting ophthalmologist.

To test whether a nonverbal or uncooperative patient can see, elicit optokinetic nystagmus. (See Chapter 29 for improvising optokinetic test equipment.) This test works in children as young as 4 to 6 months old. The presence of nystagmus with an optokinetic stimulus confirms cortical vision and the integrity of the frontal and parietal lobes and visual fields. An even simpler visual acuity test for a nonverbal or an uncooperative child is to offer him or her various toys and see how he or she reaches for and plays with them.[1]

If an eye chart is not available, use a newspaper or magazine. Begin with the fine print. Stop if the patient can read it. If not, work up to the largest print the patient can read. That gives a rough gauge of the patient's visual acuity.

Standard eye charts are easy to manufacture. Download copies from multiple internet sites, including the US National Eye Institute (www.nei.nih.gov/photo/visual-acuity-testing), or smart phone apps. If copies are available, even in miniature, local printers can enlarge them to produce standard Snellen visual acuity charts, as well as "illiterate" eye charts (Landolt ring chart and "E" chart), on heavy paper and cardboard. Mount these on a heavier board and, if possible, laminate or cover charts with a plastic sheet for protection.

For patients who present without their corrective lenses or for those who have never gotten lenses but should have, there are two ways to test visual acuity: an ophthalmoscope or a pinhole device.

To test visual acuity using an ophthalmoscope, have patients cover one eye while looking at the eye chart through the ophthalmoscope. Have the patient hold the instrument as would a practitioner; the examiner should adjust the lenses to find the optimal one for the patient. If the visual acuity examination is done after an ophthalmoscope examination, start with the lens setting with which the patient's disc is best seen. If only a wall-mounted ophthalmoscope is available, use a pocket eye chart to position the patient at the proper distance from the chart (generally 14 to 16 inches for a pocket chart and 20 feet for a standard chart). For supine patients, such as those suffering trauma, get a helper to stand on a stool and hold the eye card. Dr. Joseph Miller, a professor of ophthalmology at the University of Arizona, says that another option is to borrow someone's reading glasses and test the patient's vision with and without the glasses. (Personal written communication, September 8, 2008.)

You can also use a pinhole device to determine a patient's optimal visual acuity. Make one by cutting a 5-cm-diameter circle from opaque x-ray film and attaching it to a handle. Puncture the center of the film to produce a hole about the size of the head of a pin. Putting in more holes may improve the chance of some patients finding a hole to look through. Alternatively, use a paper cup with holes punched in the bottom (Fig. 30-1).

An even easier method is to remove the top from a salt shaker and use that as the pinhole device. While it may be little messy, a soda (e.g., Saltine) cracker with holes may also be used. Many elderly people use cracker holes to read the menu in restaurants, so we know it works.

Color Testing

Color vision testing probably will not be important in austere circumstances. But, if it becomes necessary, the only method is to ask the patient if he (nearly always a "he") can tell you the color of various objects in the room. Choose red, green, violet, and pink objects, because red-green

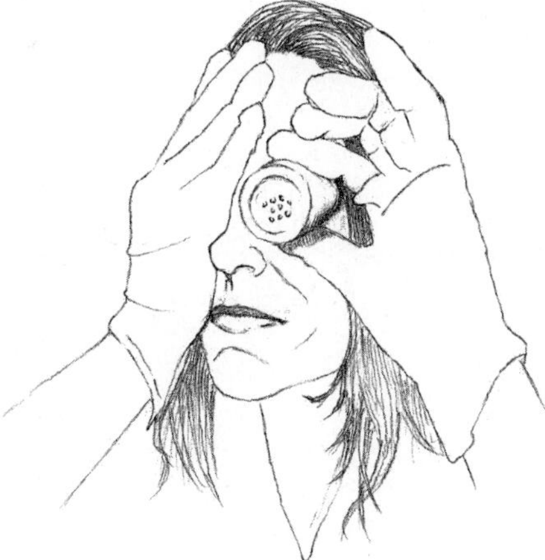

FIG. 30-1. Pinhole device improvised from paper cup.

color blindness is most common. The only caveats are (a) be certain that you have good color vision yourself to get a baseline, and (b) be aware that there is a spectrum of "normal" color vision.

Retracting Eyelids

Clinicians may need to manually open eyelids to examine or treat patients with periorbital swelling due to trauma or infection, or to look under the lids for foreign bodies.

When lifting the eyelid to examine the superior conjunctival fornix in a non-trauma patient, place a cotton-tipped applicator (e.g., Q-tip) against the lid. Then, rather than manually lifting the lid over it, roll the applicator and the eyelid will curl around it and lift.

In patients with facial trauma, retract the lids as early as possible after the patient presents; the swelling may progress enough that it may be nearly impossible to examine the eye later without surgery. Opening massively swollen eyes may reveal the most surprising result—a normal eye with normal vision. Without the examination, however, you will not know that.

The best way to open swollen eyelids is to use lid retractors. If the patient is conscious, drop in some topical anesthetic. Open a paperclip so that the small (inside the clip) and large (outer part of the clip) pieces are in the same plane (i.e., flat) (Fig. 30-2). Use a clamp to hold one end and bend it 180 degrees. (With some paperclips, this can also be done by hand, although I don't recommend it.) Bend the larger side for use in adults; the smaller side is best for children. Clean the paperclip and use it as a lid retractor. Use two if both the upper and lower lids must be retracted simultaneously, which is often the case (Fig. 30-3). Paperclip retractors can be sterilized and reused.

In the operating room (OR), tie a suture to the paperclip and secure that to the drape. If you have a sterile rubber band, secure that to the paper clip: It provides additional laxity, if you need it.

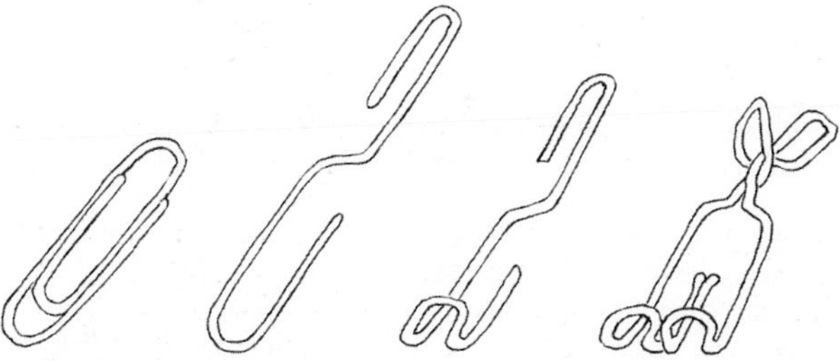

FIG. 30-2. Eyelid retractors from paperclip.

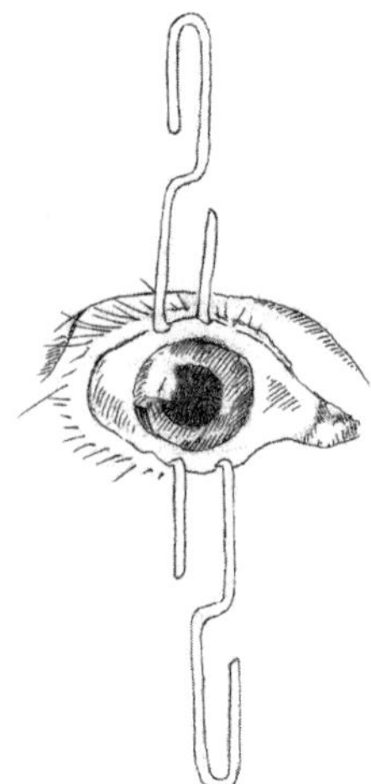

FIG. 30-3. Using eyelid retractor made from a paperclip.

Occasionally, a 7-0 (or smaller) silk or nylon suture is used for lid retraction. Pass it through the lid just above the lash line and pass it back through so it is just on the other side of the lashes. Do not penetrate the palpebral conjunctiva.

Ophthalmoscope

For a better view of the sclera and cornea during the examination, use an ophthalmoscope or put a (an additional) pair of reading glasses or a handheld magnifying lens between your eye and the patient's.

Focusing With an Ophthalmoscope

In practice, many clinicians no longer routinely use an ophthalmoscope, so using it may be challenging. This method helps you get a clear view of the fundus if you are unable to focus when using the diopter lenses. Wear your glasses and have the patient put on his or her eyeglasses. Flip the ophthalmoscope lenses until the fundus comes into focus. Then both of you remove your glasses so that you can take a closer look.[2,3]

Improvised Ophthalmoscope

A method of constructing an improvised ophthalmoscope uses a flashlight, a 2-cm diameter piece of black polyvinyl chloride (PVC) pipe, aluminum foil, glue, a drill, a small saw, and an oven (Fig. 30-4).

1. Cut a 15-cm piece of pipe; then cut one end so that it has a 45-degree angle "beveled edge" (B).
2. Cut another 10-cm piece of pipe and split it lengthwise; heat it to obtain a flat piece of PVC. (See the following "Heating PVC Pipe" section.)
3. Cut this flat piece into two discs: one disc (C) is the same diameter as the glass at the front of the flashlight, which it will replace. (If you have a small [mini-] Maglite, that may provide a better view.) Drill a 2-cm hole in its center. Cut the other disc (A) so that it fits over the beveled end of the long pipe (B).
4. Cover the inside of the pipe (B) with aluminum foil, except for the tip at the beveled end. The bright side of the aluminum foil should face the center of the pipe to increase illumination.
5. Cover one side of the flat PVC disc (A) with aluminum foil, and drill a small hole through its center (D).
6. Drill another, slightly larger, hole (E) directly opposite to where the disc's hole will be, at the end of the long piece of PVC pipe (B). This (hole E on pipe B) is the viewing port.
7. Attach the oval disc (A) to the beveled end of the PVC pipe (B) with glue.
8. Glue the "non-viewing" end of the long pipe (B) to the round piece with the 2-cm hole (C). Both PVC glue and cyanoacrylate work. Remove the flashlight's glass and replace it with the flat end

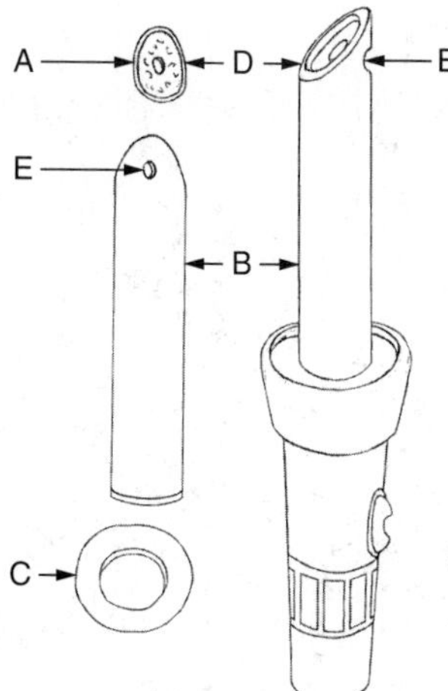

FIG. 30-4. Ophthalmoscope improvised from PVC pipe and a flashlight.

of the device. The ophthalmoscope is ready for use. This device provides enough light to observe an upright image of the optic disc without needing to dilate the eye. For refraction, use either a lens-correcting set (such as optometrists use) or various eyeglass lenses.[4]

Heating Polyvinylchloride Pipe

To flatten pieces of PVC pipe, they must be heated. Because PVC pipe emits dioxins and other toxic, potentially cancer-causing gasses, heat it in a well-ventilated area, preferably outside, while wearing a good protective mask. If possible, work on a large flat piece of wood because it acts as a good insulator, allowing the pipe to stay warmer longer. Wear gloves to protect your fingers and slowly heat the PVC with one of the following: (a) a propane torch (keep enough distance to not burn the pipe); (b) a heat gun, which will not burn the pipe; (c) very hot or boiling water (dip the piece into the water until it heats completely through and repeat as necessary); (d) an ordinary heat lamp; or (e) another heat source, such as a kerosene heater. Keep testing the pipe with a gloved finger until it becomes flexible, like rubber. Put a flat, fireproof object (like metal) on it. Once the PVC pipe is flat, cool it by spraying it with or dunking it in cool water.

Indirect Ophthalmoscopy

Ophthalmologists who want to do indirect ophthalmoscopy, but who do not have the standard equipment, may succeed in the unconscious patient with fixed, dilated pupils. Hold a ≥2-inch-diameter handheld magnifier positioned at arm's length, about 4 cm from the patient's eye. Use a direct ophthalmoscope as a light source (preferred), a transilluminator (second choice), or a Mini-Maglight (focused to the smallest possible spot, a distant third choice as it can be quite tricky). You can get a nice, wide field view of the retina and optic nerve. It is the best way to see hemorrhages. Good quality 4X and 5X magnifiers (corresponding to about 20-diopter lenses) work well, but the cheapest handheld magnifiers (3X magnification, ~ 30¢ US) produce too poor an image to use. If using the direct ophthalmoscope, set it so you can see the magnifying glass clearly and in focus. An aerial image of the retina forms about 3 inches in front of the lens. This wonderful trick does not require the fancy headlamp that ophthalmologists routinely use. (Joseph Miller, MD, PhD. Personal written communication, September 8, 2008.)

Non-Traumatic Eye Conditions

Non-traumatic eye complaints are common. Table 30-1 provides a method of differentiating among them. Some, such as an external hordeolum (sty), are usually minor problems; a corneal ulcer can be a serious, and potentially sight-threatening, condition.[5]

TABLE 30-1 Differential Diagnostic Features of Non-Traumatic Eye Complaints

Symptoms and Signs	External Hordeolum (Sty)	Internal Hordeolum	Chalazion	Conjunctivitis	Anterior Uveitis	Corneal Ulcer
Eye pain	Sensation of foreign body	Sensation of foreign body possible	Sensation of foreign body possible. After a few days, signs and symptoms resolve	Itching or burning	Moderate to severe dull ache	Moderate to severe
Vision	Normal	Normal	Normal	Normal	Blurred	Blurred
Photophobia	Possible	Absent	Absent	Absent to moderate	Present	Present
Discharge	Lacrimation	Absent	Absent	Present (purulent or watery)	Absent	Purulent
Redness/ inflammation	Usually localized, but may be diffuse	Localized	Grayish-red, freely moveable mass in lid. Conjunctiva red and elevated	Entire eye red, more pronounced away from cornea	Pink to red flush around cornea	Entire eye red, darker away from cornea
Pupil size	Normal	Normal	Normal	Normal	Constricted	Normal or constricted
Pupil shape	Normal	Normal	Normal	Normal	May be irregular	Normal
Pupil reaction to light	Normal	Normal	Normal	Normal	Diminished or absent	Normal or diminished
Special notes	Small, round, tender area of induration on lid margin	Small elevation or yellow area at site of affected gland, on conjunctival side of lid	If mass is nonmobile, it may be malignant	Rarely a serious condition	Moderately serious condition	Very serious condition

Allergic Conjunctivitis

Applying a cold compress and artificial tears most effectively reduces symptoms of allergic conjunctivitis. Unfortunately, artificial tears cannot easily be improvised.[6]

Glaucoma

If a tonometer is not available, a gross screen for glaucoma is to check visual fields. Bilateral loss of lateral vision is common with late glaucoma because of the damage to the optic nerve.

Another option to assess the intraocular pressure (IOP), known as digital ocular compression, uses fingers. While it is highly inaccurate, it is worth trying in the absence of other options. Ask the patient to close his or her eyes and try to stare straight ahead. Alternate between depressing and releasing the cornea of one eye using two index fingers placed side by side. Pushing with just one finger or somewhere else on the eye other than on the cornea simply tests how easy it is to push the eye back into the orbit. The easiest method to "calibrate" this examination is to do it on a normal subject (not yourself) and immediately do it on the patient. (Joseph Miller, MD, PhD. Personal written communication, September 8, 2008.)

Another useful tool, which has been the gold standard for more than 50 years, is the Schiøtz indentation tonometer (Fig. 30-5). It is inexpensive and does not require a power source. It measures how far a fixed, weighted plunger can indent the cornea. Although less accurate than applanation tonometers, if used correctly it provides good information about IOP. To use the Schiøtz tonometer correctly, (a) anesthetize the eye with a topical anesthetic, (b) zero it using the fixed metal piece that comes in its case, (c) open the lids widely, (d) hold it only by the "side rails" (Fig. 30-6), and (e) have the patient hold their ipsilateral thumb in front of them to stare at during the procedure. The mean IOP in normal adults is 15 to 16 mm Hg; the normal range (mean ± 2 SD) is 10 to 21 mm Hg.

Ultrasound

Ultrasound, available in many remote and austere circumstances (e.g., the International Space Station), provides an excellent diagnostic tool for intraocular abnormalities. Ultrasound may be able to define lesions that cannot otherwise be seen due to their being obscured by blood or because there is no ophthalmoscope (or the ability to use one well).

To examine the eye with ultrasound, use a linear array transducer in the 7.5- to 15-MHz frequency, which is the same one used for soft tissue examinations, line placement, and musculoskeletal examinations. Set the machine on a "small parts" setting, if there is one. Have the patient close his or her eyes, then fill the orbit you will examine with a large amount of gel—a really whopping amount. That allows an examination without any discomfort to the patient; the transducer should never touch the eyelid.[8]

To avoid a shaky image, the examiner should rest his or her arm on a bony part of the patient's face, such as the ridge of the nose or the eyebrow. The anterior and posterior chambers, the lens,

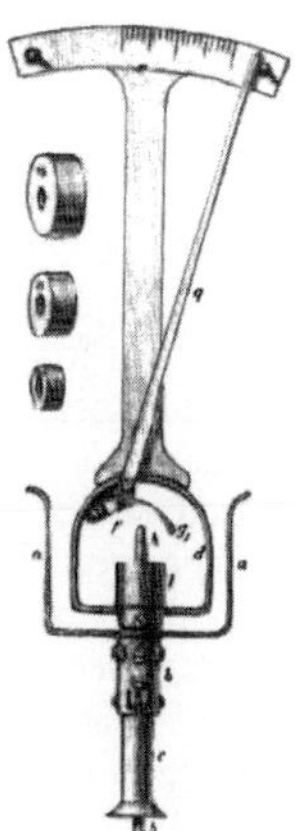

FIG. 30-5. Schiøtz indentation tonometer. *(Reproduced from Meller and Sweet.[7])*

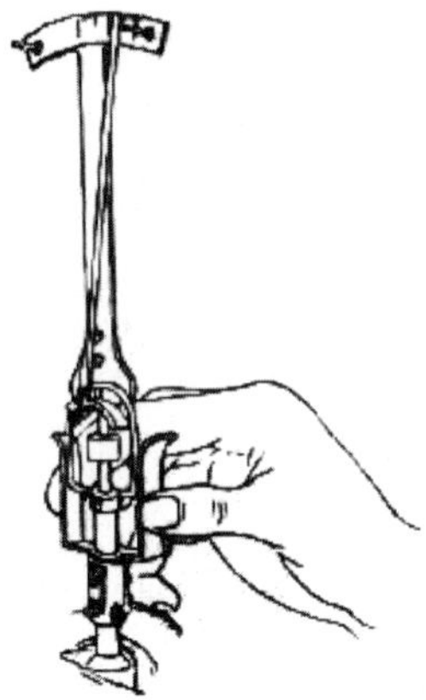

FIG. 30-6. Schiøtz indentation tonometer in use.

and the optic nerve are easily seen. During the procedure, adjust the gain to avoid artifacts. Use the transducer in the vertical and horizontal positions and sweep side to side across the eye. The patient, if cooperative, can help by moving the eye in various directions when instructed to do so.[8]

Common abnormalities that can be evaluated using ultrasound include retrobulbar hematomas; vitreous hemorrhage; globe perforations; foreign bodies; optic nerve abnormalities; lens dislocations; and vitreous, choroidal, and retinal detachments. Ultrasound can also help determine the presence of elevated intracranial pressure (ICP) by measuring the optic nerve (see Chapter 29). As with any imaging study, the more experience one has, the better one can define and understand the images.

Ultrasound and Retinal Detachments

Ultrasound has proven to be an easy and accurate tool for diagnosing intraocular disease, such as retinal detachment, lens disruption, ocular foreign bodies, increased ICP (optic nerve enlargement), or anterior chamber and vitreous hemorrhage. To use sufficient gel to eliminate the air interface while causing minimal patient discomfort, first place a transparent dressing (often used to cover intravenous [IV] sites) over the closed eye. The same quality examination is obtained through the dressing, and cleaning the gel off the patient is easier.[9] Apply a generous amount of ultrasound gel to the dressing. Then place a linear 10-MHz probe on the closed eyelid. Adjust the contrast and brightness so that small irregularities within the vitreous are visible. Finally, ask the awake patient to look left and right while watching for movements consistent with intraocular disease.[10]

Optic Nerve Sheath Diameter

Measure the optic nerve sheath diameter as a marker for elevated ICP. (See Chapter 29 for a description of the procedure.)

Problems and Treatment at Altitude

The most common eye problems at altitude result from ultraviolet light, hypoxia, cold, and low humidity. Especially in people who have had corneal refractive surgery, hypoxia or a cold, dry environment can cause refractive changes due to corneal edema. Dry eyes, exacerbated by wearing contact lenses, result from the increased evaporation of tears. Use rewetting drops more frequently. If using extended-wear lenses, decrease corneal edema and infections by not wearing them overnight. Retinal hemorrhage is common but usually asymptomatic. However, if the macula is involved, severe visual difficulties can occur. Contact lenses in a case filled with liquid solution, as well as cleaning solutions and lubricating drops, can freeze in cold weather; fluid-filled lens cases should be worn next to the skin to avoid freezing.

For symptomatic eyes, gently close the eyelids. Provide the person with sunglasses or goggles, or have him or her rest in a dark place until symptoms subside. Generally, do not apply a pad or patch, but cool the eye through the closed eyelid to reduce discomfort. For snow blindness, also administer nonsteroidal anti-inflammatory eye drops, an antibiotic ointment, and a mild analgesic. In a contact lens wearer, remove the lens, instill lubricating drops and antibiotic drops or ointment. Descend to a lower altitude if the person has not improved with treatment within 48 hours, has a serious eye injury, or has other symptoms related to acute mountain sickness (AMS), high-altitude pulmonary edema (HAPE), or high-altitude cerebral edema (HACE).[11]

Disinfecting Ophthalmological Equipment

If disposable covers are not used, applanation tonometers routinely become contaminated. In austere situations, even if tonometers are available, there probably will not be disposable covers. This poses a risk of contaminating patients with a variety of organisms, including those causing epidemic keratoconjunctivitis. Rather than the ineffective but frequent practice of wiping them with 70% isopropyl alcohol, disinfect tonometers by immersing them for 10 minutes in 0.05% sodium hypochlorite (1:100 dilution of bleach in water) or a 3% hydrogen peroxide solution. Soaking them in 70% alcohol destroys the tip.[12]

Disinfect most other ophthalmological equipment in the same manner, using 0.05% bleach or 3% hydrogen peroxide. If equipment needs to be sterile, meaning no spores are present, they should be autoclaved.[13] (See Chapter 6 for additional information.)

TREATMENT AND EQUIPMENT

Eyeglasses

Fitting for Eyeglasses

Donated or stock prescription glasses are generally available, even in austere settings. However, most clinicians are clueless about how to examine a patient for proper refraction, even if an optician is available to make the lenses. One option is to have the patient try on glasses until he or she can see objects clearly when they are held 15 inches (40 cm) from the eyes. That works for most patients.

Replacing Eyeglass/Surgical Loupe Hinges

Eyeglasses and surgical loupes (which provide magnification for both outpatient and OR procedures) often break at their hinges. If the miniscule screw holding a hinge together is lost, the loss of eyewear can render a person incapable of functioning.

A simple temporary (or not-so-temporary) fix exists: While holding the hinge in position, pass a very small needle and 4-0 (or smaller) nylon suture through the hole for the screw. Depending on the hole's size, several passes may be made with the suture before it is tied in place. Experience proves that this works well.[14]

If the hinge joint has a larger screw hole, use a paperclip, safety pin, or similar small wire to hold it in place, at least temporarily. Of course, in a pinch, duct tape also works.

Nose Pads for Eyeglasses

Eyeglasses become almost nonfunctional without their nose pads—those little discs that allow the glasses to rest, more or less comfortably, on the nose. One successful method of replacing them is to sew small shirt buttons onto the metal posts that stick out from the eyeglass rims.[15] For a balanced feel, replace both nose pads if one is missing.

Improvised Glasses

Eyeglasses generally are improvised for two reasons—to see more clearly and to protect the eyes from damage caused by glare off snow, ice, or water.

To see more clearly, apply the same principle as for pinhole visual acuity testing: If a person looks through a small hole, only the rays passing straight through to the fovea are seen. This is, theoretically, the person's best vision. To read without glasses, form a fist, leaving a small hole to look through at the reading material. For true temporary eyeglasses, punch multiple holes in a cardboard eye mask over both visual axes (Fig. 30-7, right). The person can wear the mask by attaching two paper clips or safety pins and connecting them with a rubber band. This works, but limits vision to a small area directly in front of the person.

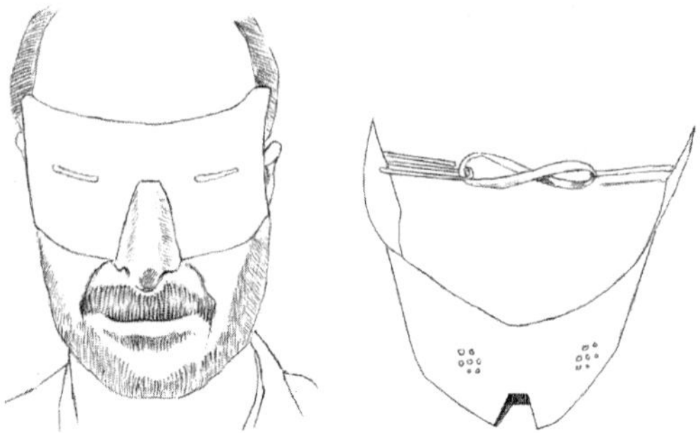

FIG. 30-7. Improvised sun-blocking eyewear, with slits (left) or holes (right).

Make similar "glasses" to protect the eyes from glare. To improve peripheral vision, make slits rather than holes in the eye mask (Fig. 30-7, left). An alternative is to stick wide black tape to itself (sticky side to sticky side) and punch holes or slits in it. Tie or tape it around the head. To make slits in eyeglasses, cover most of the lenses with black tape. Use additional tape to block the glare around the lenses and on the sides, because that can also cause eye damage. Innovative (or desperate) people have also used leaves, palm fronds, or other materials as sun-blocking glasses.

Eye Irrigation

In resource-poor situations, Morgan lenses for irrigating the eyes after chemical exposure are generally unavailable. An alternative is to use a standard nasal prong cannula attached to a saline bag. Place the patient supine with towels or other material to collect the water. Position the nasal prongs at the bridge of the nose pointing downward. Put a piece of tape over the connector between the two prongs to hold it in place. Attach the IV tubing to the end of the nasal cannula tubing and open the "IV" all the way. This irrigates both eyes. To irrigate just one, clamp one "prong" or just use the end of the IV tubing at the medial side of the affected eye. (Joe Lex, MD, FACEP, FAAEM. Personal oral communication, May 25, 2007.)

Analgesia

Most eye pain resolves with normal analgesics.

For an alternative, or to supplement the medicine, use warm moist soaks. One method is to have the patient wrap a cloth around a spoon, dip it in very hot water, and bring it as close as possible to the eye. Do not use this method in a child. The other option is to put a cloth in hot water, such as from the faucet, wring it out, and cover the eye. Put a piece of plastic over the cloth to retain the heat and moisture. Leave the cloth on until it cools; repeat as often as needed for comfort.

Prolonged Topical Anesthesia Use

Despite classic dogma, patient-administered topical tetracaine is safe. While it does not relieve pain any better than saline drops, patients think that it is much more effective.[16]

Using Eye Drops

No one likes drops placed directly in their eyes. Children squirm, and many attempts and hands are needed to accomplish the task; adults grit their teeth and bear it. Often, trying to put in eye drops (e.g., antibiotics, pilocarpine, or other medication) at home leads patients to abandon the treatment. Ease the process by always instilling eye drops at the medial canthus. This also avoids having to get the dropper close to the eyelashes; touching them contaminates the dropper.

Tell patients who need eye drops to tilt their heads back, with the affected eye up. Instruct adults and older children to close their eyes first; infants will do this automatically. Hold the medication container well above the face, and instill two drops of medication into the medial canthus. Keep patients in this position until their eye opens, even a little, and the medication will enter—without effort. At home, have adults use this technique on themselves; parents should also use this technique with their children.

Ophthalmic Antibiotics

Most ophthalmic conditions do not require antibiotic drops, even though clinicians often prescribe them. The most common example of this is most cases of conjunctivitis. Save resources and do not use unnecessary antibiotics.

If you do need antibiotics, chloramphenicol, which is still widely available around the world, works well. Dissolve two 250 mg capsules in 100 mL sterile water. Filter the solution into sterile 10-mL dropper bottles. Screw the caps loosely onto the bottles, and put them in a hot water bath at 100°C (212°F) for 30 minutes without letting the water splash over the bottles' necks. After removing them from the water, tighten the tops and check them again when they cool, because the glass may contract, causing the tops to loosen. Refrigerate at 2°C to 8°C (36°F to 46°F) for up to 2 months. Chloramphenicol, because it penetrates the eye when given systemically, is also useful for more severe eye infections.[17]

When using ophthalmic ointment, Dr. Joseph Miller says the easiest method is to place a dab on a clean cotton swab and transfer it to the inside of the retracted lower eyelid. (Personal written communication, September 8, 2008.)

Eye Shield

Make a protective eye shield from a small paper cup by cutting off the top half or top three-fourths of the cup. Put tape around the cut edges so that they do not irritate the patient's face. Tape the cup to the face, so that the bottom and sides protect the eye.

Alternatively, make a protective cone by cutting a 6-cm circle in a piece of x-ray film or lightweight cardboard and then making one cut to the center of the circle. Overlap the cut ends to form a cone. Tape the film in that form and then tape the cone over the eye.[18]

Corneal Foreign Body Removal

Rather than using an eye burr to remove a corneal foreign body, use a tuberculin or insulin needle with the syringe attached as a handle. Try to do the procedure under magnification—the needle will look enormous. Alternatively, use the sterile plastic 20- or 22-gauge catheter from an IV.

Broken Contact Lens

If a contact lens has broken while on the eye and pieces remain, identify them easily by instilling topical fluorescein dye. Then use an ultraviolet (UV) light to find them. The gel matrix in the lens quickly absorbs fluorescein dye.[19]

Corneal Ulcer

Corneal ulcers, a common problem among malnourished children in the tropics, usually respond to aggressive therapy. However, children tend to remove bandages and rub their eyes, which often results in a secondary infection and can cause blindness. So, how do you keep an uncooperative child's hands away from the eye while it is healing?

One solution is to use a splint made from an empty disposable plastic container, such as a 0.5- or 1-L bottle of bleach or irrigation solution. Cut off the top and bottom to form a uniform-diameter cylinder. Then cut the container in half lengthwise, and smooth the rough edges by covering them with a piece of plaster or duct tape. After padding the inside with soft cloth, fit the plastic bottle around the child's elbow and fix it in place with a plaster sheath and an elastic bandage. The child can still bend his or her arms slightly (for comfort), but cannot remove the eye dressings, thus preserving his or her vision.[20]

Local Anesthesia for Eye Procedures

If the normal topical anesthetic for the eye is not available, two other commonly available options exist: lidocaine and cocaine. As Boulton wrote, "Lidocaine 4% is a suitable surface analgesic for the cornea which is as efficacious as a topical analgesic, as is 2% cocaine; it does not dilate the pupil or the corneal vessels."[21]

If performing a procedure under or with the aid of topical anesthetic, apply two to three drops to the cornea and conjunctiva every 5 minutes, starting about 20 to 30 minutes before surgery. Give additional drops, as needed, throughout the procedure.[22]

Lateral Canthotomy/Cantholysis

Clinicians may need to relieve a sudden increase in IOP, which normally occurs after direct trauma. The most effective procedures are the combination of lateral canthotomy and cantholysis of the lower (and often upper) lids. The procedures include crushing the lateral canthus with a hemostat to reduce bleeding before cutting it with an iris scissors. The iris scissors are then used to spread and "strum" the tissues to locate the canthal ligaments within the orbit (by retracting the eyelids) before cutting them.

When a hemostat is unavailable, gently use a pliers, such as on a multitool, to get the same result. When an iris scissors is unavailable, use a #11 scalpel blade to cut the lateral canthus. Use one arm of the hemostat or pliers as a "backstop" to avoid cutting too deep. Use the flat/dull side of the same blade to "strum" for the tissues under the eyelid to locate the canthal ligaments. Then turn the blade to cut them.[23]

Glaucoma Treatment

If acute narrow-angle glaucoma affects someone in an austere setting, there are several options to ameliorate the problem. Apply atropine 1% topically six times a day.[24] Epinephrine also works, although it irritates the eye and may need to be used in high concentrations or frequently.[25,26] Commonly carried and used by high-altitude groups, acetazolamide (250 mg four times a day [qid]) or other carbonic anhydrase inhibitors can be used to decrease aqueous humor production, lowering the IOP. So can beta-blockers, which are generally administered twice a day (bid). However, these measures only temporize the situation until the patient can be put on a chronic medical regimen or have surgery.[25,26]

Improvising Operating Room Instruments

For cataract surgery: "If a formal operating room is not available, any clean room and a body-length table will suffice. A clean water source is necessary."[27]

Make a small-gauge intraocular surgical hook from a 27-gauge needle. Similar to fashioning a skin hook (see Chapter 22), make it by bending the tip of a $^{5}/_{8}$-inch, 27-gauge needle with a needle holder. After sterilization, this can be used alone or connected to a 1-mL syringe as a handle.[28]

A metal lid plate for eyelid surgery (provides lid support and elevation) can be made from the handle of a stainless steel soup spoon. It has the benefits of being available without alteration, its length makes it easy to handle, and it does not distort the nasal and temporal aspects of the lid.[29]

Fashion corneoscleral sutures by attaching a bent 30-gauge needle to size 9-0 monofilament nylon (or the fishing line equivalent).[30] Swag the suture onto the needle as described in Chapter 22.

Cataract Surgery

Cryoextractor

Ophthalmologists often extract cataracts—especially those that are mature, intumescent, or hypermature—by allowing the cold tip of a cryoextractor to form an adhesion with the cataract. A cryoextractor is expensive and often not available. It can, however, be improvised by passing a short length of copper electrical wire into the barrel of a 5-mL syringe (Fig. 30-8).

Most of the wire extruding from the syringe tip (~1 cm) should remain covered with insulation; only remove the insulation from a very small part of the wire at the tip. Also, remove the insulation from about 1 cm of the wire inside the syringe barrel. Invert a container of refrigerant, such as dichlorodifluoromethane (i.e., Freon, Frigen), and hang it from an IV stand. Run 1 to 2 mL of Freon through the tubing on the Freon container and into the syringe. The evaporation of the Freon immediately freezes the copper wire. Experience shows that the Freon should be

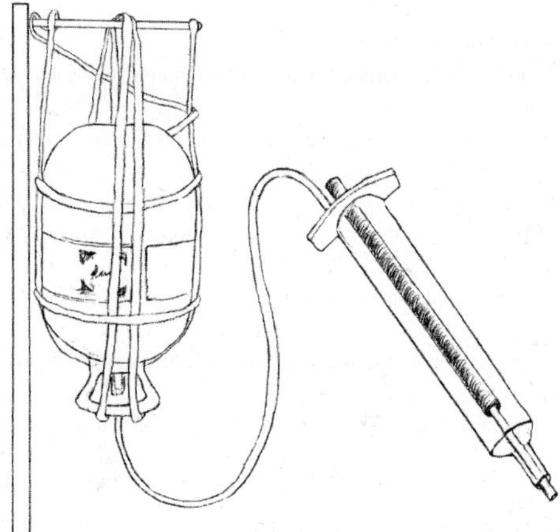

FIG. 30-8. Improvised cryoextractor.

refilled in the syringe, if necessary, so that contact with the cataract lasts 10 to 15 seconds before extraction.[31,32]

Aphakic Surgery Problems

Blindness, both from cataracts and from a lack of eyeglasses post-cataract surgery, is a common problem in areas with scarce resources.[33] Anyone doing cataract surgery should understand that the main problem with aphakic surgery (removing the lens for a cataract) is that patients often cannot get or replace their eyeglasses after the surgery. This leaves them essentially no better, or even worse, than prior to the surgery.

One solution is to hold or tape a single magnifying lens over an eye. Even better is to fit two lenses into a makeshift holder to use as a pair of glasses. Instruct the patient to move the makeshift glasses closer to or further from the eyes until the right focal distance is found. For these aphakic individuals, even a pair of reading glasses can produce an in-focus image. However, the patient must hold the glass a very long distance from his or her eye. This way, the patient gets a reduced field of view but the image is focused. (Joseph Miller, MD, PhD. Personal written communication, September 8, 2008.)

Blowout Fracture Treatment

If you suspect an orbital blowout fracture, check for extraocular muscle entrapment before rushing the patient to a surgeon. While all surgeons operate as soon as possible on patients who have extraocular muscle entrapment, most will not operate if no entrapment exists.[34]

REFERENCES

1. Yamashiroya VK. Neurologic examination. In: Yamamoto LG, Inaba AS, Okamoto JK, et al, eds. *Case Based Pediatrics for Medical Students and Residents*. http://www.hawaii.edu/medicine/pediatrics/pedtext/s18c01.html. Accessed November 15, 2006.
2. Sullivan W. Focus on the fundus. *Postgrad Med*. 2000;107(5). http://www.postgradmed.com/pearls.htm. Accessed September 23, 2007.
3. Personal written communication from Joseph Miller, MD, PhD, Professor of Ophthalmology, University of Arizona, Tucson, Ariz., September 8, 2008.
4. Maertens K, Taveire L, Matumona M. An inexpensive ophthalmoscope. *Trop Doct*. 1985;15:141-142.
5. US Air Force. *The Air Force Independent Duty Medical Technician Medical and Dental Treatment Protocols*. AFM 44-158, December 1, 1999:81.
6. Bilkhu PS, Wolffsohn JS, Naroo SA, Robertson L, Kennedy R. Effectiveness of nonpharmacologic treatments for acute seasonal allergic conjunctivitis. *Ophthalmology*. 2014;121(1):72-78.
7. Meller J, Sweet WM. *Ophthalmic Surgery*. Philadelphia, PA: P. Blakiston's & Co.; 1913:224.

8. Lyon M, Blaivas M. Ocular ultrasound. In: Ma OJ, Mateer JR, Blaivas M, eds. *Emergency Ultrasound*. 2nd ed. New York, NY: McGraw Hill; 2008:449-462.
9. Roth KR, Gafni-Pappas G. Unique method of ocular ultrasound using transparent dressings. *J Emerg Med*. 2011;40(6):658-660.
10. Shinar Z, Chan L, Orlinsky M. Use of ocular ultrasound for the evaluation of retinal detachment. *J Emerg Med*. 2011;40(1):53-57.
11. Ellerton JA, Zuljan I, Agazzi G, Boyd JJ. Eye problems in mountain and remote areas: prevention and onsite treatment—official recommendations of the International Commission for Mountain Emergency Medicine. *Wild Environ Med*. 2009;20(2):169-175.
12. Rutala WA, Weber DJ. Uses of inorganic hypochlorite (bleach) in health-care facilities. *Clin Microbiol Rev*. 1997;10(4):597-610.
13. Brouwer MR, Hardus PLL. Sterilization of ophthalmological instruments. *Trop Doct*. 1988;18(4): 174-176.
14. Fraser KE. A simple emergency method for improvising a lost surgical loupe's hinge screw. *Microsurgery*. 1994;15:611-612.
15. Raman R, Omar R. Nose pads. *Trop Doct*. 2010;40:210.
16. Waldman N, Densie IK, Herbison P. Topical tetracaine used for 24 hours is safe and rated highly effective by patients for the treatment of pain caused by corneal abrasions: a double-blind, randomized clinical trial. *Acad Emerg Med*. 2014;21(4):374-382.
17. King M, Bewes P, Cairns J, et al. *Primary Surgery, Vol. 1—Non-Trauma*. Oxford, UK: Oxford Medical; 1990:409.
18. Schwab L. *Primary Eye Care in Developing Nations*. Oxford, UK: Oxford University Press; 1987: 145-146.
19. Forson PK, Osei-Ampofo M, Ofori-Boadu L, et al. Ujuzi (Practical Pearl/Perle Pratique). *Afr J Emerg Med*. 2014;4(1):42.
20. Sauter JJM. Blindness prevention by arm-splints. *Trop Doct*. 1978;8:95-96.
21. Boulton TB. Anesthesia in difficult situations. The use of local analgesia. *Anaesthesia*. 1967;22(1):101-133.
22. Pittman JAL. Local anesthesia for eye surgery. *Update Anaesth*. 2000;12(5):1.
23. Iserson KV, Luke-Blyden Z, Clemans S. An alternative method of performing a lateral canthotomy and cantholysis. *J Wild Environ Med*. 2016;27(1). (In press).
24. Ruben S, Tsai J, Hitchings R. Malignant glaucoma and its management. *Br J Ophthalmol*. 1997;81: 163-167.
25. Block JH, Beale Jr JM. *Wilson and Gisvold's Textbook of Organic Medicinal and Pharmaceutical Chemistry*. 11th ed. Philadelphia, PA: Lippincott Williams & Wilkins; 2003:532.
26. Gifford SR. Some non-surgical aids in the treatment of glaucoma. *Br J Ophthalmol*. 1929;13(10): 481-490.
27. Schwab L. *Primary Eye Care in Developing Nations*. Oxford, UK: Oxford University Press; 1987:39.
28. Stewart MW, Landers MB. Transscleral intraocular lens fixation with a "homemade" needle and hook. *J Cataract Refract Surg*. 2006;32:200-202.
29. Schwab L. *Primary Eye Care in Developing Nations*. Oxford, UK: Oxford University Press; 1987:141.
30. Van Oosterwyk, Hodges AA. Atraumatic sutures can be made locally. *Trop Doct*. 2004;34:95-96.
31. Maertens K. Cheap and reliable cryoextractor. *Trop Doct*. 1982;12:89.
32. Schwab L. *Primary Eye Care in Developing Nations*. Oxford, UK: Oxford University Press; 1987: 138-140.
33. Absolon MJ. Cataract surgery in developing countries. *Trop Doct*. January 1986;15(1):20-22.
34. Alinasab B, Ryott M, Stjärne P. Still no reliable consensus in management of blow-out fracture. *Injury*. 2014;45(1):197-202.

31 | Obstetrics/Gynecology

GYNECOLOGY

Contraception

Contraceptive methods include medications, intrauterine devices (IUDs), surgery (e.g., vasectomy, tubal ligation, hysterectomy), spermicides, barriers (e.g., condoms), and "natural" methods. Only condoms protect against sexually transmitted diseases (STDs). Hysterectomies do not completely protect the patient, because *Chlamydia trachomatis* and *Neisseria gonorrhoeae* can still infect the urethra.

Nonmedication Methods

The so-called natural contraceptive methods are not very effective. However, without other means to control pregnancy, they have to be used. The methods include abstinence, withdrawal, breastfeeding, temperature measurement, mucous, and counting days (rhythm method).

Abstinence is hard to sustain and therefore does not work. Withdrawal is not much better, because the male often does not withdraw in time, or even know exactly when to withdraw. Breastfeeding often protects a woman from pregnancy in the first 6 months after delivery if she has not had menses, feeds the child nothing other than breast milk, and never goes more than 6 hours between breastfeedings. The temperature measurement method relies on keeping track of very small temperature changes over time, and so is unlikely to be useful in austere situations.

The mucous method requires the woman to check her vaginal mucous every day, at the same time, before she has intercourse. She wipes her vagina with a clean finger, paper, or cloth. If the mucous is clear, wet, and slippery, it means that she is fertile and should not have intercourse. If there is no mucous or if it is white, dry, and sticky, intercourse is probably safe two days later. If using this method, the woman should not douche or wash her vagina. The method is completely useless in the presence of vaginal infections.[1]

The counting days or rhythm method is somewhat effective for women with a regular menstrual cycle of 26 to 32 days. Counting from the first day of menstrual bleeding, she abstains from sex from the 8th day through the 19th day of her cycle. She can have sex again on the 20th day. Women should use a chart to mark these days or, as an alternative, a bead chain with different colors. Each bead designates 1 day. To make a bead chain, string 32 beads on a string in this order: 1 red bead followed by 6 blue beads, 12 white beads, and 13 more blue beads. Use a small string or rubber grommet to mark where she is in her cycle. The red bead marks the onset of menses. The 6 blue beads are "safe" days for sex, as are the other 13 blue beads. The white beads are her fertile days.[2]

Male and female condoms are both successful contraceptive methods, but they cannot be improvised. Buy them! They also have medical uses, as described elsewhere in this book (e.g., controlling postpartum hemorrhage, ultrasound probe covers, and improvised esophageal stethoscopes).

Emergency Contraception

Even in austere circumstances, emergency contraception may be an important issue. The medication of choice after unprotected sexual intercourse (UPSI) is levonorgestrel (LNG), which is now widely available. Table 31-1 lists specific indications for this treatment. It should be given as a single 1.5-mg dose as soon as possible and, for the most efficacy, within 72 hours. If the woman can tolerate only a 0.75-mg dose of the drug, repeat it in 12 hours.

The alternatives are to use birth control pills with adequate doses of ethinyl estradiol (EE) and LNG within the first 120 hours after UPSI or to insert a copper-containing IUD within 5 days of UPSI. If combination birth control pills are used, the dose must be ≥100 micrograms (mcg) EE plus 0.50 mg LNG or 0.75 mg LNG alone. This means the woman will have to take between 2 and 20 pills at one time. She repeats the same dose 12 hours later. Taking diphenhydramine

TABLE 31-1 Indications for Emergency Contraception

Normal Contraceptive Method	Indications for Emergency Contraception
Combined pills (21 active tablets)	If *three or more* 30-35 mcg EE or if *two or more* 20 mcg EE pills have been missed in the first week of pill taking (i.e., days 1-7) *and* UPSI occurred in week 1 or in the pill-free week.
POP	If *one or more* POPs have been missed or taken >3 hours late *and* UPSI has occurred in the subsequent 2 days.
Intrauterine contraception	If there has been complete or partial expulsion of the IUD, or if it is removed at mid-cycle *and* UPSI has occurred in the last 7 days.
Progestogen-only injectables	If the contraceptive injection is late (>14 weeks from the previous injection for medroxyprogesterone acetate or >10 weeks for norethisterone enanthate) *and* UPSI has occurred.
Barrier	If there has been failure of a barrier method.

Abbreviations: EE, ethenyl estradiol; IUD, intrauterine device; POP, progestogen-only pill; UPSI, unprotected sexual intercourse.

Data from AHRQ.[4]

(Benadryl) or a similar medication 1 hour before the contraceptive markedly reduces the frequent incidence of emesis. If emesis occurs within 2 hours of taking the contraceptives, repeat the dose.[3]

Note that if the contraceptive contains norgestrel, it is only half as effective as LNG; double the dose. Women who are using liver enzyme-inducing drugs (e.g., some antiepileptics, antibiotics, St. John's wort) must take between 2.25 and 3 mg of LNG. If necessary, women can use emergency contraception more than once during each menstrual cycle.

Physical Diagnosis: Pelvic Versus Abdominal Pain

Differentiating intra-abdominal pain from pelvic pain can be challenging, especially when few imaging resources exist. Ming-Cheh Ou described a physical examination method that helps identify the source of abdominal pain in women with an acute abdomen. The procedure, shown in Fig. 31-1, uses the non-palpating hand to physically separate the "pelvic trapezoid" from the rest of the abdomen, while the other hand palpates on both sides of the barrier hand. If pain is found only within the trapezoid and absent outside of it, this indicates pelvic disease (Fig. 31-2). If the woman has definite pain outside the trapezoid and none or equivocal pain within, it is most likely abdominal pain. Diffuse pain within and outside the trapezoid can stem from multiple causes.[5]

Vaginal Speculum

When a vaginal speculum is not available or is not the right size to examine a patient, simply revert to what our forebears used: retraction. In austere circumstances, clinicians still fashion

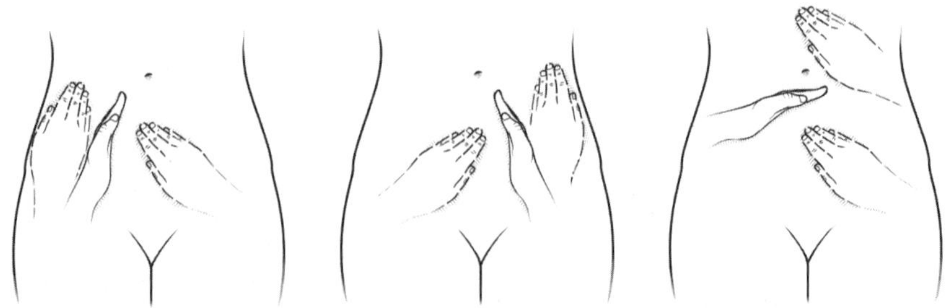

FIG. 31-1. Hand positions for isolating intrapelvic pain. *(Adapted from Ou et al.[5])*

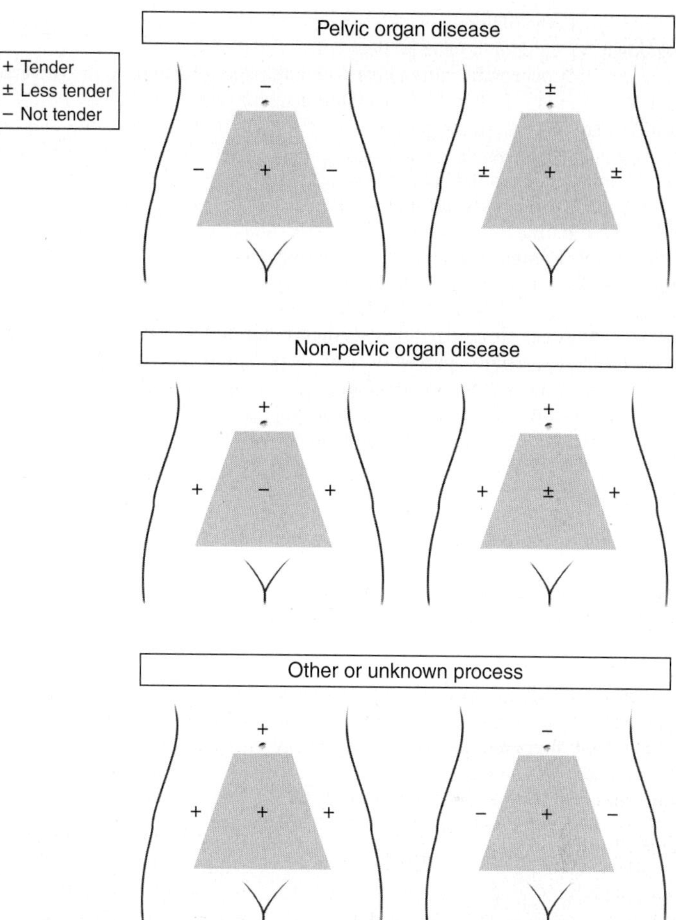

FIG. 31-2. Interpreting pain response in Ou examination. *(Adapted from Ou et al.[5])*

vaginal retractors from spoons, surgical retractors, or even barbecue tongs. (Col. Patricia R Hastings, AMEDDCS. Personal communication, April 9, 2007.) Using these instruments does, however, require an assistant to hold the posterior retractor while the examiner elevates the anterior vagina with another retractor. The only additional requirement is a light source; use a headlamp, if available.

In small girls, use test tubes of varying sizes to examine the vagina, although procedures cannot be done with this method.

Sexually Transmitted Diseases

In austere situations, syndromic treatment of STDs is the best approach to this common problem. (See the "Tests for Sexually Transmitted Diseases" section in Chapter 35.)

Bartholin's Abscess—Word Catheter

Easily treat a Bartholin's gland abscess with a small stab incision (not large enough for the catheter to fall out) and the placement of a short Word catheter. However, Word catheters are unlikely to be available in austere settings. An alternative is to use a balloon urethral catheter and run the catheter down the leg, with a gauze or plastic bag over the end to catch any pus that drains. Use an 8- or a 10-Fr pediatric catheter, if available, because they are shorter. Do not cut the catheter; it destroys the balloon port. Patients, however, do not like having this extra appendage hanging down for the time it takes to heal with a fistula.

So, make a generally acceptable alternative with a few modifications to the catheter. Once the pediatric catheter balloon is in the abscess, clamp it with a hemostat. Slowly inflate the balloon with 3 to 4 mL of saline or sterile water (do not overinflate it and cause pain), and firmly clamp the catheter with a hemostat several centimeters distal to the balloon. Then cut the catheter 2 cm distal to the clamp site to keep the balloon inflated. Using a tuberculin or insulin syringe, inject a generous amount of cyanoacrylate into the small balloon port in the remaining part of the catheter and squeeze it for a minute or so. After a few minutes, the adhesive hardens and you can remove the hemostat. The balloon will remain inflated due to the cyanoacrylate. The patient can return in 3 to 6 weeks to have the catheter removed by cutting the catheter proximal to the cyanoacrylate. The balloon deflates and the catheter drops out.[6]

There are two additional, simpler methods to modify the catheter: tying it off with a silk suture rather than occluding the balloon port with glue, or tying the catheter itself into a knot before cutting it short. Both work well in austere settings. Andy Norman, MD, tells the women to stick the end of the catheter into the vagina for comfort once it stops draining. This prevents it from getting caught on their clothes. (Personal communication, February 15, 2015.)

Cervical Dysplasia

Remarkably, an improvised test may be nearly as good as cytology (Pap smear) for detecting high-grade cervical lesions (squamous intraepithelial lesions) or invasive cervical cancers. It may also be better than cytology for detecting moderate dysplasia. In resource-poor areas, the World Health Organization (WHO) suggests that clinicians use a "visual inspection with acetic acid" (VIA) and "visual inspection with Lugol's iodine" (VILI) for detection of cervical dysplasia.

To do this, place the speculum without using gel. First do a VIA, applying 3% to 5% acetic acid (white vinegar) to the cervix with a cotton-tipped applicator. The vinegar may sting a little. After 1 minute, look for white patches. (The high-protein-content areas of premalignant and malignant cells coagulate and appear white when acetic acid is applied.) If they are there, it signifies a pathological lesion—which may be dysplasia, human papilloma virus, cervical cancer, or an STD. The test has a sensitivity of 56% and a specificity of 71% (positive predictive value 30%, negative predictive value 88%).

Then do a VILI by applying iodine to the cervix with a cotton-tipped applicator. If the entire cervix stains with iodine, it is a negative test; otherwise, it is positive. (Normal squamous cells are rich in glycogen that takes up iodine.) The test has a sensitivity of 87% and a specificity of 49% (positive predictive value 31%; negative predictive value 93%).[7]

These tests require no special magnification or tools. Patients who test positive should get further testing, if possible. If that is not possible and cryotherapy is available, use it. It is much less dangerous than letting untreated cervical cancer progress.[8]

Lacking equipment for colposcopy, gynecologists aboard the US Navy Ship (USNS) Comfort, on their Continuing Promise 2009 mission to Latin America, used eye loupes to provide sufficient magnification to view the cervix. (Commander Chris Reed, MD, USNS Comfort. Personal communication, June 3, 2009.)

Female Circumcision

Rarely encountered in industrialized countries, female circumcision comes in three forms: (a) partial or complete removal of the clitoris, (b) clitorectomy with removal of the labia minora, and (c) infibulation, the removal of the labia majora, labia minora, and clitoris with the vaginal opening sewed nearly closed. The last form causes most of the severe problems seen by health care workers. These include heavy vaginal bleeding, possibly with shock; infection (tetanus or wound infection initially, but human immunodeficiency virus [HIV] and hepatitis are common some time later); severe pain; and dysuria, urinary retention, or other urinary tract problems. Treatment is to stop the bleeding, treat pain and infection, and, if necessary, place a urethral catheter.

When a woman who has had an infibulation tries to deliver a child vaginally, problems can ensue. Be prepared to "deinfibulate" her by cutting through the scar.

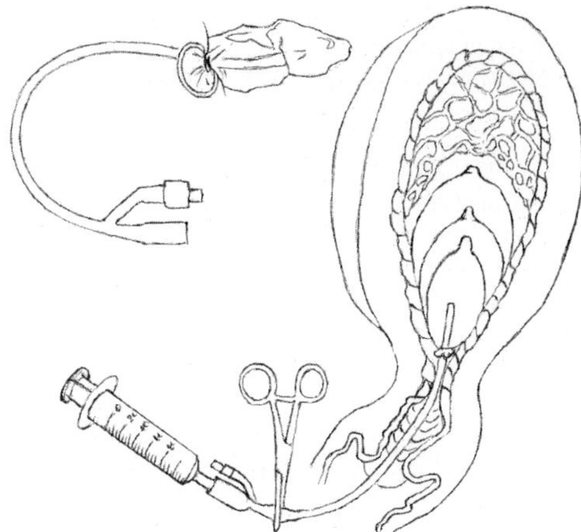

FIG. 31-3. Inflated condom-urethral balloon catheter.

Vaginal Bleeding

Acute Massive Hemorrhage

The control of acute hemorrhage from the nonpregnant uterus can be difficult, because the cervical os may not be wide open. The hemorrhage may be due to a variety of sources, including gynecologic procedures. Historically, clinicians have used curettage to halt the bleeding; when this fails, hysterectomy has often been a last resort. However, it may be prudent to try mechanical methods first.

One method that stops acute, profuse uterine hemorrhage in most patients is to insert a balloon urethral (Foley) catheter into the uterine cavity. This requires no special expertise, equipment, or anesthesia. Once the catheter is in place, inflate the catheter balloon full enough with saline to tamponade the bleeding against the semi-rigid uterine wall. Leave the catheter in place from several hours to 2 days, depending on the etiology of the hemorrhage.[9]

As described in the "Postpartum Hemorrhage Control" section below in this chapter, if the uterine cavity is larger than normal, such as postpartum, tie a condom over the end of the catheter, then insert the catheter and inflate the condom, rather than the catheter (Fig. 31-3).

Bleeding Mass

A hemorrhaging mass in the vagina is most likely cervical cancer. After placing a urethral catheter, pack the vagina to tamponade the bleeding. Placing sutures is generally futile and may make the bleeding worse.[10]

Medical Abortions

While surgical evacuation of the uterus takes special equipment, medical abortions do not. Most tested regimens use mifepristone or methotrexate plus misoprostol.

Using mifepristone, give 100 to 600 mg orally, followed in 6 to 72 hours by misoprostol 400 mcg orally or 800 mcg vaginally. Using methotrexate, give 50 mg/m^2 intramuscularly (IM) or orally, followed by misoprostol 800 mcg vaginally in about 3 days. If the pregnancy persists 1 week after the methotrexate administration, give another dose of misoprostol.

With either regimen, if the pregnancy persists, a surgical abortion is indicated.[11]

OBSTETRICS

Obstetric Emergencies

Approximately 15% of pregnant women develop complications that require special obstetric care, with up to 5% requiring surgery, including Cesarean sections (C-sections). Basic obstetric care includes the ability to assess the mother and fetus; do episiotomies; manage hemorrhage, infection, and eclampsia; deliver multiple births and breech presentations; use a vacuum extractor; and provide care for women after genital mutilation.[12]

An excellent online professional resource for routine and emergency obstetric care (with good illustrations) is WHO's *Managing Complications in Pregnancy and Childbirth: A Guide for Midwives and Doctors.* Download it in any one of seven languages at www.who.int/maternal_child_adolescent/documents/9241545879/en/.

Another excellent professional resource is from the Johns Hopkins Program for International Education in Gynecology and Obstetrics (JHPIEGO), *Emergency Obstetric Care: Quick Reference Guide for Frontline Providers*, which is available to download from the USAID website: http://pdf.usaid.gov/pdf_docs/pnacy580.pdf.

Diagnosing Pregnancy

Signs and Symptoms

Diagnosing pregnancy without a human chorionic gonadotropin (HCG) level relies on signs and symptoms, some of which can be quite nebulous. The only three physical findings of pregnancy that most clinicians can rely on are palpating the enlarged uterus, hearing the fetal heartbeat, and seeing the baby in the birth canal. If HCG test strips are available, use either urine or serum. Whole blood may also work (see Chapter 20).

Rudimentary Laboratory Tests

If you really must have laboratory test results to diagnose pregnancy in austere circumstances, use the frog test, which is much easier than the fabled rabbit test. The test, which uses a male frog (the common North American frog, *Rana pipiens*), is simple, rapid, and inexpensive. Inject 1 mL of the patient's early-morning, concentrated urine sample (or blood serum obtained at any time) into the frog's dorsal lymph sacs (back area behind the head). Blood serum is preferable, because it can be obtained any time and is less likely to cause toxic deaths in the frogs. Using a microscope, examine the frog's urine at 30-minute intervals for 3 hours. If the test is positive, the frog will have spermatozoa in its urine. During the summer, the accuracy of the test decreases, but partially compensate for this by refrigerating the frogs.[13]

How Pregnant?

Without ultrasound to date the pregnancy, you must use the less-reliable method of counting from the patient's last menses. One way to get the due date is to add 9 months and 7 days from the onset of the patient's last period. For those using lunar time for measurements rather than a calendar, and assuming that the woman's cycles are "1 moon" (4 weeks) apart, the due date would be "10 moons" after the onset of the patient's last menses.

Once the fundus is palpable, the gestational age is closely related to the fundal height (Fig. 31-4).

Fetoscope

Use any hollow tube made from wood, bamboo, plastic, clay, or metal as a fetoscope. The optimal size is a piece about 15 cm long, with a hollow core 3 to 4 cm in diameter.[14,15]

Counting the fetal heart rate with a stethoscope or Doppler is accurate and has good interobserver reliability.[16] Skilled practitioners can often hear the baby's heartbeat by the seventh or eighth month just by putting their ear to the patient's belly in a quiet room. However, the heartbeat is easier to hear with a stethoscope or a fetoscope. (For improvised stethoscopes, see Chapter 5.)

If the baby's heartbeat is heard best below the umbilicus, the baby is probably in the head-down position. If it is heard best above the umbilicus, the baby is most likely head-up (breech).

Analgesia in Pregnancy

Non-pharmacological treatment includes locally applied heat and cold. Heat can be applied as a hot water bottle, a hot bath, or a microwaved wheat pillow (see the "Heating the Bed" section in Chapter 5). Locally applied ice packs often work well for headaches. If non-pharmacological treatment is ineffective, consider using local anesthetic infiltration or regional anesthetic blocks, depending on the location of the pain. If those do not work or if they are not applicable, use acetaminophen 1 g q6hr.[17]

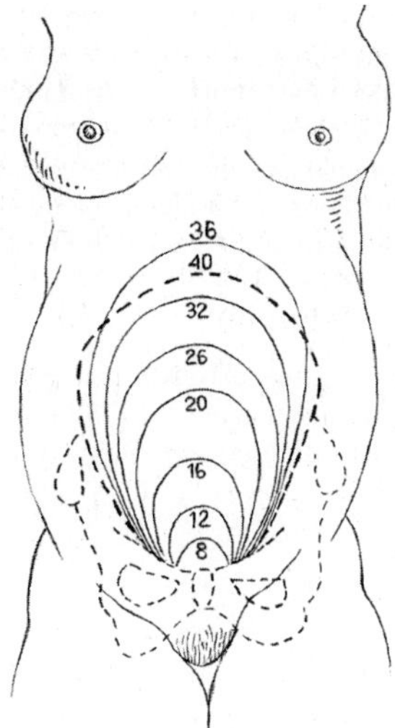

FIG. 31-4. Fundal height related to gestational age (in weeks).

Miscarriage

If a woman passes tissue during her first trimester and the os has closed again, check her vital signs and, if normal, send her home. Tell her to return if there is increased bleeding or any sign of infection.

If she is spotting, reassure her that most pregnancies with only spotting go to term without difficulty. Check her vital signs; if normal, send her home.

If she has been bleeding and the os is open, she has an incomplete or inevitable miscarriage. She can wait for passage of more tissue and for the os to close. If the os remains open, she will need the products of conception removed.

Products at Cervical Os

If vaginal bleeding occurs after a miscarriage, delivery, or abortion, and a speculum or forceps is not available, use a sterile- or clean-gloved hand to feel the cervical os. Check for products of conception that are not permitting the os to contract. If necessary, use a non-gloved, but clean, hand. If material seems to be at the os, but it is too slippery to hold, use sterile gauze or a cloth boiled in water wrapped around your fingers to try to grasp and remove the tissue.

Obstetric Checks

Simple tests can help to determine a pregnant woman's well-being.

Checking her weight may be the most difficult test to improvise without a scale. However, other observations, such as her overall body habitus (e.g., extremely thin or fat face), may help a little. You are trying to determine whether the woman is too thin due to parasites, HIV, drug use, hyperemesis, or lack of food. She should gain at least 20 lb (9 kg) during the pregnancy. You also want to be sure that she has not gained >42 lb (19 kg) during the pregnancy, or >3 lb (1.5 kg) a week or 8 lb (3 kg) in a month, especially during the last 2 months of pregnancy. If she has gained too much weight, check her for diabetes, preeclampsia, or twins.

Check the mother's vital signs. (See Chapter 7 for ways to improvise these tests.) If her blood pressure (BP) is >140/90 mm Hg, beware of preeclampsia. Also, check for very brisk reflexes (clonus) and for peripheral edema, especially in the hands and face.

Test her urine for protein. While the easiest method is to use a urine dipstick, you can also test for protein by heating the urine. (See "Protein" under the "Urinalysis" section in Chapter 20.)

If an ultrasound is available, what you can do with it depends on both the machine's and your own capabilities. Dating the pregnancy by measuring the fetus is relatively easy. Determining the sex and looking for fetal abnormalities or the placenta's position can all be done with relatively little training.

Without ultrasound, use external measurements to help determine the pregnancy's progress. The basic rule is that the fundal height increases by approximately two fingerbreadths each month. At 3 months, the fundus is just above the pubic symphysis. At 5 months, it is at the umbilicus, and at 8.5 to 9 months, it is almost up to the costal margin. One or two weeks before delivery, it drops a bit. Use a tape measure to check the fundal height and record it for each visit (see Fig. 31-4).

Most pregnant women, especially those in resource-poor situations, need to have supplemental iron. Mix ferrous salts in a palatable solvent (e.g., juice) to make an acceptable iron mixture.[18]

Ectopic Pregnancy

Ectopic pregnancies can be life threatening. Women presenting with abdominal pain, vaginal bleeding, or hypotension need to have this diagnosis excluded or treated. Four specific symptoms that can help identify (or eliminate the diagnosis of) ruptured ectopic pregnancy are:

- Vomiting during pain
- Diffuse abdominal pain
- Acute abdominal pain for >30 minutes
- Flashing/rapid shooting/lightning/shock-like pain

In a pregnant woman, the presence of any one symptom has a 93% sensitivity and 44% specificity for tubal rupture, with a negative likelihood ratio for ruling out tubal rupture of 0.16. If none of the symptoms are present, the probability of tubal rupture is <4%; if ≥3 are positive, the likelihood is 73%.[19]

While ultrasound has virtually eliminated the use of diagnostic culdocentesis from the developed world, it still is valuable for diagnosing ectopic pregnancies and pelvic infections in austere circumstances. The procedure is simple (for the clinician). Pick up the posterior cervix with a single-tooth tenaculum (Fig. 31-5). This is often when patients feel the most pain. Apply the tenaculum very slowly, counting from "1" to "30" while the teeth are applied. Then infiltrate the posterior fornix with a local anesthetic using a spinal needle. Insert a 16- or 18-gauge spinal needle into the cul-de-sac. Aspirate. If blood returns, wait 6 minutes to see if it clots. If it does, it is most probably due to the needle entering a pelvic vein. If it does not clot, the blood is from a ruptured ectopic pregnancy or ovarian cyst. If pus returns, the patient has pelvic inflammatory disease. If a small amount of straw-colored fluid is withdrawn, that is physiologic. If you cannot withdraw any fluid, the tap is non-diagnostic; repeat it.

Preeclampsia/Eclampsia Diagnosis and Treatment

Preeclampsia's hallmarks are hypertension and proteinuria after 20 weeks of gestation. Hypertension is a BP ≥140/90 mm Hg in a woman who has not previously been hypertensive. (Improvised

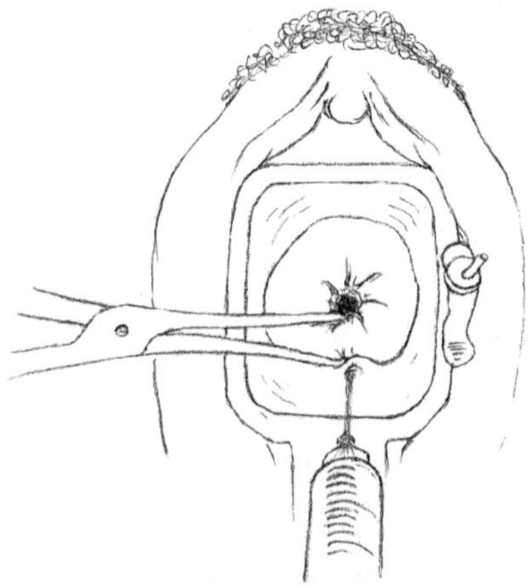

FIG. 31-5. Culdocentesis from the clinician's viewpoint.

methods to take the BP are described in Chapter 7. A qualitative urine protein test can be found in Chapter 20.) The women also frequently have sudden weight gain or the presence of swelling of the face and hands—especially upon awakening. Indicators of severe preeclampsia include the presence of severe headaches, hyperreflexia, blurred or double vision, upper abdominal pain, oliguria, and pulmonary edema. Treat women with preeclampsia using available resources.

The first drug to try—and that may be available—to treat active seizures in eclampsia is diazepam 10 mg intravenous (IV) over 2 minutes. If necessary, the IV preparation can also be given rectally.[20,21] Repeat this dose if another seizure occurs. If referral is delayed or if the woman is in late labor, start a maintenance drip of 40 mg diazepam in 500 mL normal saline (0.9%; NS) or lactated Ringer's solution and run over 6 to 8 hours at a level to keep the patient sedated, but arousable. Limit the dose to 100 mg diazepam in 24 hours. Stop the drip if respirations slow to ≤16/min.[22]

Because diazepam has erratic absorption IM and, in some situations, it may be impossible to start an IV line in edematous or seizing patients, administer diazepam via the rectal route. Demonstrating its utility in remote areas, Dr. Povey wrote,

> At Maputo Central Hospital [Mozambique] we have many times used it to control eclamptic convulsion, following which it is possible to access a vein and to continue management with magnesium sulphate … We use 20 mg of the IV preparation of diazepam in a 10-mL syringe. The needle is removed, the barrel is lubricated, and the syringe is inserted into the rectum for half its length. The contents are discharged, the syringe is left in place, and the bullocks are held together for 10 min to prevent expulsion of the drug. If convulsion is not controlled within 10 min, an additional 10 mg is instilled. Alternatively, the drug can be injected into the rectum through a urinary catheter. In circumstances in which IV administration is impossible or dangerous, as in a primary care unit that lacks the appropriate equipment or skills, we advise the rectal loading dose described above followed by an hourly rectal dose of at least 10 mg, depending upon the size of the woman and her clinical response. This method is invaluable when a patient must be transported for a long distance by human carriers, animal cart or truck.[21]

Magnesium sulfate ($MgSO_4$) is traditionally the first-line medication used for preeclampsia and eclampsia.[23] However, it is not available in many of the world's hospitals and birthing centers.[22] Magnesium sulfate treatment is expensive, not only because of the medication, but also because of the need to hospitalize and monitor the patient.

To use it, administer a loading dose of 4 g $MgSO_4$ IV over 5 minutes. (Warn the patient that she will feel warm when the drug is given.) Then, immediately give 5 g $MgSO_4$ (50% concentration is best) mixed with 1 mL 2% lidocaine in each buttock as a deep IM injection. After 15 minutes, if seizures persist or recur, give 2 g $MgSO_4$ IV over 5 minutes. If referral is delayed or the woman is in late labor, repeat the IM injections in each buttock using half the dose of $MgSO_4$ (i.e., 5 g total). Give it in alternate buttocks every 4 hours for 24 hours after delivery or the last seizure. Before every $MgSO_4$ dose, be certain that the respiratory rate is ≥16/min, patellar reflexes are present, and urine output is ≥30 mL/hr. The antidote for respiratory depression is calcium gluconate 1 g (10 mL of 10% solution) IV administered over 10 minutes.[22]

The third drug to try, if available, is phenytoin (Dilantin). It is not as effective as $MgSO_4$. Give 10 mg/kg IV at a rate of ≤25 mg/min. Two hours later, give 5 mg/kg IV. Begin a maintenance dose of 200 mg three times a day (tid) IV or orally (po) 12 hours later.[20]

Terminating the pregnancy is the definitive treatment for preeclampsia. In almost all cases, this means a term or near-term delivery.

Inducing Labor

If the woman's membranes have broken but labor has not started, labor sometimes can be inducted by administering an enema (carefully, so as not to infect the vaginal area) or by giving 60 mL castor oil po in 240 mL fruit juice.[24]

Anesthesia

Local

Boulton described the method (not often used) of using local anesthesia for the perineum and vagina: "The technique of topical analgesia of the skin of the perineum and the mucous membrane of the introitus of the vagina for spontaneous delivery, suction extraction and suturing of perineal lacerations is simple and efficacious. Lidocaine gel 2% can be used for the purpose but the 10% aerosol is superior. The dose should not exceed 200 mg lidocaine to mucous membranes and 200 mg to the surrounding skin. [More than] 90% of patients receiving spraying alone report satisfactory relief of pain; blood lidocaine did not exceed 2.4 mcg/mL, which is well below the toxic level (10 mcg/mL)."[25]

Pudendal Blocks

Bilateral pudendal blocks provide excellent anesthesia over the perineum and lower third of the vagina. They reduce pain during vaginal delivery and minor gynecological procedures, provide some introital relaxation, and are adequate anesthesia for repairing lacerations or episiotomies. A pudendal block does not, however, provide adequate anesthesia when extensive obstetric manipulation is required.

A pudendal block requires a small-gauge (e.g., 22-gauge) spinal needle, 10 mL 1% lidocaine for each side, and a needle guide/guard (e.g., Iowa trumpet) that allows the needle to protrude only 1.5 cm out of the distal end. Improvise the needle guard by cutting 1.5 cm off the end of the spinal needle's plastic sheath, as is done when making a needle guard to aspirate peritonsillar abscesses. Also use this guide when doing a paracervical block.

Then palpate the ischial spine through the vagina. Feel the spine as a distinct boney "bump" quite separate from the rest of the pelvic wall. Insert the needle guide along the palpating finger to a point on the sacrospinous ligament, about 1 cm from its insertion onto the ischial spine. Insert the needle through the guide and into the sacrospinous ligament. Aspirate and then slowly infiltrate 3 mL 1% lidocaine. Advance through the ligament and inject 3 mL more anesthetic as the plunger loses resistance. Then withdraw the needle into the guide, and move the guide just above the ischial spine; inject the rest of the anesthetic. Repeat the process on the other side. It takes 10 to 20 minutes for the block to take effect. If the block does not work on one side, administer another 5 mL of anesthetic on that side. When giving a pudendal block during labor, locally infiltrate the area for an episiotomy, in case that procedure needs to be done before the block takes effect.

Spinal

Spinal anesthesia is discussed in Chapter 15. However, giving these blocks to pregnant patients involves some special considerations. First, these women should receive at least 1.5 L crystalloid before the lumbar puncture (LP). Be careful if the woman has a bleeding disorder, such as occurs in moderate-to-severe eclampsia. In addition, pregnant patients generally need less anesthetic medication to achieve the same level of anesthesia than do women who are not pregnant. The general doses and techniques are as follows:

For a C-section, the block should extend to T6, about the level of the sternum. Use one of the following typical doses to achieve that level[26]:

2.0 to 2.5 mL hyperbaric 0.5% bupivacaine *—or–*
2.0 to 2.5 mL of isobaric 0.5% bupivacaine *—or–*
1.4 to 1.6 mL hyperbaric 5% lidocaine *—or–*
2.0 to 2.5 mL isobaric 2% lidocaine with 0.2 mL 1:1000 epinephrine.

If the spinal is for a forceps delivery, 1 mL of a hyperbaric anesthetic, given with the mother in a sitting position, is usually adequate. When removing a retained placenta, inject 1.5 mL hyperbaric solution with the mother sitting up; then lay her down.

Anesthesia for C-Sections

The methods for using spinal and general anesthetics, including ketamine for C-sections, are discussed in Chapters 15 and 16.

Dystocia

In certain cases of obstructed labor or when there is head dystocia (and a C-section is not possible and alternative maneuvers have not succeeded), two procedures might work: symphysiotomy or, if the fetus has died, fetal craniotomy.

Symphysiotomy

Recommended by WHO to avoid maternal and fetal complications during difficult vaginal deliveries, symphysiotomy entails surgically dividing the cartilage of the symphysis pubis, usually under local anesthesia.[27] Performed in the second stage of labor, it temporarily enlarges the pelvic outlet from 1 to 3 cm, permitting a vaginal delivery. Contraindications include a dead fetus (see "Fetal Craniotomy," below), incomplete cervical dilation, and a non-longitudinal lie.

The 2- to 3-minute procedure, which was commonly performed throughout the 20th century, is generally done in the labor ward. After inserting a catheter to drain the bladder, liberally anesthetize the area using local anesthesia. Place a finger in the vagina behind the pubic symphysis and make a 1.5- to 3-cm skin incision. Then divide the cartilage at the pubic symphysis. Deliver the baby.

Although women often experience more and longer postoperative pain after this procedure than with a C-section, most women can walk using a walker or chair within 2 to 4 days; 95% can be discharged from hospital within 2 weeks.

Scar tissue between the pubic bones permanently enlarges the pelvis. Post-symphysiotomy patients sometimes experience pain over the symphysis or in the sacroiliac joints or urinary incontinence—although less often than after normal vaginal deliveries. Rarely, problems with walking occur.[28]

Fetal Craniotomy

If the fetus has died or the mother's life is at risk and clinicians cannot deliver the child any other way, reduce the fetal head size with a craniotomy. This makes a vaginal delivery possible. If a fetus has hydrocephalus, passing a needle into the head to drain the fluid can reduce the head size sufficiently for vaginal delivery.

Before C-sections became common, clinicians often performed craniotomies. In poor countries, clinicians still frequently do them in cases of fetal death and hydrocephalus. Drs. Smith and Neill describe the craniotomy procedure shown in Fig. 31-6:

> In some cases, where the sutures are very loose, the evacuation of the brain is often sufficient, as the bones of the cranium collapse so much by the pressure of the womb that the child may be expelled by the natural powers. Should this not be the case, the brain must be evacuated, and extracting force applied. The instruments required are of two kinds, the one to perforate the skull, and the other to extract.
>
> It is not absolutely necessary . . . that the os uteri should be entirely dilated, although the wider the orifice is, the less danger will there be of injuring that organ. The rectum and bladder having been previously emptied, the woman is to be placed in the [lithotomy] position. The perforator should then be carefully applied upon the groove between two

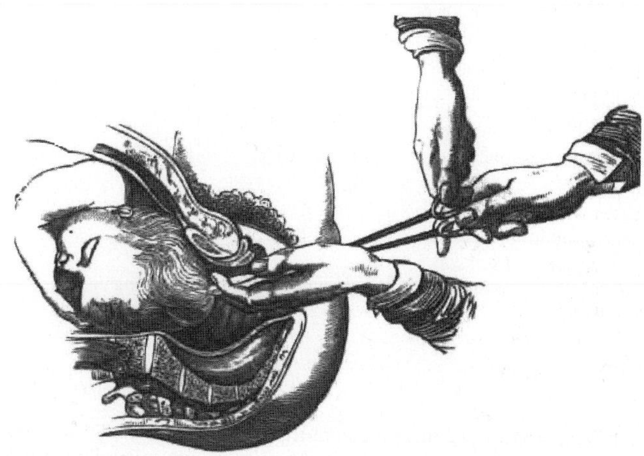

FIG. 31-6. Craniotomy for head dystocia. *(Reproduced from Smith and Neill.[29])*

> fingers of the left hand, previously introduced, and placed upon the part of the head, which it is proposed to open. It must now be passed forwards with a semi-rotatory motion until it penetrates the bone; if the scissors are used [to perforate the skull, then separate] the handles as widely as possible. The cutting edges are then to be placed at right angles to the first incision, and again separated, so as to make an [x-shaped] opening. The instrument should now be passed into the skull, and the brain broken up, after which [the instrument] should be withdrawn. Then [use an instrument to grasp] the inside or outside of the head, and [extract the fetus], being very careful to guard the soft parts of the mother. If the head cannot be delivered in this manner, recourse must be had to the craniotomy forceps and the bones broken up and extracted in pieces.[30]

Drs. Smith and Neill go on to note that the mother will need special care after this procedure.

Antepartum/Intrapartum Hemorrhage

About 4% of pregnant women experience significant antepartum hemorrhage from placenta previa, abruptio placenta, or uterine rupture.[31]

In cases of placenta previa when the mother is hemorrhaging during labor and when there is no other option (e.g., C-section), you may have to revert to older methods to save the woman's and, possibly, the child's life. These include moving the baby (i.e., version) so the foot protrudes from the vagina for traction, using a towel clip or forceps to grab the baby's scalp (if it is a vertex presentation) to apply traction, or, in less-severe cases, rupturing the membranes.

Using forceps on the fetal skull to tamponade the bleeding is very effective. It can be done even when the os has dilated only enough to admit one finger at a time. Once the forceps are applied, mild traction (1 to 1.5 lb) abruptly stops the bleeding. This method saves nearly all the mothers' lives, although the neonatal mortality varies widely. Using traction, only 44% of the children survived. This, however, was better than the 7% survival using "version."[32]

Dead Fetus—Breech

Removing a dead fetus can prove difficult if it is in the breech position. One method of removal is to pass a large balloon (Foley) catheter into the fetus's rectum, inflate it with water, and pull on the catheter. According to Verkuyl, this makes extraction easy and avoids maternal complications.[31]

Emergency Childbirth

Emergency Childbirth Kit (~1.5 lb)

This kit is designed to be carried in a 36- × 36-inch baby blanket. For births occurring outside the medical facility or in shelters or refugee camps, this portable kit may prove useful.

- One 36- × 36-inch "receiving" blanket
- Plastic to wrap around the kit
- One or two diapers
- Four sanitary napkins (wrapped)
- ID bands for mother and baby
- Short pencil
- Soap
- Sterile package containing:
  - Small pair of blunt-end scissors
  - Four pieces of white cotton tape, 0.5 inches wide by 9 inches long
  - Four cotton balls
  - Roll of 3-inch-wide gauze
  - Six 4-inch squares of gauze
  - Two to six safety pins

Additional medical supplies that may prove useful for those who know how to use them are: a syringe with oxytocin; bulb syringe; intubation equipment; ketamine; IV needles, tubing, and NS (0.9%); surgical scrub; sterile gloves; and a scalpel. These take a bit more room and double or triple the kit's weight. Most importantly, only those who have the knowledge required to use them correctly should use these items.

To prepare the kit, lay out the plastic sheet and open the blanket onto it. Put all the equipment in the center. (If additional medical supplies are included, the IV solutions and tubing may have to be carried separately.) Pull the two opposite corners of the blanket and plastic together and tie them. Do the same with the opposite corners, pulling them tight enough so that nothing will fall out. Add another knot so there is a loop to sling over the arm for carrying the kit.

Procedure

Preparation for Childbirth

1. Have the mother lie on a clean surface. Waterproof the mattress with plastic sheeting or pads made from several thicknesses of paper covered with cloth. Over this, put a clean bed sheet. Place the mother on her left side for labor, and gather available equipment for delivery and care of the neonate.
2. Prepare a bed for the baby by using a clothes basket, a box, or a dresser drawer placed on a table, stable chairs, or the floor and lined with a blanket. If possible, warm the baby's blanket, shirt, and diapers with a hot water bottle, warm bricks, or a bag of preheated salt. (See also Chapter 37.)
3. Examine the patient to determine how much the cervix has dilated. The woman should begin pushing when the cervix is completely dilated (10 cm) and no cervix can be felt on either side of the fetal head.
4. Check the fetal heart rate every 15 minutes prior to pushing and after each contraction. Normal fetal heart rate is 120 to 160 beats/min. While the heart rate often drops with the contractions, it should recover to normal prior to the next contraction.

An immediate C-section is indicated if any one of the following is present: (a) The fetal heart rate drops below 100 beats/min and stays low for >2 minutes. (b) The baby's head is not the presenting part. Use an ultrasound, if available. (c) Acute uterine hemorrhage persists for more than a few minutes (suggestive of placental abruption or previa).[33]

Delivery

1. Place the patient on her back or tilted slightly to the left. When the patient begins pushing, flex her hips to open the pelvis maximally. Have assistants support her legs when she pushes and relax them between contractions.
2. Clean her perineum with sterile antiseptic solution or soap and water. If this is the patient's first delivery, anesthetize the perineum in case an episiotomy is needed.
3. The fetal head delivers by extension. Push upward on the fetal chin through the perineum to assist this process. Control the rate of the head's delivery with the opposite hand.
4. If an episiotomy is needed, cut the posterior midline from the vaginal opening approximately half the length of the perineum, and extend about 2 to 3 cm into the vagina.
5. After delivering the head, suction the baby's mouth and nose, and then palpate the neck for a nuchal cord. If a nuchal cord is present, loop it over the child's head or clamp it twice and cut it.
6. Put your hands along the side of the child's head and have the mother push again to deliver the anterior shoulder. Apply gentle downward traction to get the shoulder to clear the pubis. Direct the fetus anteriorly to allow delivery of the posterior shoulder. The remainder of the body rapidly follows. Wrap the infant in dry towels.
7. Once the neonate is delivered, double-clamp or double-tie the cord and cut it between the ties. Use sterilized shoestrings or strips of a sheet folded into narrow bands 1 inch wide and 9 inches long to tie the umbilical cord. Boil them for about 20 minutes, or immerse them in 70% isopropyl alcohol for at least 20 minutes before use. Have four ties ready to use, in case any are dropped.
8. To cut the umbilical cord, use a sterilized knife, pair of scissors, or razor blade. Either boil these utensils (preferred) or immerse them in 70% isopropyl alcohol for no less than 20 minutes and, preferably, for 3 hours.
9. The placenta usually delivers within 15 minutes of delivery, but it may take up to 60 minutes. Delivery of the placenta is heralded by uterine fundal elevation, lengthening of the cord, and a gush of blood. While waiting, place gentle pressure on the cord, but avoid vigorous uterine massage and excessive cord traction.

10. Immediately put an ID anklet or bracelet on the child. This is especially important if the child is born in a large group shelter or refugee camp.
11. Inspect the placenta for evidence of fragmentation that can indicate retained products of conception. Following placental delivery, administer oxytocin 20 units by drip or IM, methylergonovine maleate 0.2 mg IM, or have the patient breastfeed (although breastfeeding is not that effective in helping the uterus to contract).[33]

Inspection and Repair

1. Following delivery of the placenta, inspect the vagina (especially the posterior fornix), cervix, perineum, and periurethral areas for lacerations.
2. Repair vaginal and cervical lacerations with 3-0 absorbable suture, if available.
3. If the anal sphincter is lacerated, repair it with 2-0 absorbable suture using interrupted or figure-eight stitches.
4. If the patient's rectum has torn, carefully repair the rectal-vaginal septum with interrupted absorbable 3-0 sutures. A second layer of sutures overlapping the tissue layers decreases the risk of breakdown.
5. Patients with a periurethral tear may require urethral catheterization. In addition to lacerations, hematomas in the vulva, vagina, or retroperitoneum may occur.[33]

Complications

Even in the United States under routine conditions, home deliveries have a high rate of neonatal complications: nuchal cord (12% of the time), cyanosis (9%), apnea/pulseless (6%), apnea only (4%), feet-first breech (3%), toilet bowel retrievals (3%), amniotic sac intact (1%), and twins (1%). Maternal complications are minimal.[34]

Warm Chain

A system for keeping newborns warm and for improving survival has been termed the "warm chain" or "kangaroo care." It is described in Chapter 37.

Squatting Chair for Delivery

Fashion a squatting chair for vaginal deliveries by firmly attaching strong, outward-facing legs (for stability) to the underside of a toilet seat. Figure 5-9 shows the seat in one of its alternative configurations—as a bucket toilet. Generally, these seats are made of wood, so they need to be sanded and covered with several coats of polyurethane or a similar varnish.[35]

Unusual Obstetric Presentations

Entire books describe how to manage unusual obstetric presentations. Rather than using improvised equipment, managing them takes extensive knowledge and experience. Prepare in advance: Read the books, get help, or do a C-section. (Think of a C-section as the cricothyrotomy of pregnancy. When nothing else works, it gets your patients out of trouble.)

Emergency C-Section

C-sections in a dead or dying mother have little chance of success. Because fetal distress precedes maternal hemodynamic instability, fetal survival is unlikely in hypovolemic cardiac arrests. In non-hypovolemic cardiac arrests (or in severe shock, where taking the baby may be the only way to save the mother), a C-section must be done within 4 to 5 minutes if the baby is to survive.[36] Generally, emergency C-sections are done because of problems with the pregnancy or the delivery.

Local Anesthesia for C-Section

In case you have to do a C-section without spinal or general anesthesia, you can administer local anesthesia with good effect. Make a wheal of local anesthetic 3 to 4 cm on either side of the midline, from the symphysis pubis to 5 cm above the umbilicus. Inject the anesthetic through all layers of the abdominal wall with a long needle. Keep the needle almost parallel to the skin, being careful not to pierce the peritoneum or insert the needle into the uterus, which is easy to do because the abdominal wall is very thin at term. Use up to 100 mL of 0.5% lidocaine with epinephrine 5 mcg/mL (1:200,000). Although infiltrating the abdomen may be uncomfortable for the mother, do not administer IV analgesics or sedatives; they adversely affect the baby. If necessary, you can safely give up to 0.5 mL/kg IV ketamine for analgesia. Once the baby is delivered, give the mother IV opiates, if needed.[37]

C-Section Procedure[38]

1. Place the patient with her left side up, using an IV bag or towel to displace the uterus to the left. Quickly prep her from just below the breasts to mid-thigh.
2. Enter the abdomen through a lower-midline incision.
3. Identify and incise the peritoneal reflection of the bladder transversely, and create a bladder flap to retract the bladder out of the field.
4. Carefully incise the uterus transversely across the lower uterine segment (where the uterine wall thins). See Fig. 31-7.
5. Once the amniotic membranes are visible or opened, extend the incision laterally, either bluntly or by carefully using bandage scissors. Avoid the uterine vessels laterally. If necessary, extend the incision at one or both of its lateral margins in a J-fashion with a vertical incision.

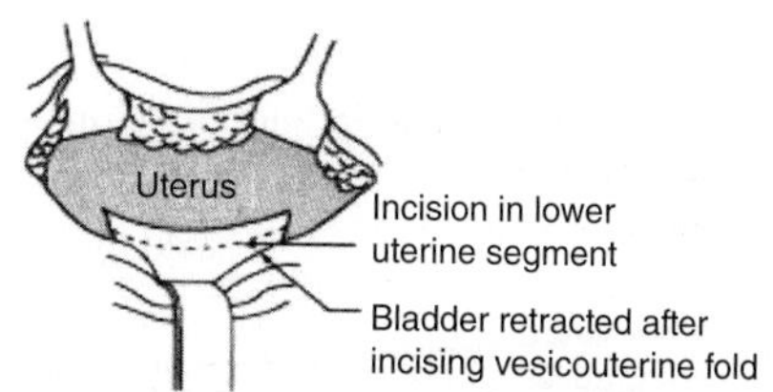

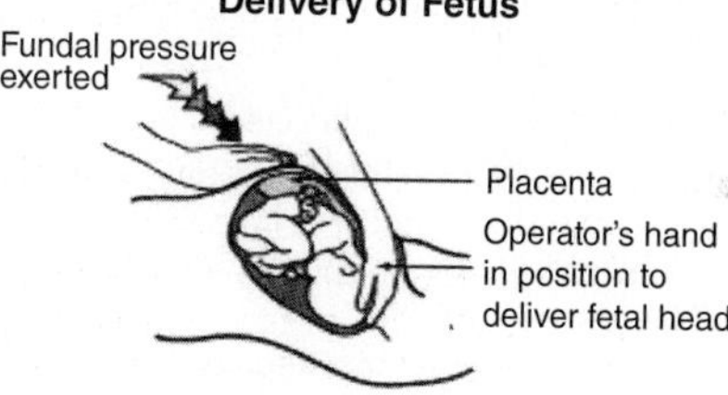

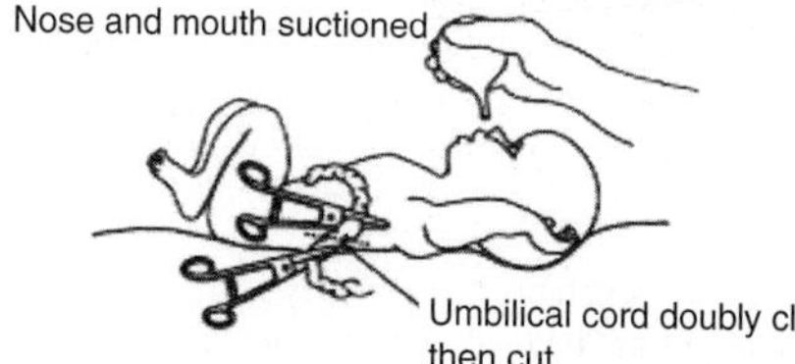

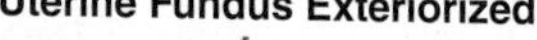

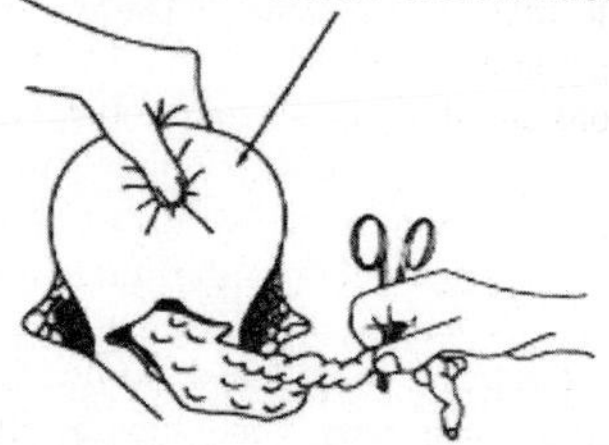

FIG. 31-7. Emergency C-section. *(Source: US Army.*[39]*)*

6. Elevate the presenting fetal part into the incision, with an assistant providing fundal pressure.
7. Deliver the fetus, suction the nose and mouth, and clamp and cut the cord. Hand the infant off for care.
8. Apply gentle traction on the cord to deliver the placenta; massage the uterus.
9. Begin oxytocin (or an alternative), if available.
10. Using a gauze sponge, clean inside the uterus, and vigorously massage the fundus to help the uterus contract.
11. Quickly close the incision with large (size 0) absorbable sutures. A single suture layer (running, locking to provide hemostasis) is adequate for transverse incisions. Avoid the lateral vessels. If the incision has a vertical extension, close it in two or three layers.
12. Once hemostasis is assured, close the fascia and abdomen.

Postpartum Hemorrhage

Hemorrhage is the underlying cause of >25% of maternal deaths in the developing world. Blood loss occurs rapidly, because the gravid uterine blood flow is 600 to 900 mL/min at term. With uterine atony, the woman loses blood at the rate of >500 mL/min. Early postpartum hemorrhage is seen in 10% of women due to uterine atony (1:20 incidence), genital lacerations, retained placenta, and uterine inversions (1:6400 incidence).[40]

Uterine Atony

Most postpartum hemorrhage stems from uterine atony (failure of uterine contracture). This bleeding may be torrential and fatal.

Initial management includes manual uterine exploration for retained placenta. Without anesthesia or with only a pudendal block, this procedure is painful. Place an open sponge (gauze) around the fingers of your dominant hand, and place the opposite hand on the patient's uterine fundus. Apply downward pressure. Gently guide your fingers through the open cervix and palpate for retained placenta. The inside of the uterus should feel smooth; retained placenta will feel like a soft mass of tissue. Remove this tissue manually or with a large curette, if available.[41]

If no tissue is encountered, use both hands to apply vigorous uterine massage to improve uterine tone. Give medications, if available. Usually, that will be oxytocin: 40 international units (IU) in 1000 cc IV or up to 10 IU given IM. Never give it IV push. If no medication is available and the bleeding is not heavy, encourage the patient to breastfeed or do nipple stimulation to increase endogenous oxytocin release.

If these measures do not stop the bleeding quickly, begin the following measures.

Postpartum Hemorrhage Control

Significant postpartum hemorrhage (>500 mL within 24 hours after delivery or enough to affect physiological functions) is not uncommon, occurring in about 3% of women in many populations and resulting in ~150,000 annual deaths worldwide. Because up to 90% of women with significant postpartum hemorrhage have no identifiable risk factors, assume that it might occur in any delivery.

The problem with treating postpartum hemorrhages effectively is that clinicians often do "too little, too late." They delay in transfusing blood, transfuse too little, and delay initiating surgical treatment. Often, the delays are due to trying different oxytocics and massaging the uterus in the hope that this will stop the hemorrhage.[42] There is also a reluctance to perform unnecessary and difficult surgery.[43]

If available, oxytocin, ergotamine, and 800 mcg of misoprostol can often successfully stop hemorrhage. Oxytocin normally works within 3 minutes. If the problem is a retained placenta, injecting 20 to 30 IU oxytocin mixed with an equal amount of NS into the umbilical vein may allow the placenta's removal without resorting to anesthesia.[44]

The key element to managing these patients is to immediately prepare for, and then quickly go on to, the next step if the current method does not immediately show results. If the patient is already in shock, use the next step—tamponading the uterus and giving blood and blood products—while giving oxytocics. Then, if the bleeding does not stop, prepare for surgery.

If the bleeding occurs while the abdomen is open for a C-section, infuse oxytocics while compressing the uterus with two longitudinal sutures along its long axis to prevent it from relaxing and filling with blood.[45] If that is not effective, use a balloon device and, if that does not immediately stop the bleeding, prepare to do a hysterectomy.

Visual estimation is an inaccurate method to determine how much blood a woman is losing intra- and postpartum. To measure the amount of blood loss, employ the same method as in cholera; that is, while the woman is in the birthing position, use a plastic sheet to funnel blood into a bucket. After about 2 hours, move her to a cholera bed (with the same bucket) so that any blood lost continues to flow into the bucket.[46] Mark several buckets in advance, inside and outside, at 500-mL increments.

Packing

Do not use uterine packing to control postpartum hemorrhage unless no other options are available.[47] Problems with using packing to control postpartum hemorrhage include the trauma inflicted by blindly placing gauze packs, the time it takes to insert them, and the need to pack them tightly enough to control the hemorrhage. Most importantly, you cannot tell whether the procedure is successful until after the blood soaks through the gauze—demonstrating that it has failed.[43]

Condom and Foley Catheters

Condom catheters can be successfully used to tamponade massive postpartum hemorrhage. Tightly tie a large condom to the end of a urethral balloon (Foley) catheter using a heavy suture, of silk if possible. Insert it through the open os until the condom is completely within the uterus and inflate it through the main catheter lumen with 250 to 500 mL NS, or until the bleeding completely stops. Clamp the catheter. If the bleeding does not stop immediately, it usually stops within 15 minutes. Most clinicians pack the vagina around the catheter (see Fig. 31-3).

A major concern is that, with the catheter in place, clinicians cannot monitor the bleeding. A simple modification solves this problem (Fig. 31-8). Cut the end off a plastic needle cap to form an open hollow tube. Insert it through the hole at the end of the Foley catheter, making sure that it is proximal to and does not obstruct the hole. Cut open the Foley balloon, and tie the condom both proximal to the balloon and distally over the area of the catheter with the plastic "bracing." The plastic prevents the suture tie from collapsing the catheter. Use a large syringe or pressurized IV to inflate the condom using the balloon inflation port (not the main catheter port). The main catheter port will be used to monitor any residual bleeding.[48]

Some clinicians have kept the balloon in place for 24 to 48 hours, depending on the initial intensity of blood loss. However, it probably only needs to be in place for 12 hours. If using the catheter modification, keep it in place for at least several hours after bleeding ceases, but no less than 12 hours. If bleeding recurs, quickly replace it in the uterus. Even with longer placements, however, no intrauterine infections usually occur.[49]

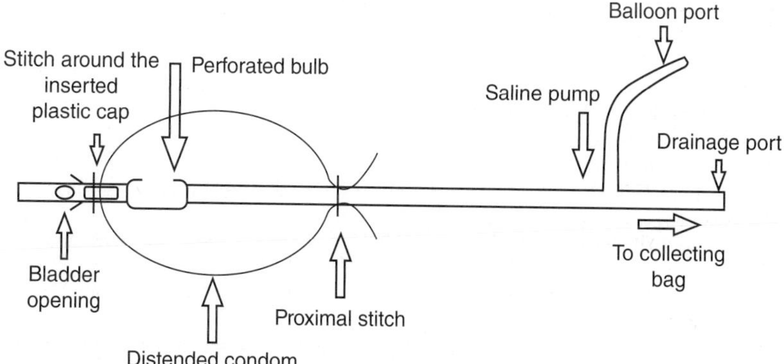

FIG. 31-8. Modified catheter system to control postpartum hemorrhage. *(Published compliments of Drs. Rishard, Galgomuwa and Gunawardane.)*

ANTI-SHOCK GARMENT

A temporizing measure while waiting to transfer the patient for surgery or transfusion is to place a pneumatic anti-shock garment (e.g., military anti-shock trousers [MAST] or a similar device). While a similar non-inflating device has been successfully tested for postpartum hemorrhages, these relatively inexpensive (<$200 US) devices are unlikely to be available when needed.[50] MAST or an improvisation to apply pressure to the pelvis and legs is worth trying, because it may help the resuscitation process.[51] Be careful not to overinflate the trousers.

Uterine Inversion

Uterine inversion is a rare cause of major postpartum hemorrhage and shock, often presenting with abdominal pain and an impalpable or vaginally appearing uterus (procidentia). It most often occurs with fundal implantation of the placenta and inappropriate traction on the umbilical cord in the presence of an atonic uterus.

Reinserting the uterus may require pharmacologic relaxation. One readily available option is to use sublingual nitroglycerin (NTG), which causes rapid uterine relaxation. Its onset is 30 to 45 seconds, with peak action at 90 to 120 seconds. It lasts up to 5 minutes. If available, IV NTG can be used, although sublingual NTG 800 mcg should completely relax a partially inverted uterus within 30 seconds, so that it can be reduced.[40]

Nipple Infections

Gentian violet (1% solution in water) is an excellent improvised treatment for *Candida albicans* nipple infections. About 10 mL is sufficient for an entire treatment. Nursing mothers with a yeast infection of the nipple may experience severe nipple pain, as well as deep breast pain. The pain is often burning, lasts throughout the feeding, and may radiate into the mother's armpit or into her back. Gentian violet nearly always brings rapid relief.

Have the patient dip a cotton-tipped applicator into the gentian violet and put it in the baby's mouth to suck on for a few seconds. If the entire mouth is not colored with the dye, have her spread the dye over the tongue and buccal mucosa. Then have the baby breastfeed. If both nipples are not purple at the end of feeding, paint the nipples with gentian violet. Repeat this treatment once a day for 3 to 4 days. If the patient is not better by the third day, consider other diagnoses.

Advise the patient that the gentian violet stains clothing, but not skin. Any skin discoloration disappears in a few days. While using this treatment, boil or stop using any artificial nipples.[52]

REFERENCES

1. Burns AA, Lovich R, Maxwell J, et al. *Where Women Have No Doctors: A Health Guide for Women.* 3rd rev. Berkeley, CA: Hesperian Foundation; 2006:313.
2. Burns AA, Lovich R, Maxwell J, et al. *Where Women Have No Doctors: A Health Guide for Women.* 3rd rev. Berkeley, CA: Hesperian Foundation; 2006:314.
3. Abramowicz M (ed.). Choice of contraceptives. *The Medical Letter.* 2015;57(1477):127-134.
4. AHRQ. *Emergency Contraception.* www.guideline.gov/summary/summary.aspx?view_id=1&doc_id=12218. Accessed August 19, 2008.
5. Ou MC, Pang CC, Ou D, Su CH. The implications of abdominal palpation with Ou MC manipulation for women with acute abdomen. *Am J Emerg Med.* 2012;30(3):421-425.
6. Wechter ME, Wu JM, Marzano D, Haefner H. Management of Bartholin duct cysts and abscesses: a systematic review. *Obstet Gynecol Survey.* 2009;64(6):395-404.
7. Qureshi S, Das V, Zahra F. Evaluation of visual inspection with acetic acid and Logol's iodine as cervical cancer screening tools in a low-resource setting. *Trop Doct.* 2010;40:9-12.
8. Pan American Health Organization. *Visual Inspection of the Uterine Cervix With Acetic Acid (VIA): A Critical Review and Selected Articles.* Washington, DC: PAHO; 2003.
9. Goldrath MH. Uterine tamponade for the control of acute uterine bleeding. *Am J Obstet Gynecol.* 1983;147(8):869-872.
10. US Army. *Emergency War Surgery.* 3rd rev. Washington, DC: Borden Institute, Walter Reed Army Medical Center; 2004:19.8.
11. Cunningham FG, Leveno KJ, Bloom SL, et al, eds. *Williams' Obstetrics.* 22nd ed. New York, NY: McGraw-Hill; 2005:246.

12. Sphere Project. *Humanitarian Charter and Minimum Standards in Disaster Response*. 2004:290. www.sphereproject.org/handbook. Accessed November 8, 2006.
13. Beacham DW, Beacham WD. *Synopsis of Gynecology*. St. Louis, MO: CV Mosby; 1972:110-111.
14. Werner D. *Where There Is No Doctor: A Village Health Care Handbook*. Berkeley, CA: Hesperian Foundation; 1977:445.
15. Lynn Johnson, photographer for National Geographic, Zambia, November 2008.
16. John AH. The accuracy of direct auscultation and the normal variation of foetal heart rate. *J Obstet Gynaecol Br Commonw*. 1966;73(6):983-985.
17. Roche SI, Goucke CR. Management of acutely painful medical conditions. In: Rowbotham DJ, Macintyre PE, eds. *Clinical Pain Management: Acute Pain*. London, UK: Arnold; 2003:369-391.
18. Bybjerg IC. Use of drugs in developing countries. *Trop Doct*. 1978;8:174-176.
19. Huchon C, Panel P, Kayem K, et al. Is a standardized questionnaire useful for tubal rupture screening in patients with ectopic pregnancy? *Acad Emerg Med*. 2012;19:24-30.
20. Shah SM, Kelly KM. *Emergency Neurology: Principles and Practice*. Cambridge, UK: Cambridge University Press; 1999:517.
21. Povey WG. Control of eclamptic convulsions with rectal diazepam. *Trop Doct*. 1998;28:175.
22. Blouse A, Gomez P, eds. *Emergency Obstetric Care: A Quick Reference Guide for Frontline Providers*. Baltimore, MD: JHPIEGO; 2003:12-13.
23. Eclampsia Trial Collaborative Group. Which anticonvulsant for women with eclampsia? Evidence from the collaborative eclampsia trial. *Lancet*. 1995;345:1455-1463.
24. Burns AA, Lovich R, Maxwell J, et al. *Where Women Have No Doctors: A Health Guide for Women*. 3rd rev. Berkeley, CA: Hesperian Foundation; 2006:342-343.
25. Boulton TB. Anesthesia in difficult situations. The use of local analgesia. *Anaesthesia*. 1967;22(1):101-133.
26. Casey WF. Spinal anesthesia: a practical guide. *Update Anaesth*. 2000;12(8):2. www.nda.ox.ac.uk/wfsa/htmL/u12/u1208_01.htm. Accessed September 13, 2006.
27. Hofmeyr GJ, Say L, Gülmezoglu AM. WHO systematic review of maternal mortality and morbidity: the prevalence of uterine rupture. *Br J Obstet Gynecol*. 2005;112:121-128.
28. Bjorklund K. Minimally invasive surgery for obstructed labour: a review of symphysiotomy during the twentieth century (including 5000 cases). *Br J Obstet Gynecol*. 2002;109:236-248.
29. Smith FG, Neill J. *Hand-book of Obstetrics*. Philadelphia, PA: Blanchard & Lea; 1852:109.
30. Smith FG, Neill J. *Hand-book of Obstetrics*. Philadelphia, PA: Blanchard & Lea; 1852:108-111.
31. Verkuyl DA. The use of a balloon catheter for breech extraction. *Trop Doct*. 2002;32(4):244-245.
32. King G, Chun D. Treatment of placenta praevia, with special reference to the use of Willett's forceps. *Br Med J*. 1945;1(4383):9-12.
33. US Army. *Emergency War Surgery*. 3rd rev. Washington, DC: Borden Institute, Walter Reed Army Medical Center; 2004:19.10-19.11 and multiple other sources, including personal experience.
34. Verdile VP, Tutsock G, Paris PM, et al. Out-of-hospital deliveries: a five-year experience. *Prehosp Disaster Med*. 1995;10(1):10-13.
35. Platt A, Carter N. *Making Health-Care Equipment: Ideas for Local Design and Production*. London, UK: Intermediate Technology Pub; 1990:73.
36. Gougelet RM. *OB-GYN Issues in Disasters: Management of Pregnancy and Related Problems*. NDMS Response Team Training Program, September 2003.
37. Dobson MB. *Anaesthesia at the District Hospital*. 2nd ed. Geneva, Switzerland: World Health Organization; 2000:91.
38. US Army. *Emergency War Surgery*. 3rd rev. Washington, DC: Borden Institute, Walter Reed Army Medical Center; 2004:19.11-19.13.
39. US Army. *Emergency War Surgery*. 3rd rev. Washington, DC: Borden Institute, Walter Reed Army Medical Center; 2004:19.12.
40. Ranasinghe JS, Lacerenza L, Garcia L, et al. Obstetric haemorrhage. *Update Anaesth*. 2006;21:19-24.
41. US Army. *Emergency War Surgery*. 3rd rev. Washington, DC: Borden Institute, Walter Reed Army Medical Center; 2004:19.13-19.14.
42. Royal College of Obstetricians and Gynaecologists. *Why Mothers Die: Report on Confidential Enquiries Into Maternal Deaths in the United Kingdom, 1997-1999*. London, UK: RCOG Press; 2001.
43. Condous GS, Arulkumaran S, Symonds I, et al. The "tamponade test" in the management of massive postpartum hemorrhage. *Obstet Gynecol*. 2003;101(4):767-772.
44. Carroli G, Bergel E. Umbilical vein injection for management of retained placenta. *Cochrane Database Syst Rev*. 2001;(4):CD001337.

45. B-Lynch C, Coker A, Laval AH, et al. The B-Lynch surgical technique for control of massive postpartum haemorrhage: an alternative to hysterectomy? Five cases reported. *Br J Obstet Gynecol.* 1997;104: 372-376.
46. Strand RT, da Silva F, Bergstrom S. Use of cholera beds in the delivery room: a simple and appropriate method for direct measurement of postpartum bleeding. *Trop Doct.* 2003;33(4):215-216.
47. Drucker M, Wallach RC. Uterine packing: a re-appraisal. *Mt Sinai J Med.* 1979;46:191-194.
48. Rishard MRM, Galgomuwa GVMP, Gunawardane K. Improvised condom catheter with a draining channel for management of atonic post partum haemorrhage. *Ceylon Med J.* 2013;58(3):124-125.
49. Akhter S, Begum MR, Kabir Z, et al. Use of a condom to control massive postpartum hemorrhage. *Med Gen Med.* 2003;5(3):38.
50. Hensleigh PA. Anti-shock garment provides resuscitation and hemostasis for obstetric hemorrhage. *Int J Gynecol Obstet.* 2002;109:1377-1384.
51. Brees C, Hensleigh PA, Miller S, et al. A non-inflatable anti-shock garment for obstetric hemorrhage. *Int J Gynecol Obstet.* 2004;87:118-124.
52. Newman J. Using gentian violet. 1998, 2009. http://www.nbci.ca/index.php?option=com_content&view=article&id=73:using-gentian-violet&catid=5:information&Itemid=17. Accessed August 8, 2011.

32 | Orthopedics

Treating orthopedic and related soft-tissue injuries can be problematic when medical equipment is scarce, especially in settings with high levels of injury (e.g., wilderness, war) or where having a disability is a threat to survival (e.g., treks, battles, subsistence economies). Extremity injuries are the primary cause of injury-related disability in many countries, especially in the developing world.[1] In developed countries, they account for about 6% of all adult emergency department visits.[2]

The World Health Organization (WHO) has developed a list of essentials for treating extremity trauma at facilities with different levels of treatment capability throughout the world (see the "Facilities" section in Chapter 5). Table 32-1 suggests what equipment and skills may need to be improvised in situations of scarcity.

This chapter discusses the diagnosis and treatment of fractures and dislocations, including emergency amputations.

DIAGNOSIS OF FRACTURES, DISLOCATIONS, AND SOFT-TISSUE INJURIES

Lacking radiographs or other imaging capability, clinicians need to rely on physical signs and symptoms to make presumptive diagnoses of fractures and dislocations. Table 32-2 lists the common signs and symptoms of fractures, with a comment about their diagnostic utility. Radiographs

TABLE 32-1 Worldwide Essentials for Diagnosing and Treating Extremity Injuries

Resources	Facility Level			
	Basic	GP	Specialist	Tertiary
Ability to recognize neurovascular and disability-prone injuries	E	E	E	E
Basic immobilization (sling, splint)	E	E	E	E
Wrap pelvic fractures for hemorrhage control	E	E	E	E
Hand injury assessment and basic splinting	E	E	E	E
Spine board availability/use	D	E	E	E
Proper management of immobilized patient	D	E	E	E
Radiology available	D	D	E	E
Closed reduction of fractures/dislocations	PR	PR	E	E
Compartment pressure measurement	I	D	D	E
Operative wound management	I	PR	E	E
External fixation (or pins and plaster)	I	PR	E	E
Skeletal traction	I	PR	E	E
Skin traction	I	PR	E	E
Tendon repair	I	PR	E	E
Hand injury debridement and repair	I	PR	E	E
Amputation	I	PR	E	E
Fasciotomy for compartment syndrome	I	PR	D	E
Internal fixation	I	I	E	E

Abbreviations: D, desirable; E, essential resources; GP, general practioners' hospital; I, irrelevant; PR, possibly required.

Modified with permission from Mock et al.[3]

TABLE 32-2 Usefulness of Clinical Information for Diagnosing Fractures (10 = Most Useful, 1 = Least Useful)

Open fracture with observable bone fragments **(10)**	When bone fragments or fat-containing blood extrude from a wound, the question is no longer whether a fracture exists, but rather its extent and how to treat it.
False point of motion **(10)**	Definitive proof of a disruption in the bone and, after acute trauma, indicates a fracture. Its absence does not indicate anything.
Palpable discontinuity in bone **(9)**	This is an excellent indicator of bony discontinuity, especially in the patella, long bones, and diastasis of the symphysis pubis. Soft-tissue defects, edema, and hematomas may limit palpation of or simulate this defect.
Results of radiograph **(9)**	Excellent, if positive. The usefulness of radiographs depends on obtaining the correct images, the radiographic technique, the practitioner's skill at interpreting radiographs, and the type of fracture. Some fractures will not be seen initially on radiographs (e.g., stress fractures, some hip fractures), so clinical evidence must always weigh more heavily with negative studies.
Examination under anesthesia **(8)**	Giving local, regional, or general anesthesia to examine the possible fracture site may aid in making the diagnosis, especially in children or uncooperative adults. Once anesthetized, test the patient for abnormal movement, deformity, and crepitus. Fractures may exist without any of these being found.
Deformity **(8)**	Presume diagnosis of fracture or dislocation if it can be discerned. Deformities are more likely to be seen if the patient presents before there is significant edema or several days later after edema has resolved, and if the fracture is away from the joints, is angular, is not a partial (e.g., stress, torus) fracture, and is not a compression fracture. Old fractures and some chronic bone deformities, such as rickets, may give the appearance of a fracture, although generally without the acute pain and skin tenting often seen after trauma.
Crepitus **(8)**	Crepitus, a grating sound caused by contact of the broken surfaces with each other, is highly suggestive of a fracture. Patients generally feel a rough, grinding sensation. In fractures with many spicules, the sensation is often that of a click. Badly comminuted or impacted fractures and those that are days or weeks old may have no crepitus [Hamilton]. Occasionally, chronic joint disease or blood clots near a suspected fracture may produce crepitus, so the sign is not perfect. .
Shortening of a limb **(7)**	This is a convincing sign of a long-bone fracture. Both extremities should be measured using easily identified landmarks (e.g., anterior iliac spine and medical malleolus). The difference may be an inch or more. Dislocations or prior injuries on either side may also cause shortening, but other signs can often differentiate between the two problems. Measurements can also be used to determine if adequate traction has been applied. The measurements must be taken accurately. For details, see the sections "Measuring Legs for Diagnosis" and "Angle Measurement Using a Goniometer" in this chapter.
Loss of function **(4)**	Many injuries can limit a patient's ability or willingness to use the extremity. There is often inability to lift the limb, owing to pain or to the separation of the bony lever upon which the muscles act, but this inability does not extend to all fractures, and especially does not exist in all partial or impacted fractures [Hamilton]. Mild, non-sedating analgesics may help make the diagnosis by allowing a patient to better test their use of an extremity.

(*Continued*)

TABLE 32-2 Usefulness of Clinical Information for Diagnosing Fractures (10 = Most Useful, 1 = Least Useful) (*Continued*)

Pain and tenderness **(1)**	Unreliable sign. Often present, even severe, with only soft-tissue injury; may be minimal or absent with a fracture.
Swelling **(1)**	Unreliable acutely. Swelling is such a common sign that it loses its diagnostic significance. If the swelling is out of proportion to the soft-tissue injury or persists longer than such apparent damage would warrant, it may indicate a fracture. If deep swelling persists after the skin edema resolves, it often indicates a displaced bone or callus.
Ecchymosis **(1)**	Although ecchymosis is more common in fractures than in dislocations [Hamilton], even if it occurs acutely, it has minimal diagnostic value. If it persists over several days, it probably indicates ongoing bleeding from a deep (probably bony) vessel.
Altered percussion **(1)**	Although highly touted, clinicians who have tried the technique of listening for changes of tone across fractures produced by either percussion or tuning fork have found it to be grossly unreliable. False-positive and false-negative results are the rule, rather than the exception.

Data from Foote[4] and Hamilton.[5]

and ultrasound are included in the list to identify their relationship with the physical examination. Many factors affect the usefulness of imaging as a diagnostic tool, including its technical quality and the skill of those interpreting the images.

Compartment Syndrome/Fasciotomy

Compartment syndrome (CS) denotes high pressure within a myofascial space, which reduces perfusion and decreases tissue viability. The role of most clinicians is to recognize the potential for CS as early as possible so that an experienced surgeon can do a fasciotomy. The most common CS occurs in the anterior leg and is associated with open tibial fractures; the most commonly missed CS occurs in the leg's anterior and deep posterior compartments.

Recognizing CS means considering the mechanism of injury, the injuries sustained, and the classic 5 Ps, although all five are rarely present. The 5 Ps are: (a) **P**ain out of proportion to that of the injury when muscles are passively stretched. This is often a sensitive, but nonspecific finding. (b) A **p**alpably tense muscle is specific but not sensitive for CS. (c) **P**aralysis, **p**aresthesias, and sensory deficits are generally late findings. (d) **P**ulselessness is rare in civilian injuries. Therefore, clinical diagnosis relies primarily on pain during passive ankle dorsiflexion, muscle palpation for tenseness, and a high index of suspicion. Use hourly serial examinations to monitor patients at high risk of CS. Pressure monitoring is unreliable in austere settings. (Pallor is often included as one of the 5 Ps, although it parallels Pulselessness.)

Note that in the absence of crush injury, fracture, multiple trauma, over-resuscitation, electrical injury, or similar indications, prophylactic fasciotomies on burned extremities may increase morbidity and mortality and are not indicated.[6]

Using Tuning Forks/Percussion

One of the most persistent myths in orthopedics is that fractures can be diagnosed using a stethoscope with a tuning fork or percussion. This fallacy continues to be sustained by experts in academia and wilderness medicine.[7-10] Yet our forebears knew that this was nonsense. Stimson, for example, wrote in 1910 that even under the best circumstances, this adds nothing to the diagnosis. "Auscultatory percussion," he wrote, "the stethoscope being moved from one fragment to the other while percussion is made upon the first, will sometimes give a marked change in the sound as the line of fracture is crossed; but it is rarely significant, except in cases in which the diagnosis can be made by other means."[11] What Stimson did not mention is that the percussion usually hurts over the fracture site: not a great finding, but enough to suggest that there might be a fracture.

No study has demonstrated the validity or reliability of the tuning fork test in detecting simple acute fractures.[12] My own tests, done with naïve optimism, used not only percussion, but also tuning forks of various recommended frequencies. These tests demonstrated that while percussive diagnosis works occasionally—usually in cases where the fracture is clinically obvious anyway—there are many false positives and false negatives, making the method virtually worthless. False negatives were especially frequent when hematomas overlaid the fracture site.

Using Ultrasound

Physicians use ultrasound successfully both to diagnose and to reduce fractures.[13] See Chapter 19 for information about how to use ultrasound for orthopedic injuries.

Physical Diagnosis

The balance of this section deals with the physical diagnosis of fractures and dislocations, which is an art seemingly lost to a reliance on imaging. Physical diagnosis consists of (a) observation, (b) measurement, and (c) palpation. Using these three modalities, the clinician can diagnose many acute orthopedic disorders without imaging.

Upper Extremity

Carpal Bone Fractures

Unlike many other fractures, carpal bone fractures may not produce much deformity, or even edema. After trauma, the patient's wrist pain, limitation of motion, and tenderness on palpation should provide enough information, without imaging, to treat an injury as a probable fracture and immobilize it. Even with imaging, some fractures, especially those of the scaphoid, may not be seen.

If all of the following signs are present, there is a 100% sensitivity and 74% specificity for a scaphoid fracture.[14] Assume that there is a scaphoid fracture, even if it appears normal on imaging, when there is:

1. Tenderness when pressing the anatomical snuffbox. The anatomical snuffbox is the groove between the tendons of extensor pollicis longus (on the ulnar side) and of extensor pollicis brevis and abductor pollicis longus (on the radial side).
2. Tenderness when pressing on the scaphoid tubercle. The scaphoid tubercle is the palpable prominence visible at the distal flexor crease when the wrist is extended and radially deviated.
3. Tenderness when longitudinally pushing the thumb toward the scaphoid while holding the wrist.

Shoulder Dislocation

Diagnosing a shoulder dislocation without a radiograph is quite simple: Just feel for the "hole" when your finger falls into the now-empty joint at the glenoid (Fig. 32-1). If there is any doubt, feel the other side. Other signs include a flattening of the shoulder, projection of the elbow with the impossibility of bringing it to the side of the body and, most important, the presence of the head of the bone in an abnormal position, usually below the coracoid process. If measured from the tip of the acromion to the external condyle of the humerus, the affected arm will be shorter than the other; this difference is increased by abducting the arm.[15]

Fracture of the Proximal Humerus

Patients with a fracture of the proximal humerus usually have localized pain, especially when the elbow is pressed upward. If the elbow is rotated slightly, the tuberosities fail to move. With marked displacement, the arm appears to be at an abnormal angle, with the axis of the humeral shaft pointing medially. Any movement usually produces pain at the groove between the pectoralis and the deltoid near the coracoid. Dislocation of the shoulder is excluded by recognizing that the humeral head is still in place.[16]

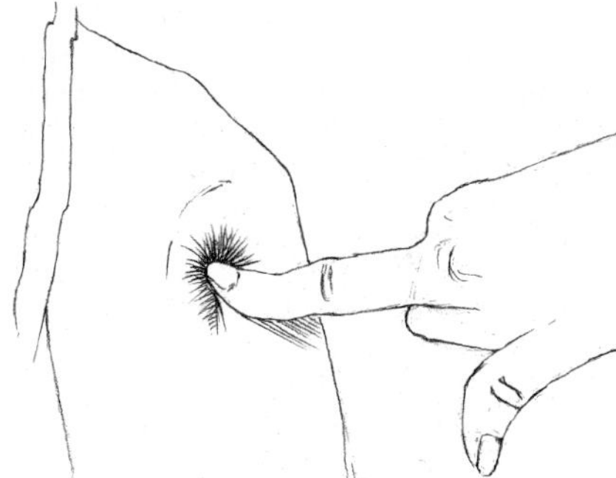

FIG. 32-1. Digital diagnosis of shoulder dislocation.

ELBOW INJURIES

With injuries at the elbow, the clinician must differentiate between fracture, dislocation, and sprain. If signs of the first two are not present, the diagnosis of exclusion—which must be given with caution—is sprain. History is usually of no help, so you must rely on the clinical examination.

Examination of the elbow is much easier if done early, before significant swelling impedes the exam. If there is swelling, try to reduce it by having the patient hold his or her arm down or by using an elastic bandage. When doing the exam, concentrate on the area where the swelling first appeared or where it remains after reducing it.

If the anatomical relationship of the olecranon and epicondyles and the radial head is normal, the elbow is not dislocated. So, begin by simultaneously holding the two epicondyles and the tip of the olecranon to determine if their relative positions are normal. At 90-degree flexion and viewed from the back (posteriorly), the three should look like an isosceles triangle—with the two equal sides being from the olecranon to the condyles. Next, palpate the radial head to determine its position.

If the exam shows no dislocation, and if the patient can cooperate, test to see what areas are painful. Grasping the elbow with one hand and the humeral shaft with the other, first press the two together and then sideways. Then, with your thumb and fingers on the epicondyles, check the distal humerus for abnormal mobility and trace the humeral shaft downward to determine its relation to the condyles. If a supracondylar fracture is suspected, confirm its presence by palpating the condyloid ridge for points of pain and irregularity.

Supracondylar fractures also have abnormal lateral mobility. If examined on an extended arm, abnormal adduction and abduction of the forearm can be demonstrated. Grasp the condyles firmly with one hand and the shaft with the other to demonstrate free mobility of one upon the other, usually with crepitus. Pressing upward with the hand under the flexed elbow causes pain. If the line of the fracture runs between the condyles (T-fracture), pressing the condyles together neither causes pain nor permits independent movement.[17]

If there is no evidence of a supracondylar fracture, press the condyles together and then hold each separately to check for pain or abnormal movement. If either moves independently, often with crepitus, a fracture is present. Local, regional, or general anesthesia may greatly facilitate this exam—for both the patient and the clinician.[18]

Pelvis/Hip

PELVIC TRAUMA

If there is any suspicion of pelvic fracture, clinicians should quickly apply a pelvic binder. Many trauma protocols require pelvic radiographs, because physical examinations for pelvic fractures are unreliable and can cause additional bleeding without providing additional vital clinical information.[19,20] Yet, in situations of scarcity, access to imaging may be limited or nonexistent. The following information is helpful to determine which trauma patients need radiographs, transfer, or the maximal possible treatment. A clinically significant pelvic fracture will exist only if a trauma patient has at least one of the following findings: (a) Glasgow Coma Score <14,

(b) complaint of pelvic pain, (c) pelvic tenderness on palpation, (d) distracting injury, or (e) clinical intoxication. One study found that if one or more of the previously listed criteria were present in adult patients after blunt trauma meeting Level 1 (serious) criteria, those patients had a 12% chance of having a significant fracture.[21] After trauma, the presence of diastasis (separation) at the pubic symphysis on palpation suggests a fracture, whether or not the patient has pain.

Hip Dislocation

Because quick recognition and treatment of hip dislocations decreases long-term disability and the treatment may depend on the type of dislocation, rely on the patient's clinical appearance to determine the type of dislocation (Figs. 32-2 and 32-3). Palpating the femoral head in the groin is also a common clue to the correct diagnosis. If there is severe pain in the hip without rotation, consider femoral neck fracture.

Hip Fracture

Unlike many other areas of orthopedics, patient history often plays a large role in the diagnosis of a hip fracture—especially in an elderly patient. As Helferich noted, "One should always think of the possibility of a fracture of the femoral neck when an old person, after a fall on the knee or side of the body, cannot stand up, and when the injured limb is shortened and rotated outward. In the diagnosis, contusions and dislocations of the hip and fractures of the pelvis have to be considered. It is hardly possible to mistake the injury for a dislocation (with outward rotation only a forward dislocation could be possible)."[24] A confounder is that elderly hip fracture patients may complain about knee, rather than hip, pain.

With hip fractures, normally, (a) the patient cannot lift his leg off the bed, (b) the leg is shortened to various extents (you may need to measure the limbs; see "Measuring Legs for Diagnosis," below), (c) passive motion of the foot laterally and medially causes hip pain, (d) crepitus is felt unless the fracture is impacted or the fragments are widely separated, (e) the leg may be

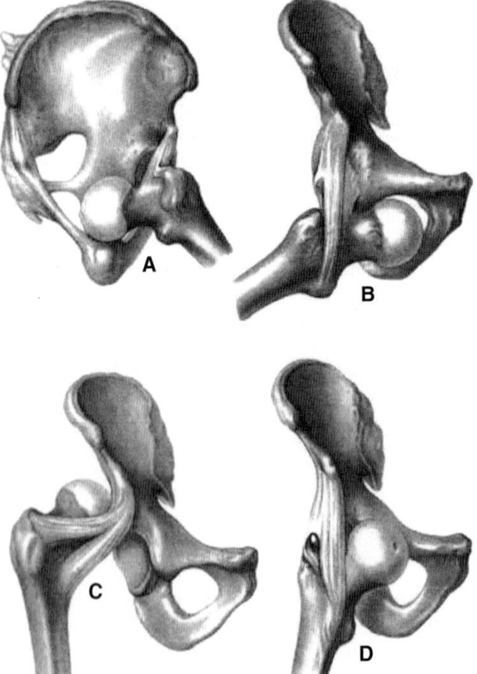

FIG. 32-2. Anatomical appearance of different hip dislocations. (A) Anterior dislocation onto the ischium. (B) Anterior-central dislocation into the obturator foramen. (C) Posterior dislocation onto the ilium. (D) Anterosuperior dislocation onto the pubic rami. *(Reproduced from Helferich.[22])*

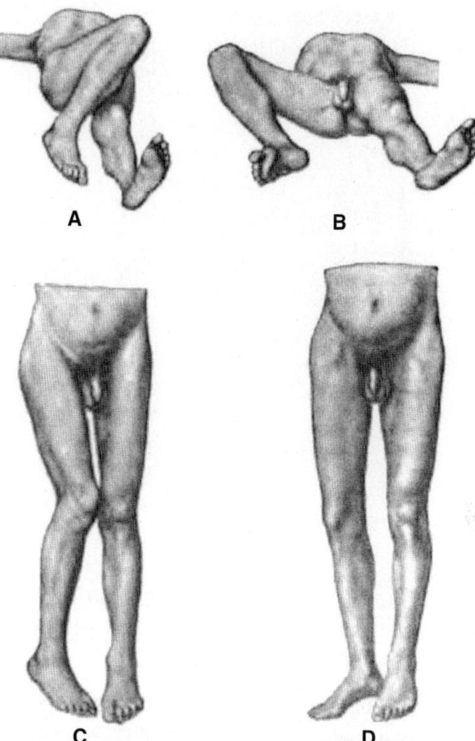

FIG. 32-3. Clinical appearance of different hip dislocations. (A) Anterior dislocation onto the ischium. (B) Anterior-central dislocation into the obturator foramen. (C) Posterior dislocation onto the ilium. (D) Anterosuperior dislocation onto the pubic rami. *(Reproduced from Helferich.[23])*

externally rotated, and (f) the greater trochanter can be felt above Nélaton's line, an imaginary line from the anterior superior iliac spine to the ischial tuberosity (Fig. 32-4).[24]

Measuring Legs for Diagnosis

Measuring limbs to detect a discrepancy between the two sides after an acute injury is a technique that has been lost over time. However, it is still useful, especially when imaging is not available and the clinician must rely solely on the physical examination to diagnose fractures and dislocations—of any extremity.

Regarding hip fractures, Stimson wrote that leg length discrepancy "may vary in extent from a small fraction of an inch to two or three inches." It may occur immediately or "appear gradually or suddenly after the lapse of a few hours or days." He added that it is vital "to have them form the same angle with the pelvis, that each is in the same position of extension and abduction. . . . The measurements are usually made between the anterior superior spine of the ileum and a malleolus."[26]

Lower Extremity

Femur, Mid-Shaft Fracture

This injury nearly always shows the typical signs of a fracture. It may, however, occasionally be confused with a large hematoma.

Knee and Ankle Fractures

The Ottawa Ankle-Foot Rule, the Ottawa Knee Rule, and the Pittsburgh Knee [Decision] Rule (discussed next) are validated diagnostic criteria for two commonly injured joints. They are useful when radiographic imaging is present, but limited. If there is no imaging, the clinician must

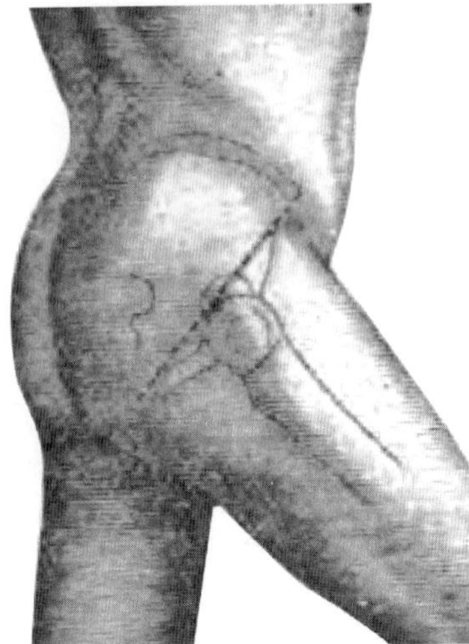

FIG. 32-4. Nélaton's line. *(Reproduced from Helferich.[25])*

assume that patients who are "positive" using these rules have a fracture that they must treat with immobilization or by providing non-weight-bearing assistance with crutches or other devices.

Use and Limitations of the Rules

These rules are for patients with blunt trauma, including twisting injuries, falls, and direct blows. They have not been validated in children <18 years old, pregnant women, or those with diminished ability to cooperate with the test (e.g., head injury, intoxication).[27]

The knee and ankle-foot rules all have nearly 100% sensitivity and are modestly specific.[28,29] The Pittsburgh Knee [Decision] Rule is 99% sensitive and 60% specific for the diagnosis of knee fractures. Of patients in whom the rule indicated a fracture, 24% had a knee fracture. For patients in whom the rule suggested no fracture, 99.8% had no fracture. The Ottawa Knee Rule was 97% sensitive and 27% specific for knee fractures.[30]

Ottawa Ankle-Foot Rule

There is a high suspicion of fracture (obtain an ankle radiograph, if available) if there is pain near a malleolus *plus* one of the following:

- Bone tenderness at the posterior edge of the distal 6 cm or at the tip of either malleolus.
- The patient could not bear weight for at least four steps immediately after the injury and still cannot at the time of evaluation.

There is a high suspicion of fracture (obtain a foot radiograph, if available) if there is pain in the mid-foot *plus* one of the following:

- Bone tenderness at the navicular or at the base of the fifth metatarsal.
- The patient could not bear weight for at least four steps immediately after the injury and still cannot at the time of evaluation.

Ottawa Knee Rule

A knee radiograph is required *only if* a knee injury patient has one of the following[31]:

- Age >55 years
- Isolated tenderness of the patella
- Tenderness at the head of the fibula
- Inability to flex to 90 degrees
- Inability to walk four weight-bearing steps immediately after the injury and at the time of the evaluation

Pittsburgh Knee [Decision] Rule

A patient with a knee injury following blunt trauma or a fall needs a radiograph *only if* they have either[32]:

- Age <12 years or >50 years, *OR*
- Inability to walk four weight-bearing steps at the time of the evaluation

Tibia-Fibula Fractures

Because the tibia is subcutaneous for much of its length, the clinician can diagnose fractures of the tibial spine by palpating the entire shin.

REDUCTION AND TREATMENT OF FRACTURES AND DISLOCATIONS

As with all procedures in this book, the techniques described for fracture and dislocation reduction and treatment are for use only by medically trained personnel who are in wilderness, isolated, developing world, or disaster settings in which more expert help, the normal equipment, or another needed resource is not available. In these settings, treating fractures and dislocations is often complicated because radiographs are not available.

The three goals of fracture treatment are:

1. *Reposition bone fragments:* Correct any bone angulation and pull the limb out to length, especially when there are no pulses below the site of the injury or when the patient must be moved and the limb's position will interfere with that effort. The best time to undertake a dislocation reduction is immediately after the injury, when there is minimal muscle spasm and resistance. Try to minimize pain during this process by using local, regional, or general sedation/anesthesia. (See Chapters 15, 16 and 17.)
2. *Immobilize the fragments:* Keep the limb at length if required (traction) and immobilize it while the bone heals.
3. *Restore function:* This requires evaluating the limb's (and the patient's) neurovascular status before and after any manipulation.

Reduction and Treatment Without X-Rays

In resource-poor settings, the closest x-ray machine may be located hours away; often radiographs are not available at all. In such cases, you will have to rely on physical signs (such as remeasuring limbs, see below) to achieve the treatment goals listed above.

Battlefield Management

As Husum and colleagues wrote, battlefield fracture management means

> Immediate reduction! Every fracture, open as well as closed, should be reduced as soon as possible after injury. . . . Early fracture reduction improves the local circulation, reduces pain and improves the general condition. During the first 1–2 minutes after the injury, manipulation of the fracture is less painful, and any fracture may be aligned without anesthesia. Reduction more than two minutes after the time of injury, should be done with local anesthesia (10–20 mL lidocaine injected into the fracture hematomas; or low-dose IV ketamine anesthesia).[33]

Remeasure

After any attempted fracture reduction where shortening of the extremity has occurred, remeasure the two extremities after reduction. Generally, if the shortening continues to be >0.5 inches, reduction is unsatisfactory: Either the fragments have not been restored to their normal position or the muscles have distracted them again. At that point, make another attempt to reduce the fracture under better anesthesia or, if that fails, splint to await additional intervention—which may include surgery.[34]

Open Fractures

For open fractures, the first step is to control bleeding. Direct pressure on soft-tissue bleeding sites usually works best. If absolutely necessary, a tourniquet can be used (see Chapter 24).

Irrigate the wound extensively: Use at least 5 to 10 L of fluid for the typical open fracture. Use the cleanest fluid possible. Tap water works well if the water supply is relatively clean (i.e., can be used for drinking). If not, boil and cool the water first. Prepackaged sterile fluids are not necessary. Because dilute iodine solution is useful for wound irrigation in open fractures, adding a single povidone-iodine pad to each liter of water is thought to provide the equivalent antibacterial efficacy; however, this has not been proven.[35,36]

A continuous fracture irrigation system (that may also be used, if desired, for continuous antibiotic instillation into a wound) can be improvised using any closed drainage system. The most commonly available, other than intravenous (IV) systems, is a urethral catheter drainage system: Just insert a small-gauge urethral catheter into the wound and hang the drainage bag to drip in fluids for irrigation.

After cleaning the wound, reduce the fracture as well as possible, and put the bone beneath the skin. Do this either by extending the limb or by pulling the skin aside with the fingers, with the handle of a metal spoon, the blunt end of a tweezers ("pickup"), or a similar firm instrument.[37] Experience shows that these methods work well to lift skin over extruding segments of bone in an open fracture. "If these measures do not succeed, the skin may be slit open freely … Enlarging the opening does not generally complicate the case—sometimes it is even advantageous."[37]

Do not close the wound in an open fracture. Pack it open with gauze; soak the gauze in a dilute iodine solution, if available. Change the packing at least twice a day and do not let the wound close until there is no sign of infection and there is good granulation tissue. Then, allow the wound to close by secondary intent—bottom-up and inside-to-outside without the skin closing over the wound, until it fills in with granulation tissue.

If available, give antibiotics, immobilize the limb using plaster or traction, and begin rehabilitation as soon as practicable.

Upper Extremity

Shoulder Reduction

Anterior shoulder dislocations are common. Clinicians need a "bag of tricks" to reduce these deformities, because any single method does not seem to work in every case. Especially in austere circumstances, methods that do not require sedation are helpful. When analgesia is needed, consider using hypnosis or intra-articular injections, both of which have worked well for joint reductions (see also Chapter 15).[38,39] Reduction methods include:

Biceps massage: Simply massaging the biceps may reduce the shoulder dislocation. If not, this technique usefully augments any of the other methods.

Stimson's method: The shoulder reduction technique first described by Stimson in 1900 may be the easiest one to use in the midst of multiple casualties or limited resources. With the patient prone, extend the affected arm vertically from the examination table. Attach a 10- to 15-lb weight to the wrist and allow it to hang there for approximately 6 to 20 minutes to achieve reduction. Stimson used a cot with a hole in it for the patient's arm to go through or "two tables placed end to end, so that the body would rest on one and the head on the other, the arm hanging down between."[40]

Snowbird traction: The easier and faster Snowbird traction technique is done while the patient sits facing the back of an armless chair, with the affected arm draped over the back. A special chair is unnecessary.[41] Place a pad under the axilla and flex the elbow to 90 degrees. Drape a stockinet or cloth loop over the proximal forearm and let it hang to the floor. Using the chair back as counter-traction, the clinician should place his foot in the loop and apply a firm, steady downward traction. This way, his hands are free to apply pressure or to rotate the arm, as needed (Fig. 32-5). This method has been reported to be successful in 97% of cases without complications; >90% can be done without sedation or narcotic analgesia.[42] Alternatively, have the cooperative patient keep his arm straight while the clinician (with strong arms and a good back) applies traction in line with the arm. As the muscles relax, have the patient stand; this increases the traction.[41,43]

Boss-Holzach-Matter autoreduction: This method allows the patient to reduce his or her own anterior shoulder dislocation.[44] The patient sits on a hard surface, clasping the hands (which are often tied together) around the flexed knee ipsilateral to the shoulder injury. The patient

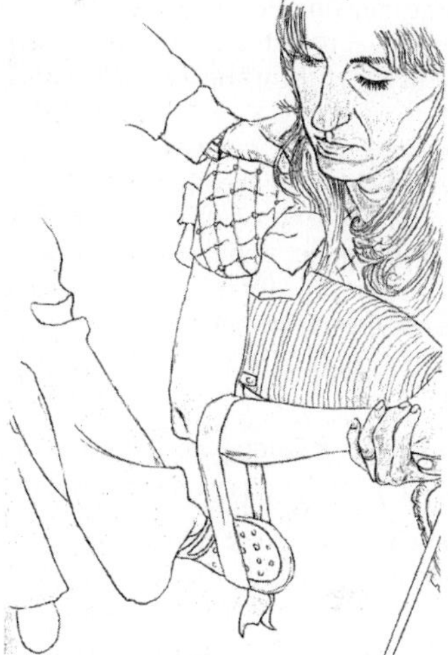

FIG. 32-5. Snowbird traction for anterior shoulder dislocation.

leans back and hyperextends the neck. This exerts anterior axial traction on the humeral head. Instruct the patient to perform an anterior shoulder shrug, increasing anteversion of the glenoid cavity and facilitating relocation (Fig. 32-6).[45]

Milch technique: Cooper first described the Milch technique in 1825. With the patient supine, the clinician abducts the affected arm while simultaneously applying pressure to the humeral head. External rotation and traction are applied when the arm is fully abducted, that is, straight "up" so that the arm is in line with the body. Few patients require sedation or analgesia for this procedure.[46,47]

Hippocratic method: This method of shoulder reduction is very old and some have suggested that the method is dangerous, because it can cause nerve damage to the axilla. However, recent studies show that the Hippocratic method may actually be safe, although it often requires sedation or significant analgesia to be successful. Place the patient supine, and put traction on the patient's hand and forearm while an assistant provides counter-traction at the axilla with a sling. Pull the arm along its axis in approximately 30 degrees of abduction to move the humeral head from its dislocated position into apposition with the rest of the joint.[48]

Scapular manipulation: The scapular manipulation/rotation method, often used along with other methods, supposedly has a success rate of >90% when used alone, although that presumes significant relaxation. With the patient sitting, have an assistant hold the affected arm straight out from the patient with the palm up (the patient's shoulder should be flexed to an angle of 90 degrees), while resting his other hand on the patient's ipsilateral clavicle. This applies gentle

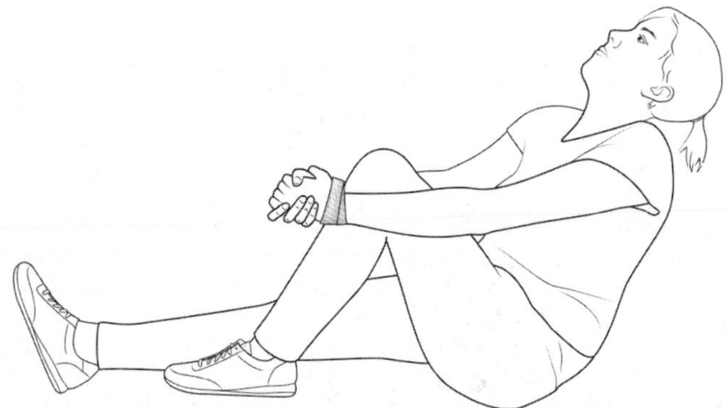

FIG. 32-6. Boss-Holzach-Matter autoreduction method to reduce anterior shoulder dislocations.

traction. The clinician then pushes the tip of the scapula medially and upward while pushing the superior part of the scapula laterally. A palpable "clunk" confirms reduction. The patient can also be positioned prone, with the arm dangling, while an assistant maintains gentle traction with the hand in supination.[49]

External rotation/Kocher maneuver: This external rotation maneuver is a modification of the Kocher maneuver. It can be performed in any position with the assistance of only one person or by the patient. If the patient is very cooperative, he or she can sit and allow the muscles to relax. Then, flex the elbow at a 90-degree angle, stabilize it against the trunk, and, slowly, externally rotate the arm at intervals. This allows time for any muscle spasms to subside. Most dislocations are reduced after about 5 minutes of external rotation.[50]

Supracondylar Fractures

Both open and closed supracondylar fractures can be successfully treated with traction and splinting. As Stimson wrote.

> In the higher fractures in adults and the late lateral angular deviation in the low ones in children, the overriding can be corrected by traction, preferably with the elbow at a right angle, and its recurrence effectively opposed by anterior and posterior molded splints, or a plaster encasement, aided sometimes by a weight attached to the forearm close by the elbow, with the wrist supported by a sling. In the low form in children. . . . even very marked deformity disappears rapidly in the young by absorption of projecting bone and the filling up of hollows, and functional limitations are rarely caused by it. In compound [open] fractures, I always use vertical suspension of the limb for about a fortnight [two weeks] unless the wound heals sooner. It is of great value in controlling reaction as well as preventing gross displacements; minor adjustments can still be made after the wound has healed or has become unimportant.[51]

Colles' (Distal Radial) Fractures

A Colles' (or similar) fracture can be reduced by suspending the arm. A hematoma block (see Chapter 15) helps relieve discomfort. Make a finger trap by forming a girth hitch with bandage material, cloth, or thick rope (Figs. 32-7 and 32-8). Loop these around the thumb and index finger, or the index and long fingers, and suspend the material from a hook or an IV pole. Traditional Chinese finger traps used as toys also work well to hold fingers aloft. Usually made of folded paper, they may not be good for more than a few patients before they need to be replaced.[52] Do not use string, wire, or anything else that might compromise circulation to the fingers, even when you are not using any added weight to assist fracture reduction. Suspend 2.3 to 4.5 kg (1 to 2 lbs) from a padded cloth at the proximal forearm to speed the reduction. After 20 to 30 minutes, return and make any necessary minor adjustments. To make life simple, keep the arm suspended while the splint or cast is applied.

Metacarpal Fractures

The usual treatment for most metacarpal fractures and dislocations is nonoperative. The goal is to preserve function. This section describes nonoperative management and refers to surgery only when that is the only option. In austere circumstances, that may mean operating outside your comfort zone, waiting or referring for treatment, or advising the patient that there may be a poor outcome.

If you cannot splint the hand or reduce the fracture, the hand can be treated using an old and less-than-optimal method, which Stimson described[53]:

> Fill the palm with a mass of tightly packed cotton or similar substance or with a ball, over which the fingers are closed and fastened down with a bandage or adhesive plaster. If there is no displacement or tendency thereto, a simple immobilizing dressing of cotton held snugly with a roller-bandage is sufficient; the fingers being left free to prevent their stiffening. The flexion of the finger over the firm mass tends to draw the knuckle downward, and thus prevent shortening. The support furnished by the adjoining bones is an additional aid against displacement, and the back of the hand can be left partly uncovered for inspection.

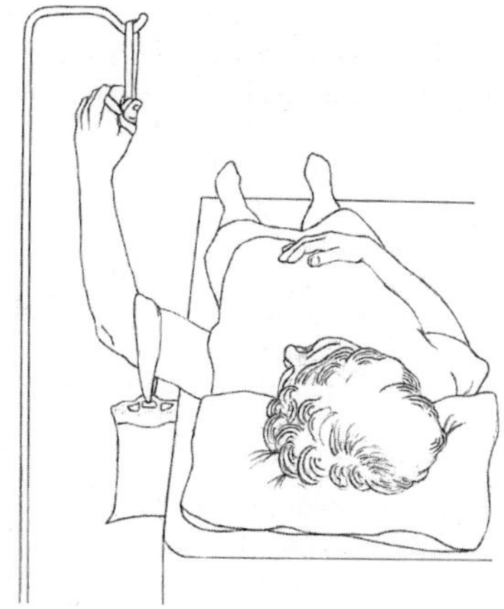

FIG. 32-7. Improvised finger trap in use.

Proximal Metacarpal (Base) Fractures

Reduce these fractures if there is >2 mm of articular surface displacement or if there is significant angular deformity or dislocation of the carpometacarpal joint. Hematoma blocks usually do not work, so a regional block or sedation may be necessary (See Chapter 15). Use traction and direct digital pressure from the clinician's thumb to reduce the fracture. Although fractures of the base of the fifth metacarpal are usually pinned, in austere circumstances, treat it like the others until or unless orthopedic services are available. Splint the wrist in 20- to 30-degree extension with the metacarpophalangeal (MCP) joints flexed for ≥4 weeks, with continued active motion of the finger interphalangeal (IP) joints.[54]

Metacarpal Shaft Fractures

Reduce metacarpal shaft fractures if there is significant palmar angulation (>10 degrees for second or third metacarpals, 20 degrees for fourth metacarpals, 30 degrees for fifth metacarpals) or any rotational angulation. To reduce the fracture, anesthetize it with a hematoma block and flex the affected finger's MCP joint and the proximal IP joints to 90 degrees. Apply upward pressure on the middle phalanx and downward pressure over the dorsal apex of the fracture. Use the finger to control or correct any rotation. Splint for <4 weeks, followed by active range of motion.[54]

Fractures at the Distal End

Splint non-displaced fractures of the metacarpal head (distal end) for 3 weeks, and follow with gentle motion. Use an ulnar gutter splint for the most common fractures, those of the fourth and

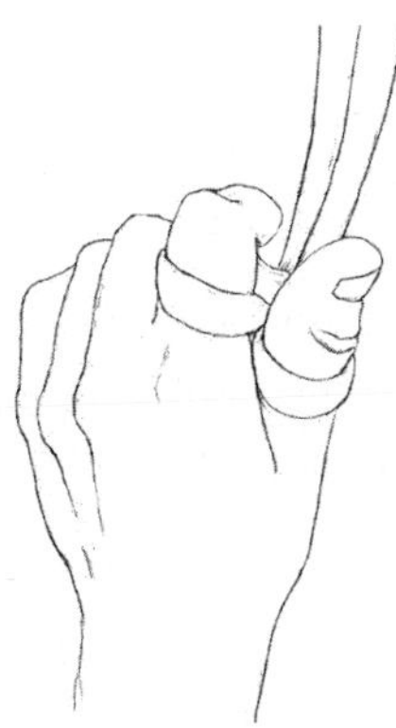

FIG. 32-8. Improvised finger trap, close-up.

fifth metacarpal heads. For fractures of the neck (just proximal to the head), such as a Boxer's fracture, you can splint most of them for 3 or 4 weeks. If there is too much palmar angulation (≥10 degrees in the second or third metacarpals, ≥20 degrees in the fourth metacarpal, and ≥30 degrees in the fifth metacarpals) or any rotational deformity, reduce it like a shaft fracture. A splint maintains about 50% of the initial correction.[54]

Metacarpophalangeal Dislocations

Attempt to reduce MCP dislocations under local or regional anesthesia. The easy ones still will be in extreme (60 to 90 degrees) hyperextension. Flex the wrist and IP joints; gently put traction on the finger and bring the joint toward the palm. If it does not go in, the only option is to wait for a surgeon, because soft tissue or the volar plate is keeping it dislocated.[54]

Splinting Metacarpal Injuries

Once these fractures or dislocations are reduced, apply a forearm-based splint that covers both the dorsal and palmar surfaces of the metacarpal, but allows the IP joints to move. The dorsal splint should extend to the IP joints; the volar aspect should end at the distal palmar crease. The wrist should be in 20 to 30 degrees of extension and the MCP joints in 70 to 90 degrees of flexion. Buddy-tape the fingers of the involved metacarpal to maintain rotational control. Encourage the patient to begin moving the IP joints immediately and, as soon as the splint is removed, encourage active movement of the fingers and wrist.[54]

Pelvis/Hip

Risk of Bleeding From Pelvic Fractures

Unstable pelvic fractures may cause life-threatening hemorrhage. Patients with a high risk (>60%) of pelvic arterial bleeding are those with a pulse of ≥130 beats/min, a hematocrit ≤30%, ≥1 cm diastasis of the pubic symphysis, and displacement of an obturator ring fracture. A patient with three or more indicators has a high (>60%) probability of major arterial pelvic hemorrhage. Those with one indicator have a 14% risk; those with two have a 46% risk.[55] An unconscious patient may be hypotensive on arrival. A conscious patient may splint the fracture with his muscles, so significant bleeding may not occur until after he is paralyzed for intubation, which causes the pelvis to fall open and the patient to become hypotensive. If pelvic fracture bleeding is a real or potential concern, apply a pelvic binder.

Pelvic Binder

A pelvic binder is used to splint the bony pelvis to reduce hemorrhage, pain, and movement during transfers, and to provide temporary pelvic stabilization.[56] Considered a treatment, rather than a method of preparing the patient for treatment, it should be applied early by people trained to do it, because it is frequently applied incorrectly.[57]

A pelvic binder tightly encircles the entire pelvis over the greater trochanters. First, fold a long sheet or other strong cloth lengthwise to get a width of 15 cm; use this as a draw sheet. Next, tightly roll a pillow, tape it, and place this behind the patient's knees. Then secure the patient's lower thighs and calves together with gauze or a similar bandage. This internally rotates both lower limbs, which act as levers on the displaced pelvis.

Ease the draw sheet beneath the patient. Whenever possible, apply the binder either directly to skin or just over thin underwear to get maximal effect.[57] The two people applying the binder should stand on either side of the patient, lean toward each other, and pull on an end of the sheet while they each simultaneously push their side of the pelvis. When it is tight, secure the sheet with a cable tie or square knot. Then place a dowel, wooden branch, or metal bar against the knot and tie another square knot. Use the rod as a windlass to tighten the sheet. A tight belt or webbing may also be used, but these usually cannot be tightened enough to get a good effect.[58]

Lower Extremity

Hip Reductions

A relatively easy way to reduce hip dislocations is to use the "Captain Morgan" technique that Lefkowitz first described in 1993.[59] Place the patient supine, with both the hip and the knee

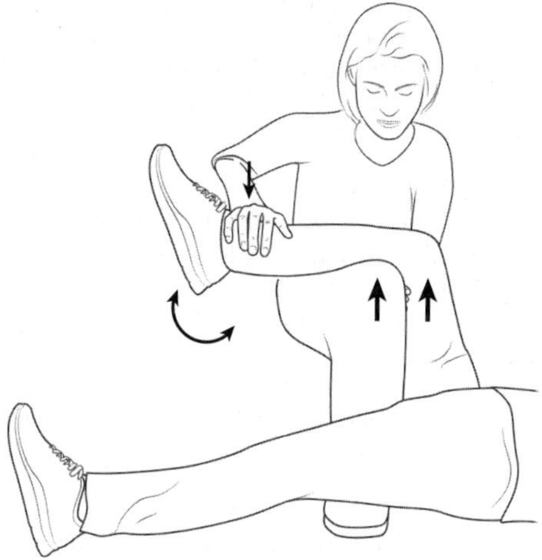

FIG. 32-9. A clinician using the "Captain Morgan" hip reduction technique.

flexed to 90 degrees. If available, put the patient on a backboard. Use an assistant or a strap to hold the patient's pelvis to keep it from lifting off the board. Place one hand and a knee under the patient's knee and another hand on the patient's ankle, then plantar flex (rise up on your toes) while lifting with the hand behind the knee and pushing down on the patient's lower leg (Fig. 32-9). If not immediately successful, internally and externally rotate, adduct and abduct the hip by rocking and rotating the patient's lower leg.[60] Take care not to apply too much force to the patient's knee, because it can cause damage.[61]

Hip Fracture

In austere conditions without the availability of x-ray or operative intervention, closed reduction and traction are the only options for treating hip fractures.

Femoral neck fractures are the most common fractures seen in the elderly. These fractures can heal with bed rest, but patients often have chronic pain and may not be able to walk. Our forebears got good results with traction. Helferich wrote that extension and inward rotation should be secured with weight extension by means of strapping. A weight of 12 to 15 lb is usually required to overcome thigh muscle spasm, with the leg slightly abducted. Maintain traction for 2 weeks; then use crutches and physical therapy for 10 weeks or so. Have the patient change position on a regular basis to avoid decubitus ulcer formation.[62]

If the patient has a non-displaced intracapsular fracture and surgery is not available, don't fret. There seems to be little difference in outcome between surgery and conservative treatment in these cases.[63,64] Fractures of the femoral head, if not displaced, usually heal fairly well with 8 to 12 weeks of bed rest. If the femoral head is displaced, the patient will probably have avascular necrosis, a loss of range of motion, and chronic hip pain. However, if there is a central fracture-dislocation (the femoral head has pushed through the acetabulum), use 25 lb or more of traction in each of two directions: pulling the hip both laterally away from the body and in line with the body. Keep the patient in traction for 6 to 10 weeks, followed by crutches. Even after this prolonged therapy, do not expect a great result from this major injury.[65]

Ankle Fracture-Dislocations

A fracture-dislocation of the ankle (Fig. 32-10) is a devastating injury that, if not properly aligned, can be disabling when healed. Use a Dupuytren's splint (Fig. 32-11) to achieve and maintain alignment. Apply the splint to the inner side of the leg; the foot will be pulled toward the splint when the bandage is wrapped around it. Note that there is no padding under the ankle joint.[66]

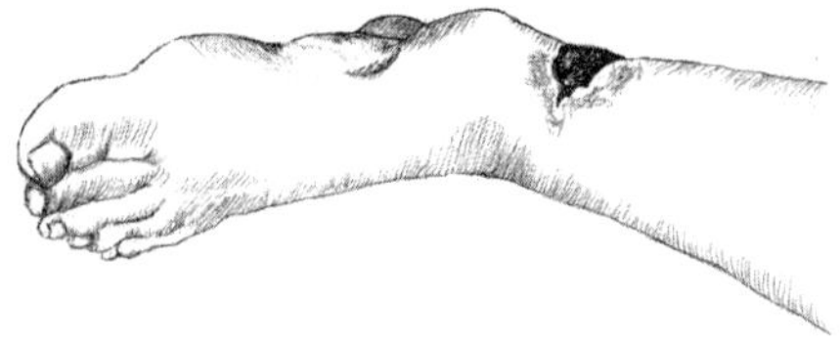

FIG. 32-10. Open ankle fracture-dislocation.

OTHER TREATMENT

Treating Soft-Tissue Injuries

To reduce edema, treat soft-tissue joint injuries with compression dressings and cold packs (usually crushed or cubed ice). Interrupt the cold application every 20 minutes, or more often if the cold causes discomfort.

Hematoma Under the Nail

Drain subungual hematomas if they are painful. Use either a sharp, sterile tool (such as a needle or pin) or a thin wire (such as a paperclip) heated with an open flame. Neither of these requires anesthetizing the digit as long as the "drilling" stops as soon as blood exudes from the hole.

Do not remove the nail to repair the nail bed, even if the hematoma occupies >50% of the nail surface. It uses additional resources and causes increased patient morbidity.[67] The original nail can be used to protect a nail bed after an injury, as can artificial nails if the original nail is gone.

Compression Dressing

For patients with major fracture dislocations who cannot have an immediate operation, apply a Robert Jones dressing to control and minimize edema. Easily improvised, this dressing makes the patient more comfortable and improves surgical results by permitting better visualization of the tissues, in addition to reducing edema and fracture blisters. The technique for applying it is described in Chapter 10 as a treatment for peripheral edema.

Improvised External Fixator

Used for the treatment of complicated lower-leg fractures with soft-tissue damage, an external skeletal fixator can be easily improvised using wood. In each of two wooden boards (3.5 cm × 2 cm × 45 cm), drill holes about 1 cm apart, the same diameter as 5-mm Steinmann pins. The apparatus has greater strength if the holes are drilled across, rather than through, the board's width. The holes in the two boards must line up exactly with each other. Under appropriate local anesthesia or sedation, cleanse the wound and reposition the fracture. Then drill two Steinmann pins through the bone on both sides of the fracture, keeping a safe distance from injured tissues. Apply the boards to both sides of the leg. Place the pins through the holes in the wooden board that most closely match the anatomical position. As soon as the wounds heal, usually within 3 to 4 weeks, remove the external fixator and replace it with a plaster cast. The primary problem with this device is that it is not strong enough to allow walking exercises and weight bearing.[68]

Vacuum Dressing

To make a vacuum (negative-pressure) dressing, pack the wound with soap-free surgical sponges retrieved from single-use scrub brushes. Make holes in a sterile suction tube or in IV tubing with

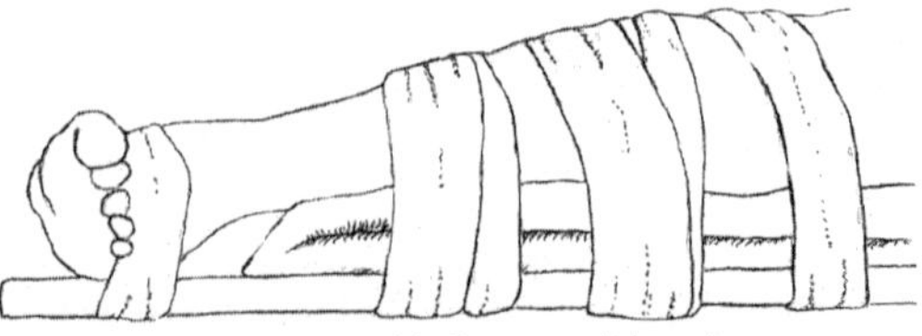

FIG. 32-11. Dupuytren's splint applied to ankle fracture-dislocation.

a small (#15 or #11) scalpel. Place the tubing over the sponges and seal the wound with a plastic adhesive dressing or similar airtight dressing. Connect the tubing to a continuous suction device.[69]

Amputation

Clinicians may need to perform emergency amputations outside a medical facility, either to extricate trapped people or to finish a nearly complete traumatic amputation.

Mass casualty situations may precipitate more amputations than might otherwise occur. As Husum wrote, "Mass casualties are different! Attempts to salvage seriously damaged limbs are time- and staff-consuming; the clinic capacity will influence the reasons to do primary amputation."[70]

Indications

According to the US Army's Medical Corps, the "goals for initial care are to preserve life, prepare the patient for evacuation, and leave the maximum number of options for definitive treatment." A combination of civilian and Medical Corps guidelines result in the following indications for amputation in field settings[71,72]:

1. Partial or complete traumatic amputation.
2. A hypotensive patient with an entrapped extremity who does not respond to initial IV fluids, and extrication will not occur rapidly.
3. A patient with an entrapped extremity that cannot be rapidly extricated and is in imminent danger of additional injury if not quickly extricated.
4. A patient with an entrapped extremity who faces an extended extrication, was initially hypotensive but responded to initial IV fluids, and currently has an adequate blood pressure. (Judgment call; patient participates in decision.)
5. A patient with an entrapped extremity who is hemodynamically normal, but the local experts believe that extrication may not be possible. (Judgment call; patient participates in decision.)

Emergency Prehospital Technique

In a dire emergency when the clinician needs to do an on-scene amputation, use the following guidelines, modified for the immediate situation. If possible, communicate with more experienced surgeons to help make the amputation decision and to guide you through the process.

1. Wear personal protective equipment (PPE), if available.
2. Control the bleeding by pressing on the pressure point, or by using a tourniquet and then tying the vessels.
3. Assess the patient and ensure vascular (IV or intraosseous [IO]) access and a stable airway.
4. Get verbal consent from conscious patients.
5. Give whatever anesthesia is available and safe for the patient. Ketamine (intramuscular [IM] or IV) or an opiate works well. (See Chapters 15 and 16 for more detailed options.) Also, infiltrate the limb with a local anesthetic, although this generally will be less than optimal.
6. Place a tourniquet as distal as possible, but proximal to the planned amputation site. Record the time when the tourniquet is tightened.
7. If available, place sterile towels around the site and secure them with towel clips.
8. Clean the area, with betadine solution if available; let it dry for 2 minutes if there is time.
9. Make an incision around or through what remains of the extremity, cutting all the soft tissue, down to bone.
10. Place a Kelly clamp underneath the bone, using a back and forth motion to allow for further dissection of the tissue. Place a laparotomy pad in the jaws of the Kelly clamp and pull the pad underneath the bone. Grab both ends of the pad, and move it back and forth to allow for further dissection and retraction.
11. If a bone saw is unavailable and a comminuted fracture is not present at the amputation site, the bone can be difficult to remove. Use a carpenter's saw, a sharp chisel, or a straight gouge to cut the bone. An alternative is to make small-caliber drill-holes close to each other around the bone at the level to be amputated, and then manually fracture the bone transversely. Another

option is to make a track in the outer cortex around the entire circumference of the bone by hitting the knife with light hammer blows, and then manually breaking the bone. Then apply a firm pressure dressing to the stump to control any bleeding.[73,74]

12. If a bone saw is available, hold both ends of the laparotomy pad in your left hand, place the saw blade perpendicular to the bone and begin sawing. You will feel release of the bone when you are completely through.
13. Use a sharp blade to cut the remaining soft tissue, completing the amputation.
14. If bleeding continues, place a second tourniquet just above or below the first and tighten it. For additional bleeding, apply direct pressure over the site and then, if necessary, selectively clamp bleeding vessels.
15. Place sterile, saline soaked gauze over the end of the limb and cover it with an Ace bandage.
16. If you can retrieve the amputated limb, place sterile, saline soaked gauze over the end and secure it in place with an elastic bandage. Place the amputated limb in a clean bag and transport to the hospital with the patient; do not place it on ice.[72-74]

Post-Amputation Care

Place a layer of fine mesh gauze over the wound and pack the recess loosely with fluffed gauze. Apply a stockinet over the stump, securing it with tape. Wrap the stump with elastic wraps (Ace bandages) using compression decreasing proximally and applying 5 to 6 lbs of traction. Continued traction results in secondary skin closure over the stump.[76]

Provide analgesics, as available, in sufficient quantities to lessen the patient's postoperative pain. To prevent possible hemorrhage from the surgical site, for the first week post-injury, keep a tourniquet at the patient's bedside and during transport.

While surgeons working in a relatively stable environment may be able to treat post-amputation patients by delayed primary closure, many patients will need to be transferred for definitive treatment. Place these patients in skin traction to leave the wound open and prevent skin retraction. Ideally, skin traction will be maintained throughout the treatment course (Fig. 32.12). One way to maintain skin traction, while also maintaining traction on the residual limb, is by using a cast. The cast should be well padded, with integral skin traction maintained by use of an "outrigger."[75]

SPLINTS AND CASTS

Outpatient treatment of fractures, sprains, and strains, as well as postoperative treatment for various soft-tissue repairs, relies on immobilization to aid the healing process. Improvised immobilizers for extremities can be divided into (a) non-rigid splints, (b) rigid splinting materials that are not suitable for circumferential casting, and (c) casting materials. Casting materials can be used for circumferential casting, and include plaster of Paris and its many alternatives.

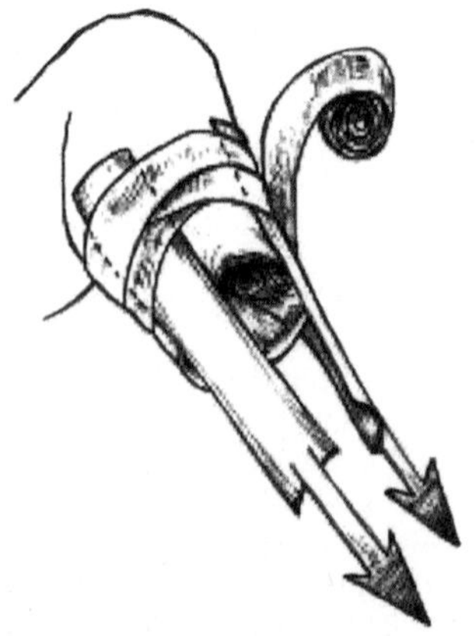

FIG. 32-12. Skin traction after an amputation. *(Source: US Army.[75])*

Non-rigid Splints

Sling (Arm)

A sling is the most basic extremity support. If nothing else is available, improvise a sling by putting the patient's wrist inside his or her shirt and buttoning the buttons around it. For more support, and if using a long-sleeved shirt, pin the sleeve containing the affected arm to the shoulder area on the opposite side of the shirt. Alternatively, double up the bottom of a short-sleeve shirt or a T-shirt over the forearm and pin it to both shoulder areas of the shirt.

Make a more formal sling from any available material. A strip of material pinned so there is a loop around the wrist and around the neck makes a "collar-cuff" sling. This sling is ideal when the patient can tolerate shoulder movement or when an elderly patient uses it to avoid a frozen shoulder. Alternatively, use any strip of cloth, webbing, or belt.

Buddy Taping

One of the simplest effective methods of splinting an injured finger or toe is to tape it to the adjacent digit. The key to success is to put absorbent cloth or gauze between the digits before taping and to change the material at least three times a day, or any time it gets wet, to avoid macerating the tissues. Keep it on until it feels better without it than with it.

Buddy taping can also be used for humerus fractures in infants. Bandage the arm to the torso and it will quickly heal. (Consider child abuse in these cases.)

A field-expedient method of stabilizing long-bone fractures in a lower extremity is to buddy tape the legs together, preferably with some padding between them. This may be more comfortable for a patient than a rigid splint.

Pillow Splints

Make splints for joint fractures, dislocations, or other injuries from pillows, blankets, sleeping bags, sleeping pads, or any similar items (Figs. 32-13 and 32-14). Wrap the pillow or multiple layers of other items around the injured part. Secure it tightly with any bandaging material. This is often a more comfortable method of splinting than using traditional materials.

Sandbag Splints

Effectively splint an extremity using a garbage bag, fanny pack, or similar soft-sided container filled with sand or dirt. Mold it to the extremity and tape or bandage it in place. Because this is heavy, the patient tends to move the extremity less than with a pillow splint.

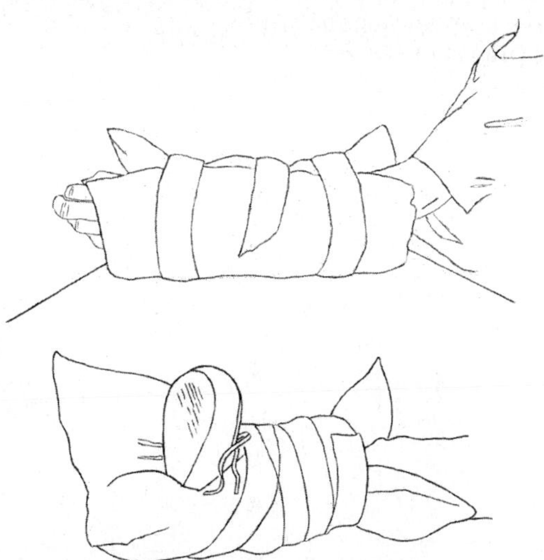

FIG. 32-13. Pillow splints on forearm and ankle.

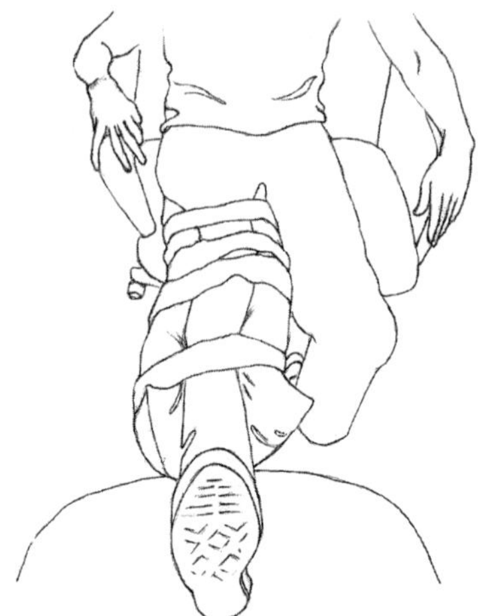

FIG. 32-14. Pillow splint on knee.

Heel Pad

Place a pad made from thick foam with a hole cut in the center in a shoe or boot beneath the heel to help ameliorate pain in the calcaneal area. Long thought to be due to exostosis (extra bone growth), this pain is probably due to nonspecific inflammation.

Rigid Splints Not for Circumferential Casting

Fixation splints may be made of plaster of Paris; celluloid; pasteboard; wood; stiffened felt, paper, or leather; gutta-percha; wire; polyvinyl chloride (PVC) pipe; aluminum; or other available materials. Keep splints in place with bandages or other similar ties.

Metal

Caused by disruption of the extensor tendon to the distal phalanx, a mallet or dropped finger can be managed by splinting the affected joint in full extension with a paperclip for 8 weeks. Have the patient wear the splint at all times. Pad the paperclip with soft cloth and tape it to the dorsal surface of the finger so the patient can still use his or her digit. A disposable plastic spoon or a section of a Popsicle stick can also be used.[77]

A metal can makes a useful splint for a broken wrist or to help support an injured knee or ankle. Carefully open the can at both ends, cut it up the side, and tape the sharp edges so they don't injure the patient. Then bend the metal to fit the patient's wrist, enclose in cloth for padding, and wrap in place with a bandage or tape. Likewise, a car's hood support is just the right length to make a long leg splint. Bandage it onto the injured leg.

Splints made of galvanized wire or tin mesh (Fig. 32-15) can easily be fashioned to support arm, knee, or ankle injuries. "They can be readily made from sheets of wire by taking a strip of

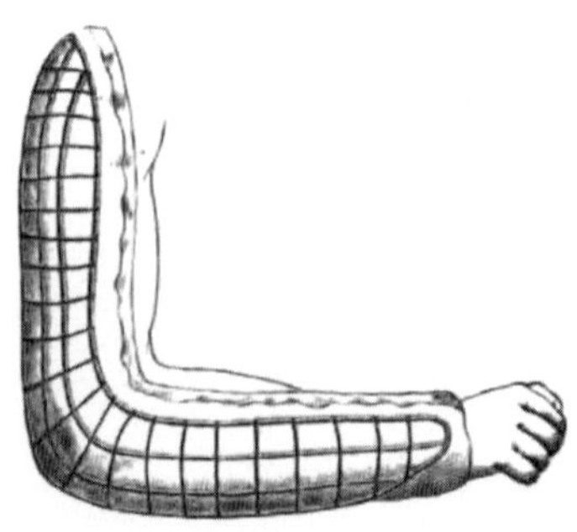

FIG. 32-15. Wire splint.

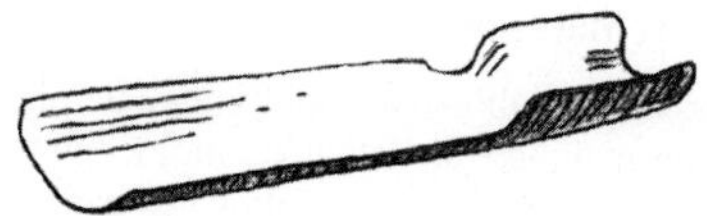

FIG. 32-16. Forearm splint made from plastic drainpipe.

suitable size and cutting it partly through at the angle, and tying together the meshes which overlap where it is bent."[78]

Plastic Pipe

Durable splints have also been made from pieces of appropriately sized PVC drainpipes (Fig. 32-16). First, saw them in half, and then shape them so they conform to the extremity. To do this, heat the pipe by placing it in boiling water or by using a welding torch or other low-intensity flame. (See the "Heating PVC Pipe" section in Chapter 30 for additional instructions.) If a flame is used, take care not to burn the plastic or to inhale the toxic fumes.[79]

Tongue Depressors

The lowly tongue depressor (or Popsicle stick) can be useful as splinting material in many situations and may also be used to make a metatarsal arch bar. These remarkably simple devices lessen toe pain, especially from injuries to the large toe (hallux), and pain from metatarsal fractures or pain over the metatarsal heads or sole of the foot. This can be invaluable when treating patients who must keep walking to survive, such as on a trek or in combat. The metatarsal arch bar functions by eliminating much of the stress of rotating and pushing off from the forefoot and hallux—a key part of walking. An arch bar to use over shoes is easy to make. (Of course, some patients may not be able to obtain shoes.)

Make an arch bar by breaking or cutting three tongue depressors or other material to the width of the widest part of the shoe or boot. Tape the tongue depressors together. Then tape the entire piece across the sole of the shoe at its widest part by wrapping the tape around the bar and outside the shoe (Fig. 32-17). If the patient has more than one pair of shoes, it is easy to re-tape the arch bar onto a different shoe or to make another bar for that shoe.

Pediatric Fracture Treatment

Removable splints may be as good as casts for minor, or "buckle," fractures of the wrist, particularly in toddlers and preschool infants. These splints even allow for the final removal at home with no further follow-up. Removable splints, either plastic or plaster, generally keep the fractures aligned as well as casts but provide greater comfort and less restriction, allowing children to bathe and participate in other activities.[80] Some orthopedic surgeons, however, are concerned that very small children will not keep their splints in place.

Reverse Sugar Tong Splint

A sugar tong splint is ideal for splinting fractures of the radius, ulna, or wrist. However, it may be difficult to apply without assistance. That is where the reverse splint comes in handy. Cut the plaster strip needed for a sugar tong splint. Then, midway down its length, cut it almost in half, leaving a small piece that will suspend the splint from the web space between the thumb and index finger. Apply the splint "in reverse," with the open ends at the elbow, which can then be folded over themselves.

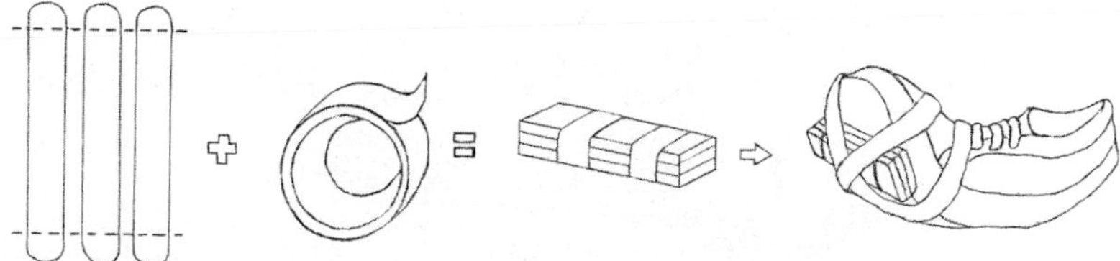

FIG. 32-17. Metatarsal arch bar made from tongue depressors.

Rigid Circumferential Casting Material

Because of its lightness, porosity, and ability to rapidly harden, plaster of Paris is the best, most commonly available material for making splints that are molded to the body. There are many ways to use plaster of Paris; some are discussed in the following paragraphs. In addition, there are a multitude of alternative materials that can be used to make casts. For how to make plaster bandages for casting and splinting, see the "Making Plaster of Paris Bandages" section in this chapter.

Some Ways to Use Plaster of Paris

Plaster Box

If no other option is available, try this old method to immobilize an extremity using liquid plaster of Paris. Make a box of cardboard or wood into which the extremity (usually the forearm) will fit. Coat the skin with oil or lubricant or, better yet, wrap it with thin cloth to protect the skin from the heat and irritation from the plaster, and to prevent it from adhering to the skin when removed. Pour enough plaster into the box to surround the arm completely. When the plaster sets, remove the box. These casts are too heavy and cumbersome for patients to be ambulatory and must be removed with a mallet and chisel.[81]

Plaster Cream

An alternative method that may be easier to use than preparing rolled plaster bandages is to immerse large pieces of cloth in a plaster cream (Fig. 32-18). Prepare this cream by sifting dry plaster into water (three parts water and four parts plaster of Paris). Take previously cut splint/cast material and either soak it in the cream or spread the cream onto it just before applying it to the limb. Note that the plaster cream must be thoroughly worked into the material.[82,83]

Hamilton described the use of plaster cream at New York's Bellevue Hospital in the 19th century: "The usual practice has been to envelop the limb with a dry roller, and to apply the plaster with a paint brush as the successive turns of the roller are laid upon the limb. It hardens very quickly, and in this regard it has an advantage over flour paste or starch; but it is heavy, and not so generally accessible, and for this reason its use is more restricted."[84]

Making Plaster of Paris Bandages

Commercial plaster bandages are excellent, but they may not be available due to general scarcity or cost. Homemade plaster bandages are about one-tenth as expensive. To make them:

1. Get plaster of Paris (dried calcium sulfate; or use hemihydrate gypsum plaster). Although it is readily available as a building material, the best type for casts and splints is dental casting plaster. (Other types work, but they set more slowly.) Because it becomes inert if exposed to moisture or cold, keep the plaster in a tightly sealed container and, if possible, in a warm, dry location. To get plaster to set more quickly, add one-twentieth-part Portland cement (1:20 mixture), which may also strengthen the cast and make it lighter.[86] Mixing the plaster with water in the proportion of 75 to 100 by weight and adding two parts of boiled starch may produce a similar result.[84]

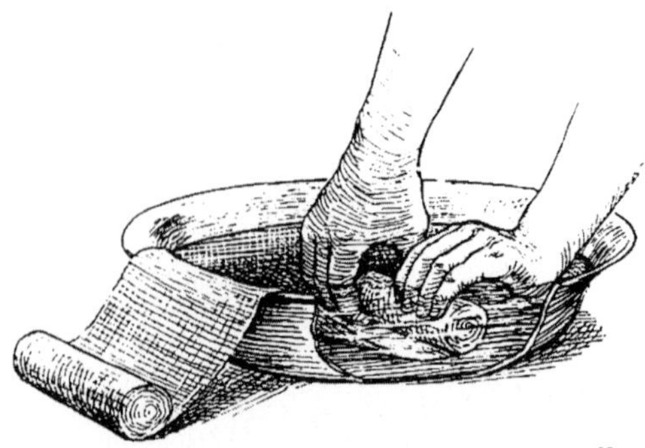

FIG. 32-18. Wetting bandage in plaster cream. *(Reproduced from Ware.[85])*

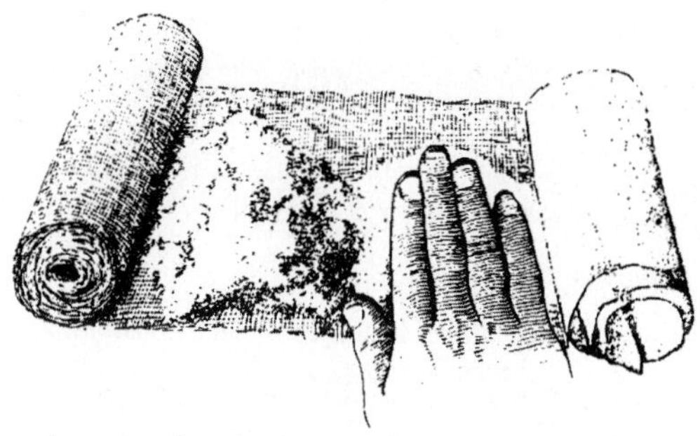

FIG. 32-19. Rubbing plaster into bandage material. *(Reproduced from Ware.[85])*

2. Obtain bandage material. Crinoline, a high-quality open-mesh cloth, or muslin (30-35 threads/inch) works best, but good quality gauze with about 8 to 10 holes/cm^2 (20 holes/inch^2) also works well. If necessary, cheesecloth also can be used.[86,87] One group in India finally found that suitable gauze has about 16 threads per inch; and that the thickness is also important. If the gauze is too thin, it does not hold the plaster powder; if it is too thick, the plaster takes too long to set and dry.[88]
3. If using gauze or cheesecloth, dip it into a weak laundry starch solution or a bucket of rice water (left over from cooking rice) and let it dry. This helps maintain the bandage's shape.[88]
4. Cut the cloth into strips of the desired length and width. Some workers have found that 12-foot lengths are easy to handle; the width will depend on the need, but generally 4 or 6 inches are sufficient.[88]
5. Rub plaster powder into the cloth by unrolling a portion of the bandage on a dry table with a smooth top and gently but firmly rubbing the powder into the cloth mesh (Fig. 32-19). Rub the plaster in by hand or scrape it in with a straight-edged knife or stick. It is important that neither too much nor too little plaster be used; the proper amount is just enough to thinly cover the fabric mesh.[86] As one section is covered in plaster, roll it up and begin the same process with the next section until the entire roll has been powdered.
6. If you are making many plaster bandages, such as for a hospital or large clinic, a simple plaster application machine is worth constructing (Fig. 32-20). Developed in India, the large inclined tray, with plaster powder at three places, allows workers to easily impregnate the bandages with plaster as they are pulled across the top. Construct an 8- to 10-inch-wide tray, on a base that is inclined at 15 degrees and that has an open-top catch box at the end. Stretch three strands of #8 rubber tubing (8-mm diameter) across the tray to hold the bandage down and distribute the plaster powder. Place strips of wood along the sides to hold the tubing in place and help keep the plaster on the tray. Place a pile of plaster powder above each length of rubber tubing. When the bandage material is pulled under the taut tubing, it becomes impregnated with plaster powder; the open box in the base will catch any loose plaster.[88]

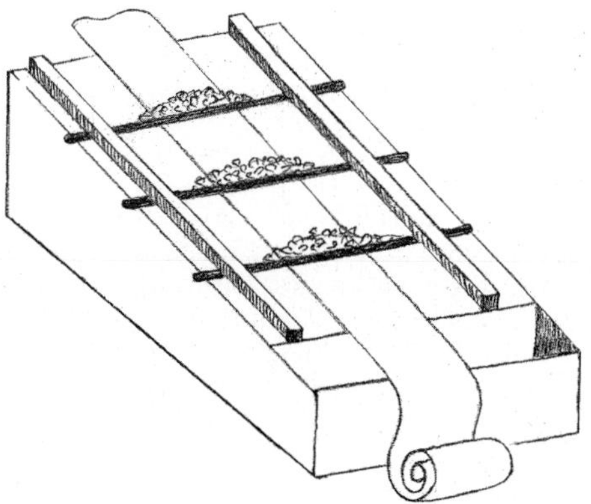

FIG. 32-20. Plaster-application device.

7. As the bandage is finished, loosely roll it up. Use immediately or store it in a dry place for future use. Be careful not to roll it too tight because this will prevent the water from penetrating it sufficiently when the bandage is dipped in water before application.[86,87]
8. To store premade bandages, roll them loosely. If you need to make slabs for splinting, double the plaster over itself in strips, wrap in old newspapers or plastic bags, and put these in an airtight container. Do not prepare too many at a time. They can absorb moisture and harden.[89]

Applying Homemade Plaster Bandages

A common problem with homemade plaster bandages is that the gauze does not hold enough powdered plaster. If enough plaster is in the bandages, rubbing each wet bandage layer into the next should make the threads of cloth disappear into the smooth, plaster surface. If this is not the case, there is not enough plaster and it will not set hard. A possible solution is to try the method used by Antonius Mathijsen, a 19th-century Dutch Army physician. Rather than soaking them in water, he used a wet sponge or brush to moisten homemade plaster-impregnated bandages as he applied them to the patient, rubbing them by hand until they hardened.[81] Another useful trick is to have some dry plaster powder ready while casting, then sprinkle it over each layer of bandage and rub it smooth with your wet hands. Add more to the final layer and rub it in to form a polished surface.

To reduce the amount of plaster lost into the water, dip the bandage gently into water and then take it out and let it drip. If you must squeeze it, hold the ends of the roll and squeeze gently toward the center. To speed drying, use hot water or else add salt or zinc oxide to the water. If the plaster has been exposed to the air before use, dry it in an oven; this may make it more useable and speed its setting.[83]

Homemade plaster casts are heavier than casts made with proprietary bandages, but they work well in all circumstances and are much cheaper.[88]

Improvised and commercial plaster bandages can be made water resistant by painting the dried plaster of Paris with a mixture of shellac dissolved in alcohol, or by varnishing them or pouring melted wax on them.[83,90]

Alternatives to Plaster of Paris

Although plaster of Paris is the preferred casting material, it may not be available in any particular situation. There are a number of alternative materials that may be used for casts. Most have the disadvantage that they take a long time to harden.

SAND

In the early 1800s, German physicians treated leg fractures by aligning them in a long box that was then filled with firmly packed moist sand.[81] Unfortunately, this is not a very practical method, because the patient must remain immobile while the fracture heals.

THICK CARDBOARD

Louis Jean Seutin, the Belgian Army's chief surgeon who fought against Napoleon, developed a rigid splint made of cardboard pieces that conformed to the injured extremity after being moistened, and which were then wrapped with wet bandages that had been soaked in a solution of laundry starch. It required 2 to 3 days to dry, but this was shortened to about 6 hours when the 19th-century French anatomist/surgeon Alfred-Armand-Louis-Marie Velpeau replaced the starch with dextrin (i.e., starch gum, vegetable gum).[91]

In his 1899 text, Stimson wrote[92]

> Pasteboard [thick cardboard] is used by softening one or two strips of suitable size by immersion in hot water, and then molding them to the limb by binding them on snugly with a roller bandage. Temporary support must usually be given by other splints until the pasteboard has become hard by drying. When it is necessary to bend the pasteboard at a sharp angle, cuts should be made in it in suitable directions and places and the overlapping portions stitched together. Leather and felt are prepared in the same manner.

PAPIER MÂCHÉ

Folklore abounds with tales of using papier mâché as a splint or a cast. Our test showed that it was time consuming and extremely messy; the resulting casts were heavy and took from many hours to days to dry. Papier mâché is useless for orthopedic purposes, but might be a fun activity for children.

TRACTION

Traction is generally applied to leg fractures, particularly the femur or hip. It can, however, also be applied to the arm or the finger.

General principles for using traction on the leg are to apply 10 to 15 lbs of weight, or the amount needed to reduce the affected leg to the same length as the other leg. Always take care to ensure that traction does not compromise the extremity's pulses, perfusion, or neurological status, especially in the foot below the ankle hitch. Traction should also maintain anatomic position, including reducing any rotation and angulation.

Improvised traction includes many of the methods taught in first-aid classes, including using ski or tent poles, canoe paddles, ice axes taped together at the handles, a piece of wood, a tree branch, or, most commonly, the foot of a litter. In reality, with many of these makeshift devices, it may be difficult to secure them proximally at the hip to ensure that they provide adequate counter-traction and do not cause the patient pain. Ankle hitches often go over the boot or shoe, and can be made from webbing or rope as long as they do not compromise blood flow to the foot. Tighten traction by winding the ankle traction with any short, rigid piece of equipment, such as a sheathed knife, wooden ruler, or solid stick. Once tightened, secure it so it does not unwind. Check this periodically, because the patient may move and loosen the traction or the neurovascular status could become compromised.

Improvised traction also includes techniques that can be used in medical facilities that lack either clinicians comfortable with doing invasive orthopedic procedures for traction or the necessary orthopedic equipment.

Improvised Traction in the Field

Sock/Plaster Boot Traction

The US Army described a field-expedient traction method (Fig. 32-21) during World War I:

> An excellent traction may be obtained by a light-weight army sock. The lower leg, ankle, and foot, with the exception of the toes and the plantar surface, are painted with glue [cyanoacrylate can be used] and the sock slipped on. The toe of the sock is cut off and a piece of light splint wood or the ladder splint material, cut the length of the foot, is inserted between the sole and the sock. Traction may then be made on this by means of pieces of bandage or cord passed through the sock and around the wood or the rods of the ladder splinting.[93]

Rather than gluing the sock to the foot (a rather drastic measure), after placing the splint to be used for traction, cover the sock with plaster or, if that is unavailable, a non-stretch bandage.

Traction Using a Crutch

A crutch makes an excellent traction device (Fig. 32-22). Use a crutch that is 8 to 12 inches longer than the affected leg (or adjusted to that length); measure it against the good leg. Remove the

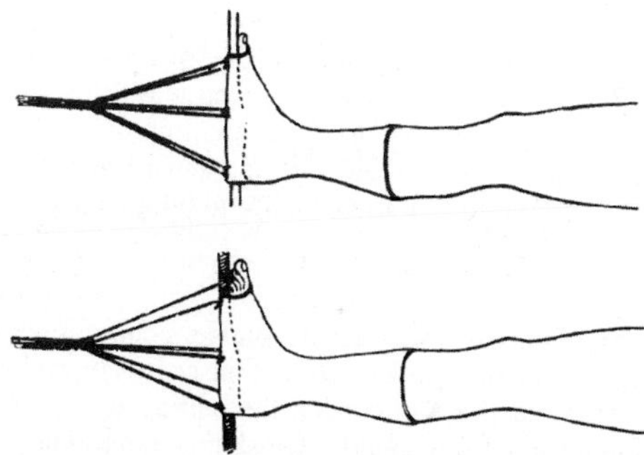

FIG. 32-21. Traction using socks. *(Reproduced from US Orthopedic Council.[93])*

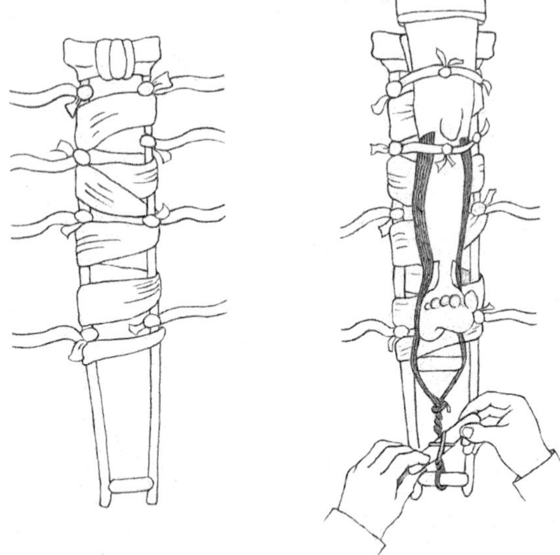

FIG. 32-22. Traction from crutch.

rubber piece from the bottom (ground end) of the crutch, and securely tape the axillary pad to the crutch. Remove the handgrip and screw it into the lowest hole at the bottom of the crutch. Securely tie four pieces of gauze, fabric, or belting material, beginning just below the axillary pad, on each side of the crutch. These should be evenly spaced and opposite each other, because they will be used to secure the leg to the splint. Next wind gauze around the crutch to support the leg. Position the crutch/splint under the patient's legs, so that the top (padded) end of the crutch lies under the ischial tuberosity, with the other end extending at least 12 inches beyond the foot.

Apply ankle traction by securing a wide piece of tape to either side of the leg, from just below the knee and extending past the end of the crutch. Use tincture of benzoin, if available, so the tape will adhere more securely to the leg. Use wide tape or an elastic bandage around the lower leg to help hold the long pieces in place. Place some gauze or fabric over both ankles, so the tape doesn't stick to them. Just below the foot, cut a small hole in each piece of tape and insert three tongue blades or small dowels through the holes to hold the two pieces of tape apart. Tape these tongue blades to the long pieces of tape. Then, below the tongue blades, bring the two long pieces of tape together and firmly attach the end of the tape to the crutch handle at the bottom of the splint. Cut a hole midway in this joined piece of tape and insert three tongue blades or an equivalent sized dowel. Twist these to provide traction on the leg. When adequate traction is achieved, tape the tongue blades to the sides of the crutch. Secure the leg to the splint with the fabric tied to each side of the crutch.[94]

Field Traction for Femur/Hip Fractures

In prehospital and austere settings, the potential benefits of traction splints include decreasing pain and potential bleeding into the thigh, stabilizing and realigning fractures, decreasing soft tissue injury, and avoiding progression to an open fracture. Improvised traction splints may need to be made from a variety of materials and are part of standard first aid training. All appear to provide stability and patient comfort when used with 5- to 6-kg weights (use saline bags).[95]

Skin Traction

The vast majority of hip and femur fracture patients in poor countries are treated in district hospitals, where the equipment and surgical expertise to insert traction pins does not exist. Skin traction requires pressure on the skin to maintain the pulling force across the bone. Apply a maximum of 5 kg of weight using this method if the skin is in reasonable condition. More than 5 kg of weight causes the tightly wrapped strapping to slip, resulting in skin excoriation with blistering and pressure sores. If the straps are wrapped more tightly to prevent slipping, it can cause a compartment syndrome.[87]

If >5 kg of weight is needed to control the fracture, use an alternate form of traction.

Do not apply traction to skin with abrasions, lacerations, surgical wounds, or ulcers. In addition, do not apply traction to areas with loss of sensation, or in patients with peripheral vascular disease or a tape allergy.

Technique[87]

1. Clean the limb with soap and water and dry it. Gather adhesive tapes, traction cords, spreader bar, and foam or other material to protect the malleoli.
2. Use adhesive bandages in place of standard traction bandages. Shave the skin and use benzoin to increase bandage adhesion to the skin. Then wrap a nonadhesive bandage around the extremity. Wrapping an adhesive bandage can make it too tight.
3. Measure the appropriate length of adhesive strapping, and place it on a level surface with the adhesive side up. The tape should extend on both sides of the limb up to, but not above, the fracture.
4. Place a piece of wood in a loop of the long wraps to keep the bandage from rubbing against the malleoli and to provide a site to secure the weights for traction.
5. Gently elevate the limb off the bed while applying longitudinal traction. Apply the strapping to the medial and lateral sides of the limb, allowing the spreader to project 15 cm below the sole of the foot.
6. Pad bony areas with felt or cotton and wrap crepe or ordinary gauze bandage firmly over the strapping.
7. Elevate the end of the bed, and attach a traction cord through the spreader with enough weight, up to 5 kg, to reduce and align the fracture (Fig. 32-23).
8. The traction cord can be any strong cord or wire. If the area that the cord drapes over is not smooth, attach a 60-cc syringe barrel to the site and run the cord through it. The weight can be bags of water or sand, bricks, or other heavy objects. Be certain that, whenever possible, the weights are measured, not just estimated. (The weight of water is 1 kg [2.2 lb] per liter; if you know the volume, you can figure out the weight.)
9. Skin traction also can be used on the arm (e.g., Dunlop's traction for supracondylar fractures) (Fig. 32-24).

"Gallows" Traction in Children

In children weighing <12 kg, vertical or "gallows" traction using skin traction works well for femur fractures. Both legs are generally kept in traction taut enough to just raise the buttocks off the bed (Fig. 32-25).

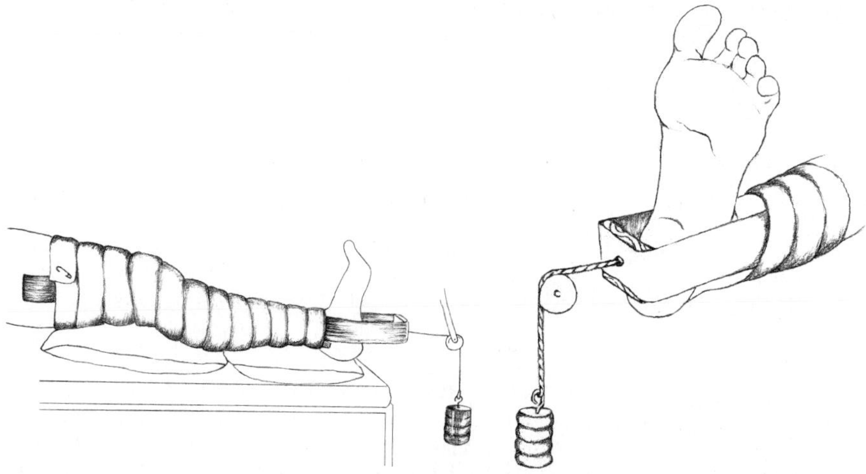

FIG. 32-23. Skin (Buck's) traction of leg. Overview (left) and close-up of weight connection (right).

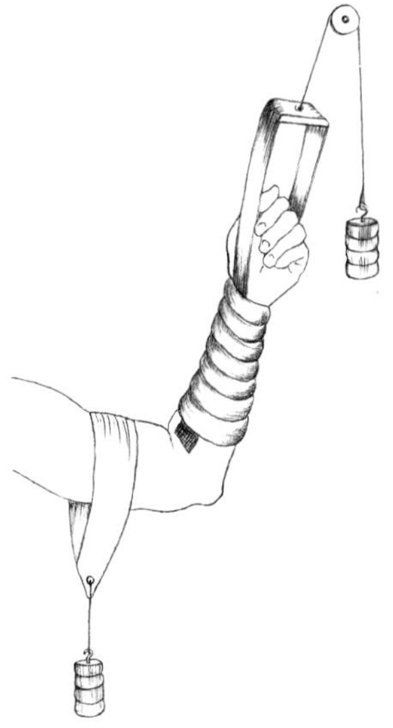

FIG. 32-24. Dunlop's traction.

Another way to treat fractures in newborns and small children, and certainly the simplest, "consists in fixing the thighs, strongly flexed upon the abdomen, by means of a broad band of strapping passed round the back and thigh."[96]

Skin Traction in Adults

There are several makeshift skin traction devices for adults. Figures 32-26 and 32-27 show the easily constructed Volkmann's apparatus, which allows the foot piece to slide as weight is applied. Obtain counter-traction by raising the foot of the bed and using a wooden block to stabilize the uninjured limb.

Traction Using Plaster

Similar in principle to skin traction, using plaster has fewer restrictions and can accommodate more weight without causing complications (Fig. 32-28). Taylor described the technique[98]:

> [Apply plaster] to the leg, which is fastened by buckles to a stirrup carrying a cord passing over a pulley to a weight, the patient being in bed ... The adhesive plasters should be evenly applied nearly to the groin; if they do not reach high enough injurious strain comes

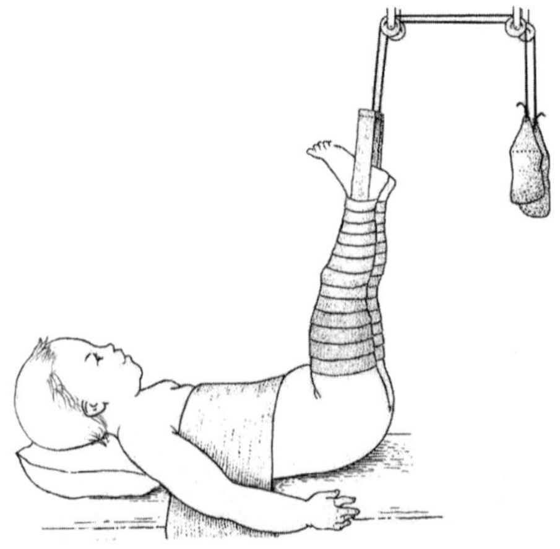

FIG. 32-25. Gallows traction.

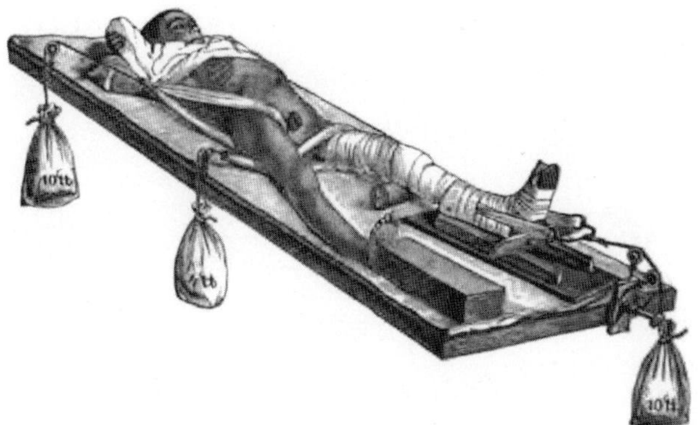

FIG. 32-26. Rudimentary leg traction device. *(Reproduced from Helferich.[97])*

> upon the knee. If the thigh is flexed or adducted, the leg is placed upon an inclined plane, and the weight and pulley so arranged as to pull in the line of the deformity; the knee should be slightly flexed. Symptoms are frequently aggravated by pulling against the hip deformity. As the muscles gradually relax to the traction, the pulley is lowered until the pull is in line with the bed and the body. Five or six pounds in a sand or shot bag, flat iron, or brick are usually sufficient for a child; ten or twelve pounds for an adult. It is important that the feet should not touch the foot of the bed or the weight touch the floor; a metal bedstead is the most convenient, and should be long enough to allow six or eight inches space below the foot; the mattress should be hard to prevent sagging. If necessary, thin boards may be placed under the mattress. To prevent the patient from being drawn downward by the pull of the weight, the foot of the bed should be elevated six to eight inches, or the patient should have counter-traction from perineal straps attached to a frame or to the bed. . . . In addition to raising the foot of the bed, a towel is pinned around the patient below the ribs, and the back of this is fastened to the head of the bed by a bandage.

Plaster of Paris traction is also useful to treat femur fractures when you need to quickly ambulate the patient, to treat patients with delirium tremens, or to treat young children. Ambulatory treatment of fractures of the femur has many detractors, but one method of doing it with some success is to ambulate patients using a Thomas splint. The Thomas splint is commonly available worldwide. In addition to its usefulness for treating femur fractures in adults and children, it can also be used as part of "ambulatory" fracture treatment after the patient has been in traction for 3 or 4 weeks. Do not attempt to do this if the fracture site is in the upper one-third of the femur.[99]

Traction Using Pins

Skeletal traction is commonly used in austere settings, because it requires few resources. The main drawbacks to this method are prolonged hospital stays (averaging 60 days), a reduction in knee range of movement, and an increased incidence of thromboemoblic events.

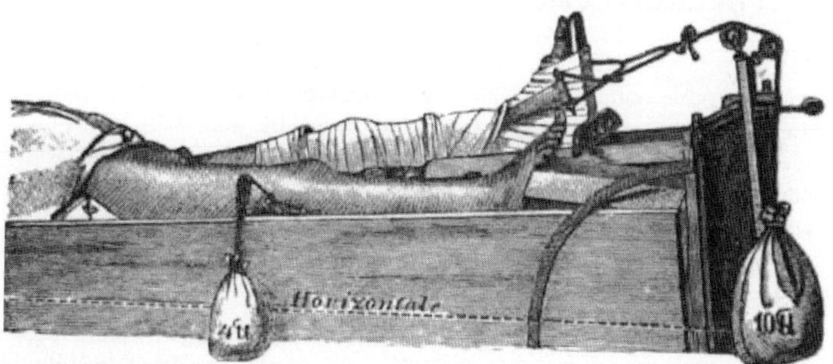

FIG. 32-27. Leg traction when there is contracture at the knee. *(Reproduced from Helferich.[97])*

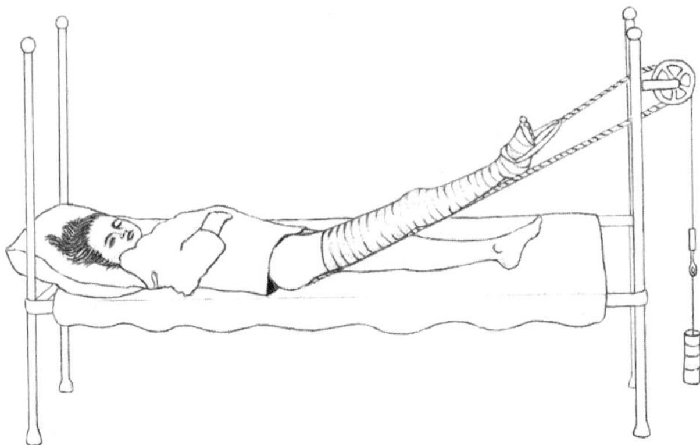

FIG. 32-28. Traction using plaster.

Husum and colleagues recommend using an ordinary awl and drill to make a hole for a traction pin. The pin itself can be a thick welding rod inserted by careful blows with a hammer. Others have suggested that any sterilized strong wire will work. Apply corks against the skin at the rod ends and attach plain ropes tied to sandbags for traction. For olecranon traction (arm fractures) and trochanter traction (pelvic acetabular fractures), Husum recommends that carpenter's eye screws be used for about 4 to 6 weeks, although they may cause some irritation.[74]

For lower extremity fractures, apply a weight equivalent to about 10% of the patient's body weight, usually 5 to 10 kg. Once the need for fracture distraction passes (usually one week), reduce any weight >5 kg by 2.5 kg.

Those with experience in this technique in austere settings recommend the following[100]:

1. Do not delay treatment to obtain radiographs; apply initial and definitive traction, and initiate physical therapy.
2. Apply skeletal traction on the day of admission. If this is not possible, apply temporary skin traction. Use a tibial pin rather than a femoral pin.
3. Use an anti-rotation splint beginning when traction is applied and leave it on at least until the fracture feels stiff. One way to do this is to place the ankle in a plaster boot with a horizontal bar to prevent rotation. This can also be made from wood (Fig. 32-29).
4. Have the patient clean the pin sites with cotton and alcohol twice daily.
5. Intensive physiotherapy should focus on the quadriceps.
6. Use mechanical thromboprophylaxis, because this may be all that is available. One method is to combine ipsilateral ankle exercises and contralateral full-limb exercises with quads physiotherapy.
7. Discharge patients when the fracture demonstrates clinical and radiological union. Keep them non-weight-bearing on crutches for at least 6 more weeks.

MANAGEMENT OF COMPLEX FRACTURES

Pseudoarthrosis

When absolutely no other option is available, treat fractures of the neck of the femur by promoting the development of a pseudoarthrosis (false joint). Inject the joint with 5 mL of 2% lidocaine, and encourage the patient to walk with crutches or a walker. The claim is that, while the result will not be perfect, it will be better than traction or inexpert nailing.[102] This treatment method is foreign to most medical standards.

FRACTURE HEALING TIMES

Healing time is the generally expected interval of time for physiological wound repair following an injury or surgery. This differs from the time to overcome injury-related disability, that is, the

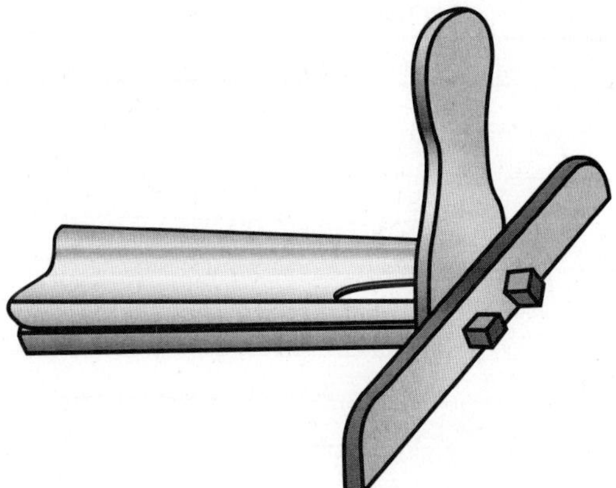

FIG. 32-29. Wooden nonrotation attachment for traction. *(Reproduced from Helferich.[101])*

time required to return to pre-injury activity levels. The time to overcome the disability is always longer than the healing time.

Fractures take varying lengths of time to heal, depending on the patient's age, physical condition, simultaneous disease or injury, and overlying soft-tissue damage. Table 32-3 shows estimated healing times in patients who do not have open reductions and fixation of their fractures.

ANALGESIA

Trigger Point Injections

This is easy: Do not bother. There is no rationale for, or benefit from, injecting the so-called trigger points, even though this has often been the cornerstone of myofascial pain treatment.[103] How you explain this to the patient who has been receiving injections for years is another matter.

Intra-Articular Injections

When oral analgesics are not readily available, intra-articular injections may be used. The injections are relatively easy to do at the knee, elbow, shoulder, and any joint that is dislocated. However, they are not very good at providing immediate analgesia.

Although immediate analgesic effects may not be significant, intra-articular morphine injections can result in up to 3 days of analgesia due to its low lipid solubility and the joint's low blood flow.[104] Intra-articular morphine instillation may also reduce postoperative pain; clonidine (1 to 2 micrograms/kilogram [mcg/kg]) adds to morphine's analgesic effect. Adding an injectable NSAID, however, is not effective.[105] After arthroscopy, the addition of bupivacaine 0.25% (20 to 30 mL) into the knee joint provides significant pain relief.

Regional Blocks and Other Analgesics

See Chapters 15 and 16 for the variety of analgesia available to fracture patients. Note particularly the use of hypnosis and the iliofascial block for hip and femur fractures.

Postoperative Infusions of Local Anesthetics

When local anesthetics are more readily available than other analgesics, postoperative infusions of local anesthetics can reduce pain. Local anesthetics provide relief following bone graft harvest when infused into the cavity made in the anterior superior iliac spine. At the end of surgery, place the infusion catheter (usually an epidural catheter) in the bed of the bone graft donor site in proximity to the periosteum. Inject local anesthetic, usually 0.25% bupivacaine, through the catheter either intermittently (10 mL q6hr) or by continuous infusion at 10 mL/hr. Clamp any

TABLE 32-3 Average Fracture Healing Times (No Surgery)

Fracture	Weeks[a]
Complex facial fractures	16-26
Clavicle	6-8; Child 4
Humerus	6-26
Elbow	6
Forearm	6
Distal radius (wrist)	6
Carpal bones	6-20
Metacarpal	4-6
Mallet finger	6-8
Phalanges (finger/toe)	4-6
Vertebral body compression (any level)	12-36
Spinal fracture	52
Pelvis (acetabulum stable)	12-26
Pelvis (one fracture)	12-26
Pelvis (two or more rami)	12-52
Hip (non-displaced impacted)	8-12
Hip displaced (no surgery)	26-52
Femoral shaft	10-12
Tibia	26-36
Ankle-trimalleolar	8
Talus	6-8
Metatarsal	6-26
Calcaneus	12-36

[a]Healing times vary widely. Open (compound) fractures, those in patients with poor nutrition, and those in elderly patients generally take longer to heal.

Data from Palmer,[106] *STEP MANUAL*,[107] and *New Brunswick General Guidelines for Expected Healing Times*.[108]

vacuum drainage tube during the intermittent boluses. Local anesthetics have provided analgesia when infused into the subacromial space after acromioplasty and rotator cuff repair. Insert the catheter close to the incision site and infuse 0.25% bupivacaine 2 mL/hr or 2% lidocaine 2 mL/hr.[105]

REHABILITATION

Angle Measurement Using a Goniometer

A goniometer measures a joint's angle during its range of motion. It can also be used on radiographs to measure the angle of fracture deformities. Acutely, the clinician can use it to assess the joint's movement and, during rehabilitation, to document improvement in range of motion. Easily construct a goniometer using a piece of wood, such as a ruler, with a hole drilled in one end (Fig. 32-30). Cut a circular piece of cardboard and mark degree gradations (0 to 350 degrees) in 10-degree increments around the side. Punch a hole in the center of the cardboard, and cement it to the wood with the 0-degree mark over the wood and the hole in the cardboard fitting over the hole in the wood. Then tie a string to the hole. The wood is placed parallel with the extremity

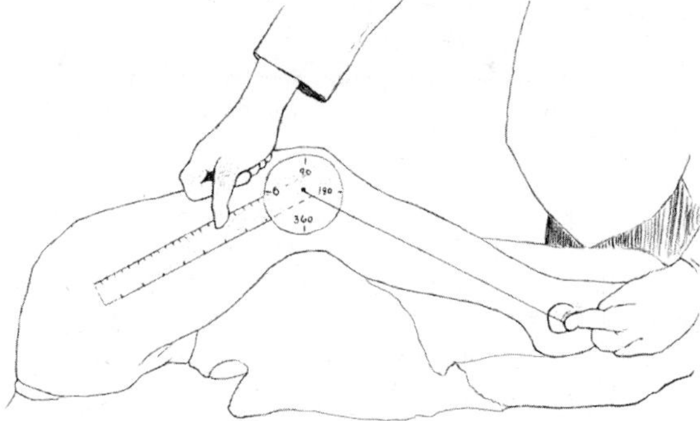

FIG. 32-30. Makeshift goniometer.

above the joint and the string follows the extremity below the joint. The string should align with the angle of flexion/extension.[109]

REFERENCES

1. Mock C, Lormand JD, Goosen J, et al. *Guidelines for Essential Trauma Care*. Geneva, Switzerland: World Health Organization; 2004:36.
2. Ault A. Sprains, strains are top reasons for adult ED visits. *ACEP News*. 2008;27(5):33.
3. Mock C, Lormand JD, Goosen J, et al. *Guidelines for Essential Trauma Care*. Geneva, Switzerland: World Health Organization; 2004:39.
4. Foote EM. *A Text-book of Minor Surgery*. New York, NY: Appleton; 1912:363-368.
5. Hamilton FH. *The Principles and Practice of Surgery*. 2nd ed. New York, NY: William Wood & Co.; 1879:236-237.
6. Joint Theater Trauma System Clinical Practice Guideline. *Compartment Syndrome (CS) and the Role of Fasciotomy in Extremity War Wounds*. US Military, March 2012:1.
7. The Remote, Austere, Wilderness and Third World Medicine Discussion Board Moderators. *Survival and Austere Medicine: An Introduction*. 2nd ed. 2005:93-94. http://www.aussurvivalist.com/downloads/AM%20Final%202.pdf. Accessed June 8, 2007.
8. Peltier LF. The diagnosis of fractures of the hip and femur by auscultatory percussion. *Clin Orthop Relat Res*. 1977;123:9-11.
9. Colwell JC, Berg EH. Auscultation as an important aid to the diagnosis of fractures. *Surg Gynecol Obstet*. 1958;106:713-714.
10. Carter MC. A reliable sign of fractures the hip or pelvis. *N Engl J Med*. 1981;305:1220.
11. Stimson LA. *A Practical Treatise on Fractures and Dislocations*. New York, NY: Lea & Febiger; 1899:54.
12. Kazemi M. Tuning fork test utilization in detection of fractures: a review of the literature. *J Can Chiropractic Assoc*. 1999;43(2):120-124.
13. Chinnock B, Khaletskiy A, Kuo K, Hendey GW. Ultrasound-guided reduction of distal radius fractures. *J Emerg Med*. 2011;40(3):308-312.
14. Parvizi J, Wayman J, Kelly P, et al. Combining the clinical signs improves diagnosis of scaphoid fractures: a prospective study with follow-up. *J Hand Surg*. 1998;23b(3):324-327.
15. Foote EM. *A Text-book of Minor Surgery*. New York, NY: Appleton; 1912:350.
16. Stimson LA. *A Practical Treatise on Fractures and Dislocations*. New York, NY: Lea & Febiger; 1899:240-241.
17. Stimson LA. *A Practical Treatise on Fractures and Dislocations*. New York, NY: Lea & Febiger; 1899:255-256.
18. Stimson LA. *A Practical Treatise on Fractures and Dislocations*. New York, NY: Lea & Febiger; 1899:269-270.
19. Grant PT. The diagnosis of pelvic fractures by 'springing.' *Arch Emerg Med*. 1990;7:178-82.
20. Graham CA. Temporary pelvic stabilization after trauma. *New Engl J Med*. 2014;370(4):388.
21. Gross EA, Niedens BA. Validation of a decision instrument to limit pelvic radiography in blunt trauma. *J Emerg Med*. 2005;28(3):263-266.

22. Helferich H. *On Fractures and Dislocations*. 3rd ed. New York, NY: William Wood; 1899:Plate 51.
23. Helferich H. *On Fractures and Dislocations*. 3rd ed. New York, NY: William Wood; 1899:Plate 52.
24. Helferich H. *On Fractures and Dislocations*. 3rd ed. New York, NY: William Wood; 1899:100.
25. Helferich H. *On Fractures and Dislocations*. 3rd ed. New York, NY: William Wood; 1899:94.
26. Stimson LA. *A Practical Treatise on Fractures and Dislocations*. New York, NY: Lea & Febiger; 1899:347-348.
27. Stiell I, Wells G, Laupacis A, et al. Multi-centre trial to introduce the Ottawa ankle rules for use of radiography in acute ankle injuries. *BMJ*. 1995;311(7005):594-597.
28. Bachmann LM, Kolb E, Koller MT, et al. Accuracy of Ottawa ankle rules to exclude fractures of the ankle and mid-foot: a systematic review. *BMJ*. 2003;326(7386):417-423.
29. Auleley GR, Kerboull L, Durieux P, et al. Validation of the Ottawa ankle rules in France: a study in the surgical emergency department of a teaching hospital. *Ann Emerg Med*. 1998;32(1):14-18.
30. Seaberg DC, Yealy DM, Lukens T, et al. Multicenter comparison of two clinical decision rules for the use of radiography in acute, high-risk knee injuries. *Ann Emerg Med*. 1998;32:8-13.
31. Stiell IG, Greenberg GH, Wells GA, et al. Prospective validation of a decision rule for the use of radiography in acute knee injuries. *JAMA*. 1996;275:611-615.
32. Bauer SJ, Hollander JE, Fuchs SH, et al. A clinical decision rule in the evaluation of acute knee injuries. *J Emerg Med*. 1995;13:611-615.
33. Husum H, Ang SC, Fosse E. *War Surgery: Field Manual*. Penang, Malaysia: Third World Network; 1995:202.
34. Foote EM. *A Text-book of Minor Surgery*. New York, NY: Appleton; 1912:369.
35. Chundamala J, Wright JG. The efficacy and risks of using providone-iodine irrigation to prevent surgical site infection: an evidence-based review. *Can J Surg*. 2007;50(6):473-481.
36. REQDOC website. November 2001. http://medtech.syrene.net/forum/showthread.php?s=349d3c19041ccaab2d90a951edc6fe34&t=1532. Accessed September 14, 2006.
37. Hamilton FH. *The Principles and Practice of Surgery*. 2nd ed. New York, NY: William Wood; 1879:248.
38. Iserson KV. Reducing dislocations in a wilderness setting: use of hypnosis and intra-articular anesthesia. *J Wild Med*. 1991;2(1):22-26.
39. Miller Sl, Cleeman E, Auerbach J, et al. Comparison of intra-articular lidocaine and intravenous sedation for reduction of shoulder dislocations: a randomized, prospective study. *J Bone Joint Surg Am*. 2002;84-A(12):2135-2139.
40. Stimson LA. *A Practical Treatise on Fractures and Dislocations*. New York, NY: Lea & Febiger; 1899:585-586.
41. Iserson KV. Improvised shoulder reduction: a useable method. *Emerg Med J*. 2014;31:255.
42. Westin CD, Gill EA, Noyes ME, et al. Anterior shoulder dislocation: a simple and rapid method of reduction. *Am J Sports Med*. 1995;23:369-371.
43. Nordeen MHH, Bacarese-Hamilton IH, Belham GJ, et al. Anterior dislocation of the shoulder: a simple method of reduction. *Injury*. 1992;23(7):479-480.
44. Boss A, Holzach P, Matter P. Eine neue Selbstrepositionstechnik der frischen, vorderenunteren Schulterluxation. [A new self-repositioning technique for fresh, anterior-lower shoulder dislocation.] *Helv Chir Acta*. 1993;60:263-265.
45. Ceroni D, Sadri H, Leuenberger A. Anteroinferior shoulder dislocation: an auto-reduction method without analgesia. *J Orthop Trauma*. 1997;11(6):399-404.
46. Cooper A. *A Treatise on Dislocations and Fractures of the Joints*. 2nd ed. Boston, MA: Lilly & Wait, Carter and Hendee; 1832.
47. Milch H. Treatment of dislocation of the shoulder. *Surgery*. 1938;3:732-740.
48. Christofi T, Kallis A, Raptis DA, et al. Management of shoulder dislocations. *Trauma*. 2007;9(1):39-46.
49. Anderson D, Zvirbulis R, Ciullo J. Scapular manipulation for reductions of anterior shoulder dislocations. *Clin Orthop Relat Res*. 1982;164:181-183.
50. Leidelmeyer R. Reduce a shoulder, subtly and painlessly. *Emerg Med*. 1977;9:223-224.
51. Stimson LA. *A Practical Treatise on Fractures and Dislocations*. New York, NY: Lea & Febiger; 1899:256-257.
52. Haywood Hall, MD, PACEMD, San Miguel de Allendé, Mexico. Personal communication with author, September 29, 2010.

53. Stimson LA. *A Practical Treatise on Fractures and Dislocations*. New York, NY: Lea & Febiger; 1899:388-389
54. Dye TM. *Metacarpal Fractures Treatment & Management*. Medscape. http://emedicine.medscape.com/article/1239721-treatment. Accessed October 8, 2015.
55. Blackmore CC, Cummings P, Jurkovich GJ, et al. Predicting major hemorrhage in patients with pelvic fracture. *J Trauma*. 2006;61(2):346-352.
56. Ofori-Boadu L, Osei-Ampofo M, Forson PK, et al. *Afr J Emerg Med*. 2013;3:88-89.
57. Scott I, Porter K, Laird C, Greaves I, Bloch M. The prehospital management of pelvic fractures: initial consensus statement. *Emerg Med J*. 2013;30(12):1070-1072.
58. Nunn T, Cosker TDA, Bose D, et al. Immediate application of improvised pelvic binder as first step in extended resuscitation from life-threatening hypovolaemic shock in conscious patients with unstable pelvic injuries. *Injury*. 2007;38(1):125-128.
59. Lefkowitz M. A new method for reduction traumatic dislocations. *Orthop Rev*. 1993;2:253-256.
60. Hendey GW, Avila A. The Captain Morgan technique for the reduction of the dislocated hip. *Ann Emerg Med*. 2011;58(6):536-540.
61. Almazroua FY, Vilke GM. The Captain Morgan technique for the reduction of the dislocated hip. *Ann Emerg Med*. 2012;60(1):135-136.
62. Helferich H. *On Fractures and Dislocations*. 3rd ed. New York, NY: William Wood; 1899:100-101.
63. Raaymakers EL, Marti RK. Nonoperative treatment of impacted femoral neck fractures: a prospective study of 170 cases. *J Bone Joint Surg Br*. 1991;73B:950-954.
64. Parker MJ, Myles JW, Anand JK, et al. Cost-benefit analysis of hip fracture treatment. *J Bone Joint Surg Br*. 1992;74(2):261-264.
65. *Remote, Austere, Wilderness & Third World Medicine*. http://medtech.syrene.net/forum/showthread.php?s=349d3c19041ccaab2d90a951edc6fe34&t=295. Accessed September 14, 2006.
66. Helferich H. *On Fractures and Dislocations*. 3rd ed. New York, NY: William Wood; 1899:125.
67. Singer AJ, Dagum AB. Current management of acute cutaneous wounds. *N Engl J Med*. 2008;359(10):1037-1046.
68. Jongen VHWM. Alternative external fixation for open fractures of the lower leg. *Trop Doct*. 1995;25(4):173-174.
69. Sechriest VF, Lhowe DW. Orthopaedic care aboard the USNS Mercy during Operation Unified Assistance after the 2004 Asian tsunami. *J Bone Joint Surg Am*. 2008;90:849-861.
70. Husum H, Ang SC, Fosse E. *War Surgery: Field Manual*. Penang, Malaysia: Third World Network; 1995:239.
71. US Army. *Emergency War Surgery*. 3rd rev. Washington, DC; Borden Institute, Walter Reed Army Medical Center; 2004:25.1.
72. Zils SW, Codner PA, Pirrallo RG. Field extremity amputation: a brief curriculum and protocol. *Acad Emerg Med*. 2011;18(9):e84.
73. King M. *Primary Surgery, Vol. 2: Trauma*. Oxford: Oxford University Press; 1987:44.
74. Husum H, Ang SC, Fosse E. *War Surgery: Field Manual*. Penang, Malaysia: Third World Network; 1995:71.
75. US Army. *Emergency War Surgery*. 3rd rev. Washington, DC; Borden Institute, Walter Reed Army Medical Center; 2004:25.4-6.
76. US Army Medical Corp. *US Special Forces Medical Handbook: 10-6 Amputations*. Washington, DC: US Dept. of Army, 1981.
77. Meals RA. Mallet finger. *Emedicine*. www.emedicine.com/orthoped/topic413.htm. Accessed September 14, 2006.
78. Stimson LA. *A Practical Treatise on Fractures and Dislocations*. New York, NY: Lea & Febiger; 1899:91.
79. Platt A, Carter N. *Making Health-Care Equipment: Ideas for Local Design and Production*. London, UK: Intermediate Technology Pub; 1990:58.
80. Abraham A, Handoll HH, Khan T. Interventions for treating wrist fractures in children. *Cochrane Database Syst Rev*. 2008;16(2):CD004576.
80. Peltier LF. *Fractures: A History and Iconography of Their Treatment*. San Francisco, CA: Norman; 1990:67-68.
82. Peltier LF. *Fractures: A History and Iconography of Their Treatment*. San Francisco, CA: Norman; 1990:69-70.

83. Stimson LA. *A Practical Treatise on Fractures and Dislocations*. New York, NY: Lea & Febiger; 1899:93-94.
84. Hamilton FH. *The Principles and Practice of Surgery*. 2nd ed. New York, NY: William Wood; 1879:246.
85. Ware MW. *Plaster of Paris and How to Use It*. New York, NY: Surgery Pub Co; 1911:2. Cited in: Peltier LF. *Fractures: A History and Iconography of Their Treatment*. San Francisco, CA: Norman; 1990:70.
86. Taylor HL, Ogilvy C, Albee FH. *Orthopedics for Practitioners*. New York, NY: Appleton; 1909:410-411.
87. Wilkinson DA, Skinner MF. *The Primary Trauma Care Manual: A Manual for Trauma Management in District and Remote Locations*. Geneva, Switzerland: World Health Organization. http://www.steinergraphics.com/surgical/manual.html. Accessed May 15, 2008.
88. Tovey FI, Tovey WE. The making of plaster bandages. *Trop Doct*. 1988;18:190.
89. King M. *Primary Surgery, Vol. 2: Trauma*. Oxford, UK: Oxford University Press; 1987:215-216.
90. Peltier LF. *Fractures: A History and Iconography of Their Treatment*. San Francisco, CA: Norman; 1990:73.
91. Peltier LF. *Fractures: A History and Iconography of Their Treatment*. San Francisco, CA: Norman; 1990:63.
92. Stimson LA. *A Practical Treatise on Fractures and Dislocations*. New York, NY: Lea & Febiger; 1899:89.
93. US Orthopedic Council. *Military Orthopaedic Surgery*. Philadelphia, PA: Lea & Febiger; 1918:uppl A:iii.
94. Burgess RD. *Community Health Aide/Practitioner Manual*. Washington, DC: Alaska Area Native Health Service; 1987:254-255.
95. Weichenthal L, Spano S, Horan B, Miss J. Improvised traction splints: a wilderness medicine tool or hindrance? *Wild Environ Med*. 2012;23(1):61-64.
96. Helferich H. *On Fractures and Dislocations*. 3rd ed. New York, NY: William Wood; 1899:107.
97. Helferich H. *On Fractures and Dislocations*. 3rd ed. New York, NY: William Wood; 1899:104-108.
98. Taylor HL, Ogilvy C, Albee FH. *Orthopedics for Practitioners*. New York, NY: Appleton; 1909:426-427.
99. Helferich H. *On Fractures and Dislocations*. 3rd ed. New York, NY: William Wood; 1899:104.
100. Doorgakant A, Mkandawire NC. The management of isolated closed femoral shaft fractures in a district hospital in Malawi. *Trop Doct*. 2012;42(1):8-12.
101. Helferich H. *On Fractures and Dislocations*. 3rd ed. New York, NY: William Wood; 1899:104, Fig. 108.
102. King M, Bewes P, Cairns J, et al, eds. *Primary Surgery, Vol. 1: Non-Trauma*. Oxford, UK: Oxford University Press; 1990:610.
103. Cohen MI. Acute rheumatological and inflammatory pains. In: Rowbotham DJ, Macintyre PE, eds. *Clinical Pain Management: Acute Pain*. London, UK: Arnold; 2003:394-404.
104. Cashman J. Routes of administration. In: Rowbotham DJ, Macintyre PE, eds. *Clinical Pain Management: Acute Pain*. London, UK: Arnold; 2003:205-218.
105. Murphy DF. Nerve blocks for acute pain: principles. In: Rowbotham DJ, Macintyre PE, eds. *Clinical Pain Management: Acute Pain*. London, UK: Arnold; 2003:267-274.
106. Palmer DD, Wolf CE. *Handbook of Medicine in Developing Countries*. Bristol, TN: Christian Medical & Dental Assoc.; 2002:412.
107. *STEP MANUAL* (Sequential Trauma Education Programs). Baltimore, MD: University of Maryland; 2007:141-200.
108. *New Brunswick General Guidelines for Expected Healing Times*. http://www.grandroundsnow.com/whscc/whscc_pdfs/Expected_Healing.pdf. Accessed May 19, 2008.
109. Taylor HL, Ogilvy C, Albee FH. *Orthopedics for Practitioners*. New York, NY: Appleton; 1909:77.

33 | Urology

Urinary drainage and penile obstructions are the two most common urological problems needing improvised treatment.

BLADDER DRAINAGE/TUBES

Urethral Lubrication/Anesthesia

Anesthetic jellies (gels), such as lidocaine 2%, reduce the discomfort of male catheterization, although this is not true in women.[1,2] Lidocaine jelly may not be available, so it helps to know about the alternatives.

Diphenhydramine (e.g., Benadryl) and promethazine (e.g., Phenergan) may be used effectively as urethral anesthetics. The dose is the same, or less, than would be used orally. Inject the drug into the urethra using a bulb syringe, and keep it in place for about 5 minutes using a penile clamp or equivalent. Some patients experience an initial burning sensation. The anesthesia lasts about 1 hour. To obtain more extensive anesthesia, coat a small urethral sound with an ointment of these medications and leave in it place about 5 minutes before passing larger sounds.[3]

Use mineral oil to lubricate urethral catheters if standard lubricating jellies are unavailable.[4] In women, apply 10% cocaine jelly with a cotton-tipped applicator for an effective urethral anesthetic. Leave this in place for 5 minutes.[5]

Difficult Urethral Catheter Placement

Passing a urethral catheter is almost routine from the clinician's perspective. Some catheters are difficult to pass, especially in older men. When calling the urologist is not an option, the following technique may make catheter insertions more successful.

In males >50 years old, use a syringe to inject 25 to 50 mL lidocaine jelly 2% into the urethra before attempting to pass any catheter. If lidocaine jelly is not available, use any sterile gel (e.g., K-Y). If you anticipate that passing a urethral catheter will be difficult, use at least an 18- to 20-Fr Foley rather than a smaller-sized catheter. Smaller catheters simply bend if they hit an obstruction, rather than passing into the bladder. Use slow, steady pressure to insert it all the way to the Foley's hub. Do not inflate the balloon until the catheter is fully inserted and urine returns.

Use a coudé catheter if you suspect that the patient may have an enlarged prostate. A coudé catheter has a gentle upward curve at its distal 3 cm that allows easier passage through an enlarged prostate. When inserting a coudé catheter, point the tip anteriorly. This means that the balloon inflation side port should be facing up (on the same side as the curve). If the patient has a red catheter in place, it generally means that it is either a coudé or a Councill (used by urologists to pass over a guidewire). In either case, beware of removing it for replacement.

If multiple attempts at catheter placement have failed, a suprapubic aspiration using a needle and large syringe can easily buy time until a suprapubic tube can be placed or an experienced clinician can use alternative methods (e.g., filiforms and followers) to drain the bladder.

Bladder Clots

Bladder clots are reasonably common and often cause painful obstructive symptoms. Assuming that you know why these are occurring (chronic infection, tumor, anticoagulant), treat the acute problem and ensure bladder drainage. To do this, put in a ≥4-Fr catheter. Do not place a three-way catheter, which is normally used for continuous bladder irrigation, until the clot is removed—the opening is too small, because two smaller catheters and an inflation port must fit into the one catheter. Advance the catheter all the way. It may pass beyond the clot and allow the urine to drain. Then use an irrigation syringe to instill 60 to 120 mL aliquots of sterile water, which is more lytic than saline (up to 300 mL total). Then withdraw the fluid and repeat the

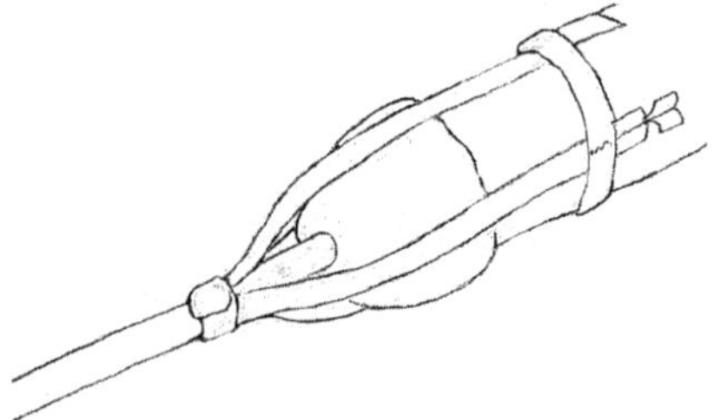

FIG. 33-1. Securing a straight, non-balloon catheter, method #1.

process. If the clot cannot be removed in this fashion, a surgical approach may be necessary. If surgery is not an option, some clinicians have instilled thrombolytics.[6,7]

Securing Non-Balloon Catheters/Tubing

If only a straight (non-balloon) catheter or a makeshift catheter (e.g., a nasogastric tube) must be placed, the trick is securing it to the penis. After inserting the tube, secure it to the penis using three long strips of adhesive tape. First, attach about 1 inch of a tape strip to the catheter just as it exits the urethra. Lay the rest of the tape along the penis. Do the same for the two other pieces of tape. Use benzoin, if necessary, to keep the pieces in place. Then wrap one or two non-constricting circular pieces of tape around the penis to secure the long strips further (Fig. 33-1).

Another method of securing a non-balloon catheter is to tie a suture around the catheter just beyond the external meatus and carry the ends along the body of the penis (Fig. 33-2). Secure the ends with a piece of tape, wrapping it in a spiral beginning at the catheter and then around the penis.[8]

In infants, using a pediatric feeding tube as a catheter is common. Matt Steinway, MD, a urologist in Phoenix, Ariz., suggests securing these with a clear adhesive dressing (e.g., OpSite) or with a suture placed through the glans and tied to the tube at the meatus. (Personal written communication, February 2008.)

In women, securing a straight catheter may be less successful. It can be taped to the labia, after shaving.[9] Alternatively, as Keyes wrote in 1917, "In the female, the (non-balloon) catheter is held in place by tying a number of silk strings to it as it issues from the vulva and fixing these to the pubic hairs in front, and by means of adhesive strapping to the lateral gluteal creases behind."[10]

External Catheter

A condom (external) catheter can easily be improvised using a normal condom and any tube that connects to the collection bottle or bag. Slip the end of the tube completely into the condom. Make a small hole at the end of condom, but don't pass the tube through it or it will rub against the penis. Tie the end of the condom tightly around the end of the tube, and invert the condom so it dangles free of the tube (Fig. 33-3). Put the condom over the penis and secure it with tape around the penis, extending the tape onto the anterior abdomen. In many cases, a Penrose drain, a glove, or other material can be used in place of a condom.

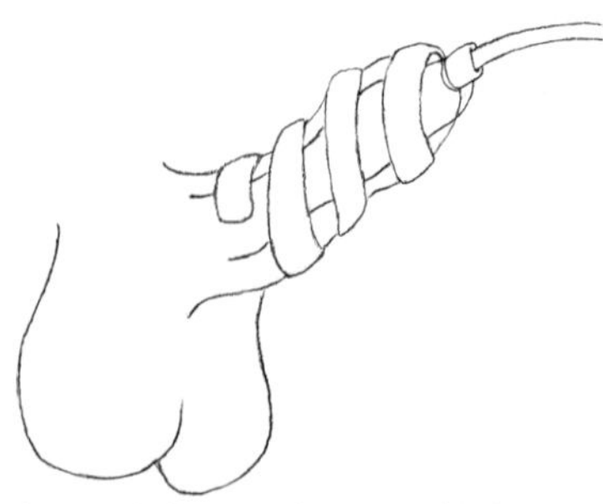

FIG. 33-2. Securing a straight, non-balloon catheter, method #2.

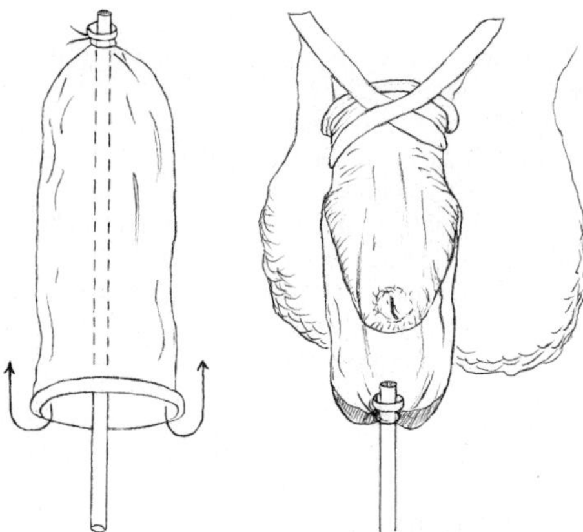

FIG. 33-3. Condom catheter. Putting it on (left) and in place (right).

Cleaning Reusable Catheters

Between intermittent catheterization of the same patient, clean catheters as follows:

Wash the catheter using plain liquid soap (without deodorant or fragrance); rinse well until the soap residue is gone. Shake out any excess fluid, air dry the catheter, and then place it on a clean paper towel or in a clean basin. Alternatively, soak the catheter for 30 minutes in a homemade vinegar solution (one part white vinegar to three parts room-temperature water). Rinse, thoroughly shake out excess water, and air dry.

Store the washed catheters in a clean zip-top bag, tampon case, toothbrush holder, small camera case, or other clean container. Discard reusable catheters when they become hard, brittle, or cracked, or when they change color.[11]

Retained Urethral Catheters

Retained urethral catheters (those that cannot easily be removed by simply deflating the balloon) are a common problem. The longer the catheter is left in place, the more chance this will occur. Most often, the inability to deflate the balloon is due to either a complete or a partial obstruction of the catheter's inflation canal.

The first step should be to cut off the balloon valve. If that is the problem, as it often is, the balloon deflates and can be removed. If not, pass a thin wire, such as a wire from a catheter introducer, through the balloon port to either burst the balloon or alter its shape so that it can be removed.

A number of methods may be used to deflate the balloon and remove the catheter. These include injecting ether,[12] liquid paraffin (kerosene), chloroform,[13] or toluene[14] to dissolve the balloon, although these may cause chemical cystitis to varying degrees.[15,16] A common practice in some developing countries has been to deflate the balloons in malfunctioning urethral catheters by injecting 2 to 3 mL of mineral oil through the balloon port.[4] The balloon deflates within about 2 hours.[17] Even though mineral oil is inert and generally considered innocuous and causes no discomfort to the patient, reports have suggested that the presence of mineral oil in the urinary tract may cause oil granulomas in a small number of patients.[18]

The balloon can also be punctured by using a suprapubic, transvaginal, or perineal approach.[19-21] Use these methods, with or without ultrasound guidance, only after other methods have failed. For the suprapubic approach, use the stylet from an 18-gauge spinal needle. With the catheter balloon pulled against the floor of the bladder, direct the stylet vertically downward until the balloon is punctured or the entire stylet has been introduced. If this is unsuccessful, withdraw the stylet and reinsert it progressively caudally or cranially, 10 to 15 degrees from vertical. In men, the mean angle for puncture is 2 degrees cephalad of vertical; in women, it is 17 degrees caudal of vertical.[20]

One concern is that pieces of the punctured balloon may be retained in the bladder, causing irritation and infection. While this seems to occur frequently with in vitro tests,[16] in practice, it is rarely seen.[22] The chances of this seem to be lessened if catheter balloons with a 30-mL capacity have ≤40 mL of fluid injected before puncture; balloons with a 10-mL capacity should have ≤15 mL before puncture.[16]

A relatively simple method of deflating these balloons is to inject the balloon with normal saline until it bursts, which may take up to 500 mL! If the inflation canal is blocked at its proximal port so no fluid can be injected, pull the catheter so that its original light brown color is visible. At that point, clamp the catheter so that it does not retract and cut it. Then carefully insert a 21-gauge needle with an attached syringe into this part of the exposed inflation canal and either deflate the balloon or, more commonly, inflate it until the balloon ruptures; then remove the catheter. This reportedly works ≥90% of the time.[22] Use this technique cautiously, because if the Foley is misplaced (such as in the urethra), overinflating the balloon could cause significant pain and, possibly, damage to the patient.

Rarely, an encrustation on the end of the catheter blocks removal. This may require surgical removal of the catheter.

Alternative Urine Collection Bags/Systems

Use old intravenous (IV) or irrigation bottles, rather than disposable urine collection bags, to collect urine from urethral catheters. Make tubing for the bottle from an old IV set (Fig. 33-4). Put a tape on the side of the bottle and mark it as you add water in 100-mL increments (Fig. 33-5). Empty the bottle, put a hole in the lid for the tube, and it is ready to collect and measure urine output.

Pediatric urine collection bags (a technique not useful for urinalysis or culture) can be made inexpensively from disposable plastic bags, adhesive tape, old IV tubing, and waxed paper or something similar.[24] (For details, see Fig. 5-10 and the "Urine Collection" section in Chapter 37.)

DIAGNOSIS

Ultrasound for Ureteral Stones

Ultrasound can discriminate between renal calculi and other causes of flank pain as well as computed tomography (CT). Up to 6 months after the examination, patients experience essentially the same incidence of serious adverse events whether they had a CT or an ultrasound examination by an emergency physician or radiologist.[25]

Cystometry

A simple cystometry can be performed with a catheter and a syringe or manometer held 15 cm above the patient's symphysis pubis. These items are inexpensive and readily available; however, exact measurements of bladder pressure and determination of compliance are not possible using

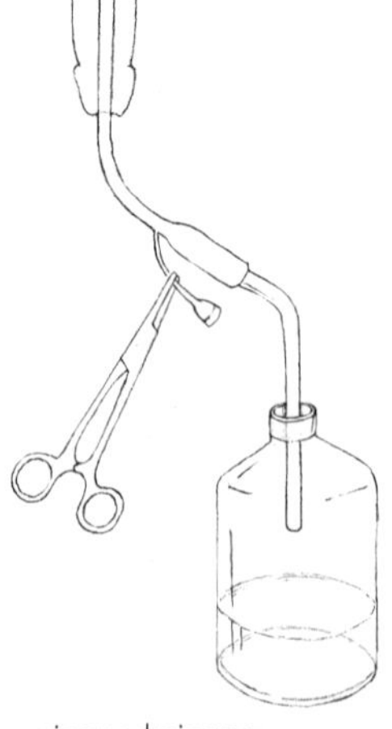

FIG. 33-4. Empty IV bottle used for urinary drainage.

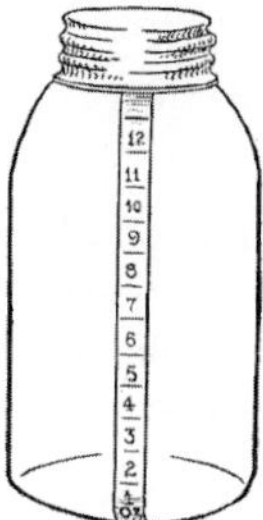

FIG. 33-5. Improvised collecting jar with volume measurements. *(Adapted from Olson.[23])*

this method. Also, this "single-channel" method increases intra-abdominal pressure that may result in elevated detrusor pressure readings.[26]

PENIS AND PROSTATE

Local Anesthesia for Penile Procedures

Anesthetizing the penis may be necessary to repair injuries, remove a zipper, do a circumcision, provide postoperative analgesia, and do other surgical procedures. Two common methods are the circumferential and the dorsal penile blocks: in both, use a long-acting anesthetic.

A circumferential block is the easiest method. It requires placing a ring of anesthetic (without epinephrine) subcutaneously and intradermally around the base of the penile shaft. However, it may cause a hematoma, and it may not be effective in every case.[27,28]

Anesthesia of the dorsal/ventral penile nerves blocks sensory nerves to the distal one-third of the penis. Insert a needle into the infrapubic space dorsally at the base of the penis; a pop is felt as the needle enters the fascia of the compartment. Aspirate and direct the needle to each side of the penile shaft; inject 5 mL of a non-epinephrine-containing anesthetic.[28] Block the paraurethral branches by injecting ventrally. Pull the penis up, aspirate, and inject into the grooves between the corpus cavernosum and corpus spongiosum.[27]

Anesthesia for a dorsal slit may be necessary for phimosis or paraphimosis. To anesthetize this area, simply inject anesthetic with epinephrine along the area of the foreskin to be cut (Fig. 33-6).

Osmosis-Reduced Paraphimosis

Paraphimosis involves venous congestion and edema of the retracted foreskin, making it impossible for the patient to return it to the normal position. Manually reducing the foreskin or making a dorsal slit is a painful procedure. If no ischemia is present, put a generous amount of granulated sugar on the foreskin and into a condom, rubber glove finger, or ultrasound probe cover. Put the sugar-filled device over the entire glans and foreskin. Leave it on without manipulating it for

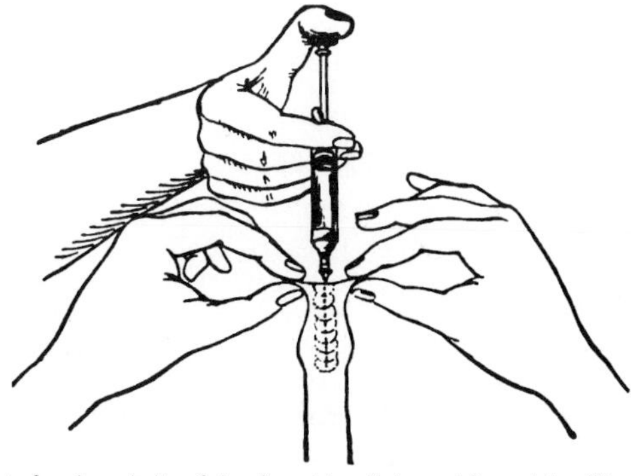

FIG. 33-6. Anesthesia for dorsal slit of the foreskin. *(Adapted from Allen.[29])*

2 hours. If the foreskin cannot be reduced at that point, continue the process a bit longer before resorting to other methods.[30]

Foreign Bodies

According to Yacobi et al., "creative thinking is essential to remove heavy metal objects" from a penis when they get stuck there after unusual sexual activities.[31]

The simplest method to remove a constricting device is to use a string wrap, as is done to remove a ring from a swollen finger. If that is ineffective, drain blood from the penis to help shrink it and allow removal of the foreign object. The patient's tolerance will determine whether sedation or anesthesia is needed. A penile block (without epinephrine) often helps.

If the only way to remove a constricting device is to cut it, always cut on opposite sides of the penis, while protecting the skin to avoid avulsions. Ordinary hospital equipment is often insufficient to do the job. Maintenance staff, the fire department, or a rescue team may have to supply bolt cutters, powered rotary tools, heavy-duty air grinders, or pneumatic saws, especially to remove heavy iron and steel objects encircling the penis. Consider letting the people supplying these tools operate them, because they are more experienced. The operating room may be able to supply portable dental drills and power surgical saws. When nothing else is available, a hammer and chisel may have to be used. To help cool and protect the area, continuously pour large volumes of water over the area being cut. The entire process often takes up to 90 minutes. If any question about penile tissue viability exists once the object has been removed, inject fluorescein (15 mg/kg) IV, wait 20 minutes, and examine the penis under a Wood's lamp. Doppler flow ultrasound may also be used.[31]

REFERENCES

1. Siderias J, Guadio F, Singer AJ. Comparison of topical anesthetics and lubricants prior to urethral catheterization in males: a randomized controlled trial. *Acad Emerg Med.* 2004;11:703-706.
2. Tanabe P, Steinmann R, Anderson J, et al. Factors affecting pain scores during female urethral catheterization. *Acad Emerg Med.* 2004;11:699-702.
3. Naranjo P, Naranjo EB. Los antihistaminicaos como anesthesicos locales. [Antihistamines as local anesthetics.] *Bol Inform Cient Nac.* 1957;9:33-41.
4. Jain BK, Agrawal CS. Safety of mineral oil in urological procedures. *Trop Doct.* 1999;29(2):116-117.
5. Fitzpatrick FJ, Orr LM. Antihistamines as local anesthetic agents for urethral manipulation. *JAMA.* 1952;150(11):1092-1094.
6. Pautler SE, Luke P, Chin JL. Upper tract urokinase instillation for nephrostomy tube patency. *J Urol.* 1999;161(2):538-540.
7. Olarte JL, Glover ML, Totapally BR. The use of Alteplase for the resolution of an intravesical clot in a neonate receiving extracorporeal membrane oxygenation. *ASAIO J.* 2001;47(5):565-568.
8. World Health Organization. *Surgical Care at the District Hospital.* Geneva, Switzerland: WHO; 2003:9.2.
9. Smith DR. *General Urology.* Los Altos, CA: Lange, 1972:106.
10. Keyes EL. *Urology: Diseases of the Urinary Organs, Diseases of the Male Genital Organs, the Venereal Diseases.* New York, NY: D. Appleton; 1917:674.
11. National Association for Continence (NAFC). http://www.nafc.org. Accessed October 6, 2015.
12. King M, Bewes PC, Cairns J, et al, eds. *Primary Surgery, Vol. 1: Non-Trauma.* Oxford, UK: Oxford Medical Publishing; 1990:11.
13. Gulmez I, Ekmekcioglu O, Karacagil M. Management of undeflatable Foley catheter balloons in women. *Int Urogynecol J Pelvic Floor Dysfunct.* 1997;8(2):81-84.
14. Khanna S. Preliminary results with toluene for retained urinary catheters. *Eur Urol.* 1991;19(2): 169-170.
15. Lebowitz RB, Effmann EL. Ether cystitis. *Urology.* 1978;12:427.
16. Hamdi JT. Management of retained Foley catheters. *J Roy Coll Surg Edinburgh.* 1995;40:290-291.
17. Murphy GY, Wood Jr DP. The use of mineral oil to manage the nondeflating Foley catheter. *J Urol.* 1993;149:89.
18. Albers DD, Hosty TA, Prakhurst JD, et al. Oil granulomas of the ureter. *J Urol.* 1984;132:114.
19. Rees M, Joseph AEA. Guided suprapubic puncture: a new simple way of releasing a blocked Foley balloon. *Br J Urol.* 1981;53:196.

20. Moscovich R. Suprapubic puncture for nondeflating urethral balloon catheters. *J Roy Coll Surg Edinburgh.* 1984;29:181-183.
21. Vandendris M. How to deflate refractory balloon of a bladder catheter. *Urology*. 1985;26(3):300.
22. Bowa K. Removing a retained urinary catheter. *Trop Doct*. 2007;37:205-206.
23. Olson LM. *Improvised Equipment in the Home Care of the Sick*. Philadelphia, PA: W.B. Saunders; 1928:26-27.
24. Kuhan N, Azhmad ZA, Lip TQ. Improvised urine bag. *J Singapore Paediatr Soc*. 1977;19(3):212-215.
25. Osterweil N. Medscape Medical News from the American Urological Association 2014 Annual Scientific Meeting, May 17, 2014. www.medscape.com/viewarticle/825323?nlid=57715_1361&src=wnl_edit_medn_emed&uac=50765FZ&spon=45.
26. Ellsworth PI. Bladder pressure assessment technique. http://emedicine.medscape.com/article/2113529-technique. Accessed May 20, 2014.
27. Dobson MB. *Anaesthesia at the District Hospital*, 2nd ed. Geneva, Switzerland: World Health Organization; 2000:91-92.
28. New York School of Regional Anesthesia. Peripheral nerve blocks for children. http://www.nysora.com/techniques/. Accessed May 11, 2008.
29. Allen CW. *Local and Regional Anesthesia*. 2nd ed. Philadelphia, PA: W.B. Saunders; 1918:386.
30. Kerwat R, Shandall A, Stephenson B. Reduction of paraphimosis with granulated sugar. *Brit J Urol.* 1998;82(5):755.
31. Yacobi Y, Tsivian A, Sidi AA. Emergent and surgical interventions for injuries associated with eroticism: a review. *J Trauma*. 2007;62(6):1522-1530.

V NONSURGICAL INTERVENTIONS

34 | Gastroenterology

TREATMENT

Hiccups

Hiccups (singultus), an involuntary diaphragmatic spasm with a sudden closure of the glottis, is considered persistent when it lasts more than 48 hours. Its etiology can be organic, psychogenic, or idiopathic. Usually, the initial problem is to stop the hiccups, even if an organic cause is being investigated. In austere settings, some of the safer non-pharmacological remedies (Table 34-1)

TABLE 34-1 Non-drug Treatments for Hiccups and Their Proposed Physiological Bases

Interruption or Stimulation of Respiration
• Gasping with sudden fright
• Breath holding
• Valsalva maneuver
• Hyperventilation
• Rebreathing into paper bag
• Sneezing induced with snuff or pepper
Irritation of Uvula or Nasopharynx
• Forcible tongue traction
• Gargling
• Drinking pineapple juice
• Sipping ice water
• Drinking water while covering ears tightly
• Swallowing hard bread or crushed ice
• Drinking water rapidly
• Pharyngeal stimulation with nasal catheter
• Swallowing mixture of honey and vinegar
• Drinking water from the "wrong side" of a glass
• Granulated sugar swallowed dry
• Lifting the uvula with a spoon or cotton-tipped swab
Counter-Irritation of Vagus Nerve
• Rectal massage
Disruption of the Phrenic Nerve
• Vapocoolant sprays or ice over C5 vertebra
• Percussion over C5 vertebra
Counter-Irritation of the Diaphragm
• Mustard plaster to lower chest
• Tightly pulling knees to chest or leaning forward
Relieve Gastric Distention—Especially After Overeating
• Gastric lavage
• Emetic-induced vomiting
• Nasogastric aspiration

Adapted from Friedman.[1]

may be the most helpful. One of the most interesting is continuous tapping, usually for a few minutes, over the C5 vertebra until the hiccups cease. Another is self-compression of the chest by either pulling one's knees to one's chest or leaning forward. While some of these methods have a sound physiological base, their effectiveness is uncertain, especially with protracted hiccups.

Multiple drugs have also been successfully used. If hiccups persist, prescribe chlorpromazine (Thorazine) 25 to 50 mg orally three or four times a day. Haloperidol, 2 to 5 mg intramuscularly (IM), is a safer and possibly more successful alternative. If it works, prescribe 1 to 4 mg orally three times a day. Other drugs used for hiccup treatment include many anticonvulsants (e.g., phenytoin, phenobarbital, carbamazepime, valproic acid), benzodiazepines, metoclopramide, various sedatives, and narcotics.[2]

Another method of treating hiccups that is relatively benign, generally available, inexpensive, and simple to use is IV lidocaine. On multiple occasions, it has worked successfully when other medications have failed. Reported successful procedures with lidocaine doses, in both children and adults, have involved loading the patient with 1 to 2 mg/kg and then generally beginning a 2 mg/kg (sometimes up to 4 mg/kg) drip for 4 to 12 hours. This often had to be repeated within 24 hours.[3-6] My personal experience with this technique was in a remote location with an adult who had had several severe and debilitating hiccup attacks over the prior decade. I used an infusion of 2 mg/kg lidocaine over 20 minutes, which stopped the hiccups as the infusion was ending. Although they did not recur, I gave him a 20-minute infusion of 1 mg/kg on each of the next 2 days. He did not have a recurrence over the next 5 months.

Nausea and Vomiting

Treatments for the common complaint of nausea and vomiting vary around the globe. Some medications, such as the phenothiazines that are commonly used in some countries, are unavailable for this use in other countries. Other common treatments, such as metoclopramide and ginger root, are no better than placebos.[7]

Generally available and inexpensive medications that have been shown to be effective for nausea and vomiting include dexamethasone, 5 to 10 mg IV (pediatric dose: 0.5 to 1.5 mg/kg); droperidol, 0.625 to 1.25 mg IV; dimenhydrinate, 1 to 2 mg/kg IV; and ephedrine, 0.5 mg/kg IM.[8] A side benefit of using dexamethasone is that it often relieves bowel obstruction along with the accompanying nausea and vomiting in cancer patients.[9]

Acupressure, as both a preventive (anesthesia and pregnancy) and a treatment, has shown mixed results. Acupressure may be more effective in controlling nausea symptoms than in preventing emesis.[10] But, because it costs nothing, has no side effects, is simple to use, and is available in any situation, it is probably worth trying. The Pe6 Neiguan point where acupressure is applied can be located on the volar forearm about 2 inches proximal to the distal wrist crease (in adult males) between the tendons of the flexor carpi radialis and palmaris longus. For others, it is one-sixth the distance between the distal wrist crease and the elbow flexor crease (Fig. 34-1). Apply pressure to this site using a marble, ball bearing, or similar object placed beneath an armband, such as used for a venous tourniquet, or an elastic bandage. Begin by compressing the sphere intermittently for a few minutes; then apply the pressure constantly under the band.[11]

Diarrhea

Diarrhea afflicts nearly everyone at some point. Among the Bataan prisoners of war (POWs), physician–prisoners "created pills for dysentery from cornstarch, guava leaves and charcoal."[12] Pepto Bismol tablets are frequently used for symptomatic treatment of non-dysenteric diarrhea.

Probiotics (live nonpathogenic microorganisms, usually bacteria or yeast) may benefit patients

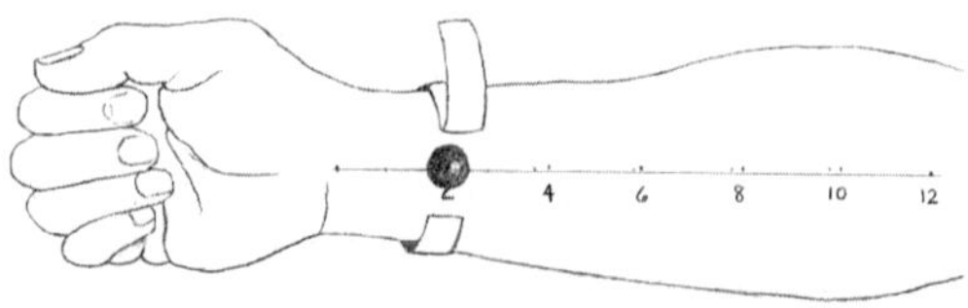

FIG. 34-1. Acupressure site for nausea and vomiting.

TABLE 34-2 Glasgow-Blatchford Criteria

Risk Indicator	Value
Blood Urea	
≥6.5 to <8.0	2
≥8.0 to <10.0	3
≥10.0 to <25.0	4
≥25	6
Hemoglobin (g/L) for Men	
≥12.0 to <13.0	1
≥10.0 to <12.0	3
<10.0	6
Hemoglobin (g/L) for Women	
≥10.0 to <12.0	1
<10.0	6
Systolic Blood Pressure (mm Hg)	
100 to 109	1
90 to 99	2
<90	3
Other Markers	
Pulse ≥100 (beats/min)	1
Presentation with melena	1
Presentation with syncope	2
Hepatic disease	2
Cardiac failure	2

From Blatchford O, et al. *Lancet*. 2000;356(9238):1318-21. Reprinted with permission from Elsevier.

with infectious and antibiotic-associated diarrhea, including *Clostridium difficile*–associated disease. Yogurt with *Lactobacillus* species and *Saccharomyces boulardii* has been shown to be effective.[13,14] However, the optimal bacterial species and dose to prescribe remains unclear.[15]

Gastrointestinal Bleed Scoring

When resources are limited, use the Glasgow-Blatchford bleeding score (Table 34-2) to help determine which patients with an acute upper gastrointestinal bleed can be safely discharged and which will need advanced medical interventions, such as a blood transfusion or endoscopy. If the patient has none of the criteria, he or she can be discharged. Those with a score >6 have at least a 50% chance of needing a significant intervention.[16]

Helicobacter pylori Treatment

While the 'test before treatment' policy is the recommended way to eradicate *Helicobacter pylori* in young patients with uninvestigated dyspepsia, if the prevalence of *H. pylori* is high, immediately initiating proton pump therapy may be a better option for these patients.[17]

Irritable Bowel Syndrome

Irritable bowel syndrome (IBS) is characterized by mild-to-severe abdominal pain, discomfort, bloating, and alteration of bowel habits. In some adult patients with IBS, administering

TABLE 34-3 Readily Available Oral Agents to Treat Constipation

Mechanism/Class	Agent	Typical Adult Dose	Time to Action (Hours)
Bulking or hydrophilic agents	Dietary fiber (most often, bran)	20-40 g[a]	12-72
Osmotic agents	Magnesium hydroxide (milk of magnesia)	15-60 mL	0.5-6
	Sorbitol syrup (10.5 g/15 mL)	15-60 mL	0.5-3
Stimulant laxative	Senna (standardized concentrate)	15-60 mg	0.25-1
	Cascara sagrada (fluid extract)	5 mL	0.25-1
	Castor oil (ricinoleic acid)	30-60 mL	0.25-1
Lubricating agent	Mineral oil	15-30 mL	6-8

[a]Given in divided doses.

Data from Schiller.[19]

intrarectal lidocaine (300 mg) jelly may reduce rectal pain. It works within 15 minutes of administration and is reported to be safe and effective.[18]

Constipation

Constipation is a common complaint, especially in postoperative and pregnant patients, the elderly, those on several types of medications, and those with diabetes, hypothyroidism, depression, and inflammatory bowel disease.

Treatment for constipation can be either mechanical (i.e., enema) or with oral agents. Table 34-3 lists some inexpensive, readily available oral agents that have been shown to be effective. There is good evidence to suggest that increased dietary fiber and increased physical activity can also reduce the incidence of constipation.

Constipation can also be treated with enemas. Enemas, of course, may also be used to administer medications and to provide parenteral fluids, as described in the "Rectal Hydration/Proctoclysis" section in Chapter 12. Multiple types of improvised equipment can be used to give an enema. With an improvised connection, nearly any tubing can be attached to a tea or coffee pot, an IV bag, or a funnel.

Rectal Pain

Proctalgia Fugax

Rectal pain from intermittent spasm is often a chronic condition. Patients can be taught to relieve the spasm by using a few ounces of warm water as an enema. The pain usually resolves within a minute.[20]

Hemorrhoids

Common and painful, hemorrhoids are enlarged vascular cushions in the anal canal. They most commonly present with painless rectal bleeding, but patients often have pruritus, swelling, prolapse, discharge, or soiling. Hemorrhoids normally appear at 3 o'clock (when patients are in the lithotomy position), 7 o'clock, and 11 o'clock positions around the anus. Severe pain occurs when hemorrhoids are thrombosed or strangulated. Note that anal cancer presents very much like prolapsed hemorrhoids.

Those familiar with the technique can use rubber band ligation on all prolapsed hemorrhoids except those that cannot be reduced. Up to three hemorrhoids can be banded at each visit. Make the bands by cutting a Foley catheter into $^{1}/_{16}$-inch-wide segments. Up to 150 bands (which also can be used to band esophageal varices) can be made from one catheter. Use thread seal to fasten the bands to the application cylinder on the scope.[21] To minimize pain, banding should be done above the dentate line (transition from squamous to columnar epithelium). Most patients are happy with the outcome, but delayed bleeding 5 to 10 days after the procedure is possible.[22]

Submucosal injection of 5% oily phenol (sclerotherapy) is an inexpensive and easily performed alternative to treat first- and second-degree hemorrhoids. The difficulty is that this does not seem to have any better result than fiber supplementation, and it has a relatively high failure rate.[23] Opening thrombosed hemorrhoids under less-than-ideal circumstances may initially relieve the pain, but it soon leads to bleeding, increased pain, and increased incidence of infection.

Anal Fissures

Painful anal fissures are often treated with surgery. They are thought to be due to increased internal sphincter pressure causing an ischemic ulceration distal to the dentate line. Usually, they lie in the posterior midline and can progress to chronic fissures. Acute anal fissures often persist because the pain causes spasm of the internal anal sphincter, which results in more pain and bleeding. Without surgery, acute fissures can often be successfully treated with topical nitroglycerine or by using a "frozen finger."

Topical nitroglycerine cures about 60% of adult patients with acute fissures; it does less well treating chronic fissures. How well it works in infants and children is unknown. Make a 0.2% glyceryl trinitrate ointment by mixing 2 g glyceryl trinitrate (standard preparation) with 20 g fatty yellow petroleum jelly. Tell the patient to keep the ointment refrigerated. The patient should apply it to the anus and in the anal canal three times daily for 4 weeks.[24]

Another simple and effective treatment is to use a "frozen finger" to reduce the symptoms and promote healing.[25] To make a frozen finger, fill an ordinary rubber examination glove with water and tie off the fingers with string. Empty the rest of the glove and cut off each of the fingers, leaving a generous margin of glove. Put them in a freezer and leave them there until needed.

To use a frozen finger, apply 5% lidocaine jelly to the anus and insert the frozen finger through the anal ring, leaving the strings used to tie it closed and a small part of the finger outside the anus so that it can be removed easily. Leave it in place until it is no longer cold and stiff—about 7 minutes. Once shown how to do this, patients can place the fingers themselves once a day. Fingers work very well when accompanied by the standard patient recommendations to eat a high-fiber diet, hydrate well, and use anesthetic creams, laxatives, and sitz baths, as possible, for 3 months. They generally provide immediate temporary pain relief and significant ongoing pain relief within 2 weeks; 60% of the fissures heal within 2 weeks (as opposed to only 10% in the "non-finger" group).[25] This technique also works well for symptomatic relief from thrombosed external hemorrhoids.[26]

PROCEDURES

Insertion of a Nasogastric Tube Using a "Peel-Away" Endotracheal Tube

Inserting a nasogastric (NG) tube can be especially difficult in intubated patients. One effective technique is to use a standard tracheal tube, split down one side, as an introducer. However, with this method, the tube may kink, making NG insertion difficult; the NG may pass through the slit; or the cut edges may traumatize the esophageal mucosa. An alternative method is to use the "peel-away" endotracheal (ET) tube, made by removing the connector, the cuff, and the pilot tube from a standard ET tube. First, use a scalpel to make perforations along opposite sides of the axis of the tube's curve (at the "6 o'clock" and "12 o'clock" positions). About 4 cm from the proximal end, completely split the tube so that it can be firmly gripped when peeling it away from the NG tube. Carefully insert the NG tube into the nasopharynx and retrieve it through the mouth, using Magill forceps. Lubricate the "peel-away" ET tube and insert it through the mouth into the esophagus. Pass the lubricated NG tube (or orogastric tube directly) into the "peel-away" ET tube. Once the NG is in the stomach, peel the ET tube and simultaneously remove it from the esophagus, as an assistant holds the NG tube in place (Fig. 34-2).[27]

Securing a Nasogastric Tube

To secure an NG tube, tie a suture around it close to the nares. Leave the suture ends long and tape them to the outside of the nose (Fig. 34-3).

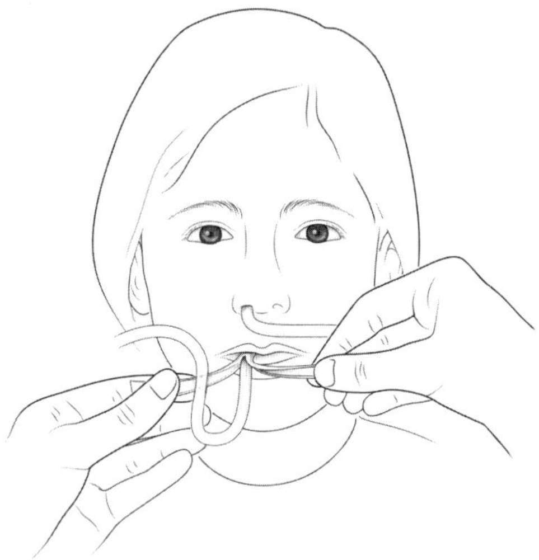

FIG. 34-2. Insertion of an NG tube using a "peel-away" ET tube.

Rigid Intravenous Bottles as Nasogastric Suction Devices

If IV fluids come in semirigid plastic bottles, squeeze the bottle to create suction and connect the IV port of an empty bottle to an NG tube (Fig 34-4). If the connection is loose, it can be sealed with tape, producing portable NG suction. Replace the bottles as they fill.

Esophageal Foreign Bodies

Esophageal foreign bodies most commonly get stuck at the cricopharyngeal constriction (Fig. 34-5). In adults, who usually have food impactions, rather than foreign bodies, objects often lodge in the mid-esophagus or at the gastroesophageal junction. The safest and simplest solution may be simply to observe whether the patient can still swallow liquids.[28]

A safe, fast, and inexpensive method for removing coins (and probably other non-sharp objects) from the pediatric esophagus is to push them through to the stomach using an

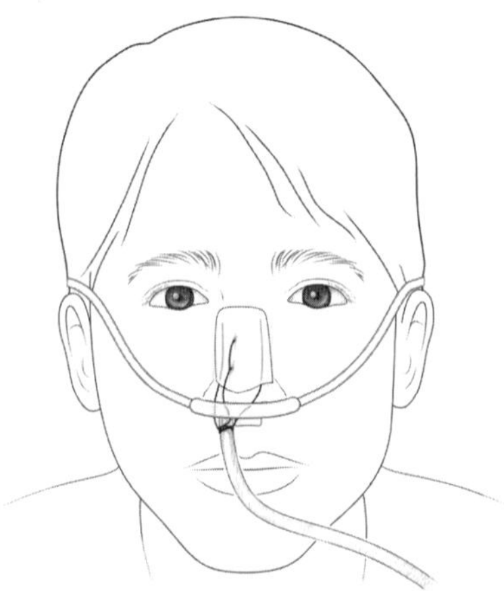

FIG. 34-3. Securing an NG tube with ties and tape.

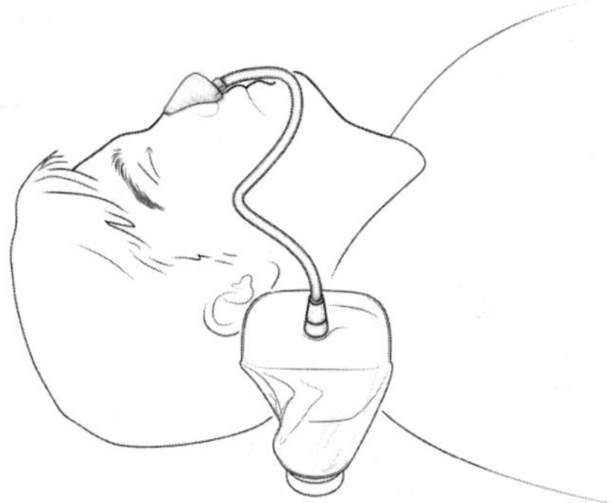

FIG. 34-4. Plastic IV bottle used as NG tube suction and collection device.

esophageal dilator. First, take a radiograph to be sure that a non-sharp foreign body is present in the esophagus. Select an appropriate esophageal dilator size, and measure the proper depth by using the distance from the tip of the nose to the ear and then to the epigastrium. To maintain airway reflexes, and because the procedure is so brief, no sedation is used and no IV is started. Topical anesthetic can be applied to the posterior pharynx, but that is not necessary. Lubricate the dilator tip with water-soluble gel. Seat the child on a parent's or an assistant's lap. Wrap the child in a sheet and have the parent hold him or her in a "bear hug." Put a stack of tongue depressors between the anterior-lateral teeth as a bite block and quickly pass the dilator to the premeasured depth; immediately remove it. This "bougienage" takes less than 5 seconds. Tell the parents to watch the stool; if a radio-opaque foreign body doesn't appear within 2 weeks, they should return for a follow-up examination and a repeat abdominal radiograph.[29]

If a child has a coin stuck in the esophagus and can still swallow water without difficulty, the following method has been successful at getting most coins with diameters from 2.5 to 3.2 cm

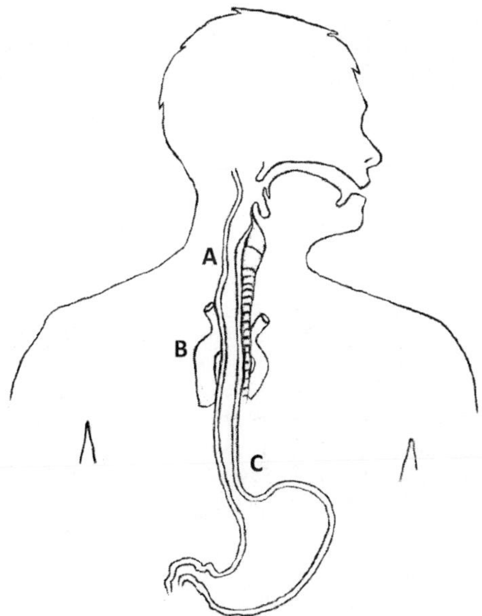

FIG. 34-5. Areas of esophageal constriction: (A) cricopharyngeal area, (B) bronchial constriction, (C) diaphragm/gastroesophageal junction.

to pass (including those stuck at the cricopharyngeal constriction). Spray the pharynx three times with local anesthetic and have the child swallow the spray. Then give the child another test dose of water to be sure he or she can swallow normally. If so, have him or her swallow 10 to 20 mL of cooking oil, followed by eating a solid meal. (In the article cited here, they used meals of vegetables and cereal.) If the foreign body has been in place ≥15 days prior to seeking medical care, this method will probably not work; removal by esophagoscopy may be the only option.[30]

Use a balloon (e.g., Foley) catheter to remove a proximal foreign body—with or without fluoroscopy. First, put the patient in a lateral decubitus-head-down (Trendelenburg) position to avoid aspiration. To remove an object, gently pass a urethral catheter with balloon past the obstruction. Inflate the balloon with water and withdraw the catheter using steady traction. Success has been as high as 98%, but there is a risk of the patient aspirating the foreign body.[31,32] If the foreign body does not come out easily, consider another method.

Esophagoscopy

If available, a sigmoidoscope or bronchoscope of the appropriate size can be used for esophagoscopy.[33] If not, improvise a crude pediatric esophagoscope by slipping a curtain rod over the straight blade of a pediatric laryngoscope. The thin tube (or equivalent) should have an outer diameter of ~15 mm and a thickness of 1 mm. Its length can be 30, 40, or 50 cm, depending on the child's size and what needs to be examined. The distal end of the pipe is beveled at 45 degrees with the cut edges filed smooth. Used in children primarily around 5 years old for various indications, it provides moderately bright illumination.[34]

Paracentesis Drainage System

Construct a paracentesis system using a standard Foley catheter kit, IV tubing, a spinal needle, and some suture removal scissors. Cut the proximal end off the collecting tube connected to the urine bag. Insert the "spike" on the IV tubing into that end. Place the Foley bag below the patient or on the floor. Puncture the abdomen (using ultrasound visualization, if available) with a 20-gauge spinal needle (most angiocatheters are too short and too flexible) and a "Z-track" to prevent post-procedure leaking. To perform a Z-track, push the needle halfway through the abdominal wall. Then, while keeping it at a right angle to the abdomen, move the needle 1 to 2 cm away and finish the puncture. Leave the plastic needle guard on, but cut it to match the abdominal wall thickness (also determined from the ultrasound). This prevents inadvertently pushing it too deeply into the abdomen. Connect the needle to the IV tubing and bolster the needle with gauze and tape. Add a three-way stopcock, if available.

Rectal Foreign Bodies

Rectal foreign bodies can lead not only to partial obstruction, but also to mucosal erosions and perforations. So, if they do not pass spontaneously, they must be removed. If sedation is available, removing them can often be done outside the operating room. There are several common makeshift methods. One method uses a urethral balloon catheter that is passed beyond the object so that the liquid-inflated balloon pushes the object out (from behind). This technique also has the benefit, even if it doesn't work, of helping break the vacuum seal that often prevents the object from passing by itself. Another method is to use a rigid sigmoidoscope or an infant/adult pelvic speculum (with internal light, if available) to visualize and grab the object.

Actually keeping hold of the usually slippery object can be difficult. The best method depends on the object's shape, size, and consistency. Irregular objects may be held with any clamp. Rubber objects can be firmly grasped with a single-toothed tenaculum (used in gynecologic surgery or culdocenteses to grasp the cervix). This allows the object to be rotated, if necessary, and extracted without difficulty.

Anoscopy/Sigmoidoscopy

A standard test tube can be used as an anoscope for infants. For adults, an improvised proctoscope (anoscope) can be easily made from the container for a 10-mL syringe and the container

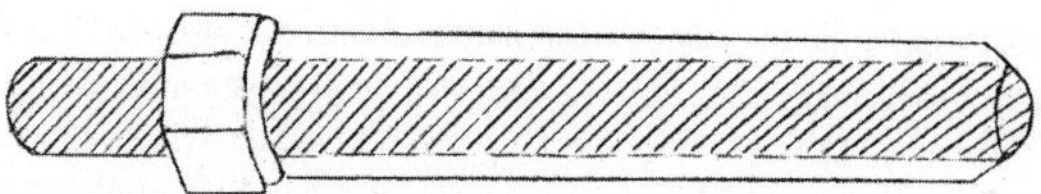

FIG. 34-6. Improvised proctoscope/anoscope.

for a chest tube. Cut off the end of the syringe container and insert the rounded end of the chest tube container as an obturator; cut it just a little longer than the length of the syringe container (Fig. 34-6). Use a headlamp or penlight to provide illumination.[35]

Replacing a Percutaneous Endoscopic Gastrostomy Tube Without Endoscopy

Replacing a percutaneous endoscopic gastrostomy (PEG) tube is often possible when endoscopy is unavailable, too costly, or dangerous. The most common method is to replace it using a Foley catheter. An alternative, when the PEG tube's proximal few centimeters near the stomach wall are preserved, is to cut off the degraded portion of the tube and connect the residual portion to a urobag. The urobag tube fits snugly into the original PEG tube, and the twist lock and adapters can be refitted onto it. This method avoids the risks and costs of a repeat endoscopy. Moreover, the urobag is 20 times cheaper than a replacement PEG tube.[36]

REFERENCES

1. Friedman NL: Hiccups: a treatment review. *Pharmacotherapy*. 1996;16(6):986-995.
2. Kolodzik PW, Eilers MA. Hiccups (singultus): review and approach to management. *Ann Emerg Med*. 1991;20:565-573.
3. Landers C, Turner D, Makin C, Zaglul H, Brown R. Propofol associated hiccups and treatment with lidocaine. *Anesth Analg*. 2008;107(5):1757-1758.
4. Boulouffe C, Vanpee D. Severe hiccups and intravenous lidocaine. *Acta Clin Belg*. 2007;62(2): 123-125.
5. Dunst MN, Margolin K, Horak D. Lidocaine for severe hiccups (letter). *N Engl J Med*. 1993;329: 890-891.
6. Cohen SP, Lubin E, Stojanovic M. Intravenous lidocaine in the treatment of hiccup. *South Med J*. 2001;94(11):1124-1125.
7. Tramèr MR. A rational approach to the control of postoperative nausea and vomiting: evidence from systematic reviews. Part I. efficacy and harm of antiemetic interventions, and methodological issues. *Acta Anaesthesiol Scand*. 2001;45:4-13.
8. Gan TJ, Meyer T, Apfel CC, et al. Consensus guidelines for managing postoperative nausea and vomiting. *Anesth Analg*. 2003;97:62-71.
9. Glare P, Pereira G, Krisjanson LJ, Stockler M, Tattersall M. Systematic review of the efficacy of antiemetics in the treatment of nausea in patients with far-advanced cancer. *Support Care Cancer*. 2004;12: 432-440.
10. Roscoe JA, Matteson SE. Acupressure and acustimulation bands for control of nausea: a brief review. *Am J Obstet Gynecol*. 2002;186(5 suppl):S244-S247.
11. Fan C-F, Tanhui E, Joshi S, et al. Acupressure treatment for prevention of postoperative nausea and vomiting. *Anesth Analg*. 1997;84:821-825.
12. PBS. *American Experience: Bataan Rescue*. http://www.pbs.org/wgbh/amex/bataan/peopleevents/e_disease.html. Accessed September 29, 2006.
13. Van Niel CW, Feudtner C, Garrison MM, et al. *Lactobacillus* therapy for acute infectious diarrhea in children: a meta-analysis. *Pediatrics*. 2002;109(4):678-684.
14. Anon. Probiotics. *The Medical Letter*. 2007;49(1267):66-68.
15. Allen SJ, Martinez EG, Gregorio GV, et al. Probiotics for treating acute infectious diarrhoea. *Cochrane Database Syst Rev*. 2010;(11):CD003048.
16. Stanley AJ. Update on risk scoring systems for patients with upper gastrointestinal haemorrhage. *World J Gastro*. 2012;18(22):2739-2744.
17. Kashyap B, Kaur IR, Garg PK, Das D, Goel S. 'Test and treat' policy in dyspepsia: time for a reappraisal. *Trop Doct*. 2012;42(2):109-111.
18. Verne GN, Robinson ME, Vase L, et al. Reversal of visceral and cutaneous hyperalgesia by local rectal anesthesia in irritable bowel syndrome (IBS) patients. *Pain*. September 2003;105(1-2):223-230.

19. Schiller LR. Review article: the therapy of constipation. *Aliment Pharmacol Ther*. 2001;15:749-763.
20. Soholt RL. Remedy for proctalgia fugax. *Postgrad Med*. www.postgradmed.com/pearls.htm. Accessed September 23, 2007.
21. Wijewickrama ES, Wanigasuriya IWMP, Jayaratne SD. Banding of oesophageal varices using locally improvised materials. *Ceylon Med J*. 2005;50(2):79-80.
22. MacRae HM, McLeod RS. Comparison of hemorrhoidal treatment modalities. A meta-analysis. *Dis Colon Rectum*. 1995;38:687-694.
23. Senapati A, Nicholls RJ. A randomized trial to compare the results of injection sclerotherapy with a bulk laxative alone in the treatment of bleeding haemorrhoids. *Int J Colorectal Dis*. 1988;3:124-126.
24. Bacher H, Mischinger H-J, Wekgartner G, et al. Local nitroglycerin for treatment of anal fissures: an alternative to lateral sphincterotomy? *Dis Colon Rectum*. 1997;40(7):840-844.
25. Chintamani, Tandon M, Khandelwal R. 'Frozen finger' in anal fissures. *Trop Doct*. 2009;39:225-226.
26. Kaufman HD. Outpatient treatment of haemorrhoids by cryotherapy. *Br J Surg*. 2005;63:462-463.
27. Dobson AP. Nasogastric tube insertion: another technique. *Anaesthesia*. 2006;61:1127.
28. Conners GP, Cobaugh DJ, Feinberg R, et al. Home observation for asymptomatic coin ingestion: acceptance and outcomes. The New York State Poison Control Center Coin Ingestion Study Group. *Acad Emerg Med*. 1999;6:213-217.
29. Arms JL, Mackenberg-Mohn MD, Bowen MV, et al. Safety and efficacy of a protocol using bougienage or endoscopy for the management of coins acutely lodged in the esophagus: a large case series. *Ann Emerg Med*. 2008;51(4):367-372.
30. Du QH. Non-surgical management of coins lodged in the oesophagus in Tanzanian children. *Trop Doct*. 1998;28:234.
31. Bigler FC. The use of a Foley catheter for removal of blunt foreign objects from the esophagus. *J Thorac Cardiovasc Surg*. 1966;51:759-760.
32. Harned RK, Strain JD, Hay TC, et al. Esophageal foreign bodies: safety and efficacy of Foley catheter extraction of coins. *Am J Roentgenol*. 1997;168:443-446.
33. King M, Bewes P, Cairns J, et al, eds. *Primary Surgery, Vol. 1: Non-Trauma*. Oxford, UK: Oxford Medical Publishing; 1990:440-441.
34. Oyewole EA. Improvised rigid oesophagoscope. *Trop Doct*. 2006;36:214.
35. Williams JG. A disposable proctoscope. *Lancet*. 1982;2(8309):1228.
36. Khaliq A. Percutaneous endoscopic gastrostomy tube replacement. *Trop Doct*. 2012;42:85.

35 | Infectious Diseases

EPIDEMICS/OUTBREAKS

Confirming an Outbreak

Confirming that an epidemic is occurring is not always straightforward. In part, that is because clear definitions of outbreak thresholds do not exist for all diseases. For some diseases, a single case may indicate an outbreak. These include cholera, measles, yellow fever, shigella, and the viral hemorrhagic fevers.

General guidelines for meningococcal meningitis are that for populations >30,000, 15 cases/100,000 persons/week in 1 week indicates an outbreak. However, with a high outbreak risk (i.e., no outbreak for 3+ years and vaccination coverage <80%), this threshold is reduced to 10 cases/100,000 persons/week. In populations <30,000, an incidence of 5 cases in 1 week or a doubling of cases over a 3-week period confirms an outbreak.

For malaria, an increase in the number of cases above what is expected for the time of year among a defined population in a defined area may indicate an outbreak.[1]

Post-Disaster Infectious Diseases

Following natural disasters, multiple factors increase the risk of contracting a communicable disease. These include inadequate sanitation, crowded conditions, food shortages, contaminated water, and inadequate immunization. Take all preventive measures possible and be alert for signs of potential epidemic diseases to avoid or quell a secondary disaster.

The diseases listed in Table 35-1 are common following disasters. All but tetanus have the potential of developing into epidemics. The best strategy is prevention, because adequate resources may not be available for treatment—or there may be no good treatment. Unfortunately, some preventive measures, such as hand washing, may not be easy to abide by in austere circumstances.

Conserve scarce resources for those who can benefit from them by limiting treatment to those who have a reasonable chance of surviving. The definition for "reasonable" depends on the amount of resources available in relation to the number of patients.

PREVENTION

Immunizations

Individuals who are not used to giving intramuscular (IM) injections, including physicians, dentists, pharmacists, and emergency medical technicians (EMTs), may be needed to help during mass immunizations or for routine immunizations when trained personnel are scarce or busy elsewhere. As a reminder, IM injections and immunizations can be given in the lateral arm in the deltoid muscle; in the anterior thigh, especially with infants or struggling psychiatric patients; or in the upper outer-quadrant of either buttock (to avoid hitting the sciatic nerve). Do not give flu shots or rabies vaccine anywhere but in the arm. Administer as much rabies immune globulin as possible at the bite site and the rest in the arm that does not get the vaccine.

Cholera

Acidification of water rapidly kills *Vibrio cholerae* organisms. Adding the juice of one lime to a liter of drinking water rapidly kills *Vibrio*, although its efficacy depends on the type of lime. This technique has been successful in multiple locations around the world where the local limes' pH is <2.5. In any cholera outbreak, it is prudent to first test the local limes' ability (i.e., pH level) to kill *Vibrio* before suggesting this to the population.[4,5]

Decontamination

Many diseases are transmitted through contact with body fluids, including hepatitis B virus, hepatitis C virus, and human immunodeficiency virus (HIV). Use hypochlorite concentrations

TABLE 35-1 Infectious Diseases Frequently Seen Post-Disaster

Disease	Transmission	Prevention/Control	Clinical Features	Incubation Period
Waterborne				
Cholera	Fecal/oral, contaminated water or food	Hand washing, proper handling of water/food and sewage disposal	Profuse watery diarrhea, vomiting	2 hr-5 days
Leptospirosis	Fecal/oral, contaminated water	Avoid entering contaminated water; safe water source	Sudden-onset fever, headache, chills, vomiting, severe myalgia	2-28 days
Hepatitis	Fecal/oral, contaminated water or food	Hand washing, proper handling of water/food and sewage disposal; hepatitis A vaccine	Jaundice, abdominal pain, nausea, diarrhea, fever, fatigue, loss of appetite	15-50 days
Bacillary dysentery	Fecal/oral, contaminated water or food	Hand washing, proper handling of water/food and sewage disposal	Malaise, fever, vomiting, blood and mucus in stool	12-96 hr
Typhoid fever	Fecal/oral, contaminated water or food	Hand washing, proper handling of water/food and sewage disposal; mass vaccination in some settings	Sustained fever, headache, constipation	3-14 days
Acute Respiratory				
Pneumonia	Person-to-person by airborne respiratory droplets	Isolation; proper nutrition. If cause is *Streptococcus*, give polyvalent vaccine to high-risk populations	Cough, dyspnea, tachypnea, retractions	1-3 days
Direct contact				
Measles	Person-to-person by airborne respiratory droplets	Rapid mass vaccination within 72 hr of initial case report (priority to high-risk groups if limited supply); vitamin A in children 6 months to 5 years old (prevents complications, reduces mortality)	Rash, high fever, cough, runny nose, red/watery eyes. Serious post-measles complications (5%-10% of cases) are diarrhea, croup, pneumonia	10-12 days
Bacterial Meningitis (meningococcal meningitis)	Person-to-person by airborne respiratory droplets	Rapid mass vaccination	Sudden-onset fever, rash, nuchal rigidity; altered consciousness; bulging fontanel if <1 year old	2-10 days

(*Continued*)

TABLE 35-1 Infectious Diseases Frequently Seen Post-Disaster (*Continued*)

Disease	Transmission	Prevention/Control	Clinical Features	Incubation Period
Wound-Related				
Tetanus	Soil	Thorough wound cleaning, tetanus vaccine	Difficulty swallowing, trismus, muscle rigidity and spasms	3-21 days
Vector-Borne				
Malaria	Mosquito (*Anopheles* spp)	Mosquito control; insecticide-treated nets, bedding, and clothing	Fever, chills, sweats, head and body aches, nausea, and vomiting	7-30 days
Dengue fever	Mosquito (*Aedes aegypti* spp)	Mosquito control, isolation of cases, mass vaccination	Sudden-onset severe flu-like illness, high fever, severe headache, pain behind the eyes, and rash	4-7 days
Japanese encephalitis	Mosquito (*Culex* spp)	Mosquito control, isolation of cases, mass vaccination	Quick onset, headache, high fever, neck stiffness, stupor, disorientation, tremors	5-15 days
Yellow fever	Mosquito (*Aedes* spp, *Haemagogus* spp)	Mosquito control, isolation of cases, mass vaccination	Fever, backache, headache, nausea, vomiting. Toxic phase: jaundice, abdominal pain, kidney failure	3-6 days

Data from Waring and Brown[2] and World Health Organization.[3]

ranging from 500 (1:100 dilution of household bleach) to 5000 ppm (1:10 dilution of household bleach) to clean spills of blood or body fluids such as cerebrospinal fluid and peritoneal fluid. The concentration depends on the amount of organic material that must be cleaned and the area to be disinfected. During *Clostridium difficile* outbreaks, disinfecting environmental surfaces with dilute sodium hypochlorite solutions (between 500 and 1600 ppm) effectively reduces the levels of environmental contamination.[6]

Stability of Hypochlorite (Bleach) Solutions

When 1:100-dilution hypochlorite solutions are stored in non-opaque spray or wash bottles, they retain 40% to 42% of their initial activity 30 days later. Solutions diluted 1:50 or 1:5 that are stored in closed brown opaque bottles retain their original activity at 30 days.

Either store hypochlorite solutions in sealed brown opaque bottles or prepare the initial hypochlorite dilutions at twice the final concentration of the chlorine level desired following 1 month of storage. For example, to have a solution containing 500 ppm of available chlorine on day 30, prepare an initial solution containing 1000 ppm of chlorine.[6]

Method to Preserve Possibly Infected Medical Records

The World Health Organization personnel developed a system to preserve the presumably infected medical records in treatment rooms for Ebola patients in West Africa. The system, which can be used in similar situations, is: Write the data on paper; then, when you leave, just before the sprayer begins disinfecting ("Show me your hands," "Spread your fingers," "Turn over your hands," "Put your arms out"), somebody meets you with a camera phone and takes a picture of the paper with all its crucial data. They can also photograph the record through a window.

Infection Prevention Among Health Care Workers—Personal Hygiene

Hand Washing

Recent reports found that improved hand hygiene was associated with reduced health care–associated infections.[7] However, hand washing may not be necessary before donning nonsterile gloves, because it does not decrease the already low bacterial counts on gloves—unless they are punctured with sharp instruments.[8]

When there are limited hand drying options, vigorously shake your hands 12 times. One folded paper towel or even a pants leg can finish the job.[9]

Emergency Medical Service Basic Hygiene Guidelines

Optimally, emergency medical service (EMS) personnel observe seven hygiene behaviors: (a) Disinfect hands with an alcohol-based hand cleaner before and after patient contact; (b) Correctly use gloves when faced with risk of contacting blood or other biological fluids; (c) Change gloves between treatment interventions; (d) Use gowns when there is risk of contact with blood or other biological fluids; (e) Wear short-sleeved uniforms when possible; (f) Do not wear rings, watches, or bracelets during patient care; and (g) Have short or tied-back hair.[10]

Fist Bump

Because of decreased surface area and time of contact, the fist bump, in place of a handshake, may further help reduce transmission of nosocomial infections in health care settings.[11]

Surgical Hand Scrub

Two alternatives that exist for cleaning your hands before a surgical procedure are:

1. Alcohol preparation
   a. Wash hands and arms and clean fingernails; then dry them.
   b. Apply alcohol solution containing emollient, rubbing until dry. Use approximately 3 to 5 mL per application; continue applications for approximately 5 minutes, using a total of 9 to 25 mL.
2. Traditional 5-minute scrub with an agent containing chlorhexidine or an iodophor.

Homemade Soap

While soap is generally cheap and available, there may be times when you must make it. Here is a very basic recipe for hand soap:

½ ounce (14 g) lye
¼ cup cold water
½ cup lukewarm fat
1 tablespoon lemon juice (optional)

In a plastic container, gently stir the lye into cold water with a wooden spoon. Slowly add lukewarm fat. Continue to stir until slightly thickened. Add lemon juice, stirring to mix thoroughly. Pour mixture into plastic molds. Cover with plastic wrap and leave for 24 hours. Remove soap from molds and allow to air dry for 14 days. This will make one to two medium-sized bars.

Homemade Hand Sanitizer

Either use 100% isopropyl alcohol as a hand sanitizer or make one that is a little gentler on the skin, using the formula below. In both cases, the active ingredient is alcohol, so use lotion on your hands to keep your skin from getting irritated. Put liquid in a small spray bottle or an old hand soap pump bottle and keep it on the counter.

⅓ cup aloe vera gel
⅔ cup 99% rubbing alcohol
Optional 8-10 drops essential oil (e.g., vanilla, lavender, grapefruit, peppermint, Thieves oil)

Mix ingredients. Use a funnel when pouring the mixture into a bottle.[12]

Additional Standard Precautions

Table 35-2 lists standard precautions to use when the necessary resources or improvised resources are available.

DIAGNOSIS

Syndromic Treatment

Clinicians use the constellation of patient-reported symptoms and observed physical signs to diagnose and treat patients. They often add imaging and laboratory testing, but these may not exist in austere situations. Therefore, clinicians have to go back to the basics, relying on their knowledge and experience. International medical groups call this "syndromic treatment." In the old days, we called it good medical practice. The primary disadvantages of using this approach are overdiagnosis and overtreatment.[13]

Syndromic treatment regimens must be adapted to the local disease prevalence, antibiotic susceptibility, medication availability, and the patient's ability to follow-up.

Exposure and Incubation Periods

A history of specific exposure, and the interval until disease onset, can often suggest the diagnosis, as illustrated in Table 35-3.

Pattern Recognition

Only awareness and reasonable suspicion can help signal the presence of an epidemic, a new disease, or the use of a biowarfare agent in the civilian community. Alerting authorities to any of the following problems may get you assistance; it may also signal the onset of some austere times ahead. Clues are:

- Previously healthy people present with severe diseases, including severe pneumonia, sepsis (possibly with coagulopathy), fevers, rashes, and diplopia with progressive weakness.
- Multiple patients with similar complaints present from a common location.
- Many more patients than normal present with fever plus respiratory or gastrointestinal complaints.

TABLE 35-2 Precautions Against Infectious Agents for Health Care Personnel

	Standard Precautions (SP)	Airborne Precautions	Droplet Precautions	Contact Precautions	Drug-Resistant Organism Precautions
When to use? (disease examples)	For all patients	TB, chickenpox, disseminated zoster, measles (only immune staff care for patient), smallpox, SARS (also use droplet precautions)	Bacterial meningitis, *Neisseria*, *Haemophilus*, diphtheria, *Mycoplasma*, pneumonia, pertussis, pneumonic plague, group A *Streptococcus* (in children), mumps, rubella, serious viral disease	Gastroenteritis (incontinent patient), *Clostridium difficile* (active diarrhea), RSV, skin infections, herpes simplex, impetigo, non-contained wounds, lice, scabies, zoster (localized), smallpox, SARS, varicella (chickenpox or disseminated)	MRSA, VRE, gram-negative rods resistant to multiple drugs, hemorrhagic fevers
Infectious material	All moist body substances and mucous membranes	Small droplet nuclei	Large droplets	Body secretions and skin, possibly the environment/equipment	Body secretions and skin, possibly the environment/equipment
Private room	No	Yes, negative pressure	Yes	Preferred	Yes
Visitors	No restriction	Wear TB-grade mask	Wear surgical mask	Hand hygiene; barriers for patient care	Hand hygiene; barriers for patient care
Gloves; hand hygiene (most important)	Use gloves when touching body substances, mucous membranes, open wounds, between patients, when contaminated; routine	SP; routine	SP; routine	For direct patient contact; mandatory	For room entry if touching the patient or room environment; mandatory

(*Continued*)

TABLE 35-2 Precautions Against Infectious Agents for Health Care Personnel (*Continued*)

	Standard Precautions (SP)	Airborne Precautions	Droplet Precautions	Contact Precautions	Drug-Resistant Organism Precautions
Gowns	When soiling of clothing is likely	Per SP	Per SP	For direct patient contact	For room entry if clothing may touch environment/patient
Masks; eye protection	When splash to face or eyes is likely	TB-grade mask; per SP, use eye protection for SARS	Surgical mask within 3 feet of patient; per SP	Per SP	Surgical mask within 3 feet of patient. With respiratory case or infected site, per SP
Waste, linen, equipment	Per normal policy; follow sharps safety guidelines	Per normal policy	Per normal policy	Disinfect all reusable equipment leaving room; waste/laundry per normal policy	Disinfect all reusable equipment leaving room; waste/laundry per SP
Transport	Hand hygiene For all patients: Wash hands between patients and if patient contact; notify receiving dept of precautions needed	Discouraged; patient wears surgical mask	Discouraged; patient wears surgical mask	Gown and gloves for direct contact. Wear clean gloves/gown for transport in hall/public area. Disinfect all surfaces patient has contact with	Gown and gloves for direct contact. Mask, as above under "Mask." Wear clean gloves/gown for transport in hall/public area. Disinfect all surfaces patient has contact with

Abbreviations: MRSA, methicillin-resistant *Staphylococcus aureus*; RSV, respiratory syncytial virus; SARS, severe acute respiratory syndrome; TB, tuberculosis; VRE, vancomycin-resistant enterococci.

TABLE 35-3 Simplified Guide to Possible Infectious Disease: History and Incubation Periods

	Incubation Period With Possible Infections			
Exposure	<21 days	~21 days	>21 days	Variable
Untreated water, unpasteurized dairy products	Typhoid fever Yellow fever Salmonellosis Shigellosis Hepatitis C Brucellosis		Amebic liver abscess Leishmaniasis	Hepatitis A, B, E Amebiasis
Raw/undercooked meat or fish	Enteric infections Cestodiasis Trichinosis			
Mosquitoes	Dengue fever			Malaria
Ticks	Viral hemorrhagic fever (Crimean-Congo) Rickettsial diseases Tularemia			
Reduviid bugs	American trypanosomiasis (Chagas' disease)			
Tsetse flies	East African trypanosomiasis		African trypanosomiasis	
Animal contact	Tularemia		Q fever Brucellosis Echinococcus	Rabies
Freshwater contaminated			Schistosomiasis Leptospirosis	
Barefoot exposure				Strongyloidiasis Cutaneous larva migrans
Sexual contact	Gonorrhea Herpes *Chlamydia*	Acute HIV infection	Hepatitis B	Syphilis
Infected person	Viral hemorrhagic fever SARS Enteric fever Meningococcal disease		TB	

Abbreviations: HIV, human immunodeficiency virus; SARS, severe acute respiratory syndrome; TB, tuberculosis.

Data from Centers for Disease Control and Prevention.[14]

- An endemic disease appears during an unusual time of year.
- The occurrence of an unusual number of rapidly fatal cases.

Sexually Transmitted Diseases

Tests for Sexually Transmitted Diseases

Sexually transmitted diseases (STDs) constitute a huge healthcare problem. In developing countries, because of technical and cost constraints, the most useful healthcare tests to confirm the diagnosis of STDs are the Gram stain (gonorrhea, bacterial vaginosis), wet mount (*Trichomonas*), and rapid plasma reagin (RPR; syphilis) tests. Even these tests may not be available in many locations, so the syndromic treatment described in the following paragraphs is the best option.

Sexually Transmitted Disease Syndromes

Treating presumed STDs using the following criteria leads to treating a higher proportion of patients and, in some cases, a lessening of the disease's prevalence in communities. Clinicians usually treat patients with these syndromes on their first visit. If possible, treatment is a single dose of antibiotics taken immediately. Patients must return after 7 days if treatment fails (i.e., symptoms persist or return).[14]

Vaginal Discharge

Treat for gonorrhea, chlamydia, *Trichomonas vaginalis*, and bacterial vaginosis whether or not pruritus is present. If it appears to be *Candida albicans*, treat only for that. Three non-medication treatments often are effective against vaginal yeast infections. The first is to have the patient sit in a pan of clean, warm water containing vinegar or yogurt twice a day until she feels better. Or, have her mix three tablespoons of vinegar in 1 L of boiled, cooled water; then soak a piece of cotton in this liquid and insert it into her vagina each night for three nights. Remove the cotton each morning. The third alternative is to insert the cotton as above, but soak it in 1% gentian violet.[15]

Lower Abdominal Pain (Female)

In a female patient with painful cervical motion that is not a surgical/obstetric emergency, treat for pelvic inflammatory disease: gonorrhea, chlamydia, anaerobic bacteria, *T. vaginalis*, and bacterial vaginosis.

Urethral Discharge Syndrome (Male)

Discharge is spontaneous or present after "milking" the urethra. First, treat for gonorrhea and chlamydia. If the treatment fails, treat for *T. vaginalis* or, if antibiotic-resistant gonorrhea is suspected, add second-line therapy. Consider treating the patient's sexual partner(s).

Genital Ulcer Syndrome

If patients present with genital ulcers (but excluding typical herpes blisters), treat for chancroid and syphilis. In countries with a high prevalence of granuloma inguinale (donovanosis), treat for that. Improvised treatment for typical vaginal herpes lesions is to treat the discomfort, rather than to cure the problem. Other than analgesics (see the "Transdermal" section in Chapter 14), locally applied agents can often help. Tell the patient to apply ice directly to the area as soon as it feels like a new outbreak is occurring. The patient can also hold a wet cloth soaked in cooled black tea or clove tea on the lesions. Other options are to apply witch hazel or a paste of baking soda or cornstarch in water to the lesions.[16]

Epididymo-Ochitis (Male)

The patient has a hot, tender, painful scrotum. If there is no evidence of surgical (trauma, tumor, torsion) or medical (mumps) causes, treat for gonorrhea and chlamydia.

Inguinal Bubo

Patients have painful swollen inguinal lymph nodes without an ulcer. If there is no other infection causing regional lymphadenopathy, treat for chancroid and lymphogranuloma venereum.

Community-Acquired Pneumonia

Community-acquired pneumonia is both common and a leading cause of death. The CURB-65 score helps clinicians predict which patients may need aggressive therapy due to increased 30-day mortality, but it is not sensitive enough to use as an absolute rule. The CURB-65 Score gives one point each for confusion, uremia >19, respiratory rate ≥30 breaths/min, blood pressure <90 mm Hg systolic or ≤60 mm Hg diastolic, and age ≥65 years.[17] A CURB-65 score >2 predicts 30-day mortality with a sensitivity of 0.62, a specificity of 0.79, and a positive likelihood ratio of 3.

Pharyngitis

Group A beta-hemolytic *Streptococcus* (GABHS) causes only about 10% of adult pharyngitis cases, although this may be higher in children.[18] Antibiotic treatment benefits only those patients with GABHS infection. To determine which patients should get antibiotics, use Centor's criteria[19]: no cough, tender anterior cervical lymphadenopathy, a history of fever, and tonsillar exudates. Each of these equals 1 point. (Remember them as "CAFE" criteria: **C**ough absent, **A**denopathy, **F**ever, **E**xudate.) Without the ability to test for streptococcal pharyngitis (including cultures in children), treat only those patients with three or more criteria (points).[20] Always treat patients who have four criteria.

Bacterial Meningitis Mortality

When deciding how to allocate scarce resources, consider that the risk of death among patients with a single episode of community-acquired meningitis is twice as high for patients ≥60 years old as it is for patients <60 years old. The risk of death is three times higher for those with obtunded mental status on admission than for those who are awake, and four times greater for those in whom seizures began within 24 hours of admission.[21] This trend can be extrapolated to other causes of meningitis.

SKIN LESIONS

Diagnosis and Communicating With Consultants

Describing lesions correctly helps make dermatological diagnoses, either when using the algorithms found in many texts or when speaking with consultants. Table 35-4 gives the standard nomenclature for skin lesions. Figure 35-1 illustrates some of these lesions.

With the lesions described, use a standard algorithm, such as the one in Figure 35-2, to narrow the possible diseases.

TABLE 35-4 Standard Description of Skin Lesions

Lesion	Description	Size (Diameter)	Position
Petechia	Blood in skin; does not blanch when pressed	<0.5 cm	Flat
Macule	Discoloration, color varies; like a freckle	<1 cm	Flat
Papule	Solid, color varies; like a mosquito bite	<0.5 cm	Raised
Plaque	Circumscribed, solid; may be confluence of papules; like psoriasis	>0.5 cm	Raised
Nodule	Solid; like a lymph node	>0.5 cm	Raised
Wheal	Firm, transient	Varies	Raised
Vesicle	Circumscribed, fluid filled	<0.5 cm	Raised
Bulla	Circumscribed, fluid filled; like a blister	>0.5 cm	Raised
Pustule	Circumscribed, pus filled; like a pimple	Varies	Raised
Erosion	Skin breakdown; does not penetrate below dermal-epidermal junction	Varies	Depressed
Ulcer	Focal epidermal and dermal loss; heals with scarring	Varies	Depressed

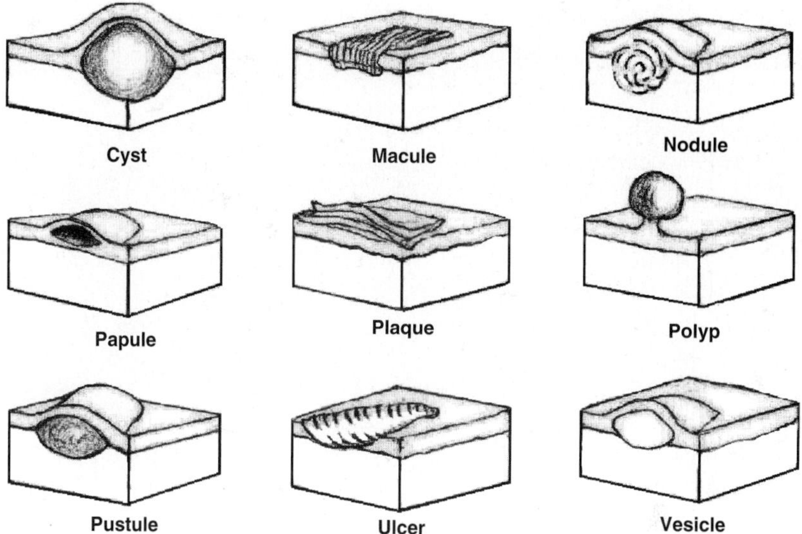

FIG. 35-1. Common skin lesions.

After making a diagnosis, clinicians may find documenting the patient's condition problematic, especially when trying to identify specific lesions. Measure the lesion and then localize it. One way to localize it is to mentally place the center of a clock face over a specific, identifiable point on the patient's anatomy (e.g., right tragus, left nasal ala, right nipple) and then describe the lesion(s) in relation to that point. For example, to document a lesion 2 inches above and behind the left eye (Fig. 35-3), write "0.4-cm lesion at 5 cm 1 o'clock from left lateral canthus." For a lesion 2 inches behind and below the left side of the nose, write "0.6-mm lesion at 5 cm 4 o'clock from left ala." This pinpoints the lesion and facilitates a later comparison by you or another clinician. This is especially helpful when there are several lesions in the same area. In addition, this system is easily understood.[22]

Teledermatology

Clinicians in austere settings now often consult electronically with dermatologists, a practice called teledermatology. To do this successfully, provide the consultant with the patient's history, examination findings, and digital images of the skin condition via email (as secure as possible). The teledermatologist responds via email or telephone and can nearly always provide a correct diagnosis and treatment plan.[23] This has proven to be an excellent tool for me when practicing in both Antarctica and the Arctic.

Tinea Versicolor

Tinea versicolor is a common skin condition caused by an overgrowth of yeast on the skin, primarily in oily areas such as the neck, upper chest, and back. It results in an uneven skin color (dyspigmentation) and scaling, and it may be pruritic.

To treat this condition, use an antifungal cream. If one is not available, make a cream with sulfur and lard (1 part sulfur to 10 parts lard) and apply it to the whole body every day until the lesions disappear. Although treatment of the infection lasts a few weeks, it takes a few months for the pigmentation to return as the epidermis replaces itself. Even better is to treat the lesions with sodium thiosulfate, which anyone still developing photographic film will have on hand. Dissolve a tablespoon of this in a glass of water and apply it to the whole upper body. Then rub the skin with a piece of cotton dipped in vinegar. Many patients must repeat the treatment every 2 weeks to keep the spots from returning. Selenium sulfide (in dandruff shampoo) or Whitfield's ointment may also help, but it must be applied 5 to 10 minutes before getting into the shower. Use it daily from the neck down for 4 to 6 weeks. (Julie Dixon, MD, Tucson, Ariz. Personal

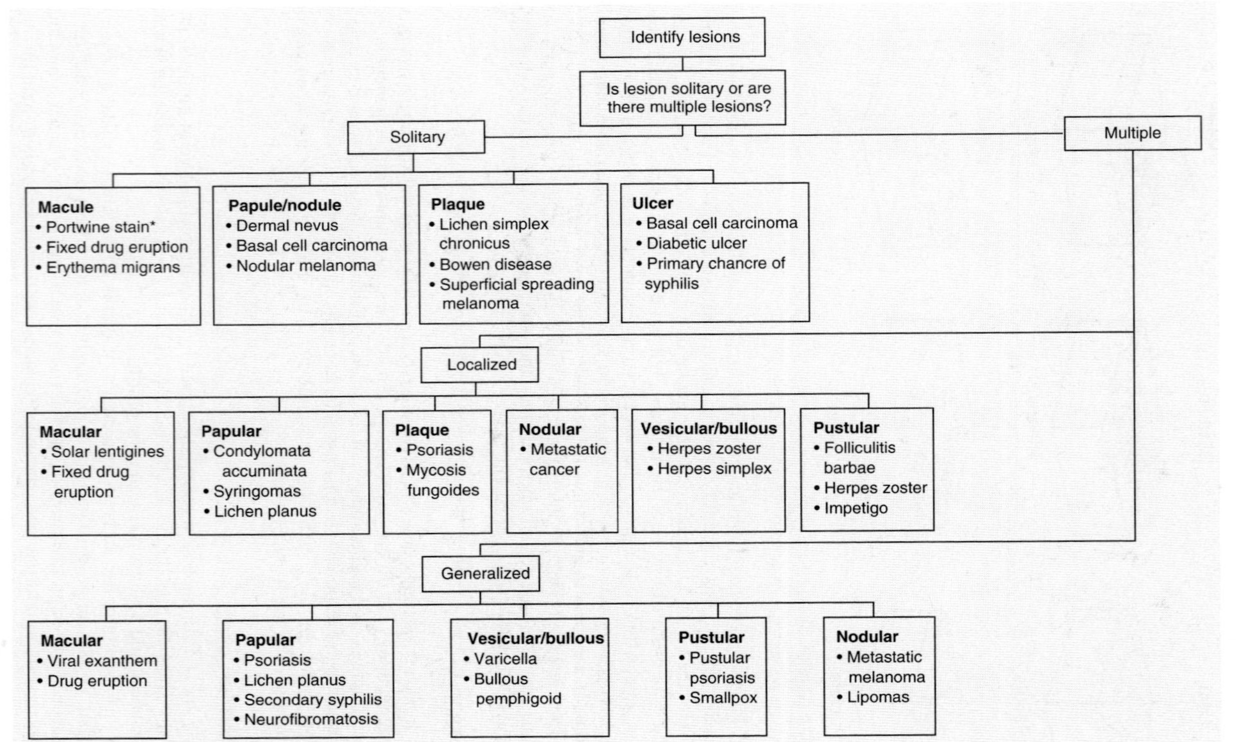

FIG. 35-2. Algorithm for narrowing possibilities for skin lesions. The listed diseases represent some of the most common disorders. *(Reproduced with permission from Wolff et al.[24])*

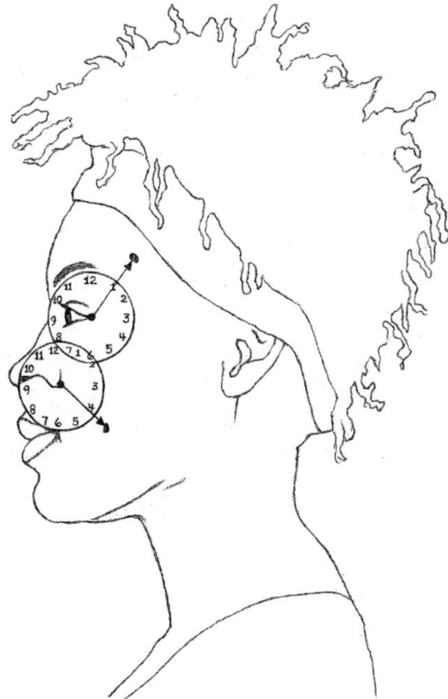

FIG. 35-3. Clock-face identification of lesions.

communication, September 4, 2008.) Whitfield's ointment is a mixture of 6% salicylic acid and 12% benzoic acid (or 6% benzoic acid plus 3% salicylic acid) in a lanolin or petroleum jelly base. All these ingredients are readily available and inexpensive. Although effective, treatment with Whitfield's ointment can be uncomfortable, because the patient feels a burning sensation.

Herpes Zoster

Herpes zoster is a reactivation of the varicella zoster virus along any dermatome in the body, although it rarely occurs on the extremities. To ease the discomfort of herpes zoster, use a light bandage over the area so that it does not rub on or stick to clothing. Zoster pain and post-herpetic neuralgia often respond to tricyclic antidepressants (e.g., amitriptyline) better than to narcotics. Post-herpetic neuralgia sometimes responds to hypnotherapy. Patients would need to do self-hypnosis, which is not difficult. See the "Hypnosis" section in Chapter 15 for details.

Topical lidocaine under occlusive patches works well both for acute pain and for post-herpetic neuralgia; its action may last up to 1 week. Use it as a cream, gel, ointment, jelly, or solution. In general, place about 700 mg lidocaine under a 10-cm × 14-cm occlusive dressing. See also the "Topical Anesthetics" section in Chapter 15.

Both the acute attacks of zoster and post-herpetic neuralgia have been successfully treated with a topical licorice (*Glycyrrhiza glabra, Glycyrrhiza uralensis*) gel. While safe topically, it can be dangerous if given orally.[25]

Verruca (Warts)

Duct tape seems to work on common warts if applied continuously (24 hours at a time; change after bathing) for 6 (out of 7) days of the week. This treatment takes weeks or months to work, but the wart eventually becomes macerated and then stimulates a host immune response and eliminates the virus. (Julie Dixon, MD, Tucson, Ariz. Personal communication, September 4, 2008.)

For those using liquid nitrogen to freeze a wart, it helps to have steady hands. An alternative is to funnel the liquid nitrogen spray directly onto the lesion using a plastic earpiece from an otoscope. This removes any fear of damaging the surrounding tissue.[26] Another method is to dip

TABLE 35-5 Factors Predicting the Failure of Outpatient Antibiotic Treatment of Cellulitis

Factor	Odds Ratio
Initial fever (Temp >38°C [100.4°F])	4.3
Chronic leg ulcers	2.5
Chronic edema or lymphedema	2.5
Prior cellulitis in the same area	2.1
Cellulitis at the wound site	1.9

Adapted from Peterson et al.[29]

a cotton-tipped applicator into the liquid nitrogen and press it into the tip of an otoscope earpiece held above the lesion. As you press harder on the applicator, more liquid nitrogen is released.[27] These treatments also likely require a number of applications over a few months.

TREATMENT

Nonsteroidal Anti-Inflammatory Drugs for Treating Urinary Tract Infections

When antibiotics are unavailable—and even when they are available—consider using nonsteroidal anti-inflammatory drugs (NSAIDs) in adult women with uncomplicated urinary tract infections (UTIs). After both 4- and 7-day treatment with NSAIDs, patients had the same symptom relief as with ciprofloxacin.[28]

Failure of Empiric Antibiotics for Cellulitis

Empiric treatment with oral or topical antibiotics for cellulitis is the norm. Factors that predict when this treatment will fail are listed in Table 35-5.

Cutaneous Myiasis

Cutaneous myiasis, caused by botfly (*Dermatobia hominis*) maggots under the skin, may be the one parasitic disease amenable to alternative treatments. Botflies have strong hooked spine rings around their midsections, and so cannot be removed easily while alive.

Many folk methods supposedly remove the larvae, including by using venom extractors (which are of no use for extracting venom); by occluding the skin hole with petroleum jelly, beeswax, or pork fat or sealing the hole with duct tape to reduce their air supply; or by applying native tobacco leaf, injecting ether or chloroform, or topically applying 5% chloroform in olive oil to immobilize the larvae. Natives of endemic areas claim that putting a small piece of meat over the affected area will eventually cause the larvae to burrow through the meat to gain access to oxygen, at which point the meat may be removed with the larvae trapped inside.

Two certain methods to remove the larvae exist. The safest and surest method is to wait for the botfly to develop and leave the body on its own, a process that takes about a month. While this is both uncomfortable and a bit discomfiting, there may be no other option. If surgical skill and equipment exist, and the lesion is in an area without vital superficial structures, remove the botfly by excising an ellipse of skin and subcutaneous tissue, including the larva's subcutaneous burrow. Leave the wound open to heal by secondary intention. No antibiotics are necessary.[30]

Cholera

Cholera treatment consists of measuring output and replacing that amount with electrolyte-containing fluids. This treatment is extremely effective in reducing the case-fatality rate (CFR) in outbreaks that can otherwise be as high as 50%. The first trick is to measure the massive output.

To determine the volume of "rice water" stool output, place patients on cholera beds, if possible. These are cots with a hole in the middle; buckets to collect the output are placed beneath the hole (Fig. 35-4). Using these beds allows patients, in their weakened state, to stay in their beds and avoid possible cross-contamination of others, rather than going to a latrine. This practice also simplifies nursing care. In an epidemic, however, such beds may be at a premium.

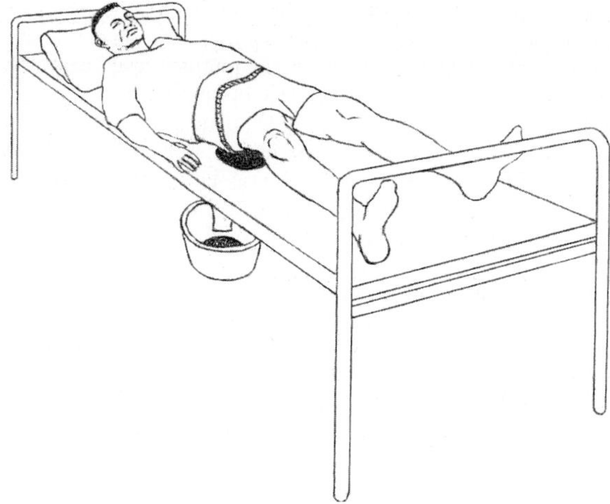

FIG. 35-4. Cholera bed.

Rather than putting two patients in one bed, a common practice that makes the bed much less useful and much more uncomfortable, improvise these beds using military stretchers. Cut a circular, 40-cm-diameter hole in the middle to fit the patients' buttocks. (Cut a smaller hole for children.) Then put the stretcher on blocks with a bucket underneath the hole.[31]

Once you have determined the output, begin treatment by rehydrating the patient. Oral rehydration therapy (ORT) is amazingly effective. For patients presenting in shock, limited intravenous (IV) therapy precedes ORT. See Chapter 11 for additional information on ORT and on making oral rehydration solutions.

Malaria—Alternative Treatment Routes

The best treatment for malaria is prevention. However, the disease is endemic in the tropics. Although antimalarial drugs are widely available, increasing resistance makes the choice of medication a moving target. When treating malaria, an alternative to administering quinine intramuscularly or intravenously in children is to administer it intrarectally. The dose of the injectable quinine dihydrochloride administered via intrarectal tube is 20 mg/kg twice a day (bid) diluted in 2 mL water.[32] This method works well in children with severe malaria or with malaria with severe emesis and no diarrhea.

To avoid death, young children with severe or complicated malaria need treatment with antimalarial drugs as quickly as possible. If transfer to a medical facility will take more than 6 hours, use rectal artesunate (or another available antimalarial). Rectal artenusate saves lives in children <72 months old. However, this route may be harmful in older children and adults.[33] Use a 10-mg/kg body weight single dose of artesunate rectal suppository as soon as the presumptive diagnosis of severe malaria is made. If the child expels the suppository within 30 minutes of insertion, insert a second suppository and, especially in young children, hold the buttocks together for 10 minutes to ensure retention of the rectal dose. The child should receive subsequent doses parenterally. The outcome of using rectal artemether 10 to 40 mg/kg body weight (at 0, 4 or 12, 24, 48, and 72 hours) is less certain. Occasionally, the maintenance dose has been one- to two-thirds of the initial dose.[34]

In patients diagnosed with *falciparum* malaria, hematuria on the urine dipstick is highly sensitive and specific for impending renal failure. Use this method in conjunction with or in the absence of appropriate blood tests. The presence of urine protein does not have the same correlation.[35]

Convalescent Serum

In situations where no antibiotics or, more likely, no antiviral agents are available or effective, transfuse serum or the blood from a patient who has recovered from the disease. Without adequate treatment for some viral illnesses that have high CFRs, the use of convalescent serum as a treatment may be the only option—if blood-banking facilities are available.

In the early, pre-antibiotic 20th century, clinicians routinely used convalescent serum taken from patients who had just recovered from the same disease to treat patients with scarlet fever, measles, poliomyelitis, erysipelas, mumps, and pneumonia. Clinicians obtained this serum at various times (e.g., 4 to 7 weeks after patients had scarlet fever). The results of treatment depended on the timing of the treatment and the disease. For measles, small aliquots of serum (5 to 10 mL) injected into susceptible contacts of an active case within 6 days of exposure prevented the disease. If the serum was given 6 to 9 days after exposure, it modified the disease. After that, it provided no benefit.[36]

More recently, convalescent serum has been used to treat hemorrhagic fevers in animals and humans with good results.[37] For the human cases, the serum was obtained from patients discharged from the hospital after recovering from Ebola virus 4 to 6 weeks earlier. Their blood was typed, tested, and anticoagulated per standard blood bank protocols. Adults received an infusion of between 250 and 400 mL of blood. Children received 150 mL infusions. While only one of eight patients receiving convalescent serum died (much lower than the normal CFR), it is unclear what role the serum played in this.[38]

Clinicians have successfully used this "old medical trick" to treat severe cases of H1N1 flu. In those cases, clinicians gave plasma donated from patients who had recovered from H1N1 to severely ill patients with the disease. The treatment markedly reduced their mortality compared to those receiving standard therapy. None suffered any adverse effect from the transfusion.[39] Dr. John A. McLean of Australia used this technique for decades to cure typhoid fever.[40]

Sepsis (or Systemic Inflammatory Response Syndrome)

When limited resources are available to monitor and treat sepsis, such as during epidemics, use the following basic methods, which do not require expensive equipment, to evaluate patients' progress. If a patient fails to improve or deteriorates at any stage, promptly reassess the patient (e.g., airway, breathing, and circulation [ABC], history, examination). Consider whether the original diagnosis was correct, whether new problems have arisen, and if the current treatment is appropriate. Signs of deterioration may include:

- Persistent or worsening tachycardia
- Persistently elevated or swinging temperature
- Rising white blood cell (WBC) count or C-reactive protein (CRP)
- Falling blood pressure, or increasing vasopressor requirement
- Deteriorating renal output
- Deteriorating level of consciousness
- Deteriorating respiratory function[41]

Because no scoring system accurately predicts the outcome for individual patients with severe SIRS/sepsis, survival depends on the patient's age, previous health, delay before medical intervention, and medical care provided. In epidemic situations, resources are limited, so physicians must face difficult decisions concerning which patients should receive potentially lifesaving treatments. (Find an extensive discussion of this in the short videos, *The Most Difficult Healthcare Decisions*, available free at https://www.youtube.com/channel/UC-KrAtJ_TCLv05NgZUNlUuQ [English] and www.reeme.org [Spanish].[42])

Neglected Tropical Diseases

Eliminating or treating some common tropical diseases may actually be easier than many clinicians think. The "neglected tropical diseases" comprise 17 diseases found in the poorest parts of the world; they afflict 1 billion people. Seven of these diseases—ascariasis, trichuriasis, hookworm infection, schistosomiasis, lymphatic filariasis, trachoma, and onchocerciasis—can be treated (and probably controlled or eliminated if an entire population were to be treated) using a rapid-impact package of drugs. Called "rapid-impact" because community-based workers can quickly distribute them, these drugs result in rapid physical improvements and, in some cases, interruption of disease transmission. These packages include four of six drugs: albendazole or mebendazole, praziquantel, ivermectin or diethylcarbamazine, and azithromycin. They are readily available in many developing countries and generally cost about 50 cents a package, because individuals and companies routinely subsidize some of the medications. An additional benefit is that this drug combination also effectively treats scabies, strongyloidiasis, pediculosis, tungiasis, and cutaneous larva migrans.[43,44]

REFERENCES

1. Sphere Project. *Humanitarian Charter and Minimum Standards in Disaster Response*. 2004:282. www.sphereproject.org/handbook. Accessed November 8, 2006.
2. Waring SC, Brown BJ. The threat of communicable diseases following natural disasters: a public health response. *Disaster Manag Response*. 2005;3:41-47.
3. World Health Organization. Infectious diseases. www.who.int/topics/infectious_diseases/en/. Accessed August 12, 2008.
4. Rowe AK, Angulo FJ, Tauxe RV. A lime in a litre rapidly kills toxigenic *Vibrio cholerae O1*. *Trop Doct*. 1998;28(4):247-248.
5. D'Aquino M, Teves SA. Lemon juice as a natural biocide for disinfecting drinking water. *Bull Pan Am Health Organ*. 1994;28:324-330.
6. Rutala WA, Weber DJ. Uses of inorganic hypochlorite (bleach) in health-care facilities. *Clin Microbiol Rev*. 1997;10(4):597-610.
7. Boyce JM. Update on hand hygiene. *Am J Infect Control*. 2013;41(5):S94-S96.
8. Rock C, Harris AD, Reich NG, Johnson JK, Thom KA. Is hand hygiene before putting on nonsterile gloves in the intensive care unit a waste of health care worker time?—a randomized controlled trial. *Am J Infect Control*. 2013;41(11);994-996.
9. Smith J. *How to Use a Paper Towel*. TedX 2012. www.ted.com/talks/joe_smith_how_to_use_a_paper_towel. Accessed January 2, 2015.
10. SOSFS. *The National Board of Health and Welfare regulations of basic hygiene routine in health care, etc*. [in Swedish]. Stockholm, Sweden: Socialstyrelsen; 2007.
11. Ghareeb PA, Bourlai T, Dutton W, McClellan WT. Reducing pathogen transmission in a hospital setting. Handshake verses fist bump: a pilot study. *J Hosp Infect*. 2013;85(4):321-323.
12. Anon. *Homemade Hand Sanitizer Recipe*. www.livingonadime.com/homemade-hand-sanitizer-recipe/. Accessed July 14, 2014.
13. Mayaud P, Mabey DC. Managing sexually transmitted diseases in the tropics: is a laboratory really needed? *Trop Doct*. 2000;30(1):42-46.
14. Centers for Disease Control and Prevention. *Yellow Book, 2007-2008*. New York, NY: Elsevier, Inc.; 2007.
15. Burns AA, Lovich R, Maxwell J, et al. *Where Women Have No Doctors: A Health Guide for Women*. 3rd ed. Berkeley, CA: Hesperian Foundation; 2006:327.
16. Burns AA, Lovich R, Maxwell J, et al. *Where Women Have No Doctors: A Health Guide for Women*. 3rd ed. Berkeley, CA: Hesperian Foundation; 2006:332.
17. Loke YK, Kwok CS, Niruban A, et al. Value of severity scales in predicting mortality from community acquired pneumonia: a systematic review and meta-analysis. *Thorax*. 2010;65:884-890.
18. Cooper RJ, Hoffman JR, Bartlett JG. Principles of appropriate antibiotic use for acute pharyngitis in adults: background. *Ann Intern Med*. 2001;134:509-517.
19. Centor RM, Witherspoon JM, Dalton HP, et al. The diagnosis of strep throat in adults in the emergency room. *Med Decis Making*. 1981;1:239-246.
20. Hall MC, Kieke B, Gonzales R, et al. Spectrum bias of a rapid antigen detection test for group A beta-hemolytic streptococcal pharyngitis in a pediatric population. *Pediatrics*. 2004;114(1):182-186.
21. Durand ML, Calderwood SB, Weber DJ, et al. Acute bacterial meningitis in adults: a review of 493 episodes. *N Engl J Med*. 1993;328:21-28.
22. Quan LT. Surgical pearl: accurate documentation of facial lesions using only one landmark. *J Am Acad Dermatol*. 2001;44(6):1043-1044.
23. Muir J, Xu C, Paul S, et al. Incorporating teledermatology into emergency medicine. *Emerg Med Australasia*. 2011;23(5):562-568.
24. Wolff K, Johnson RA, Suurmond D. *Fitzpatrick's Color Atlas & Synopsis of Clinical Dermatology*. 5th ed. New York, NY: McGraw-Hill; 2005:xxxi.
25. Bedi MK, Shenefelt PD. Herbal therapy in dermatology. *Arch Dermatol*. 2002;138:232-242.
26. Healy C. Help for unsteady hands. *Postgrad Med*. 200;108(1). http://www.postgradmed.com/pearls.htm. Accessed September 23, 2007.

27. Faber WK. Warts—an easy freeze. *Postgrad Med.* http://www.postgradmed.com/pearls.htm. Accessed September 23, 2007.
28. Bleidorn J, Gágyor I, Kochen MM, Wegscheider K, Hummers-Pradier E. Symptomatic treatment (ibuprofen) or antibiotics (ciprofloxacin) for uncomplicated urinary tract infection—results of a randomized controlled pilot trial. *BMC Med.* 2010;8(1):30.
29. Peterson D, McLeod S, Woolfrey K, McRae A. Predictors of failure of empiric outpatient antibiotic therapy in emergency department patients with uncomplicated cellulitis. *Acad Emerg Med.* 2014;21(5): 526-531.
30. Sampson CE, MaGuire J, Eriksson E. Botfly myiasis: case report and brief review. *Ann Plastic Surg.* 2001;46:150-152.
31. Heyman SN, Ginosar Y, Shapiro M, et al. Diarrheal epidemics among Rwandan refugees in 1994: management and outcome in a field hospital. *J Clin Gastroenterol.* 1997;25(4):595-601.
32. Niger N. Is intrarectal injectable quinine a safe alternative to intramuscular injectable quinine? *Trop Doct.* 1994;24(1):32-33.
33. Okebe J, Eisenhut M. Pre-referral rectal artesunate for severe malaria. *Cochrane Database Syst Rev.* May 2014;5:CD009964. doi: 10.1002/14651858.CD009964.
34. World Health Organization. *Guidelines for the Treatment of Malaria.* 2nd ed. Geneva, Switzerland: WHO; 2010:40-41.
35. Pati SS, Mishra SK. Can urine dipstick tests detect renal impairment in *Plasmodium falciparum* malaria in a rural setup? *Trop Doct.* 2010;40:106-107.
36. Long PH. Biological products in their prophylaxis and treatment. *Am J Nurs.* 1933;33(4):303-311.
37. Penruddocke E, Levinson SO. Human convalescent serum. *Am J Nurs.* 1936;36(2):121-123.
38. Mupapa K, Massamba M, Kibadi K, et al. Treatment of Ebola hemorrhagic fever with blood transfusions from convalescent patients. *J Infect Dis.* 1999;179(suppl 1):S18-S23.
39. Hung IFN, To KKW, Lee C-K. Convalescent plasma treatment reduced mortality in patients with severe pandemic influenza A (H1N1) 2009 virus infection. *Clin Infect Dis.* 2011;52:447-456.
40. McLean JA. Direct blood transfusion: its history, with special reference to the Alfred Hospital, Melbourne. *Med J Aust.* 1979;2:625-628.
41. Mackenzie I. The management of sepsis. *Update Anaesth.* 2001;13(8):2.
42. Iserson KV. *The Most Difficult Healthcare Decisions.* Part 1: Resource allocation—the ethical justification (video); Part 2: How to ration healthcare resources (video); Part 3: Who allocates scarce healthcare resources? (video). 2007. https://www.youtube.com/channel/UC-KrAtJ_TCLv05NgZUNlUuQ (English); Las decisiones más difíciles en la asistencia sanitaria, Parta 1 a 3. www.reeme.arizona.edu (Spanish). Accessed October 6, 2015.
43. Hotez PJ, Molyneux DH, Fenwick A, et al. Control of neglected tropical diseases. *N Engl J Med.* 2007;357:1018-1027.
44. Campagna AM, Patnaik MM, Walker PF. Neglected tropical diseases: challenges, progress, and hope. *Minn Med.* July 2008. www.minnesotamedicine.com/PastIssues/PastIssues2008/July2008/Commentary-CampagnaJuly2008/tabid/2639/Default.aspx. Accessed 20 June 2009.

36 | Malnutrition

Malnutrition is a huge problem throughout the world, and it worsens in disaster situations. Estimates are that moderate-to-acute malnutrition affects around 10% of children <5 years old in low- and middle-income countries,[1] and contributes to more than half (54%) of the deaths in this group (Fig. 36-1). Among elderly patients in the US general population, the prevalence of malnutrition ranges from 12% to as high as 85% among the institutionalized elderly.[2] Malnutrition usually occurs in resource-poor situations. The keys are both to recognize it and to treat it effectively.

RECOGNIZING MALNUTRITION

Malnutrition can be identified using mid-arm circumference (MAC) or by comparing a child's weight and height with standard charts.

Mid-Arm Circumference

Measuring a child's MAC helps to determine the degree of malnourishment. This technique is at least as good at predicting mortality from malnutrition as is a child's position on a weight/height growth chart. Measure MAC, in centimeters, at the midpoint of the left upper arm, halfway between the point of the shoulder and the elbow. From 1 to 5 years of age, the mid-arm circumference remains fairly stable because the increasing growth in muscle mass is balanced by a decrease in arm fat. The median value for this age group is 16.5 cm. In the first 12 months of life, MAC changes so rapidly that it is not a reliable indicator of malnutrition. And, while skin thickness over the scapula or triceps can be measured, this requires the use of calipers and provides little additional information.[3]

To make the measurement, have the child keep the arm hanging straight down by his side (Fig. 36-2). If the MAC of a child between the ages of 1 and 5 years is <12.5 cm, he is severely malnourished. If it is between 12.5 and 14 cm, he is moderately malnourished. Above 14 cm is normal.[4,5]

If a measuring tape is not available, one of the easiest measuring tools is to see which finger touches your thumb when wrapped around the child's mid-arm. Predetermine measurements for each of your finger-to-thumb distances. Then you will know which combination indicates severe malnutrition (<12.5 cm), moderate (12.5-14 cm) and normal (>14 cm). Practice and teach this to others, using a roll of gauze as a surrogate arm.[6] A marked piece of non-stretchable cloth or a string with knots at the appropriate distances can be used, although it may stretch a little. Another method is to use a strip of x-ray film. Scratch or paint the film at the 0-cm mark, and

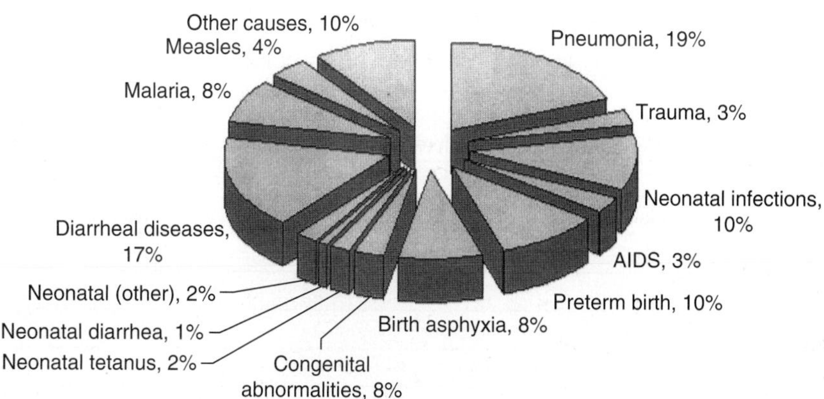

FIG. 36-1. Causes of death in children, worldwide.

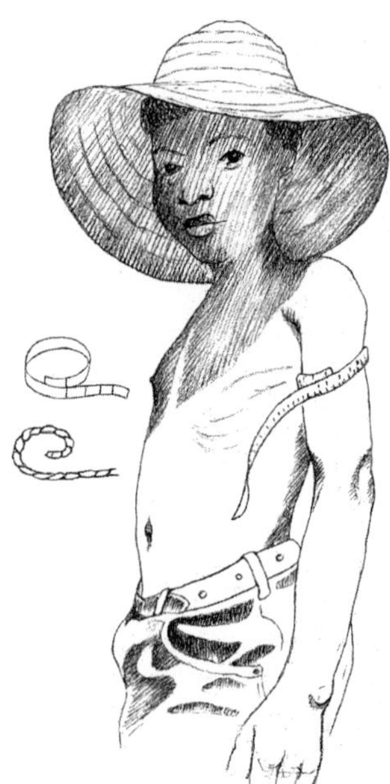

FIG. 36-2. Measure the mid-upper arm circumference to assess malnutrition.

again at the 12.5- and 14-cm marks. For clarity, the area between the 0- and 12.5-cm marks can be colored red; the area between 12.5 and 14 cm, yellow; and the area above 14 cm, green.

MALNUTRITION IN ELDERLY ADULTS

The best parameters to determine nutritional risk in adults ≥65 years old are MAC and calf circumference.

Measure MAC as in a child. The standards for people at the 5th and 50th percentile are listed in Table 36-1. Those below the 50th percentile are at risk for malnutrition; those at or below the 5th percentile are seriously malnourished. For calf circumference, both the knee and ankle should be at 90-degree angles. In a sitting person, pass the measuring tape around the calf and move it along the calf to locate the largest circumference. If the person is supine, bend the knee to a 90-degree angle and support the foot so that it is also at 90 degrees before measuring the calf.[7] The calf circumference which indicates that this group is at malnutrition risk is ≤31 cm.[8]

CLASSIFICATION OF PEDIATRIC MALNUTRITION

A child's classification as malnourished depends on his or her position on the standard weight-height-for-age charts, which can be accessed at the Centers for Disease Control and Prevention:

TABLE 36-1 Percentiles for Mid-Arm Circumference (cm): Older Adults

Age (years)	5th Percentile		50th Percentile	
	Men (cm)	Women (cm)	Men (cm)	Women (cm)
65-69	20.6	21.2	26.0	26.4
70-74	20.9	20.1	25.5	25.5
75-79	19.7	19.3	24.5	24.9
80-84	19.3	17.9	23.7	23.5
85+	18.9	16.4	23.0	22.1

Adapted from Burr and Phillips.[9]

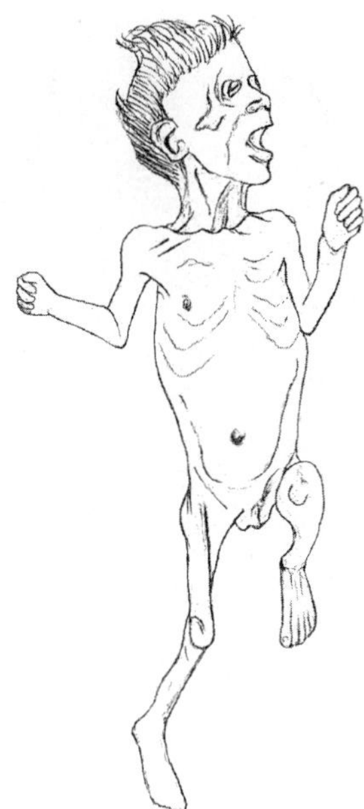

FIG. 36-3. Marasmus.

Growth Charts (www.cdc.gov/growthcharts/). Height (length for a supine infant) and weight can be measured using standard means or by the improvised methods described in Chapter 7. Interpret the results using the Welcome Classification system:

Percentage of Standard	Edema Present	Edema Absent
60-80	Kwashiorkor	Underweight
<60	Marasmic-kwashiorkor	Marasmus

MALNUTRITION MANAGEMENT IN CHILDREN

Severe malnutrition takes the form of either marasmus (wasting; Fig. 36-3) or kwashiorkor (edema; Fig. 36-4), or a combination of the two. The reasons for a progression of nutritional deficit into one form rather than the other are unclear and cannot be explained solely by the composition of the deficient diet.[10]

Moderate Malnutrition

A child has moderate malnutrition if he or she is at 60% to 80% of expected weight, with a flat or falling position on the weight chart and there is no edema. Treat the child as an outpatient. Discuss one or two of the following "nutrition messages" with the child's parent(s).[11]

1. Start giving soft food as well as breast milk when your child is 4 months old. If you do not know the child's age, start this when he or she can roll over.
2. Add extra coconut cream, pan drippings, or margarine to the child's food.
3. Feed your child four to six times a day.
4. Feed your child cooked and mashed peanuts, beans, or fish every day.
5. Continue to feed your child when he or she is sick and give extra food after sickness.
6. Eat plenty of food when pregnant or breastfeeding.

Check and treat the child for diseases that cause malnutrition, such as worms, anemia, chronic diarrhea, other infections, resistant malaria, and tuberculosis (TB). Admit only if another illness is present or if there is no improvement after 1 month of outpatient treatment.

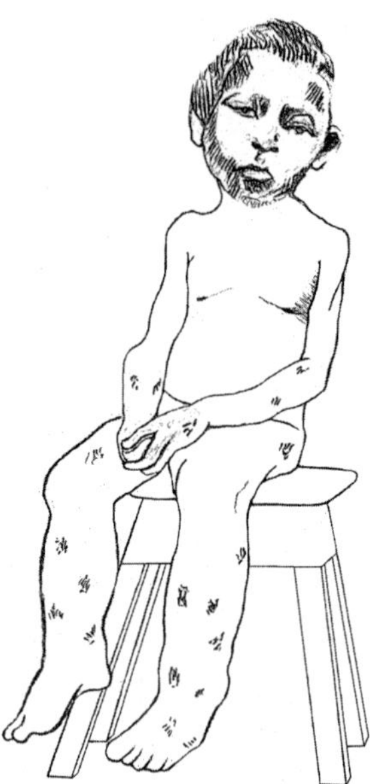

FIG. 36-4. Kwashiorkor.

Severe Malnutrition

A child has severe malnutrition if the weight-for-height is <70% for the population, with a flat or falling position on the standard weight chart; if there is obvious severe wasting; or if the child has edema of both feet. Admit the child to the hospital and treat any infection and anemia. Rule out resistant malaria and TB.

Severely malnourished hospitalized children die primarily from hypoglycemia, hypothermia, cardiac failure (over-hydration and potassium deficiency), and missed or untreated infections. The basic steps, and a timeline, for treating severely malnourished children are described in Table 36-2.

TABLE 36-2 Caring for Severely Malnourished Children (Approximate Timeline)

	Stabilization		Rehabilitation
	Days 1-2	Days 3-7	Weeks 2-6
1. Prevent/treat hypoglycemia	→		
2. Prevent/treat hypothermia	→		
3. Treat/prevent dehydration	→		
4. Correct electrolyte imbalance	→	→	→
5. Treat infections	→	→	
6. Correct micronutrient deficiencies	No Iron →	→	With Iron →
7. Start cautious feeding	→	→	
8. Rebuild wasted tissues (catch-up growth)		→	→
9. Provide loving care and play	→	→	→
10. Prepare for follow-up/counsel parents		→	→

Data from Ashworth et al[12] and Parry et al.[13]

Feeding Severely Malnourished Children[14]

Immediately give 50 mL of 10% glucose or sucrose solution (one rounded teaspoon of sugar in 3½ teaspoons water) orally or by nasogastric (NG) tube. If it will be quicker, give Starter formula (Table 36-3) or Formula-75 (F-75; see Table 36-4 for homemade F-75). Always use boiled water.

1. Prepare the F-75 formula by adding the dried skimmed milk, sugar, cereal flour, and oil to some water and mix. Boil the mixture for 5 to 7 minutes. After the mixture cools, add the mineral mix and vitamin mix, and mix the solution again. Add enough boiled water to bring the volume up to 1000 mL.
2. Alternatively, make a similar formula with 35 g dried whole milk, 70 g sugar, 35 g cereal flour, 17 g oil, 20 mL mineral mix, 140 mg vitamin mix, and enough water to make 1000 mL. Another alternative is to use 300 mL fresh cows' milk, 70 g sugar, 35 g cereal flour, 17 g oil, 20 mL mineral mix, 140 mg vitamin mix, and enough water to make 1000 mL.
3. If cereal flour is not available or if there are no cooking facilities, make a comparable formula with 25 g dried skimmed milk, 100 g sugar, 27 g oil, 20 mL mineral mix, and 140 mg vitamin mix in enough water to make 1000 mL. Note that this formula has a high osmolarity (415 mOsmol/L) and may not be well tolerated by all children, especially those with diarrhea.
4. Commercially available isotonic versions of F-75 (280 mOsmol/L) contain maltodextrins to replace cereal flour and some of the sugar.

TABLE 36-3 Formulas for Milk-Based Starter and Catch-Up Feeding

	For Full-Cream Milk Powder, Use	
	Starter	Catch-up
Full-cream milk powder	35 g	110 g
Sugar	100 g	50 g
Vegetable oil	20 g (or mL)	30 g (or mL)
Electrolyte/mineral solution	20 mL	20 mL
Bring volume up to 1000 mL with cooled, boiled water.		
	For Dried Skimmed Milk, Use	
	Starter	Catch-up
Dried skimmed milk	25 g	80 g
Sugar	100 g	50 g
Vegetable oil	30 g (or mL)	60 g (or mL)
Electrolyte/mineral solution	20 mL	20 mL
Bring volume up to 1000 mL with cooled, boiled water.		
	For Fresh or Long-Life Cows' Milk, Use	
	Starter	Catch-up
Fresh or long-life milk	300 mL	880 mL
Sugar	100 g	75 g
Vegetable oil	20 g (or mL)	20 g (or mL)
Electrolyte/mineral solution	20 mL	20 mL
Bring volume up to 1000 mL with cooled, boiled water.		

To prepare solutions: Place the ingredients in a 1-L electric blender. Add water up to the 1-L mark and blend. (Do not add 1 L of water because this makes solution too dilute.) If a blender is not available, mix the oil and sugar thoroughly, then mix in the milk and electrolyte/mineral solution and bring volume up to 1 L. Whisk thoroughly to prevent the oil from separating out.

Data from Ashworth et al[15] and Parry et al.[16]

TABLE 36-4 Recipes for Homemade F-75 and F-100 Formulas

Homemade F-75 Formula	
Ingredient	**Amount**
Dried skimmed milk	25 g
Sugar	70 g
Cereal flour	35 g
Vegetable oil	27 g
Mineral mix[a]	20 mL
Vitamin mix[a]	140 mg
Potable water	1000 mL
Homemade F-100 Formula	
Ingredient	**Amount**
Dried skimmed milk	80 g
Sugar	50 g
Vegetable oil	60 g
Mineral mix[a]	20 mL
Vitamin mix[a]	140 mg
Potable water	1000 mL

[a]Usually a commercial mix, but pharmacies can also make them.

Data from World Health Organization.[17]

If the child will eat, give him or her food and, if needed, start rehydration immediately. Feed every 2 to 3 hours, day and night, to prevent hypoglycemia and hypothermia.

For the first 1 to 7 days (stabilization phase), give small frequent feedings of commercial or homemade F-75 or milk-based Starter formula. The norm is 130 mL/kg/day, or 100 mL/kg/day if the child has severe edema.

As the child's appetite returns, switch to Formula-100 (F-100) solution (see Table 36-4) or to Catch-up formula (see Table 36-3). Add 10 mL to each feeding until some remains uneaten. This should provide about 200 mL/kg/day.

1. To prepare the F-100 diet, mix dried skimmed milk, sugar, and oil into warm water that has been boiled. Add the mineral mix and vitamin mix, and stir the solution. Add more boiled water to make 1000 mL.
2. Make a similar formula using 110 g whole dried milk, 50 g sugar, 30 g oil, 20 mL mineral mix, 140 mg vitamin mix, and boiled water to make 1000 mL. Alternatively, use 880 mL fresh cows' milk, 75 g sugar, 20 g oil, 20 mL mineral mix, 140 mg vitamin mix, and sufficient boiled water to make 1000 mL.

After 1 to 2 days, the child normally regains his or her appetite. At that point, give him or her frequent feedings of unlimited amounts of either F-100 or the Catch-up formula. If the child is still being breast-fed, continue this after providing the F-100, which has more protein. For children on solid foods, use peanut butter (paste) or commercial ready-to-use therapeutic food (RUTF), such as Plumpy'Nut, in place of some or all the formulas.[18] Encourage the child to eat; good foods are mashed ripe banana, bread or wheat meal with margarine, ground-up roasted or boiled peanuts, sweet potato, rice, or similar local foods.[11]

Supplement feedings with snacks: Children love to eat snacks. That they are healthy is a side benefit. Available high-carbohydrate, high-protein snacks may include high-protein biscuits, peanut paste, peanut balls, banana, pawpaw, other appropriate local foods, and egg or milk balls.[11]

- *Peanut balls:* Mix 2 cups mashed sweet potato (or taro, yam, or sago) and ¼ cup peanut paste. Roll into balls of about 1 teaspoonful and allow to dry.
- *Milk balls:* Mix 6 tablespoons milk powder, one tablespoon sugar, and 1 tablespoon cocoa. Then mix in 3 tablespoons boiled water. Roll into balls of about 1 teaspoonful and let dry.

Treat hypothermia in infants and neonates using methods as described in the "Hyperthermia," "Hypothermia," and "Frostbite" sections in Chapter 23, or in the "Neonatal Hypothermia" section in Chapter 37.

Do not overhydrate the child; confusing dehydration with malnutrition is a common problem. Use parenteral fluids only if necessary.

Give vitamin A (<6 months, 50,000 IU; 6-12 months, 100,000 IU; >12 months, 200,000 IU) immediately. Repeat if there is xerophthalmia. Give daily doses of multiple-vitamin liquid, folic acid (5 mg immediately, then 1 mg/day), zinc (2 mg/kg/day), and copper (0.3 mg/kg/day), or give an electrolyte mixture that contains these elements. Wait to give iron until the child has a good appetite, and then give 3 mg Fe/kg/day.[14]

Treat infections or presumed infections. Administer vaccines (if due or overdue), especially against measles.

Discharging the Patient

Both the child and the parent/caregiver must be ready before discharge. Do not discharge the child until he or she is stable and the parents/caregivers have been taught how to prevent a recurrence.

Discharge only if the child:

- Has completed antibiotic treatment
- Has no edema
- Is eating very well
- Shows good weight gain
- Has had 2 weeks of potassium and vitamin supplements (or can continue them at home)

Discharge only if the parents/caregivers know the following:

- When and how to follow up with neighborhood clinics
- What to feed the child, and how much and how often, using foods that will support continued catch-up growth and are affordable and culturally acceptable
- How to keep their child healthy at home
- How to provide play and stimulation to promote development
- To take their child for follow-up at 1, 2, and 4 weeks, then monthly, and for booster immunizations and vitamin A (every 6 months)

PREVENTABLE NUTRITIONAL DISORDERS

Early recognition and innovation can overcome problems of nutritional deficiencies.

Vitamin A

Vitamin A deficiency is one of the most common vitamin deficiencies. Vitamin A deficiency indicators that occur at the following prevalence levels in children aged 6 to 71 months signify a serious public health problem: Night blindness present at 24 to 71 months (≥5%), Bitot spots (foamy-appearing conjunctival lesions) (>0.5%), corneal xerosis/ulceration/keratomalacia (>0.01%), or corneal scars (>0.05%).[19] Vitamin A deficiency can be treated by providing oral or parenteral supplements. Because adequate vitamin A contributes to disease-fighting capability, it is given to every severely malnourished child.

Iodine Deficiency

Iodine is an essential element for thyroid function and is necessary for normal growth, development, and functioning. A diet deficient in iodine is associated with a wide spectrum of illnesses, collectively known as iodine-deficiency disorders. The most obvious result is goiter. If ≥30% of school-age children (6 to 12 years old) have a goiter, the severity level of the public health problem is high. If 20% to 29.9% have a goiter, the problem is moderate, and it is mild if 5% to 19.9% have a goiter.[19] To treat iodine deficiency, add iodized salt to the diet; eat milk, egg yolks, and saltwater fish; add iodine to the water source; or inject iodized oil.

REFERENCES

1. Lazzerini M, Rubert L, Pani P. Specially formulated foods for treating children with moderate acute malnutrition in low- and middle-income countries. *Cochrane Database Syst Rev*. 2013;6:CD009584. DOI:10.1002/14651858.
2. John BK, Bullock M, Brenner L, McGaw C, Scolapio JS. Nutrition in the elderly: frequently asked questions. *Am J Gastroenterol*. 2013;108(8):1252-1266.
3. Seear MD. *Manual of Tropical Pediatrics*. Cambridge, UK: Cambridge University Press; 2000:22.
4. Berkley J, Mwangi I, Griffiths K, et al. Assessment of severe malnutrition among hospitalized children in rural Kenya: comparison of weight for height and mid-upper arm circumference. *JAMA*. 2005;294(5):591-597.
5. King M, King F, Martodipoero S. *Primary Child Care: A Manual for Health Workers*. Oxford, UK: Oxford University Press; 1978:89.
6. Pollach G, Mndolo S. A semiquantitative way to measure MUAC in anaesthesia. *Trop Doct*. 2011;41(2): 68-70.
7. World Health Organization. *Physical Status: The Use and Interpretation of Anthropometry: Report of a WHO Expert Committee*. Geneva, Switzerland: WHO; 1995:398.
8. Saka B, Kaya O, Ozturk GB, Erten N, Karan MA. Malnutrition in the elderly and its relationship with other geriatric syndromes. *Clin Nutrition*. 2010;29(6):745-748.
9. Burr ML, Phillips MK. Anthropometric norms in the elderly. *Br J Nutr*. 1984;51:165-169.
10. Shann F, Biddulph J, Vince J. *Paediatrics for Doctors in Papua New Guinea: A Guide for Doctors Providing Health Services for Children*. 2nd ed. PNG Dept Health; 2003:213.
11. Shann F, Biddulph J, Vince J. *Paediatrics for Doctors in Papua New Guinea: A Guide for Doctors Providing Health Services for Children*. 2nd ed. PNG Dept Health; 2003:216.
12. Ashworth A, Jackson A, Khanum S, Schofield C. Ten steps to recovery. *Child Health Dialogue*. 1996;(3-4):10-12.
13. Parry E, Godfrey D, Mabey D, et al. *Principles of Medicine in Africa*. 3rd ed. Cambridge, UK: Cambridge University Press; 2004:185.
14. Parry E, Godfrey D, Mabey D, et al. *Principles of Medicine in Africa*. 3rd ed. Cambridge, UK: Cambridge University Press; 2004:185-189.
15. Ashworth A, Khanum S, Jackson A, et al. *Guidelines for the Inpatient Treatment of Severely Malnourished Children*. New Delhi, India: World Health Organization; 2003:38-39.
16. Parry E, Godfrey D, Mabey D, Gill G. *Principles of Medicine in Africa*. 3rd ed. Cambridge, UK: Cambridge University Press; 2004:189.
17. World Health Organization. *Management of Severe Malnutrition: A Manual for Physicians and Other Senior Health Workers*. Geneva, Switzerland: WHO; 1999:13.
18. Briend A, Lacsala R, Prudhon C, et al. Ready-to-use therapeutic food for treatment of marasmus. *Lancet*. 1999;353:1767-1768.
19. Sphere Project. *Humanitarian Charter and Minimum Standards in Disaster Response*. 2011:225. www.sphereproject.org/handbook. Accessed October 7, 2015.

37 | Pediatrics and Neonatal

GENERAL APPROACH TO CHILDREN

"Little Adults"

Clinicians who do not regularly care for children often are fearful of them, particularly because many are nonverbal and may not cooperate with an examination. While children are not just "little adults," they will be much more willing to cooperate with the examination, and even procedures, if you spend a few minutes interacting with them, rather than interacting only with the parent. As much as possible, talk with children directly as if they were an adult patient. Also, tell children the truth. If a procedure is going to hurt, tell them. They may not like that it hurts, but they will trust that when you do something else and you tell them it will not hurt, you are telling the truth.[1]

Pediatric Developmental Milestones

Failure to progress through normal developmental milestones may indicate underlying medical problems, including malnutrition, anemia, human immunodeficiency virus (HIV), hearing loss, chronic infections, lung disorders, and chronic toxicity (e.g., lead poisoning).[2] To determine how well children are progressing, remember the four important milestones listed below.

Action	50% Do It By	97% Do It By
1. Sits unsupported	6 months	9 months
2. Walks 10 steps unsupported	12 months	18 months
3. Speaks three or four single words	14 months	20 months
4. Says phrase ("Daddy go work")	24 months	36 months

For more complex testing, use the developmental assessment provided in Table 37-1, which was initially created to assess children in rural India.

HOSPITALIZED AND VERY ILL CHILDREN

Parents Caring for Children in the Hospital

In many cultures, a parent, usually the mother, traditionally helps to care for her own child in the hospital. While this should be encouraged in nearly all instances, in situations of scarcity, it has several advantages. It provides (a) low-cost bedside care, (b) continued breastfeeding, (c) emotional support from a known caregiver, (d) warmth for babies if mother and child sleep together, and (e) an opportunity to teach the mother important health care practices.

When to Refer Patients

In remote areas or in situations with scarce resources, it is important to know which children you must immediately refer to a hospital for admission or, possibly in a less urgent manner, to specialists. The following rules (Table 37-2) were developed for practitioners in Papua-New Guinea, which has a chronic scarcity of health resources.[3] However, the rules can be applied to all scarce-resource circumstances.

NEONATES/INFANTS

Normal Vital Signs

Knowing the normal neonatal vital signs for preterm infants (Table 37-3) helps to determine whether a neonate needs resuscitation (assuming that the resources to do this are available) and whether you have successfully resuscitated the infant.

TABLE 37-1 Pediatric Developmental Assessment

Age	Test Type	Behavior
3 months	T	Visually very alert, particularly interested in human faces.
	T	Moves head deliberately to look around.
	T	Definite response to mother's voice, either by becoming quiet or by smiling.
6 months	A, T	Can roll over from belly to back.
	T	If placed face down (prone), will lift head and chest, supporting herself on extended arms.
	T	If held standing with feet touching a hard surface, the baby bears his weight on his feet and bounces up and down actively.
	A, T	Reaches for and grasps small objects.
9 months	A, T	Sits alone for 10-15 minutes on a firm surface.
	A, T	Moves on the floor by rolling or squirming.
	A, T	Tries to crawl on hands and legs.
	T	If the baby is held standing, she steps on one foot then the other.
	A, T	Can distinguish strangers from known persons. May become distressed with strangers.
12 months	A, T	When lying down, can get into a sitting position.
	A, T	Pulls himself to standing and lets himself down again, holding on to furniture.
	A, T	If the baby's hands are held, she will walk, and may even walk without help.
	T	Gives objects to an adult on request.
15 months	T	Walks unevenly with feet wide apart and arms raised for balance.
	A, T	Speaks two to six recognizable words. Understands more.
	T	Points to familiar persons, animals, toys when asked to do so.
18 months	T	Picks up a toy from the floor without falling.
	T	Shows his own hair, nose, and eyes when asked to do so.
	A, T	Demands desired objects by pointing and making a noise.
	A, T	Explores her surroundings energetically.
2 years	T	Runs safely on whole feet, easily stopping and starting to avoid obstacles.
	A, T	Puts two or more words together to form a simple sentence.
	A, T	Refers to himself by name.
	A, T	When asked, correctly shows her hair, hands, feet, nose, eyes, and mouth, and repeats their correct names.
2.5 years	T	Jumps with two feet together.
	T	Can stand on tip-toe if shown how to do so.
	A, T	Uses the pronouns I, me, and you.

(*Continued*)

TABLE 37-1 Pediatric Developmental Assessment (*Continued*)

Age	Test Type	Behavior
3 years	T	Stands for a short time on one foot when shown how to do so.
	T	Can have simple conversations and talk about past experiences.
	A	Likes to help with adult activities.
	A	Plays with other children.
4 years	T	Hops on one foot.
	A	Climbs ladders and trees.
	T	Gives a connected account of recent experiences.
	A	Needs other children to play with, and is alternatively cooperative and aggressive.
5 years	T	Runs lightly on his toes.
	T	Can stand on one foot for 8 to 10 seconds.
	T	Can hop 2 to 3 meters forward on each foot.
	A	Undresses and dresses alone.

Abbreviations: A, ask the mother, although this may be unreliable; T, test by putting the child in a situation where the desired activity is likely to be undertaken.

Data from Milestones suggested by Penelope Hubley[4] and Shann et al.[5]

Which Newborns Need Resuscitation?

As soon as an infant is delivered, evaluate the baby's condition condition to determine if additional intervention is needed. To do this, I devised the simple mnemonic, "BoTToM," which stands for the status of the normal newborn: **B**reathing spontaneously (Bo), **T**erm infant (T), normal muscle **T**one (T), and no **M**econium staining (oM). If the baby does not meet the BoTToM criteria, have other practitioners (preferably two) take the child to a heated area of the room for further evaluation and, if necessary, resuscitation. If the baby meets all these criteria, dry the child and put him or her on the mother's chest for "kangaroo care." (See below for an explanation of kangaroo care.)

Successful Infant Position for Lumbar Puncture

In infants <12 months old, clinicians' first-attempt success rate for lumbar punctures is higher with the sitting-flexed position (odds ratio: 2.74), rather than with the lateral-flexed position. Their ultimate success in obtaining cerebrospinal fluid (CSF) for culture, cell count, and in obtaining non-traumatic CSF is the same in both positions.[6]

Stimulation

In most cases, neonates begin breathing without any stimulation. If not, drying and suctioning them is sufficient stimulation.

Suction

For neonates, sucking the mucous and meconium may require mouth suction. The easiest way to make a mouth-operated suction device is to punch two holes in the top of a sealed container, insert two rubber tubes through these holes, and begin sucking on one of the tubes (Fig. 37-1). The suction pressure is easily controlled by how hard the clinician sucks. Once common, use of these devices has decreased due to the risk of infection posed to health care workers. Yet mouth-operated suction devices have many advantages: They are easy to make, inexpensive, disposable, and portable; need only one hand to operate; and do not require a power source other than the

TABLE 37-2 When to Send and Admit Children to the Hospital

• Born with an imperforate anus	• <4 weeks old with meningitis, severe jaundice, or sepsis who are not improving after 2 days of treatment	• Neonates with any sign of infection, including fever in infants <28 days old
• Moderate to severe dehydration	• Fever and not sucking	• Babies with bile-stained vomit
• Intercostal retractions	• Newborns with frequent vomiting and marked salivation in the first few hours of life	• <6 months old with whooping cough
• Stridor	• Suspicious injuries that do not fit the history	• Edema
• Continued abdominal pain and vomiting	• Convulsion with fever (tropical setting with concern for TB, malaria, HIV)	• Sudden onset of paralysis
• Weight <60% of predicted for age, and flat or falling weight curve	• Mid-upper-arm circumference <12.5 cm	• Snakebite with evidence of envenomations (edema, ecchymosis, hematologic or systemic signs)
• Poison ingestion	• Child in coma	• Distended, tender abdomen
• Suspected meningitis who are not improving after 2 days of treatment	• Hematuria, with or without edema, who do not improve after 2 days of treatment	• Hematochezia
• History of unconsciousness after head injury and not back to normal when seen	• Fever, tenderness, and swelling of a limb or a joint that does not improve after 2 days of treatment	• Suspected diabetes mellitus
• [a]Malnourished children not responding to treatment	• [a]Not responding to standard medical/surgical treatment	• [a]Babies with ambiguous genitalia
• [a]Slow development	• [a]Poorly responsive w/umbilical hernia	• [a]Persistent heart murmur

Abbreviations: HIV, human immunodeficiency virus; TB, tuberculosis.

[a]Important, possibly not emergent, pediatric referrals.

Data from Shann et al.[3]

clinician. Some studies found that using these devices is a relatively safe procedure, although others have found that they occasionally can transmit pathogens.[7,8]

In some regions, mothers of older children, in what is a type of reverse mouth-to-mouth procedure, suck the mucus out of their babies' noses with their mouths.[9] The danger of passing pathogens from baby to mother is probably a moot point.

Neonatal Hypothermia

Hypothermia can be devastating to neonates, especially those who are premature or small-for-dates. In fact, all infants <12 months old are highly susceptible to hypothermia, as are any children with marasmus (previously termed "protein-energy malnutrition"), with large areas of damaged skin, or who have serious infections. Hypothermia is defined as a rectal temperature <35.5°C (95.9°F) or an axillary temperature <35.0°C (95.0°F). Also, treat all hypothermic children for hypoglycemia and for serious systemic infection.

The "warm chain" for infants (as opposed to the "cold chain" for vaccine preservation) is a set of interlocking procedures designed to minimize the likelihood of hypothermia around the

TABLE 37-3 Normal Pediatric Vital Signs at Various Ages

	Preterm	Term	6 months	1 year	3 years	6 years
Weight (lb)	3	7.5	15	22	33	44
Weight (kg)	1.5	3.5	7	10	15	20
Heart beats/min	140	125	120	120	110	100
Respirations/min	40-60	40-60	24-26	22-30	20-26	20-24
Systolic BP (mm Hg)	50-60	70	90 ± 30	95 ± 30	100 ± 25	100 ± 15
Fluid challenge (mL)	30	70	140	200	300	400
	8 years	**10 years**	**11 years**	**12 years**	**14 years**	
Weight (lb)	55	66	77	88	99	
Weight (kg)	25	30	35	40	45	
Heart beats/min	90	90	85	85	80	
Respirations/min	18-22	18-22	16-22	16-22	14-20	
Systolic BP (mm Hg)	105 ± 15	110 ± 20	110 ± 20	115 ± 20	115 ± 20	
Fluid challenge (mL)	500	500	500	500	500	

Abbreviation: BP, blood pressure.

From Canadian Air Division.[10]

time of birth.[11] These include ensuring that the place of delivery is draft-free and is stocked with the appropriate materials to immediately dry and wrap the infant, including a warm cap for the head. In addition, cover the mother and baby together, and start early breastfeeding.

"Kangaroo Care" for Very-Low-Birth-Weight Infants

"Kangaroo care" means keeping mothers and their small or premature infants together, skin-to-skin, over the first days and weeks of life.[12] Developed for resource-poor areas, kangaroo care provides an appropriate heat source (mother) that helps maintain neonates' temperatures, improves survival rates, and spurs weight gain.[13]

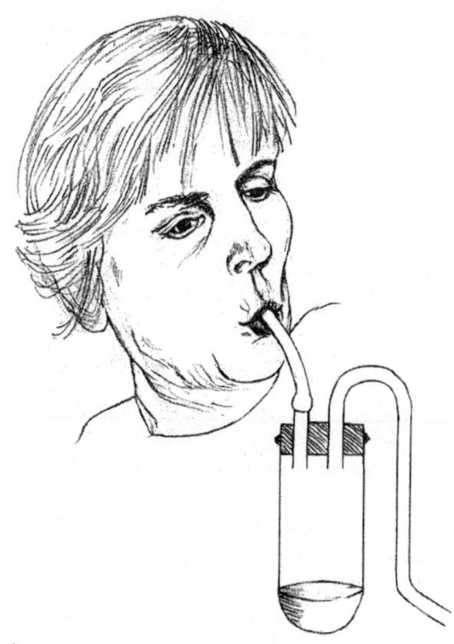

FIG. 37-1. Mouth-operated suction.

It allows low-birth-weight (<1500 g) babies, some as small as 700 g, to be safely fed, warmed, and bonded to their mothers. The technique is to breastfeed the infant with skin-to-skin contact. Place the child on the mother's bare chest or abdomen (skin-to-skin) and cover both of them. Alternatively, clothe the child well, including the head, cover with a warmed blanket, and place him or her in an incubator with an incandescent lamp over, but not touching, his or her body. Even in a public setting, mothers can continue such care under a loose dress. After the infant is discharged home, they should continue to use kangaroo care.[14,15]

Kangaroo care reduces the risk of reflux and aspiration, reduces apnea and infection, and shortens the hospital stay. It also encourages bonding between mother and baby, improves lactation, decreases the amount of time health care workers must spend with the family, and apparently improves the infant's psychological adjustment.[16,17]

Baby Bags

A simple way to maintain the neonatal warm chain is to swathe the child in a plastic "baby bag" immediately upon birth.

Make "baby bags" by loosely swaddling the infant in polyethylene doubled over on itself, with one thickness above and two below the infant. This retains the neonate's body temperature and moisture. Dry the head, *but do not cover the baby's head with plastic wrap*! This material, often used as household plastic wrap and industrial packing, is inexpensive (<5¢ US) and lightweight (<20 g for a piece to cover an infant). Optimally, use it in conjunction with a radiant warmer. Similarly, a thermal blanket laid over an infant helps preserve heat and moisture. Covering the baby's large head with a hat might further maintain heat.[18-20]

Incubators and Covers

Commercial incubators often do not work in developing countries, usually because they lack proper maintenance. Consider making improvised incubators rather than using one incubator for several infants, which only serves to facilitate cross-infections, or electric heating pads, which tend to overheat them, may produce burns, and has led to deaths[19] (see the "Equipment" section below in this chapter). Use homemade incubator covers to reduce light by completely covering the incubator. Closed-weave quilted and flannel covers perform similarly to commercial covers. Crocheted covers and receiving blankets are markedly inferior.[21]

Airway/Ventilation

Oxygenated Mouth-to-Mouth Resuscitation

Without equipment, successfully resuscitate neonates using mouth-to-mouth breathing. The best way is to run an oxygen tube into the corner of the child's mouth, with oxygen flowing at 3 to 4 L/min. The clinician uses his or her cheeks as bellows and "puffs" into the neonate's mouth. Observe chest rise to determine if the ventilation is adequate.[22]

Frog Breathing

The ventilation technique, known as "frog breathing" is suitable only for temporary use in babies weighing under about 5 kg.[23] However, this is true ventilation, not apneic oxygenation.

1. Insert an 8- or 10-Fr nasogastric (NG) tube through one nostril into the stomach. Drain it to gravity to prevent the stomach from overinflating.
2. Give nasopharyngeal oxygen at 2 L/min. Insert the oxygen cannula to a depth equal to the distance between the side of the baby's nose and the tragus (front of the ear). Do not insert it farther than this, or it may go into the esophagus.
3. With one hand, slightly lift the baby's chin, extend the neck, and pinch the mouth shut. With the other hand, pinch the baby's nose for about 2 seconds so that oxygen fills the lungs. Then release the nose for about 2 seconds and allow the elastic recoil of the lungs to empty them; you must allow adequate time for the exhalation phase. Watch the chest expand and deflate.
4. Give 12 to 15 breaths/min. Ensure that the stomach does not inflate. If ventilation is inadequate, intubate the infant. (See Chapter 8.)

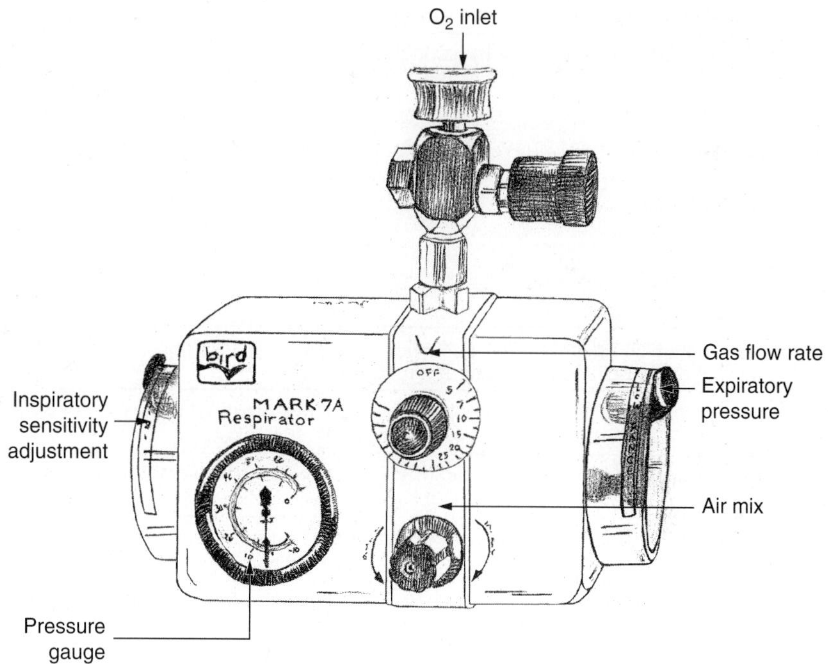

FIG. 37-2. Bird pressure-cycled ventilator.

Using a Bird Ventilator for Children

In situations with limited resources, use ventilators only for those patients who have a good prospect of benefitting, generally quickly, from mechanical ventilation, such as those with acute poisoning and some neonates. The Bird "green box" pressure-cycled ventilator (Figs. 37-2 and 37-3), while relegated to museums in developed countries, is commonly used in remote areas. It is easy to disassemble and clean, requires relatively few parts, and has been a reliable piece of medical equipment for more than 50 years. Also, use it for intermittent positive-pressure ventilation (IPPV). To ventilate a child <12 months old, use an infant breathing circuit, which is usually supplied with the ventilator.[24]

Pressure-cycled means that the patient's inspiratory effort triggers the respirator and gas flows at the rate determined by the gas flow-rate control. Gas continues to flow into the patient's lungs until the pressure in the system rises to the level set on the expiratory pressure control, then the flow stops until the patient triggers the respirator again. If the patient is too small or too weak to

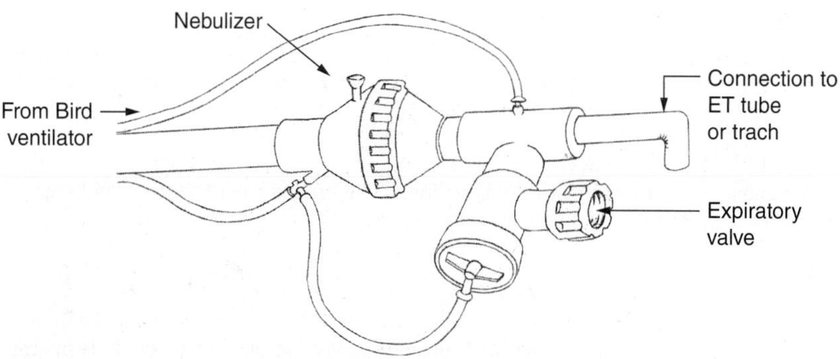

FIG. 37-3. Breathing circuit on Bird ventilator.

TABLE 37-4 Using the Bird Pressure-Cycled Ventilator

1. Before connecting the patient, adjust the controls (see Fig. 34-2) so that: — Expiratory pressure control sets the depth of inspiration. Start at a setting of 15. — Air-mix: PULL OUT AND LOCK. This gives 40% oxygen. — Expiratory time for apnea: OFF. (This control is not present on all models.) — Inspiratory sensitivity effort control determines the inspiratory effort from the patient that is required to begin gas flow. Start at a setting of 10. — Gas flow-rate control: OFF. This sets the length of inspiration. — Negative-pressure generator: OFF. (This control is not present on all models.)
2. Check that the breathing circuit is connected correctly, with no leaks (Fig. 34-3).
3. Remove the nebulizer cap and instill 2 mL sterile water. Check that fine mist appears in the nebulizer with each inspiration. Add water every hour.
4. Connect the ventilator to an oxygen supply, if available. It uses about 1.7 L/min O_2 with the air-mix control out (40% oxygen) and the flow-rate control on 10 L/min.
5. Turn the gas flow-rate control to 15, then immediately connect the breathing circuit to the patient's endotracheal tube.
6. If the patient breathes in but gas does not flow, adjust the inspiratory sensitivity effort control lower, e.g., 5-10.
7. Alter the expiratory pressure control by observing chest excursion. Adjust it until it is on the lowest setting that gives full excursion, e.g., 10-15.
8. Adjust the gas flow-rate control to alter the length of inspiration. A lower setting (e.g., 5-10) gives a longer inspiration than a higher setting (e.g., 10-15). If the patient is too weak to breathe at all, turn on the expiratory time control to set the desired time of expiration. In an older child or an adult (without lung disease), inspiratory and expiratory times should be at a ratio of about 1:2 and the respiratory rate should be about 12 breaths/min. (Patients with lung disease may need an expiratory time that is much longer than the inspiratory time.) In the absence of blood gas analysis and noninvasive pCO_2 monitors, adjust the ventilation using clinical observations, such as skin color, pulse rate, and blood pressure, as well as the timing, character, and magnitude of chest movements.

Data from Shann et al.[25]

make even the minimal effort required to trigger the flow of gas, automatically start the gas flow by turning on the expiratory time control. The air-mix control adjusts the concentration of expired oxygen to 40% (knob out) or 100% (knob in).

Set the controls on the Bird ventilator as described in Table 37-4.

Fluids

Storing Breast Milk

Breastfeeding is the norm in resource-poor areas. Yet pumping the breast and storing breast milk introduce the problems of contamination and bacterial growth. Table 37-5 describes various storage methods and their potential safe periods.

Newborn Fluid Requirements

Fluid requirements relate to a neonate's weight. Table 37-6 gives the normal daily fluid requirement, in mL/kg/day, for each birth weight.

EQUIPMENT

Nasogastric Tube

Make neonatal-sized NG or feeding tubes from the insulation on an electrical cord (2- to 2.5-mm external diameter). To remove the insulation, make a cut in the insulation at the length needed

TABLE 37-5 Human Milk Storage for Healthy Infants

Location	Temperature	Duration	Comments
Countertop, table	Room temperature <77°F (<25°C)	6-8 hours	Cover containers and keep as cool as possible; covering container with a damp towel may keep milk cooler.
Insulated cooler bag	5°F to 39°F (−15°C to 4°C)	24 hours	Keep ice packs in contact with milk containers at all times; limit opening the cooler bag.
Refrigerator	39°F (4°C)	5 days	Store milk in the back of main part of refrigerator.
Freezer compartment of refrigerator	5°F (−15°C)	2 weeks	Store milk toward the back of freezer, where temperature is most constant.
Freezer section of refrigerator/freezer with separate doors	0°F (−18°C)	3-6 months	Milk stored for 3-12 months is safe, but some lipids degrade, resulting in lower quality.
Chest or upright manual-defrost freezer	−4°F (−20°C)	6-12 months	

Data from Eglash et al.[26]

and slip it off the wire core. Smooth out the patient's end by passing it over a flame. Clean it before use.[28] Note that this can also be used as a pediatric urinary catheter.

Neonatal Incubator

A neonatal incubator is one of the easiest pieces of medical equipment to improvise. Use one of the following methods, or your imagination, to construct an incubator from existing supplies.

One disaster team wrote, "The nurses made cribs out of cardboard boxes lined with cotton and covered with plastic-lined incontinent pads. . . . Each infant was placed in the makeshift bassinet with two warmed intravenous fluid bags placed on either side of the baby's body."[29]

Improvisations over the years have included a wash boiler, a broiler, and a large metal pan, such as a turkey roaster. To use, place a layer of hot bricks in the bottom and cover them with wire mesh. Then place a pillow and blanket over the mesh, leaving about 4 inches on all sides for warm air to circulate. Make small ventilation holes by cutting openings in the cover and at each end. To supply moist air, use a vat of hot water in place of the bricks. Be sure to keep the air holes open, or leave the top partially open.[30]

Another method is to line a clothes basket with flannel or soft padding that has sewn-in pockets to hold 10- or 12-oz bottles. Fill the bottles with hot water and put them in the pockets. Keep the temperature even by refilling every other bottle at regular intervals.[30]

Yet another method is to use a laundry basket and make a support for two or three electric lightbulbs to fit over the top (Fig. 37-4). Cover the basket with a blanket or comforter. Shield the baby's eyes from the light.[30] (See the "Incubators and Covers" section, above.)

TABLE 37-6 Newborn Fluid Requirements (mL/kg/day)

Birth Weight	Day 1	Day 2	Day 3	Day 4	Day 5	Days 6-7
Preterm <1000 g	80-90	90-110	110-130	120-150	130-160	160-180
Preterm >1500 g	60-80	75-100	90-120	110-150	130-160	135-160
Term neonate	60-120	80-120	100-130	120-150	140-160	160-180

Data from Anon.[27]

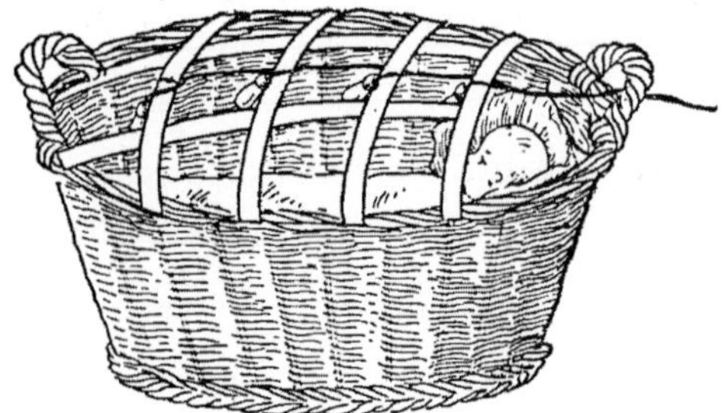

FIG. 37-4. Infant incubator from a laundry basket, with electric lights to provide heat. *(Reproduced from Olson.[31])*

Crib/Playpen

Make a basic crib or playpen by inverting a table and draping mosquito netting over it (Fig. 37-5). Be sure that the table's underside is smooth; if not, cover it with a blanket or piece of canvas. Tack it down well. Note that this also protects the child from mosquitoes, which is highly desirable, and even lifesaving, in many regions.[32]

Phototherapy Box

Light therapy is often needed for neonatal jaundice, which arises due to a transient deficiency in bilirubin conjugation combined with an increased turnover of red cells, or in exclusively breastfed infants when the breastfeeding results in poor caloric intake. The goal of light therapy is to lower the concentration of circulating bilirubin or to keep it from increasing by converting it to molecules that can be excreted even when normal conjugation is deficient.[33]

Construct a simple phototherapy device for neonatal jaundice from a wooden box and six 40-watt daylight fluorescent tubes (Fig. 37-6). Cut the box to a depth about double the diameter of the light tubes. Mount the tubes parallel to each other on the inside of the box lid, and line the inside lid with a white reflecting surface to direct the light downward. Then, mount the box on supports so that it sits about 18 inches above the baby. Use a box 140 cm × 75 cm × 20 cm (55 inches × 30 inches × 8 inches) over three cots or two incubators; the size and materials can vary to meet local needs. Cover the baby's eyes during phototherapy.[34]

Infant Bathtub

Make a baby's bathtub by attaching a piece of canvas, tarp material, or plastic sheeting to the outside edge of a wooden box about the baby's size (Fig. 37-7). Leave some slack in the center. Fill with water before placing the baby in the bathtub.[35]

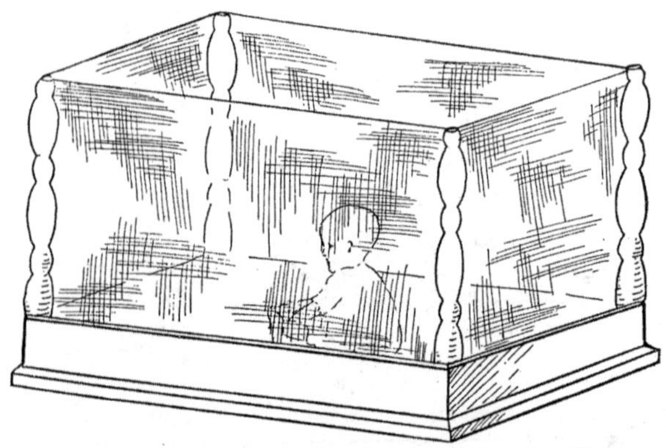

FIG. 37-5. Improvised mosquito-proof playpen. *(Reproduced from Olson.[32])*

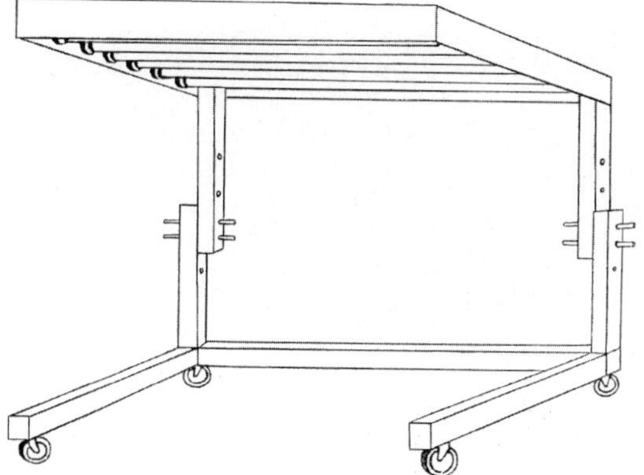

FIG. 37-6. Phototherapy device.

PROCEDURES

Urine Collection

For an improvised infant urine collection bag, see Chapter 5.

Midstream Urine Sample in Neonates

Quickly obtain a neonatal midstream urine sample by combining fluid intake and noninvasive bladder stimulation. Twenty-five minutes after either breastfeeding or providing formula, clean the infant's genitals with warm water and soap, and dry them with sterile gauze. Administer nonpharmacological analgesia, such as nonnutritive sucking or 2% sucrose syrup, to diminish crying. Then, while one person holds the baby under the armpits with their legs dangling, the other stimulates the bladder with a gentle tapping (100/min) in the suprapubic area for 30 seconds. Next, stimulate the lumbar paravertebral zone in the lower back with a light circular massage for 30 seconds. Repeat both maneuvers until micturition starts. This technique was successful in 86.3% of infants, with a median time to sample collection of 45 seconds.[36]

Measuring Volume

In neonatal units with limited nursing staff, it can be valuable to constantly measure urine output in noncatheterized infants. To do this, first make an acrylic (Perspex) V-shaped tray that fits into an incubator. The tray should have a downward slope, so that the point of the V is in the center. Cover this with a fine (100 threads/inch) mesh (georgette) that is stretched over the tray's frame and attached with Velcro strips—two 2-cm strips on either side and three strips at either end (Fig. 37-8).

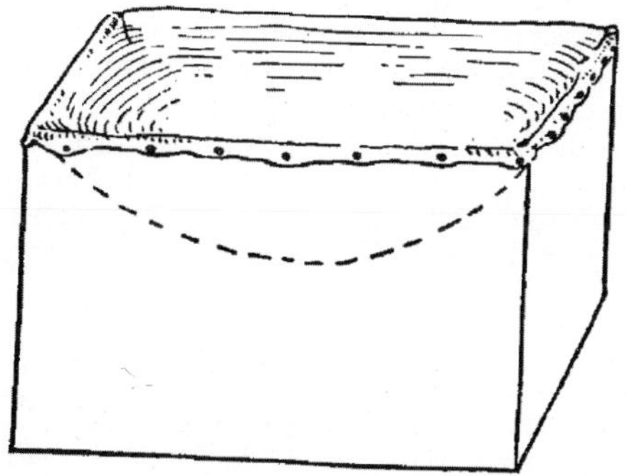

FIG. 37-7. Improvised bathtub for infant. *(Reproduced from Olson.[35])*

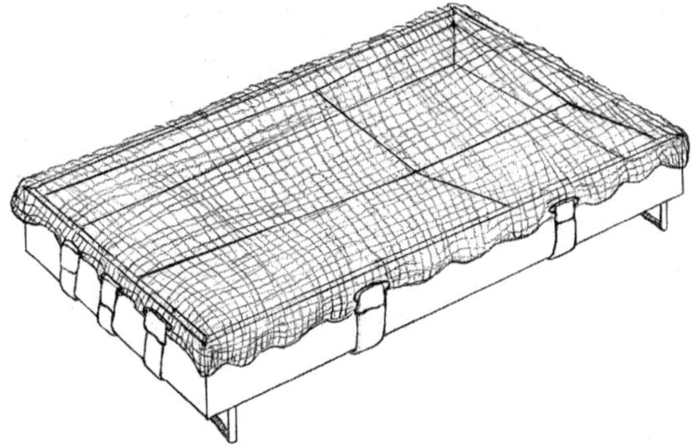

FIG. 37-8. Neonatal constant urine collector.

The mesh covering keeps neonates suspended above the bottom on this tray. Only urine and the most-liquid stools will pass through the mesh into the tray, collect in the tray's most dependent area, and drain out of the incubator through one of the low hood ports into a collecting/measuring bag.[37]

Restraint Devices/Methods

Sedation is not always available, safe, or appropriate. Therefore, you may need to restrain infants and children. Figures 15-7 and 15-8 show methods to restrain a child. Note that children may need to be restrained simply for safety if under light ether anesthesia or ketamine.

Infant Peritoneal Dialysis

Perform improvised peritoneal dialysis in a young child using a suprapubic aspiration catheter with additional small side holes cut into it distally. Place the catheter into the peritoneal cavity through a small incision using local anesthesia. Prepare peritoneal dialysis fluid using 250 mL of 5% dextrose solution, 750 mL of 0.9% normal saline, 40 mL of 8.4% sodium bicarbonate, 7.5 mL of 10% calcium gluconate, 1000 units of heparin, and 250 mg of ceftriaxone. As an example, an 18-month-old boy with kwashiorkor and renal failure had a dwell time of 30 minutes for the first exchange, 2 hours for the subsequent two exchanges, and 6 hours after that. Dwell volumes were 250 mL for the first two exchanges, and 200 mL for subsequent exchanges. He received ceftriaxone 500 mg at the onset of dialysis each day. The child did well and had the catheter removed on day 7.[38]

Proctoscopy

Complaints of fecal blood are relatively common in infants and are usually due to anal fissures. However, investigating them, and the less frequent complaint of frankly bloody stools, may be difficult due to a lack of adequate equipment. Make an infant proctoscope to get a better view of an infant's rectosigmoid than can be obtained with an ear speculum (the commonly used method).

To make an infant proctoscope, take an appropriate length of rubber or plastic tubing, 1 to 2 inches, depending on the child's size, and slip it over the end of a nasal speculum attachment or directly onto the end of an otoscope without an ear speculum attached. Use a large-size NG, rectal, or similar tubing. Immerse the end of the tube in hot water and stretch it onto the speculum using a hemostat. Smooth the cut edge with an open flame. With the child in a knee-chest position, lubricate the tube and carefully insert it under visualization.[39] As with sigmoidoscopy, always aim for the lumen when it is advanced. If you cannot see a lumen, do not advance it further (Fig. 37-9).

Inguinal Hernias

Inguinal hernias are common in infants and children. Reducing them is generally the first maneuver; surgery may not even be an option in austere circumstances. While it helps to provide some type of mild analgesic, a warm bath may work as well. An old maneuver, similar to the acute Trendelenburg position in which clinicians place adults for reduction, is to "lift the patient

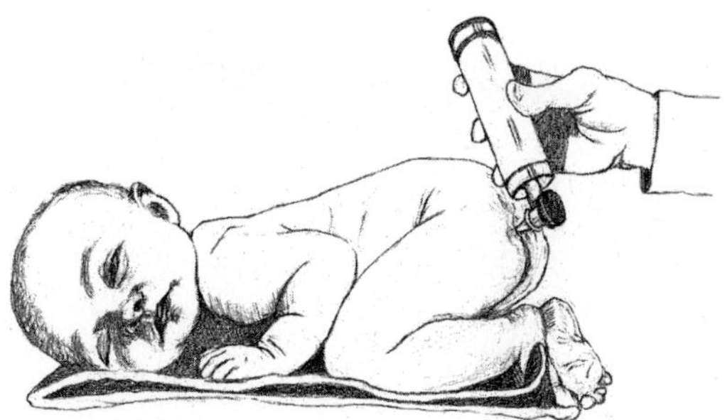

FIG. 37-9. Pediatric proctoscope.

straight up by the legs, letting the body hang down; then pull the scrotum up and shake the contents back into the abdominal cavity."[40]

Value of Clinical Signs in Pediatric Meningitis

The diagnostic accuracy is relatively poor for nuchal rigidity, Kernig's sign (flexing the patient's hip 90 degrees and then extending the patient's knee causes pain), and Brudzinski's neck sign (flexing the patient's neck causes flexion of the patient's hips and knees) in children 3 months to 17 years old with suspected bacterial meningitis, no matter the severity or causative organism (Table 37-7).[41] However, their utility is far better in children than in adult patients.[42]

Subdural Effusions: Meningitis & Trauma

Subdural effusions are particularly likely in children <2 years old with meningitis due to *Haemophilus influenzae*; it occurs in up to 20% of children <1 year old. In neonates with meningitis, measure the head circumference twice a week. Suspect an effusion if most of the following symptoms are present[43]: (a) fever persists for >3 days, (b) vomiting persists or recurs, (c) difficulty with feeding occurs, (d) head circumference increases, (e) papilledema appears, (f) focal neurological signs appear, (g) CSF protein rises, and (h) there is persistent or increased bulging of the fontanel (Fig. 37-10). Also consider a subdural bleed in critical neonates doing poorly after neonatal trauma (or suspected trauma) with a bulging fontanelle.

In resource-poor situations, ultrasound or transillumination may be the only available confirmatory tests. For best results, do transillumination in a dark room using a standard two-cell flashlight held tightly to the anterior fontanelle or, even better, a powerful narrow-beam flashlight with a rubber adapter over the lighted end to form a tight seal over the skull. If it produces >2 cm transillumination around the edge of the beam or if there is asymmetry of the transillumination, it suggests underlying pathology. With unilateral intracranial fluid or swelling, the two sides appear different. However, this may not be true with bilateral pathology. Because findings may vary with the child's prematurity and age, the light source used, and the operator's technique, perform the procedure on a normal infant if there is any question about the results.[44]

Subdural Tap

If imaging or transillumination suggests a subdural effusion or if the clinical situation is dire and there is no time or ability to do any testing, perform the remarkably simple subdural tap. This is one of those times when, to save a life, you may need to "suck it up" and proceed.

TABLE 37-7 Value of Clinical Signs in Pediatric Meningitis

	Sensitivity (%)	Specificity (%)	+Likelihood Ratio	−Likelihood Ratio
Nuchal rigidity	64.5	53.5	1.4	0.7
Kernig's sign	52.6	77.5	2.3	0.6
Brudzinski's neck sign	51.4	95.0	10.3	0.5

Data from Bilavsky et al.[41]

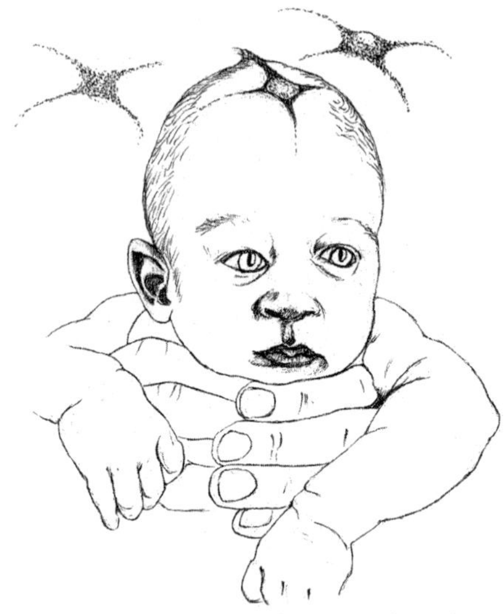

FIG. 37-10. A sunken (top left inset), normal (center), and bulging (top right inset) fontanel.

Subdural Puncture Technique[43]

1. Shave the anterior half of the scalp and swab it with iodine.
2. Scrub as for surgery and put on sterile gloves, cap, and mask.
3. Drape the child's head but allow adequate space for breathing.
4. Have someone else hold the child's head firmly.
5. With a 19-gauge or 20-gauge short-bevel needle, puncture the scalp obliquely at the extreme lateral corner of the anterior fontanel, at least 3 cm from the midline. Advance the needle until the resistance gives at a depth of 0.5 to 1 cm. *DO NOT GO DEEPER THAN THIS*. Allow up to 15 mL of fluid to drain. *DO NOT ASPIRATE FLUID*. If necessary, rotate the needle, but do not move it from side to side (Fig. 37-11).
6. Unless there is definite proof (computed tomography scan or an excellent ultrasound interpretation) that there is no fluid collection on the other side, repeat the puncture there.
7. Repeat the procedure over the next several different days until there is no further drainage. Up to 15 mL per side each day may be safely removed.

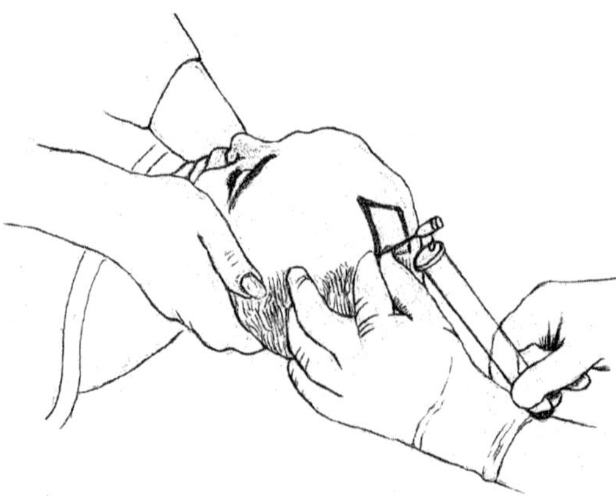

FIG. 37-11. Subdural tap for subdural effusion (or hematoma).

CHILDREN

Pediatric Vital Signs

You must know the normal vital signs for a child's age to appreciate and to treat deviations. Table 37-3 has the normal vital signs (and the amount of initial fluid bolus) for children from preterm (3 kg) to 14 years old.

Pneumonia

You do not need a radiograph to ascertain that a child does not have pneumonia. Large studies have shown that clinicians can reliably rule out a diagnosis of pneumonia if the child has no tachypnea, no increased work of breathing, and clear lungs on auscultation. This avoids doing a chest radiograph and using antibiotics.[45]

For clarity, an increased work of breathing is flaring at the nostrils, retraction, or grunting. This suggests the presence of pneumonia.

Tachypnea (with the respiratory rate counted for 60 seconds) is as follows:

0 to 2 months old: >60 breaths/min
2 to 12 months old: >50 breaths/min
>12 months old: >40 breaths/min

Also, in children <5 years old presenting with respiratory complaints, an oxygen saturation <93% helps predict the presence of radiographically evident pneumonia.[46]

Interpret abnormal auscultation with caution, because it has only fair inter-rater reliability, except for patients with wheezing.

Diagnosis of Urinary Tract Infection Without Laboratory Tests

In verbal children >24 months old, use a simple algorithm and basic urine dipsticks to make a presumptive diagnosis of urinary tract infection (UTI) (Table 37-8). While a urinalysis and

TABLE 37-8 Determining the Probability of UTI Using Symptoms and Dipstick

Verbal females and uncircumcised male[a] children with urinary or abdominal symptoms

⇓

Dysuria or Frequency?

⇓	⇓		
YES	NO		
Obtain urinalysis and culture, if available	Abdominal pain, back pain, or new-onset incontinence?		
⇓	⇓		⇓
⇓	YES		NO
⇓	Obtain urinalysis and culture, if available		UTI unlikely; consider other conditions
⇓	⇓	⇓	
Urine dipstick nitrite *AND* Leukocyte esterase **Negative**	Urine dipstick nitrite *OR* Leukocyte esterase **Positive**	Urine dipstick nitrite *AND* Leukocyte esterase **Positive**	
Prob of UTI = 4%-8%	Prob of UTI = 60%-80%	Prob of UTI = 80%-92%	

Abbreviation: UTI, urinary tract infection.

[a]Circumcised males: consider a urinalysis and culture if multiple signs and symptoms of UTI or if the child has had prior UTIs.

Data from Shaikh et al.[47]

culture are optimal, treatment can begin before performing these laboratory tests (or without them, if they are unavailable).

Hypoglycemia With a Decreased Level of Consciousness

Hypoglycemia is common in critically ill children. Treat it by wetting your finger, dipping it into granulated sugar (so that sugar sticks on the finger), and rubbing the sugar-coated finger on the inside (buccal portion) of the child's cheek or inside the lip. Repeat as often as necessary. Do not put your fingers between the teeth, because the patient may bite down as they awaken.

Give oral rehydration solution (ORS) or sugar water, generally with an NG tube, to provide sugar. See Chapter 11 for more information about these solutions.

Disabilities

Childhood disabilities present in situations of scarce resources as frequently as in other circumstances. You cannot send all children to specialists for evaluation. The following questions form a simple screening method to determine whether a child has developmental disabilities. A positive answer to any one question suggests the need for further screening by specialists.[48]

General Questions for All Children

1. Compared with other children, was there a major delay in your child's sitting, standing, or walking?
2. Compared with other children, does your child have difficulty seeing at any time—day or night?
3. Does your child have problems hearing?
4. Does your child understand you when you tell him/her to do something?
5. Does your child have any stiffness or weakness in his/her arms or legs or difficulty walking?
6. Does your child ever have fits, become rigid, or lose consciousness?
7. Can your child learn to do things as well as other children his/her age?
8. Does your child speak any recognizable words and is he/she understood?
9. Does your child appear dull or slow compared with children of his/her age?
10. For 3- to 9-year-olds, also ask: Is your child's speech clear enough to be understood by people outside your immediate family?

    Or

    For 2-year-olds, also ask: Can your child name at least one object (such as an animal, a toy, a cup, a spoon)?

REFERENCES

1. Iserson KV. Little adults: successful strategies for treating children. *Resident & Staff Physician.* 1997;43:(6):45-47.
2. Shann F, Biddulph J, Vince J. *Paediatrics for Doctors in Papua New Guinea: A Guide for Doctors Providing Health Services for Children.* 2nd ed. PNG Dept of Health: Port Moresby; 2003:99-100.
3. Shann F, Biddulph J, Vince J. *Paediatrics for Doctors in Papua New Guinea: A Guide for Doctors Providing Health Services for Children.* 2nd ed. PNG Dept of Health; 2003:286-287.
4. Milestones suggested by Penelope Hubley for Indian village children. In: Morley D, Woodland M, eds. *See How They Grow: Monitoring Child Growth for Appropriate Health Care in Developing Countries.* London, UK: Macmillan; 1979.
5. Shann F, Biddulph J, Vince J. *Paediatrics for Doctors in Papua New Guinea: A Guide for Doctors Providing Health Services for Children.* 2nd ed. PNG Dept of Health; 2003:99.
6. Hanson AL, Ros S, Soprano J. Analysis of infant lumbar puncture success rates: sitting flexed versus lateral flexed positions. *Ped Emerg Care.* 2014;30(5):311-314.
7. Josse E, Connelly J. Mucus extractors: an infection risk? *Nurs Times.* 1988;9:84.
8. Penman DG, Band DM. Orally operated mucus extractors made safe (comment). *Lancet.* 1990;336(8721):1009.
9. King M, King F, Martodipoero S. *Primary Child Care: A Manual for Health Workers.* Oxford, UK: Oxford University Press; 1978:17.

10. Canadian Air Division. *Search and Rescue Technician: Pre-Hospital Protocols and Procedures*. 1st Canadian Air Division, A1 Division Surgeon; June 2003:8.7.
11. World Health Organization. *Thermal Control of the Newborn: A Practical Guide*. Geneva, Switzerland: WHO; 1993.
12. Ludington-Hoe SM, Nguyen N, Swinth JY, et al. Kangaroo care compared to incubators in maintaining body warmth in preterm infants. *Biol Res Nurs*. 2000;2:60-73.
13. Ellis M. Temperature measurement and thermal care in low income countries. *Trop Doct*. 2002;32(3): 129-130.
14. Whitelaw A, Heisterkamp G, Sleath K, et al. Skin-to-skin contact for very low birth weight infants and their mothers. *Arch Dis Child*. 1988;63:1377-1381.
15. World Health Organization. *Management of Severe Malnutrition: A Manual for Physicians and Other Senior Health Workers*. Geneva, Switzerland: WHO; 1999:8.
16. Charpak N, Ruiz-Peláez JG, de Calume ZF. Current knowledge of Kangaroo mother intervention. *Curr Opin Pediatr*. 1996;8(2):108-112.
17. Charpak N, Ruiz-Peláez JG, Figueroa de CZ, et al. Kangaroo mother versus traditional care for newborn infants ≤2000 grams: a randomised controlled trial. *Pediatrics*. 1997;100(4):682-688.
18. Marks KH, Friedman Z, Maisels MJ. A simple device for reducing insensible water loss in low-birth-weight infants. *Pediatrics*. 1977;60(2):223-226.
19. van den Bosch CA, Nhlane C, Kazembe P. Trial of polythene tobacco-wrap in prevention of hypothermia in neonates less than 1500 grams. *Trop Doct*. 1996;26(1):26-28.
20. Cramer K, Wiebe N, Hartling L, et al. Heat loss prevention: a systemic review of occlusive skin wrap for premature neonates. *J Perinatol*. 2005;25:763-769.
21. Ludington-Hoe SM, Abouelfettoh A. Light reduction capabilities of homemade and commercial incubator covers in NICU. *Int Schol Rsrch Notices Nursing*. 2013:502393.
22. Robinson R. Resuscitation of the newborn. *Br J Hosp Med*. 1977;17(3):260-271.
23. Shann F, Biddulph J, Vince J. *Paediatrics for Doctors in Papua New Guinea: A Guide for Doctors Providing Health Services for Children*. 2nd ed. PNG Dept of Health; 2003:139.
24. Shann F, Biddulph J, Vince J. *Paediatrics for Doctors in Papua New Guinea: A Guide for Doctors Providing Health Services for Children*. 2nd ed. PNG Dept of Health; 2003:46-49.
25. Shann F, Biddulph J, Vince J. *Paediatrics for Doctors in Papua New Guinea: A Guide for Doctors Providing Health Services for Children*. 2nd ed. PNG Dept of Health; 2003:47.
26. Eglash A, Chantry CJ, Howard CR. *Human Milk Storage: Information for Home Use for Healthy Full-Term Infants (Protocol #8)*. New Rochelle, NY: Academy of Breastfeeding Medicine; 2004. http://bfmed.org/Resources/Protocols.aspx. Accessed September 25, 2007.
27. Anon. Fluid and electrolytes (Na, Cl and K). *J Ped Gastroenterol Nutr*. 2005;41(suppl 2):S33-S38.
28. Remis R. Improvisation of medical equipment in developing countries. *Trop Doct*. 1983;13:89.
29. Owens PJ, Forgione A, Briggs S. Challenges of international disaster relief: use of a deployable rapid assembly shelter and surgical hospital. *Disaster Manag Resp*. 2005;3(1):11-16.
30. Olson LM. *Improvised Equipment in the Home Care of the Sick*. Philadelphia, PA: W.B. Saunders; 1928:56-58.
31. Olson LM. *Improvised Equipment in the Home Care of the Sick*. Philadelphia, PA: W.B. Saunders; 1928:58.
32. Olson LM. *Improvised Equipment in the Home Care of the Sick*. Philadelphia, PA: W.B. Saunders; 1928:63.
33. Maisels MJ, McDonagh AF. Phototherapy for neonatal jaundice. *N Engl J Med*. 2008;358(9): 920-928.
34. Mee J, Scott D. Phototherapy for neonatal jaundice in rural Africa. *Trop Doct*. 1977;7(1):33-34.
35. Olson LM. *Improvised Equipment in the Home Care of the Sick*. Philadelphia, PA: W.B. Saunders; 1928:28.
36. Fernández MLH, Merino NG, García AT, et al. A new technique for fast and safe collection of urine in newborns. *Arch Dis Child*. 2013;98:27-29.
37. Coulthard MG. Device for continuous urine collection in the newborn. *Arch Dis Child*. 1982;57(4):322.
38. Fredrick F, Valentine G. Improvised peritoneal dialysis in an 18-month-old child with severe acute malnutrition (kwashiorkor) and acute kidney injury: a case report. *J Med Case Rep*. 2013;7(1):168.
39. Furnas DW. Improvised infant proctoscope. *Am J Dis Child*. 1959;97(6):868-869.
40. Campbell WF, Kerr LG. *The Surgical Diseases of Children*. New York, NY: D. Appleton; 1912: 479-480.

41. Bilavsky E, Leibovitz E, Elkon-Tamir E, et al. The diagnostic accuracy of the 'classic meningeal signs' in children with suspected bacterial meningitis. *Eur J Emerg Med.* 2013;20(5):361-363.
42. Thomas KE, Hasbun R, Jekel J, Quagliarello VJ. The diagnostic accuracy of Kernig's sign, Brudzinski's sign, and nuchal rigidity in adults with suspected meningitis. *Clin Infec Dis.* 2002;35(1):46-52.
43. Shann F, Biddulph J, Vince J. *Paediatrics for Doctors in Papua New Guinea: A Guide for Doctors Providing Health Services for Children.* 2nd ed. PNG Dept Health; 2003:225-226.
44. Barozzino T, Sgro M. Transillumination of the neonatal skull: seeing the light. *Can Med Assoc J.* 2002;167(11):1271-1272.
45. Margolis P, Gadomski A. Does this infant have pneumonia? *JAMA.* 1998;279:308-313.
46. Modi P, Munyaneza, RBM, Goldberg E, et al. Oxygen saturation can predict pediatric pneumonia in a resource-limited setting. *J Emerg Med.* 2013;45(5):752-760.
47. Shaikh N, Morone NE, Lopez J, et al. Does this child have a urinary tract infection? *JAMA.* 2007;298(24):2895-2904.
48. Adapted from: Zinkin P, McConachie H. *Disabled Children & Developing Countries.* Cambridge, UK: Cambridge University Press; 1995:4.

38 | Psychiatry

All medical practitioners should be able to recognize stress-induced psychiatric illness and be prepared to do basic interventions. Psychiatric help is often not immediately available in austere situations.

BASIC APPROACH

In austere medical situations, mental health professionals and psychiatric facilities are usually inadequate or nonexistent. Psychiatric medications may be scarce or of limited variety. The first step for the non-psychiatrist working with patients who have psychiatric disorders is to review Table 38-1. It describes the general approaches for common psychiatric presentations.

The most critical patients are those with new presentations of psychiatric disorders, including delirium. These symptoms represent serious disease states, often from a systemic disease or drug effect, that may respond to rapid treatment.

TABLE 38-1 Common Psychiatric Presentations and Clinical Responses

Patient Presentation	Clinical Response
Patient <40 years old with new-onset psychiatric symptoms and normal vital signs. (If ≥40 years old, do as complete a medical evaluation as possible.)	Brief medical workup and, if available, admit to psychiatric facility. Begin atypical antipsychotics, if available. The presentation of new-onset psychiatric symptoms usually warrants inpatient care or the use of antipsychotics.
Any patient with an altered mental status whose condition appears to vary over time without an obvious cause.	Look for causes of delirium, including alcohol or drug withdrawal. Sedate or medicate the patient only if absolutely necessary and with the smallest dose possible.
Cooperative patient with known psychotic illness but taking no medication.	Try to find "last known good" regimen and restart, if possible. Otherwise, prescribe effective agent based on side-effect profile matched to patient factors.
Uncooperative manic bipolar patient with known organic disease.	Ensure everyone's safety; use restraints, if necessary. If available, use disintegrating tabs of antipsychotics. Oral medications may work; use parenteral agents when necessary.
Agitated and dangerous patient with unknown pathology in need of sedation.	Use antipsychotics, benzodiazepines, or both. Choose agents based on degree of sedation desired. Use enough medication.
Elderly patient with psychosis or dementia and possibly ill.	Evaluate for delirium. Use low-dose antipsychotics. Atypicals are presumed safe for limited exposure. Avoid benzodiazepines.
Elderly patient with known psychiatric illness and psychotic symptoms.	Evaluate for delirium or causes of psychosis. Antipsychotics are useful. Avoid benzodiazepines.
Agitated patient on alcohol.	If available, use lorazepam or clonidine. If not, antipsychotics are safe for sedation; benzodiazepines are drug of choice for withdrawal.
Agitated patient on other psychoactive agents.	Antipsychotics are drugs of choice. Use benzodiazepines if more sedation is needed.

Data from Angelino and Cordover.[1]

DIAGNOSIS

Disaster Triage: Psychological Simple Triage and Rapid Treatment

Disasters represent a special case for psychiatric evaluation and treatment because, no matter their scope, they may generate psychiatric problems for both rescuers and victims. Table 38-2, which is specifically designed for use in disaster settings, helps identify key behavioral symptoms that often signal problems. This model parallels standard triage systems, so is easy to learn.

The colors in the table correspond to those on the psychological simple triage and rapid treatment (PsySTART) triage tag. This tag has specific questions that help categorize patients according to the severity of their event exposures and post-event ongoing stressors. The questions assess the intent to harm oneself or others (Purple Category); perceived threats to one's own life or threats to or recent deaths among one's family or friends (Red Category); and separation from one's family or having a prior mental health history (Yellow Category).[4]

Table 38-2 is more detailed than the triage tag and explains what clinicians may see in each group. The columns focus on three observable elements of personality, the ABCs: **A**, Arousal; **B**, Behavior; and **C**, Cognition. Arousal refers to one's general level of alertness, which may be abnormal by being overly activated, such as in mania, or underactive (retarded), as in severe depression. Behavior refers to how we act and cognition refers to thought and understanding, that is, orientation, judgment, memory, attention, concentration, and insight.

Using this table, identify the phrases that describe the patient's general behavioral patterns. If *any* of these behaviors falls into the "Caution" (Red) or "Danger" (Purple) zones, follow the recommended speed of intervention for further psychiatric evaluation and treatment. If the person falling into the caution or danger zones is part of the disaster team, immediately relieve the team member from his or her duties.

Short Posttraumatic Stress Disorder Screen for Trauma Patients

The four-question Primary Care-Posttraumatic Stress Disorder screen (PC-PTSD) is a simple, useful tool to identify trauma patients at risk for PTSD symptoms. Much shorter than the standard test, it identifies the same percentage of at-risk patients. The questions are:

1. Do you have repeated, disturbing memories, thoughts, or images of a stressful experience from the past?
2. Do you avoid activities or situations because they remind you of a stressful experience from the past?
3. Have you felt emotionally numb or unable to have loving feelings for those close to you?
4. Are you "super-alert" or watchful or on guard?

A positive screen result is an affirmative answer to any three of the four questions.[5]

Stress Disorders

Recognizing Crisis-Induced Psychiatric Illness

People in stressful situations fall into one of three categories: adequately functioning, anxious and agitated, or shocked and subdued.[6]

Adequately Functioning

This category includes the vast majority of people. However, be aware that some people in this group will suppress their feelings until they return to a more normal setting or environment. Thus, they may need counseling after the acute event. If there is any question that they are "on the edge," move them for a short period to a separate rest area so they will not feel the need to assist others. If you are not able to move them, assign them less-stressful tasks.

Anxious and Agitated

These individuals demonstrate obvious distress by loud or unmistakable crying and screaming, fainting, rapid pacing, and other signs of panic and histrionic behavior. Some may convert their distress into physical symptoms, such as nausea, dizziness, or confusion. They should be isolated from any work environment and buddied with someone who can "talk them down" and monitor their behavior. Restrain or sedate these people only if absolutely necessary, because this may only increase the amount of work necessary to care for them.

TABLE 38-2 Disaster Mental Health TRIAGE

Triage Priority Categories	Observations: Arousal	Behavior	Cognition
0. DOING WELL (**GREEN**) Currently *NO* specific behavioral needs.	Not particularly increased or decreased	No specific functional or safety issues Coping well	Cognitive functions intact
1. OKAY FOR NOW (**YELLOW**) Behavior indicates mild impairment of ability to function in this setting. At present, *NO* significant indication of direct harm to self/others due to psychological state.	*Increased:* Upset but can be comforted Some anxiety/agitation Some increased vigilance *Decreased:* Mildly withdrawn	Disturbed sleep but some rest Crying at times Irritable, then apologetic Clings to family/helpers Needy, but can be alone	Aware of circumstances Needs extra effort to maintain attention/concentration Some decreased memory Aware of needs/responsibilities and able to perform with effort and resolve Judgment generally intact
2. CAUTION (**RED**) INTERVENTION LIKELY APPROPRIATE Behavior indicates moderate to very substantial impairment of ability to function in this setting. At present, *NO* significant indication of direct harm to self/others due to psychological state.	*Increased:* Significant agitation/anxiety Occasional panic Able to be calmed or comforted for brief time Hyper-vigilance *Decreased:* Withdrawn Reduced responsiveness Detached	Disturbed sleep with little rest Fleeting self-harm ideation possible Crying often Irritable, but able to control self Isolates self from family/helpers Very needy	Generally aware of circumstances Some decreased attention/concentration possible Some decreased memory Aware of needs and responsibilities but impaired ability and impetus to organize efforts (disturbed goal-directed behavior) Judgment mostly intact
3. DANGER! (**PURPLE**) INTERVENTION REQUIRED IMMEDIATELY Behavior indicates serious impairment of ability to function in this setting *OR* significant potential for harming self or others based on present psychological state.	*Increased:* Extreme agitation/anxiety Constant panic Cannot be calmed or comforted Active mania *Decreased:* Severe withdrawal Catatonia	No sleep or rest Specific self-harm plan or action Pacing incessantly Bizarre behaviors Brought in by security Fighting, yelling Intrusive, "out of control" Mute Constant crying	Not able to appreciate reality of circumstance Generally confused/disoriented Denies obvious needs Markedly deficient memory or attention Markedly disturbed judgment Hopeless/helpless

Adapted from Hipshman[2] and Hipshman.[3]

SHOCKED AND SUBDUED

Often attracting the least attention, these individuals may wander aimlessly or sit and stare. Physical signs may include confusion and disorientation, and even signs consistent with shock. After a medical evaluation to determine whether they are seriously injured, treat them the same as the "anxious and agitated" group.

Panic Disorder

Panic "attacks" are common and can be disabling. Panic attacks occur in 1% to 3% of the population and in up to 8% of primary care patients. Twice as common among women as among men, the incidence of panic attacks peaks in late adolescence and again in the mid-30s.[7]

Diagnosis

Patients often present with typical symptoms that appear suddenly without an obvious cause. This can be disabling and, if it occurs in a health care worker, can diminish vital personnel resources. These patients often carry a diagnosis of or have had recurrent symptoms consistent with a panic disorder, simplifying the diagnosis and treatment course. Table 38-3 lists the criteria to make a diagnosis of panic disorder.

Treatment

Medications and cognitive behavior therapy (CBT) have equal success in treating panic disorder, although trained personnel will probably not be available to do CBT. Benzodiazepines

TABLE 38-3 Criteria for Diagnosing Panic Disorder

A. Recurrent unexpected panic attacks. A panic attack is an abrupt surge of intense fear or intense discomfort that reaches a peak within minutes, and during which time four (or more) of the following symptoms occur: **Note:** The abrupt surge can occur from a calm state or an anxious state.
   1. Palpitations, pounding heart, or accelerated heart rate
   2. Sweating
   3. Trembling or shaking
   4. Sensations of shortness of breath or smothering
   5. Feelings of choking
   6. Chest pain or discomfort
   7. Nausea or abdominal distress
   8. Feeling dizzy, unsteady, light-headed, or faint
   9. Chills or heat sensations
   10. Paresthesias (numbness or tingling sensations)
   11. Derealization (feelings of unreality) or depersonalization (being detached from one's self)
   12. Fear of losing control or "going crazy"
   13. Fear of dying

Note: Culture-specific symptoms (e.g., tinnitus, neck soreness, headache, uncontrollable screaming or crying) may be seen. Such symptoms should not count as one of the four required symptoms.

B. At least one of the attacks has been followed by 1 month (or more) of one or both of the following:
   1. Persistent concern or worry about additional panic attacks or their consequences (e.g., losing control, having a heart attack, "going crazy").
   2. A significant maladaptive change in behavior related to the attacks (e.g., behaviors designed to avoid having panic attacks, such as avoidance of exercise or unfamiliar situations).

C. The disturbance is not attributable to the physiological effects of a substance (e.g., a drug of abuse, a medication) or another medical condition (e.g., hyperthyroidism, cardiopulmonary disorders).

D. The disturbance is not better explained by another mental disorder (e.g., the panic attacks do not occur only in response to feared social situations, as in social anxiety disorder; in response to circumscribed phobic objects or situations, as in specific phobia; in response to obsessions, as in obsessive-compulsive disorder; in response to reminders of traumatic events, as in posttraumatic stress disorder; or in response to separation from attachment figures, as in separation anxiety disorder).

From American Psychiatric Association.[9]

TABLE 38-4 Symptoms of Seasonal Affective Disorder (SAD)

• Depressed mood most of the day	• Irritability	• Eat more than usual
• Excessive sleepiness	• Lethargy	• Weight gain
• Difficulty concentrating	• Anxiety	• Decreased libido
• Crave carbohydrates		

(e.g., diazepam 5 to 30 mg/day), tricyclic antidepressants (e.g., imipramine 100 to 300 mg/day), and selective serotonin reuptake inhibitors (SSRIs) (e.g., sertraline 25 to 100 mg/day) can be used to treat panic disorder. While psychiatrists now rarely use benzodiazepines and tricyclic antidepressants for this disorder, their low cost and ready availability may make them the first-line medication in austere situations.[7,8]

Seasonal Affective Disorder Depression

Seasonal affective disorder (SAD), a type of severe "wintertime blues," diminishes one's ability to function in the autumn and winter. It becomes more prevalent the farther people live from the equator, as there are fewer hours of daylight.

Patients generally have the symptoms listed in Table 38-4. However, unlike patients with typical depression, they are less likely to have feelings of worthlessness or suicidal thoughts.

Treatment consists of self-help therapy (Table 38-5) or light therapy, with or without fluoxetine (Prozac) 20 mg/day. Patient self-help and light therapy can both be used in austere situations when mental health professionals are a scarce resource.

Light Therapy (Phototherapy)

Exposure to bright artificial light improves symptoms in about 50% to 80% of people with SAD. Light therapy and fluoxetine (Prozac) seem to have equivalent effectiveness, and they may be synergistic if used together.[10] Devices for delivering bright light include (a) light-emitting caps or visors that are worn on the head like a baseball hat; (b) dawn simulators, such as bedside lights connected to an alarm clock, which mimic a sunrise and gradually awaken the user; and (c) specially made light boxes that provide ≥10,000 lux (measure of light intensity at least 10 times stronger than that emitted by normal lightbulbs) and emit white, not blue, light.

An effective dose, if administered as soon as possible after awakening, is 5000 lux/day, either as 2500 lux for 2 hours or as 10,000 lux for 30 minutes. Most people notice an improvement in symptoms within 3 to 4 days, although they need to continue therapy until spring.

Sedative-Hypnotic Interview

Patients may present with complaints of sudden, non-traumatic paresis or paralysis of the extremities and in catatonia-like states. Usually, such patients consume an inordinate amount of resources. The use of sedative-hypnotic interviews (also called "amobarbital interviews") can quickly alleviate acute symptoms, confirm or rule out a psychiatric basis for the symptoms, and assist with treatment and disposition. In other words, these interviews can be both diagnostic and therapeutic.[11,12]

An easy procedure that takes about 20 minutes, the sedative-hypnotic interview quickly resolves conversion-reaction symptoms, preventing them from becoming permanent. Sedative-hypnotic interviews have also been used (a) to treat acute panic states following traumatic events, such as rape, catastrophic loss, or disaster; (b) to diagnose and treat benign stupor (mute and

TABLE 38-5 Patient Self-Help Behavior for SAD

• Go outside every day	• Sit near windows while inside
• Learn relaxation techniques	• Do regular, moderate exercise
• Eat a well-balanced diet	• Use light colors to decorate the house
• Avoid stress whenever possible	
• Leave any major projects until summer and plan ahead for winter	

unresponsive patients) or acute hysterical amnesia; (c) to diagnose malingering; (d) to reveal suicidal ideations; (e) to gain information in criminal cases (of dubious merit or legal worth); and (f) to differentiate between organic illness or psychosis and functional psychosis.

Do not use this interview technique for the commonly seen patient with psychogenic unresponsiveness who is usually hysterical and whose symptoms last only several minutes. Experienced clinicians can quickly identify such patients, because they actively resist anyone trying to open their eyelids and, when opened, the eyelids close rapidly rather than with the smooth motion seen in coma. These patients normally respond quickly to noxious stimuli and a firm approach by the clinicians. Patients in a catatonic-like state, however, often present either in a state of mute wakefulness without response to verbal or tactile stimuli, or in a mildly stuporous condition. The former will often track the observer with his or her eyes (coma vigil, akinetic mutism) and may show a waxy flexibility of the extremities.

While most of the experience with this technique has been using amobarbital, some clinicians have used thiopental, mixtures of thiopental and amobarbital, chloroform, *Cannabis indica*, paraldehyde, scopolamine, chloral hydrate, most modern barbiturates, benzodiazepines, or other sedative-hypnotic agents for the same purpose.

Interview Technique

Place the patient in a relatively quiet room with a relative or chaperone in attendance. Having relatives observe the interview is helpful, because it is often difficult for them to comprehend that certain symptoms, such as paralysis, have a psychogenic basis. Through an intravenous line of D_5W, administer sodium amobarbital (10% solution) at 50 mg (0.5 cc)/min. Carry on a conversation (or monologue, in the stupor cases) with the patient during induction. Limit this to benign, nonthreatening topics. The clinician's calm, reassuring attitude and suggestions similar to hypnotic inductions are useful; the interview effect sometimes is as great as that of the medication.

The stages of narcosis are: (a) fully alert and responsive patients; (b) Stage I, when patients describe their first symptoms—fatigue, light-headedness or dizziness, blurring or double vision; (c) Stage II, when patients become euphoric or drowsy, or when the unresponsive patient begins answering questions; and (d) Stage III, the absence of corneal reflexes in the patient, which should be avoided.

It usually requires 100 to 500 mg of amobarbital to reach Stage II. At that point, ask the patient questions about personal identification data (when necessary), his or her current situation and predisposing factors, and any further medical history needed (including drug ingestion). Then suggest that the patient again has the ability to use the affected part, or, for the previously mute/unresponsive patient, that he or she must remain responsive once the medication wears off.

In patients with conversion reactions causing paralysis or other physical symptoms, once the symptom, such as paralysis, resolves, the interviewer should reinforce the fact that the extremity is now back to normal and that it will continue to be normal after the patient leaves the hospital. This is analogous to the familiar posthypnotic suggestion. Do not confront the patient with a psychiatric diagnosis at this time. When spontaneous speech or movement returns to the catatonic or unresponsive patient, emphasize that such a responsive state is normal and desirable.

Patients with organic/toxic psychoses will not respond verbally and will merely fall asleep or become more sedated during the interview. If this occurs, terminate the interview and presume that the patient has an organic etiology that needs further evaluation.

Patients only need their respirations monitored during the procedure; the patients need to be observed for 2 to 4 hours post-interview. Refer the patient for psychiatric treatment, if available.[11,12]

Psychosis—Treatment in Crisis Situations

Easily and quickly elicit psychiatric symptoms by asking a person to write down his or her thoughts. Psychosis will often immediately become evident, including suicidal and homicidal ideations. Patients may be much more willing to write down these thoughts than to discuss them with a clinician. Table 38-6 lists a general way to classify major psychiatric conditions by their presenting symptoms.

TABLE 38-6 Symptoms of Major Psychiatric Conditions

Syndrome	Behavior	Speech	Thought Content	Perception	Affect	Orientation and Memory	Onset and Duration	Physical Findings
Delirium	Agitation (occasionally quiet) carphologia	Nonspecific	Variable, delusions	Illusions Hallucinations	Fear, anxiety	Disoriented, memory impaired, clouded consciousness	Acute with fluctuating symptoms	Abnormal vital signs
Dementia	Apathy, apraxia, echopraxia	Echolalia, aphasia	Variable, few, if any, delusions	Few, if any, hallucinations	Lability	Disorientation, memory impairment	Insidious	Frontal lobe release signs (such as grasp reflex)
Schizophrenia	Social withdrawal, agitation	Rambling, mutism	Bizarre, persecutory delusions, ideas of reference	Hallucinations	Blunt, flat, inappropriate affect	Intact	Symptoms for 6 months	None
Mania	Hyperactivity, gregariousness	Rapid, forceful	Delusions of grandeur Paranoia	Hallucinations (possible)	Elation, frequent irritability	Intact	Symptoms for 1 week	None
Depression	Motor retardation, occasional agitation	Lack of spontaneity, slow pace and monotone	Helplessness, hopelessness, delusions of guilt, somatic delusions	Few, if any, hallucinations	Depression, sadness, despondence	Intact	Symptoms for 2 weeks	None

From US Air Force.[13]

TABLE 38-7 Six-Item Screen for Cognitive Impairment

Tell the patient the following:
I would like to ask you some questions that require you to use your memory. I am going to name three objects. Please wait until I say all three words; then repeat them. Remember what they are because I am going to ask you to name them again in a few minutes. Please repeat these words for me: APPLE—TABLE—PENNY. (Interviewer may repeat words three times if necessary.)
1. What year is this?
2. What month is this?
3. What day of the week is this?
What were the three objects I asked you to remember? (They should answer:)
4. Apple
5. Table
6. Penny

Three or more incorrect answers strongly correlate with cognitive impairment.

Data from Callahan et al.[15]

Dementia

Formal mental status testing is time consuming and often unnecessary for general medical evaluations. However, if a patient with reasonable hearing looks at his or her companion more than twice before answering direct questions during history taking, there is a strong likelihood of incipient dementia.[14] In these cases, administer a cognitive screening test. The prevalence of cognitive impairment is 23% to 40% in older emergency department (ED) patients.

Studies have shown that when time is limited, a rapid (1- to 2-minute) assessment of dementia can produce results comparable to those from much longer, more complex testing. The combination of an abnormal Six-Item Screen for Cognitive Impairment score (Table 38-7) with an abnormal score on the cAD8 Cognitive Screen (Table 38-8) had a positive likelihood ratio of 19.9 for identifying patients with potential cognitive impairment. Three or more errors in the Six-Item Screen score suggest dementia (88% sensitivity and specificity). Getting more items wrong correlates with a greater chance of cognitive impairment.[15]

When using the cAD8 Cognitive Screening test, ask a reliable informant about the patient, using the questions in Table 38-8. If only the patient is present, ask him or her the questions. Emphasize that these questions relate to *changes over the past several years* caused by thinking and memory problems. Each positive answer is one point, with two or more positive answers considered high risk for cognitive impairment. Note that these are *behavioral changes*. If the person could never balance a checkbook and still cannot do it, there has been no change.

TABLE 38-8 cAD8 Cognitive Screening Test

Does the person

1. Have a problem with judgment (e.g., makes bad financial decisions, falls for scams, buys inappropriate gifts)?
2. Have a reduced interest in hobbies and other activities?
3. Repeat questions, stories, or statements?
4. Have trouble learning how to use tools, appliances, or gadgets (e.g., smart phone, computer, microwave)?
5. Forget the correct month or year?
6. Have difficulty handling complicated financial affairs (e.g., paying bills, balancing checkbook)?
7. Have difficulty remembering appointments?
8. Consistently have a problem with thinking or memory?

Data from Carpenter et al.[16]

Once the clinician recognizes that a patient has cognitive impairment, the challenge becomes to differentiate dementia from delirium, depression, or acute psychosis. Each has a different prognosis, as well as different methods of evaluation and treatment. Table 38-9 lists some of the clinical factors that can help differentiate these disorders.

Intimate Partner Violence—Perpetrator Identification

About 29% of women experience some form of intimate partner violence (IPV) in their lifetime. The PErpetration RaPid Scale (PERPS) is a short screening tool to identify the perpetrators, rather than the victims. It consists of three simple Yes or No questions:

1. Have you ever forced your partner to have sex or hurt your partner during sex?
2. Have you ever pushed or shoved or poked your partner violently?
3. Have you ever hit or punched your partner's arms, body, head, or face?

The PERPS is considered positive if any of the three questions are answered "yes." The test has an accuracy of 85% in identifying IPV perpetrators. Age, gender, and race do not predict positive results.[20]

TREATMENT

Psychological First Aid

It is useful to teach basic psychological treatment techniques, termed psychological first aid, to all health care workers (and non-health care workers). The techniques, essentially those listed in

TABLE 38-9 Clinical Features Helpful in Distinguishing Dementia, Delirium, Acute Psychosis, and Depression

Characteristic	Delirium	Dementia	Acute Psychosis	Depression
Onset	Acute; sudden	Usually insidious	Acute	Acute, often with prior history
Course over 24 hours	Marked fluctuations	Stable	Stable	Stable
Long-term course	Transient	Progressive decline	Fluctuating	Variable duration
Consciousness	Reduced	Normal	Normal	Normal
Attention	Usually impaired globally	Normal, unless dementia severe	May be disturbed	Slowed
Cognition	Impaired	Impaired	Unimpaired if cooperative	Appears impaired; fluctuates
Orientation	Impaired	Often impaired	May be impaired	Normal
Hallucinations	Visual, ± auditory	Rare	Mostly auditory	Absent
Delusions	Transient, poorly organized	Usually absent	Sustained	Usually absent
Psychomotor activity	Increased or reduced, varies unpredictably	Often normal	Increased or reduced; does not shift rapidly	Usually slowed
Tremor	Asterixis; tremor may be present	Usually absent, unless from other condition	Absent	Absent
Speech	Incoherent, slow, or rapid; disorganized	Word finding impaired, normal pace	Normal, slow, or rapid	Usually slow or normal

Data from Basten and McGuire,[17] Lipowski,[18] and Wells.[19]

TABLE 38-10 Modern Crisis Intervention Techniques—Initial Steps

1. Establish rapport. Introduce self and develop relationship.
2. Rapid assessment. Determine the level of distress and identify problems.
3. Stabilize situation. Take control of the situation; protect person and others.
4. Contain situation. Remove antagonists; set boundaries; avoid spread to others.
5. Lower stimuli. Cut visual, auditory, and olfactory stimuli.
6. Reduce symptoms. Calm the person and provide reassurance that help is there.
7. Lessen impact of event. Be active, calm, and in control; inform victim.

Data from Mitchell and Thoumaian.[6]

Table 38-10, combined with the following principles of crisis intervention, ameliorate acute distress following exposure to trauma[21]:

- *Simplicity:* Use simple, rather than complex, approaches to the patient.
- *Brevity:* Do brief interventions over a short time period.
- *Innovation:* Use whatever methods work.
- *Pragmatism:* Advise patients to do only what is possible in their current situation.
- *Proximity:* Conduct the intervention in a safe area close to where the person works/lives.
- *Immediacy:* A key to recovery is providing help soon after the event.
- *Expectancy:* Promote patient expectations that they will recover. Patients who believe this have a much better chance to recover fully.

Table 38-10 lists the initial crisis intervention techniques that any health care professional should be able to use. A mental health professional may later need to provide in-depth follow-up.

Using Restraints

Although safety is rarely an issue, staff may need to use physical or chemical restraint, or both, to restrain patients (or others) if they become violent and threaten other people's safety. The rule is to keep yourself safe, to keep your staff safe, and then to worry about your patient's safety. Remember that most violent patients who are still aware, that is, not on an illicit stimulant or alcohol, do not want to hurt anyone. Try a "show of force": Gather a group of really big people and approach the patient in a nonthreatening manner. Ask, and then tell, the patient to lie down to be restrained. This technique often works well—and no one gets hurt.

If needed, most health care workers can easily improvise restraints in a crisis. The most common method is to use a web-type bandage (e.g., Kerlix) to form a slip knot and then put the loop over the patient's wrists and ankles. An alternative in some centers is to tape two fingers together and slip the restraint between the tape and the hand. Restrain the entire body with sheets or the stretcher straps. Rather than straps for extremities, use socks. (Col. Patricia R Hastings, AMEDDCS. Personal communication, April 9, 2007.) Any patient in restraints should not be lying on his or her back; this is the death-from-aspiration position.

Outside the confines of medical facilities, the idea of restraint gets a bit dicier. "Fearful that extensive training on airline violence would adversely affect their image, several major US airlines refuse even to carry plastic handcuffs on the plane. In the case of an emergency, the flight crew is left to devise makeshift restraints from their neckties, headset wires, seatbelt extensions or even pantyhose."[22]

When available, chemical restraint, such as haloperidol, chlorpromazine (beware postural hypotension), or other sedatives, may be used. If a psychiatric patient is supposed to receive a sedating medication for treatment, try to use that drug.

Depression

Major depression (vegetative signs) is common and often difficult to treat. Antidepressants often take weeks to work and have significant side effects. They also may be expensive and unavailable.

Ketamine, commonly used around the world for conscious sedation, analgesia, and anesthesia, is a rapid-acting treatment for depression.

In 2000, Berman et al showed that ketamine has a rapid antidepressant effect in patients with major depression.[23] We now know that a single intravenous infusion of ketamine hydrochloride (0.5 mg/kg diluted in 40 mL of saline given over 40 minutes) has a significant and immediate effect on patients with bipolar and unipolar treatment-resistant depression. Note that if the dose is 1 mg/kg, >5% of patients become hypotensive.[24] Nearly two-thirds of the patients have a reduction in suicidal thoughts within 6 hours of the infusion[25] and have significantly reduced depressive symptoms within 24 hours. The duration of this antidepressant response is highly variable, ranging from hours to several weeks, with most patients eventually relapsing. However, the treatment produces significant dissociative symptoms in about one of six patients.[26] More sustained effects have resulted from repeated ketamine infusions over 2 weeks.[27]

Administration via the intranasal route is also effective. In adults, a 50-mg dose of intranasal ketamine alleviates depressive symptoms within 24 hours, with few side effects in people with treatment-resistant depression.[28] At doses ranging from 30 to 120 mg every 3 to 7 days, depending on their response and tolerance, it has also proven effective in refractory bipolar disorders in children 6 to 19 years old.[29]

Posttraumatic Stress Disorder

Posttraumatic stress disorder (PTSD) is a catch-all term that encompasses stress caused by any traumatic event. Usually, PTSD is discussed in the context of situations where the individual or group (a) was exposed to dead, dying, or mutilated bodies or too many injured people; (b) felt that their own or a loved one's life was in danger; (c) heard the screams of those in pain or who were dying; (d) was trapped; (e) was lost or became separated from loved ones; (f) witnessed a devastating event (e.g., mutilating deaths); (g) suffered or was at risk of suffering a severe illness or injury; or (h) lost major possessions. Posttraumatic stress disorder also can occur when the disaster is unexpected (e.g., earthquake), is human-made (e.g., terrorist attack), or leads to prolonged stress. Particularly in children, the loss of or separation from a parent or the fear of such a death or separation, or of a recurrence of the disaster can lead to PTSD.[30]

Often, there are not enough mental health professionals to help the large numbers of people suffering from PTSD or to help those whose PTSD could have been prevented by early intervention. Many health care workers and members of the helping professions may feel—incorrectly—that they are too strong to suffer from PTSD or that seeing a mental health professional would be stigmatizing. Because of this, colleagues may need to step in.

The first step for health care and rescue workers is to try to avoid PTSD through pre-event counseling, engaging in specific behaviors while on-scene (Table 38-11), and participating in critical incident stress debriefing (CISD). Lumped together, these actions constitute critical incident stress management (CISM).

In general, CISD follows the format shown in Table 38-12. Remember two key points: (a) some, or even many, PTSD victims cannot tolerate any reminder of the incident, and (b) referring to participants as patients and to their responses as symptoms indicates that they are ill and may alienate participants. Lawrence Hipshman, MD, of Oregon Health Sciences University, says that, in fact, participants are generally not ill, but rather are having predictable responses to severe stress. (Personal written communication, October 4, 2008.)

TABLE 38-11 On-Scene Posttraumatic Stress Disorder (PTSD)-Avoidance Strategies

Concentrate on the task at hand
Concentrate on your work's benefit to society
Avoid humanizing dead bodies
Do not look at corpses' faces
Do not learn victims' names

Adapted from Oster and Doyle.[30]

TABLE 38-12 Phases of Critical Incident Stress Debriefing

1. *Introduction phase*: CISD team members introduce themselves and explain the purpose of the group meeting and the process they will follow. Hopefully, this will create an environment in which participants feel comfortable, can overcome their resistance, and cooperate during the debriefing intervention. Team members answer questions to alleviate anxiety, encourage participants to help each other, and start the process by asking the first questions.
2. *Fact phase*: Participants are asked to describe the traumatic event from their perspective. They are asked to describe themselves, their role during the incident, and what they saw happen.
3. *Thought phase*: The CISD team asks participants to state the first or most prominent thought they had once they stopped functioning on "autopilot." This helps participants begin to identify their emotional, rather than fact-based, reactions to the event by describing their response on a more personal level.
4. *Reaction phase*: Each member is asked to identify the aspect of the event that was most personally traumatic and his or her emotional reactions. This part of the debriefing tends to be the most emotionally powerful.
5. *Symptom phase*: To diffuse the emotions before ending the debriefing, participants are asked to describe any affective, behavioral, cognitive, or physical reactions they may have encountered while working at the scene or afterward. To get the group moving in this direction, team members may need to give several examples of stress-related symptoms, such as angry feelings, trembling hands, difficulty making decisions, or severe fatigue.
6. *Teaching phase*: The entire CISD debriefing process helps teach the most common symptoms of stress and provides a variety of stress survival and management strategies. This part of the debriefing is didactic and designed to distance participants from the emotional content in the reaction phase. This phase continues until participants exhaust the topics that are most important to them.
7. *Reentry phase*: This summary phase helps clarify issues, answers questions, and reviews the CISD intervention. This provides closure on the debriefing discussions and allows the session to end on a positive note.

Abbreviation: CISD, critical incident stress debriefing.

Data from Mitchell et al.[31]

Immediate PTSD Patient Care

Once you identify a probable PTSD patient, focus on demonstrating that the person is (a) safe; (b) secure; (c) can connect with significant others; and then (d) listen to the person's description of what occurred, if he or she wants to talk about it.

Do *not* force the person to talk about the event immediately. Counseling at a later time is helpful—but not initially. (Barry Morenz, MD. Personal communication, August 15, 2014.) In resource-poor settings, an SSRI may be used, if necessary and available.

Suicide Risk

Initial Assessment

The three-question Emergency Department Safety Assessment and Follow-up Evaluation (ED-SAFE) is a simple, validated way to quickly screen for patients at risk for committing suicide. Any positive answers warrant a more in-depth assessment. The three questions are[32]:

1. Over the past 2 weeks, have you felt down, depressed, or hopeless?
2. Over the past 2 weeks, have you had thoughts of killing yourself?
3. Have you ever attempted to kill yourself? If "yes," when did this happen? (A recent attempt is one occurring within the past 6 months.)

TABLE 38-13 Criteria for Releasing Patients With Suicidal Ideations[a]

- No need for inpatient medical treatment.
- No history of suicide attempt, psychiatric disorder, or substance abuse.
- No evidence of suicide intent or plan (not actively suicidal).
- A competent adult agrees to remove all potentially lethal substances and means from the patient's environment.
- A competent adult agrees to monitor the patient until follow-up.
- Follow-up with a health care (preferably mental health) professional within 48 hours.
- Patient demonstrates understanding of and agreement with the plan.
- The patient may sign a "contract" agreeing not to harm self (unclear whether this is helpful).

[a]Criteria must be appropriately applied to each patient.

Disposition

Many patients initially classed as "suicidal" may be released into the community for later treatment. Table 38-13 lists some suggested criteria (that will never be 100% correct).

Tranquilizing Medications

Be familiar with parenteral chlorpromazine, diazepam, and haloperidol. In Africa and most other resource-poor regions, these are the medications psychiatrists and other clinicians commonly use to rapidly tranquilize patients with severe behavioral disturbances.[33]

REFERENCES

1. Angelino AF, Cordover MD. *Psychosis in the Emergency Department* (monograph). Oklahoma City, OK: University of Oklahoma; 2006.
2. Hipshman L. Behavioral health triage in disaster settings (presentation). http://www.slideserve.com/shubha/behavioral-health-triage-in-disaster-settings. Accessed October 9, 2015.
3. Hipshman L, MD, MPH, Dept. Psychiatry, OHSU, Portland, OR. Personal written communication, received October 4, 2008.
4. Schreiber M. PsySTART rapid mental health triage and incident management system. *The Dialogue*. 2005:68. http://www.cdms.uci.edu/PDF/PsySTART-cdms02142012.pdf. Accessed October 9, 2015.
5. Hanley J, DeRoon-Cassini T, Brasel K. Efficiency of a four-item posttraumatic stress disorder screen in trauma patients. *J Trauma Acute Care Surg*. 2013;75:722-727.
6. Mitchell JT, Thoumaian AH. *Maintaining the Balance: A Strategic Support System for Operations Personnel and Survivors*. NDMS Basic Training Course, September 2003.
7. Katon WJ. Panic disorder. *N Engl J Med*. 2006;354(22):2360-2367.
8. Gorman JM. A 28-year-old woman with panic disorder. *JAMA*. 2001;286(4):450-457.
9. American Psychiatric Association. *Diagnostic and Statistical Manual of Mental Disorders*, 5th ed, text rev. *(DSM-V-TR)*. Washington, DC: APA; 2013:208-209.
10. Lam RW, Levitt AJ, Levitan RD, et al. The CAN-SAD study: a randomized controlled trial of the effectiveness of light therapy and fluoxetine in patients with winter seasonal affective disorder. *Am J Psychiatry*. 2006;163:805-812.
11. Iserson KV. The emergency amobarbital interview. *Ann Emerg Med*. 1980;9(10):513-517.
12. Iserson KV. The sedative-hypnotic interview. In: Roberts JR, Hedges JR, eds. *Clinical Procedures in Emergency Medicine*. 3rd ed. Philadelphia, PA: W.B. Saunders; 1998:1214-1218.
13. US Air Force. *The Air Force Independent Duty Medical Technician Medical and Dental Treatment Protocols*. AFM 44-158, December 1, 1999:90.
14. Van Gerpen JA. Heeding a clue to possible dementia (pearls). *Postgrad Med*. www.postgradmed.com. Accessed September 23, 2007.
15. Callahan CM, Unverzagt FW, Hui SL, et al. Six-item screener to identify cognitive impairment among potential subjects for clinical research. *Med Care*. 2002;40(9):771-781.

16. Carpenter CR, DesPain B, Keeling TN, Shah M, Rothenberger M. The six-item screener and AD8 for the detection of cognitive impairment in geriatric emergency department patients. *Ann Emerg Med.* 2011;57(6):653-661.
17. Basten CJ, McGuire BE. Delirium: the role of the psychologist in assessment and management. *Austral Psychol.* 2000;(35)3:201-207.
18. Lipowski Z. Delirium in the elderly patient. *N Engl J Med.* 1989;20:578.
19. Wells CE. Pseudodementia. *Am J Psychiatry.* 1979;136(7):895-900.
20. Ernst AA, Weiss SJ, Morgan-Edwards S, et al. Derivation and validation of a short emergency department screening tool for perpetrators of intimate partner violence: the Perpetrator RaPid Scale (PERPS). *J Emerg Med.* 2012;42(2):206-217.
21. Salmon TW. The war neuroses and their lessons. *NY Med J.* 1919;59:993-994.
22. Budden L. Airlines are inviting disaster with 'see no evil' approach to air rage. *Insight on the News.* March 12, 2001. http://findarticles.com/p/articles/mi_m1571/is_10_17/ai_72328670. Accessed July 23, 2008.
23. Berman RM, Cappiello A, Anand A, et al. Antidepressant effects of ketamine in depressed patients. *Biological Psych.* 2000;47(4):351-354.
24. Kudoh A, Takahira Y, Katagai H, et al. Small-dose ketamine improves the postoperative state of depressed patients. *Anesth Analg.* 2002;95:114-115.
25. Diamond PR, Farmery AD, Atkinson S, et al. Ketamine infusions for treatment resistant depression: a series of 28 patients treated weekly or twice weekly in an ECT clinic. *J Psychopharmacol.* 2014;28:536-544.
26. Murrough JW, Iosifescu DV, Chang LC, et al. Antidepressant efficacy of ketamine in treatment-resistant major depression: a two-site randomized controlled trial. *Am J Psychiatry.* 2013;170:1134-1142.
27. Aan het Rot M, Collins KA, Murrough JW, et al. Safety and efficacy of repeated-dose intravenous ketamine for treatment-resistant depression. *Biol Psychiatry.* 2010;67:139-145.
28. Lapidus KA, Levitch CF, Perez AM, et al. A randomized controlled trial of intranasal ketamine in major depressive disorder. *Biol Psychiatry.* 2014;76(12):970-976.
29. Papolos DF, Teicher MH, Faedda GL, Murphy P, Mattis S. Clinical experience using intranasal ketamine in the treatment of pediatric bipolar disorder/fear of harm phenotype. *J Affective Disorders.* 2013;147(1):431-436.
30. Oster NS, Doyle CJ. Critical incident stress. In: Hogan DE, Burstein JL, eds. *Disaster Medicine.* 2nd ed. Philadelphia, PA: Lippincott-Williams Wilkins; 2007:64-71.
31. Mitchell AM, Sakraida TJ, Kameg K. Critical incident stress debriefing: implications for best practice. *Disaster Manag Response.* 2003;1(1):46-51.
32. Boudreaux E, Camargo C, Miller V. Emergency Department Safety Assessment and Follow-up Evaluation (ED-SAFE). www.emnet-usa.org/EDSAFE/edsafe.htm. Accessed January 3, 2015.
33. James BO. Rapid tranquillization agents for severe behavioural disturbance: a survey of African psychiatrists' prescription patterns. *Trop Doct.* 2011;41(1):49-50.

39 | Rehabilitation

When health care resources are limited, rehabilitation services are rare. You may need to improvise rehabilitation equipment for use in therapy or to help patients with mobility and activities of daily living (ADLs). Therapy devices help patients gain or regain activity levels as close to normal as possible. Equipment used for mobility and ADL helps patients function better in their daily lives, despite decreased physical ability. For convenience, I will discuss each of these separately.

THERAPY

Transfer Belt

Use transfer belts (aka walking belts or gait belts) for people who have difficulty walking. These belts enable helpers to lift patients safely and without straining their backs into and out of beds and chairs.

To make a transfer belt, place a 3-inch-wide webbing (or several loops of it), a wide clothing belt or a sturdy, wide piece of cloth, such as canvas, with a buckle around a patient's waist, and use it as a handhold while transferring them or helping them to walk.

Parallel Bars

Patients use parallel bars to practice walking. Fashion these from two long, sturdy poles set into Y-shaped supports at each end. Place the poles parallel to one another and low enough so that patients can use their arms to steady themselves as they walk. Fix the apparatus solidly in place, because patients depend on it if their legs give out.

Child's Walker

When children need to use walkers or to practice walking, such as when they are healing from a leg fracture, it helps to make it fun. Use your imagination to craft these devices. Girls especially enjoy using a baby buggy, with a doll in it if possible. For boys, decorate a walker with cardboard or paint to make it look like a car or boat. When using a baby buggy, be sure to put enough weights in the bottom so that it provides the child with support and will not tip over.

Cervical Traction

Cervical traction helps lessen the pain for patients with cervical disc disease. It can be applied in a clinic for 30 minutes twice a day, or at home more frequently for shorter periods of time.

To make a cervical suspension device

1. Build an overhead suspension frame using a flat 2-inch × 12-inch metal bar bent so that it can hook over a door.
2. Bend a 0.5-inch diameter × 6-inch-long rod into a horseshoe shape and then weld both ends to the flat bar.
3. Fashion a head harness from leather, jeans, or khaki clothing material and fasten with sandal buckles. Pad it well with soft cloth. Use a cotton cord or rope purchased from a local market. Tie one end of the cord to the support.
4. Make two hooks from 0.25-inch metal rods shaped into an "S." Tie these to both ends of the cord.
5. Loop the cord from the head harness through the metal loop on the door hanger and attach it to a bag, bucket, or jar, which acts as a weight. As shown in Fig. 39-1, wrap the cord around the door hanger to reduce the tension. One alternative to the weight is to use a clothesline tightener between the head harness and the door hanger. Another alternative is to hang the weight over the end of a bed, as is done when using cervical traction for spinal injuries (see Fig. 29-9).
6. When water is used as weight, start with 2 L for an adult and add water until the patient is comfortable and no longer has pain.[1]

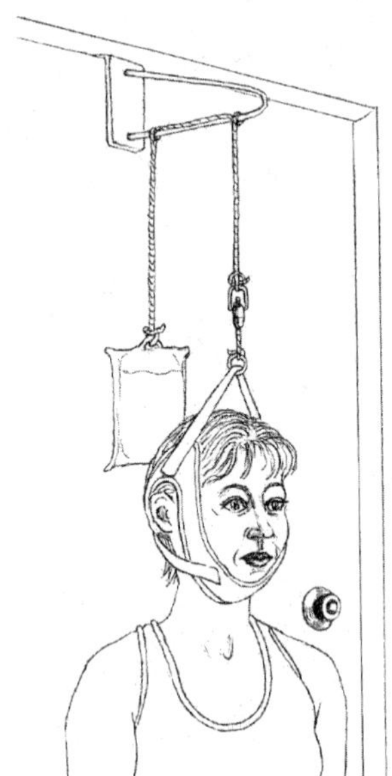

FIG. 39-1. Cervical traction, improvised.

MOBILITY AND ACTIVITIES OF DAILY LIVING

A wide variety of devices can be improvised to assist patients' mobility or to help them perform their daily activities.

Canes

The cane is the easiest mobility device to improvise. Patients often do not use their cane because it is the wrong size for them or because they are not told how to use it correctly.

To use a cane, patients should hold it in the hand *opposite* to their injury or weakness. In addition, they need sufficient upper-extremity strength to bear 20% to 25% of their body weight on the cane. (If they use it in the wrong hand, they need to support >50% of their weight.)

To determine the correct size of cane, measure the cane against the patient while he or she is standing. Turn the cane upside down and rest it on the ground next to the standing patient. Cut the bottom of the cane at the level of the patient's flexor wrist crease and apply a rubber tip to the end.

You can make canes from a tree limb or small tree that has a small sturdy branch that extends at a right angle. It should be light enough so that the patient can easily use the cane. Remove any bark, extra branches, or leaves, and smooth the surface. Patients use canes and walking sticks for balance rather than to support an injured limb.[2] Fashion a cane with an arm brace by attaching a piece of polyvinyl chloride (PVC) pipe to the tree limb (Fig. 39-2).

Crutches

Crutches must be used when the patient's leg, ankle, or foot injury requires that he or she bear no, or only minimal (that is, toe-touching), weight on it. Crutches can be used individually or in pairs. Not everyone needs two crutches. When crutches are in short supply, give only one crutch to those patients for whom one will suffice. This allows another patient to use the extra crutch.

To fit crutches correctly, align the axillary pad three fingerbreadths below the axilla. When crutches are in use, the patients should slightly bend their elbows.

To make crutches, start with one sturdy tree branch (or a matched pair of branches if two crutches are needed). Use the "Y" formed by the branches (Fig. 39-3A). Remember that the crutch must support the patient's weight but still be light enough that the patient can use it. You

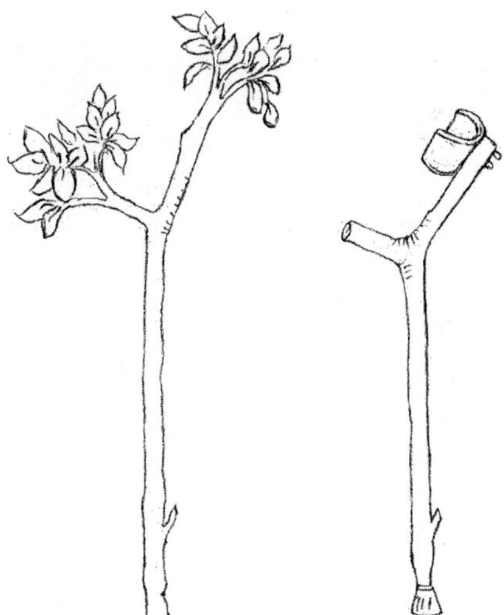

FIG. 39-2. Makeshift cane with PVC arm brace.

can also use a straight green sapling (2.5-cm diameter if hardwood, 3-cm diameter if soft wood). Split it halfway down its length (Fig. 39-3B) and then insert a crosspiece (2.5- to 3.5-cm-diameter dowel or similar piece of wood) as a handhold for the patient about a third of the way down; firmly secure the crosspiece to the two sides using screws or cement. Tape the area where the split ends to prevent the sapling from continuing to split on its own. To finish the crutch, secure a padded crosspiece at the top and put a piece of rubber at the bottom.[2] Hang a basket from one of the crosspieces, so the patient can carry items (e.g., phone, keys) that they need to access quickly.

Wheelchairs

Although there are kits to transform plastic lawn chairs into wheelchairs,[3] the materials for makeshift wheelchairs most often need to be scrounged locally. Alternatives include removing the legs from an easy chair and fastening the chair to the frame of a baby carriage (Fig. 39-4, left),

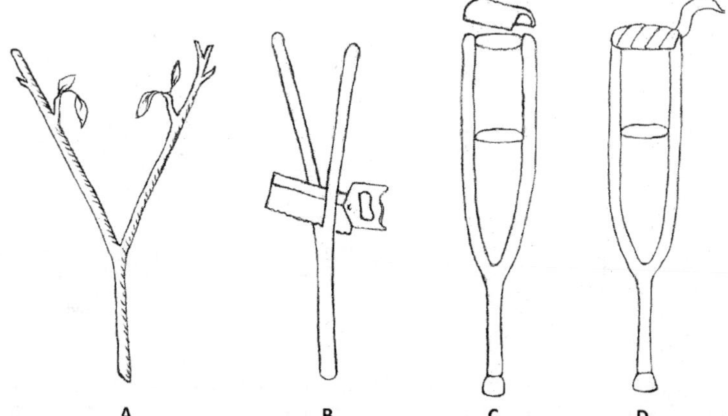

FIG. 39-3. Making a crutch: Begin with either a "Y" tree limb (A) or by cutting a straight pole (B). Add padding to the top (C), then wrap the padding and add a rubber piece to the bottom (D).

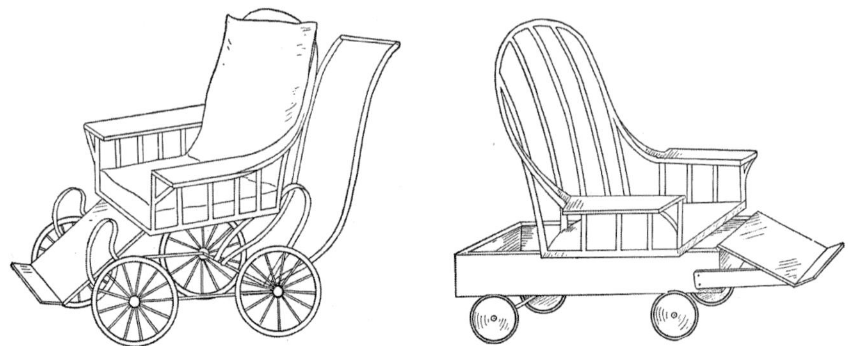

FIG. 39-4. Multiple conversions of chairs to wheelchairs. *(Reproduced from Olson.[4])*

fastening the upper half of a chair to a child's wagon (Fig. 39-4, right), and fastening a pair of roller skates onto a rocking chair's runners.[4]

A simple alternative is to use a child's wagon to transport small children or small adults. However, using a wagon as a wheelchair for long periods is not recommended because (a) there is no support for the patient's back, although one can easily be fashioned; (b) patients must keep their legs extended rather than dependent; and (c) this method of transport is difficult for patients to use on their own.

Another way to make a wheelchair is to use a chair as the base, and attach bicycle wheels (especially those from mountain bikes) and an axle to the back legs. Simply fitting the wheels onto the back legs of most chairs will not work; you must use the axle as well. Fit smaller wheels that swivel, such as from a grocery cart, to the bottom of the chair's front legs—metal chairs work best because they are stronger. Fashion a handle out of metal or wood to fit onto the back of the chair to assist in moving the patient.

Enhancing Zipper Pulls

A common problem for patients is not being able to hold a zipper pull to zip it closed, or, the pull has fallen out and you need a substitute. To remedy this, you can slide a jumbo paper clip, a large safety pin, a string, a twist tie, or a ribbon through the hole at the end of the existing zipper pull or on the slider to make it easier to grip.

Toilet Accommodations

Bedside Commode

Many patients need a bedside commode to avoid climbing stairs or going out to the latrine. Remove the seat from a metal kitchen-type chair, cut a hole in the seat of a wooden chair, or use a toilet seat with legs attached. Place a bucket underneath.[5] (See Figs. 5-7 through 5-9.)

Raised Toilet Seat

Patients in spica casts find sitting on a normal toilet seat impossible. Solve this problem by cutting the bottom off a tapered plastic waste can so that it just fits into the top of the toilet bowl. Then use a heat gun to soften the plastic and mold the can top so there is an indentation two-thirds of the way toward the front and also a pointed spout at the front (Fig. 39-5). To use it, wedge the bottom firmly into the toilet bowl. For an elderly patient who simply needs a raised seat, attach a standard toilet seat to this device.

Raised Bed

Patients with limited mobility often have difficulty using low beds or cots. To raise the bed safely, drill holes into four wooden blocks of the same size and insert the bed frame legs. Use this method to raise cots for use as cholera beds; these have a hole cut in the center of their plastic-sheet mattress and a bucket placed underneath (see Fig. 35-4).

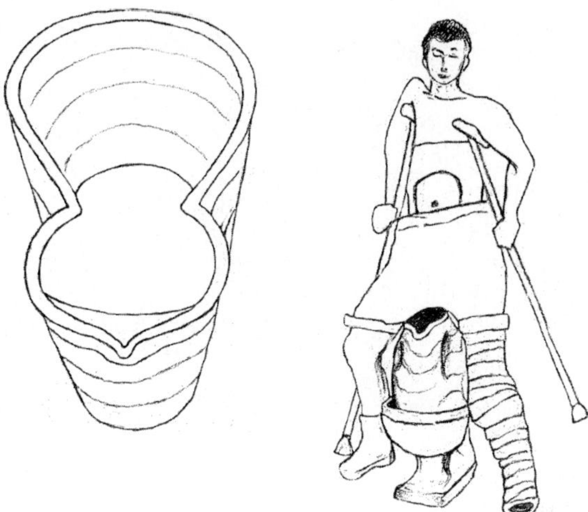

FIG. 39-5. Raised toilet seat. *(Redrawn from Ford.[6])*

Protective Sandals

Thick-soled protective sandals may be needed for patients with severe peripheral neuropathy, such as from diabetes or leprosy. To make an inexpensive sandal that will last about a year, have the patient step on a piece of soft insulating/microcellular/foam rubber (such as that used as packing material) and draw a pattern of his foot on it, about 1.5 cm away from the foot (Fig. 39-6). Make holes for the straps, which are made from leather or cut from a tire's inner tube. Securely sew the straps onto the foam. Cut a piece of automobile tire and glue it to the bottom of the foam. After the glue completely dries, cut the tire to match the foam's shape. If desired, sew on buckles (or attach them with rivets).

Thoracic Brace

A chest, or thoracic, brace is useful for multiple purposes, including protecting chest and thoracic spine injuries while healing occurs. Figure 39-7 shows a chest brace fashioned from PVC pipe. See the "Heating PVC Pipe" section in Chapter 30 for how to work with PVC pipe.

Pads for Pressure Sores

Filling a rubber air mattress with water forms a cushion for the beds of patients prone to develop decubitus ulcers.[7] To make a pad to use on a chair, wheelchair, or hard bed, tie inner tubes together (see Fig. 5-28). Use one inner tube pad on a chair or several linked together to form a mattress (Fig. 39-8).

Sitting Support

Patients may need support to sit upright in a chair because of weakness or instability. (Do not sit or prop them up if their difficulty sitting is due to hypotension! They will simply pass out—or maybe have a stroke.) Use sheets, folded towels, or pieces of cloth to fashion a harness similar to that shown in Fig. 39-9.

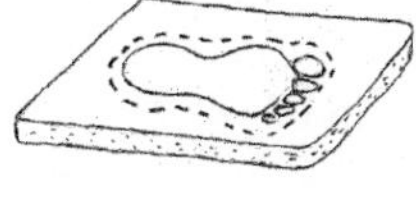 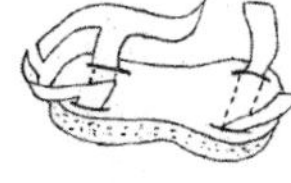 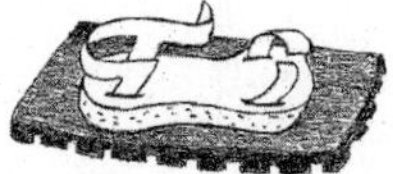 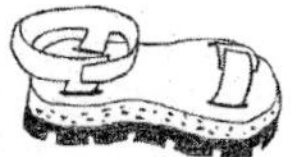

FIG. 39-6. Protective sandals.

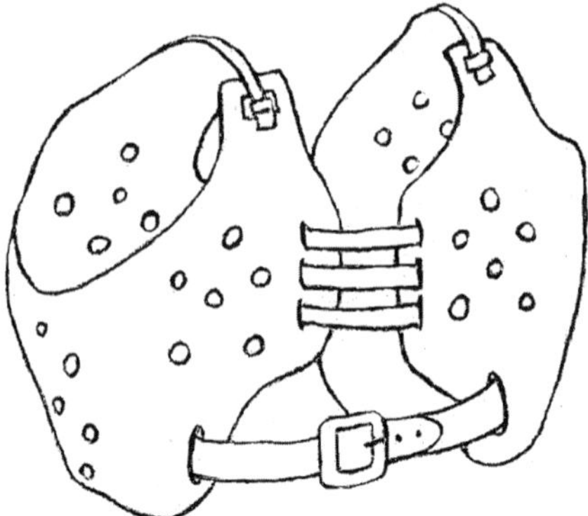

FIG. 39-7. Chest brace from polyvinyl chloride pipe.

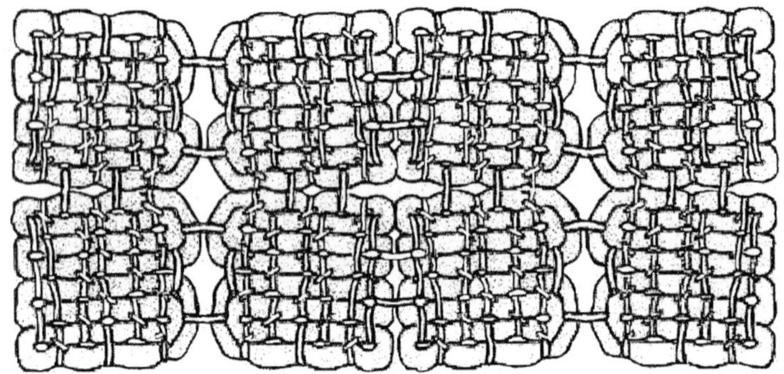

FIG. 39-8. Improvised mattress.

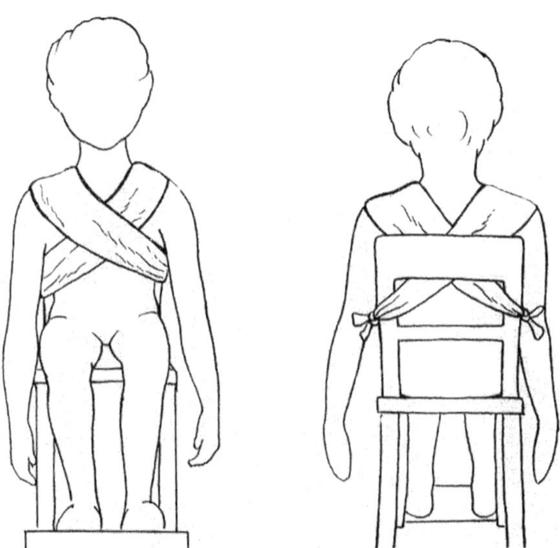

FIG. 39-9. Support harness. *(Redrawn from Arey.[8])*

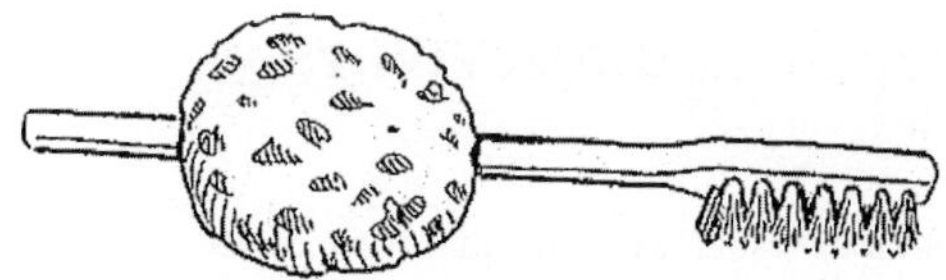

FIG. 39-10. Toothbrush with sponge-ball handle grip. *(Reproduced with permission from Arey.[10])*

Handles for Utensils

Patients with a weak hand grip after a stroke, with other neuromuscular diseases, and with arthritis often have trouble holding eating utensils, writing implements, and toothbrushes. Patients often do well if a handle is enlarged so that they can grip it with their entire hand closed over the handle in a fist.

For an eating utensil, cut a hole in a large sponge or rubber ball and shove the item or its handle through it (Fig. 39-10). For a pen or pencil, push it through the hole in a spool of thread. Enlarge the hole and tape it in place, if necessary.[9]

Prostheses for Amputees

In resource-poor environments, you will need to fashion the prosthesis. One way to do this is, after padding the stump well, to form a plaster cast around the stump, remove the cast, and fit it with a sawn-off, thinned-down crutch. Then fix it in place with additional plaster. This works for both above-the-knee (AK) and below-the-knee (BK) amputations. (It looks similar to pirates' peg legs in the movies and works fine.)

If both legs must be amputated above the knees, consider making short, the so-called "stumpy" prostheses. These can simply be boots pulled over the stumps and held on by cords over the shoulders. They are easier for the patient to balance on, although he or she will need two short walking sticks to assist him.[11]

REFERENCES

1. Iyor FT. A simple design for cervical traction kit. *Trop Doct*. 2002;32:216-217.
2. Werner D. *Disabled Village Children—A Guide for Community Health Workers, Rehabilitation Workers, and Families*. Berkeley, CA: Hesperian Foundation; 1999.
3. Levy M. Charity meets ingenuity. *USA Today*. December 19, 2006:7D.
4. Olson LM. *Improvised Equipment in the Home Care of the Sick*. Philadelphia, PA: W.B. Saunders; 1928:108-109.
5. Brown AR, Mulley GP. Do it yourself: home-made aids for disabled elderly people. *Disabil Rehabil*. 1997;19(1):35-37.
6. Ford VR. Improvised raised toilet seat. *Phys Ther*. 1969;49(9):993.
7. Blass RA. Improvised cushions. *Am J Nurs*. 1970;70(7-12):2605.
8. Arey MS. *Improvised Equipment for the Physically Handicapped*. New York, NY: JONAS NOPHN and NLNE; 1944:30.
9. Arey MS. *Improvised Equipment for the Physically Handicapped*. New York, NY: JONAS NOPHN and NLNE; 1944:23.
10. Arey MS. *Improvised Equipment for the Physically Handicapped*. New York, NY: JONAS NOPHN and NLNE; 1944:10.
11. King M. *Primary Surgery, Vol 2: Trauma*. Oxford, UK: Oxford University Press; 1987:48.

40 | Death and Survivors

Maximizing the utilization of resources means that some deaths will be unavoidable, especially in resource-poor situations. When resources are limited, you may have to forego trying to save patients whose deaths are imminent or unavoidable. Considerable improvisation may be required to fashion body bags, equip holding areas, set up a body-identification system, and even embalm a body or perform an autopsy.

RISK OF DISEASE FROM CORPSES

The myth that all human and animal corpses pose a public health threat following natural or human-made disasters continues to lead to the misallocation of many scarce resources needed to help the living. Corpses pose only a limited health threat when the person did not die from an infectious disease, because most bacteria and viruses die quickly in a dead body as the internal temperature drops and the body desiccates. This limits any microbe's ability to transfer to vectors that could infect humans. In fact, corpses pose a much lower risk of infecting people than do the living who are harboring an infection.[1]

For those corpses of people who died from infectious diseases, the Centers for Disease Control and Prevention (CDC) guidelines require standard precautions for personnel involved in handling the bodies. These include using a surgical scrub suit, a surgical cap, an impervious gown or apron with full-sleeve coverage, a form of eye protection (e.g., goggles or face shield), shoe covers, and double surgical gloves with an interposed layer of cut-proof synthetic mesh. Those doing autopsies should wear N95 respirators and, if available, consider using powered air-purifying respirators equipped with N95 or high-efficiency particulate air (HEPA) filters. Much of this equipment cannot be easily improvised.[2]

General Population

Dead bodies from natural disasters do not cause epidemics. Because they do not have infections when they die, they do not spread diseases. Despite the hysteria from the media and politicians, the risk to the public from even masses of corpses is negligible. However, corpses can leak fecal material that can contaminate rivers or other water sources, causing diarrheal illness. Do not drink untreated water that has had dead bodies in it. In reality, routine disinfection of drinking water is sufficient to prevent waterborne illness.

In cases in which people died of an endemic, communicable disease (e.g., cholera, hemorrhagic fevers), see that the populace uses the best hygiene possible. Also, try to prevent direct contact between corpses and family members. One way to do this is to give the family the body in an airtight box for rapid burial.[3] Spraying bodies with disinfectant or lime powder does not hasten decomposition or provide any protection to the living against disease.[4]

Body Handlers

Those handling corpses have a small, but real, risk of contracting diseases through the bodies' blood and feces, particularly when the individual died of an infectious disease. (There is little risk from corpses resulting from natural disasters.) Handlers are especially at risk for contracting hepatitis B and C, human immunodeficiency virus (HIV), tuberculosis (TB), hemorrhagic fevers, and diarrheal diseases. However, the infectious agents responsible for these diseases do not last more than 2 days in a dead body, except for HIV, which may survive up to 6 days, and Ebola virus, which may last even longer.[4,5] Tuberculosis can pose a hazard during an autopsy or for those handling a body when air is expelled from the respiratory tract. To reduce this risk, place a cloth over the corpse's mouth, ensure adequate ventilation in any temporary morgue, and, if handling hemorrhagic fever bodies, use complete personal protective equipment (PPE).[2,6]

Precautions

In austere circumstances, body-recovery workers can wear normal clothing, along with rubber gloves and boots, if available. However, they must adhere to basic hygiene practices, such as washing their hands with soap and water after handling bodies and before eating, and not wiping their face or mouth with their hands. They should wash and disinfect all equipment, clothes, and vehicles used when transporting bodies.

The primary function of facemasks is to lessen the smell from decaying bodies. The smell is unpleasant, but it is not a health risk in well-ventilated areas. There is no danger of contamination through the respiratory tract (unless the patient had TB) because there is no respiratory function in dead bodies. Even though wearing a facemask is not required for health reasons, it may help lessen workers' anxiety. However, normal facemasks do not filter the air or provide protection against most things (except bad smells) for very long. The problem with wearing masks is that they limit ventilation and increase the work effort.[4,7]

If entering potentially hazardous structures, body recovery personnel should use the same protective gear as search and recovery personnel. If recovering bodies from confined, unventilated spaces, first ventilate the area, because after several days of decomposition, potentially hazardous toxic gases can build up. Body recovery teams should also receive priority status for tetanus immunization because of the hazardous locations in which they often work.[8]

BODY RECOVERY AND DISPOSITION

Immediately after disasters, rather than prioritizing help for survivors, officials usually expend great efforts and resources collecting corpses. While rapid retrieval helps when trying to identify the dead, this effort should never take priority over or use resources that are needed to care for survivors.

Place recovered bodies and body parts (e.g., limbs) in body bags along with non-perishable personal belongings, such as jewelry. If body bags are unavailable, use plastic sheets, shrouds, bed sheets, or other locally available material. Place personal documents in a plastic bag and keep them with the body.

Transporting Bodies

Generally, take bodies either to a short-term holding area or to a site for long-term storage or final disposition. While mortuary workers normally use specialized mortuary vehicles to transport dead bodies, in major disasters, these may be in short supply or unavailable, so you may need to improvise. (Always check to see if local regulations prohibit using certain vehicles for this purpose.)

While workers often collect bodies using open flatbed trucks, it is preferable to use closed trucks or vans and to cover the floors with plastic. If possible, use refrigerated trucks normally used to transport perishable items. Try to cover any lettering or symbols, including license plates, that identify the companies or individuals who own the vehicles. This avoids any negative repercussions for the vehicles' owners when the public sees them being used in this way. When finished using any vehicles to transport bodies, thoroughly clean them. Any commercial vehicles should then be inspected and approved by government officials as being safe to transport their normal cargo.[9]

Never use ambulances to transport the dead; they are valuable resources designed to help the living. While this practice is common (and inappropriate) during minor incidents, using ambulances in this way when there are mass fatalities is dangerous and potentially harms survivors. Even in mass casualty situations with few survivors (e.g., airplane crash), use alternative vehicles such as trucks, pickups, hearses, and vans to transport the remains of the dead.

Short-Term Holding Areas

Initially, take bodies to a short-term holding area (temporary morgue). Ideally, this site will have controlled access, sufficient space, good ventilation, and be air-conditioned—or at least be out of the sun—to avoid rapid decomposition. It should also have facilities for the staff and areas in which to counsel relatives and, if necessary, to do limited autopsies and embalming. Planning the site layout as soon as the site is chosen is a key element in organizing body identification.

Good on-site organization is essential. Sorting bodies by category helps workers easily locate specific bodies when the family arrives or identifying information becomes available. Place the remains in groups by gender and age (e.g., elderly men) and then further divide them into subgroups, such as by skin color, and then by hair color. For example, there may be six initial parts of the holding area for groups of men and women, each divided into elderly, adult, and child/teenager. With a sizable number of casualties, subdivide each of these areas for bodies of a different skin color (e.g., black, white, other) and hair color (e.g., black, brown, blond, other). If the number of bodies is substantial, further subcategorize these groups by height and hair length. Then, even with hundreds or thousands of bodies, the small subset with the six characteristics can be easily located. Computer programs may be useful to help sort and identify remains.

Storage

Several methods may be available to store bodies. Use any or all of these as the situation requires. Before storing bodies, put each body or body part in a body bag or wrap it in a sheet. Because these will often be unidentified bodies, give each a unique identification number matched to a master list of bodies. Put any identifying information with the body or part, and put their identification number on waterproof labels (e.g., paper in sealed plastic). Do not write the identification numbers directly on the body, body bag, or covering sheet, because the numbers can rub off during storage.

Refrigeration

Cold storage is optimal, especially in hot climates where decomposition advances so rapidly that facial recognition is not possible after 12 to 24 hours. The optimal temperature for storage is between 2°C and 4°C (35.6°F and 39°F). If available, the refrigerated transport containers used by commercial shipping companies can each store up to 50 bodies. Because sufficient refrigeration is rarely available immediately at a disaster site, try to obtain commercial refrigerator trucks. Move them close to the site for use as temporary storage and, later, to transport remaining corpses.

Burial

Use burial either as temporary storage or as a permanent disposition.

Temporary burial provides a good option for immediate storage, sometimes at the disaster site itself, when no other method is available or when longer-term temporary storage is needed. Use this method for individual deaths in remote areas when the body cannot safely be removed at that time. One benefit is that temperatures are lower underground than at the surface; this helps to preserve the body. Design temporary burials so that it is possible later to locate and recover the bodies. To ensure retrieval, use individual burials for a smaller number of bodies and trench burial for a larger number. All bodies should have waterproof identification tags on them and in the body bags or sheets.

However, do not use common mass graves. Rushing to dispose of bodies without proper identification traumatizes families and communities, cannot be justified as a public health measure, and violates important social norms. It also wastes scarce resources and may make it difficult or impossible to recover and identify remains later.[4,10] Likewise, mass cremations are not only technically and logistically difficult, but also waste tremendous amounts of scarce resources (mainly fuel and usually wood). They also destroy evidence for any future identification. Complete incineration is difficult, usually resulting in partially incinerated remains that must be buried.[11]

Grave Construction

If possible, bury human remains in clearly marked, individual graves, although after very large disasters, communal graves may be unavoidable. When digging the graves, consider what the prevailing religious practices say about the bodies' orientation, such as that the head must face east or toward Mecca. Bury each body with its unique reference number on a waterproof label. This number must be clearly marked at ground level and mapped for future reference.

The following are the general guidelines for constructing graves, although the distances may have to be increased depending on soil conditions. Graves should be ≥1.5 meters (5 feet) deep. Communal trench graves should consist of a single row of bodies placed parallel, ≥0.4 meters (1.5 feet) apart. Bury them in one layer—never stack the bodies on top of each other. Graves with fewer than five bodies should allow for ≥1.2 meters (4 feet) between the bottom of the grave and the water table or any level to which groundwater rises; allow ≥1.5 meters (4.5 feet) if the burials are in sand. Communal graves should have ≥2 meters (6 feet) between the bottom of the grave and the water table or any level to which groundwater rises.[12]

Grave Location

When choosing any burial site, consider (a) the number of bodies needing burial—allow some leeway, (b) soil conditions, (c) the highest water-table level, (d) the location's acceptability to nearby communities, and (e) the distance from nearby water sources. Clearly mark burial sites and surround them with a buffer zone ≥10 meters (30 feet) wide to allow the community to plant deep-rooted vegetation and to separate it from inhabited areas.

For public health reasons, place burial sites at least 200 meters (600 feet) from any water source, such as wells, streams, lakes, springs, waterfalls, beaches, and the shoreline. The distance, in part, will vary with the number of bodies being buried, soil porosity, and the water-table level. The more porous the soil and the higher the water table, the farther the grave should be from the water source.[12] The suggested distances between burial sites and drinking-water sources are:

- 200 meters (600 feet) if there are 4 or fewer bodies per 100 m^2.
- 250 meters (750 feet) if there are 5 to 60 bodies per 100 m^2.
- 350 meters (383 yards) if there are more than 60 bodies per 100 m^2.[13]

Ice and Dry Ice

Ice is not the optimal method for preserving bodies in warm climates. It melts quickly and large quantities are needed. When it melts, ice produces large amounts of dirty wastewater that must be disposed of so that it does not seep into the water supply system. In cold regions, using the ambient cold temperatures or existing ice and snow may be an option.

Dry ice, solid carbon dioxide (CO_2) frozen at −78.5°C (−109.3°F) may be suitable for short-term storage. To use it most effectively, build a low wall of dry ice (i.e., 0.5 meters high [1.5 feet]) around groups of about 20 bodies and cover them with a plastic sheet, tarpaulin, or tent. Do not place dry ice on top of bodies, even when wrapped—it damages them. You will need about 10 kg of dry ice per body per day, depending on ambient temperature. Use dry ice preservation only in well-ventilated areas (e.g., outdoors), because it produces carbon dioxide gas when it melts. Use gloves to handle dry ice to avoid "cold burns."[14]

Long-Term Disposition

Generally, the simplest body disposition is to release all identified bodies to relatives or their communities for disposal according to local custom and practice. Long-term storage is required for the remaining unidentified and unclaimed bodies.

Embalming

Embalming requires skills acquired through special training. However, when necessary, any clinician with basic surgical skills can accomplish rudimentary embalming using the steps[15] outlined here. The goal is to inject approximately the person's blood volume (~70 mL/kg) of embalming fluid. Of course, some of the blood will normally have to be drained out and disposed of (safely) first.

Place the body supine and extend the extremities. Incise the inside of the upper left arm and expose the brachial artery. Pass two ligatures, 5 cm apart, under the artery. Then make a transverse incision just large enough to insert a trocar, feeding tube, or very large needle pointing distally. Tighten the proximal ligature and inject embalming fluid. Loosen the ligature and redirect the trocar proximally, tie the distal ligature, and tighten the proximal ligature around the trocar. Inject most of the embalming fluid in this direction. Then remove the trocar, tie off the vessel, and close the incision. Repeat this procedure through the carotid or femoral arteries.

A less effective but simple alternative or supplement to this procedure is to insert a trocar into the abdomen (Fig. 40-1) and then into the chest at multiple points, and aspirate any gas or liquids. Then, inject at least 16 oz (~500 mL) of embalming fluid into each cavity. Repeat this procedure in a male's genitals. Sew the trocar holes closed. To embalm the cranial cavity, inject

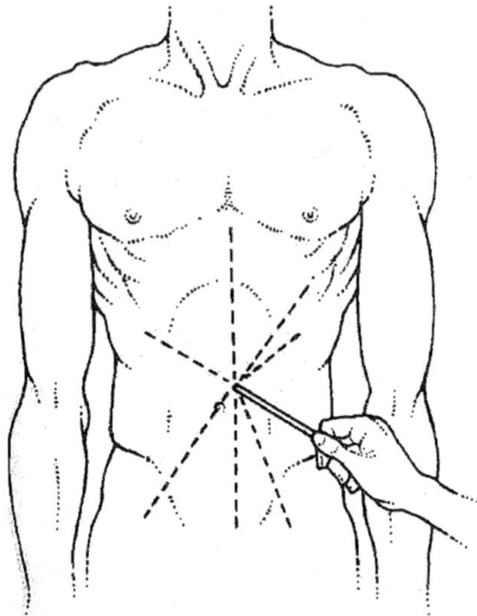

FIG. 40-1. Cavity embalming using a trocar. *(Reproduced with permission from Iserson.[17])*

embalming solution through the carotid arteries or insert a trocar through the cribriform plate via the nose.[16]

Make embalming solution from 40% formaldehyde (formol) and carbolic acid. The more common solution is 10% formaldehyde plus alcohol and glycerin: For each liter of formaldehyde, use 0.5 L alcohol. If formaldehyde is not available, use 20% zinc chloride in alcohol or glycerin. One formula, recommended by the Pan American Health Organization (PAHO), uses the following ingredients[18]:

30% formaldehyde, 300 mL
80-proof ethanol, 700 mL
Glacial acetic acid, 5 mL
Phenol, 20 g

To embalm body fragments, first attempt to suture them together, and to the body, if available. Then inject them with preservative. Alternatively, preserve the fragments using powdered forms of calcium hydroxide (lime), zeolite, or formalin that will adhere to the surface. Then place the fragments in plastic bags wrapped tightly with adhesive tape. This generally prevents fluid leaks and reduces odors during handling.

Embalm a fetus by instilling preservative fluid through the umbilical vein. Use gravity to instill ~1 L of fluid. For a newborn, either use this method or inject 1 to 2 L of preservative through the brachial, axillary, or femoral artery and fill the abdominal and thoracic cavities with preservative-soaked material.

In cases of rapid putrefaction and bloating, puncture the affected areas to release the gasses. This is most common in the perineum, scrotum, and the female mammary folds. Lessen facial swelling by incising the mucosa on the interior cheeks and compressing them with gauze.

Contaminated Bodies

Bodies may have radiological, biological, or chemical contamination. These bodies should generally not be embalmed, and those handling the bodies and performing autopsies should take special precautions, including wearing the appropriate PPE. In these cases, cremation is the preferred method of disposition, although local health officials may permit burial in sealed containers.

Officials can generally permit family to view most bodies if the death was due to a disease that requires a vector (e.g., tularemia, Rocky Mountain spotted fever) or to radiological contamination (they are generally not "contaminated," but rather affected by radiation). Viewing should not be permitted when death was due to a chemical warfare agent or an infectious disease with person-to-person transmission (e.g., anthrax, hemorrhagic fever, smallpox).[19]

Animal Corpses

Three factors that determine whether animal bodies can harm humans are as follows:

1. If the animal carcasses have specific infectious agents, particularly *Cryptosporidium*, *Campylobacter*, and *Listeria,*
2. If the pathological microbe can survive the animal's death, and
3. If the corpse is leaking contaminating material into drinking water.[20]

Unless all three of these elements are present, the dead animal presents no threat to humans. Note that the microorganisms mentioned survive only briefly if the animal's carcass is on dry land.

Three methods for disposing of animal remains exist: bagging, burying, and burning. Usually, the easiest method is to bag the body. The University of Virginia's protocols for disposing of animal remains after natural death or disasters recommend putting animal bodies in sealed, thick plastic bags until they can be taken to an area designated for final disposal.[21]

Burying animal remains is more labor intensive, especially when there are large numbers of dead animals. The danger is that other animals may unearth these burials. Place a layer of a thorny plant, such as cactus or brambles, over the burial site. This discourages dogs, foxes, and other canines from digging up the site. In the case of herbivores that have a large amount of grass in their four stomachs, putrefaction often swells the body, causing the soil over the animal to rise. Puncture the stomach to allow gas to escape before interring the animal. To be effective, bury animal carcasses at least 3 feet deep. Initially, spray the remains with oil and then cover them with soil to protect them from predators until there are resources available to destroy or bury them.[22]

Cremating animals in austere circumstances is generally a bad idea. Not only does it waste valuable resources, but it also often fails to incinerate the body fully, which makes it more difficult to inter the body at a later time.[22]

POST-DISASTER FORENSICS

Post-disaster forensics usually means identifying the bodies. Rarely are there significant questions about the mechanism of death.

Body Identification Process

Even in the worst conditions, any physician who uses common sense can organize the procedures for victim identification and markedly advance the process. On-site health care professionals have the best opportunity to identify victims before the bodies decompose. When trying to identify victims, the basic principle is that the sooner the process is started, the more successful it will be. Once bodies have decomposed, they are much more difficult to identify, often requiring forensic expertise. Mobilizing forensic resources may take several days. This means that in the absence of forensic specialists, many types of health care professionals may need to help with the identification process. Others who may be a valuable part of the process are veterinarians, biologists, pharmacists, funeral administrators, and even gravediggers. The last have the psychological preparation to carry out the work under supervision.

Identify dead bodies by matching the deceased through physical features, clothes, and so forth with similar information about individuals who are missing or presumed dead. To do this, use photographs, fingerprints, and forensic dental comparisons. These rapid, inexpensive, and efficient methods of identification use relatively few resources. Transmission of visual information via the Internet or telephone has speeded long-distance identification of remains.

There are five key steps to identification: (a) assign unique reference numbers, (b) label items, (c) photograph, (d) record, and (e) secure.[23]

Assign Unique Reference Numbers

Perhaps the most important part of the identification process is to assign a unique identification number to each body and body part, so that workers can catalog any materials or information connected to it using that number. This allows information to be found quickly and is useful when trying to identify the remains. Why also assign a number to body parts? Any part that proves a person is dead can aid in identification and subsequent closure for relatives, and therefore we should manage it in the same way as a whole body.

Forms to use when recovering bodies can be downloaded (MSWord or PDF file formats) at www.paho.org/english/dd/ped/DeadBodiesFieldManual.htm. This site also has forms to use to inventory corpses, to assign sequential numbers (up to 500) to recovered bodies, and to collect data on missing persons.

Label Items

Write the unique reference number on a waterproof label (e.g., paper sealed in plastic), then securely attach it to the body or body part. Attach a waterproof label with the same unique reference number to the container for the body or body part (e.g., body bag, cover sheet, or bag for the body part).

Photograph

Visual identification of fresh bodies on-scene or using photographs is the simplest and most efficient identification method during the early, nonspecialist identification process. However, visual identification and photographs can result in mistaken identification. Clean the body sufficiently to fully demonstrate facial features and clothing in the photographs. Identification errors increase with injuries to the decedent or with the presence of blood, fluids, or dirt, especially around the head.[23]

For each corpse or body part, complete a set of photos to use for identification (Fig. 40-2). When taking photographs, always include a clearly visible and readable label that includes the corpse's unique ID number. Take at least the following shots: (a) full length of the body, front view; (b) whole face; and (c) any obvious distinguishing features. If circumstances permit, or at a later time, take additional photographs (including the unique reference number) of (a) upper part of the body, (b) lower part of the body, and (c) all clothing, personal effects, and distinguishing features.

When taking photographs, remember the following tips:

- Steady the camera or use a tripod—blurred photographs are useless.
- Take close-ups. The face should fill most of the frame.
- Stand at the middle of the body when taking the picture, not at the head or feet.
- The photo is useful only if the unique ID number is clearly visible and readable.

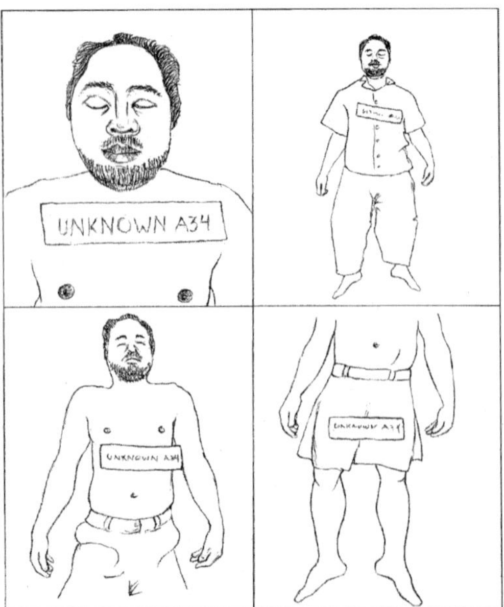

FIG. 40-2. Typical set of photographs for identification.

Record

Even if photographs have been taken, record the following data on a sheet with the unique ID number[23]:

- Gender (look at genitals to confirm)
- Age range (infant, child, adolescent, adult, elderly)
- Personal belongings (jewelry, clothes, identity card, driver's license, and so forth) on or near the body
- Obvious specific skin marks (e.g., tattoo, scar, birthmark) or deformity
- Where body or belongings were found
- The exact burial location, if buried for temporary storage

If no photographs are taken, also record the following:

- Race
- Height
- Color and length of hair
- Color of eyes

Secure

Personal belongings should be securely packaged, labeled with the same unique ID number, and stored with the body or body part. Keep data sheets and photographs in a secure site; PAHO recommends also sending data via the Internet to one or more secure sites, if possible.

Identification and Release of the Body

Although there may be no alternative following large disasters, the psychological impact of viewing dozens or hundreds of dead bodies may reduce the validity of the identification. Rather than further traumatizing relatives by having them personally identify bodies, have them view photographs. This also increases the reliability of visual identification.

Confirm visual identification by other information, such as identification of clothing or personal effects. Release a dead body only when identification is certain. Never expect children to help visually identify corpses.

Record the name and contact details of the person who claimed the body, together with the body's unique ID number. Consider retaining bodies that are not intact, because this may complicate subsequent management of body parts. Properly store bodies that cannot be recognized by visual identification (see the "Storage" section earlier in this chapter) until forensic specialists can investigate.

Information Management

For early data collection, you may use paper forms, but enter the information later into an electronic database. To optimally use collected information, it is essential to coordinate all data through one central processing point. This increases the possibility of finding a match between missing person reports and known information about dead bodies. To do this, establish information centers at regional and local levels that feed their data into a central data bank. Local centers are particularly necessary for receiving requests, acquiring photographs and information from relatives, and releasing information about found or identified persons.[24]

Information can also be transmitted using the Internet, public information boards, and the media (newspapers, television, radio).

Tentative Identifications

Once there is a general idea of a body's identity, search for the information needed to create identification files corresponding to the case.[25] Interviews with people having close ties to the victim are common sources of basic information. In addition to the interviews, use available documents and personal articles to obtain essential information.

Couple the physical characteristics gleaned from examining the remains with known physical attributes. These include age, gender, race, and stature; scars, blemishes, birthmarks, or tattoos; hair color (natural and dyed) and characteristics; presence of moustache or beard and their characteristics; dental prostheses, dental chart, and other dental studies; blood type and other genetic information; x-rays and other relevant laboratory tests; data about any ante-mortem trauma, abnormalities, and orthopedic and other prostheses; known illnesses; surgery experienced and special consequences, if any; and any other particular information for each case.[25,26]

Secure ID Tags

Consider placing an additional ID tag inside the mouth within a few hours of death, because rigor mortis will cause the mouth to remain tightly shut so that the tag cannot be lost. In austere circumstances, that may be beneficial. The disadvantage of putting the ID tag in the mouth is that workers may later need to incise the tissue to extract the tag and check the code.[27]

DNA Samples

DNA analysis, while slow and expensive, is now available after disasters in most regions of the world, through either local sources or nongovernmental organizations (NGOs).

DNA can help to identify individuals even when on-scene investigators cannot. The keys are to collect the correct type of samples and to package them correctly. Label all samples with any reference number referring to the body, the type of sample, where it was taken, and who is sending it. Table 40-1 lists the samples generally needed to help identify corpses in different states of decomposition.

TABLE 40-1 DNA Evidence

	State of Corpse			Transport Method
	Well-preserved	Charred	Decomposed	
Blood	10 mL in an anticoagulant (EDTA) tube	Semisolid blood from inside heart	N/A	Protective container; refrigerate if possible.
Skeletal muscle	Two fragments ~10 grams each and 2 cm wide; use plastic screw-cap container	N/A	Any tissue remaining on bone	Jar with screw-on lid or air-tight closure; seal with tape. Refrigerate, if possible.
Teeth	Four teeth, preferably molars; do a dental chart first	N/A	Four teeth, preferably molars; do a dental chart first	Cardboard box or paper bag; seal with tape. Refrigeration not necessary.
Bone	N/A	Fragments from deep in body	An entire long bone—femur, if possible	Cardboard box or paper bag; seal with tape. No refrigeration.
Hair, Scabs, Skin, Nails, etc.	N/A	N/A	N/A	Collect in small pieces of paper; carefully fold and put in paper bag; seal with tape. No refrigeration.
Dry, sterile swabs	N/A	N/A	N/A	Put in small cardboard box, or label with identifying information and dry completely at room temperature in protected area. Seal in a shipping container. Refrigeration not needed.

Abbreviation: DNA, deoxyribonucleic acid; EDTA, ethylenediaminetetraacetic acid.

Adapted from Pan American Health Organization.[28]

TABLE 40-2 Protocol to Support Disaster Survivors

Meet survivors as they arrive at the morgue waiting (or other gathering) area. Staff should wear identification: Armbands color-coded to an individual's job, such as support, medical, counselor, clergy, etc., are optimal.
After identifying the survivors, give them all information currently available. (Accurate information is priceless in disaster situations.)
If there are enough counselors on each shift, assign them specific survivor family groups to monitor.
Keep track of which survivors are present or where they have gone.
Give survivors an overview of the identification process, the forms they need to complete, and the required autopsy or other forensic investigations. Assist them with the necessary formalities and paperwork.
Assess survivors involved in the disaster for injuries.
Provide a means of communicating with distant relatives, and comfortable rest areas, bathrooms, and eating facilities while survivors wait to hear news of their loved ones. (This may require logistical support from local hospitals, the National Guard, Red Cross, Salvation Army, or similar local agencies.)
Have a staffed play area for small children. (Surviving children's need for immediate psychological support is often neglected.)
Support emotionally distressed relatives who are waiting to identify bodies.
Provide a liaison with the disaster scene and local hospitals.
Accompany survivors to any mass briefings held for them.
Protect survivors from the media and, when desired, act as their spokesperson or intermediary. (The media can help to publicize that mental health services are available for survivors who were not at the morgue.)
Support survivors through the process of identification. Assure them that they have not misidentified their loved one or otherwise made an error (a common fear). This may be particularly stressful, because the bodies are often burned, dismembered, or mutilated and may have begun decomposing for lack of refrigeration.
Give survivors information about available funerary facilities, if asked.
Provide crisis psychiatric intervention, as necessary.
Help identify the survivors' normal support system to further assist them.
Collect survivors' identifying information so follow-up can be done.
During the event (usually at each change of shift) and after the event, the notifier/mental health team should hold debriefings to share information and to relieve their own stress.

Reproduced with permission from Iserson.[29]

SURVIVORS

We often neglect survivors in the hubbub of a crisis. Yet these patients are the ones for whom we can do the most. The first task is to deal with them compassionately, both during and subsequent to the identification or notification process. They may need counseling for posttraumatic stress disorder (see the "Posttraumatic Stress Disorder" section in Chapter 38). Inevitably, they will want to follow their religio-cultural rituals for parting with their loved ones. The following protocol (Table 40-2) provides a model to use when dealing with large numbers of disaster survivors.[29]

REFERENCES

1. Pan American Health Organization. *Management of Dead Bodies in Disaster Situations*. Washington, DC: PAHO; 2004:73, 171.

2. Centers for Disease Control and Prevention. Guidance for safe handling of human remains of Ebola patients in US hospitals and mortuaries. www.cdc.gov/vhf/ebola/healthcare-us/hospitals/handling-human-remains.html. Updated February 11, 2015. Accessed February 19, 2015.
3. Pan American Health Organization. *Management of Dead Bodies in Disaster Situations*. Washington, DC: PAHO; 2004:74.
4. Morgan O, ed. *Management of Dead Bodies After Disasters: A Field Manual for First Responders*. Washington, DC: PAHO; 2009:14-15. www.paho.org/English/dd/ped/DeadBodiesFieldManual.pdf. Accessed October 7, 2011.
5. Centers for Disease Control and Prevention. Review of human-to-human transmission of ebola virus. www.cdc.gov/vhf/ebola/index.html. Accessed October 9, 2015.
6. Healing TD, Hoffman PN, Young SE. The infectious hazards of human cadavers. *Commun Dis Rep CDR Rev*. 1995;5:61-68.
7. Pan American Health Organization. *Management of Dead Bodies in Disaster Situations*. Washington, DC: PAHO; 2004:21.
8. Morgan O, ed. *Management of Dead Bodies After Disasters: A Field Manual for First Responders*. Washington, DC: PAHO; 2009:15.
9. Pan American Health Organization. *Management of Dead Bodies in Disaster Situations*. Washington, DC: PAHO; 2004:19-20.
10. Sphere Project. *Humanitarian Charter and Minimum Standards in Disaster Response*. 2004:269. www.sphereproject.org/handbook. Accessed November 8, 2006.
11. Iserson KV. *Death to Dust: What Happens to Dead Bodies?* 2nd ed. Tucson, AZ: Galen Press, Ltd.; 2001:323-324.
12. Morgan O, ed. *Management of Dead Bodies After Disasters: A Field Manual for First Responders*. Washington, DC: PAHO; 2009:30.
13. Morgan O, ed. *Management of Dead Bodies after Disasters: A Field Manual for First Responders*. Washington, DC: PAHO; 2009:31.
14. Morgan O, ed. *Management of Dead Bodies After Disasters: A Field Manual for First Responders*. Washington, DC: PAHO; 2009:20.
15. Pan American Health Organization. *Management of Dead Bodies in Disaster Situations*. Washington, DC: PAHO; 2004:62-65.
16. Iserson KV. *Death to Dust: What Happens to Dead Bodies?* 2nd ed. Tucson, AZ: Galen Press, Ltd.; 2001:251-257.
17. Iserson KV. *Death to Dust: What Happens to Dead Bodies?* 2nd ed. Tucson, AZ: Galen Press, Ltd.; 2001:257.
18. Pan American Health Organization. *Management of Dead Bodies in Disaster Situations*. Washington, DC: PAHO; 2004:64.
19. Tun K, Bucher B, Sribanditmongkol P, et al. Panel 2.16: Forensic aspects of disaster fatality management. *Prehosp Disaster Med*. 2005;20(6):455-458.
20. Pan American Health Organization. *Management of Dead Bodies in Disaster Situations*. Washington, DC: PAHO; 2004:78-81.
21. University of Virginia, Office of Environmental Health and Safety. *Waste Management Decision Tree*. http://ehs.virginia.edu/biosafety/bio.waste.html#e and www.phclab.com/resource%20centre/rclinks.htm. Accessed October 9, 2015.
22. Jiménez EF, as cited in: Pan American Health Organization. *Management of Dead Bodies in Disaster Situations*. Washington, DC: PAHO; 2004:79-80.
23. Morgan O, ed. *Management of Dead Bodies After Disasters: A Field Manual for First Responders*. Washington, DC: PAHO; 2009:22-26.
24. Morgan O, ed. *Management of Dead Bodies After Disasters: A Field Manual for First Responders*. Washington, DC: PAHO; 2009:28.
25. Pan American Health Organization. *Management of Dead Bodies in Disaster Situations*. Washington, DC: PAHO; 2004:34-36.
26. Pan American Health Organization. *Management of Dead Bodies in Disaster Situations*. Washington, DC: PAHO; 2004:40.
27. Iserson KV. *Autopsies: More Than You Ever Wanted to Know*. Tucson, AZ: Galen Press, Ltd.; 2012.
28. Pan American Health Organization. *Management of Dead Bodies in Disaster Situations*. Washington, DC: PAHO; 2004:54-55.
29. Iserson KV. *Grave Words: Notifying Survivors About Sudden, Unexpected Deaths*. Tucson, AZ: Galen Press, Ltd.; 1999:249.

VI APPENDICES

Appendix 1

Hospital Disaster Plan

Generic All-Hazard Hospital Disaster Resource-Allocation Plan

Kenneth V. Iserson, MD, MBA, FACEP, FAAEM, FIFEM

This plan is designed for health care facilities in normally resource-sufficient regions. **It may need to be adapted for facilities in resource-poor areas.**

"Triggers" indicate the situations that should initiate the **"Actions"** and associated "**Treatment Priorities**."

The Triggers change with each **"Level."** Within each Level, all Actions or Treatment Priorities are in addition to or modify those listed for the preceding Levels.

In resource-poor institutions:

- **"ICU"** beds and treatment mean any beds and treatment used for the sickest patients
- **"ED beds"** are beds in the facility's intake or reception area
- **"ED physician or equivalent"** is the clinician with the most experience in quickly evaluating patients to make difficult triage decisions
- The institutional disaster plan should be used when the facility does not use the **"Hospital Incident Command System"**

	Level 0
Triggers	"Normal" demand-to-available-resource ratio.
Actions	Normal activity.
Treatment Priority	Five-level nurse-run triage in emergency department (ED). Immediately lifesaving surgeries before urgent surgeries before elective surgeries. ICU bed allocation based on greatest need. Patients' attending physicians and intensivist make decisions.
	Level 1
Triggers	50% of ED (A&E[a]) beds are filled with admitted patients.[b] *- or -* Staffed inpatient beds are 98% filled.[b] *- or -* External incident(s) is likely to generate or has already generated a combination of critical and/or noncritical patients exceeding 30% of normal ED or reception-area bed capacity in a short period of time. *- or -* Only 75% of any critical resource[c] will be available for a significant period during the next 24 hours.

(*Continued*)

Level 1, *continued*	
Actions	Notify the Hospital Incident Command System (HICS) leadership.[d] Stop all elective admissions and do not begin any elective surgeries.[e] Refuse to accept transfers from other facilities if patients can be treated elsewhere.[e] Whenever possible, transfer admitted patients who are not yet inpatients to other institutions.[f] Immediately discharge all patients from the hospital (a) whose discharge is planned to occur within 12 hours and (b) who can be safely managed at home or in another available facility. The vacated bed must be available for new patients within 2 hours of discharge papers being signed.[e] Fill all physical beds, use all levels of nursing personnel (expand their scope of practice to the extent that safety and the law permit), and, if necessary, decrease nurse-to-patient ratios.[g] Discharge all ambulatory patients. Send them to other appropriate facilities, if available.[e] If the situation is caused by an infectious agent or other contaminant, institute protective measures, including isolation and quarantine. Activate "over-capacity" plan(s), including opening pre-identified locations to accommodate "surge capacity."[h] Consider implementing disaster plan.[i] Consider using a trained risk-communicator to inform the public about the situation.[i,j]
Treatment Priority	The most experienced ED physician or the equivalent triages incoming patients. Do not start any elective surgeries. Physician Crisis Triage Officer (CTO)[k] asks individual attending staff to discharge ICU/critical care patients who will probably not benefit from that level of care.
Level 2	
Triggers	75% of ED beds are filled with admitted patients.[b] *- or -* Staffed adult inpatient beds are >100% filled.[b] *- or -* External incident is likely to generate patients rapidly or has already generated 6 to 20 critical and/or 31 to 100 noncritical patients. *- or -* Only 50% of any critical resources[c] will be available for a significant period during the next 24 hours.
Actions	[Take actions as described for prior Levels, modifying them as described for this Level.] Refuse to accept transfers except for those that are immediately life-threatening and that cannot be treated elsewhere.[e] Divert noncritical ambulance traffic if other hospitals are open. Immediately discharge all patients from the hospital as listed in Level 1, plus those who do not require acute care hospitalization.[e] Implement disaster plan, including opening pre-identified locations to accommodate "surge capacity."[i] Consider asking for assistance from local, regional, or national authorities.[i] ICU beds and ventilator use may be rationed. Use a trained risk-communicator to inform the public of the situation and, if possible, work with the local and regional authorities to establish an area-wide risk-communication system.[j]

(Continued)

	Clinics outside the institution are asked to take "Triage Level 4 and 5" patients (those requiring the least resources for treatment).
Treatment Priority	Physician CTO[k] decides, in conjunction with patient's primary treating physician, about ICU bed allocation (continued use and new admissions) and the use of ventilators, other critical equipment, and medication in short supply. These decisions are based on greatest need - *and* - the probability of benefit from ICU treatment based on current knowledge.
	Level 3
Triggers	76% to 95% of ED beds are filled with admitted patients.[b] *- or -* External incident is likely to generate rapidly or has already generated ≥21 critical and/or ≥101 noncritical patients.
Actions	[Take actions as described for prior Levels, modifying them as described for this Level.] Refuse to accept all transfers.[e] Fill all physical beds, stretchers, and cots; use all nursing personnel, decreasing the nurse-to-patient ratios as necessary.[g]
Treatment Priority	Ask for assistance from local, regional, or national authorities, if not already done.[i]
	Level 4
Triggers	>95% of ED beds are filled with admitted patients.[b] *- or -* Disaster plan activated and already have maximum number of inpatients under the plan.[b] *- or -* Only 25% of any critical resources[c] will be available for a significant period during the next 24 hours.
Actions	[Take actions as described for prior Levels, modifying them as described for this Level.] Ask for additional assistance from local, regional, or national authorities.[i]
Treatment Priority	The Physician CTO[k] informs all clinical staff that, until further notice, all medical resources will be distributed to all patients using the following treatment priorities: –Those with a high probability of successful medical intervention. –Those who perform essential emergency response roles, especially if they may quickly return to work after treatment. –Those not needing excessive resources. –Those in caretaker roles. –Those with essential community roles.
	Level 5
Triggers	Contamination (including radiation); fire, flood, structural damage, or bomb threat requiring evacuation. *- or -* The disruption of a major support service (pharmacy, food service, supply/distribution, power, water). *- or -* Dangerous police-related situation within the institution.[l]

(*Continued*)

Level 5, *continued*	
Actions	[Take actions as described for prior Levels, modifying them as described for this Level.] Transfer current patients. Stop all admissions from any source and do not begin any surgeries.[e]
Treatment Priority	No treatment of new patients within the facility until situation stabilizes. Physician CTO[k] determines evacuation priority and, if necessary, which patients will not be evacuated.[m] Ambulatory first aid rendered, if possible.
Level 6	
Triggers	No hospital services available—for whatever reason. *- or -* At least one critical resource[c] will be completely unavailable for a significant period during the next 24 hours.
Actions	[Take actions as described for prior Levels, modifying them as described for this Level.] All patients evacuated from hospital and ED.[e] Physician CTO[k] determines evacuation priority and, if necessary, which patients will not be evacuated.[m]
Treatment Priority	Inpatient facility closed.

[a]Accident & Emergency

[b]This information should be assessed frequently (elegant markers) and represents the institution's current ratio of patient demand to available resources (personnel, equipment, and space). The "number of ED beds" must be determined in advance, but should include only those beds that can safely accommodate admitted patients under normal circumstances. The "number of inpatient beds" should include only those beds that can be used for acute adult or pediatric medical-surgical patients (not neonatal beds).

[c]Critical Resources are: essential medical gasses (e.g., oxygen and nitrous oxide), electricity, water (including a method to purify before use), natural gas (used for heating and cooking), ventilation system, food, key pharmaceuticals for the event, waste and garbage disposal, linen, and essential computer systems (admission, discharge, transfer [ADT] system; pharmacy information system; radiology information system; laboratory information system; network; telephone and paging; and interface engine). Those responsible for providing and maintaining critical resources must provide their best estimate of the percentage of the resource that will be available over the next 24 hours.

[d]The Hospital Incident Command System (HICS) is an emergency management system that employs a logical management structure, defined responsibilities, clear reporting channels, and a common nomenclature to help integrate hospital operations with other emergency responders. There are advantages to all hospitals using this particular emergency management system. It is designed to minimize the confusion and chaos commonly experienced by the hospital staff at the onset of a medical disaster. HICS is the standard for health care disaster response and offers the following features:

–Predictable chain of management

–Flexible organizational chart allows quickly tailoring the response to emergencies

–Prioritized response checklists

–Accountability of position function

–Enhanced documentation for improved accountability and cost recovery

–Common language to promote communication and facilitate outside assistance

–Cost-effective emergency planning within health care organizations

(*Continued*)

The HICS, to work effectively in disasters, must also be used during lower-Level situations. The site(s) used as the Command Center must have excellent, redundant internal and external communication systems. (For an overview of the HICS, see: www.emsa.ca.gov/media/default/HICS/HICS_Guidebook_2014_10.pdf.)

[e]Hospital Chief Medical Officer (CMO) or designate(s) must approve all admissions and surgeries and must enforce hospital discharge policies, as specified for each Level. At Levels 5 and 6, he or she also enforces the "no admission/no surgery" and "transfer all patients" policies.

[f]Social Services will assist with these arrangements.

[g]Hospital Chief Nursing Officer (CNO) or designate(s) modifies staffing patterns to use all physically available beds. (All nursing staff, including those who often function in a "Case Manager" role, will be assigned tasks to maximize their clinical effectiveness.)

[h]Pre-identified surge-capacity locations may include clinical (e.g., ambulatory surgery, gastrointestinal [GI] laboratory, minor treatment areas, cardiac catheterization laboratory) or nonclinical (e.g., cafeteria, waiting room) areas.

[i]Decision made by institution's Incident Commander, or the CMO, CNO, and Chief Operating Officer (COO) or their designates. They are also responsible for downgrading to a lower Disaster Plan Level, when appropriate.

[j]Risk-Communication provides timely, accurate information through multiple sources, with the chief communicators being credible spokespeople. In health crises, these will usually be physicians. Knowledgeable risk-communications specialists must educate this team in these techniques (i.e., using scripts, how to work with the press) in advance of any crisis. The same professionals will work with the designated key communicators throughout the crisis.

[k]Crisis Triage Officer (CTO) is a member of the medical staff who allocates critical resources using the criteria of best outcome related to the resources needed (amount of resources times length of time used). Whenever possible, these decisions will be consistent with evidence-based medical literature. The CTO will never be the primary physician of the patient for whom a resource-allocation decision is being made. Decisions are made, whenever possible, with input from the treating team and, when necessary and if possible, other expert consultants. These decisions should be reassessed if the demand-to-resource ratio changes. However, the CTO's decisions may not be overruled.

This is the most difficult position in the triage system and, without proper experience and education, the CTO will not function effectively. CTOs, in some cases, will need to ration or deny resources to patients who, under normal circumstances, would probably survive. This includes, at Level 6, abandoning some patients whose transfer would be too dangerous or would consume too many resources. (This is analogous to triaging patients into the "Expectant" category.)

CTOs will be designated in advance. The cadre of CTOs must become familiar with the triage criteria, participate in frequent discussions with the Bioethics Committee to understand the moral basis for these resource allocation decisions, and practice this role in lower-Level situations. The senior medical and nursing staff, as well as the senior hospital administrators, must understand the CTO's role and be prepared to fully support his decisions—no matter how painful.

CTOs should be relieved every 4 to 6 hours and have an 8- to 12-hour rest period without other duties (as should others in high-stress positions during a disaster). Their rest areas should be quiet and away from any disturbance. It is essential that excellent communication (e.g., a log book with vital details and decisions) is maintained among CTO team members. (For more information, see: www.youtube.com/watch?v=w2qFjRNmtX4.)

[l]Lockdown of the facility or evacuation of all or part of the facility may be done immediately by any senior clinician or administrator or at the direction of the law enforcement authorities. This may require moving to Disaster Level 6. Follow other parts of the plan for this Level, if possible and if required by the situation.

[m]If moving a patient places staff at risk or if the time and resources it would take to move that patient would compromise the lives of other patients, the CTO will decide if the patient is to be evacuated or not.

Appendix 2 | Medical Kits

The contents of your medical kit can range from Minimalist, which will have only the most basic first aid items, to Advanced Life Support, with all the drug and equipment "bells and whistles." Most people will pack something in between these extremes, depending on the answers to the following questions:

- *Who:* The skill of the practitioner(s) and the number, ages, and chronic illnesses of potential patients.
- *What:* The type of activity and the space/weight limitations for the kit.
- *When:* The time of year and the trip length.
- *Where:* Is the activity in the mountains, tropics, or ocean?
- *Why:* Is the purpose work or play?
- *How far* and *how long* to reach definitive medical care?

To assess the need for each item, ask the following questions: What is the chance you will need an item? Can you improvise without it? Will someone die/be disabled without it? Do you have space/energy to carry it? Do you know how to use it?

An appropriate medical kit should be durable, padded, weatherproof, a bright color, and easy to carry.[1] Even an automobile kit will need straps to tote it to where it is needed. Ideally, it will open completely to be able to identify and access everything in an emergency. Use plastic bags (e.g., Ziploc) to keep similar items together.

If you carry medications, include a weatherproof/laminated drug-treatment card for each, because a wide variety of practitioners may end up using the same kit. These cards should include (a) correct pediatric and adult doses for specific conditions, (b) information on how to reconstitute (if powder) and administer the medication, and (c) contraindications and adverse effects.

FIELD MEDICINE KIT

A "one-man mobile forward clinic" consists of a clinician carrying a backpack with a complete basic life support kit and simple surgical instruments. "In skilled hands and with support from the local population, the one-man mobile forward clinic may handle close to 80% of all casualties."[2]

Dr. Matthew Lewin, who equips scientific teams for remote expeditions, suggests that some of the basics for any kit are ear plugs, nail clippers, superglue (small wounds), suture stapler (larger wounds), thermometer (to determine if there really is a fever), duct tape (lots of uses), condoms (no need for pregnancy or STDs in the field), pregnancy tests (to know if care must be modified), zip ties (to prevent tampering with the kit, but allows it to be opened if the clinician is the patient), adrenaline (envenomations and allergic reactions), and antibiotics. For any other medications, use pills rather than capsules, which may crack in an arid environment; even better are vacuum-sealed medications. What Dr. Lewin *does not include* are venom suction extractors (worthless), rehydration salts (use salt and sugar), or unnecessary narcotics (abuse potential is great).[3]

AUTOMOBILE MEDICAL KIT

The most common situation in which health care professionals may need to provide medical treatment with few resources is while driving. I believe that all advanced health care professionals should carry medical supplies in their vehicle. Not to do so is more than irresponsible: It is a repudiation of the healer's moral codes. If your services are gratis and you have no preexisting requirement to intervene, at least in the United States, you are completely protected from liability.

I stop and ask if help is needed in two situations: when (a) people seem to be in distress and no one else seems to be helping, or (b) prehospital personnel seem to need help. (A clue to this is when one or more of them are kneeling next to a patient.) I have intubated, performed cricothyrotomies, put in chest tubes, and done other advanced procedures at the roadside over the years. Use what you know, the equipment you carry, and lots of improvisation. It will be appreciated.

The equipment you should carry depends, in part, on the skills and knowledge you have. Note that this medical kit should not contain your own personal medical supplies and equipment (e.g., daily medications, first aid creams), but rather supplies to save lives and reduce suffering when no one else can help. Over many decades, I have found the equipment listed in Table A-1 to be adequate. The number of each item in the kit depends on your expected needs and resources.

FIRST AID EQUIPMENT FOR A MASS GATHERING

What do you stock to anticipate illness and injuries in a large group of rambunctious teenagers (or similar groups)? The list in Table A-2 was compiled based on actual injuries among a large number of Boy Scouts (nearly 4000 person-days) in a wilderness setting. Note that this is a first aid, rather than a medical, kit. The quantities are designed for 2 weeks with 12 individuals in the party (168 person-days).[4]

TABLE A-1 Health Care Professional's Automobile Medical Kit

General Equipment		
• Personal protective equipment (PPE, e.g., masks, gloves, gown, booties)	• Nasogastric tube	• Stethoscope
• Headlamp (to see and be seen)	• Trauma shears (heavy scissors)	• Roadside flares
• Grease pencil (to write vital information on bandages or patient's forehead—such as "T" for tourniquet applied and the time)	• Blood pressure cuff (Also used as a tourniquet if tubing is clamped and tape wrapped around it so that it doesn't come loose)	• Foley catheter and drainage bag (the bag is also useful for nasogastric tube and chest tube drainage)
• Gloves (sterile—also useful as Heimlich valve, wound drain, hand dressing, and pediatric distraction/analgesia)	• Adhesive tape—heavy (rubberized, electrical, or duct)	• Scalpels (#10 & #15)
• Small notepad and pencil	• Short dowel (for tourniquet)	• Lubricant (water soluble)
• Emergency thermal (metallic) blanket	• Sheet (to help move person or cover body)	• Alcohol-based hand cleaner gel or wipes
• Chemical heat/cold packs	• Eye wash	• Glucometer
• Biohazard bag	• Sterile sheet	• Multi-Tool
• Smart phone with medical apps, translator and interpreter programs	• Copy of *Improvised Medicine*	• Safety pins (2 sizes: 2.7 cm & 5.1 cm)
Airway/Breathing (Know How to Use the Equipment You Carry)		
• Nasal airways	• Oral airways	• Pocket mask
• Bag-valve-mask	• Bulb or other manually operated suction	• Pulse oximeter (finger)
• Alternative airway devices—Adult and pediatric (e.g., esophageal-tracheal tube, laryngeal mask airway)		• Laryngoscope
• Spare batteries & bulbs	• Endotracheal cuffed tubes (sizes 4-0, 6-0, 7-0, 8-0)	• 10-cc syringe
• Stylet	• Bougie/tube introducer	

(Continued)

TABLE A-1 Health Care Professional's Automobile Medical Kit (*Continued*)

	Bone/Joint Injuries	
• Malleable padded splints	• Triangular bandages	• Cervical collar or sandbags
• Elastic bandage with Velcro closure or safety pins	• Collapsible long-leg splint (optional and expensive)	• Chemical ice pack
	Wound Treatment (This Is for Emergencies, Not for Plastic Closures)	
• Disposable wound stapler	• Suture kit	• Staple remover/suture removal kit
• Sutures (4-0 nylon) on large needle	• Dressings (gauze, non-adherent, ABD pad, or trauma dressing)	• Bandages (roller gauze, self-adherent, and pressure bandage)
• Liquid soap	• Wound closure tape and benzoin	• Cyanoacrylate (as wound adhesive)
• Hemostat		
	Intravenous (IV) Supplies	
• Normal 0.9% saline	• IV catheters	• Butterfly catheters
• IV tubing	• 14- and 16-gauge needles for intraosseous (IO) infusion	• IV start kits
	Medications	
• Benzodiazepine (orally [PO] and parenteral)	• Syringes (1-, 3-, & 5-cc)	• Needles (25-, 21-, & 18-gauge)
• Benadryl	• Aspirin	• Acetaminophen/Panadol
• Butorphanol (or other agonist-antagonist parenteral narcotic. It is unlikely that this will be a target for drug addicts.)		
• Naloxone	• Epinephrine (1:1000)	• Lidocaine 1%
• Albuterol inhaler	• Antiemetic (parenteral)	• Glucose (paste, granules, and $D_{50}W$)
• Ketorolac (parenteral)	• Imodium	• Dexamethasone
• Ketamine	• Oral rehydration salts	• Succinylcholine
• Antibiotics (e.g., ceftriaxone, amoxicillin/clavulanic acid)		

TABLE A-2 First Aid Kit for 2-Week Trip (12 people)

Item/Quantity
Dressings and Wound Care
• Adhesive bandages (Band Aid), 12
• Adhesive tape (2-inch roll), 2
• Conforming gauze bandage (3-inch roll, Kling), 2
• Elastic bandage (3-inch wrap, Ace), 1
• Moleskin sheets, 2
• Spenco 2nd Skin (3- × 4-inch pads), 4
• Sterile gauze compresses (4 × 4 inch), 6
Oral Over-the-Counter (OTC) Preparations
• Antacid (chewable tablet), 6
• Antihistamine (diphenhydramine 50 mg), 6
• Bismuth subsalicylate (Pepto Bismol, chewable), 6
• Ibuprofen (200-mg tablets), 6
Topical OTC Preparations
• Alcohol swabs (for cleaning equipment), 10
• Antibiotic ointment (Neosporin, 0.9-g packets), 6
• Hydrocortisone 1% cream (30-g tube), 1
• Povidone/iodine solution (individual swabs), 8
• Tincture of benzoin (30-mL bottle), 1

Adapted from Welch.[4]

REFERENCES

1. Jackson AS. Emergency care of the trauma patient in remote regions of Papua New Guinea. *PNG Med J.* 2002;45(3-4):222-232.
2. Husum H, Ang SC, Fosse E. *War Surgery: Field Manual.* Penang, Malaysia: Third World Network; 1995:36.
3. Vance E. The field medic. *Nature.* 2010;466:22-23.
4. Welch TP. Data-based selection of medical supplies for wilderness travel. *Wilderness Environ Med.* 1997;8:148-151.

Index

Page numbers followed by "f" and "t" indicate figures and tables, respectively.

Q

R

S